PATHOLOGY

The mechanisms of disease

PATHOLOGY
The mechanisms of disease

Roderick A. Cawson, M.D., B.D.S., F.D.S., R.C.S. (England), R.C.P.S. (Glasgow), F.R.C.Path.

Emeritus Professor of Oral Medicine and Pathology, University of London, Guy's Hospital Medical School, London, England; Visiting Professor of Pathology, Baylor College of Dentistry, Dallas, Texas

Alexander W. McCracken, M.D., F.C.A.P., D.Clin.Path. (London), D.T.M&H (Liverpool), F.R.C.Path.

Chief, Department of Pathology and Director of Laboratories, Methodist Hospitals of Dallas, Texas; Clinical Professor of Pathology, The University of Texas, Southwest Medical School; Adjunct Professor of Pathology, Baylor College of Dentistry, Dallas, Texas

Peter B. Marcus, M.B., Ch.B., F.C.A.P., M.Med.Path.

Director of Anatomic Pathology and Associate Director of Laboratories, Methodist Hospitals of Dallas; Adjunct Associate Professor of Pathology, Baylor College of Dentistry, Dallas, Texas

Ghazi S. Zaatari, M.D., F.C.A.P.

Associate Director of Anatomic Pathology, Methodist Hospitals of Dallas; Lecturer in Pathology, Baylor College of Dentistry, Dallas, Texas; Visiting Professor of Pathology, American University, Beirut

SECOND EDITION

with 631 illustrations

The C. V. Mosby Company
ST. LOUIS • BALTIMORE • PHILADELPHIA • TORONTO   1989

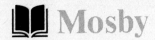

Editor: George Stamathis
Assistant Editor: Valerie Gardiner
Book Designer: Susan E. Lane
Editing and Production: Top Graphics

SECOND EDITION

Copyright © 1989 by The C.V. Mosby Company

All rights reserved. No part of this publication may be
reproduced, stored in a retrieval system, or transmitted, in
any form or by any means, electronic, mechanical, photocopying,
recording, or otherwise, without prior written permission from
the publisher.

Previous edition copyrighted 1982

Printed in the United States of America

The C.V. Mosby Company
11830 Westline Industrial Drive, St. Louis, Missouri 63146

Library of Congress Cataloging in Publication Data

Pathology: The mechanisms of disease.

    Rev. ed. of: Pathologic mechanisms and human
disease / Roderick A. Cawson, Alexander W. McCracken,
Peter B. Marcus. 1982.
    Includes bibliographies and index.
    1. Pathology. 2. Histology, Pathological.
I. Cawson, R. A. II. Cawson, R. A. Pathologic
mechanisms and human disease. [DNLM: 1. Disease.
2. Pathology. QZ 4 P29856]
RB111.P34 1989   616.07′1   88-34513
ISBN 0-8016-1246-2

GW/MV/MV 9 8 7 6 5 4 3 2 1

We dedicate this second edition to our wives
Diana, Terry, Brenda, and ***Balkis***

Preface

The response to this text has been sufficiently encouraging to justify a second edition. For this purpose, in addition to updating it, some changes had to be made both to take into account the many helpful comments of reviewers and to keep the text within an acceptable size.

In particular, the description of physiologic immune responses had to be omitted, as have the principles of genetics and molecular biology. These are subjects that we would expect currently to be taught in other parts of the reader's course of study, as part of the essential content of the biologic sciences. Nevertheless, it has been essential to expand slightly the chapters on the biology of the cell and its reactions to disease, to take into account the many recent developments in this area and because an understanding of these processes is essential to the understanding of pathologic processes and their microscopic appearances.

Otherwise, our primary aim remains unchanged, namely, to provide a concise account of important aspects of the pathology of human disease, with emphasis on the clinical implications.

However, we have two other major objectives. The first is to keep this text within such a length as to enable the reader to gain as clear as possible an idea of the scope of the human pathology without being overwhelmed by detail. Authoritative texts more than 1000 pages are, of course, invaluable but to a newcomer to pathology are likely to prove discouraging or even confusing. Second, there is undoubtedly a need for a pathology text of a size and at a price accessible to as wide a range of health care workers as possible. Much therefore had to be compressed into a relatively small space, and for medical students in particular, this text may best serve as an introduction to large, standard texts or for review purposes. Nevertheless, the curriculum has also become so crowded that in many schools, pathology, even though it forms the basis for the understanding and practice of the whole of clinical medicine, has been forced into little more than a subsidiary position with too few hours allowed to it. Where this applies, undesirable though it may be, a short text such as this may be particularly appropriate.

No pretense is made that this text is comprehensive, and we would certainly not dispute any suggestion that too little attention has been given to one particular subject and too much to another, but as mere mortals we have had to make arbitrary decisions on this matter. We also wonder, if 100 experts were asked to arbitrate in such a controversy, whether we would not get at least 50 different answers.

With these limitations in mind, we sincerely hope that as many readers as possible will find this text to be a useful introduction to the understanding of human disease. Perhaps we might also be permitted to hope that this text might also kindle, in some readers, an interest in pathology.

Roderick A. Cawson
Alexander W. McCracken
Peter B. Marcus
Ghazi S. Zaatari

Acknowledgments

As with the previous edition of this book, we must express our appreciation of those on both sides of the Atlantic who helped bring this second edition to fruition.

Our thanks are due to Dr. Donna Wilson, Dr. Dewey Long, and Dr. Walt Davis, who reviewed sections of the text and made many helpful suggestions, and to Dr. William Hayes and his colleagues in the Radiology Department of Methodist Medical Center, Dallas, for providing the additional radiographs for this edition.

We gratefully acknowledge Dr. D.W. Day and Dr. S.M. Jamal, who generously provided chromosome preparations. Dr. Rolland Reynolds, Dr. James Martin, and Mr. George Bridges, M.S., gave valuable assistance with microscopy and also, along with Mr. Stephen Moser, with the photography. We also thank Miss Claire McCracken, B.A., for providing several of the new line drawings.

We are indebted to Miss Cynthia Bury, B.A., and Mrs. Eunice Melzer for their typing and secretarial skills, and a special thanks is due to Mr. Sydney Luck for his untiring help, over a very long period, in retrieving relevant current literature.

Contents

CHAPTER 1

The normal cell and extracellular matrix

The structural elements of the body are its *cells* and the *extracellular matrix* they secrete about them. The average normal human cell is a dynamic membranous sac permeated by a complex system of constantly changing channels and compartments in which, largely under the direction of nuclear deoxyribonucleic acid (DNA), the varied activities of life go on. The extracellular matrix is the cell's morphologic environment, and practically all the cells of the body (not only the so-called connective tissue cells) contribute toward its production; as with the cell, the molecules of the extracellular matrix are not fixed or static but are subject to constant turnover. The major components of both the cell and matrix are the subject of this chapter.

The language of cell biology and pathobiology is complex and, to the newcomer, even bewildering. In recent years, many new terms have come into use. To assist the reader in becoming familiar with this terminology, much of this nomenclature is included in summary form in the Glossary at the end of the book.

The cell
Structural-functional organization

The cell in all higher forms of life (eukaryotes—i.e., those with nucleated cells) is compartmentalized by a system of membranes into several anatomic and functional units (Fig. 1-1). Aside from the surface membrane (plasmalemma or cell membrane), the eukaryotic cell has two membrane systems: the major one is the cytocavitary network and the smaller is represented by the mitochondria. Although they differ functionally, all the membranes of the cell share a similar trilaminar ultrastructure (Fig. 1-2). This organization of the cell is assisted and maintained by cytoskeletal and cytocontractile elements found in the nuclear and cytoplasmic matrices, which lie outside these membrane systems.

The *cytocavitary network* (see Fig. 1-1) is a series of membrane-bound sacs, channels, and vesicles that are in continuity with one another and with the extracellular environment, either directly, or indirectly by means of vesicles that bud off from or fuse with components of the system. The nuclear envelope, the parent portion of the cytocavitary network, houses the genetic archives of the cell, except when the cell is dividing. Its outer surface is studded with ribosomes, which are used in protein synthesis and enable it to generate membranes. The nuclear envelope thus gives rise to the granular endoplasmic reticulum and, through it, the other components of the cytocavitary network. During secretion the membranes of secretory vesicles fuse with the plasmalemma, and in this manner used or worn plasmalemma is continuously replaced. The cytocavitary network has diverse functions that include:

1. Protein synthesis
2. Hormone and enzyme secretion
3. Intracellular digestion
4. Drug metabolism and detoxification

Mitochondria arose, during the course of evolution, as bacterial (probably gram-negative) endosymbionts within some ancestral type of eukaryotic cell. Aside from housing the enzymes of the Krebs cycle, they possess their own separate synthe-

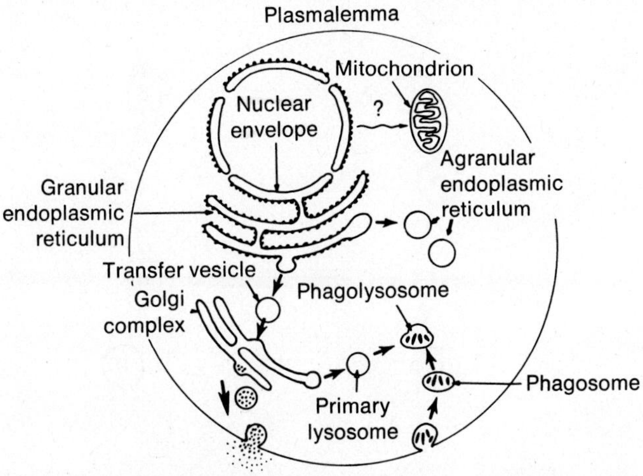

FIG. 1-1. Structural-functional relations between the major components of the cytocavitary network. The mitochrondria comprise a separate system. Neither is found in prokaryotic cells.

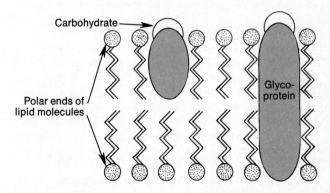

FIG. 1-2. The unit membrane of the cell consists largely of a double layer of lipid molecules—phospholipids or glycolipids plus cholesterol—with their hydrophilic (polar) heads facing outward on either side, in contact with the aqueous medium. On or in the bilayer are glycoproteins that serve as enzymes, or as receptors, or as histocompatibility antigens. Also included are transmembrane proteoglycans, important in the cell's interaction with the extracellular matrix. The carbohydrate portions of all of these molecules contribute to the formation of the glycocalyx at the cell surface.

sizing apparatus for proteins and fatty acids and undergo self-replication by budding. Like gram-negative bacteria they are bounded by a double membrane, their DNA is in a circular form, and they are severely damaged by chloramphenicol.

The *cytoplasmic matrix* (cytosol) contains the "free" (non-membrane-bound) ribosomes, which mainly synthesize proteins that are retained by the cell (nonexport protein); chief among these are the enzymes for anaerobic glycolysis and the components of the cytoskeleton (filaments and microtubules). The cell matrix also houses varying quantities of glycogen and lipid.

The different parts of the cell are discussed in greater detail in the next section of this chapter.

The nucleus

The major components of the nucleus, lying internal to the nuclear envelope, as identified on both light and electron microscopy, are as follows:

1. Chromatin
2. Nucleolus
3. Nuclear matrix

Most of the description that follows focuses on the *chromatin*, the study of which is currently at the cutting edge of medical research; the practical applications of this research have led to exciting advances in the diagnosis and treatment of disease. Aside from routine morphology, there are three main methods for studying the chromosomal material of the cell in the clinical laboratory: (1) cytogenetic study by karyotyping, (2) recombinant DNA technology ("genetic engineering"), and (3) quantitative DNA analysis (flow cytometry, static cytometry).

Chromatin consists of nucleoprotein (i.e., nucleic acids bound to an equal weight of protein). The nucleic acids are mainly DNA and the protein is mainly histones. The sequence of the nitrogenous bases in the DNA (Fig. 1-3) is unique in every individual and constitutes the genetic code. The term *chromatin* originates from the observation that most nuclear material stains blue-black with hematoxylin in routine histologic sections or cytologic smears. Only the protein constituents of chromatin stain with hematoxylin; for the specific staining of DNA, special stains, such as the Feulgen stain, are required.

The varying morphology of chromatin

During mitotic division, chromatin assumes a highly compact form and becomes recognizable as discrete, broad, thread-like structures termed *chromosomes* (Fig. 1-4). At other times (the interphase), chromosomes are no longer identifiable as discrete structures, and what is seen is simply referred to as *chromatin*. The chromatin in the average interphase nucleus is seen in two main forms: a densely staining, distinctly particulate form and a very lightly staining, amorphous or very faintly particulate form (Fig. 1-5). In order to explain how it is possible for chromatin to assume these different appearances, it is necessary to briefly review its structural organization as brought to light by high resolution analytic techniques.

The DNA from a human cell is about 1 m in length and must be condensed into a nucleus whose diameter is only in the realm of 10 μm. The packaging must, however, allow accessibility of DNA constituents to bases for nucleoprotein synthesis and must prevent tangling during replication. Eukaryotic cells achieve this condensation by a series of *packaging mechanisms* (Fig. 1-6). The fundamental unit of DNA packaging in higher organisms is the *nucleosome*. Under the electron microscope, nucleosomes can be visualized as beads about 10 nm in diameter. With spreading of preparations for electron microscopy, chromatin becomes stretched and the nucleosomes assume a "beads-on-a-string" configuration. In the living cell, however, the nucleosomes touch each other, forming a 10 nm–diameter chain.

Each nucleosome consists of a spool-like octamer of *histones* around which the double helix takes two full turns; the octamer consists of two of each of histones H2A, H2B, H3, and H4. A fifth histone, called H1, occupies the site at which DNA enters and leaves the nucleosome. Nucleosomes are interconnected by short stretches of double helical DNA termed *linker DNA*. A single nucleosome with one attached stretch of linker DNA comprises about 200 base pairs. Linker DNA stretches are more exposed to the action of nucleases (nucleotide-cleaving enzymes) than is nucleosomal DNA; these therefore are the sites of action of (1) the bacterial restriction endonucleases employed in recombinant DNA technology and (2) the endonucleases that mediate apoptosis (Chapter 2).

Packing of DNA in chains of nucleosomes with their intervening linker DNA results in a fivefold to sevenfold compaction of the double helix. These chains are themselves subject to further coiling, with the formation a *solenoid* (cylindrical coil), having six nucleosomes per turn. This results in the formation of a 30 nm–diameter chromatin chain and represents about a 40-fold compaction of the double helix. The histone H1 molecules are essential to the formation of the solenoid, which is maintained by cross-linkages between H1 molecules of adjacent nucleosomes. Both the 10 nm nucleosome chain and the 30

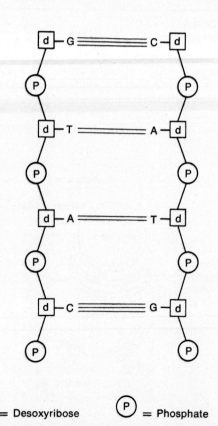

d = Desoxyribose P = Phosphate

FIG. 1-3. Simplified diagram of segment of DNA molecule showing the selective pairing of the bases thymine *(T)* with adenine *(A)* and guanine *(G)* with cytosine *(C).*

nm nucleosome solenoid are further organized in a series of *loops* which extend radially from an axial scaffold composed of nonhistone protein filaments, termed *lamins*, belonging to the nuclear matrix. Such loops average 20 to 100 kilobase (thousand base) pairs each.

The tightest packing of chromatin is found in metaphase chromosomes, in which the DNA is compacted 5000-fold to 10,000-fold, due to yet further folding of the matrix protein scaffold with its attached loops.

The geography of the human genome

The total genetic repertoire of the organism is called its *genome*. The genome of a human cell carries some 2.5 billion base pairs; a leading scientist has estimated that printing one entire haploid genomic base sequence would require the equivalent of about 13 sets of the Encyclopedia Britannica! A group of base sequences responsible for specifying the structure of a particular product, usually either an enzyme or a structural protein of the cell, is termed a *gene* (cistron). There are an

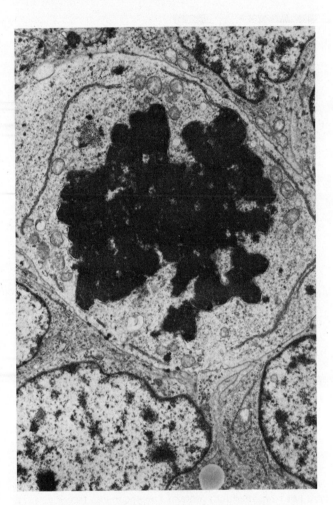

FIG. 1-4. Electron micrograph of a cell in mitosis. Fragmentation of the nuclear envelope is clearly demonstrated.

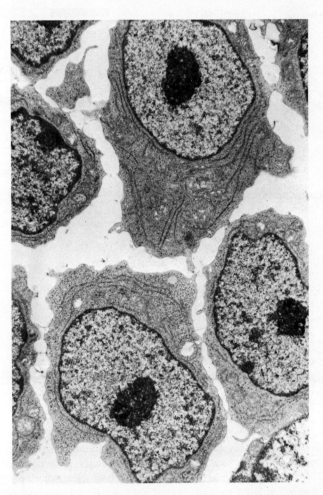

FIG. 1-5. Electron micrograph of typical blast cells showing nuclei with finely dispersed chromatin and large nucleoli. The cytoplasm contains occasional long strands of rough endoplasmic reticulum as well as numerous free ribosomes.

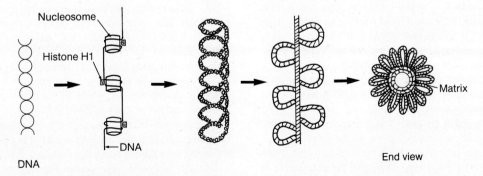

FIG. 1-6. Diagram of the different levels of chromatin organization, with increasing degrees of compaction from left to right. The central figure depicts the nucleosome solenoid, shown here partly uncoiled.

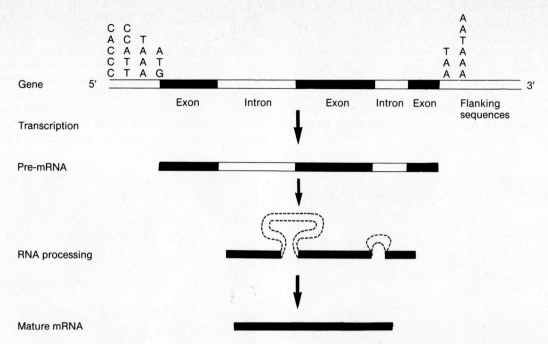

FIG. 1-7. Diagram depicting the anatomy of a typical gene. Transcription proceeds from the 5′ end of the gene toward the 3′ end. During RNA processing, the introns are "spliced out" of the pre-mRNA chain. Only the exons are translated into polypeptides. *C*, Cytosine; *A*, adenine; *T*, thymine; *G*, guanine.

estimated 50,000 to 100,000 genes in the human genome; those coding for the synthesis of known proteins comprise only a small percentage of these.

A gene-sized portion of DNA can be conveniently regarded as being 1000 nucleotide base pairs, or one kilobase in length (i.e., encompassing approximately 5 nucleosomes). Most genes are much longer (seven times or more), however, because of the presence of one or more *introns* (intervening base sequences) that separate *exons* (coding base sequences) (Fig. 1-7). The genes of some large proteins have over 50 introns. At either end—as integral parts of individual genes—are *flanking sequences* of base pairs, which play important roles in "switching genes on and off". Interspersed among the genes are *highly repetitive DNA sequences*, accounting for half or more of the entire genome. The function of these seemingly redundant DNA sequences is unknown, for they do not appear to undergo transcription into protein.

The genetic code and protein synthesis

The sequence of bases in DNA (see Fig. 1-3) specifies the order in which amino acids are assembled to form proteins. When the information in a gene is read out *(expressed)*, its base sequence is copied *(transcribed)* into a strand of ribonucleic acid (RNA). Messenger RNA (mRNA) serves as a template for the synthesis of protein: its base sequence is translated into the amino acid sequence of a protein.

Transcription. In this process a class of enzymes (the *RNA polymerases*) construct an RNA copy of the DNA sequence of one strand (the coding strand).

At the upstream end of the gene, where transcription begins, are the flanking base sequences known as *promoter regions*; these are DNA regions to which RNA polymerases bind when initiating transcription. Following binding of the polymerase to the promoter, the double helix undergoes a local denaturation, or untwisting, that separates the two DNA strands and thus makes it possible for transcription to proceed. In addition, nucleosomes are disrupted in the promoter regions of genes that are being transcribed. The polymerase "reads" the gene until it encounters certain *terminating base sequences* at the downstream end of the gene, where transcription is thus terminated. Yet other base sequences, the *enhancer sequences*, the location of which varies within the gene, are important for increased or tissue specific expression of genes. Promoters, enhancers, and terminating sequences are not transcribed.

Processing of the transcript. Most of the RNA transcribed is mRNA, which contains the appropriate base sequences for proteins destined to be synthesized in the cytoplasm. Both exons and introns are transcribed in a *pre-mRNA*, but the exon sequences are processed, or spliced out of the pre-mRNA, and are not *translated* into proteins (polypeptides) (see Fig. 1-7). Although the function of the introns is still far from clear, it has been observed that, by and large, they separate regions of genes that code for different functional domains of proteins.

Translation. In addition to mRNA, at least two further forms of RNA are transcribed on the DNA molecule. One is ribosomal RNA, from which the tiny cytoplasmic granules known as ribosomes are assembled. The other is amino acid–specific transfer RNA (tRNA) molecules, which carry their specific amino acids to the ribosomes, where ribosomes function in linking amino acids together to form proteins.

The *nucleolus* is the site of ribosomal RNA transcription. It is absent during mitosis, when all the cell's resources are oriented toward the process of division. The bulk of the nucleolus may appear on electron microscopic examination as an anastomosing network (the nucleolonema) (Fig. 1-8), or the entire organelle may appear solid and compact. The nucleolus stains a distinct cherry-red color due to the acidophilia of ribosomal RNA.

The control of gene expression

The expression of different genes—and the resulting synthesis of different proteins—distinguishes one type of cell from another, for example, a brain cell from a muscle cell. Generally speaking all cells in an individual organism contain the same DNA, but not all genes are active in every cell. As well as genes that can be turned on and off, such as those regulated by hormones, human cells have many permanently shut-down genes; thus, for example, a muscle cell does not express the genes encoding proteins found only in a brain cell.

Gene expression is controlled at multiple levels. Activation of transcription is probably the most common mechanism used; thus substances (mainly proteins) specifically binding to promoter or enhancer regions of genes may influence the frequency with which the gene is transcribed. Among the better understood are steroid hormone–protein complexes that enter the nucleus from the cytoplasm and control the expression of steroid hormone–responsive genes. *DNA rearrangements* may also alter gene expression at the transcriptional level; transposition of "silent genes" to expression sites permits their transcription.

Transcriptionally active chromatin is believed to be predominantly in the form of 10 nm nucleosome chains rather than in the more coiled or compact forms. This arrangement presumably permits greater spatial exposure of DNA base sequences for transcriptional activity. Conversely, most compact chromatin is believed to be transcriptionally inactive. Transcriptional control may thus also be under the influence of factors controlling chromatin conformation.

The *nuclear matrix* (interchromatin areas, parachromatin) is the nuclear equivalent of the cytoplasmic matrix (cytosol) and has an unimpressive ultrastructural appearance. Most of the stainable constituents are finely filamentous, granular, or amorphous and include finely dispersed chromatin elements enmeshed within the matrix. The nuclear matrix, like the cytosol, consists of water, solutes, and a delicate network of filaments termed *lamin filaments* that serves a scaffolding function. Lamin filaments, which are members of the *intermediate filament* group (discussed later), are also found aggregated along the inner aspect of the nuclear envelope, where they form the *nuclear fibrous lamina*, important in anchoring chromatin to the nuclear envelope. These filaments are closely related biochemically, and connect physically, to certain intermediate filaments of the cytoplasmic matrix.

The cytocavitary network
The nuclear envelope

The nuclear envelope is the parent portion of the cytocavitary network. It consists of two membranes that enclose a space (the perinuclear cistern) and are continuous with each other around the nuclear pores. The outer layer is continuous with the rough endoplasmic reticulum and may itself be studded with ribosomes (see Fig. 1-1). The nuclear envelope is broken up during cell division and is subsequently reformed around the chromatin of the newly formed cells; polymerization of lamin filaments along the inner aspect of the nuclear envelope accompanies its reassembly.

In addition to its role in the formation of new membranous organelles, the nuclear envelope has a variety of functions. The outer layer, like the membranes of the granular endoplasmic reticulum, may synthesize not only proteins that form parts of membranous organelles but also proteins destined for transport outside the cell (export proteins). This is most striking in primitive cells (such as embryonal and some tumor cells) where the newly formed protein is deposited in the perinuclear cistern. Finally, the different forms of RNA enter the cytoplasm by traversing the nuclear envelope so that the nuclear envelope plays a role in the regulation of protein synthesis in the cytoplasm. The nuclear pores are important in this process—the greater the rate of protein synthesis in a cell, the more numerous are the nuclear pores.

The endoplasmic reticulum

There are two types of endoplasmic reticulum, rough (granular) and smooth (agranular). They are morphologically and functionally quite distinct.

Rough endoplasmic reticulum (Fig. 1-9) owes its name to the ribosomes attached to the outer surface of its constituent membranes. It consists of a system of vesicles and tubules that frequently expand to form flat saccular structures called *cisternae*. In most cells cisternae are solitary or form loosely arranged groups and appear collapsed and almost empty. In cells that are highly active in the production of protein destined for export (e.g., plasma cells), the cisternae tend to be arranged as closely packed, parallel stacks and often appear distended with secretory products.

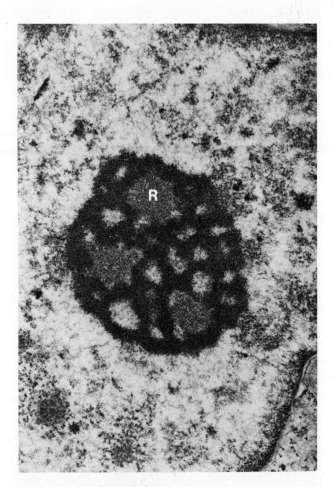

FIG. 1-8. Electron micrograph of a nucleolus with a well-developed nucleolonema. Three fibrillar centers consisting of collections of early ribosome precursors *(R)* are present.

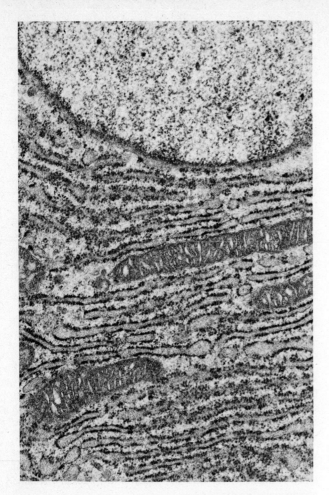

FIG. 1-9. Portion of a plasma cell showing parallel cisterns of rough endoplasmic reticulum interspersed with mitochondria.

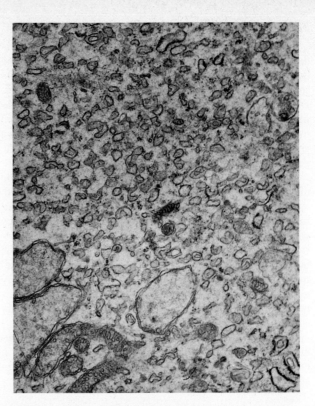

FIG. 1-10. A cluster of smooth endoplasmic reticulum vesicles in a hepatocyte.

ever, most conspicuous in cells that synthesize steroidal hormones such as testicular Leydig cells and those of the adrenal cortex and corpus luteum. The rich concentration of membranes imparts a striking ground-glass, eosinophilic quality to the cytoplasm of such cells.

The Golgi complex and its products

The Golgi complex receives the newly made glycoprotein products of the rough endoplasmic reticulum and, through enzymic action, chemically *modifies* these glycoproteins as they pass through the organelle. Depending on the specific product being manufactured, the enzymes may add or remove sugar molecules or add phosphate groups, sulfate groups, or even fatty acids to the glycoprotein molecules. The finished products are then packaged into membrane-bound vesicles and made ready for secretion by the cell or, in certain instances, for use by the cell itself.

The Golgi complex, like the smooth endoplasmic reticulum, is composed of smooth membranes but appears otherwise quite different (Fig. 1-11). It consists of a stack of membranous sacs, often curved, with vesicles fusing with, or budding off, the periphery. The organelle has three distinct portions, each with its own specific complement of enzymes. The medial portion of the stack consists of flattened sacs (cisternae) that often show slightly dilated ends. The sacs always appear almost, if not completely, empty and tend to be smaller than those of the rough endoplasmic reticulum. On the convex (cis) face lie numerous protein-containing transfer vesicles that have budded off the rough endoplasmic reticulum. On the concave (trans) face of the stack are vacuoles containing material that has been condensed and packaged and is leaving the Golgi complex.

The *ribosomes* that stud the membranes of this system are approximately 15 nm in diameter and exist either singly as monoribosomes or in groups as polyribosomes. A polyribosome resembles a string of pearls in which the ribosomes represent the pearls and a fine strand of mRNA (about 1 nm in thickness) represents the string. Polyribosomes form rows, loops, spirals, or rosettes and, unlike monoribosomes, are actively engaged in protein synthesis. Many ribosomes are involved in synthesizing a single protein molecule; there is roughly one ribosome to every thirty amino acids. The rough endoplasmic reticulum adds an oligosaccharide chain, consisting of 14 sugar molecules, to every protein it synthesizes; thus, specifically, the rough endoplasmic reticulum is engaged in the synthesis of *glycoproteins*.

The *smooth endoplasmic reticulum* usually appears as a meshwork of fine, branching tubules or vesicles and seldom forms cisternae. Cells with abundant rough endoplasmic reticulum usually have little smooth endoplasmic reticulum and vice versa. An exception is the hepatocyte, where both forms are fairly well represented (Fig. 1-10). The smooth endoplasmic reticulum in the hepatocyte is involved in a variety of metabolic functions that include bilirubin conjugation, drug detoxification, and lipoprotein synthesis. In striated muscle cells this organelle is known as the *sarcoplasmic reticulum* and functions in the release and capture of calcium ions during muscle contraction and relaxation. Smooth endoplasmic reticulum is, how-

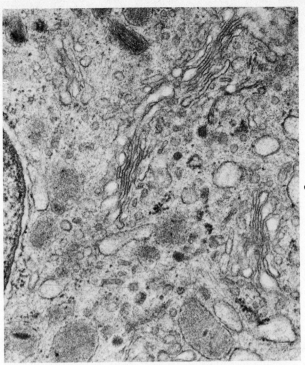

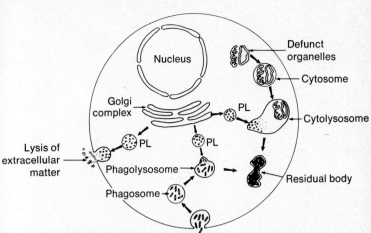

FIG. 1-12. Diagram depicting the formation and use of primary lysosomes by the cell. The limiting membrane of the primary lysosome fuses with that surrounding different kinds of particulate matter, thus bringing its enclosed enzymes into direct contact with that matter. *PL*, primary lysosome.

FIG. 1-11. Several Golgi complexes seen in an active glandular secretory cell.

The morphology and functions of the packaged Golgi products vary considerably. Among the more important products thus formed are the following:

1. Secretory granules of both exocrine and endocrine glands
2. Mucus
3. Collagen
4. Immunoglobulins
5. Milk
6. Melanosomes
7. Primary lysosomes
8. Vesicles containing clathrin (receptor site membrane protein)
9. Perforin (membrane-pore-forming protein)

When the contents of these various vacuoles are released at the cell surface, the membranes surrounding them fuse with the cell surface membrane, thus replenishing it. Membranes leaving the Golgi complex are rich in carbohydrates, which are added to the glycocalyx at the cell surface.

Lysosomes

Lysosomes are membrane-bound vesicles that function as the "digestive system" of the cell and are sometimes released to perform related functions outside the cell (Fig. 1-12). They owe this digestive capability to their powerful arsenal of enzymes, of which more than 60 are known. These enzymes function in an acid medium and are capable of hydrolyzing most classes of macromolecules found in mammalian tissue.

There are two major types of lysosomes. *Primary lysosomes* are "virgin" lysosomes in that their enzymes have not yet come into contact with substrate (Fig. 1-13). Some cells, such as histiocytes and neutrophils are particularly well endowed with primary lysosomes. The enzymes of *secondary lysosomes* have already come into contact with the substrate. Depending on the origin or composition of the substrate concerned, various sub-

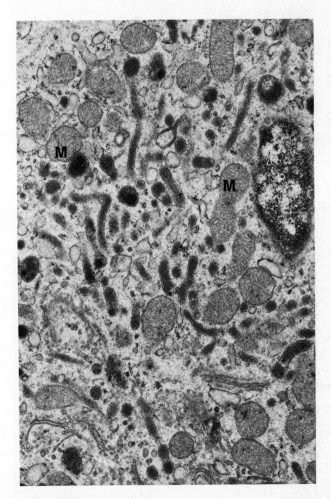

FIG. 1-13. Electron micrograph of cytoplasm of a histiocyte showing primary lysosomes and mitochondria *(M)*.

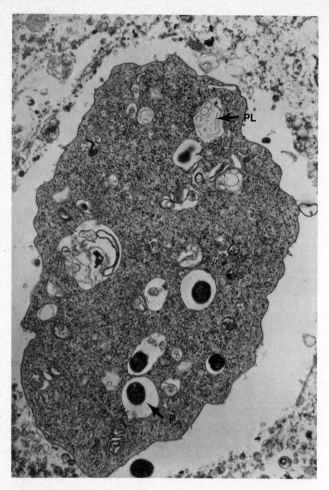

FIG. 1-14. Electron micrograph showing part of a macrophage. Phagosomes *(P)* contain newly ingested cocci, and phagolysosomes *(PL)* contain debris from partially degraded cocci.

classes of secondary lysosomes are recognized. Lysosomes degrading particulate material ingested by the cell (heterophagy) are termed *phagolysosomes* (Fig. 1-14). Those which act as the "trash can" of the cell by enzymatically digesting its defunct or damaged components (autophagy) are called *autolysosomes* (cytolysosomes).

Lipopigments (Fig. 1-15) are lipid-rich lysosomal structures, of which three types are recognized:

1. *Ceroid pigment* consists of lysosomes that develop as a consequence of heterophagy of fatty substances or lipid-containing tissue material (e.g., during resolution of the corpus luteum) and is therefore found in macrophages.
2. *Lipofuscin pigment* (Fig. 1-16) consists of lysosomes that develop as a consequence of autophagy, generally as a result of the normal turnover of membranous organelles, and is found in parenchymal organs, neurones, and muscle cells.
3. *Residual bodies* (telolysosomes) are late-stage lipopigments, in which the oxidation of lipid has reached the point where only undigestible, polymerized unsaturated lipids remain. Residual bodies accumulate with age in long-surviving cells and have for this reason been termed "aging pigment."

Lipopigments lend a yellow or brown appearance to tissues; the significance of these and other forms of lysosomes in pathologic processes is discussed in Chapter 2.

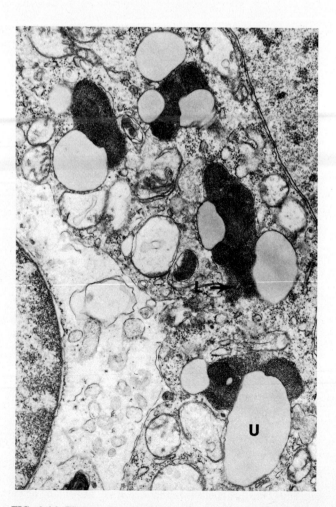

FIG. 1-16. Electron micrograph of lipofuscin granules *(L)*. The pale areas are unoxidized lipid *(U)*.

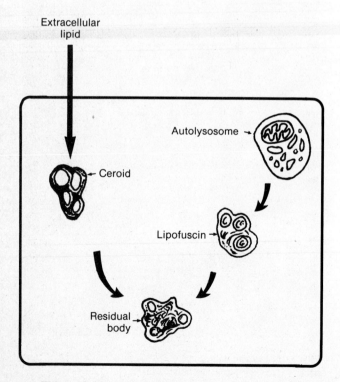

FIG. 1-15. Diagram depicting the genesis of lipopigments.

Mitochondria

Mitochondria (see Fig. 1-9) are usually drug capsule-shaped and are bounded by two separate membranes, the innermost being folded inward to form shelflike structures termed *cristae*. Mitochondria are the power plants of the cell; they are the major source of adenosine triphosphate (ATP), which is generated by the process of oxidative phosphorylation. The enzymes for oxidative phosphorylation, as well as those for electron transport, lie in or on the inner limiting membranes, whereas most of the enzymes of the Krebs cycle are found in the space called the matrix chamber, which is enclosed by this membrane. The matrix contains a few tiny granules that function as accumulators of divalent cations, mainly calcium. In calcifying tissues the mitochondria probably function as the chief site in the cell for the accumulation of calcium before the latter is finally released into the extracellular matrix.

The mitochondrial matrix has a high content of basic proteins and is therefore strongly eosinophilic. Thus cells rich in mitochondria characteristically show an eosinophilic (pink-red) cytoplasm. Examples of such cells are the parietal cells of the stomach and the oxyphil (acidophil) cells of the thyroid, parathyroid, pituitary, and salivary glands.

Because they provide high-energy phosphates, the mitochondria tend to be intimately associated with structures that urgently require this source of energy. In striated muscle cells, for instance, rows of mitochondria are found between the myofibrils. In cells that are actively synthesizing protein, cisterns of rough endoplasmic reticulum are sometimes seen to have mitochondria closely applied to their sides. Certain quantitative and qualitative features of mitochondria also correlate with cell activity. The mitochondria of cardiac muscle cells are therefore far more numerous and have many more cristae than those of skeletal muscle, which has long rest periods.

The cytoplasmic matrix and its contents

The cytocavitary network and the mitochondria are separated by their investing membranes from the cytoplasmic matrix, the nuclear matrix, and the non-membrane-bound structures that are contained in them. The following are chief among the microscopically identifiable elements that populate the cytoplasmic matrix:

1. Cytoskeletal and cytocontractile components (filaments and microtubules)
2. Glycogen
3. Free ribosomes
4. Lipid

Filaments are fine, fibrous protein threads that can be resolved individually only with the aid of the electron microscope. They become visible with the high power of the light microscope when they form aggregates or bundles, which are then called fibrils. Aggregates of fibrils visible with the low power of the light microscope or with the naked eye are called fibers. Filaments, fibrils, or fibers, when plentiful, impart a striking eosinophilic quality to cells or tissues.

The cytoskeletal and cytocontractile elements

The cytoskeletal and cytocontractile elements are the following:

1. *Intracytoplasmic filaments*
   a. *Myofilaments*
      (1) Thick (12 to 15 nm in diameter): myosin
      (2) Thin (6 to 8 nm in diameter): actin
   b. *Intermediate filaments* (diameter of 8-11 nm—i.e., intermediate between those of the actin filaments and the other filaments or the microtubules)
2. *Microtubules*

The term *cytoskeleton*, used to refer to these structures collectively, is unfortunately misleading, as it implies a lack of dynamic activity, which, as will be seen, is certainly not the case. Many of these elements exert a cytocontractile function, and some serve both as scaffolding and motile elements. All of the major classes of cytoskeletal elements may be found in virtually all of the body's cells.

In addition to the major proteinaceous subunits making up the backbone or core of the cytoskeletal elements (e.g., tubulin in microtubules), there are also numerous *associated proteins* that are thought to be involved in such functions as cross-linking and polymerization. These proteins include tropomyosin (associated with actin), intermediate filament-associated proteins (IFAPs), and the microtubule-associated proteins (MAPs).

The following discusses each of the cytoskeletal-cytocontractile elements in more detail.

Myofilaments. Myofilaments (thin actin and thick myosin) are present in virtually all vertebrate cells, being found in greatest quantity in muscle cells, in which they are diffusely distributed. In striated muscle, actin and myosin filaments are set side by side in a highly orderly fashion giving striated muscle its striated appearance (Fig. 1-17). In smooth muscle, only rare myosin filaments are identified, but many well ordered (par-

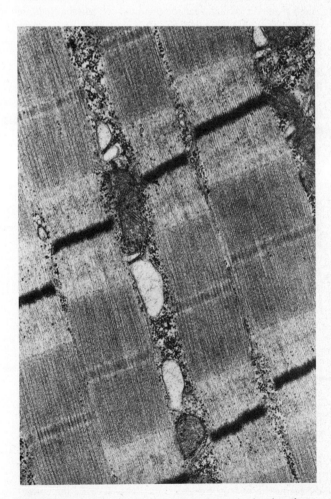

FIG. 1-17. Electron micrograph of skeletal muscle showing characteristic banding pattern.

allel) actin filaments with focal densities are present. Myosin molecules in nonmuscle cells are not polymerized into thick filaments and are difficult to detect.

Nonmuscle cells display a much larger repertoire of motility than do muscle cells. In the latter the myofilaments have a regular geometry that changes during contraction in a predictable manner along only one axis. By contrast, in nonmuscle cells, actin filaments are concentrated, in parallel arrays, in those parts of the cell in which they perform motile functions, particularly the cell periphery; there they may be linked to extracellular filaments through connecting protein complexes in the plasma membrane. Their preference for the cell periphery is due to their involvement in activities (such as pinocytosis, cell division, or cell migration) that involve plasma membrane movements.

Actin filaments consist of a double helical array of globular actin molecules with a width of 6 nm. In nonmuscle cells, actin filaments are transient structures and are only seen when actin molecules are polymerized. Myofilament-associated proteins of actin, such as tropomyosin and profilin, play a role in promoting or inhibiting polymerization. In contraction, myosin binds reversibly to actin filaments and catalyzes the hydrolysis of ATP.

Intermediate filaments. Intermediate filaments are true cytoskeletal elements. They maintain cell shape, the positioning and distribution of organelles including the nucleus, and the integrity of cell-to-cell contacts. These filaments are usually found distributed throughout the cytoplasm in radiating networks from the juxtanuclear region to the cell surface, lending credence to the idea that they provide a cytoskeletal framework upon which other structures and molecules may be organized. However, the functions of intermediate filaments are still hypothetical, because, at least under laboratory conditions, it appears that an intact cytoskeleton is not vital to the cell.

Intermediate filaments lack the tremendous lability of myofilaments and microtubules. The subunits of intermediate filaments are probably polymerized as soon as they are synthesized and remain, for the most part, polymerized until they undergo proteolysis and therefore form stable structures. All intermediate filaments have (1) a similar ultrastructural appearance, and (2) with x-ray diffraction, an alpha-helical protein secondary structure. Chemically, however, intermediate filament subunits represent a very large and diverse family of proteins. Their location in different cell types implies that they are related to cellular differentiation. This property is used to classify neoplasms of uncertain differentiation: sections can be stained to determine which types of filaments the tumor cells contain. Six major types of intermediate filaments have been identified:

1. Cytokeratins
2. Vimentin
3. Desmin
4. Neurofilaments
5. Glial filaments
6. Lamins

Cytokeratins. Cytokeratins are largely confined to epithelial or epithelial-derived cells, but are sometimes expressed in cells of mesenchymal derivation, such as smooth muscle cells.

Although many cell types contain cytokeratins, it is only squamous epithelial cells that form keratin, i.e., which keratinize. *Keratinization* is seen as a physiologic phenomenon in the formation of hair, nails, and the horny layer of the epidermis. In the course of this process, virtually the entire content of the cell is replaced by the accumulation of cytokeratin bundles termed *tonofibrils* (Fig. 1-18), and there is concurrent autolysis of cellular organelles, including the nucleus, by a process of limited proteolysis. *Fillagrins* are IFAPs specifically associated with keratinization and function in the aggregation of cytokeratin filaments into tonofibril bundles. Keratin appears as glassy, refractile material on light microscopy and is strongly eosinophilic.

Vimentin. Vimentin filaments are the predominant class of filaments found in mature nonmuscle cells of mesenchymal derivation. They are also found in immature cells of other types, including epithelial, muscle, and glial cells. They sometimes form tonofibrils, such as those found in meningothelial cells.

Desmin. Desmin (skeletin) filaments are found chiefly in smooth muscle, skeletal, and cardiac muscle cells.

Neurofilaments. Neurofilaments are found in most neurons of the central and peripheral nervous systems.

Glial filaments. Glial filaments, consisting of glial fibrillary acidic protein (GFAP), are found in astrocytes.

Lamins. Lamins have been discussed earlier in connection with the nuclear matrix.

Microtubules. Microtubules are hollow, noncontractile structures with an exterior diameter of 24 nm and measuring up to many micrometers in length. Like myofilaments, their subunits are in dynamic equilibrium between assembly and disassembly; disassembly into their subunits *(tubulin dimers),* as well as reassembly, can take place very rapidly, giving rise to a dynamic cellular scaffold rather than a rigid skeleton. Microtubules are involved in various types of cell movement, including ciliary beating, phagocytosis, movement of secretory granules and other organelles, and mitosis. Microtubules are sensitive to low temperature and high concentrations of calcium, which may be important in the regulation of their assembly.

Cytoskeletal components seem to be structurally coordinated in the cell, with microtubules appearing to play a dominant role as coordinators. Probably central to this role are the *microtubule-associated proteins (MAPs)*, which form fine filamentous projections on the microtubule surface and which connect with other structures. MAPs are of different types and function in different ways. Some appear to guide the distribution of actin filaments by linking actin filaments with microtubules, thus giving rise to a network of microtubules crosslinking with myofilaments. Yet others appear to be involved in determining the distribution of intermediate filaments.

In cilia (Fig. 1-19), centrioles, and sperm tails (collectively termed *microtubular organelles),* two groups of MAPs have been defined. The ATPase *dynein* allows the sliding movement of microtubules along each other, inducing a beating movement. Static structural linkers termed *nexin links* and *radial spokes* serve to maintain the correct spatial relationships between microtubular doublets (in cilia and sperm tails) and triplets (in centrioles). Dyneinlike MAPs may be found in other sites than cilia, functioning in the cytoplasm to "propel" organelles along the length of the microtubules at great speeds. In neurons, high molecular weight MAPs and MAPs termed *tau protein* link microtubules with neurofilaments and also appear to catalyze tubulin polymerization into microtubules.

Centrioles, which are barely visible with the light microscope, are pairs of hollow, open-ended cylinders lying at right angles to each other near the Golgi complex. Their walls consist of nine parallel microtubule triplets, and they function as sites of initiation of microtubule production. Thus they give rise to the pole-to-pole microtubules of the mitotic apparatus, as well as to the microtubules of cilia.

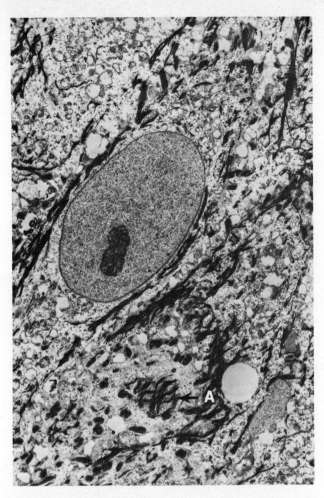

FIG. 1-18. Squamous epithelial cells containing tonofibril bundles *(A)*.

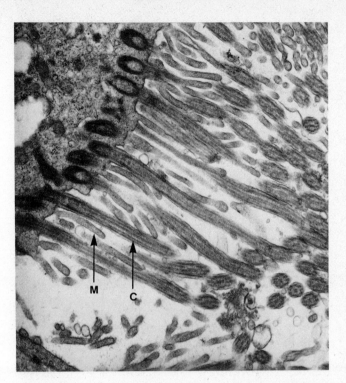

FIG. 1-19. Electron micrograph of nasal mucosal epithelium demonstrating the contrasting appearances of cilia *(C)* and microvilli *(M)*. The latter are more slender than the former and lack a content of microtubules. *(Courtesy Dr Rolland C Reynolds, University of Texas, Southwestern Medical School, Dallas.)*

Glycogen

Glucose is stored in cells as the polysaccharide glycogen. Most of the enzymes involved in its synthesis and degradation are located in the cytoplasmic matrix, where glycogen is usually found. Glycogen is present in greatest amounts in cells (such as striated muscle cells and hepatocytes), which constantly require large quantities of fuel for energy. At the ultrastructural level, glycogen is seen as dark-staining granules twice the size of ribosomes and tends to form caviar-like clusters unlike ribosomes, which are generally widely dispersed in the cell (Fig. 1-20). Glycogen is usually washed out during the processing of routine histologic sections. For this reason, the cytoplasm of cells rich in glycogen may appear clear or vacuolated in such preparations.

Free ribosomes

Both monoribosomes and polyribosomes are not only bound to the membranes of the rough endoplasmic reticulum but also are found lying free in the cytoplasmic matrix (see Fig. 1-4). These so-called free ribosomes are in other respects similar to the membrane-bound variety. Whereas membrane-bound ribosomes are largely involved in the synthesis of export protein, free ribosomes take part in producing protein intended for use by the cell itself. Examples of the latter proteins are filaments, the globin portion of hemoglobin, and the enzymes of the cytoplasmic matrix.

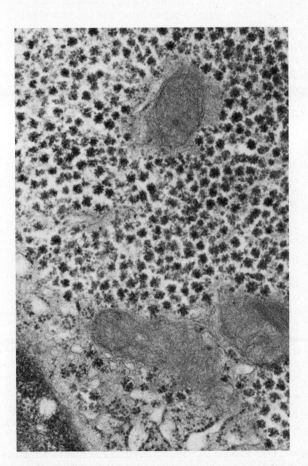

FIG. 1-20. Electron micrograph of liver cell with numerous glycogen rosettes, each consisting of clusters of glycogen monoparticles.

When present in large qualities, ribosomes (whether free or membrane-bound) impart the qualities of pyroninophilia (orange-red staining with methyl green pyronin) and hematoxyphilia to the cytoplasm. There is a correlation between the level of protein synthesis and the ribosomal content of the cell. This is exemplified in the maturing red cell, where the ribosomes diminish in number as hemoglobin synthesis nears completion and finally disappear altogether. Reticulocytes are nearly mature red cells in which the few remaining ribosomes can be demonstrated by appropriate stains.

Lipids of the cytoplasmic matrix

Lipids form an important part of biologic membranes. They may also be seen as amorphous droplets in the cytoplasmic matrix, not only in fat cells but also, in lesser quantities, in a variety of other cell types. The removal of lipid from the cell during histologic processing may, as in the case of glycogen, impart a clear appearance to the cytoplasm. Intracellular mucus is a third class of substance that may give cells this appearance in routine paraffin sections.

The cell surface
Cell surface projections and invaginations

The cell surface may be modified in several ways. This and the following sections deal with those parts of the cell surface that show specialization of various kinds.

Cilia (see Fig. 1-19) are structurally the most specialized cell surface projections. They are formed from long microtubules that extend from centrioles at right angles to the cell surface, with evagination of the plasma membrane. Each cilium contains 9 outer pairs of microtubules and one central pair, all parallel. The centriole remains at the base of the cilium as its so-called basal body. Cilia are abundant in the epithelia of the respiratory tract, fallopian tube, ductuli efferentes, and cerebrospinal fluid pathways and are essential for transport of their contents, namely mucus, ova, spermatozoa, and cerebrospinal fluid respectively. Protozoan flagella are structurally and functionally similar to cilia.

Microvilli (see Fig. 1-19) are more widely distributed in the body than cilia, but unlike the latter, they are not individually discernible under the light microscope because of their smaller size. They consist of simple projections of plasma membrane that contain only a fine core of myofilaments but no microtubules. Microvilli are much less motile than cilia; their main function is to enhance the absorptive and secretory capabilities of the cell by vastly increasing the area of its surface. They are most numerous in epithelia that have important absorptive and secretory functions, that is, those lining the intestines and the proximal renal tubules. In these sites they form so-called brush borders (Fig. 1-21), discernible with the light microscope, since the microvilli there are so densely packed that they resemble the bristles of a brush. It may be relevant that helminths that parasitize the intestines also have a brush border covering which may enhance their absorptive capacity.

Endocytosis and exocytosis

The transport of ions or small molecules into or out of the cell only occasionally requires modifications in the configuration of the surface membrane of the cell. Transport of macromolecules or insoluble (particulate) matter, by contrast, very commonly involves transient changes of cell surface morphology. This is aptly termed *vesicular transport*. There is incorporation of extraneous matter into membrane vesicles that form at the cell surface *(endocytosis)*, or there is release of matter

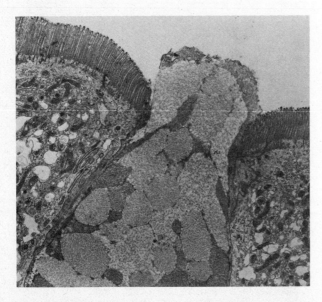

FIG. 1-21. Electron micrograph of small intestine showing a mucus-filled goblet cell flanked by absorptive cells with brush borders.

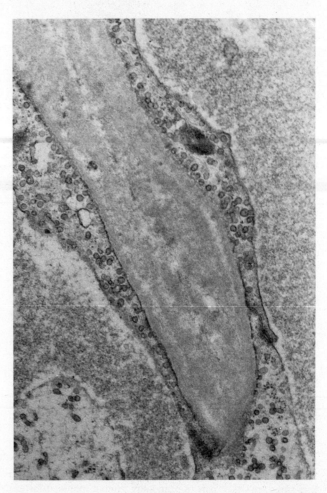

FIG. 1-22. Portions of several capillary endothelial cells containing numerous micropinocytotic vesicles.

from vesicles at the cell surface into the surrounding environment *(exocytosis)*. Vesicles formed by endocytosis become part of the cytocavitary network, and those from which matter is released (secreted) at the cell surface are, of course, derived from it.

Because of the continual membrane recycling as a result of endocytosis and exocytosis, the term *endocytic cycle* is employed. In nonmotile cells, this cycling is a random process, going on in many different directions in different parts of the cell. In cells migrating in tissues, however, the endocytic cycle demonstrates a well-defined polarity, with endocytosis taking place at the rear end of the cell, and exocytosis at the leading edge. This produces a continual "flow" of plasma membrane from front to rear, and the cell moves forward.

Endocytosis of coarse particles such as bacteria involves their entrapment by large, blunt, temporary cell surface projections called *pseudopodia*. This process is called *phagocytosis*. En-

gulfment of finer particulate matter and/or fluid is accomplished with the aid of projections more slender than pseudopodia and termed *filopodia*. The term used to describe this process is *pinocytosis* (Gr., drinking cell). Pinocytic vesicles are smaller than phagosomes. In *micropinocytosis* (Fig. 1-22), extremely fine particles (e.g., iron micelles) and/or fluid are taken into the cell in tiny flasklike invaginations of the plasma membrane that subsequently "pinch-off," toward the interior of the cell, as micropinocytic vesicles. The latter form of endocytosis involves little alteration of the cell surface configuration.

A variation on the theme of micropinocytosis is *receptor-mediated endocytosis*, most of which takes place at sites on the cell surface known as *coated pits* (Fig. 1-23, *A*); these are shallow surface indentations where a fibrous protein called *clathrin* is intimately associated with the cytosol-facing aspect of the plasma membrane. "Pinching-off" of these pits results

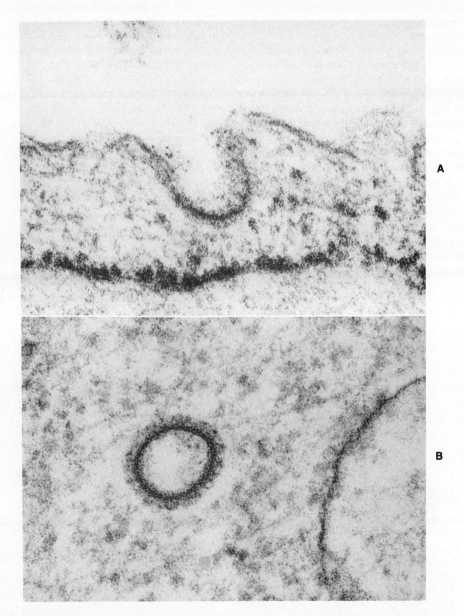

FIG. 1-23. A, Electron micrographs depicting the formation of a coated pit at the cell surface; **B,** with transformation into a coated vesicle. *(Courtesy Dr RGW Anderson, University of Texas Health Science Center at Dallas, and Journal of Cell Biology.)*

in the formation of *coated vesicles* in the cytoplasm (Fig. 1-23, *B*). Among the more important compounds taken into the cell by this mechanism are the low-density lipoproteins (LDL), an important source of cholesterol needed for the synthesis of most cellular membranes. The role of LDL and LDL receptors in the pathogenesis of atherosclerosis is discussed in Chapter 10.

Intercellular connections

Cells can be connected to one another in many ways (Fig. 1-24), all of which may be seen in a wide variety of tissues, especially epithelia. The following are the most common:

1. Cells may be held together through *fusion* of their adjacent glycocalyces but with a fairly regular narrow gap remaining between them.
2. There may be *interdigitation* of the cell's opposing membranes in the fashion of a jigsaw puzzle.
3. Cells may be connected by *cell junctions* that are localized structural modifications at certain points between adjacent cells. Cell junctions provide an exceptional degree of mechanical resilience.

Essentially, there are three types of cell junctions: tight junctions, gap junctions, and desmosomes. *Tight junctions* are seen especially around the lumenal margins of cells forming ducts and glands and serve to seal the lumen off from the surrounding extracellular environment. Tight junctions involve actual fusion of the outer lamellae of the plasma membranes of the adjacent cells.

In the vicinity of *gap junctions* the cells are separated by a narrow space that is seen (by specialized electron microscopy techniques) to be crossed by a series of minute channels that permit the passage of ions and small molecules between adjacent cells. Gap junctions are found especially in cardiac and smooth muscle, and they facilitate the transmission of electrical impulses that involve the movement of ions.

In the *desmosome* there is a localized increase in intervening cell coat material, and the space between the opposing plasma membranes remains relatively wide. In addition, a bunch of tonofibrils (cytokeratin in most cells, vimentin in meningothelial cells) is anchored to the cytoplasmic aspect of each opposing

membrane at this point. Although fairly widely distributed in the body, desmosomes are especially large and numerous in squamous epithelia. So-called intercellular bridges, seen with the light microscope in tissues with well-developed desmosomes, are areas where desmosomes continue to hold cells together that have elsewhere been pulled apart by the action of fixatives.

The extracellular matrix

The major components of the matrix are (1) the *fibrous component* (collagen fibers and elastic fibers) and (2) the largely amorphous *interfibrillary matrix* (mainly proteoglycans, non-collagenous glycoproteins, solutes, and water). In the formation of bones and teeth the extracellular matrix becomes calcified.

Collagens

The term *collagen* represents not a single protein species, but a family of closely related glycoproteins, each of which is genetically, biochemically, and functionally distinct. At least 15 types of collagen molecules, indicated with Roman numerals, have been identified to date. For the purposes of this chapter, note the following classification of collagens.

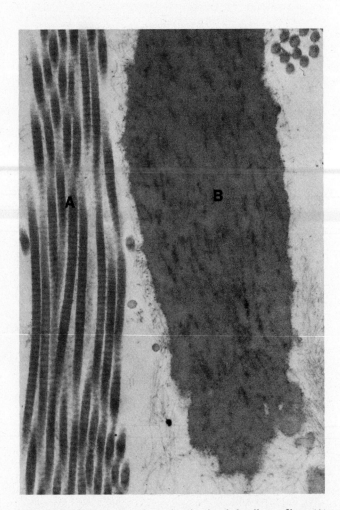

FIG. 1-25. Electron micrograph showing banded collagen fibers *(A)* and a single elastic fiber *(B)*.

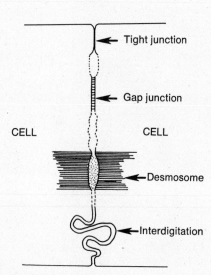

FIG. 1-24. Diagram showing the major ways in which cells may be connected.

Fibrillar collagens. These collagens form fibrils with uniform periodic cross-striations (Fig. 1-25). Also termed the *interstitial collagens*, this group includes types I, II, and III. Type I is the most abundant and is present in most connective tissues. Type III is a less abundant collagen that is usually distributed in association with type I. The fibrillar collagens are largely responsible for the rigidity of connective tissue matrices. Tissues rich in types I and III collagens appear grossly white and have a tough, fibrous nonelastic character. Type II collagen is a major component of hyaline cartilage.

Nonfibrillar collagens. Included in this group are most of the remaining collagen types. The most common nonfibrillar collagen is type IV, a major constituent of all basement membranes.

The major steps in *collagen synthesis* are depicted diagramatically in Fig. 1-26.

Collagen nomenclature. In a given collagen molecule, the triple helix may be composed of any combination of α_1 and/or α_2 chains or their subtypes. A type designation is assigned to each combination. The common type I collagen molecule, for example, contains two $\alpha_1(I)$ chains and one $\alpha_2(I)$ chain.

Basement membrane

The basement membrane consists of two layers: the basal and reticular laminae. The *basal lamina (external lamina)* is the ultrastructurally distinctive component of the basement membrane and lies almost immediately adjacent to the basal aspect of epithelial and endothelial cells and around muscle and Schwann cells. It consists of a discrete, usually thin zone of amorphous, noncollagenous glycoprotein matrix (including laminin and entactin) in which proteoglycans and tiny filaments of unbanded type IV collagen, barely discernible with the electron microscope, are embedded. Basal laminae exhibit a strong affinity for silver stains. The *reticular lamina* lies external to the basal lamina. Its major components are fibronectin and type III collagen fibrils.

Reticulin fibrils

So-called *reticulin fibrils* are found in a wide variety of tissues, including lymph nodes and bone marrow, and consist of a variety of amorphous and fibrillar matrix components (chiefly collagens) that, like basal laminae, avidly bind silver stains. Reticulin fibrils are not specific ultrastructural entities but are defined by their staining properties.

Elastic fibers

Elastic fibers are considerably broader than collagen fibers (see Fig. 1-25). They tend to have a jagged outline and consist of a meshwork of fine, noncollagenous glycoprotein fibrils in which an amorphous protein, elastin, is embedded. Elastic fibers confer an elastic flexibility on tissues. To the naked eye, elastic tissue appears opaque and yellow.

Proteoglycans

All the *glycosaminoglycans* in the body, with the possible exception of hyaluronic acid, are found in the native state covalently bound to proteins (i.e., they exist as *proteoglycans*). These are defined as macromolecules that contain a core protein to which at least one glycosaminoglycan is covalently linked. Proteoglycans differ greatly in protein content and molecular size and in the number and/or types of glycosaminoglycan side chains per molecule; those with many side chains resemble a bottle brush. The molecular heterogeneity of proteoglycans may imply distinct functions in the organization of the extracellular matrices of connective tissues. Aside from their role as major structural elements of the extracellular matrix, some proteoglycans are bound to plasma membranes and appear to be involved in adhesiveness and receptor binding, among other functions. Examples of major proteoglycans, their distribution, and functions are listed in Table 1-1.

Proteoglycans appear with the electron microscope as polygonal electron-dense granules, 10 to 50 nm in diameter, lying in an abundant, poorly staining amorphous background.

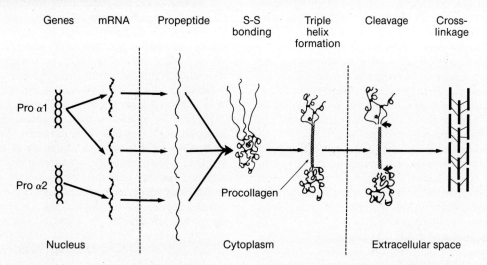

FIG. 1-26. Diagram depicting major steps in collagen synthesis. One or both of two types of pro α polypeptide chains are synthesized in the rough endoplasmic reticulum, where they are wound together to form pro α triple helices. Following secretion via the Golgi complex, there is enzymatic splitting off of globular polypeptide sequences from either end of the pro α chains. The result is the formation of α triple helices, which (except in the case of basement membrane collagen) subsequently undergo spontaneous polymerization into long fibrils that aggregate alongside one another with covalent cross-links to form mature banded collagen fibrils.

TABLE 1-1. Distribution and functions of major proteoglycans

Type	Location	Functional roles
Chondroitin sulfate proteoglycan	Cartilage	Resilience, water-binding
	Vessel wall	Maintenance of viscoelasticity, regulation of permeability
Dermatan sulfate proteoglycan	Tendon, skin	Regulation of fibrillogenesis and fibril diameter, maintenance of normal architecture
Heparan sulfate proteoglycan	Cell surface	Cell recognition, cell attachment
	Basement membrane	Permeability, filtration of macromolecules
Keratan sulfate proteoglycan	Corneal stroma	Maintenance of corneal transparency, refractive properties

On light microscopy, tissues rich in proteoglycans have a pale, loose-textured appearance, stain light blue-gray with hematoxylin and eosin, and stain with cationic dyes such as Alcian blue; when examined grossly, such tissues tend to appear translucent and feel slimy or gelatinous or (in the case of cartilage) resemble plastics. The distinctive gross characteristics of such tissues are attributed to the tremendous water-binding capacity of proteoglycan molecules. Historically, the term *mucopolysaccharide* was applied to these substances in order to describe a polysaccharide material that was viscous or mucuslike.

Noncollagenous glycoproteins

Although most normal cells in the body keep their places, a few cell types routinely move through the extracellular matrix; during embryonic development and wound healing, certain cells migrate extensively. This movement is highly organized, and most of the cells reach their destination unerringly. This organization of cells, both fixed and dynamic, is at least in part maintained by a variety of large noncollagenous glycoproteins that bind cells to the extracellular matrix. The best understood of these are the *fibronectins*; others include the *laminins*, *chondronectins*, and *osteonectins*.

The fibronectins, collectively known as *fibronectin*, are found almost ubiquitously in the extracellular matrix. They are synthesized by many different cell types. There is also a circulating form, known as plasma fibronectin, produced mainly by hepatocytes. Fibronectin molecules are versatile and can assemble into 2 to 5 nm diameter filaments, bind to cells, and link cells to other kinds of filaments or fibrils in the extracellular matrix. Fibronectin's adhesive character makes it a crucial component of blood clots (Chapter 13) and of pathways followed by migrating cells. Fibronectin-rich pathways guide and promote the migration of many kinds of cells (e.g., neural crest cells) during embryonic development.

Cytoskeletal actin filaments and the extracellular fibronectin are physically connected across the cell membrane. This connection is mediated by a complex of proteins termed the *fibronexus*. Presumably the same proteins that make the transmembrane connection also interact with fibronectin during cell adhesion and migration.

Calcified extracellular matrix

Calcified tissue is radiopaque, appears black in electron micrographs (Fig. 1-27), and stains blue-black with hematoxylin.

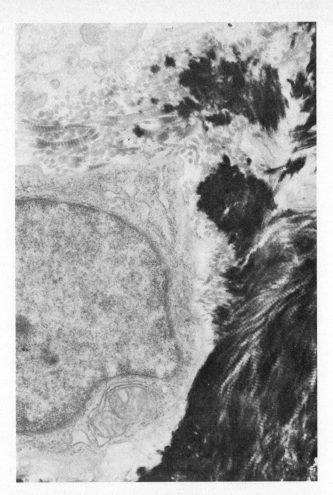

FIG. 1-27. Electron micrograph of calcifying cartilage showing banded collagen fibers with varying degrees of calcium phosphate deposition.

Calcification of the extracellular matrix takes place in the formation of bones and teeth. It involves, as the terminal event, the formation of insoluble, crystalline, calcium-phosphate mineral in the form of *hydroxyapatite*. The calcification process has two major phases, an initiation (nucleation) phase and a mineral growth phase.

Initiation phase. A major role in the *initiation phase* has been attributed to structures termed *matrix vesicles* (Fig. 1-28). These are submicroscopic, membrane-invested, extracellular particles, about 200 nm in diameter. They probably form by budding from the plasma membrane of cells, such as osteoblasts, which control the calcification process. There is also evidence that they may form as a result of a process akin to *apoptosis*, a type of energy-dependent cell death in which the cell disintegrates into multiple, tiny, discrete bodies (for full discussion, see Chapter 2). There is evidence that apoptosis may, for instance, be the mode of cell death in the cartilage growth plate during bone formation. Matrix vesicles probably function as follows:

1. Calcium is attracted by acidic phospholipids concentrated in the matrix vesicles.
2. This is followed by the concentration of phosphates in the matrix vesicle by means of phosphatases located in the vesicle membrane.
3. High calcium and high phosphate within the protected microenvironment of the matrix vesicle are then probably

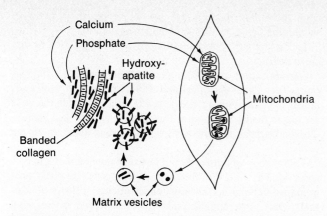

FIG. 1-28. Possible pathways of apatite deposition in bone, dentin, and cementum.

sufficient to promote deposition of calcium phosphate mineral, first as an amorphous compound and later as highly insoluble hydroxyapatite.

Sometimes, matrix vesicles do not appear to be involved in the nucleation process. In these cases, proteoglycans may act as initial calcification sites. In this regard, the sulfur contained within sulfated glycosaminoglycans and released from proteoglycan molecules appears to promote the binding of calcium and phosphorus, with resulting apatite crystal formation.

Mineral growth phase. The second phase, that of *mineral growth,* is brought about by exposure of preformed apatite crystals to the extracellular fluid. The *rate* of mineral propagation is controlled by factors outside matrix vesicles in the extracellular space. Two groups of controlling factors have been identified.

First, there are natural *inhibitors* of crystal proliferation that include pyrophosphates, magnesium, citrate, gamma-carboxyglutamic acid-rich proteins, and inadequate concentrations of calcium and phosphate. Second, there are factors that act as *promotors* of crystal proliferation. Among these are (1) collagen, which also spatially orientates hydroxyapatite in bone; (2) the noncollagenous glycoproteins chondronectin and osteonectin, which may serve to link collagen and apatite deposits; and (3) elevated levels of calcium and/or phosphate.

There is evidence that *mitochondria* may function as the earliest storage site of amorphous calcium and phosphorus. This stored mineral is subsequently made available extracellularly to support the mineral growth phase (see Fig. 1-28). This is still, however, hypothetical.

In summary, cells control skeletal mineralization, not only by regulating the composition of the matrix in which calcification takes place but also by depositing matrix vesicles at the sites where calcification will begin. The role of the mitochondria in these cells in mineralization is uncertain.

Remodeling of the extracellular matrix

The remodeling of the connective tissue matrix is an essential process in human physiology and depends on a precise balance between (1) the breakdown of existing connective tissue and (2) the deposition of newly synthesized matrix elements. In most tissues, the same cell is responsible for the regulation of the two arms of the process, and this cell is generally a differentiated mesenchymal cell (such as a chondrocyte or fibroblast). In certain tissues (e.g., bone), different cells are re-

sponsible for each of these components of remodeling. In other types of tissues (basement membrane), the remodeling process is orchestrated by epithelial or endothelial cells. Thus, the resident connective tissue cells possess the enzymic potential for degrading the individual components of the extracellular matrix. This is controlled by strict regulatory mechanisms, breakdown of which may result in disease. A discussion of this aspect is found in Chapter 2.

The normal cell and matrix at the borderland of pathology

The classic, prototypic appearance of cells, as described in standard histology texts, represents a steady state of biologic activity in a healthy, nonstressed environment. Besides this, there exists a spectrum of cell morphology (varying from appearances reflecting heightened cellular activity to changes indicating decreased cell function) that can also be regarded as being completely within normal limits. These variations on the theme of cellular normality are important to emphasize because (1) they highlight the essentially dynamic nature of the human organism and (2) overlap with certain important pathologic processes which, to some extent, represent an exaggeration of normal functional states. It is also timely, in this highly litigious world in which health care practitioners function, to stress the principle that functional deterioration and death (at both the cellular and whole body levels) are very much a part of normal life.

Increased cellular activity

Normal cell populations are occasionally subjected to stimuli that call for a great increase in function. Under such circumstances, cells respond either by increasing in number (*hyperplasia*), increasing in size (*hypertrophy*), or both. The size of the organ or body part often increases concomitantly. When cellular enlargement is seen under such circumstances it is due to changes that reflect increased protein synthesis on the part of the cell. These changes include the following:

1. Increase in the nuclear envelope's surface area in order to effect increased passage of RNA from nucleus to cytoplasm—the nucleus may be strikingly enlarged, or less obviously so due to folding of the nuclear envelope.
2. Increase in nucleolar size and/or number, for increased ribosomal RNA synthesis.
3. Changes in the conformation and distribution of chromatin, with the formation of enlarged chromatin aggregates (chromatin "clumping") and consequent decreased density ("clearing") of the parachromatin areas—these changes presumably promote the transcription process, but the exact mechanism is unclear.
4. Increased numbers and/or size of cytoplasmic organelles—among the more constant changes seen is an increase in the number of ribosomes, imparting an increased hematoxyphilia to the cytoplasm.

Examples of greatly increased cellular activity in physiologic circumstances include the dramatically enlarged smooth muscle cells of the myometrium that prepare the uterus for labor, the enlarged cells of the biceps muscle of the lumberjack, and the changes that breast lobular epithelium undergoes in preparation for lactation. In addition, in order to give rise to cells that form antibodies, lymphocytes undergo transformation to large blastic cells (blast transformation) (see Fig. 1-5) following exposure to antigens, a process that takes place in all individuals except those housed in an artificial, germ-free environment from birth. In individuals at high altitudes with low atmospheric oxygen tension, there is a dramatic increase in red cell production by the marrow, coupled with an increased number of marrow erythroblasts, in response to erythropoietin secretion by the kidneys.

In order to facilitate tissue molding, the extracellular matrix produced by embryonal cells tends to be very rich in proteoglycans and sparse in collagen. For this reason, embryonal connective tissue has a "myxoid" look. This appearance in postnatal life generally reflects a pathologic state (see "Connective Tissue Activation," Chapter 2).

Changes reflecting increased cellular activity may be seen in an exaggerated form in several pathologic states (Chapters 2 and 9). Whether normal or pathologic, they are potentially reversible if the stimuli producing them are removed.

Decreased cellular activity: physiologic cell death and the biology of aging

Physiologic cell death. Perhaps the most dramatic example of physiologic cell death is the daily loss of blood cells, calculated to be about 370,000,000,000! Most of this cell loss appears to take place through a process by which effete cells rupture and are rapidly sequestered by phagocytically active organs such as the spleen.

A special form of cell death, the importance of which has only recently come to be recognized, is *apoptosis* (Gr. dropping off, as of leaves from trees). This is a morphologically distinct, energy-dependent process affecting isolated cells in living tissue and is seen in a wide range of physiologic, as well as pathologic, circumstances. Its mechanisms, morphology, and role in disease are discussed in Chapter 2.

Apoptosis as a physiologic phenomenon. Apoptosis is the chief mechanism that the normal body has for the elimination of unwanted cell populations. This is the process by which the molding of tissues takes place during embryologic development. Thus, for example, apoptosis is responsible for the elimination of interdigital webs during the formation of fingers.

Apoptosis plays a role in the process termed *atrophy*, which may be a normal event or a manifestation of a pathologic process. The term atrophy means a decrease in size in a body part due to loss and/or shrinkage of its cells and/or matrix. In addition to apoptosis, which appears to be the chief mode of cell deletion in atrophy, there is increased cellular autodigestion (autophagy), which, in turn, is responsible for the shrinkage of surviving cells; such cells tend to show increased numbers of autolysosomes. Examples of *physiologic atrophy* include the regression (due to trophic hormone withdrawal) of the corpus luteum of the ovary and the cyclical involution of breast lobules. Whether apoptosis plays a part in the atrophy of aging (see following section) is unknown, although observations made in tissue culture studies suggest that it does.

Apoptosis also serves an opposite function to mitosis in the *regulation of tissue size* and is especially obvious in rapidly proliferating, mitotically active cell populations, such as intestinal crypt epithelium or the seminiferous tubular germ cells.

Apoptosis may also play a role in the *elimination of cells with mutations*; random mutations due to changes, such as breaks in DNA strands, appear to develop in all individuals, especially in cells with a naturally high proliferative activity. Such mutations may be corrected by the cell's own repair mechanisms. However, where there are irreparable genetic abnormalities, those cells appear to be selectively eliminated through apoptotic self-destruction. The passing on of genetic errors to succeeding cell generations is thus prevented.

Lastly, apoptosis plays a role in matrix calcification as discussed earlier.

Keratinization as a physiologic phenomenon. Keratinization is yet another example of physiologic cell death. However, unlike the case with the previous examples in which the cells are lost to the body as useful, functioning entities, the keratinized cell serves a protective, waterproofing function to the body.

The biology of aging. Aging is a fundamental biologic process, which, like the molding of embryos, involves programmed cellular self-destruction; it affects virtually all animals. Only those animals (some fish and reptile species) that continue to increase in size after reaching adulthood do not age; they are not immortal, however. As in animals that do age, these animals will die from disease, accidents, or predators.

The discipline of cytogerontology, the study of aging at the cellular level, is a relatively new one. Despite the fact that many, if not most, of the secrets pertaining to cellular aging in humans still need to be revealed, certain fundamental principles, based chiefly on study of serial cell cultures or transplants, have already been established. These may be summarized as follows.

Aging is inevitable. Cell immortality is defined as continuous serial cultivation in vitro or in vivo in which there are at least 100 population doublings over a minimum of at least 2 years. It has been repeatedly demonstrated that when normal human embryonic cells are grown under the most favorable conditions, functional decline and death is the inevitable consequence after about 50 population doublings.

The number of population doublings of cultured human cells is inversely proportional to donor age. For instance, cultured fibroblasts derived from older humans are found to replicate fewer times than those derived from embryos.

There is a direct relationship between maximum species lifespan and population doublings of their cultured cells. The cells of the mouse, for instance, replicate fewer times in culture than do human cells, which in turn replicate fewer times than those of the Galapagos tortoise. This relationship suggests the presence of a chronometer or pacemaker within all normal cells that is characteristic for each species. The postulated chronometer may or may not be the same one that has been suggested to control the inverse relationship between donor age and population doubling potential.

Cells remember. Viable normal human cells taken from culture after a specific number of doublings and stored in the frozen state for as long as 23 years remember at which population doubling level they were frozen and, upon reconstitution, undergo the number of population doublings that would normally have remained to them had cell culture not been interrupted.

Immortal cells are abnormal. Cancer cells, along with other derangements in the genetic control of growth and replication, lose the capacity to undergo aging. Cancer cell populations behave like immortal cell lines and can be serially cultured indefinitely. Still in use today in research laboratories throughout the world are cell lines such as the HeLa cells (derived from a human cervical carcinoma in 1952) and the L cells (derived from mouse mesenchyme in 1943).

A progressive decline in cell function heralds the cell's approaching loss of ability to divide. To date, almost 200 functional changes have been found in cultured normal human cells before their loss of replicative capacity. The reported changes cover virtually all aspects of cell biochemistry, morphology, and behaviour. Many of these same changes that are known to take place in cultured normal human cells as they age in vitro are identical to changes found in cells in vivo as humans age. They include, among many other changes, increased autophagy. It is likely that these changes underlie the clinical expression of aging and result in the death of the individual well before his or her cells reach their potential for division. Cessation of mitotic activity is probably only one functional decrement that succeeds many others in the aging process; all of these may share a similar genetic basis.

A model for precocious aging may be the very rare disease *progeria*. Afflicted individuals manifest, at the end of the first decade of life, the physical signs of aging typical of their normal counterparts at the seventh decade of life. Cultured fibroblasts taken from these donors exhibit from 2 to 18 doublings, whereas normal values for the same chronological age are between 20 and 40. The full clinical picture of progeria consists of early graying and loss of hair, short stature, juvenile cataracts, proneness to diabetes, atherosclerosis and calcification of the blood vessels, osteoporosis, and a high incidence of malignancy.

Future research in cytogerontology will be directed toward yielding information on the molecular nature of the pacemakers or chronometers that are thought to be present in the nuclei of normal cells. Although "clock tampering," as researchers themselves acknowledge, could be a time bomb, with the potential for very undesirable consequences, new information of this kind might unlock the key to the understanding and possible treatment of diseases (such as cancer) related to cellular aging.

Selected readings

Adams LP et al, editors: The biochemistry of the nucleic acids, ed 10, London and New York, 1986, Chapman & Hall, Ltd.

Basic molecular and cell biology, Series of articles in Br Med J 295, 1987.

Bretscher MS: How animal cells move, Sci Am 257:72, 1987.

Cormack DH, editor: Ham's histology, ed 9, Philadelphia, 1987, J.B. Lippincott Co.

De Robertis EDP and De Robertis EMF, editors: Cell and molecular biology, ed 8, Philadelphia, 1987, Lea & Febiger.

Frost JK: The cell in health and disease, ed 2, Basel, 1986, S Karger.

Ghadially FN: Ultrastructural pathology of the cell and matrix, ed 2, London, 1982, Butterworth & Co (Publishers), Ltd.

Hayflick L: Cell death in vitro. In Bowen ID and Lockshin RA, editors: Cell death in biology and pathology, London and New York, 1981, Chapman & Hall, Ltd.

Hayflick L: The cell biology of aging, Clin Geriatr Med 1:15, 1985.

Hynes RO: Fibronectins, Sci Am 254:42, 1986.

McDonagh J: Fibronectin: a molecular glue, Arch Pathol Lab Med 105:393, 1981.

McKusick VA: The morbid anatomy of the human genome: part 1, Medicine (Baltimore) 65:1, 1986.

The molecules of life, Series of articles in Sci Am 253(4), 1985.

Rothman JE: The compartmental organization of the Golgi apparatus, Sci Am 253:74, 1985.

Rubin RP et al, editors: Calcium in biological systems, New York and London, 1985, Plenum Publishing Corp.

Uitto J and Perejda AJ, editors: Connective tissue disease: molecular pathology of the extracellular matrix, New York and Basel, 1987, Marcel Dekker, Inc.

Wang E et al, editors: Intermediate filaments, Ann NY Acad Sci 455:1, 1985.

Wright AF: DNA analysis in human disease, J Clin Pathol 39:1281, 1986.

Yang D et al: Mitochondrial origins, Proc Natl Acad Sci USA 82:4443, 1985.

CHAPTER 2

The cell and extracellular matrix in disease

Injury to tissue, whatever the cause, can produce changes at any or all levels of its organization, ranging from the molecule at one end of the scale to the whole patient at the other. This chapter deals with the basic morphology and pathobiology of disease, emphasizing its molecular and ultrastructural alterations. Read in conjunction with Chapter 1, it should provide a basis for understanding the gross and microscopic changes in diseased tissues.

In very simple terms, *cells* in disease may:
1. Die
2. Be injured but not die
3. Become hyperactive
4. Become hyperactive and exhibit bizarre growth patterns

In summary, the *matrix* may be:
1. Improperly formed
2. Deposited in excessive quantities
3. Destroyed
4. The site of deposition of unwanted material

THE CELL IN DISEASE

As stated previously, most of the cellular changes in disease can be placed in one of four categories that can be present alone or in combinations in a particular disease. In pathologic terms they are as follows:
1. Cell death (lethal cell injury, usually acute)
2. Sublethal cell injury (usually chronic)
3. Inappropriate increase in cell activity
4. Malignant neoplasia

Cell death

Cell death, also termed acute lethal cell injury, is the permanent cessation of the life functions of the cell. The term *acute* describes cellular events that take place in a short period of time.

Two forms of cell death important in disease are to be distinguished morphologically:
1. *Apoptosis,* which has physiologic functions (Chapter 1) as well as being implicated in many disease processes
2. *Necrosis,* which has no physiologic function and is virtually always associated with disease

Apoptosis

When apoptosis takes place in disease a biologically meaningful role is usually evident. This may be seen, for instance, when apoptosis is induced by cell-mediated immunity. In the latter, the process appears to be aimed at the elimination of antigenically altered cells, which benefits the host. Regrettably, this same process can also lead to the elimination of important cell populations, such as liver or thyroid cells in viral hepatitis or autoimmune thyroiditis.

The following are examples of apoptosis in pathologic states:
1. Lymphocyte-mediated cell killing
    a. Autoimmune disease
    b. Graft rejection
    c. Graft-versus-host disease
    d. Lichenoid skin diseases
    e. Tumor regression
    f. Viral infections
2. Cell deletion in low-grade ischemia
    a. Ischemia-induced atrophy
    b. Tumors
3. Cell deletion by physical agents
    a. Ionizing radiation
    b. Transient mild hypothermia (seminiferous tubules)
    c. Ultraviolet light (epidermis)
4. Hormone-induced tissue atrophy
    a. Decreased trophic hormone levels (e.g., adrenal cortex after ACTH withdrawal)
    b. Glucocorticoid-induced lymphoid tissue atrophy
5. Other
    a. Atrophy associated with glandular duct obstruction
    b. Cell deletion by radiomimetic cytotoxic drugs
    c. Pathologic calcification (apoptotic matrix vesicles)
    d. Regression of non-necrotizing granulomas
    e. "Spontaneous" (non-lymphocyte-mediated) tumor regression

Morphology of apoptosis. The cellular events associated with apoptosis are depicted in Fig. 2-1. The process begins with fragmentation of the nucleus (karyorrhexis) and clumping (compaction) of chromatin, which aggregates in discrete, dense, often crescent-shaped masses against the nuclear envelope. Concurrently, there is compaction of the cytoplasm, which leads to the formation of dense clusters of organelles. As this process continues, broad, often pedunculated, protuberances form on the surface of the cell and the nucleus often becomes convoluted or shaped like a cloverleaf, eventually breaking up into discrete fragments.

Subsequently, the cell disintegrates into *a variable number of membrane-bound bodies of different sizes,* some of which contain nuclear material (Fig. 2-2). Organelles within these apoptotic bodies appear to be well preserved at this stage. As seen by phase-contrast microscopy, this early stage of apoptosis lasts only a few minutes and is accompanied by violent cell movement.

Most apoptotic bodies are rapidly *phagocytosed* and *degraded* by intralysosomal digestion by adjacent epithelial cells or macrophages, although a few are extruded into lumina. In a few hours, only a little indigestible material remains within lysosomal residual bodies.

As the apoptotic bodies are removed, the surviving cells close ranks; thus many cells can be eliminated without disorganizing the tissue architecture.

Apoptosis Normal cell Necrosis

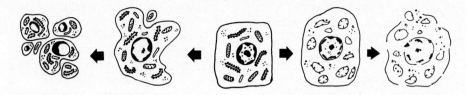

FIG. 2-1. Diagram contrasting the changes in apoptosis and necrosis. In apoptosis, there is condensation and fragmentation of cells, whereas in necrosis there is usually cell swelling and disintegration.

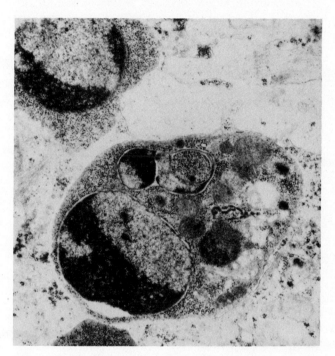

FIG. 2-2. Electron micrograph of two apoptotic bodies. Both consist of cytoplasm containing membrane-bound nuclear fragments showing the typical crescentic chromatin clumping.

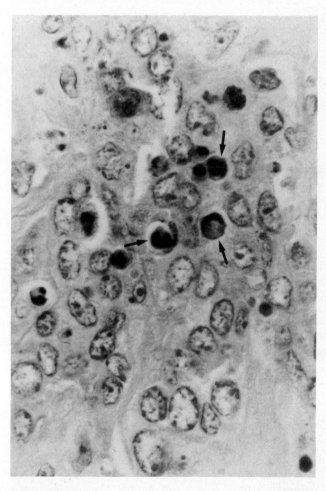

FIG. 2-3. Histologic section from a malignant lymphoma showing multiple apoptotic bodies *(arrows).*

Microscopic appearance of apoptosis. As seen by light microscopy, apoptosis affects scattered single cells. By contrast, necrosis is conspicuous and affects groups of contiguous cells or tracts of tissue.

Light microscopic evidence of apoptosis consists of (1) anuclear cytoplasmic fragments or (2) small, condensed nuclear fragments found singly or in groups; only the larger apoptotic bodies and those containing nuclear chromatin are readily seen (Fig. 2-3). In the latter, crescentic aggregates of chromatin surrounded by a thin rim of eosinophilic cytoplasm are characteristic.

Examples of apoptotic bodies include the following:
1. Acidophilic or Councilman bodies in the liver (Chapter 15)
2. Civatte bodies of lichen planus
3. Tingible bodies found in lymphoid germinal centers

Mechanisms of apoptosis. Apoptosis appears to be a process of rapid, active, energy-dependent cell destruction rather than a degeneration. Experimentally, nuclear fragmentation results from cleavage of nuclear deoxyribonucleic acid (DNA) at the linker regions between nucleosomes by an endogenous *endo-*

nuclease. This specific enzymatic change in DNA is quite different from the nonselective DNA degradation that is typical of the later stages of necrosis.

Activation of the endonuclease is due to slightly increased intracellular levels of calcium and magnesium that might follow slight alterations of cytoplasmic membrane permeability. A greater influx of cations would be likely to initiate sufficient phospholipase activity to cause membrane lysis and necrosis.

Reaction to apoptosis. Since apoptosis appears to be essentially a physiologic mechanism, it is not surprising that there is neither an inflammatory nor a connective tissue response to the process. The failure to attract neutrophil leukocytes, which are often found in areas of tissue necrosis, may be explained by the intact membranes that surround apoptotic bodies. In apoptosis-associated conditions that are immunologically mediated—such as chronic active hepatitis (Chapter 15), the fibrous tissue reaction is probably the result of lymphokine stimulation of fibroblasts and is not due to apoptosis.

Necrosis

Necrosis is morphologically the more commonly recognized form of cell death. Typically, it is the *destruction of many contiguous cells en masse* and, unlike apoptosis, is always pathologic. In fact, necrosis is one of the most significant events in disease.

Although the clinical effects of necrosis may be minimal, as for example, in an aphthous ulcer in the mouth, its consequences can be devastating in cerebral or myocardial infarction. The following are important examples of diseases or lesions of which necrosis is a major feature:

1. Abscesses
2. Acute pancreatitis
3. Amebiasis
4. Chemical burns
5. Frostbite
6. Gangrene
7. Histoplasmosis
8. Infarcts
9. Neoplasms (many)
10. Thermal burns
11. Tuberculosis
12. Ulcers
13. Viral diseases (many)

Etiology and pathogenesis of necrosis. The biochemical events and changes in organelles that take place in the evolution of necrosis due to different causes are diverse, complex, and often interrelated. Cell injury leading to necrosis can be divided into two phases:

1. An early *reversible* phase characterized by fairly subtle morphologic changes.
2. If the injurious stimulus persists, a late *irreversible* phase follows in which the cell undergoes striking morphologic changes and dies.

The *reversible phase*, whatever its cause, is characterized by an increase in cytoplasmic membrane permeability leading to an influx of cations (Na^+, Ca^{++}, Mg^{++}) moving down concentration gradients. The mechanisms causing increased permeability vary with the cause of cell injury.

In the *irreversible phase*, there is denaturation of cell proteins and destruction of cell membranes due to a varying degree of (1) activation of calcium-dependent phospholipases, (2) production of oxygen radicals leading to lipid peroxidation, and (3) hydrolysis by lysosomal enzymes.

Several of the better studied examples of mechanisms leading to necrosis are as follows:

1. Hypoxia, anoxia, or ischemia
2. Oxygen radicals and lipid peroxidation
3. Complement-mediated attack
4. Lytic enzymes
5. Cytolytic viruses
6. Massive physical or chemical cell membrane trauma

Necrosis due to tissue hypoxia, anoxia, or ischemia. The progression of events in cell injury due to oxygen depletion is well established. When the cell is subjected to a *decreased*

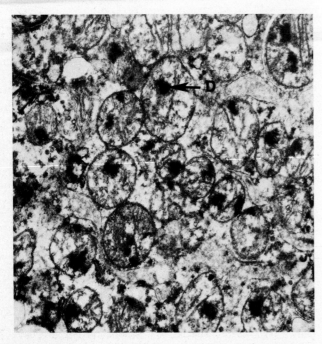

FIG. 2-4. Electron micrograph of irreversibly injured cell. The mitochondria contain matrical flocculent densities *(D)*.

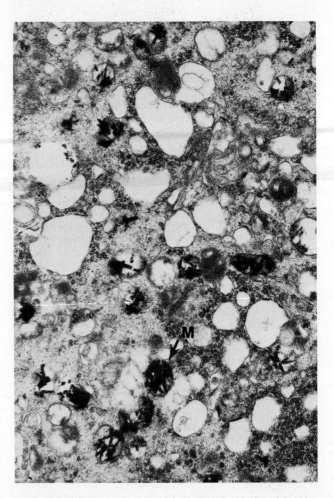

FIG. 2-5. Hydroxyapatite crystal deposition in mitochondria *(M)*.

oxygen supply, there is depression of mitochondrial oxidative phosphorylation, which results in a compensatory increase in anaerobic glycolysis to provide cell energy. This raises intracellular lactic acid levels with a fall in pH. The low pH induces depression of ribonucleic acid (RNA) synthesis, and consequently, protein synthesis stops. Ultrastructurally, at this stage, chromatin no longer has a granular appearance and appears as solid zones of electron-dense material.

Depression of mitochondrial oxidative phosphorylation also results in decreased synthesis of adenosine triphosphate (ATP), which provides essential energy for membrane transport. As a consequence, membrane transport mechanisms fail, causing increased membrane permeability to solutes. In a hydrated environment, this results in the flooding of the membranous organelles and/or the cell matrix with water, leading to *cell swelling.* If little fluid is available, the cell loses water and shrinks. If the oxygen supply is restored at this point, the cell may revert to normal. Beyond this point, however, the process is irreversible and the cell dies.

The changes associated with transition to the irreversible stage are first seen only by electron microscopy. They consist of the appearance of flocculent, electron-dense accumulations of denatured matrix protein in the inner chamber of mitochondria (Fig. 2-4). Clumping of chromatin progresses and becomes visible by light microscopy.

A steep rise in free cytosolic calcium due to anion influx activates calcium-dependent phospholipases (which cause breakdown of cellular membranes) and production of cytotoxic free fatty acids and lysophospholipids. Excessive intracellular calcium increases calcium ATP-ase activity and utilization of ATP, which is already depleted in ischemic cells. Raided levels of calcium also inhibit mitochondrial oxidative phosphorylation, which further depletes cellular energy.

Mitochondrial calcium and phosphate loading may also lead to deposition of hydroxyapatite and dystrophic calcification (Figs. 2-5 and 2-6). Cytoplasmic protein coagulation, which also accompanies calcium levels in the cytosol, results in increased cytoplasmic affinity for eosinophilic stains.

Greatly increased membrane permeability leads to leakage of enzymes from lysosomes and lysis of the nucleus *(karyolysis)* and cytoplasm; this process is known as *autolysis.* Ultimately, there may be total disruption of cell membranes, releasing phospholipids, which form large, concentric lamellar bodies called myelin figures (Fig. 2-7).

Necrosis due to free radicals. Free radicals, formerly thought to be produced only in tissues subjected to ionizing radiation, are now known to be normal intermediate products of oxygen metabolism. They appear to play a role in both lethal and nonlethal cell injury due to a variety of causes. In addition to radiation injury, they are believed to mediate cell damage caused by neutrophils, macrophages, iron overload, cigarette smoke, and most drugs and chemicals, including alcohol.

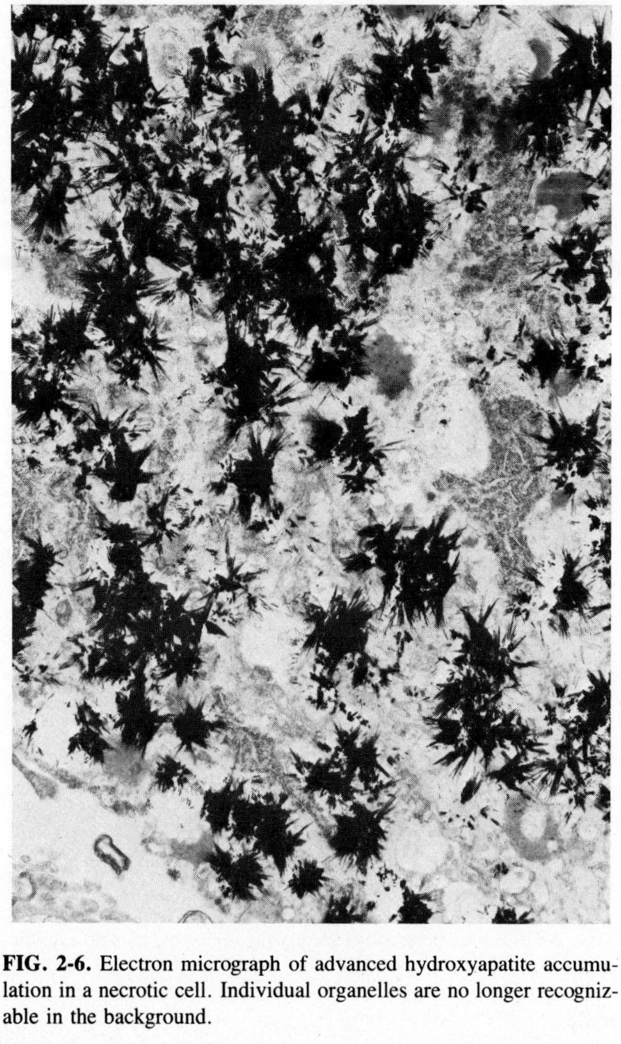

FIG. 2-6. Electron micrograph of advanced hydroxyapatite accumulation in a necrotic cell. Individual organelles are no longer recognizable in the background.

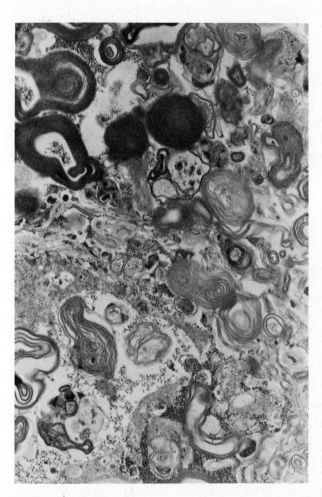

FIG. 2-7. Myelin figure accumulation in an acutely injured cell.

A *free radical* is any chemical species that has one or more unpaired electrons and thus is unstable. In oxygen metabolism, sequential univalent reduction of oxygen leads first to formation of superoxide anion radicals (O^-), which are converted to hydrogen peroxide by superoxide dismutase; hydrogen peroxide (H_2O_2) is, in turn, converted to water and oxygen. Thus:

$$2O_2^- + 2H^+ \xrightarrow{\text{superoxide dismutase}} H_2O_2 + O_2$$

$$2H_2O_2 \xrightarrow{\text{catalase}} 2H_2O + O_2$$

$$H_2O_2 + H_2 \xrightarrow{\text{peroxidase}} 2H_2O$$

If superoxide anions and hydrogen peroxide accumulate, hydroxyl ions (OH^-) can be formed. Since there are no enzymes to metabolize these anions, extensive cell destruction can take place. The exact mechanism of free radical toxicity is not known, but there is evidence that peroxidation of cell membrane lipids leads to abnormal membrane structure and cell death.

Necrosis due to complement-mediated cell lysis. Cell death can also be caused by proteins of the complement system (Chapter 6), as for example, in immune complex–mediated cell injury. Molecules of the late complement complex (C5789) can polymerize within the plasma membrane of the target cell to form the *membrane-attack complex,* * a doughnutlike structure sited across the cell membrane. This complex has a hydrophobic outer surface (which associates with membrane lipids) and a hydrophilic center, through which small ions can pass.

In complement-mediated attack, the cell cannot maintain its osmotic and chemical equilibrium, and as a consequence, it swells and bursts. This process is seen, for example, in lupus nephritis (Chapter 16), and immune hemolysis (Chapter 13). Complement may cause cell injury indirectly by promoting chemotaxis of neutrophils, which are capable of releasing oxygen radicals.

Necrosis due to hydrolytic enzymes of cells and microorganisms. Powerful enzymes capable of tissue destruction can be released by some cells in the body. In acute pancreatitis, pancreatic secretions are released into peritoneal fat, causing *enzymic fat necrosis* due to the action of lipase on triglycerides and formation of highly irritant calcium soaps.

Lytic enzymes released by macrophages are thought to be one cause of necrosis seen at the center of various *granulomas,* particularly those in tuberculosis and histoplasmosis (Chapter 6). Free oxygen radicals released by macrophages may also contribute to this process.

Clostridium perfringens, a bacterium that can cause gas gangrene, produces many toxins, including phospholipase C, which splits off diglycerides from membrane phospholipids. Cell membranes damaged in this way allow leakage of ions and influx of water. This soon leads to necrosis by mechanisms similar to those already described for anoxia-ischemia.

Necrosis due to cytopathic viruses. Most viruses kill cells by one of two mechanisms. Many (such as poliovirus) are directly cytopathic, whereas others (hepatitis B virus, for example) require participation of the host immune system to produce irreversible cell injury.

Viruses that are directly cytopathic are thought to cause cell death, in part by the incorporation of viral proteins into the host cell membranes. This disrupts ionic gradients between the outside and inside of the cell, leading to the series of events described in necrosis from other causes. In addition, cellular metabolic activity ceases as the virus switches off host cell nucleoprotein production in favor of viral synthesis. Viral-induced lethal cell injury may be accompanied by the formation of viral inclusions (Chapter 8).

Necrosis due to heat, cold, chemical, or mechanical trauma. The lethal destructive effects of these agents on cells is the result of major damage to cell membranes and requires no further description.

Light microscopic features and gross appearance of necrosis. The light microscopic features of necrosis are readily related to the ultrastructural changes already described.

In the early reversible phase of acute cell injury, there is *cell swelling,* if the cell environment is sufficiently hydrated. Cells affected in this way often appear granular, foamy, or have cloudy, vacuolated cytoplasm, and the tissue or organ appears swollen and pale. If little fluid is available, as in "dry gangrene" (described later), the cells appear condensed and shrunken.

The most obvious changes of necrosis involve the nucleus, where the chromatin first forms clumps of hematoxyphilic material around the periphery of the nucleus, leaving the remainder

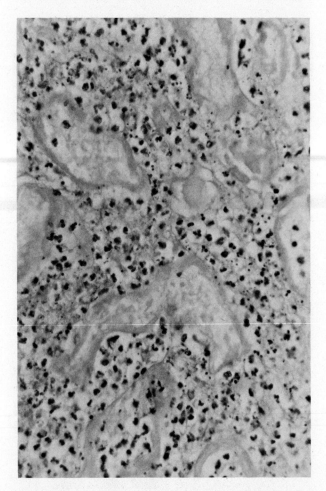

FIG. 2-8. Necrotic neutrophils seen lying among the ghosts of tubules at the periphery of a renal infarct. Many specks of nuclear dust, consisting of karyorrhectic debris from disintegrated neutrophils, are seen.

---

*This complex is structurally and functionally similar to the pore-forming protein perforin 1 released from cytotoxic T and natural killer lymphocytes during lymphocyte-mediated apoptosis. The protozoon, *Entamoeba histolytica,* causes cell damage by the same mechanism (Chapter 14).

of the nucleus empty. This appearance is called *karyorrhexis* (literally, nuclear breakup) (Fig. 2-8). If chromatin clumping is accompanied by nuclear shrinkage, the latter appears as a solid, dark blue mass. This process is called *pyknosis* (literally, a condensation). *Karyolysis,* which is enzymatic digestion of the nucleus, follows chromatin clumping and results in disappearance of the nucleus. Thus a very striking microscopic feature of necrotic tissue is the *absence* of nuclei (Fig. 2-9), while the remaining tissue stains deep pink with eosin.

Grossly, necrotic tissue is typically paler and more friable than normal. Associated hemorrhage produces red discoloration. *Fat necrosis* appears as chalky white deposits, while enzymatic lysis is capable of producing cavities in tissues and organs.

Morphologic subtypes of necrosis

Liquefactive necrosis. The degree of enzymatic destruction of tissue can vary with the cause. In its most extreme form, tissue lysis results in *liquefaction* and formation of a *cavity.* This process of liquefactive necrosis is characteristic of necrosis in the central nervous system. It is also typically seen in the center of abscesses in which proteolytic enzymes released during phagocytosis have lysed the tissue.

Coagulative necrosis. Necrosis in which liquefactive changes are not present is called *coagulative necrosis.* In many instances, the gross architecture of the necrotic tissue is pre-served for some time, although cellular detail is lost. In two special examples of coagulative necrosis, however, autolysis is more rapid and complete:

1. *Caseation* is typical of tuberculosis and is named for its cheese-like appearance.
2. *Gummatous necrosis* is characteristic of the late stages of syphilis. The affected tissue has a rubbery texture. Loss of tissue architecture is not so pronounced as in caseation and probably because the extracellular matrix is better preserved.

Infarct. An *infarct* is an area of necrosis that results from impaired blood supply (ischemia). The process is termed *infarction.*

Gangrene. *Gangrene* is an old clinical term originally applied to any black, foul-smelling area of tissue in the living body. It is the result of extensive necrosis together with putrefaction caused by microorganisms. The black color is the result of oxidation of hemoglobin and myoglobin in the dead tissues.

Dry gangrene or *mummification* does not strictly conform to the original definition of gangrene. Typically, the process affects the extremities of people with occlusive vascular disease, particularly those who are diabetic. There is little or no putrefaction, and the dead tissue appears black, dry, and shriveled, and is sharply demarcated from the adjacent viable tissue. Variants of true (wet) gangrene include gas gangrene (Fig. 2-10)

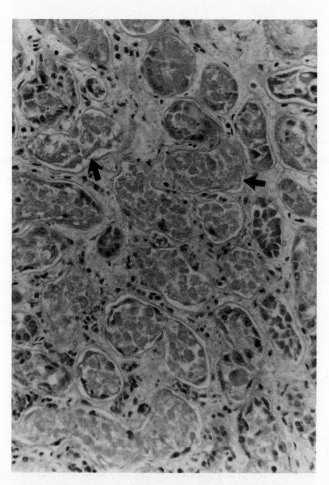

FIG. 2-9. Histologic section showing necrotic renal tubules *(arrows)* contrasted with viable-appearing tubules. The absence of stainable nuclei distinguishes the former from the latter. In this case, the tubular necrosis was caused by vascular occlusion from humoral rejection in a transplanted kidney.

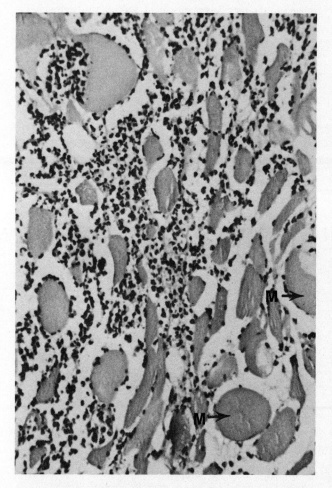

FIG. 2-10. Gas gangrene. Microscopic appearance of muscle infection by *Clostridium perfringens.* The muscle fibers *(M)* are necrotic and widely separated by gas produced by the bacteria and large numbers of inflammatory cells.

in which bubbles of gas from carbohydrate-fermenting bacteria are formed in the dead tissues.

Reactions of the body to necrotic tissue. The body treats necrotic tissue as a foreign body and attempts to remove it by an inflammatory response. The dead tissue, in some instances, is replaced by tissue of the same type (regeneration). More often, however, this cannot be accomplished, and the necrotic tissue is replaced by unspecialized connective tissue (fibrous repair). On occasions it may become calcified and cannot be removed.

Clinicopathologic correlations

Reversibility of the early stages of potentially lethal cell injury has an important clinical application. If, after cardiopulmonary arrest, the oxygen supply to the brain can be maintained artificially, anoxic injury to the brain, which will reach the irreversible stage in about 5 minutes after oxygen has been cut off, can be prevented. This is the great value of cardiopulmonary resuscitation and why speedy action by bystanders is critical in these circumstances.

Lethally injured cells release their cytoplasmic enzymes into the circulation, some of which are diagnostically useful in the detection of myocardial, hepatic, and skeletal muscle injury.

Another effect is alteration of the electrical activity of the injured cell, which can be revealed by the electrocardiogram and electroencephalogram. These electrical abnormalities are related to the membrane alterations and ion shifts already discussed.

Lastly, products of damaged cells can stimulate specific macrophages to initiate the mechanisms of fever (Chapter 8).

Summary

The terms cell death and necrosis are often used interchangeably in the literature, despite the fact that they are not synonymous. Cell death means irreversible injury; necrosis is the morphologic effect of denaturation and hydrolysis of cell components following cell death.

Apoptosis is a recently recognized process that leads to death of cells in both physiologic and pathologic states. However, terms such as *individual cell necrosis* and *piecemeal necrosis,* which usually signify apoptosis, have long been used and are still common in the literature.

Apoptosis and necrosis are compared in Table 2-1.

TABLE 2-1. Comparison of necrosis and apoptosis

Necrosis	*Apoptosis*
Always pathologic	Physiologic or pathologic
Disruption of cell's vital functions by factors extrinsic to cells	Active process of cellular self-destruction
Usually involves groups of contiguous cells	Affects single cells scattered throughout a tissue
Usually cell swelling and disruption, often followed by phagocytosis by inflammatory cells	Cell condensation and fragmentation, followed by rapid phagocytosis by local parenchymal or inflammatory cells
Excites an inflammatory response	Does not excite an inflammatory response

Sublethal cell injury

A variety of factors cause long-term changes in the structure and function of the cell but do not kill it. The "degenerations" and "infiltrations" described in older texts fall into this category. In sublethal cell injury, the affected cells often show changes that directly reflect the injury. These changes frequently consist of an accumulation in the cell of substances or organelles. Examples include the following:

1. Lipids
2. Glycogen
3. Lysosomes
4. Cytoskeletal-cytocontractile elements

Lipids in sublethal cell injury

The terms *fatty degeneration* or *fatty change* have been used to describe the accumulation of visible intracytoplasmic lipids (mainly triglycerides) in parenchymal cells such as those in the heart, kidney and liver (Figs. 2-11 and 2-12). It is controversial whether—and to what degree—fat accumulation impairs cell function. Nevertheless, it indicates an underlying metabolic disturbance or toxic injury, and it is these—rather than the mere presence of fat—which present the greater threat to the cell.

Fatty change has many causes. However, the liver is the most important and best studied site of fatty change; its mechanisms (Fig. 2-13) are often complex and poorly understood. In general terms, dietary, toxic, and anoxic causes are recognized.

Dietary causes. Malnutrition associated with a decreased intake of essential nutrients may result in fatty change through several mechanisms. First, fat in body depots is mobilized, and as a consequence, increased amounts of fatty acids reach the cells, (particularly the hepatocytes). Second, lack of choline and other lipotropic agents results in diminished biosynthesis of phospholipid, which together with a lack of dietary protein, interferes with the formation of transportable lipoprotein molecules. Third, dietary protein deficiency also inhibits lipoprotein synthesis, which interferes with triglyceride transport and promotes its retention in the cell.

Malnutrition associated with a diet high in saturated fats may also cause fatty change through a higher supply of triglycerides to the cell. Fatty livers are commonly seen in those who are *morbidly obese* or who suffer from *protein-calorie malnutrition (kwashiorkor).* Fifty percent of patients with type 2 (adult-onset) diabetes have fatty livers, but this is the result of obesity rather than of diabetes itself.

Toxic causes. Many different substances can cause fatty change. Some, such as carbon tetrachloride, chloroform, and phosphorus, do so chiefly by blocking synthesis of proteins, particularly oxidative enzymes and low-density lipoproteins.

Fatty change in the liver due to *alcohol abuse* is related to increased triglyceride synthesis and lipid peroxidation and to reduced activity of the citric acid cycle, so that the rate of oxidation of fatty acids decreases. Alcohol also decreases lipoprotein synthesis. As a result, the liver cells become swollen and laden with triglycerides; but although their appearance is greatly altered, the hepatocytes can exist in this form for long periods without any appreciable impairment of liver function. Once alcohol intake has stopped, the fatty liver reverts to normal in 3 to 4 weeks. The necrosis of liver cells occasionally seen

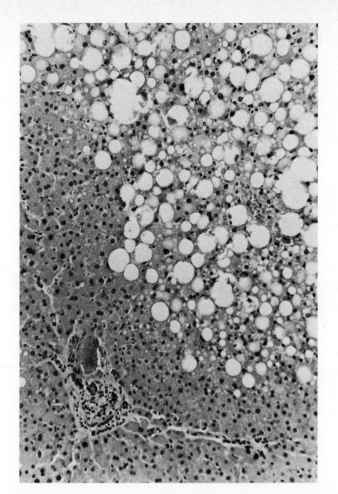

FIG. 2-11. Fatty liver. The cytoplasms of most liver cells in the upper right of the section are distended with fat.

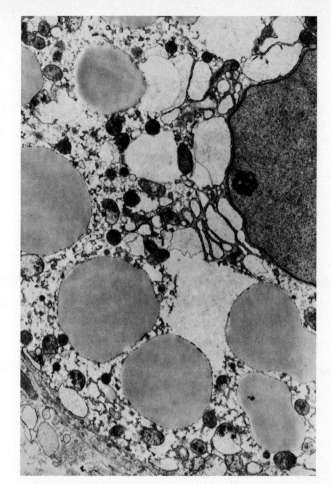

FIG. 2-12. Electron micrograph of fatty liver. Numerous fat droplets are present throughout the cytoplasm.

in alcoholics is not an effect of fat accumulation but rather the result of mitochondrial membrane damage, possibly due to acetaldehyde, an oxidation product of ethanol.

Fatty liver caused by ethanol intake is generally of the *large droplet type*. However, accumulation of *small droplet fat* in the liver and other organs is characteristic of certain potentially lethal disorders, which include Reye's syndrome (Chapter 15), acute fatty liver of pregnancy, and toxic effects of the anti-epileptic drug, valproic acid. The cause and pathogenesis of this form of fatty change are not fully understood, although viral, toxic, and nutritional factors have been implicated.

The accumulation of triglycerides in microvesicles within hepatocytes reflects interference with the exit of lipid from the cell through inhibition of synthesis of apoprotein (a very low-density lipoprotein) (Chapter 10). There is also mitochondrial injury which also inhibits oxidation of fatty acids.

Anoxic causes. Anoxia leads to decreased ATP synthesis which causes decreased lipoprotein synthesis, and results in inadequate export of lipid from the cells.

Fatty change versus infiltration. Fatty change should be distinguished from *fatty infiltration (adiposity),* which is seen in obese persons and in whom there is an increased amount of fatty tissue in parenchymal organs (Fig. 2-14). However, fatty infiltration is rarely associated with tissue injury.

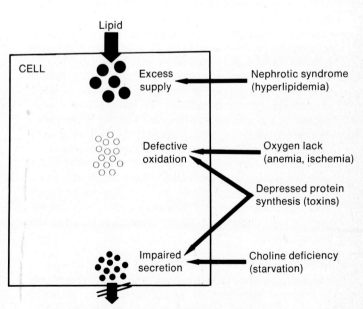

FIG. 2-13. Mechanisms of intracellular lipid accumulation.

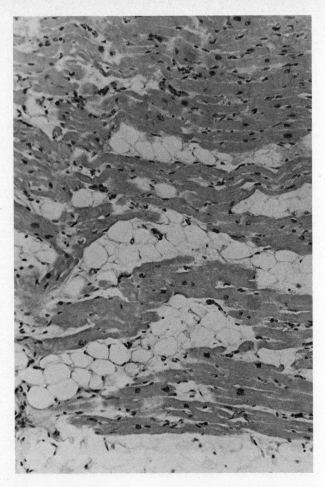

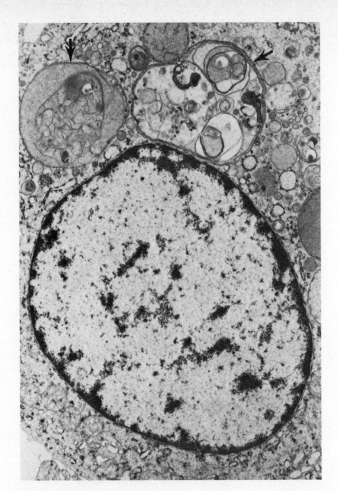

FIG. 2-14. Interstitial fat cell accumulation in subepicardial portion of right ventricle.

FIG. 2-15. Large cytolysosomes *(arrows)* containing membranous organellar debris in a sublethally injured cell.

Glycogen in sublethal cell injury

The *glycogen storage diseases*, of which 12 types have been described, result from inherited deficiencies in the enzymes necessary for the metabolism of glycogen. Pathologically, there is accumulation of glycogen in the cytoplasm and/or nuclei of cells; the nuclei appear pale and swollen by light microscopy. The tissues involved vary according to the specific enzyme deficiency. For example, in *von Gierke's disease,* in which glucose-6-phosphatase is deficient, excessive glycogen accumulates in the cells of the liver and kidney. In *McArdle's disease* (myophosphorylase deficiency) the skeletal muscles have an abnormally high glycogen content. These excessive glycogen stores are metabolically unavailable, and as a consequence, patients with von Gierke's disease are hypoglycemic, while those with McArdle's disease have pronounced muscle weakness. *Pompe's disease* (lysosomal alpha-glucosidase deficiency) particularly affects the myocardium, and this may lead to heart failure.

Lysosomes in sublethal cell injury

Autophagocytosis (literally eating of the self) appears to be an important mechanism for normal intracellular turnover of cytoplasmic contents. Increased autophagocytosis, on the other hand, is a frequent reaction when cellular organelles are injured sublethally (Fig. 2-15). It is seen, for example, following irradiation, mild hypoxia, or ischemia and as a response to a

variety of toxic chemicals. Autophagocytosis is characterized by an accumulation of *lipofuscin* pigment. This pigment appears (1) in the liver following mild viral hepatitis, (2) in the kidney in resolving acute renal failure, and (3) in the colon following the prolonged use of anthracene cathartics, where the resulting brown discoloration of the mucosa has been incorrectly called "melanosis coli" (Fig. 2-16).

Vitamin E deficiency. Cell membrane degradation, including that of lysosomes, is partly accomplished by lipid peroxidation. Vitamin E, a biologic antioxidant, inhibits this process, so that in its absence, lipid peroxidation proceeds unhindered and membrane breakdown is accelerated. As a result, there can be massive accumulation of lipofuscin in smooth muscle, particularly of the intestines, which for unknown reasons, become deep brown in color. Vitamin E deficiency is most likely to be seen in intestinal malabsorption (Chapter 14) but surprisingly is rarely of clinical importance.

Lysosomal storage disease. The accumulation of indigestible material in autophagic vacuoles (Fig. 2-17) in lysosomal storage disease is caused by complete or partial lack of one of the lysosomal hydrolytic enzymes. The enzyme deficiencies may be inherited (hereditary lysosomal enzyme deficiency) or acquired following the use of certain drugs (such as the antiarrhythmic drug amiodarone) that block the action of lysosomal enzymes.

The hereditary forms are mainly recessive disorders and par-

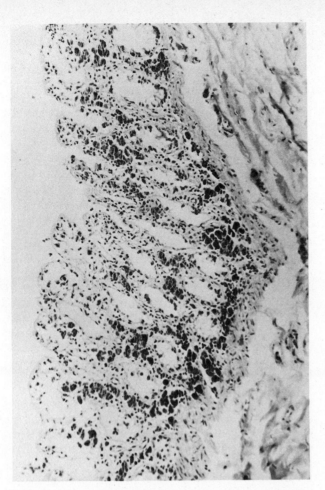

FIG. 2-16. Clusters of lipofuscin-filled macrophages in the colonic mucosa in so-called melanosis coli.

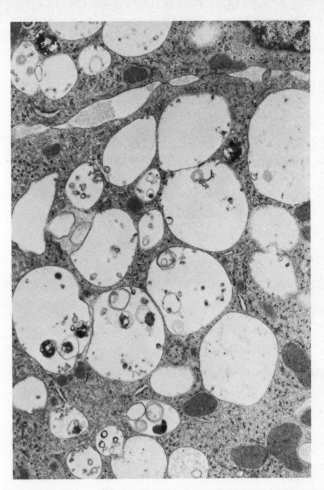

FIG. 2-17. Electron micrograph of proximal renal tubular cell showing lysosomes overloaded with proteoglycan in mycopolysaccharidosis.

ticularly affect the nervous system of infants and young children. Neurons and histiocytes are the cells most affected by these abnormalities which cause the lysomes to become more numerous and distended with indigestible cellular material.

The following is a list of the lysosomal storage diseases:

1. Glycoproteinoses
   a. Aspartyl-glycosaminuria
   b. Fucosidosis
   c. Mannosidosis
   d. Sialidosis
2. Mucolipidoses
   a. I cell disease
   b. Mucolipidosis IV
   c. Pseudo-Hurler polydystrophy
3. Mucopolysaccharidosis
   a. Hunter's disease
   b. Maroteaux-Lamy syndrome
   c. Morquio disease
   d. Mucopolysaccharidosis I
   e. Multiple sulfatase deficiency
   f. San Filipo disease
   g. Sly syndrome
4. Sphingolipidoses
   a. Fabry's disease
   b. Farber's disease
   c. GM1 gangliosidosis
   d. GM2 gangliosidosis
   e. Gaucher's disease
   f. Krabbe's disease
   g. Metachromatic leukodystrophy
   h. Niemann-Pick disease
5. Other lysosomal storage diseases
   a. Cholesteryl ester storage disease
   b. Cystinosis
   c. Pompe's disease
   d. Wolman's disease

Cytoskeletal-cytocontractile elements in sublethal cell injury

Myofilaments. The term *myofibrillary degeneration* describes a spectrum of nonspecific changes affecting myofilaments and the Z-lines of striated muscle cells undergoing degeneration and atrophy from various causes. These include denervation, ischemia, cachexia, and primary muscle diseases, such as muscular dystrophy and myositis.

The chief ultrastructural changes include disintegration and disorientation of microfilaments, including Z-line structures (Fig. 2-18) with shrinkage and even loss of cells.

Erythrocyte shape. The shape of red cells is maintained by a submembranous network of myofibrils consisting chiefly of a spectrin-actin lattice. In hereditary disorders, such as in elliptocytosis (Chapter 13), the defective cell shape is probably

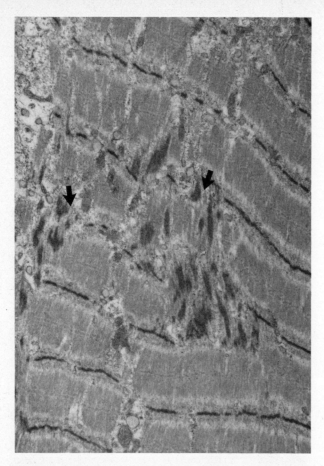

FIG. 2-18. Electron micrograph showing portion of a skeletal muscle cell from a case of muscular dystrophy. The arrows point to zones of Z-line disruption. *(Courtesy Dr James H Martin, Department of Pathology, Baylor University Medical Center, Dallas.)*

due to an abnormal spectrin molecule, which fails to form tetramers and leads to insufficient actin cross-linkage and subsequent instability of the membrane skeleton.

Intermediate filaments. A variety of disorders affecting various organs are associated with alterations of intermediate filaments. Those involving cytokeratins and neurofilaments are best understood.

Mallory bodies. Mallory bodies are focal cytoplasmic accumulations of cytokeratin filaments that are usually haphazardly arranged and accompanied by an amorphous component, possibly intermediate filament-associated protein. The cytokeratin filaments are abnormally shaped and chemically altered. In cells with large Mallory bodies, the intermediate filament cytoskeleton of the cell is severely deranged.

Mallory bodies are typical morphologic features of some liver diseases, particularly alcoholic hepatitis, where the term *alcoholic hyalin* is often used to describe these bodies. Mallory bodies are not, however, restricted to hepatocytes and are found in pulmonary alveolar cells in, for example, asbestosis and other diseases associated with pulmonary fibrosis.

Neurofilaments. Abnormalities of neurofilaments may be implicated in several neurologic diseases. In Alzheimer's disease (Chapter 19) and related forms of dementia, the typical pathologic features are the presence of the following:

1. Neurofibrillary tangles
2. Neuritic plaque amyloid
3. Vascular amyloid

These are found predominantly in the cerebral cortex, and their concentration appears to correlate with the degree of dementia. Tangles are entirely intracellular, consisting of morphologically abnormal fibrillar bundles. These are composed of two filaments, each about 10 nm in diameter, twisted helically about each other. These paired helical filaments are thought to be transported to nerve terminals, where they are released and polymerized in the extracellular space to form amyloid-like material. Accumulations of this material form the so-called neuritic plaques (senile plaques), and its uptake by blood vessels gives rise to cerebrovascular amyloid.

Microtubules. A variety of ultrastructural aberrations in the microtubular apparatus (Chapter 1) are found in the *immotile cilia syndrome*. This syndrome is an autosomal recessive disorder of the microtubules of ciliated cells and spermatozoa—and possibly of neutrophil polymorphs—that affects about 1 in 20,000 people.

The most common ultrastructural abnormality is a deficiency of dynein arms, which leads to immotility or erratic movement of spermatozoa and respiratory tract cilia. The result is male sterility, accompanied by chronic or recurring respiratory infections caused by absence of mucociliary clearance (Chapter 12) and leading to bronchiectasis in some cases.

In *malakoplakia*, there is inadequate or defective digestion of bacteria by the phagolysosomes of macrophages and the incompletely digested bacterial fragments form the organic matrix for intracytoplasmic deposition of calcium salts. Malakoplakia usually involves the urinary tract as a chronic inflammatory process, which, because of heavy macrophage infiltration, may sometimes mimic a neoplasm. The abnormal lysosomal function has been related to low levels of cyclic guanosine phosphate (cGMP), which is required by the cell to initiate microtubule assembly, a process essential for the release of lysosomal granules into phagosomes. A similar defect is thought to be the underlying cause of the Chediak-Higashi syndrome (Chapter 13) in which granulocytes have giant lysosomes, combined with impairment of lysosomal degranulation and bacteriocidal activity.

Drugs. Vinca alkaloids (such as vincristine), used in the treatment of several forms of cancer, prevent the assembly of microtubules, thus preventing mitosis and inhibiting cell division. Colchicine, used to treat gout, inhibits mitosis in a similar manner.

Increased cellular activity in disease

Increased cellular activity reflecting increased protein synthesis is found (1) following necrosis, (2) in the early stages of viral infection of the cell, (3) in hyperplasia or hypertrophy, and (4) in the malignant neoplastic cell.

Following necrosis

In a cell population, following necrosis, the remaining viable cells tend to exhibit increased compensatory proliferative and/or functional activity. Thus regenerating cells, such as the epithelial cells covering a healing peptic ulcer, tend to show enlarged nuclei and/or nucleoli, with larger chromatin aggregates and pronounced cytoplasmic hematoxyphilia that is due to increased numbers of ribosomes. Regenerating uterine cervical epithelial cells with this appearance in cytologic preparations are known as "repair cells."

With continued cell death and regeneration in a cell population over a long period, as in ulcerative colitis (Chapter 14), the morphologic changes just described may become greatly exaggerated and give rise to the use of descriptive terms such as *atypia* or *dysplasia* (Chapter 9).

In viral infection

In the early stages of viral infection of a cell, the morphologic changes reflect the increased burden placed on the cell's protein synthetic mechanisms by viral reproduction. Thus there is considerable enlargement of the nucleus and/or nucleolus and of chromatin aggregates in early viral synthesis. With viruses thought to be carcinogenic, such as certain papillomaviruses, these changes may with time become exaggerated and reflect a transition to a neoplastic process. In the later stages of some viral infections, nuclear enlargement may also be a degenerative process or may sometimes be the result of inclusion body formation (Chapter 8).

In hyperplasia or hypertrophy

When cell hypertrophy or hyperplasia is the result of disease, the processes may progress to and merge with, neoplastic states. One example is in endometrial hyperplasia in which morphologic changes similar to those already described can be seen.

In the malignant neoplastic cell (cancer cell)

The chief biologic property of the cancer cell is its ability to grow outside the normal bodily controls and to metastasize. The properties of cancer cells are discussed in Chapter 9.

THE EXTRACELLULAR MATRIX IN DISEASE

Connective tissue is the most ubiquitous component of the human body and the largest by weight. With the advent of electron microscopy and recombinant DNA technology, pathology of the extracellular matrix has assumed great importance. In the category of heritable disorders of connective tissue alone, over 140 diseases are now recognized. Some of these, together with some acquired disorders of connective tissue, are discussed in this section. They include some of the most common and debilitating diseases that affect humans.

Abnormalities of the extracellular matrix can be divided into four main categories, as follows:
1. Defective formation
2. Excessive formation
3. Abnormal degradation
4. Abnormal deposits

Defective formation of extracellular matrix

Fibrillar collagen defects. *Inherited* disorders of collagen synthesis comprise a large group of conditions that are evidenced clinically in many different ways. Among the best known are (1) osteogenesis imperfecta (Chapter 17), (2) Ehlers-Danlos syndrome (Chapter 19), and (3) Marfan's syndrome (Chapter 10).

In these three disorders, different steps in collagen biosynthesis may be defective or the synthesis of different types of collagen may be decreased (Table 2-2).

Two important examples of *acquired* disorders of collagen synthesis are (1) vitamin C deficiency (scurvy) and (2) the effects of persistently elevated levels of glucocorticoids. In *scurvy,* the absence of vitamin C impairs the activity of the enzymes involved in hydroxylation of proline and lysine, which in turn, results in defective intermolecular cross-linkages in the collagen molecule. The consequences of the poor matrix formation include defective wound healing, a tendency to bleed, osteoporosis, and loosening of the teeth (Chapter 4).

A much more common cause of defective matrix formation in Western society is persistent elevation of glucocorticoids as a result of long-term administration of glucocorticoids. There is general depression of protein synthesis and increased protein catabolism. Collagen production is therefore decreased and collagenolysis is increased, resulting in decreased bone formation (see "Osteoporosis," Chapter 17), fragility of tendons, and thinning (atrophy) of the dermis with abnormal expansion of small blood vessels (telangiectasis).

Proteoglycans. Defective proteoglycan synthesis in glomerular basement membranes appears to be the underlying defect in several diseases that are characterized by *increased glomerular permeability* (Chapter 16).

Basement membranes defects. The prototype example of defective synthesis of basement membrane components is *hereditary glomerulonephritis (Alport's syndrome).* In this disease, there appears to be an inherited metabolic defect leading

TABLE 2-2. Examples of molecular defects in inherited disorders of collagen synthesis

Disease	*Defect*	*Consequences*
OI type I	Decreased synthesis proα1(I) chains	Decreased type I collagen
OI type II	Shortened proα1(I) chains	Unstable triple helices
OI types I and III	Shortened proα2(I) chains resulting in defective cleavage of terminal sequences	Abnormal packaging of collagen fibrils
EDS type IV	Abnormal α1(III) chains	Unstable triple helices, decrease type I collagen
EDS type VI	Lysyl hydroxylase deficiency	Defective cross-linkage
EDS type VII	Procollagen peptidase deficiency, resulting in defective cleavage of terminal sequences	Abnormal packing of collagen fibrils
EDS type IX	Lysyl oxidase deficiency caused by abnormal copper metabolism	Defective cross-linkage
Marfan's syndrome (variant)	Abnormally long proα2(I) chains	Defective cross-linkage

KEY: *OI,* Osteogenesis imperfecta; *EDS,* Ehlers-Danlos syndrome.

to abnormal assembly of the basement membrane components, with the result that the glomerular basement membrane is both biochemically and structurally defective. Its two component layers, synthesized by the epithelial and endothelial cells respectively, fail to fuse, resulting in characteristic "splitting" of the basement membrane. The basement membrane is abnormally fragile and permits the passage of blood into the urine. Patients suffering from Alport's syndrome generally evidence this same abnormality of the basement membranes elsewhere in the body, and this may, for example, be responsible for the nerve deafness commonly associated with the syndrome.

Elastic fiber abnormalities. There are several inherited disorders of elastin synthesis. All of these may result from decreased activity of lysyl oxidase, the enzyme crucial to the cross-linking of elastin polypeptide chains. This group of disorders includes *cutis laxa, Menkes kinky hair syndrome,* and *type V Ehlers-Danlos syndrome.* In cutis laxa, the disorder is manifested as loose, redundant, pendulous folds of skin on the face. The patients also demonstrate signs of more generalized connective tissue weakness (such as hernias or diverticula of the gastrointestinal and urinary tracts) and often pulmonary emphysema (Chapter 12).

Impairment of elastin synthesis by persistently high levels of glucocorticoids results in the formation of striae, which are linear cutaneous lesions characterized histologically by the loss of elastic fibers.

Defective mineralization of extracellular matrix. This may be seen in such conditions as rickets and osteomalacia (Chapter 17).

Excessive synthesis of extracellular matrix

Proteoglycans and fibrillar collagen: connective tissue activation. Connective tissue activation is an extremely common but nonspecific reaction to various forms of injury. Sometimes, as in wound healing, it fulfills a useful function; it can, however, in some circumstances have serious adverse effects. The following lists examples of conditions in which connective tissue activation is seen:

1. Benign laryngeal nodules (singer's nodes) (Chapter 12)
2. Diffuse injury to parenchymal organs
   a. Lung (diffuse alveolar damage) (Chapter 12)
   b. Liver (cirrhosis) (Chapter 15)
3. Mitral valve prolapse (Chapter 11)
4. Myxedema (Chapter 18)
5. Nodular fasciitis (Chapter 17)
6. Palisaded granulomas
   a. Granuloma annulare (Chapter 19)
   b. Rheumatic and rheumatoid nodules (Chapter 19)
7. Stroma of invasive cancers (Chapter 9)
8. Tendon sheath ganglion (Chapter 17)
9. Vascular
   a. Intimal thickening after endothelial injury (Chapter 10)
   b. Atherosclerosis (Chapter 10)
10. Wound healing and repair (Chapter 4)

There are two phases of connective tissue activation: the first is mainly characterized by increased proteoglycan synthesis; in the second, fibrillar collagen synthesis predominates.

In the *early (lytic) phase,* connective tissue cells (fibroblasts, capillary pericytes) become hyperplastic and hypertrophic and are transformed into the following:

1. Cells with histiocytic (phagocytic) properties—these cells release enzymes that digest the fibrillar components of the stroma.
2. Stellate or swallow-tailed cells *(myofibroblasts)* that can elaborate the following:
   a. A proteoglycan-rich extracellular matrix that replaces the lysed fibrillar stroma
   b. Small quantities of type III collagen fibers

Myofibroblasts combine cytoplasmic features of both smooth muscle and fibroblasts, hence their name. The lytic phase is accompanied by increased vascularity and capillary permeability often with the leakage of plasma proteins; activation of the clotting process results in the extracellular deposition of fibrin, which, together with exuded plasma fibronectin, forms a gel matrix.

Synonyms for the early phase include "active fibrosis" and "young connective tissue formation." Again, because the proteoglycan-rich matrix is particularly abundant, the descriptive term *myxoid change* is also used.

Along with proteoglycans, type III collagen makes up much of the extracellular matrix normally produced in the *embryo* and *fetus.* It is apparently more distensible than type I collagen, which is lysed and which it partially replaces during early connective tissue activation. Of all collagen types, type III interacts most strongly with fibronectin, with which it is secreted both in developing connective tissues and in early connective tissue activation. Fibronectin (Chapter 1) plays an important role in cell migration. Thus the early matrix changes in connective tissue activation are of more primitive type and produce a hydrated environment that favors metabolic activity and cell migration and growth.

If the causes of tissue injury are removed, the lytic phase is potentially reversible. In the *late (desmoplastic) phase* of connective tissue activation, the myofibroblasts first secrete type III, then progressively greater amounts of type I collagen. These abundant collagen fibers replace the proteoglycan-rich matrix, which tends to be resorbed. There is lysis of the fibrin-fibronectin gel matrix; once their secretory activity has subsided, the cells resume the appearance of "resting" fibroblasts.

The late phase of connective tissue activation is sometimes termed "mature fibrosis" or "fibrous scarring." Where collagen deposition is abundant and the tissue as a result is hard and leathery, the term *sclerosis* may be used.

Contraction of connective tissue during the late phase appears to be related to the movement of myofibroblasts anchored to the collagen matrix. Contraction can cause, for example, cosmetically unsightly wounds. The late phase of connective tissue activation is rarely if ever reversible. Its purpose may be reparative or an attempt by the body to wall off an injurious agent.

Morphology of connective tissue activation. Connective tissue activation can have several morphologic appearances. Excessive deposition of fibrin in the lytic phase, with defective fibrinolysis, accounts for the "fibrinoid" material seen, for example, in rheumatic and rheumatoid nodules (Chapter 17). The same process can be seen in arterial walls following endothelial injury or deposition of immune complexes. The terms *fibrinoid change* or *fibrinoid necrosis* are often used to describe these connective tissue or vascular lesions.

During the lytic phase, after injury to tendon sheaths, failure of resorption of the abundant proteoglycans produced is responsible for the "myxoid" (mucoid) appearance of tendon sheath ganglia.

The striking connective tissue activation that accompanies

infiltrating carcinoma of the breast, is to a large degree, responsible for the hardness of the breast lump. For this reason these tumors are called *scirrhous* (Gr., *skirrhos,* hard) carcinomas.

Chemical mediators of connective tissue activation. Many substances found in tumors and wounds, have been shown to have a chemotactic effect on fibroblasts. These include lymphokines, complement components, native collagens types I through V, fibronectin, degradation products of collagen and fibronectin, and a variety of growth factors (including oncogene products). Among the latter, platelet-derived growth factor has a potent chemotactic effect on fibroblasts, as well as stimulating DNA synthesis and mitosis in these cells. Growth factors derived respectively from monocytes, alveolar macrophages, and endothelial cells can have similar effects on fibroblasts.

Basement membrane material. Generalized thickening of vascular basement membranes throughout the body is one of the main histologic features of *diabetes mellitus.* This abnormality contributes to diabetic nephropathy, retinopathy, and premature atherosclerosis (Chapter 18). The basement membranes in diabetes mellitus contain less proteoglycans but more type IV collagen and laminin than their normal counterparts. The turnover of basement membranes is also reduced in diabetes mellitus, with the result that the basement membrane is thicker than normal.

In diabetes mellitus, there is also a reduced content of proteoglycan in the glomerular basement membrane, which, as a consequence, is a far less effective barrier to the passage of plasma proteins. In addition, albumin and IgG molecules may become trapped in the glomerular basement membrane, further impairing its function and reducing the glomerular filtration rate (Chapter 16).

Elastic fibers. Several heritable and acquired disorders involve accumulation of elastic material in different tissues. Included among these are the following.

Endocardial fibroelastosis. Endocardial fibroelastosis is a recessively inherited abnormality (possibly autosomal) disorder in which there is thickening of the endocardium with proliferation of elastic tissue, leading to congestive cardiac failure.

Pseudoxanthoma elasticum. Pseudoxanthoma elasticum (PXE) is a group of inherited disorders in which the basic abnormality is in elastic tissue throughout the body. The abnormal elastic fibers, which tend to calcify, form particularly in skin, in the retina, and in arterial walls. The skin lesions are small, yellow papules, whereas the retinal changes may impair vision. The vascular lesions can cause gastric hemorrhage, angina pectoris, and intermittent claudication (Chapter 10).

Elastofibroma. Elastofibroma is a benign tumorlike lesion, usually evidenced as a mass in the soft tissues in the subscapular region in adults. It probably results from mechanical friction between the scapula and the chest wall.

Actinic (solar) elastosis. Actinic elastosis is the most common condition in this group and is characterized by thickening and furrowing of the skin in sun-exposed areas of the body. The most striking morphologic finding is deposition in the dermis of elastic material that differs ultrastructurally (and in its staining properties) from the elastic fibers seen in normal skin. More important, however, is the susceptibility of skin, chronically damaged by the sun, to the development of several types of malignant neoplasia (Chapter 19). In the skin there is a great increase in the concentration of desmosine, which is involved in cross-linking of polypeptide chains of elastic fibers.

Abnormal degradation of extracellular matrix

Fibrillar collagen and proteoglycans. Enzymatic degradation of collagen and proteoglycans, together with loss of the latter's capacity to retain water, is thought to be important in the pathogenesis of both idiopathic and secondary forms of *osteoarthritis* (degenerative joint disease) (Chapter 17). In the normal turnover of cartilage matrix, proteases, particularly chondrocytic collagenases, are normally modulated by protease inhibitors such as α-2-macroglobulin. It has been postulated that osteoarthritis may be initiated by increased proteolytic activity (or reduced inhibition of proteolysis) brought about by lymphokines such as interleukin 1, released in response to low-grade synovial inflammation of unknown cause. This, in turn, is thought to result in the characteristic fibrillation (fracturing) of articular cartilage that progressively leads to destruction of the smooth joint surface. Proteases released by neutrophils and macrophages in inflamed joints can also contribute to destruction of articular cartilage.

Recessive dystrophic epidermolysis bullosa is a heritable disorder of skin and mucous membranes characterized by extensive blistering after minor trauma. In this condition, there is increased synthesis of collagenase by skin fibroblasts, and electron microscopy reveals breakdown and phagocytosis of collagen fibrils by macrophages in the areas of blistering.

Basement membranes. Basement membranes can be attacked by proteolytic enzymes produced by various tumors, microorganisms, and inflammatory cells.

Basement membranes bar the passage of *cancer cells* to and from the circulation and into connective tissues. However, cancer cells can attach to basement membranes, chiefly through cell membrane receptors for laminin. Once attached, secretion of proteolytic enzymes such as type IV collagenase results in localized degradation of the basement membrane, allowing the cancer cell to migrate through it and metastasize.

Microorganisms can cross host basement membranes in a similar way. *Staphylococcus aureus* and *Pseudomonas aeruginosa* have, for instance, been shown to attach specifically to laminin, which is susceptible to enzymatic bacterial lysis. This can disrupt tissue integrity and promote the spread of infection.

Injury to glomerular basement membranes by neutrophils in *immune complex–mediated diseases* is discussed in Chapter 16.

Elastic fibers. Enzymatic degradation of pulmonary elastic fibers is basic to the pathogenesis of *emphysema* (Chapter 12), a common, debilitating lung disease. Normal pulmonary structure and function is dependent on the maintenance of a dynamic balance between elastase and antielastase activity within the lung. α-1-anti*trypsin* (α-1-AT), which is produced by the liver and circulates in the plasma, is an enzyme responsible for the inhibition of neutrophil elastase. If the action of α-1-AT is impaired or lost, unopposed elastase activity can destroy the elastic fibers of the respiratory bronchioles and interalveolar septae. The products of elastin breakdown attract inflammatory cells capable of releasing enzymes and oxygen radicals that subsequently cause collagen breakdown. The result is a loss of pulmonary parenchyma and its elastic recoil. α-1-AT deficiency is inherited in about 2% of cases of emphysema. In the acquired form, the oxidant effects of cigarette combustion are thought to be responsible for the inactivation of α-1-AT and the development of emphysema.

Calcified extracellular matrix. Throughout life, the skeleton is continuously being removed by osteoclasts and replaced by osteoblasts. Where bone mass is constant, as in the young adult, osteoclastic and osteoblastic activities are balanced. When resorption of bone predominates over its deposition, the result is *osteoporosis.* Endosteal resorption in long bones outstrips periosteal formation, and the cortical thickness decreases; major trabeculae are thinned in the vertebrae and elsewhere, and minor trabeculae perforated by osteoclasts may be permanently lost. As a result, bones become thin, weak, and prone to fracture with minimal trauma. The main causes of osteoporosis are old age, menopause, immobility, hyperparathyroidism, and prolonged elevation of glucocorticoid levels. Osteoporosis is discussed further in Chapter 17.

Abnormal deposits in the extracellular matrix

The extracellular matrix may be the site of deposition of many materials not normally found there, such as microorganisms and fibrin (already discussed) immune complexes (Chapters 7, 10, and 16), amyloid, and crystals. The last two are discussed in this and the following sections.

Amyloid

Amyloid is a collective term for certain filamentous materials—with similar physical properties, but diverse chemical composition—that are deposited in the extracellular matrix. Amyloid can be deposited in small amounts in normal individuals with no consequent pathologic effects. When amyloid deposits cause disease the term *amyloidosis* is employed.

The term *amyloid* can be applied to any substance with the following properties:

1. *Light microscopic appearance*—Amyloid appears glassy and eosinophilic and stains orange with Congo red. Under polarized light, formalin-fixed, Congo-red stained material has a vivid, apple green birefringence.
2. *Ultrastructural appearance*—Amyloid consists of haphazardly arranged, fluffy aggregates of straight, unbranched, unbanded filaments (Fig. 2-19).
3. *Physicochemical properties*—Amyloid deposits are composed mainly of material with a double helical polypeptide backbone with a cross-beta (beta-pleated sheet) x-ray diffraction pattern, in which the molecules are arranged in a concertina-like fashion (Fig. 2-20). It is thought that the longitudinal grooves act as binding sites for the Congo red dye.

Amyloid (literally, starchlike) was so called because, like starch, it can stain blue with iodine because of interaction between iodine and certain carbohydrate residues among the polypeptide chains. However, the carbohydrates are not always present, and therefore iodine staining is unreliable. Grossly, amyloid deposits have a waxy appearance.

Classification of amyloidosis. Amyloid deposits may be found in various organs and tissues throughout the body *(generalized amyloidosis)*, or they may develop at a specific site *(localized amyloidosis)*. Further classification employs two letters: the first of which is A (for amyloidosis), and the second denotes a biochemical or clinical type (L, for light chains, for example).

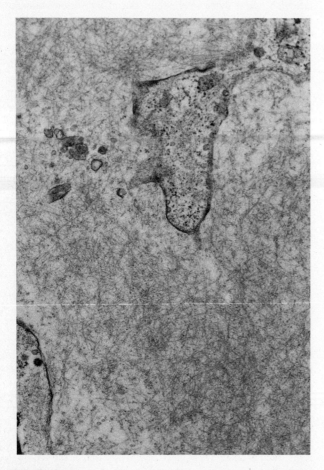

FIG. 2-19. Electron micrograph showing typical appearance of amyloid filaments arranged in haphazard fashion. From a case of cardiac amyloidosis.

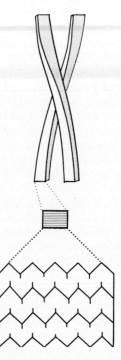

FIG. 2-20. Diagram depicting the concertina-like β-pleated sheet configuration of amyloid filaments.

Systemic amyloidosis

AL amyloidosis. AL amyloidosis includes idiopathic (primary) and myeloma-associated forms of the disease. Myeloma (Chapter 13) is a malignant proliferation of plasma cells, which almost always produce immunoglobulin light chains. These chains have polypeptide chains from which amyloid is produced. This form of amyloid has also been termed *immunoamyloid*.

Amyloid may be deposited locally among the malignant plasma cells or transported as precursor molecules in the blood to be deposited at other sites—mainly those of mesodermal origin such as skeletal and heart muscle, skin, tongue, and gums (Fig. 2-21). Often amyloid deposition is the first clinical feature of myeloma and such cases may be mistaken for idiopathic (without antecedent cause) amyloidosis.

AA amyloidosis. AA amyloidosis is a secondary response to an underlying inflammatory disorder or infectious disease, such as rheumatoid arthritis, tuberculosis, or chronic suppurative osteomyelitis. The amyloid filaments consist of so-called amyloid A protein.*

AA amyloidosis is referred to clinically as "secondary" amyloidosis and is typically distributed in the liver, spleen, kidneys, and adrenal glands.

AF amyloidosis. In the inherited form of amyloidosis, often called familial (F) amyloid polyneuropathy, the amyloid filaments are deposited in peripheral nerves and are composed of a mixture of normal and variant prealbumins.

---

*Amyloid A protein is chemically related to the acute phase reactant serum AA protein. AA protein is produced in the liver in response to interleukin 1 which is secreted by macrophages during the inflammatory response.

AH amyloidosis. AH amyloidosis is a recently described form of amyloidosis that affects patients on long-term hemodialysis for chronic renal failure. β-2-microglobulin, which is catabolized by the normal kidney, is greatly increased in the plasma of these patients and is the main constituent of AH (H, for hemodialysis) amyloid filaments. This type of amyloid has a predilection for the carpal synovium, where its deposition causes the *carpal tunnel syndrome.*

Localized amyloidosis

Endocrine amyloidosis. There is a close relationship between certain amyloid filament proteins and endocrine secretions. For example, amyloid deposits found in the pancreatic islet tissue in most cases of type 2 diabetes (Fig. 2-22), may have a causal role in this disease. The amyloid filaments found in medullary carcinoma of the thyroid, a neoplasm of C cells, share polypeptide sequences of calcitonin or precalcitonin molecules.

Age-related amyloidosis. Small deposits of amyloid in the heart, lungs, brain, pancreas, and spleen are common in old age and appear to be related to the aging of tissues in certain individuals. A derivative of prealbumin is the major component of the senile type of amyloid found in the heart; such deposits, if extensive, may be associated with congestive cardiac failure.

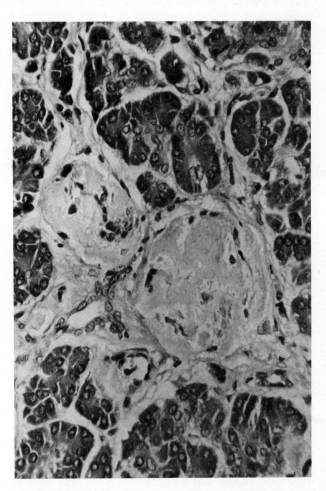

FIG. 2-22. Displacement of pancreatic islet cells by amyloid. Case of type II diabetes mellitus.

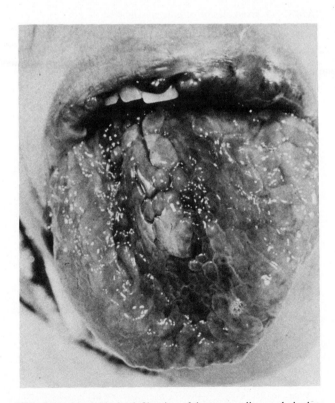

FIG. 2-21. Amyloidosis. Infiltration of the tongue, lips, and gingivae in generalized amyloidosis. *(Courtesy Curator of the Gordon Museum, Guy's Hospital, London, England.)*

The amyloid deposits in Alzheimer's disease, as discussed earlier in this chapter, appear to be derived from abnormal neurofilaments. The clinical importance of age-related amyloid is still unclear.

Primary cutaneous amyloidosis. In primary cutaneous amyloidosis, degenerative changes in the epidermis result in transformation of cytokeratin filaments into dermal amyloid deposits.

Pathogenesis of amyloid. It is generally believed that the filament protein in all types of amyloid has a precursor molecule. Two key processes appear to be involved. First, there is a mechanism whereby a stimulus alters the serum concentrations or primary structure of the amyloid precursor proteins; second, there is a step that involves processing or conversion of the precursors to amyloid filaments. In the case of AL and AA forms of amyloid, the protein molecules in tissue deposits are mostly smaller than their serum precursors and it is likely that controlled proteolysis precedes filament formation.

In AH and AF amyloidosis filaments may develop in a different way, possibly by aggregation of precursor proteins. In these forms of amyloid, the filament proteins are whole proteins similar to their presumed serum precursors.

Clinical effects of amyloidosis. Amyloid is deposited among and displaces the elements of the normal extracellular matrix. The extent of the amyloid's interference with function depends on the amount of amyloid deposited and its site. Its deposition in the kidney, which can take place in virtually all forms of amyloidosis, is particularly important. It may lead to nephrotic syndrome or renal failure (Chapter 16). Whether amyloid filaments, once deposited, can subsequently undergo degradation has never been conclusively demonstrated. For practical purposes, amyloid is irreversible.

Crystal deposition disorders

Crystal deposition disorders are a heterogeneous group of conditions that have in common the formation of crystals of various types in a variety of tissues. Crystals frequently cause a local inflammatory response, particularly when they are released into joint spaces, as in the case of urates, pyrophosphates (Chapter 17), and hydroxyapatite crystals. The last, however, is not merely a potential cause of arthritis, but is largely responsible for calcification in general.

Pathologic calcification. Pathologic calcification, a diverse collection of disorders (also termed *ectopic calcification* or *calcinosis*), involves growth of hydroxyapatite deposits in the extracellular matrix, usually in inappropriate extraskeletal sites. The molecular and cellular mechanisms that give rise to these deposits are very similar to those of physiologic calcification. Usually, the initial deposition of hydroxyapatite crystals is associated with membranous structures, especially mitochondria or matrix vesicles, and probably follows the deposition of amorphous calcium phosphate in these structures.

The terms *dystrophic* and *metastatic calcification*, which have long been used by pathologists as types of ectopic calcification, require some clarification. Metastatic calcification describes calcification in previously *undamaged* tissue when serum levels of calcium and phosphate are abnormally high. Dystrophic calcification affects *injured* tissue and does not require high calcium and phosphate levels. In both forms of ectopic calcification, the cell or the extracellular matrix, or both, may become calcified.

Metastatic calcification. This process develops in hypercalcemic states (Table 2-3). The increased calcium in the extracellular milieu promotes uptake of calcium by the cell across concentration gradients, leading to overloading of the mitochondria, which then cease to supply enough ATP. Failure to provide the plasma membrane with its energy needs leads to further ingress of calcium from the extracellular fluid, and ultimately the cell dies.

The preformed mineral in the mitochondria serves as nucleation sites for mineral crystal proliferation that calcifies the cell and extends into the extracellular spaces. The distribution of metastatic calcification is usually widespread in the body compared with most examples of dystrophic calcification, which is generally related to localized disease.

Dystrophic calcification. This form of pathologic calcification follows cell injury in tissues bathed by extracellular fluid containing normal levels of calcium and phosphate. For example, ischemia may initiate mineralization in the mitochondria of damaged cells. The cell injury also renders the plasma membrane more permeable to calcium, and the same sequence of events described for metastatic calcification ensues. Alternative mechanisms for dystrophic calcification include mineralization starting in apoptotic cell fragments (that in effect act as matrix vesicles) and calcification initiated in bacterial membranes in relation to fibrillar matrix components (Table 2-3).

Clinical importance of crystal deposition disorders. Deposits of hydroxyapatite affect the function of heart valves and arteries, impairing their elasticity and making them more

TABLE 2-3. Examples of ectopic calcification

Condition	Initial site of calcium deposition
Metastatic calcification	
Hyperthyroidism	MV or m
Milk-alkali syndrome	MV or m
Vitamin D toxicity	MV or m
Dystrophic calcification	
Atherosclerotic plaques	MV
Calcific aortic valve disease	MV
Calcific coating of IUDs	Bacterial membranes
Calcification of abnormal elastic fibers (e.g., pseudoxanthoma elasticum)	Matrix fibrils
Calcifying tendonitis	MV
Carcinoma and other breast lesions	MV or m
Cardiovascular prosthetic grafts	MV
Degenerative uterine leiomyomas	MV or m
Dental plaque and calculus	Bacterial membranes
Lithopedion (calcified retained fetus)	m
Medial sclerosis of Monckeberg	MV or m
Michaelis-Gutmann bodies in malakoplakia	Bacterial membranes
Old necrotizing granulomas	MV or m
Osteoarthritic articular cartilage	MV
Psammoma bodies in meningiomas, thyroid papillary carcinoma and other neoplasms	MV
Tympanosclerosis	MV

KEY: *MV*, Matrix vesicles; *m*, Mitochondria; *IUD*, Intrauterine device.

prone to hydrodynamic injury. Metastatic calcification can cause conduction abnormalities in the heart and impair renal function.

By contrast with these harmful effects, ectopic calcification can be helpful in diagnosis, for example, in detection of early carcinoma of the breast where there is also dystrophic calcification.

Calculi

A *calculus* (literally, a pebble) is a solid mass of precipitated, crystalline material, that forms in biologic fluids (urine, bile, saliva) from one or more constituents of those fluids. Crystals are, however, a common finding especially in the urine of healthy individuals, and their presence does not necessarily indicate that calculi have formed or will form.

If increasing amounts of a crystallizable substance are added to a fluid, eventually a high enough concentration is reached to saturate the fluid, and crystals begin to form. In biologic fluids, however, certain factors can prevent crystallization even if a substance is in a supersaturated state. These factors, which include certain chemical substances and low pH, may also inhibit the growth or promote the dissolution of crystals that have already formed. In normal persons, these *crystallization inhibiting factors* combine to maintain a balance between crystal formation and dissolution, thus preventing the formation of calculi. The following mechanisms, acting singly or in concert, are those known to be important in promoting the formation of calculi.

Excessive supersaturation of biologic fluids with crystallizable substances. This may result from a variety of causes including diet, hormonal imbalance, inherited enzyme defects, or fluid superconcentration resulting from stasis or dehydration.

Presence of nucleation-promoting matter. Calculi form as a result of continued aggregation of crystals, initiated by a process termed *nucleation* (Fig. 2-23). Nucleation is the process by which a crystal nidus (point of origin) is formed and is the result of either of the following:

1. *Homogeneous nucleation*—The random coalescence of molecules of a crystallizable substance forms a nidus large enough to permit continued crystal precipitation.
2. *Heterogeneous nucleation*—Precipitation occurs around some particle other than a pure crystal of the substance in question. Such particles effectively lower the threshold for crystal formation. Thus crystal formation can then take place at much lower levels of saturation than required for homogeneous nucleation. This is the usual process of calculus formation and examples of particles that may initiate the process include desquamated epithelium, bacterial colonies, fibrin, and mucus.

Lack of crystallization inhibitors. A decrease in one or more of the crystallization factors may result from various metabolic disturbances (some diet-induced) or from local disease such as inflammation.

Retention of crystallizing material. When the rate of crystallization exceeds that of dissolution, the crystals formed may be excreted and thereby rendered harmless. However, adherence of crystallizing material to damaged epithelium or disease causing stasis or obstruction to the outflow of fluids can allow the crystals to be retained and continue to form.

Macroscopic stone formation. Macroscopic stone formation results from several processes: (1) continued crystal growth; (2) epitaxial growth, whereby crystals of two different substances with similar molecular structure organize themselves as lattices on one another's surfaces; and (3) crystal aggregation, by which preformed crystals aggregate into large clusters.

Most (although not all) calculi contain calcium and are thus radiopaque. The etiology, pathogenesis, and clinical effects of calculi are discussed further in Chapters 14, 15, and 16.

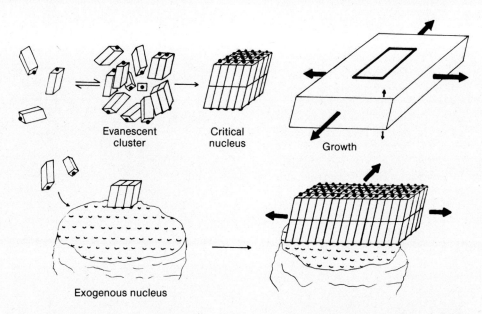

Evanescent cluster — Critical nucleus — Growth

Exogenous nucleus

FIG. 2-23. Diagram depicting homogeneous nucleation *(upper portion)* and heterogeneous nucleation *(lower portion)* of cholesterol molecules, forming crystals. *(Courtesy Donald M Small, MD; Reprinted by permission of The New England Journal of Medicine 302:1305, 1980.)*

Selected readings

Abrahams DR: Recent studies on the structure and pathology of basement membranes, J Pathol 149:257, 1986.

Anderson HC: Calcific diseases: a concept, Arch Pathol Lab Med 107:341, 1983.

Anderson HC: Matrix vesicle calcification: review and update. In Peck WA, editor: Bone and mineral research, vol 3, New York, 1985, Elsevier Science Publishing Co, Inc.

Cohen AS, and Connors LH: The pathogenesis and biochemistry of amyloidosis, J Pathol 151:1, 1987.

Constantinides P: Ultrastructural pathobiology, New York, 1984, Elsevier Science Publishing Co, Inc.

Dieppe PA: Crystal deposition and inflammation, QJ Med Summer:12, 1984.

Duvall E and Wyllie AH: Death and the cell, Immunology Today 7:115, 1986.

Farber JL: Membrane injury and calcium homeostasis in the pathogenesis of coagulative necrosis, Lab Invest 47:114, 1982.

Frank MM: Complement in the pathophysiology of human disease, N Engl J Med 316:1525, 1987.

Frost JK: The cell in health and disease, ed 2, Basel, 1986, S. Karger.

Ghadially FN: Ultrastructural pathology of the cell and matrix, ed 2, London, 1982, Butterworth & Co (Publishers), Ltd.

Goldwasser B, Weinerth JL, and Carson CC III: Calcium stone disease: an overview, J Urol 135:1, 1986.

Halliwell B: Oxidants and human disease: some new concepts, FASEBJ 1:358, 1987.

Hill RB Jr and LaVia MF: Principles of pathobiology, ed 3, New York & Oxford, 1980, Oxford University Press.

Hirsimaki P et al: Autophagocytosis. In Trump BF and Arstila AU, editors: Pathobiology of cell membranes, vol 3, San Diego, 1983, Academic Press, Inc.

Holzbach RT: Recent progress in understanding cholesterol crystal nucleation as a precursor to human gallstone formation, Hepatology 6:1403, 1986.

Iozzo RV: Proteoglycans: structure, function, and role in neoplasia, Lab Invest 53:373, 1985.

Kerr JFR, Bishop CJ, and Searle J: Apoptosis, Recent Advances in Histopathology 12:1, 1984.

Kim KM: Pathological calcification. In Trump BF and Arstila AU, editors: Pathobiology of cell membranes, vol 3, San Diego, 1983, Academic Press, Inc.

Martinez-Hernandez A and Amenta PS: The basement membrane in pathology, Lab Invest 48:656, 1983.

Perez-Tamayo R: Mechanisms of disease: an introduction to pathology, ed 2, Chicago, 1985, Year Book Medical Publishers, Inc.

Prockop DJ and Kivirikko KI: Heritable diseases of collagen, NEJM 311:376, 1984.

Proceedings of symposium on osteoarthritis: proteases, J Rheumatol Special issue 14:May, 1987.

Reed R: Connective-tissue activation, Am J Dermatopathol 4:365, 1982.

Rubin RP et al, editors: Calcium in biological systems, New York and London, 1985, Plenum Publishing Corp.

Rungger-Brandle E and Gabbiani G: The role of cytoskeletal and cytocontractile elements in pathologic processes, Am J Pathol 110:361, 1983.

Searle J, Kerr JFR, and Bishop CJ: Necrosis and apoptosis: distinct modes of cell death with fundamentally different significance, Pathol Annu 17(2):229, 1982.

Smith BF, LaMont JT, and Small DM: The sequence of events in gallstone formation, Lab Invest 56:125, 1987.

Smith LH: Pathogenesis of renal stones, Miner Electrolyte Metab 13:214, 1987.

Smith R: Osteoporosis: cause and management, Br Med J 294:329, 1987.

Uitto J and Perejda AJ, editors: Connective tissue disease: molecular pathology of the extracellular matrix, New York and Basel, 1987, Marcel Dekker, Inc.

Wewers MD and Gadek JE: The protease theory of emphysema, Ann Int Med 107:761, 1987.

Young JD and Cohn ZA: How killer cells kill, Sci Am 258:38, 1988.

CHAPTER 3

Genetic disease

Genetic disease has become a subject of ever-growing clinical importance, particularly as a result of the application of the techniques of gene mapping and recombinant deoxyribonucleic acid (DNA) technology. It is becoming increasingly possible to identify individual genes or their structural defects responsible for genetic disease, to identify healthy carriers, and to cure some of these diseases by transplantation of normal cells—or in animals, at least, by gene transfer. The haplotypes of the human leucocyte antigen (HLA) system (Chapter 7) are also important in relation to *organ transplantation* and probably in affecting susceptibility to various diseases. In addition, there is great interest in genetic aspects of cancer. Some types of cancer, particularly chronic myelogenous leukemia, are associated with chromosomal abnormalities. Also, intensive research is being carried out into *oncogenes*—genes with tumorigenic potential (Chapter 9). It must be emphasized that many problems remain unsolved, but there have been significant successes in the early diagnosis and often the management of serious genetic disorders.

As a consequence of recent developments in genetic investigative techniques, much more is known about the mechanisms underlying many genetic diseases but at the same time the subject has become considerably more complex.

Although genes determine the intrinsic characteristics of each individual, environmental factors are also important. Body height particularly is only partly genetically determined, and environmental factors, especially nutrition, can have an overwhelming effect. A genetic defect may also be completely unsuspected until an environmental influence makes it apparent. A person with mild hemophilia, for example, can lead a completely normal life until an injury and uncontrollable bleeding make the disorder obvious. In glucose-6-phosphate dehydrogenase deficiency, severe hemolytic anemia (favism) results from a combination of the defective gene and eating fava beans.

Types of genetic disease

Genetic disease is caused by an abnormality of one or more genes. Genetic disease can be (1) inherited according to mendelian principles, (2) the result of a new mutation and then heritable according to mendelian principles, or (3) caused by abnormality of a chromosome and not usually heritable.

Familial diseases are often but not necessarily heritable, as they may result from a common environmental influence acting on the family. An example is multiple sclerosis (Chapter 20) where there is a suggestion of a familial tendency but little or no evidence of a genetic factor. Instead there are features suggestive of exogenous causative factors such as a virus.

Genetic disease is *congenital* in that the underlying defect is present at birth but may not be apparent. *Huntington's chorea* (Chapter 20), for example, is inherited as an autosomal dominant trait but develops so slowly as not to become evident until

adult life is reached. Hemophilia, a sex-linked recessive trait, may similarly remain unsuspected throughout childhood (especially if mild) until an injury such as extraction of a tooth causes abnormally prolonged bleeding and hematologic investigation then indicates the cause.

The term *congenital disease* is used for any disease present at birth and, as well as clinically apparent genetic disorders, includes nongenetic defects resulting from injury to the fetus *in utero*. Examples of the latter include intrauterine infections (such as cytomegalovirus, rubella, or—in the past especially—syphilis) and the fetal alcohol syndrome (Chapter 20).

Genetic diseases can be transmitted according to simple mendelian principles, but many others are polygenic and involve more than one gene.

As mentioned earlier, genes can undergo mutation with the result that new cases of heritable disease appear unexpectedly in a previously healthy family. No fewer than 35% to 40% of hemophiliac cases have a negative family history. The most famous example, which may in some small way have contributed to the establishment of the communist regime in Russia, was the appearance of hemophilia (Chapter 13) in the Tsar's son, the grandson of Queen Victoria. For the most part, such mutations are apparently spontaneous, but there is a variety of possible causes, such as ionizing radiation, as discussed later.

Phenotype, expressivity, and penetrance

The *phenotype* is the outward manifestation of a genetic trait. Such traits may however, have variable *expressivity*, namely, a variable degree of overt manifestation of the trait. This can differ even within members of the same family who can show an inherited disease in an incomplete form. An example is the rare autosomal dominant disorder, *leopardism* (cardiocutaneous or Moynahan's syndrome*) the name of which is an acronym of the main features, namely *l*entigines, *e*lectrocardiogram (ECG) abnormalities, *o*cular hypertelorism, *p*ulmonary stenosis, *a*bnormal genitalia, *r*etardation of growth, and *d*eafness. Not surprisingly, few individuals are unfortunate enough to have the gamut of these abnormalities, and the majority of those affected show a diversity of clinical presentations as a result of expressing some but not all of the features of the disease.

Expressivity can also vary in degree. In hemophilia, for example, the hemorrhagic tendency can be so severe as to be life-threatening in childhood or so mild as not to become apparent until, as mentioned earlier, there is some severe injury late in life.

Penetrance is a statistical term and refers to the frequency with which the gene is expressed in the offspring. Historically, the most striking example of extreme penetrance and expressivity of a trait was the grossly protrusive mandible seen in

---

*E.H. Moynahan, contemporary British dermatologist.

successive portraits of the Spanish Hapsburg royal family over a period of no less than three centuries. A contributory factor was, at least in part, the repeated close intermarriages in which this family indulged.

Cytogenetics

In the past, genetics could only be investigated by clinical means and, in particular, family studies. *Cytogenetics* is the study of genetics at the cellular level.

Transmission of the special characteristics of each cell during replication depends on the genetic information in the nucleus. The *genome* is the complete set of hereditary factors contained in the (haploid) chromosomes while the *karyotype* is the chromosomal constitution of the cell nucleus. The genome determines the characteristics of the individual (except those modified by the environment), including the different functions of all tissues.

Inherited characteristics are determined by the genes, which are arranged along the chromosomes (Chapter 1). Chromosomes are only seen in characteristic form during the metaphase of mitosis or in meiosis. During this period each chromosome consists of a pair of chromatids joined together by the centromere. During interphase chromosomes are not recognizable as distinct structures.

The genetic code

The structure and function of DNA and ribonucleic acid (RNA) have been discussed in Chapter 1. Their function can be summarized in the Crick-Watson formula:

$$DNA \circlearrowleft \rightarrow RNA \rightarrow Protein$$

The genetic code is determined by the sequences of bases along the DNA helix, and because there are at least 10^7 nucleotides* in the DNA of each human chromosome, the number of possible sequences is practically endless. Any change in these sequences of bases causes failure of production of the corresponding protein. Such changes, known as mutations, cannot be recognized microscopically. Another possibility is that part of a chromosome can break off to cause a chromosomal anomaly as in Down's syndrome.

Mitosis

When the cell is performing its normal metabolic functions, it is said to be in *interphase*. Interphase ends when mitosis begins. Mitosis starts with a stage of synthesis known as *prophase*, during which the chromosomes develop their characteristic symmetrical shapes and the nuclear envelope breaks up. At the same time, the two halves of the centriole pair separate, and the mitotic spindle forms between them.

In *metaphase* the centromeres of the chromosomes become attached to the microtubules of the spindle fibers and, in side view, appear to lie along the equatorial plane.

The onset of *anaphase* is marked by symmetrical splitting of each chromosome along its axis at the centromere to form two chromatids. Each half (daughter) chromosome is drawn, one to each pole of the cell, along the spindle. The daughter chromosomes (chromatids) thus become clustered around each pole, and at the same time, the cytoplasm starts to divide. A nuclear envelope also forms around each mass of chromosomal material in this final stage known as *telophase*. Two cells are thus formed; the chromosomes are no longer identifiable as morphologically distinct bodies, and interphase starts again.

Meiosis

Meiosis takes place only during gametogenesis. Meiosis has two effects. The first is that the zygote has the same number of chromosomes as the parent cell. The second is that it ensures genetic variation because one set of chromosomes comes from the father and the other from the mother.

Meiosis involves two cell divisions. In the first division the process begins as in mitosis, but prophase is prolonged. The chromosomes line up side by side in homologous pairs *(synapsis)*. Each synapsed pair of chromosomes is known as a *tetrad* because it consists of four chromatids. One limb of each chromatid then crosses over near the centromere, and each part thus replaces its opposite number. As the chromosomes separate again, the point of cross-over *(chiasma)* becomes visible. When separation of the two chromosomes has been completed, each chromosome contains part of the other.

In metaphase a spindle forms as in mitosis, but the chromosomes do not divide into chromatids. One complete member of each pair moves intact to each pole. Telophase is then the same as in mitosis, but each daughter nucleus now contains only 23 chromosomes (i.e., is haploid).

The second meiotic division is the same as in mitosis. The diploid state of 46 chromosomes is restored at fertilization.

Normal human chromosomes

There are 46 chromosomes, comprising one pair of sex chromosomes and 21 pairs of autosomes. The chromosomes can be identified by specific techniques and are classified in pairs according to their length and the position of the centromere.

The X chromosome is large and has attached to it both the genes that control the development of the ovary and others not associated with sexual development. Nevertheless, the loss of one X chromosome has relatively little effect compared with loss of an autosome because only one X chromosome is needed for protein synthesis during interphase. Complete absence of an X chromosome is incompatible with life.

The Y chromosome is one of the smallest. The only significant gene known to be located on the Y chromosome determines the development of the testis and, hence, maleness. However absence of the Y chromosome is compatible with life as in Turner's syndrome.

The X chromosome and sex determination. The male's sex chromosomes are XY, and it appears that the male-determining properties of the Y chromosome dominate. Even when there is an excess of X chromosomes, as in Klinefelter's syndrome,* the phenotype is obviously a male.

The female has two X chromosomes and therefore has, in theory, two sets of X-linked genes. According to the *Lyon hypothesis*, however, one of the X chromosomes is inactive; it can be seen under the microscope as a compact mass of chromatin known as the *Barr body*. This can be visualized in cells scraped from the buccal mucosa. Because only the inactive X chromosome is visible as a Barr body, each cell also contains one invisible (active) X chromosome. In the abnormal XXX condition, therefore, there are two Barr bodies.

---

*Nucleotides consist of the phosphate of a purine or pyrimidine base with a sugar and form the basic components of nucleic acids.

*H.F. Klinefelter (b. 1912), American physician.

The inactive X chromosome can also be seen as a drumsticklike appendage to the nucleus of polymorphonuclear leukocytes. Although all cells containing more than one X chromosome should theoretically show a Barr body, in practice it can be seen only in 20% to 60% of cells, since cells are seen in only two dimensions.

Single gene (mendelian) disorders

Nearly 3000 mendelian disorders have now been identified, although many of them are exceedingly rare. Some of the more important examples are shown in Table 3-1, but only the more common ones can be discussed in this chapter.

Mendelian disorders result from defective single genes and can be inherited as simple dominant or recessive traits or as sex-linked recessive or (rarely) dominant traits. The results of these disorders are to give rise to the formation of defective enzymes (the inborn errors of metabolism), defective or abnormal quantities of nonenzyme proteins, defects of membrane receptors, or other diseases.

Autosomal dominant disorders

In autosomal dominant disorders, one of a pair of alternative genes at the same locus is dominant over the other. The characteristics, therefore, express themselves in the phenotype and are thus clinically evident in the heterozygote. Transmission is by an affected parent; there is a 50% chance that the offspring of such a parent will be affected, but the chances are greatly increased in the rare event that both parents are affected.

Many of what were once regarded as simple dominant traits, such as osteogenesis imperfecta (brittle bone syndrome) or Marfan's syndrome can be inherited in other ways though the dominant type may be more common.

Important examples of autosomal dominant disorders, some of which are discussed in later chapters, include:
1. Achondroplasia (Chapter 17)
2. Hereditary hemorrhagic telangiectasia (Chapter 13)
3. Huntington's chorea (Chapter 20)
4. Marfan's syndrome (not all cases) (Chapter 17)
5. Osteogenesis imperfecta (not all subtypes) (Chapter 17)
6. Polycystic disease of the kidneys (Chapter 16)
7. Polyposis coli (not all types) (Chapter 14)
8. Von Willebrand's disease (some types) (Chapter 13)

Autosomal recessive diseases

When there is a dominant normal allele but an abnormal recessive allele the latter cannot express itself in heterozygotes. The recessive gene is however transmitted in latent form through successive generations until there is the chance event of two heterozygotes mating. When this happens, one in four of the offspring (statistically speaking) will be homozygous and express the disease.

Recessive diseases can be severe or even lethal in childhood. Cystic fibrosis and most of the inborn errors of metabolism, such as phenylketonuria, are recessive disorders.

Some mild recessive traits are relatively common. If they do not adversely affect marriageability or reproduction, the chances of heterozygotes mating are significant and are greatly increased by marital consanguinity—usually the marriage of two first cousins. This hazard may explain the ancient taboo against incest. Nevertheless, it was the practice of the Pharaohs

TABLE 3-1. Examples of inherited metabolic diseases

Disorder	Disease
Disorders of carbohydrate metabolism	Galactosemia
Exocrine gland abnormality	Fibrocystic disease*
Lysosomal storage diseases	
Mucopolysaccharidoses	Hurler's syndrome
Sphingolipidosis	Tay-Sachs disease
Glycogen storage diseases	Von Gierke's disease
Hemoglobinopathies	Sickle cell disease
Defects of amino acid metabolism and other enzyme deficiencies	Phenylketonuria
	Albinism
	Lesch-Nyhan syndrome
	Glucose 6-phosphate dehydrogenase deficiency (G6PD)
Defective plasma coagulant factors	Hemophilia

*Fibrocystic disease (Chapter 21) affects 1 in 1500 white births in the United States and is the most common inherited metabolic disease in Great Britain.

of Egypt, thousands of years ago, to marry their sisters without any apparent ill effect!

Codominance

Autosomal and recessive traits have been described above as being quite distinct but in practice the difference may rather be one of degree. Thus the β-thalassemic trait (Chapter 13) may be codominant as the heterozygote expresses a mild form of the disease (thalassemia minor) characterized by a mildly reduced hemoglobin level and microcytosis. It is also apparent that heterozygote carriers of recessive traits can have some marker or minor abnormality that can be detected by appropriate tests.

Sex-linked inheritance

In sex-linked recessive disorders, the alleles are on the X chromosomes only, and the abnormal trait is recessive to the normal gene on the other X chromosome in females, in whom it is not therefore expressed. Males lack such protection; if they inherit an X chromosome carrying the abnormal gene, males suffer from the disease.

One of the most important sex-linked recessive traits is *hemophilia* (Fig. 3-1) in which the symptomless carriers are females but their male offspring can have the characteristic hemorrhagic tendency. Carrier females may, however, have a detectable marker for the defect. The female carrier is healthy but gives the disease to the male offspring. Many of the latter have, as is well known, had the additional misfortune of acquiring acquired immunodeficiency syndrome (AIDS) (Chapter 7) from contaminated blood products.

Fragile X syndrome (Fig. 3-2) is thought to be the second most common form of mental deficiency, after Down's syndrome, in males. It was previously thought to be a typical sex-linked recessive disorder; however, it has become apparent that a third of carrier females have demonstrable mental retardation and that there is a significant but small number of phenotypically normal carrier males in affected families. It therefore seems that fragile X syndrome is inherited as a sex-linked

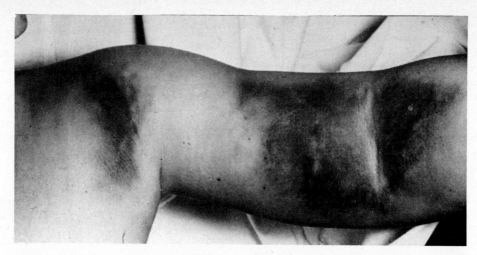

FIG. 3-1. Hemophilia. In this sex-linked recessive disease there has been severe bleeding into the soft tissues adjacent to the joints after minor injury. (See Chapter 13.) *(Courtesy Curator of the Gordon Museum, Guy's Hospital, London, England.)*

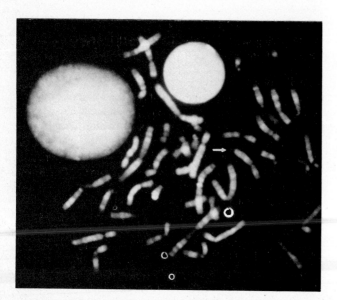

FIG. 3-2. Fragile X. Chromosome preparation showing QFQ banding. The arrow indicates the fragile site of the X chromosome.

dominant trait with variable penetrance but the nature of the genotype-phenotype interaction is not clear.

Fragile sites are somewhat mysterious features of chromosomes. They appear as little more than a thread of material joining two chromosome bands in special preparations of metaphase cells. Their association with the fragile X syndrome however demonstrates their clinical importance.

Polygenic inheritance and multifactorial disorders

Polygenic traits are determined by the combined action of several genes at different loci. Characteristics that appear to be polygenic include height, body weight, hair color, and blood pressure. In addition to the genetic component affecting these bodily features, environmental factors such as the level of nutrition clearly play an important part, and such characteristics are therefore also said to be multifactorial. Some types of diabetes mellitus may also depend on polygenic inheritance and be multifactorial.

Polygenic inheritance is difficult to confirm. Usually the attribute or disease has a familial tendency, but study of the family tree fails to confirm the pattern of inheritance as a simple dominant or recessive trait.

Mutations

A mutation is a sudden change in the structure of a gene, which, in turn, results in a change in the phenotype. Mutations in germ cells are transmissible and give rise to heritable diseases. Also new cases of heritable disease appearing in a family are the result of such mutations. As mentioned earlier, nearly 40% of cases of hemophilia result from new mutations.

Somatic mutations, unlike those in germ cells, affect the tissues but are not transmissible. Somatic mutations are, however, of interest because of their possible role in the development of cancer.

Causes of mutations

Most mutations appear to be spontaneous, but they can also be induced by several identifiable factors and, in particular, the following:
1. Ionizing radiation
2. Drugs and chemicals
3. Viruses

Ionizing radiation. Ionizing radiation is the most important known cause of mutations. Its role has been established in the laboratory, in patients who have had large doses of x-rays, and in the survivors of the atomic bombs at Hiroshima and Nagasaki. In women pregnant at the time of the explosions, a high proportion of the fetuses had chromosomal breaks and other genetic abnormalities.

These unfortunate victims also had a greatly increased incidence of cancer, which was possibly due to somatic mutations caused by the irradiation. Therapeutic irradiation (usually for cancer) can also cause chromosomal damage and be carcinogenic, as can ultraviolet irradiation. The role of irradiation in carcinogenesis is discussed in Chapters 4 and 9.

Drugs and chemicals. The main mutagenic drugs are the cytotoxic agents, particularly alkylating agents such as the nitrogen mustards, methotrexate, and azathioprine. This mutagenic effect may be clinically important as these types of drugs are used for immunosuppression, particularly for organ transplant patients, and such patients have an increased susceptibility to certain kinds of cancer. In vitro, chemicals such as nitrous acid, 5-bromouracil, and acridine are mutagenic for microbes.

The problem of the relation of somatic mutation to cancer is exceedingly difficult. Many mutagenic agents are carcinogenic, and it is widely believed that all carcinogens are mutagenic. This has lead to in vitro testing for mutagenicity as a screening test for possible carcinogenicity of drugs. However, whether an agent thus shown to be mutagenic is carcinogenic for humans is problematic; but as mentioned earlier, cytotoxic drugs, which are mutagenic, are known to increase the frequency of certain types of cancer.

Viruses. Many viruses are mutagenic and can cause a genetic change known as transformation in cells, which may then undergo neoplastic change. Most of the animal tumor viruses are mutagenic. The RNA tumor viruses (the retroviruses—formerly known as oncornaviruses) have been shown to cause genetic change and tumors in animals; other members of this group (the human T-cell lymphotropic viruses—HTLV) also incorporate themselves into the human genome, and several are strongly suspected of being carcinogenic. In addition, chromosomal abnormalities have been detected after numerous other viral infections such as hepatitis, poliomyelitis, and measles, although the significance of such findings is uncertain.

Mutagenicity and teratogenicity

It is important to appreciate the distinction between these two types of abnormality that can affect the fetus. A *mutagen* causes chromosomal changes that can be expressed in various ways but are mediated via the altered gene. A *teratogenic agent* does not operate in this way and in general, teratogenic agents, such as the drug thalidomide, or maternal rubella infection directly affect the cells of the fetus. Furthermore, their effects are not mediated by the genes. Rubella, for example, appears to inhibit mitosis of developing fetal cells.

Inherited metabolic diseases (inborn errors of metabolism)

The inherited metabolic diseases, which were first described at the beginning of this century, gave rise to the concept of "one gene, one enzyme." This is perhaps more precisely expressed now as "one gene, one polypeptide chain." The effects of these diseases are generally severe, and most are inherited as autosomal recessive traits (Table 3-2).

Most of these diseases are caused by mutations of genes coding for enzymes, and usually an excessive accumulation of substrate or of intermediate metabolic products results. The sheer bulk of these accumulations can impair normal function or development, in addition, the intermediate products may be harmful in themselves.

Phenylketonuria

Phenylketonuria (PKU) is one of the most common inborn errors of metabolism and in northern Europe affects 1 in 10,000 births. It is transmitted as an autosomal recessive disease in which there is a deficiency or absence of the hepatic enzyme phenylalanine hydroxylase. Therefore dietary phenylalanine fails to convert to tyrosine, but several mutants account for the variable expression of the disease.

A phenylketonuric baby has normal phenylalanine levels in the blood at birth, but these reach high levels after the second week. There is delay in myelination of neurons together with gliosis and fat accumulations in the central nervous system. Mental retardation becomes apparent in 98% of untreated children, who often also show psychotic behavior, uncoordinated movements, tremors, epileptic seizures, and eczematous rashes. Because tyrosine formation is blocked, melanin production is correspondingly reduced, and the skin and hair of affected infants is typically pale. Abnormal metabolic pathways lead to the formation of by-products that are excreted in sweat and urine, giving these infants a characteristic mouselike odor. Early diagnosis by determination of serum phenylalanine levels is essential because mental retardation and other abnormalities can be prevented by early treatment with a diet of minimal phenylalanine content. In the United States most infants are tested for phenylketonuria shortly after birth. However, because the newborn infant has had no opportunity to ingest phenylalanine, a false negative test can result in 15% to 20% of newborns. Ideally, testing should be carried out a few days after feeding has started.

TABLE 3-2. Important examples of mendelian enzyme disorders

Disease	*Enzyme defect*	*Typical features*
Glycogenoses		
von Gierke's (hepatorenal)	Glucose 6-phosphatase	Gross hepatorenomegaly, stunting, hypoglycemia, hyperlipidemia, hyperuricemia
Pompe's disease	Lysosomal glucosidase	Gross cardiomegaly, hypotonia, early cardiorespiratory failure
Sphingolipidoses		
Gaucher's disease	Glucocerebrosidase	(1) Splenomegaly, pathologic fractures
		(2) Hepatosplenomegaly, brainstem degeneration
Tay-Sachs disease	Hexosaminidase A	Severe mental retardation, blindness, early death
Niemann-Pick disease	Sphingomyelinase	Mental retardation, hepatosplenomegaly, early death
Mucopolysaccharidoses	Various (subtypes)	Abnormal facies, dwarfism, skeletal abnormalities often, mental
Hurler's and related syndromes		defect, and cataracts
Others (fucosidosis, mannosidosis, acid lipase deficiency, acid phosphatase deficiency)	Various	Various

More than 50% of PKU carriers can now be identified, and the various other mutants are likely to be identifiable in the foreseeable future.

The ability to control the effects of this genetic disorder by an early modification to the diet is a good example of the interactions between genes and environment.

Albinism

Albinism is a defect of tyrosine metabolism inherited as an autosomal recessive trait. Tyrosinase is absent or defective so that melanin is not formed. The skin is pale, and the hair is characteristically almost creamy white. Often there is photodermatitis caused by extreme sensitivity of the skin to sunlight. Ocular abnormalities include hypopigmentation of the fundus and translucency of the iris, and defective vision may result.

In addition to the psychologic handicap caused by the appearance, there is a greatly increased susceptibility to skin cancer, especially in those persons living in the southern United States and in tropical or semitropical areas.

Lesch-Nyhan syndrome

This rare sex linked recessive syndrome is mentioned mainly because of its relationship to adult gout (Chapter 17). Lesch-Nyhan syndrome* is characterized by hyperuricemia as a result of deficiency of the enzyme hypoxanthine-guanine phosphoribosyltransferase. As a consequence of hyperuricemia, affected children have gouty arthritis and renal damage. There is also severe mental retardation, spasticity, and involuntary movements. The most bizarre feature, however, is the compulsive self-mutilation that is often so extreme that these children chew or bite off their own lips or fingers in spite of the obvious pain that these actions cause.

Lysosomal storage diseases†
Glycogenoses (glycogen storage diseases)

The glycogenoses are rare enzyme deficiencies usually inherited as autosomal recessive traits and characterized by accumulations of glycogen in the tissues. The tissues chiefly affected are largely determined by the particular enzyme that is deficient. Glucose-6-phosphatase deficiency (von Gierke's disease) (Fig. 3-3) for example, is characterized by gross enlargement of the liver and kidneys, but stunted growth. Deranged glucose metabolism leads to hypoglycemia, but hyperlipidemia and hyperuricemia. The last two conditions can give rise to skin xanthomas and gout, and there is early death in about 50% of cases.

In lysosomal glycosidase deficiency (Pompe's disease), glycogen accumulation is generalized but the main features are gross cardiomegaly, hypotonia but only mild hepatomegaly. Death resulting from cardiorespiratory failure within 2 years is the usual outcome.

Sphingolipidoses

Gaucher's disease. Gaucher's disease,‡ which is inherited as an autosomal recessive disorder, results from a deficiency of the enzyme, glucosylceramidase, which cleaves glucose from the lipid portion of sphingolipids and leads to excessive

---

*M. Lesch (b. 1939), American physician; W.L. Nyhan (b. 1926), American pediatrician.

†See also Chapter 2.

‡P.C.E. Gaucher (1854-1918), French physician.

accumulation of glucocerebroside in the macrophages and possibly in neurons. The chief effects are hepatosplenomegaly along with neurologic and skeletal lesions. The latter may lead to spontaneous fractures. A variety of other effects may result from displacement of functional tissues in such sites as the bone marrow by the lipid-laden cells.

The severity of the disease ranges from death in childhood to mild and slowly progressive forms that allow a normal life expectancy.

It is estimated that there are at least 20,000 patients with Gaucher's disease in the United States. However, among Ashkenazi Jews, the carrier rate may be as high as 1 in 12, and the frequency of the disease about 1 in 2500.

There are three subtypes of Gaucher's disease. In *type 1* there is splenomegaly and bone pain or pathologic fractures, which can lead to permanent crippling. In about 5% the liver is enlarged. The spleen can be so large as to account for half the weight of a baby.

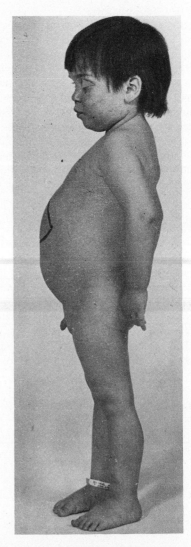

FIG. 3-3. Glycogen storage disease. This group of inborn errors of metabolism comprises many variants, each the result of deficient activity of specific enzymes involved in glycogen metabolism. Abnormal glycogens, as a result, accumulate in many organs including the liver, causing gross hepatomegaly, as shown here. *(Courtesy Curator of the Gordon Museum, Guy's Hospital, London, England.)*

In *type 2* disease, which is much more rare, neurologic symptoms develop within the first year of life, as well as hepatosplenomegaly. Brainstem degeneration leads to difficulty in swallowing and breathing with the result that respiratory complications are usually fatal within 2 years.

In *type 3* disease there is splenomegaly. However, neurologic disease develops later, typically between 5 and 20 years, and ranges from inability to control or coordinate eye movements to dementia, convulsions, and poor coordination of body movements.

Both management of and screening for Gaucher's disease are difficult. In type 1 disease, splenectomy may become necessary, especially to control thrombocytopenia and anemia secondary to hypersplenism. However, removal of the spleen tends to worsen bone involvement. Currently, therefore, partial splenectomy is being assessed. Bone marrow transplantation is a possible alternative to supply normal macrophage stem cells, but the procedure has a 20% to 50% mortality rate in this disease.

Prenatal diagnosis is easier when the parents have already borne an affected child. Usually prenatal diagnosis is difficult because of the different mutations in the relevant genes. More recently it has been found that a single base substitution accounts for the loss of enzymic activity and that the mutation is accompanied by the formation of a new restriction site, in one or both genes in type 2 and 3 disease but rarely in type 1 disease. Those with this particular mutation probably have at least an 80% chance of developing neurologic disease, and the mutation may soon be detectable in carriers and by prenatal screening.

Niemann-Pick disease. Niemann-Pick disease* is a rare autosomal dominant disorder characterized by excessive accumulation of phospholipids in the monocyte-macrophage system.

The chief effects, apparent in early infancy, are involvement of the central nervous system causing mental retardation and convulsions together with hepatosplenomegaly, but there are various other manifestations.

Diagnosis depends on liver or marrow biopsy to detect sphingomyelin-laden foam cells and abnormally raised levels of sphingomyelin in the tissues. There is no specific treatment, and the usual outcome is death in early childhood.

Tay-Sachs disease† (amaurotic familial idiocy). Sachs described the clinical and pathologic features of this disease in great detail in 1887 but was unaware that Tay, working in the East End of London, had reported a typical case (including a color plate of the changes in the retina) 6 years earlier.

Tay-Sachs disease is inherited as an autosomal recessive trait and chiefly affects Jewish persons from northeastern Europe. It is not surprising therefore that the first case reported by Tay in 1881 was in an area where there was an exceptionally large Jewish community. The carrier rate in such immigrants in New York may be as high as 1 in 30. The disease results in the accumulation of a ganglioside (GM_2 ganglioside) in the ganglia and destruction of the ganglion cells. Glial proliferation and myelin degeneration follow.

The chief effects are severe mental retardation and other neurologic effects, together with blindness associated with a cherry-red spot on the retina. Death in early childhood is the invariable result.

Hurler's syndrome and related mucopolysaccharidoses. Seven related lysosomal storage disorders of this type have now been defined. Hurler's syndrome* is perhaps the best known and is characterized by a grotesque facial appearance, dwarfism, skeletal malformations, and severe mental deficiency. There are various patterns of inheritance, and the abnormality is brought about by excessive accumulation of glycosaminoglycans (mucopolysaccharides) such as dermatan sulfate and heparan sulfate in the cells.

Galactosemia. Galactosemia is an inherited metabolic defect in which, in the homozygous form, there is excessive accumulation of galactose in the blood and tissues. This is caused by a deficiency of either galactose 1-phosphate uridyl transferase or galactokinase. These defects are transmitted as autosomal recessive traits and affect about 1 in 100,000 live births.

Galactotransferase deficiency, particularly if complete, has severe effects that include vomiting, failure to thrive, jaundice, liver enlargement, increased blood levels of galactose, and galactosuria. Kinase deficiency is more benign: cataract formation is typical, but mental deficiency may be associated. Absence of galactokinase from red blood cells is diagnostic. Because milk is the source of galactose, galactose-free milk substitutes are given to affected infants, and a diet free of galactose is often maintained for life. Neonatal testing for galactosemia is a legal requirement in many parts of the United States.

Mendelian defects of nonenzyme proteins of the blood

The most common mendelian defects affect the formation of hemoglobin, namely sickle cell disease and the thalassemias, of which there are heterozygous and homozygous forms, with partial expression in heterozygotes (Chapter 13). Other defects are in the production of clotting factors, of which the main examples are the sex-linked recessive disorders, hemophilia A and B resulting from defects or deficiencies of factors VIII and IX respectively. Von Willebrand's disease is more complex and results in deficiency of von Willebrand factor causing platelet dysfunction and a variable degree of factor VIII deficiency. There are several subtypes that may be inherited as dominant or recessive traits.

Glucose 6-phosphate dehydrogenase deficiency

Glucose 6-phosphate dehydrogenase (G6PD) deficiency affects some millions of people worldwide, but many remain asymptomatic. The disease is common in Africa, in the Mediterranean area, and among blacks in the United States.

G6PD deficiency leads to fragility of the red cell membrane and hemolytic anemia when the affected individual is exposed to oxidant drugs such as many antimalarials and sulfonamides.

These hematologic diseases are discussed more fully in Chapter 13.

Mendelian disorders of collagen synthesis

Genetic disorders can affect most of the many stages of collagen synthesis (Chapter 2). The involvement of collagen in bone formation means that some of these disorders have

---

*A. Niemann (1880-1921), German pediatrician; L. Beck (1868-1935), German pathologist.
†W. Tay (1843-1927), English ophthalmologist; B.P. Sachs (1858-1944), German neurologist.

---

*Gertrud Hurler, German pediatrician.

profound effects on the skeleton. Noncollagen proteins can also affect collagen formation as in the case of homocystinuria, which was long thought to be a variant of Marfan's syndrome.* Important examples of these disorders are shown in Table 3-3 and discussed more fully in Chapter 17.

Homocystinuria

The homocystinurias are genetically heterogeneous and are found in approximately 1 in 200,000 live births. The most common form is the result of deficiency of an enzyme, cystathionine β-synthase, which leads to accumulation of excess methionine in the blood and tissues. The disorder is characterized by defective collagen formation and its results. The central nervous, cardiovascular, and musculoskeletal systems are particularly affected. Deformities of the eyes and skeleton, mental retardation, and seizures are common. Death may result from thrombosis as a result of increased platelet stickiness. About half the patients respond to massive doses of pyridoxal (vitamin B_6). Many parts of the United States require neonatal testing for homocystinuria.

Miscellaneous inborn errors of metabolism
Malignant hyperpyrexia

Malignant hyperpyrexia is an inborn error of metabolism affecting skeletal muscle and inherited as an autosomal dominant trait of high penetrance. The disorder is characterized by sustained abnormal contracture of skeletal muscle triggered, particularly, by general anesthetic drugs. The enhanced metabolic activity of the muscle causes hyperpyrexia, which can be fatal. Abnormal muscular contraction is associated with raised concentration of calcium ions in the myoplasm and raised serum levels of the muscle enzyme creatine phosphokinase, but the precise nature of the abnormality is not known.

In the United States, this disease has been estimated to complicate 1 in 20,000 cases where anesthetics are used. One patient had no fewer than 14 relatives die while under general anesthesia as a result of malignant hyperpyrexia and was less than enthusiastic about being subjected to general anesthesia himself. This family seems otherwise to have been slow to appreciate the dangers of this condition.

There is as yet no single reliable diagnostic test; the family history remains the most useful guide. When the latter is positive, raised serum creatine phosphokinase (CPK) levels are of predictive value, but CPK levels are frequently normal in susceptible patients.

Xeroderma pigmentosum

Xeroderma pigmentosum is usually inherited as an autosomal recessive disorder with an estimated incidence of between 1 in 65,000 and 1 in 100,000 of the population. Patients have a high incidence and precocious development of malignant tumors of the skin in areas exposed to sunlight. Histologically, the skin develops changes essentially similar to those of senility, but at an early age, and changes similar to those of actinic keratosis (Chapter 19) are seen. There is also an increase of melanin in the basal layers of the epidermis, with or without proliferation of melanocytes.

Freckling and abnormal dryness of the skin usually become apparent in infancy. Pigmentation develops in exposed areas

*E.J.A. Marfan (1858-1942), French pediatrician.

and at first fades during the winter months but typically becomes permanent, darker, and increasingly extensive. Other types of skin lesions are frequently associated.

Tumors typically develop in childhood and comprise, in order of frequency, basal cell carcinomas, squamous cell carcinomas, and malignant melanomas. The rate of progress of the disease is variable but can lead to death before the age of 10; about 60% of these patients die before the age of 20.

Protection of an affected child by every possible means from exposure to sunlight and maintenance of such protection for life are essential. Tumors should be adequately excised as soon as they are detected.

Defects of membrane receptors or transport systems

The transport of many substances across cell membranes frequently depends first on binding to a specific membrane receptor and carriage across the membrane by a protein. The most important example of this type of genetic defect is familial hypercholesterolemia, which leads to accelerated atherosclerosis and a high risk of premature death from myocardial infarction. It is discussed more fully in Chapter 10.

Chromosomal disorders

Abnormalities of the chromosomes give rise to another type of disease affecting the genes. Typically, these are not hereditary diseases but are usually the result of an abnormality of meiotic division of the germ cell. Such abnormalities may affect the number or structure of the chromosomes and can apparently develop spontaneously during cell division. Environmental agents can also damage the chromosomes as discussed earlier.

The best known chromosomal disorder is Down's syndrome (trisomy 21, "mongolism"). This is an abnormality of an autosome, but other chromosomal abnormalities involve the sex chromosomes as discussed later in this chapter.

Abnormal number of chromosomes (chromosomal aneuploidy)

Chromosomes can be lost or gained during cell division as a result of failure of separation (*nondisjunction*) of chromosomes on the spindle. Both members of a chromosome pair go to the same pole and enter the same daughter cell. The corresponding daughter cell is, therefore, short of one chromosome.

If this aberration happens during meiosis, the cell will either have only one chromosome (monosomy) or three (trisomy) after fertilization. When there is trisomy of chromosome 21, Down's syndrome results. Other recognized anomalies of this type are trisomies 13 and 18, the features of which are summarized in Table 3-4.

Chromosomal breakage: deletions, translocations, and inversions

Chromosomes can apparently break spontaneously or as the result of the same factors that cause mutation of genes. Breakage of chromosomes can be followed by loss of a fragment and its constituent genes (deletion). The larger fragment can sometimes reunite in a ring form. The effects of this anomaly are severe. Alternatively, the fragments can reunite but with the sequence of genes reversed (*paracentric inversion*). This

TABLE 3-3. Mendelian diseases affecting collagen formation

Disease	Inheritance	Typical features
Osteogenesis imperfecta (brittle bone syndrome) (Chapter 17)	AR or AD (4 subtypes)	Multiple fractures, deformities, blue sclerae, deafness, hypermobile joints
Marfan's syndrome (Chapter 17)	AD	Elongated extremities and fingers; ocular, cardiac and aortic defects
Homocystinuria	AR	Skeletal and ocular defects, thrombotic tendency, cardiac and aortic defects, mental retardation often
Epidermolysis bullosa (Chapter 19)	AR, AD or X linked (10 subtypes)	Blistering of skin and mucous membranes, scarring and sometimes deformities
Ehler-Danlos syndrome (Chapter 19)	AD or AR	Hypermobile joints, lax skin; weak blood vessel walls or ocular fragility

KEY: *AR*, Autosomal recessive; *AD*, Autosomal dominant.

TABLE 3-4. Chromosomal disorders

Disease	Chromosomal defect	Typical features
Disorders affecting the autosomes		
Down's syndrome	Trisomy 21	Abnormal facies, mental retardation, floppy joints, immune defects, premature aging
Edward's syndrome	Trisomy 18	Mental defect, abnormal facies, hypertonicity
Patau's syndrome	Trisomy 13	Mental retardation, microcephaly; skeletal, cardiac, and visceral defects
Cri-du-chat syndrome	Deleted short arm of chromosome 5	Mental retardation, microcephaly, miewing cry
Disorders of the sex chromosomes		
Klinefelter's syndrome	47,XXY	Eunuchoid habitus, testicular atrophy, gynecomastia, mental retardation
Klinefelter's syndrome variants	48,XXY 49,XXXY	More severe mental defects, cryptorchidism
Turner's syndrome	45,XO 46,XX	Primary amenorrhea, infertility, neck webbing, increased carrying angle
Multiple X females	47,XXX 48,XXXX	Mental retardation, menstrual irregularities, but often fertile
Double Y males	47,XYY	Tall, possibly psychopathic personality

may have no serious effects. A third possibility is breakage of both arms of a chromatid. This can lead to union of each fragment to the wrong arm (pericentric inversion).

The phenotype depends on the total content of genes rather than their sequence. Balanced translocations, where the full set of genes is present but the genes are no longer in their original positions, may not have any effect on the phenotype.

Down's syndrome (trisomy 21)

Down's syndrome* is the most common cause of mental retardation associated with recognizable physical defects, particularly the so-called mongoloid appearance. The incidence of trisomy 21 is approximately 1 in 700 live births, and it causes 6% to 10% of all mental deficiency.

Pathogenesis. The risk of this anomaly during meiosis increases sharply with maternal age. The chance of a woman over age 45 producing a child with Down's syndrome may be as high as 1 in 50.

Occasionally, a person can have part of chromosome 21 translocated to another chromosome. Because the total genetic

content is unchanged (balanced translocation), there is no physical abnormality. At gametogenesis, however, the translocated chromosome 21 can enter a gamete that contains a free chromosome 21 (Fig. 3-4). At fertilization a third chromosome 21 is then added, and Down's syndrome results. Down's syndrome can thus be an isolated abnormality or, less commonly, a heritable disorder.

When a young woman produces a child with Down's syndrome, it is usually the result of the heritable type of translocation defect. Therefore, antenatal cytogenetic examination should be carried out because of the risk of another affected child being born.

Pathology. The brain in Down's syndrome is usually smaller than normal, and there are anomalies of the convolutions. Many immature neurons and acellular areas are present in the cortex. In addition, associated congenital heart disease may lead to cerebral embolism and abscess formation.

Affected children are mentally retarded to a variable degree, and motor development is also slowed. Unlike many other mentally defective persons, these children are typically affectionate and good natured.

The characteristic facial appearance is the result of a short

---

*J.L.H. Langdon Down (1828-1896), English physician.

face with a large forehead, widely spaced eyes, and a flat sunken nose (Fig. 3-5). The palpebral fissures slant upward and outward, and the medial corner of the eye is covered by a prominent epicanthic fold. The tongue is fissured and often large and protrusive. Ligaments are lax, and the joints are often hypermobile.

The extremities, particularly the fingers, are short, and there is a single transverse crease across the palm. Congenital defects of the heart and other organs are common.

Children with Down's syndrome are vulnerable to intercurrent infections as a result of multiple immunologic defects. There is also a greatly increased tendency to leukemia associated with the presence of the Philadelphia chromosome (Chapter 13).

Down's syndrome and Alzheimer's disease. Victims of Down's syndrome, if they live long enough, develop brain damage with formation of plaques containing amyloid, an abnormal protein (Chapter 2). Amyloid accumulation in similar plaques is also characteristic of Alzheimer's disease, the most common cause of dementia (Chapter 20). The gene for β-amyloid protein has also been found to be on chromosome 21, and both patients with Alzheimer's disease and those with Down's syndrome have three copies of this gene. In Alzheimer's disease, aging and environmental factors probably also contribute to the pathogenesis.

Other trisomic disorders. Trisomy 9, 18, and 13 and other autosomal abnormalities have been described. They are characterized by a variety of physical abnormalities (see Table 3-4) and are less common than Down's syndrome. All affected persons are mentally defective, commonly have cardiac defects, and usually die in infancy.

The physical syndrome associated with trisomy 13, a prominent feature of which is often bilateral cleft lip and palate, was described over 300 years ago.

Anomalies affecting sex chromosomes

Additional sex chromosomes can be present as a result of failure of disjunction. If the X chromosomes fail to separate at the first meiotic division of the germ cell, both may enter the primary oocyte, and fertilization will produce an XXY or

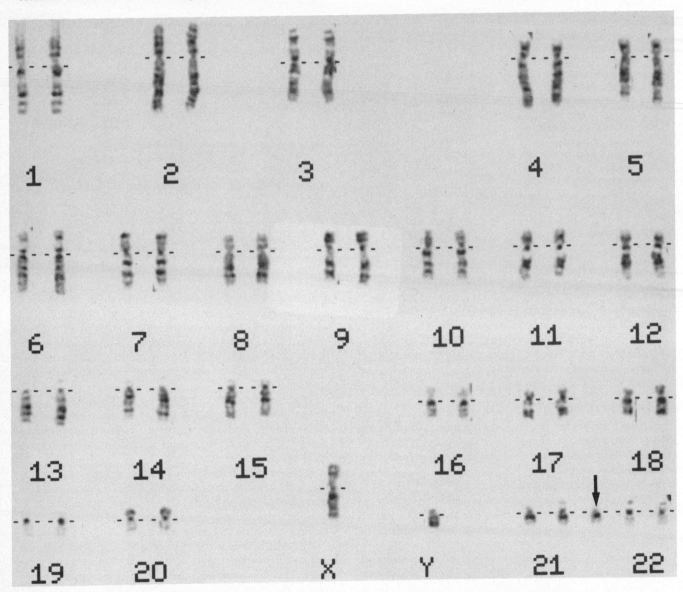

FIG. 3-4. Down's syndrome (47, XY +21). Chromosome preparation showing additional chromosome 21 *(arrow)*.

XXX distribution. Alternatively, both chromosomes can enter the polar body, and the primary oocyte receives none. An X chromosome from the sperm then produces an XO fertilized ovum. The main diseases resulting from abnormalities in the number of sex chromosomes are summarized in Table 3-4.

Turner's syndrome. Turner's syndrome* has an XO chromosome constitution (Fig. 3-6). It is estimated that only about 2% are live births (Fig. 3-7). XO fetuses have normal ovaries for about half the period of intrauterine life; but germinal cells die and the ovaries are replaced by fibrous tissue. However, the external genitalia are morphologically female.

The most constant physical features are short stature, frequent webbing of the sides of the neck, and an increased carrying angle of the arms. Intelligence is often mildly subnormal.

*H.H. Turner (b. 1892), American physician.

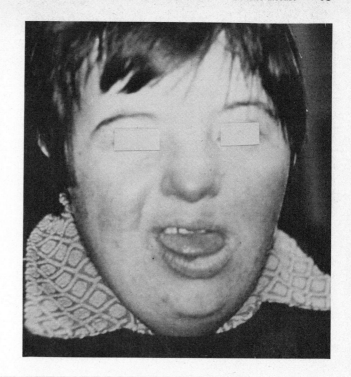

FIG. 3-5. Down's syndrome. The characteristic facial features are instantly recognizable in this chromosomal disorder. *(Courtesy Dr. Crispian Scully.)*

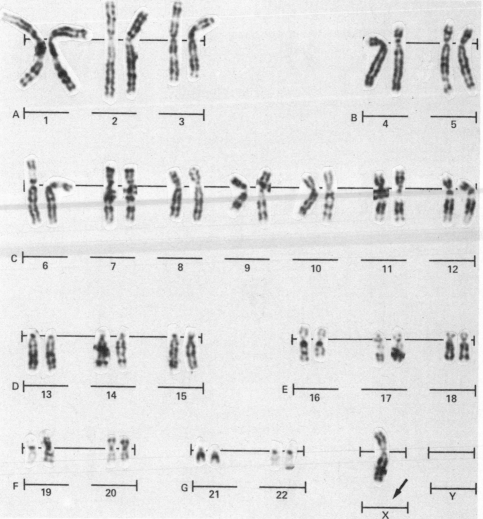

FIG. 3-6. Turner's syndrome (45, X). Chromosome preparation showing deletion of one X chromosome *(arrow).*

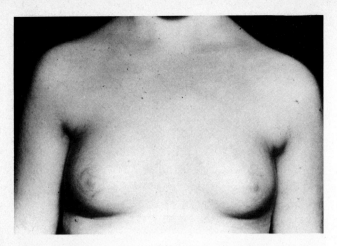

FIG. 3-7. Turner's syndrome. The outward appearance is feminine, but the patient had amenorrhea and was infertile as a result of failure of the sex organs to develop. The webbing of the neck is also typical. *(Courtesy Curator of the Gordon Museum, Guy's Hospital, London, England.)*

Klinefelter's syndrome. Males with an additional X chromosome (Fig. 3-8) are relatively common (nearly 1 in 2000) and a Barr body can be demonstrated. Most of these configurations are XXY, but several additional X chromosomes may sometimes be present.

Clinically, Klinefelter's syndrome* is rarely noticed until after puberty. However, fusion of the epiphyses is delayed so that patients are abnormally tall, but their build is eunuchoidal with narrow shoulders and broad hips.

There are no germ cells in the testis; the seminiferous tubules atrophy and the interstitial cells proliferate (Fig. 3-9). These men are infertile and may show mild enlargement of the breasts (gynecomastia). Intelligence is usually reduced.

XXX females. About 1 in 800 females have an additional X chromosome. These "superfemales" show no special physical characteristics and appear to be normally fertile, but are often of slightly subnormal intelligence.

---

*H.F. Klinefelter (b. 1912), American physician.

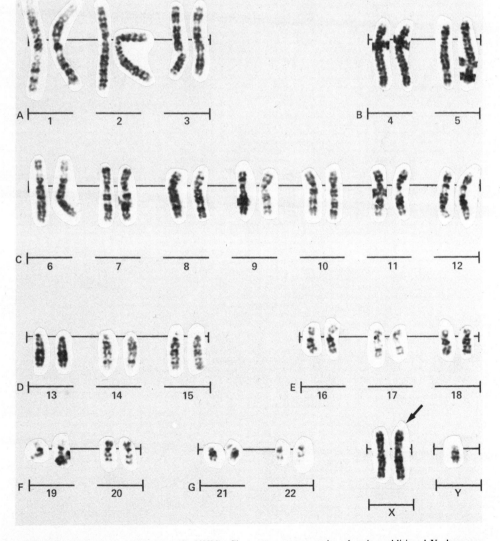

FIG. 3-8. Klinefelter's syndrome (47, XXY). Chromosome preparation showing additional X chromosome *(arrow)*.

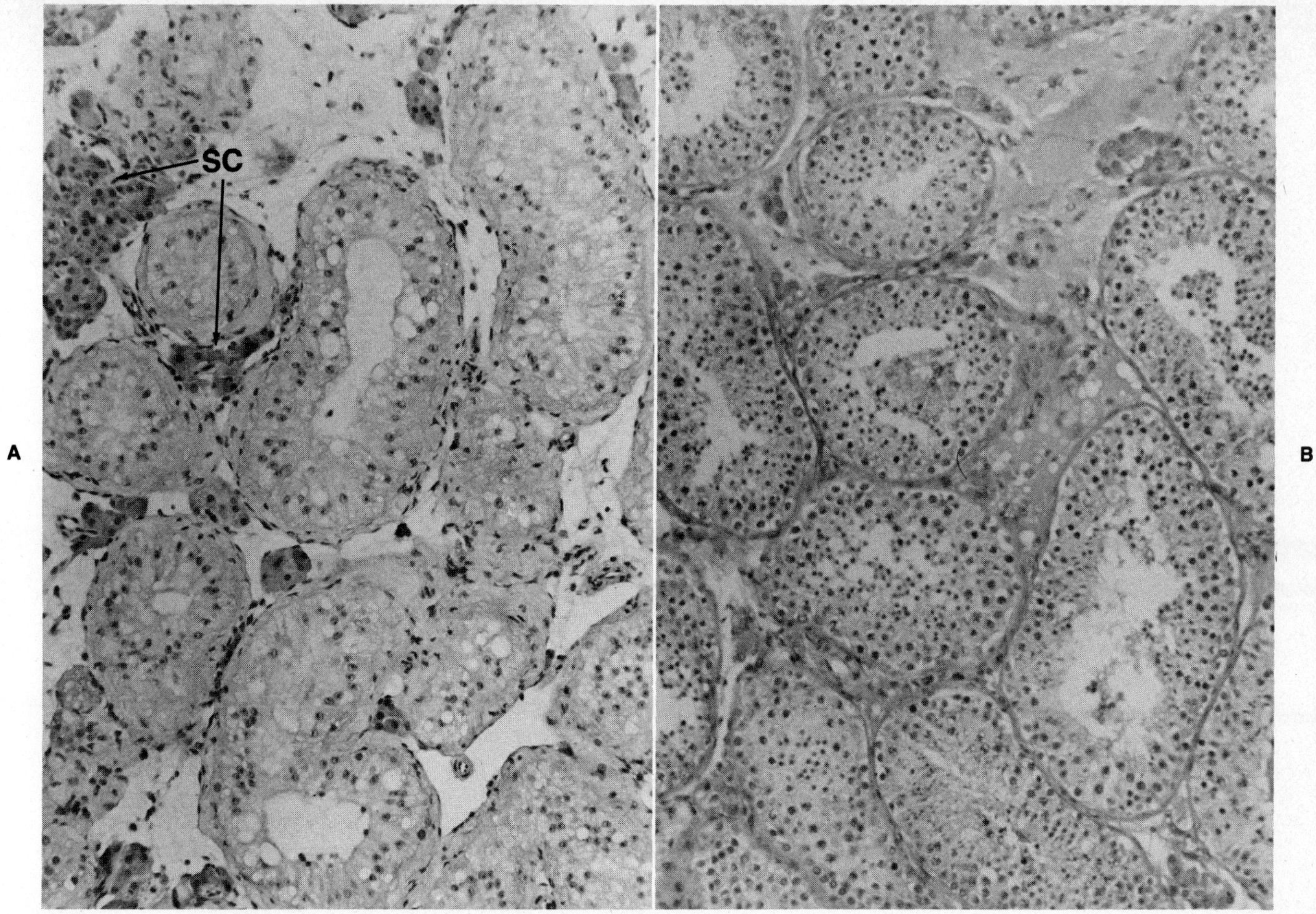

FIG. 3-9. A, Tubular atrophy with prominent Sertoli cells in Klinefelter's syndrome. **B,** Normal testicular structure.

XYY males. The incidence of this anomaly is similar to that of XXX females. These men are usually over 6 feet tall. Some have psychopathic personalities and may become habitual criminals. However, the majority are probably normal.

• • •

It seems curious, in view of the present importance attached to sex, that loss of or excess of sex chromosomes has (relative to the abnormalities of the autosomes) so little effect on sexual behavior and that the feature common to most sex chromosome abnormalities is reduced intelligence.

Oncogenes, oncogenesis, and DNA probes

Oncogenes, as mentioned earlier, are genes which may contribute to tumor formation. DNA probes and some of the techniques described above are currently being used to investigate possible inherited disposition to cancer as well as DNA changes associated with initiation and progression of tumor growth.

Selected readings

Elias S and Annas GJ: Routine prenatal genetic screening, N Engl J Med 317:1407, 1987.

De Lellis RA and Wolfe HJ: New techniques in gene product analysis, Arch Pathol Lab Med 111:620, 1987.

Fenoglio-Preiser CM and Willman CL: Molecular biology and the pathologist, Arch Pathol Lab Med 111:601, 1987.

Hirschhorn R: Therapy of genetic disorders, N Engl J Med 316:623, 1987.

Krivit W and Whitley CB: Bone marrow transplantation for genetic diseases, N Engl J Med 316:1085, 1987.

Lilford RJ and Irving HC et al: Transabdominal chorion villus biopsy: 100 consecutive cases, Lancet I:1415, 1987.

Orkin SH: Genetic diagnosis by DNA analysis, N Engl J Med 317:1023, 1987.

Pope FM and Dorling J et al: J Royal Soc Med 76:1050, 1983.

Prockop DJ and Kivirikko KI: Heritable diseases of collagen, N Engl J Med 311(6):376, 1984.

Pueschel SM: Maternal alpha-fetoprotein screening for Down's syndrome, N Engl J Med 317(6):376, 1987.

Scott J: Molecular genetics of common diseases, Br Med J 295:769, 1987.

Shapiro LJ and Comings DE et al: New frontiers in genetic medicine, Ann Intern Med 104:527, 1986.

Thomsen M: Immunogenetics of disease, mechanisms and clinical aspects: Eur J Clin Invest 15:235, 1985.

Weatherall DJ: Human molecular pathology, Q J Med 63:461, 1987.

CHAPTER 4

Disease caused by physical agents

Ionizing radiation

Two main forms of ionizing radiation are recognized. The first consists of rays (photons) that form part of the *electromagnetic wave spectrum* (x-rays, gamma rays) (Fig. 4-1). The second form includes certain types of *particulate* radiation (alpha and beta particles, neutrons, protons, and deuterons). X-rays and gamma rays penetrate matter easily and are potentially far more damaging than particulate rays.

Sources of radiation

Radiation comes from both *natural and artificial sources*. Natural sources include radioactive rock and soil formations and cosmic radiation from outer space. Artificial sources include nuclear power plants, nuclear weapons, tobacco smoke, radioisotopes, and rays used in medical diagnosis and treatment. Humans are constantly exposed to *background radiation*, which emanates from several of these sources. This is generally very small but has a cumulative effect. Sources of ionizing radiation are listed as follows:

1. Natural sources
   a. Cosmic rays
   b. Radioactive rock formations
2. Artificial sources
   a. Diagnostic radiology
   b. Laboratory and medical use of radioisotopes
   c. Industrial use of radioactive materials and x-rays
   d. Accidents releasing radioactive materials
   e. Atomic explosions
   f. Fallout from atomic explosions

Domestic radon exposure. Several centuries ago and long before cigarette smoking started, miners in Schneeburg and Joachimsthal in central Europe were known to develop a peculiar type of lung disease. This was later recognized as lung cancer (a rare disease then) and to have resulted from exposure to radon released from the surrounding rocks. Currently, there is concern that lung cancers in nonsmokers, and possibly other tumors, may result from the same cause, as homes in some areas of the United States have levels of radon 100-fold greater than in other areas and far exceeding the "safe" limits. The main source of this radon (radon 222 and its decay products) is the underlying soil, especially where houses are built on mine tailings. Grand Junction, Colorado, for example, proudly proclaimed itself "The Uranium Capital of America," but vigorous efforts are being made to change this image, both symbolically and literally, by removing the excess of radioactive mine tailings.

Radon chiefly enters the air and is inhaled; a lesser amount may be ingested in drinking water. Estimates of its effects are based on extrapolations, but some suggest that 1000 to 20,000 cases of lung cancer may be at least partly due to this cause. It must be emphasized, however, that any carcinogenic effect of this domestic exposure to radon is unproven.

By contrast, it may be noted that many people, with a variety of ills, are willing to pay for the "benefits" of inhaling radon in worked-out uranium mines in such areas as Montana.

Radiation exposure in radiotherapy. The two major types of radiation used in the radiotherapy of tumors are photons (x-rays and gamma rays) and electrons (beta particles). The linear accelerator produces beams of both types. Acceleration of electrons to high speeds produces a high-energy electron beam; if the electron beam is allowed to hit an appropriate target, x-ray beams will be produced.

The power of x-rays to penetrate tissues depends on the generating voltage. Formerly, conventional x-ray equipment (up to 300 kVp) had been used to irradiate deeply placed tumors, but this injured the skin and other intervening structures. The linear accelerator largely avoids this effect by producing high-energy x-rays that have their maximum effect below the surface. The gamma rays produced by the isotope cobalt 60 are also a deeply penetrating form of radiation.

Other isotope-containing materials, such as cesium-137 needles or iridium-192 wire, can be inserted directly into an accessible tumor, such as carcinoma of the tongue. In this way

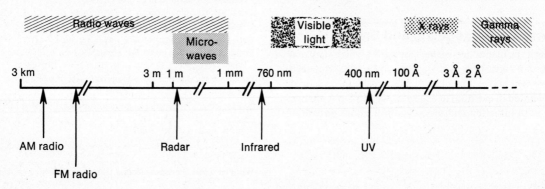

FIG. 4-1. The electromagnetic spectrum.

a high dose of radiation can be delivered directly into the tumor, with a small radius of effect on surrounding tissues.

Ionizing radiation is indiscriminating in its effects on cells. The treatment of cancer depends on determining a dose and method of delivery that cause maximal damage to the tumor and minimal damage to the host. Although these aims are theoretically incompatible, it is sometimes possible to eradicate tumors partially or completely, particularly when they are small, localized, and accessible. Cancers of the lip and skin therefore have a high chance of being cured.

Radiation exposure in diagnostic radiology. Exposure to ionizing rays employed for diagnosis generally entails little risk and, when appropriately used, the benefits should outweigh the dangers. As with radiotherapy, patients and workers alike are subjected to precautionary measures to minimize these dangers. Thus lead shielding and concrete walls are employed, as well as fast film, which keeps the time of exposure as low as possible.

Aside from x-rays, which are well known, a number of synthetic radioisotopes (radionuclides) have also been used for diagnostic work, particularly for assessing the ability of an organ or tissue to function (i.e., by demonstrating uptake of the isotope). Technetium-99m, gallium-67, iodine-123, and phosphorus-32 are a few of the many isotopes used for this purpose.

A recent innovation in diagnostic radiology, the computerized tomography (CT) scanner subjects a patient to large numbers of short bursts of x-rays, and therefore carries the usual risks that attend ionizing radiations. The magnetic resonance imaging (MRI) scanner, by contrast, employs powerful magnetic fields and operates without these dangers.

Biologic measurement of irradiation

In radiotherapy, it is obviously important to know the dose of radiation reaching a region compared with that of the surrounding tissues. The amount of energy absorbed by irradiated tissues can be measured by a dosimeter placed in the field, although this may be difficult because of the problem of placing detectors deep in the tissues and because of factors such as scattering of the rays within the body and differential absorption by the various tissues. In practice, dosimetric calibration of radiation sources, while employing water bath phantoms, is commonly employed to administer predictable amounts of radiation to tissues at fixed distances. The traditional measurement unit is the rad, which is 100 ergs of absorbed energy per gram of irradiated tissue. The système internationale (SI) unit for absorbed dose is the *gray, (Gy)* after a British radiologist, Harold Gray. It equals 1 joule (J) of energy absorbed per kilogram of tissue. One centigray (CGy) is equal to 1 rad.

People who work around radioactive sources carry a dosimeter containing photographic film, which becomes fogged by radiations. The degree of fogging, which is related to exposure, can be measured.

Mechanisms of cell injury

Although exact mechanisms are not always known, it is generally thought that ionizing radiation injures cells in both (1) direct and (2) indirect ways.

Direct effects. Direct effects on cells are the result of reaction between the high-energy radiation beam and vital molecules in the cell, chiefly deoxyribonucleic acid (DNA). Two types of changes result from injury to DNA, namely *point mutations* (i.e., changes in DNA molecular structure), and *chromosomal*

breaks. The chief effects of DNA injury may be any or all of the following:

1. Prevention of mitotic division
2. Cell death by apoptosis
3. Congenital malformations in offspring irradiated in utero
4. Carcinogenesis (Chapter 9).

Direct effects are related to two main factors, namely irradiation dosage and the proliferative activity of irradiated cells.

Dosage. Whether an irradiated cell dies or merely stops dividing depends partly on the dose of radiation it receives. The high doses of ionizing radiation used in radiotherapy are designed primarily to prevent cell division, and the irradiated cancer cells do not necessarily die. They may still retain some biologic functions, such as synthesis of certain proteins. However, if the dose of radiation is high enough, all cellular activity is extinguished and the cell is killed, probably by apoptosis.

The induction of point mutations appears to take place at a rate that is directly proportional to the radiation dose. Even the smallest dose of radiation has a finite possibility of causing such a mutation, and researchers are discovering that there may not be a dose of radiation below which carcinogenic change in cells cannot take place.

Cellular proliferative activity. Different types of cells are affected by radiation in essentially the same way but differ in the dose of radiation needed to produce the same effect. Cells are most vulnerable to the effects of radiation when dividing, and tissues where mitoses are frequent and cells are constantly being renewed are particularly sensitive. There are, however, exceptions to this general rule. Thus lymphocytes and vascular endothelium, which show little or no cell renewal, are also sensitive. The relative radiosensitivity of some important tissues is summarized in Table 4-1.

The basis of radiotherapy of tumors is that tumor cells in general proliferate more rapidly than most normal cells and tend as a consequence to be more radiosensitive. The type of cellular damage produced by radiation is, however, the same, regardless of whether it falls on a tumor or normal tissue. As a consequence, the latter is always injured during a course of radiotherapy.

Indirect effects. Indirect effects on cells take place through the ionization of water and the formation of toxic free radicals (Chapter 2). Endothelial cells are particularly vulnerable to this form of injury. Endothelial cell swelling takes place, as well as necrosis followed by thrombosis (Fig. 4-2). Capillaries and small arteries are most severely affected because the small lumens are most readily occluded by such damage. Ischemia, and perhaps necrosis, of tissues supplied by affected vessels results. Bone and central nervous system are especially vulnerable to this mode of injury.

TABLE 4-1. Radiosensitivity of tissues in relation to their mitotic activity

| *Radio resistant ⟶ Radiosensitive* | | |
No mitoses	*Few mitoses*	*Frequent mitoses*
Neurons	Endocrine glands	Bone marrow
Specialized sense organs	Liver	Intestinal epithelium
	Endothelium	Hair follicles
	Connective tissue	Gonads
		Oral epithelium
		Epidermis

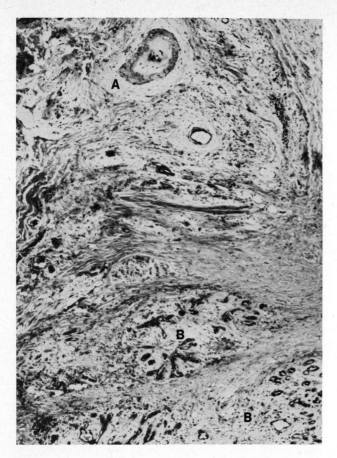

FIG. 4-2. Radiation damage to oral tissues. The main changes seen here are obliterative endarteritis of an arteriole *(A)* and destruction and fibrous replacement of salivary acini *(B)* leaving only duct tissue.

Effects of radiation on tissues and organs

Radiation effects on tissues and organs may be classed as *early or late* and as *systemic or local.*

Early effects. The effects of radiation on tissues and organs may be felt soon, or relatively soon, after irradiation (i.e., immediately, or within hours, days, weeks, or perhaps months). Early effects involving whole body systems (systemic effects, acute radiation syndrome) are chiefly the result of total body irradiation, for example, irradiation following a nuclear explosion or an accident at a nuclear power plant. Localized irradiation of a body part, such as follows radiotherapy of a cancer, generally results in a different series of effects, the nature of which varies somewhat according to the part irradiated.

Late effects. Late (delayed) effects can be experienced months, years, or even decades, after exposure, whether this involved total body irradiation or only localized irradiation of a body part. The chief late effects of radiation are carcinogenic effects and the development of genetic defects in offspring.

Systemic effects of radiation (acute radiation syndrome)

Acute radiation syndrome. Acute radiation syndrome is the term given to the effects of heavy doses of ionizing radiation to a localized area or of lesser doses to the whole body. These effects, ranging from self-limiting malaise to rapid death, were seen on an enormous scale after the dropping of atomic bombs on Hiroshima and Nagasaki. Although this happened in 1945,

TABLE 4-2. Effects of radiation on humans

Whole body exposure	Effects
1 to 2 Gy (100 to 200 rads)	Survival almost invariable with little or no treatment
2 to 5 Gy (200 to 500 rads)	Death after a variable period, survival only with optimal treatment
5 to 20 Gy (500 to 2000 rads)	Usually rapidly lethal but, exceptionally, optimal treatment may allow survival
50 Gy (5000 rads) or more	Death within 24 hours

the effects on survivors are still being felt. Since then, the nuclear accident at Chernobyl in 1987, when the results of irradiation injury and possible methods of treatment were better appreciated, has added to the knowledge in this field. However, the effects of accidents of this nature are complicated by the association of other types of injury, particularly thermal burns, with the radiation. Pure radiation injuries have been seen only in a few individuals as a result of limited accidents with radioactive material. Furthermore, experimental evidence of the effects of radiation must be interpreted in the light of the fact that different species of mammals differ in their responses; even in humans there appears to be considerable variation between individuals in their susceptibility to radiation injury.

The quantitation of the effects of radiation on humans is also difficult to assess because, after an accident such as that at Chernobyl, the precise amount of radiation received by a victim (in terms of intensity and duration of exposure and amount of body area exposed) is unknown. Management of these patients has therefore to be governed largely by the clinical features and their progress. An approximate guide, however, is shown in Table 4-2.

The most vulnerable body systems are the (1) central nervous system, (2) gastrointestinal tract, and (3) bone marrow. Death can result from sufficiently heavy radiation damage to any of these.

Radiation sickness. Radiation sickness is the term given to symptoms that result from exposure of the whole body to more than 5 to 20 Gy or from heavier doses to part of the body, particularly the upper trunk. This therefore is a common effect of irradiation of cancer of the breast.

Symptoms can start within hours and usually include headache, debility, anorexia, and nausea. With heavier doses there is usually vomiting, diarrhea, tachycardia or arrhythmias, hypotension, and dyspnea. The peripheral blood shows leukopenia, thrombocytopenia, and increased erythrocyte sedimentation rate. Anxiety, irritability, and insomnia are usually associated.

Following prodromal symptoms, particularly nausea and vomiting, acute syndromes affecting the three main body systems follow after periods of time, varying with the total dose of radiation received and the type of radiation; for example, neutrons are more damaging than gamma rays. If, however, the dose has been relatively small, the prodromal phase lasting a few days is likely to be followed by a latent period of apparent recovery. The third phase starts abruptly with recurrence of nausea and vomiting, bleeding, infections, and loss of hair; but gradual recovery takes place over a period of weeks or months. Generally speaking, the greater the dose, the greater is the rapidity of onset and severity of the symptoms. Damage to the central nervous system, gastrointestinal tract, or bone marrow follows after different latent periods. According to the main site of injury, damage dominates the picture and may be the cause of death.

Central nervous system (neurovascular) syndrome. Massive doses of radiation (20 or more Gy), as at Hiroshima or Nagasaki, are followed, within minutes or hours, by the central nervous system (CNS) syndrome. However, the neurons of the brain (which, experimentally, appear resistant to radiation) show little or no morphologic change, and the cause of death is probably widespread capillary damage leading to edema of the brain and raised intracranial pressure.

Clinically, apathy and prostration may be followed by convulsions or hypotension, arrhythmias, shock, and death within minutes or hours. Ataxia may result from cerebellar damage.

Gastrointestinal syndrome. The crypts, which are the site of cell renewal and mitotic activity, are the most sensitive areas. Radiation causes cessation of mitosis; nuclei fragment, and the cells die. Without replacement activity, the villi lose their covering of cells, so that proteolytic enzymes can damage the underlying tissue. The normal barrier function of the intestinal mucosa is thus destroyed, water and electrolytes escape into the lumen of the intestine, and bacteria and their toxins can spread into the submucosa and beyond.

Clinically, damage to the intestinal epithelium typically causes symptoms within a few days. There is loss of appetite (anorexia), nausea, and vomiting. Severe disturbance of fluid and electrolyte balance results from the combined effects of vomiting and loss of the normal barrier function of the bowel. Severe bloody diarrhea quickly follows, the abdomen distends, and paralysis of peristalsis (ileus) develops. Fluid replacement and antibiotics can lessen these effects and, if damage is not too severe, allow the bowel to recover. Otherwise, dehydration leads to peripheral circulatory failure and death.

The hemopoietic syndrome. The bone marrow is irreversibly damaged by lower doses of radiation than those needed to produce the gastrointestinal syndrome. Radiation injures or kills the marrow stem cells and causes leukopenia, thrombocytopenia, and anemia.

The rapidly dividing stem cells are affected within hours, but their successors may continue to mature for several days afterward. Replacement of mature peripheral blood cells therefore continues for 4 or 5 days before the effects of death of the stem cells are felt.

The first sign, within a few hours, is a fall in the lymphocyte count, which persists for periods related to the dose of radiation. The granulocyte count also falls, and the lowest white cell counts are found by the second to fifth weeks. Severe granulocytopenia, which develops within the first 7 to 10 days after exposure, indicates a poor prognosis. The platelet count does not usually decline until after about 1 or 2 weeks but takes months to recover. Again, massive radiation exposure can cause rapid and severe thrombocytopenia and hemorrhage.

The erythrocyte count falls more slowly and there is reticulocytopenia. Anemia is often worsened by loss of blood from the gastrointestinal tract and as a result of the thrombocytopenia.

Clinically, there are the usual prodromal symptoms, including malaise and nausea; with moderately high doses of radiation the acute gastrointestinal syndrome can develop but may respond to treatment. There may then be a period of apparent recovery for a week or more, but this is followed by malaise, fever, and loss of appetite.

The leukopenia results in increased susceptibility to infection and causes pharyngitis, tonsillar or oral ulceration, and sore throat. Depression of the lymphocyte count leads to depressed immune responses, which increases susceptibility to infection.

Thrombocytopenia causes purpura (spontaneous bruising) and bleeding, especially from the gums and from any areas of gastrointestinal ulceration.

Anemia causes fatigue and breathlessness (dyspnea) on mild exertion.

The peripheral lymphocyte count is an indicator of the severity of the injury. The count starts to fall approximately 24 hours after exposure and if greater than 1200 lymphocytes/μL, recovery is likely. A count below 300 lymphocytes/μL indicates almost certain death.

Radiation damage to the hemopoietic system is critical to survival in that, if untreated it may be fatal; but if facilities are available, the amount of damage sustained will, to a large extent, determine whether bone marrow transplantation will be feasible, as discussed later.

Prognosis of acute radiation syndromes

Exposure of the whole body to superlethal levels of radiation (50 Gy or more) is usually followed by death within 24 to 48 hours with symptoms of the CNS syndrome. Exposure to somewhat lower amounts of radiation (20 to 50 Gy) is typically followed, within hours or minutes, by acute radiation sickness then, within hours or days, intractable vomiting, diarrhea, dehydration, fever, and coma. Death usually follows before hemopoietic signs become apparent. No effective treatment is available, and palliation of symptoms is the best that can be achieved.

In those that have received 5 to 20 Gy (500 to 2000 rads), the early CNS syndrome tends to be less severe and long-lasting and is followed by a period of apparent recovery for a week or two. Symptoms resulting from the gastrointestinal and hemopoietic syndromes, and still later loss of hair, then follow. With optimal treatment, including fluid replacement, blood cell transfusions, and antimicrobial therapy, recovery is possible. Alternatively, marrow transplantation may be indicated if other injuries are compatible with survival.

In those that have been exposed to 2 to 5 Gy (200 to 500 rads) symptoms are generally similar to those sustained by more heavily exposed groups but tend to be less severe and prolonged. Survival is likely if optimal supportive treatment (as outlined above) is given, but bone marrow transplantation is not indicated.

Bone marrow transplantation for radiation injury

Several problems attend the use of bone marrow transplantation (Chapter 7) for the treatment of radiation accidents.

In those that have received relatively low doses of radiation, the resulting degree of immunosuppression is insufficient to allow acceptance of the graft without additional immunosuppressive treatment. At intermediate, midlethal levels of exposure (2 to 5 Gy) bone marrow transplantation may be associated with decreased expectation of survival (the so-called midzone effect). However, if T cells can be removed from the donor tissue, temporary engraftment may allow recovery of host hemopoietic tissue.

In extreme cases where there has been total destruction of the bone marrow, even histoincompatible donor marrow may be successfully engrafted.

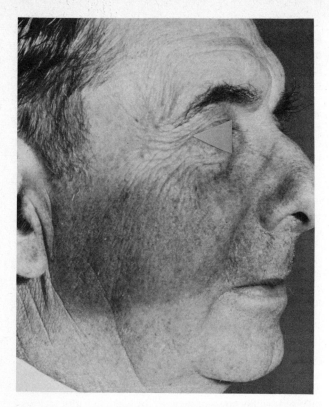

FIG. 4-3. Early radiation reaction. The early inflammatory reaction is exceedingly well demarcated, as can be seen.

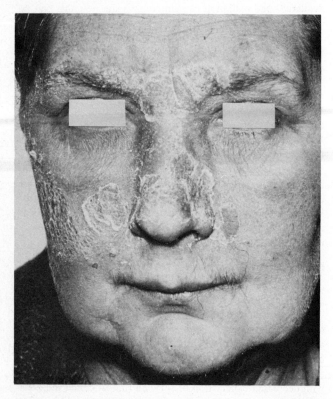

FIG. 4-4. Early radiation reaction. The patient has received radiation for carcinoma of the maxillary sinus from a conventional x-ray source. The affected side is darker because of inflammatory erythema, whereas the superficial dead epithelial cells form a thin crust that is being shed. *(Courtesy Curator of the Gordon Museum, Guy's Hospital, London, England.)*

Problems which further complicate this form of treatment include the following:

1. It is difficult to assess the level of radiation exposure to determine whether bone marrow transplantation is indicated or likely to be of benefit.
2. Finding histocompatible donors is also difficult. Apart from those whose bone marrow has been totally destroyed, histoincompatibility leads either to failure of engraftment or fatal graft-versus-host disease (Chapter 7). Large pools of human leukocyte antigen (HLA)–typed volunteer donors now exist in Europe and the United States, and this made it possible to find histocompatible donors for many Chernobyl victims within a few days of the accident.
3. Radiation-induced lymphocytopenia may make HLA typing of potential recipients impossible.

Effects of localized radiation and complications of radiotherapy

The radiation syndromes usually result from exposure of the whole body. Radiotherapy for the treatment of cancer, on the other hand, is directed toward specific sites; however, damage to the surrounding tissues also produces effects, and these depend on the radiation dose and the size of the area irradiated. Most patients have systemic symptoms, particularly malaise, loss of appetite, and often nausea, unless the area treated is exceedingly small.

General morphology of radiation injury. In acute lesions, varying degrees of apoptosis are commonly seen, with consequent loss of parenchymal cellular elements. Connective tissue activation tends to be prominent in irradiated tissues, with the lytic phase gradually merging with the late, sclerotic phase. There is often striking fibrin deposition that persists for long periods of time because of a failure in the local fibrinolytic system. Occlusive vascular intimal lesions follow endothelial injury and thrombosis. Nuclear enlargement and asymmetry, affecting both stromal and parenchymal cells, is the result of chromosomal breaks and continued DNA synthesis in the absence of mitotic division and may suggest the presence of persisting cancer cells to the unwary. None of these changes is pathognomonic of radiation injury, but taken together they present a characteristic picture.

Changes in different tissues or organs as a consequence of localized irradiation are described in the following paragraphs.

Skin. In most cases radiation comes from external sources and therefore often damages the skin to a degree depending on the dose and on the powers of penetration of the radiation used. The epithelial cells of the skin have a relatively rapid turnover rate and are moderately vulnerable. Radiation damage to skin cells provokes an inflammatory reaction (Fig. 4-3). This is followed by desquamation of dead cells (Fig. 4-4). An overdose of radiation can destroy the full thickness of the epithelium and produce a radiation burn. This resembles a thermal burn except that vascular damage causes greatly delayed healing. Microscopically, the late effects of radiation injury to the skin are thinning of the epithelium with increased keratosis and obliterative changes in the capillaries. Dermal appendages, particularly hair follicles and sweat glands, are most readily destroyed, and loss of hair is therefore a common complication (Fig. 4-5). Destruction of these specialized organs is followed by replacement fibrosis.

With heavier doses, the vascularity of the connective tissue is further impaired so that there are few fibroblasts, and the

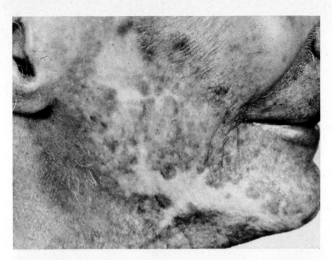

FIG. 4-5. Chronic radiation dermatitis. The skin in the affected area is recognizable by the areas of pigmentation and depigmentation (vitiligo). Hair follicles and sweat glands have been destroyed, and the skin has a thin and papery texture. *(Courtesy Curator of the Gordon Museum, Guy's Hospital, London, England.)*

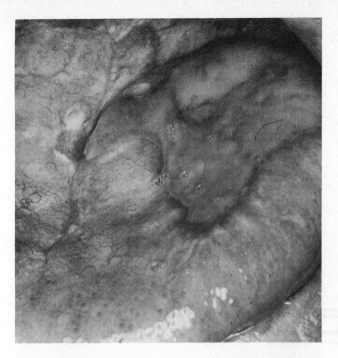

FIG. 4-6. Radiation mucositis. The epithelium has been destroyed leaving a fibrin-covered ulcer. *(From Cawson RA: Essentials of dental surgery and pathology, ed 3, Edinburgh, Scotland, 1978, Churchill Livingstone.)*

collagen assumes a hyaline appearance. The lumen of many small blood vessels is obliterated or destroyed, but superficial, dilated, thin-walled vessels form visible telangiectases.

Oral mucous membranes. The changes in oral mucous membranes are similar to those affecting the skin. With low doses, there is initially inflammation, seen as an area of redness; after about 1 week, superficial cells that have been killed form a yellow-white pseudomembrane on the surface. The pseudomembrane is usually shed after about 1 week. Minor salivary glands in the underlying connective tissue are damaged and may be destroyed. After moderate doses, the mucous membrane recovers its normal appearance in about 1 week. These changes are known as radiation mucositis (Figs. 4-6 and 4-7).

Heavier doses can destroy the full thickness of epithelium and produce an area of ulceration. This also eventually heals and usually leaves a smooth featureless area of mucosa (Fig. 4-8). Overdoses of radiation to the mucoperiosteum can destroy both epithelium and connective tissue and expose the underlying bone. This bone usually becomes infected as a consequence, and healing typically takes many years as a result of the radiation-induced ischemia, unless vigorous treatment is instituted.

Salivary glands. Glandular tissue in general is vulnerable to irradiation, and the salivary glands are particularly at risk during radiotherapy of cancers in the head and neck region (Fig. 4-9). Since saliva-secreting glands are restricted to a relatively small area, irradiation damage to this region can result in severe dryness of the mouth (xerostomia) and susceptibility to infections, including ascending (bacterial) parotitis.

The lungs. The lungs can be damaged as a result of irradiation of cancers of the bronchi or of the breast, both of which are common. Irradiation causes *diffuse alveolar damage* (Chapter 12), which is demonstrated either as an acute radiation pneumonitis or as a chronic fibrotic process, depending on the stage of the tissue response. Most patients recover unless large volumes of lung are affected.

The gonads. The ovaries and testes are particularly vulnerable to ionizing radiation, and relatively small doses (5 Gy) can cause permanent sterility.

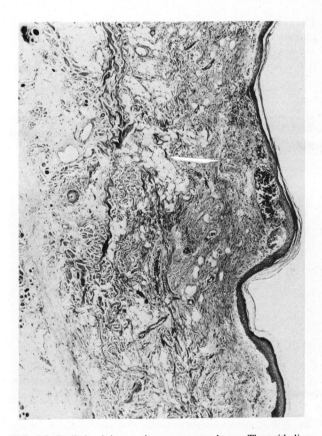

FIG. 4-7. Radiation injury to the mucous membrane. The epithelium is thin and flattened. Immediately beneath the epithelium are dilated thin-walled vessels (telangiectases), but the deeper tissues are poorly vascularized and consist only of irregular collagenous connective tissue.

The kidneys. Inadvertent irradiation of the kidney during radiotherapy of intraabdominal neoplasms may cause renal failure, frequently complicated by malignant hypertension. The pathologic changes may affect predominantly glomeruli and arteries, with changes of intravascular coagulation (acute radiation nephritis). Alternatively, the tubules may bear the brunt of the injury and a chronic interstitial nephritis may result (chronic radiation nephritis).

Bone. There are few areas of the body where there is no bone in the field of irradiation, and in the past the relatively high absorption of radiation by bone made complications common. Megavoltage therapy has largely overcome this problem

of incidental damage, but the high doses of irradiation necessary for treatment of bone tumors has severe effects, especially in the period before bone growth is complete. Damage to the epiphyses then causes the bone to become stunted.

In adults, periosteal new bone formation can be arrested, and the bone becomes ischemic, osteoporotic, and brittle. Pathologic fractures may therefore result.

Ischemia of bone is a common delayed effect of radiation damage to the vessels and obliterative endarteritis. This may have no obvious effect unless injury allows access of infection, which is then followed by intractable osteomyelitis (Chapter 17). The danger is particularly great when the jaws are in-

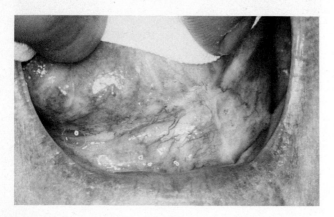

FIG. 4-8. Chronic radiation damage to the oral mucosa. Following irradiation for cancer of the tongue, the mucosa is pale and fibrotic and shows superficial telangiectases.

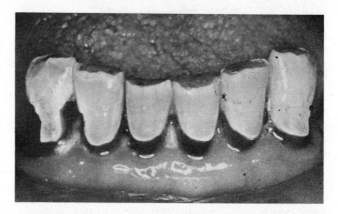

FIG. 4-9. Radiation-associated dental caries. Rampant caries following irradiation seems mainly to be caused by the reduced salivary flow but frequently shows this unusual distribution, primarily involving the necks of the teeth.

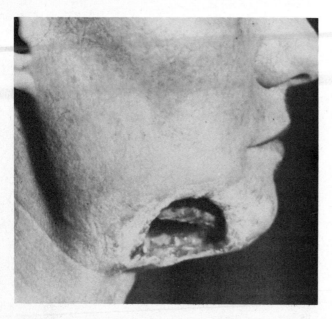

FIG. 4-10. Radiation necrosis of the jaw. The combination of a heavy dose of radiotherapy together with infection from a tooth has led to chronic osteomyelitis. The overlying skin has sloughed away, exposing the lower border of the necrotic mandible. (*Courtesy Curator of the Gordon Museum, Guy's Hospital, London, England.*)

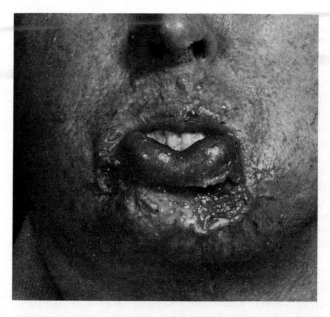

FIG. 4-11. Carcinomatous change following irradiation. The patient, a woman of 55, had received radiotherapy for lupus vulgaris some years earlier. There is fibrosis around the irradiated area and an area of ulceration below the lower lip in which a carcinoma has developed. (*From Cawson RA: Essentials of dental surgery and pathology, ed 3, Edinburgh, Scotland, 1978, Churchill Livingstone.*)

volved, since tooth extraction opens up the bone to a heavy mixed bacterial infection from the pockets that form around the teeth (Fig. 4-10).

The gastrointestinal tract. The mucosa of the gastrointestinal tract is highly radiosensitive, and damage to the intestine usually results from irradiation of other abdominopelvic structures, including the uterus and ovaries. In such cases there is typically painful diarrhea, which, if uncontrollable as a result of heavy doses of irradiation, leads to death from the gastrointestinal tract syndrome; otherwise, it eventually subsides. Radiation reaching the large bowel can also be followed by delayed reactions, with bloody and mucous diarrhea, starting after 6 months to 2 years.

The eyes. The orbit is inevitably affected when tumors of nearby structures such as the lacrimal glands or eyelids are irradiated. Effects include loss of eyelashes, distortion of the eyelids by fibrosis, and dryness of the eye, with its associated risks, as a result of radiation damage to the lacrimal glands. The last is particularly a hazard in treatment of cancer of the lacrimal gland. The lens is also sensitive and must be protected to prevent radiation-induced cataract. Other important structures such as the retina and optic tract are surprisingly radioresistant, and damage to sight after radiotherapy is mostly a result of damage to accessory structures as described.

Carcinogenic effects of radiation

Promotion of tumor formation (carcinogenesis) by radiation is characterized by a long latent period (sometimes 25 years or more) between exposure and development of a tumor (Fig. 4-11). Examples of this effect include cancers developing as a result of occupational exposure, therapeutic radiation, and, most strikingly, among survivors of the atomic explosion at Hiroshima and Nagasaki. Possible mechanisms pertaining to radiation carcinogenesis are discussed in Chapter 9.

Genetic effects of radiation

Experimentally, doses of irradiation too small to stop mitosis can induce chromosomal abnormalities and mutations. The relevance of these findings in humans is difficult to evaluate. However, exposure of the fetus to radiation is followed by a high incidence of congenital abnormalities and an increased susceptibility to leukemia or other cancers. Abdominal x-ray examination should not be carried out on pregnant women, especially during the first 2 weeks of pregnancy.

At Hiroshima, pregnant women exposed to relatively low doses of radiation have produced a high proportion of children with congenital abnormalities, particularly microcephaly, mental subnormality, and retardation of growth.

Effects and hazards of lasers and microwaves
Lasers

The term *laser* is an acronym of light amplification by stimulated emission of radiation. Whereas ordinary light is composed of a mixture of waves of different wavelengths (and therefore different colors), the light beam produced by a laser consists of waves of a single wavelength (and therefore color). This monochromatic, phase-coherent light contains tremendous energy, and a laser beam can travel in a perfectly straight line for incredible distances and can also be brought to precise focus at a chosen point.

The applications of the laser are numerous. Aside from its many uses in industry, communications, entertainment, and warfare, there is a steadily growing list of surgical applications. The *tissue effects* depend on the wavelength of the laser employed, as well as the duration of exposure. Laser beams in the ultraviolet portion of the spectrum have principally a photochemical effect rather than a thermal effect; they act by breaking intramolecular bonds and thus creating tissue incisions. The main effect of beams in the visible portion of the spectrum is to cause heating of tissues, an effect mediated by absorption of radiation by various pigments, chiefly melanin and hemoglobin, in tissue. The effect desired by the surgeon may be controlled thermal *coagulation*, as in retinal surgery or the control of gastrointestinal bleeding, or the *vaporization* of tissue, producing an incision while adjacent vessels are occluded by endothelial cell swelling and thrombi to provide a largely bloodless operating field. Vaporization is also effectively employed in the selective removal of skin or mucosal lesions, chiefly neoplasms, and in the destruction of atheromas (laser angioplasty).

Hazards created by laser use are primarily short term. Direct laser radiation may damage the retina, cornea, and skin, depending on laser type. Use of lasers may be associated with electric shock, fire, explosion of volatile gases in the operating room, and ultraviolet radiation from discharge tubes. Noxious fumes from vaporized tissue may be an environmental hazard. Laser medical devices are regulated in the United States by the Food and Drug Administration (FDA).

Microwaves

Microwaves are another form of electromagnetic radiation and have a wavelength ranging from 1 mm to 1 m. Although many radar, radio, and television signals fall into this range, certain low-frequency waves have the ability to penetrate deeply into solid media, producing internal heating. This thermal effect is due to the absorption of these waves by polar molecules, such as water, and is employed in microwave cooking ovens and the diathermy apparatus used by physical therapists. The organs most susceptible to thermal microwave injury are the eyes and the testes. The absorbed microwave energy readily produces elevated temperatures as a result of the limited amount of blood flow available in these organs for removal of heat. Cataracts and testicular tubular atrophy are said to result if the eyes and testes have not been protected during diathermy.

There is at present much disagreement regarding the nonthermal effects of microwaves on living tissue. The problems include inability to measure accurately the microwave energy absorbed by exposed biologic specimens, which is in part due to the interaction of the microwave field with the detectors. Furthermore, the cellular reactions that follow exposure to the microwaves are poorly understood, and there is even some disagreement as to whether any nonthermal effects are produced by low-energy microwaves.

Most reports on the nonthermal effects of microwave radiation come from the Soviet Union and emphasize involvement of the central nervous system. Many of the symptoms described are of a subjective nature and include fatigue, dizziness, and memory impairment. The United States embassy in Moscow is alleged to have been bombarded with microwaves, not only for the purpose of electronic surveillance, but also to induce mental aberrations in embassy employees.

Teratogenic effects are also listed among the nonthermal

effects of microwave radiation, and recent work suggests that this may be caused by separation of DNA strands.

Effects and hazards of video display terminals

At least 15 million video display terminals (VDTs) are in use in offices and homes in association with computers in the United States. Video display terminals operate in the same way as television receivers. In addition to emission of light (which forms the image on the screen), excitation of the phosphors by the electron beam also gives rise to emission of minute amounts of ultraviolet and infrared rays and low-energy x-rays.

Measurement of the radiation from VDTs has shown the level to be exceedingly low and often lower than from some domestic appliances. Cataracts, reproductive disorders, and facial dermatitis allegedly resulting from working with VDTs have been shown to be no more frequent than in those who are not exposed to VDTs. Since this text is being written on word processors with just such VDTs the writers sincerely hope that this information is correct!

Actinic (ultraviolet) radiation

Tissue damage is usually caused by excessive exposure to sunshine or ultraviolet lamps. Ultraviolet radiation (about 300 nm wavelength) has little power of penetration and causes no more than superficial damage to the skin. The retina is vulnerable, and ultraviolet damage can cause blindness.

The main effects of ultraviolet irradiation of the skin are as follows:

1. Sunburn
2. Increased pigmentation
3. Photodermatoses, including aberrations of connective tissue synthesis
4. Carcinogenesis

Sunburn

Sunburn causes mild superficial inflammation with erythema, edema, and, in severe cases, blistering. Clinically there is burning and tenderness, which improve after a few days with subsidence of inflammation. Later the damaged superficial epithelium desquamates.

Suntanning is the result of more prolonged exposure and is due to oxidation of melanin in the prickle cell layer. Pigmentation may be uniform, as in darker skinned people, or spotty, in the form of freckles (epheles) in the fair skinned.

Increased pigmentation

Freckles form in fair or red-haired people, but the tendency to freckling may also be determined by an autosomal dominant gene.

A freckle is the result of an increase in melanin production by a localized population of melanocytes in the skin. Rounded pigmented macules thus form. These may become confluent in some areas, but there are always other areas that remain unpigmented.

Photodermatoses

Many types of photodermatoses have been described. They may (1) affect otherwise normal people, (2) be allergic, (3) be the result of photosensitization by drugs, such as tetracyclines, or (4) may exacerbate preexisting dermatoses, such as lupus erythematosus. Premature degenerative changes develop in the skin of albinos.

Degenerative changes in the dermis after excessive exposure cause the extracellular matrix to appear homogeneous and hematoxyphilic. The appearance is due to the synthesis of abnormal elastic fibers (Chapter 2).

Vitiligo is the name given to patchy lack of pigmentation due to destruction of epidermal melanocytes. Vitiligo produces a piebald appearance, especially in those who are otherwise dark skinned.

Carcinogenesis

Squamous cell carcinoma, basal cell carcinoma, and malignant melanoma are significantly more frequent as a result of prolonged exposure to sunshine (Fig. 4-12). Basal cell carcinoma is more common than squamous cell carcinoma or malignant melanoma. The intraepidermal precursor lesion of squamous cell carcinoma arising in sun-damaged skin is termed *actinic keratosis*. Squamous cell carcinomas arising in this setting rarely metastisize, unlike those arising, for example, in chronic leg ulcers or burn scars. There is also an increased tendency for *keratoacanthomas* to develop in sun-damaged skin. Malignant melanomas that develop following actinic injury are typically of the *lentigo maligna* type.

Risk factors for the development of cancers are the intensity of the sunshine, duration of exposure, and skin hypopigmentation. Albinos can therefore develop skin cancers during adolescence. In the hereditary disorder *xeroderma pigmentosum*, however, there is abnormal sensitivity to sunshine, in spite of pigmentation. The pigmentation is patchy and distributed as freckles. Cancer can develop in early childhood. The ozone layer in the atmosphere filters the ultraviolet light reaching the earth, and there is concern that the incidence of skin cancers may rise with depletion of this layer as a result of industrial pollutants and other factors.

Each of these skin lesions is discussed in more detail in Chapter 19.

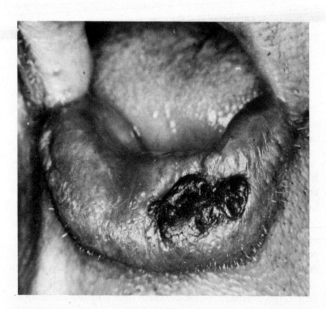

FIG. 4-12. Carcinoma of the lip. This is an important example of the carcinogenic effect of excessive exposure to sunlight. The patient was an outdoor worker (a riverboatman) and had neglected the tumor for 1 year.

Thermal burns

Burns are among the most serious and feared injuries that can afflict humans. The risk of being burned has increased greatly with the advent of many of the advances of modern civilization. These include petroleum products, gas, electric appliances, and sadly, the many weapons of war, particularly napalm and flame throwers.

Classification

The severity of burns can be determined by (1) the size of the burned area and (2) the depth to which the skin has been damaged or destroyed. The estimation of both the size and depth of a burn is important in determining the prognosis and treatment.

The size of a burn expressed as a percent of total body area can be determined from a number of tables or formulae. Such a method is shown below.

Surface burns are classified as follows with respect to depth:

1. Superficial partial thickness (first degree) burns injure or destroy the epidermis, with little injury to adnexa.
2. Deep partial thickness (second degree) burns cause necrosis of both the epidermis and dermis, along with some of the adnexal structures, but the capacity for regeneration from remaining adnexal structures is still present.
3. Full thickness (third degree) burns produce necrosis of the entire thickness of the epidermis and dermis and usually extend into the subcutaneous fat. The capacity for regeneration is lost, and skin grafts are required.

Partial thickness burns can be expected to heal on their own if properly cared for.

The size of a burn can be estimated by the following "rule of nines":

Head		9%
Arms	9% +	9%
Legs	18% +	18%
Trunk		36%
Perineum		1%
TOTAL		100%

Pathology: local changes

Most of the pathologic processes initiated by burns are inflammatory in nature (Chapter 6). The mildest burns, such as those caused by exposure of virgin skin to the sun's rays in early summer, are characterized by mild redness (erythema) and edema of the skin, which subside in a few days with desquamation of the superficial epidermis. In more severe burns there is vesiculation (blistering) of the skin. This is due to separation of the epidermis from the dermis by plasma-rich fluid exuding from damaged blood vessels. Vesiculation is followed in several days by eschar (crust) formation as the exudate dries. In the most severe burns of the skin there is necrosis of the epidermis, dermis, and the neurovascular supply of the area.

Systemic effects and complications

A variety of systemic effects complicate severe and extensive burns. These are shock, pulmonary edema, stress ulcers, and infection.

Shock. Shock (Chapter 10) is mainly the result of a severe reduction in circulating blood volume, common in burned patients. Later, systemic infection by gram-negative bacteria and release of their endotoxin may also cause shock. Renal failure is the most serious complication of shock in burned patients and accounts for about 10% of their deaths.

Pulmonary edema. Pulmonary edema (Chapter 11) may develop in burned patients as a result of smoke inhalation or hemodynamic derangements that are poorly understood or in association with congestive cardiac failure. Pulmonary edema begins between 6 and 72 hours after burning and lasts about 48 hours. However, a serious risk of pneumonia develops in these patients at this time.

Stress ulcers. Stress ulcers (Chapter 14) are acute multiple ulcers of the stomach, duodenum, and upper jejunum. Their pathogenesis is obscure, but they may result in perforation or hemorrhage. They have been reported as the immediate cause of death in about 3% of severely burned patients.

Infection. Infection, either septicemic or pneumonic, is by far the most common serious complication of burned patients. The environment provided by burned skin provides an ideal site for microbial contamination, proliferation, and the development of superficial infection, with subsequent spread to the bloodstream. Pulmonary edema, as already noted, predisposes to the development of bacterial pneumonia.

The most important organism infecting burned patients is *Pseudomonas aeruginosa.* Others are *Staphylococcus aureus, Streptococcus pyogenes, Klebsiella, Enterobacter,* and *Clostridium* species, and *Candida albicans.*

P. aeruginosa is very common in the environment of the modern hospital, especially in units taking care of burned patients. Contamination of the burn site by *P. aeruginosa* is common. The organism appears to progress through the margins between unburned tissue and eschar, spread via superficial lymphatics, and infiltrate around blood vessels. This leads to thrombosis and occlusion of the vessels with localized tissue ischemia and necrosis. The progress of *P. aeruginosa* infection is aided by its secretion of exotoxins. Finally, the organism may invade the bloodstream and produce hemorrhagic and necrotic lesions in the skin *(ecthyma gangrenosum)* and internal organs.

Survival and causes of death

Survival in burned patients depends on the patient's age and the size and depth of the burn. Infants and children have a poorer survival rate than adults with equivalent burns. The main causes of death are (1) septicemia, (2) pneumonia, and (3) renal failure.

Clinical aspects

The management of burns is highly specialized and complex. The basic principles of management follow:

1. Immediately following the injury, first aid or resuscitation to maintain respiration and circulation; the relief of pain; fluid replacement
2. In the acute phase, the detection, prevention, and treatment of complications, especially infection; care of the wound
3. In the restorative phase, reconstructive and cosmetic surgery, mainly by skin grafting

The emotional support of the severely burned patient throughout is almost as important as physical methods.

Heat stroke and related syndromes

Syndromes resulting from exposure to, and particularly, violent exercise in, excessively high temperatures are graded

clinically into (1) *heat cramps*, (2) *heat exhaustion*, (3) *exertional heat injury*, and (4) *heat stroke*. However, there is considerable overlap between them. In the past, and particularly among the lay public heat injury syndromes have been confused with overexposure to the sun. In the nineteenth century, an excessive amount of clothing, including spine pads, was worn by Europeans working in the tropics to protect against the alleged dangers of the sun, but in fact it contributed to heat stroke. Experience in World War II quickly showed that it was not even necessary to wear head protection in the tropics (in peaceful areas), provided that precautions were taken against sunburn.

Susceptibility to environmental heat injury depends very much on acclimatization, age, physical fitness, and humidity. The last determines the rate at which sweat evaporation will induce compensatory heat loss. As to acclimatization, an extreme example of what is possible is the fact that stokers on steamships in the tropics were able to adapt to immensely heavy physical labor in ambient temperatures of at least 150° F. Such adaptation is possible only as a consequence of peripheral vasodilation and increased sweating. There is also decreased circulating volume, renal blood flow, and renal sodium excretion. Pulse and respiration rates and secretion of antidiuretic hormone and aldosterone are increased.

Heat cramps

Heat cramps is the term given to painful paroxysms of muscle contractions which are precipitated by heavy sweating, usually as a consequence of violent exercise by otherwise fit individuals, in high environmental temperatures. There is hemoconcentration and decreased plasma sodium chloride levels but the body temperature is not abnormally raised.

The treatment is to replace water and salt.

Heat exhaustion

Heat exhaustion (heat prostration or collapse) is the term given to failure of normal cardiovascular responses to high environmental temperatures for a relatively brief period. Heat exhaustion therefore particularly affects the elderly, can develop even in the sedentary and is probably the most common type of heat syndrome.

The onset of heat exhaustion is typically sudden, but there may be prodromal symptoms such as weakness, headache, nausea, or dizziness followed by loss of consciousness. The patient appears ashen gray and has a cold clammy skin and low blood pressure. Body temperature is not raised in typical cases, but there may be incipient hemoconcentration.

Loss of consciousness is usually brief and the only treatment needed is to lay the person down in a cool place and to give water and salt to make up for the circulatory deficiencies.

Exertional heat injury

Exertional heat injury is in effect a severe form of heat cramps. It typically affects those who, without acclimatization, are exercising or performing athletics at ambient temperatures over about 80° F where there is high humidity. Obesity and age increase susceptibility; but as with all heat injury syndromes, there is wide individual variation.

Clinically, body temperature is usually raised to between 102° and 104° F. Symptoms may include headache, nausea, gooseflesh (piloerection), shivering, muscle cramps, and unsteady gait or ataxia. Symptoms may occasionally progress to loss of consciousness. There is also tachycardia, hypotension, and decreased peripheral vascular resistance.

Laboratory findings include hemoconcentration and hypernatremia, hypocalcemia, hypophosphatemia, and sometimes hypoglycemia. Liver and muscle enzymes are also abnormal.

Treatment is immediate cooling, to lower the core body temperature, and infusion of hypotonic glucose-saline.

Heat stroke

Heat stroke ("sunstroke") mainly affects the elderly and particularly those with cardiovascular disease. In the exceptionally hot summer of 1987, 700 persons were reported to have died from this cause over a period of a few days in the city of Athens, Greece. As implied earlier, exposure to the sun is not necessarily a prerequisite, but diabetes mellitus, alcoholism, or other factors may contribute.

Clinically, the signs and symptoms of heat stroke are similar to those of heat exhaustion but the body temperature is greatly raised and internal temperatures as high as 112° F have been recorded. Typically, the skin is hot and dry as there is no sweating, but whether this is a cause or effect of the syndrome is unknown. Pulse and respiration are rapid, and the blood pressure is low. Muscles are flaccid. Depression of consciousness to a degree related to the severity of the disorder may progress to coma and death.

Laboratory findings usually include hemoconcentration, leukocytosis, proteinuria, and raised blood urea nitrogen. There is frequently respiratory alkalosis followed by metabolic acidosis and often lactacidemia, hypocalcemia, and hypophosphatemia. Hematologic abnormalities are, particularly, disorders of hemostasis, which may progress to disseminated intravascular coagulation (Chapter 13). In addition, there may be electrocardiographic abnormalities, occasionally with progression to diffuse myocardial necrosis or myocardial infarction. Both liver and renal damage are common, and widespread parenchymal damage may be found at autopsy.

The pathologic basis of heat stroke is uncertain, but, in part at least, some of the cellular damage is the direct result of overheating. There is also considerable disturbance of the electrolyte balance and probably cellular hypoxia.

Patients may die within a few hours from heart failure or later of acute renal failure; a few patients die only after several weeks, from similar causes or other complications.

Treatment, preferably by immersion in an ice-water bath, can be life saving if the symptoms are recognized early. Frequently, however, treatment is delayed several hours: when this happens, treatment of dehydration, heart failure, or renal failure is likely to be necessary, but the prognosis is poor.

Diseases caused by cold

Cold may cause both localized and systemic disease in humans. The most severe form of localized cold injury is frostbite; a profound fall in overall body temperature (hypothermia) is the most serious systemic effect.

Localized cold injuries

Localized cold injuries arise in three ways. First, severe cold acts on the outer layers of the body causing (1) the formation of cellular ice crystals and subsequent cell death and (2) freezing of the extracellular fluid. Second, cold causes ischemic tissue damage by slowing of the peripheral circulation and

occlusion of small blood vessels by promoting aggregations of red and white blood cells. Third, vasoactive amines may be released in tissues affected by cold, causing many of the changes seen in the microcirculation in acute inflammation. Thus there may be vasodilation and increased vascular permeability.

These effects are most striking in frostbite, when feet, hands, and face are severely damaged by cold. In addition to the changes already described in cells and blood vessels, there is often localized damage to the skin and separation of the epidermis from the dermis. In mild frostbite the vascular changes are often reversible. In severe frostbite, gangrene of toes, fingers, nose, or ears may develop because of irreversible vascular occlusion and prolonged severe tissue anoxia.

Hypothermia

Hypothermia can be defined as a fall in core body temperature to below 35° C. It may be caused by (1) prolonged exposure to cold, especially in the elderly, (2) a number of endocrine diseases, including hypothyroidism and adrenal insufficiency, or (3) artificial cooling of the body before cardiac or neurologic surgical procedures when temperatures as low as 10° C may be achieved.

Hypothermia resulting from prolonged exposure to cold is now recognized as a cause of death in elderly and debilitated persons during cold weather. The mechanisms are unclear, but profound biochemical changes, particularly in the control of acid-base balance and oxygenation, are known to take place.

Hypothermic patients are cold and stiff. Their pulse rate is slow and weak, and their blood pressure is low. Death is common, especially in the elderly.

Currently, the basis of treatment of both frostbite and hypothermia is to raise the core temperature of the body. In the latter condition, the method of choice is by hemodialysis and to warm the blood as it circulates through the artificial kidney.

Pathology of weightlessness

Space travel and weightlessness seem unlikely to be a major cause of ill-health in the foreseeable future; however, some of the findings may be noted here.

The early symptoms are usually nausea and vomiting, which presumably result from the loss of gravitational orientation of the otoliths in the semicircular canals. This is sometimes followed by disorientation.

In the absence of gravitational stress on the musculoskeletal system, there is progressive muscle wasting and loss of calcium from the skeleton. Astronauts experience negative nitrogen balance during spaceflight.

Less easy to explain are hematologic changes, namely declining numbers of red and white cells leading to depressed immune function and increased susceptibility to infection.

Also reported have been minor cardiac arrhythmias. The emotional stress of existence in such an environment is obviously also considerable. The long-term effects of residence in outer space are of course, not known as, to date, the longest period in space has been 10 months.

For a discussion of a related topic, the *decompression syndrome,* see Chapter 10.

Selected readings

Anonymous: Consequences of new radiation dosimetry, Lancet 2:1245, 1987.

Berry RJ: The radiologist as guinea pig: radiation hazards to man as demonstrated in early radiologists and their patients, J Royal Soc Med 79:506, 1986.

Black D: New evidence on childhood leukaemia and nuclear establishments, Br Med J 294:591, 1987.

Demling RH: Burns, N Engl J Med 313:1389, 1985.

Fajardo LF: Pathology of radiation injury, New York, 1982, Masson Publishing USA, Inc.

Finch SC: Acute radiation syndrome, JAMA 258:664, 1987.

Foster KR and Guy AW: The microwave problem, Sci Am 255:32, 1986.

Fry, RJM and Sinclair WK: New dosimetry of atomic bomb radiations, Lancet 2:845, 1987.

Gale RP: Immediate medical consequences of nuclear accidents: lessons from Chernobyl, JAMA 258:625, 1987.

Gillies NE: Effects of radiations on cells, Br Med J 295:1390, 1987.

Goldman M: Chernobyl: a radiobiological perspective, Science 238:622, 1987.

Hopewell JW and Campling D et al: Vascular irradiation damage: its cellular basis and likely consequences, Br J Cancer 53(Suppl):181, 1986.

Jones RJ: Ozone depletion and cancer risk, Lancet 2:443, 1987.

Kohn HI and Fry RJM: Radiation carcinogenesis, N Engl J Med 310:504, 1984.

Lasers in medicine and surgery: report of Council on Scientific Affairs, AMA, Chicago, JAMA 256:900, 1986.

Lindell B: Radiation and health, Bull WHO 65:139, 1987.

Lindelof B and Eklund G: Incidence of malignant skin tumors in 14,140 patients after grenz-ray treatment of benign skin disorders, Arch Dermatol 122:1391, 1986.

Maclean D: Emergency management of accidental hypothermia: a review, J Royal Soc Med 79:528, 1986.

McRee DI: Potential microwave injuries in clinical medicine, Annu Rev Med 27:109, 1976.

Panke TW and McLeod CG Jr: Pathology of thermal injury: a practical approach, Orlando, FL, 1985, Grune & Stratton, Inc.

Prosnitz LR, Kapp DS, and Weissberg JB: Radiotherapy, N Engl J Med 309:771, 1983.

Radon in homes: report Council on Scientific Affairs, AMA, Chicago, JAMA 258:668, 1987.

Smith PJ and Douglas AJ: Mortality of workers at the Sellafield plant of British Nuclear Fuels, Br Med J 293:845, 1986.

Vasquez TE, Pretorius HT, and Rimkus DS: Space medicine: a review of current concepts, West J Med 147:292, 1987.

Wheater RH: Health effects of video display terminals: report Council on Scientific Affairs, AMA, Chicago, JAMA 257:1508, 1987.

Wieman TJ: Lasers and the surgeon, Am J Surg 151:493, 1986.

CHAPTER 5

Disorders of nutrition

Malnutrition as a result of an inadequate diet remains a major problem in developing countries, particularly parts of Africa. Countless numbers have died from starvation in recent famines, and there are probably half a billion undernourished infants in these and other areas. There are also countless persons in countries such as India who live on the borderline of starvation.

By contrast, in affluent countries, the chief problem is that of overnutrition and obesity, which contribute to hypertension, diabetes mellitus, and other disorders. Statistically, obesity is associated with a decreased expectation of life, and currently there is an obsession with dietary prevention of ischemic heart disease and of other disorders, real or imagined.

The nutritional requirements for humans are well established, but there are widespread misapprehensions and bizarre beliefs. A common idea is that even in fully nourished persons, vitamins have mysterious tonic qualities. There is therefore ample scope for entrepreneurial adventurism for those who peddle diets of dubious value. However, many responsible physicians believe that low fiber, but high animal fat and high salt intake, are important contributory factors in the pathogenesis of atherosclerosis and ischemic heart disease as discussed later.

Malnutrition

Malnutrition is present when there are physical effects caused by deficiencies in the diet that can be repaired by providing the missing foods. *Primary malnutrition* is the consequence of lack of food (Fig. 5-1). There may be deficiency of protein and calories, or there may be selective deficiencies of vitamins. Commonly, however, deficiencies are combined, and the types of malnutrition are varied.

Secondary malnutrition develops when the diet is adequate but absorption or metabolism of food is defective. Alternatively, as a result of psychiatric disease, food intake is sometimes grossly reduced. This is seen in its most extreme form in young girls with anorexia nervosa but the main causes of secondary malnutrition are summarized in the following list:

1. Abnormal eating habits
   a. Alcoholism
   b. Food faddism
   c. Drug addiction
   d. Depression
   e. Anorexia nervosa
2. Impaired ingestion (dysphagia)
   a. Oropharyngeal disease
   b. Myasthenia gravis
   c. Esophageal stricture and other obstructions
3. Defective absorption
   a. Obstructive jaundice
   b. Pancreatic insufficiency
   c. Gluten-sensitive enteropathy (celiac disease)
   d. Crohn's disease
   e. Chronic atrophic gastritis
4. Impaired use or metabolism
   a. Diabetes mellitus
   b. Severe liver disease
   c. Drug-induced
5. Increased metabolic requirements
   a. Growth, pregnancy, lactation
   b. Fever
   c. Hyperthyroidism
   d. Illness or injury

Protein-calorie malnutrition

Information on the effects of severe dietary deficiencies comes from studies on volunteers, famine conditions in underdeveloped countries, and starvation in concentration camp victims in World War II. In all of these cases the picture varies partly because starvation is rarely complete and also does not affect all essential dietary components to the same degree. Other factors such as intercurrent infection, which increases the effect of dietary deficiencies, also complicate the picture.

Effects of protein-calorie malnutrition. In an attempt to combat deficiencies, the body undergoes adaptive changes. Fat from the body stores is quickly mobilized and metabolized; later muscle is lost. The liver also loses glycogen and shrinks. By contrast, there is minimal change in the brain and skeleton.

Functional changes include a fall in the basal metabolic rate, which conserves energy. The heart rate and blood pressure both fall, and heart size decreases. There is usually moderate anemia and delayed wound healing.

Clinically, in states of complete starvation, hunger is not felt, but in semistarvation hunger is severe. In established states of malnutrition the patient is tired, weak, irritable, depressed, and apathetic. The low metabolic rate causes a feeling of coldness, and unless there is hunger edema, the body becomes thin and bony. The muscle tone is poor, and the skin is lax, thinned, and wrinkled. The pulse is weak and slow; hair is lost.

Hunger edema. Usually after about a month of semistarvation, edema, either local or generalized, starts to appear. The mechanism varies and is not entirely clear. In protein-calorie malnutrition (described later), edema is severe and appears to be caused by hypoalbuminemia. In other forms of malnutrition hypoalbuminemia is absent. Although cardiac function is impaired, edema is not necessarily a result of cardiac failure, and the venous pressure in starved patients is usually low.

Starvation edema may not be caused by excessive accumulation of fluid in the tissues but, rather, by retention of a normal extracellular fluid volume in relation to severe tissue loss.

Protein-calorie malnutrition of childhood

The two main forms of protein-calorie malnutrition of childhood, *kwashiorkor* and *marasmus*, presumably represent the ends of a spectrum.

Kwashiorkor. Kwashiorkor is seen most frequently in parts of Africa. The main precipitating factors are (1) shortage of protein, (2) excessive carbohydrate intake, (3) the effects of parasites, and (4) intercurrent childhood infections.

The most striking effect is severe edema, which often masks the underlying malnutrition and is caused by hypoalbuminemia. Because carbohydrate intake is high, some body fat is retained, and the infant may even be obese. Other features are muscle weakness, retardation of growth, and rashes. The liver often contains an excessive accumulation of fat and is detectably enlarged. Anemia and other deficiencies, particularly of vitamin A and folic acid are associated.

Nutritional marasmus. Marasmus (literally, a dying away) means extreme wasting and emaciation, especially of infants; it differs from kwashiorkor in that there is a very low intake of all nutrients, including carbohydrates. Quite simply, it is starvation.

Infants in the first year of life are predominantly affected and, unlike those with kwashiorkor, are not edematous. Clinical signs include complete loss of fat stores, wasting of muscle, and retardation of growth; the child appears shrunken, wizened, and prematurely aged.

When malnutrition is severe, the intake of vitamins is also inadequate. Clinically, however, avitaminoses do not become apparent because of the greatly reduced level of tissue activity.

Secondary malnutrition

Secondary malnutrition can be highly selective, is sometimes associated with loss of weight, and can be temporary. Thus folic acid deficiency can be caused by prolonged treatment of epilepsy with diphenylhydantoin, while vitamin deficiency can result from a variety of liver diseases.

Anorexia nervosa. Anorexia nervosa is a psychiatric disorder usually of young women who so severely restrict their diet as to become emaciated (Fig. 5-2). The disorder sometimes starts as dieting by an overweight girl, who then continues the process to excess. Patients often seem unaware of their cachectic appearance and many practice complex deceptions to

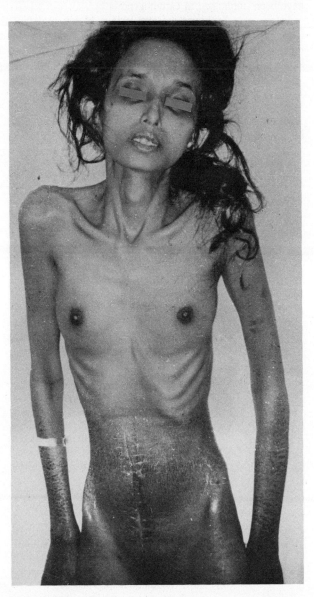

FIG. 5-1. Starvation. *(Courtesy Curator of the Gordon Museum, Guy's Hospital, London, England.)*

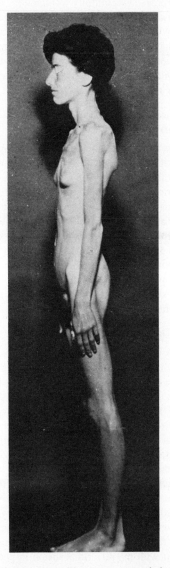

FIG. 5-2. Anorexia nervosa. The extreme emaciation caused by refusal to eat is typical. *(Courtesy Curator of the Gordon Museum, Guy's Hospital, London, England.)*

limit their eating. Malnutrition may become so severe that it occasionally threatens life. A variant of anorexia nervosa is *bulimia* in which the person deliberately induces vomiting after eating.

A variety of psychiatric disorders may be associated, but the psychiatric basis of the disease is unclear. Treatment is rarely effective, but the disease may eventually terminate spontaneously.

Malnutrition and susceptibility to infection

It is widely believed that malnutrition increases susceptibility to infection; indeed the Four Horsemen of the Apocalypse are traditionally pictured as War, followed by Famine, Pestilence, and Death. However, the situation is complicated by the fact that in conditions where there is a severe shortage of food, as in many developing countries, there are also many other factors that contribute to disease. Such factors include poor sanitation, insect-borne infections, and living conditions that promote the transmission of contagious diseases.

Unexpectedly, recent clinical studies of malnourished communities have not entirely supported the hypothesis that malnutrition increases susceptibility to infection. Indeed the incidence of some infections such as malaria increased when nutrition improved. The reason for such apparently anomalous findings is unknown, but it is suggested that malnutrition may be harmful to some pathogenic microorganisms that are in effect competing with the host for nutrients, but *severe* malnutrition appears to depress immune responses.

Avitaminoses

Inadequate intake of vitamins inevitably implies a defective diet, and avitaminoses are rarely seen in pure form. Often vitamin deficiencies are multiple and may be associated with protein-calorie malnutrition. In affluent countries avitaminoses are diagnosed more frequently than they exist. Such deficiencies are now rare except in special groups. These include food faddists, chronic alcoholics, and those with disease causing secondary malnutrition. The main features of vitamin deficiencies are summarized in Table 5-1.

Vitamins, unlike other components of the diet, are required in only very small amounts and act, in effect, like catalysts on a variety of metabolic processes.

Vitamin A deficiency

Vitamin A is a fat-soluble factor, and the best known effect of deficiency is inability to see in weak light (night blindness).

β-carotene is provitamin A, and the various vitamin A compounds have a complex nomenclature. Retinol, for instance, is vitamin A alcohol, while retinoic acid is vitamin A_1 acid. Vitamin A is usually present as retinyl ester in foods. It is hydrolyzed in the intestine and absorbed as retinol. Vitamin A is mainly concentrated in the liver but also found in other viscera and the retina.

Currently, vitamin A deficiency is rarely the result of inadequate diet but is usually the result of disorders of fat absorption, particularly obstruction of the biliary tract.

Pathology. One of the earliest effects of vitamin A deficiency is to impair the formation of the visual pigments, rhodopsin and iodopsin, with the result that vision in poor light deteriorates and later degenerative changes develop in the retina.

Secretory epithelia are, however, predominantly affected. These include the epithelia of the mouth, the respiratory tract,

the eye, lacrimal and salivary glands, and genitourinary tract. The main change is keratinization of normally unkeratinized epithelium and degeneration of glandular acini to squamous epithelia.

There is currently interest in the retinoids in relation to cancer as a result of experimental work in animals which suggests that retinoids may reduce or inhibit the carcinogenic effects of certain hydrocarbons or even depress the growth of established, experimentally induced tumors. However, to achieve these effects, retinoids usually have to be given in toxic doses. Moreover, there are also reports of vitamin A enhancing tumor growth or promoting metastases under experimental conditions.

There is epidemiologic evidence that vitamin A deficiency may be a factor in the pathogenesis of cancer, particularly of the lung, in humans. In the case of lung cancer, low serum retinol levels appear to be associated with an increased risk of developing the disease. A possible mechanism may be that vitamin A may inhibit squamous metaplasia preceding malignant change. β-carotene also deactivates free radicals, which have been implicated in carcinogenesis.

In the case of hyperkeratotic lesions of the oral mucosa (leukoplakia), which sometimes progress to carcinoma, treatment with cisretinoic acid will, reportedly, cause many such keratoses to regress.

TABLE 5-1. Deficiencies of vitamins and other essential food factors

Vitamin or other factor	Result of deficiency
Vitamin A	Epithelial hyperkeratosis or squamous metaplasia of glands; xerophthalmia; cessation of endochondral growth (children)
Thiamine	Degenerative changes in nervous system, peripheral and central (dry beriberi); cardiac failure (wet beriberi)
Riboflavin	Dermatitis, cheilitis, glossitis
Nicotinamide (niacin)	Symmetric dermatitis; cheilitis and glossitis; degenerative changes in alimentary tract and peripheral and central nervous systems (pellagra)
Folic acid	Megaloblastic anemia and glossitis
Vitamin B_{12}	Megaloblastic anemia and glossitis; subacute combined degeneration of spinal cord (pernicious anemia)
Vitamin C	Purpura, dermatitis, mental changes; subperiosteal bleeding in children (scurvy)
Vitamin D	Failure of calcification of osteoid (rickets) in children; loss of calcium and accumulation of uncalcified osteoid (osteomalacia) in adults
Vitamin K	Depressed production of clotting factors; hypoprothrombinemia; hemorrhages
Calcium	Rickets
Iron	Microcytic, hypochromic anemia
Zinc	Delayed wound healing; acrodermatitis enteropathica (infants)
Iodine	Thyroid enlargement (goiter); hypothyroidism; cretinism (infants)
Fluoride	Increased susceptibility to dental caries

Currently, large prospective trials are in progress to test whether β-carotene (which raises plasma retinol levels with less toxic effects than high dosage of vitamin A) reduces susceptibility to lung cancer. Plasma retinol levels, however, do not appear to correlate well with susceptibility to many other cancers.

Vitamin A appears also to contribute to resistance to infection. In malnourished children, vitamin A supplements significantly reduced the incidence of such infections as measles even in those with no signs of preexisting vitamin A deficiency. The role of vitamin A in susceptibility to infection may be related to the finding that deficiency is associated with impaired B and T lymphocyte function.

Clinical aspects. Clinically, vitamin A deficiency causes xerophthalmia (dry eyes) as a result of failure of tear secretion and night blindness. Xerophthalmia can lead to infection and inflammation of the eye and sometimes total destruction of the lens.

Skin lesions are caused by keratinization of the hair follicles together with atrophy of the sebaceous glands. The skin is generally dry. Pancreatic and other glandular secretions may also be deficient; in the respiratory tract this can cause tracheitis, bronchitis, and pneumonia.

In view of the importance of vitamin A or its analogs in the treatment of a variety of conditions that may be related to

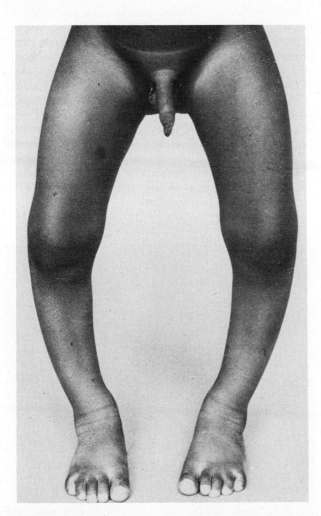

FIG. 5-3. Gross bowing of the legs caused by rickets. *(Courtesy Curator of the Gordon Museum, Guy's Hospital, London, England.)*

vitamin A deficiency, as discussed earlier, the introduction of less toxic derivatives, the retinoids, aroused great expectations. However, even these newer agents also have significant toxic effects.

Vitamin D deficiency—rickets and osteomalacia

Vitamin D plays an essential role in the absorption of calcium and phosphorus from the intestinal tract and, hence, in calcification of the skeleton. Deficiency can therefore cause rickets or osteomalacia (Chapter 17).

The main source of vitamin D is fish liver oils, but a little is present in eggs and butter. In strong sunlight vitamin D is synthesized in the skin. Rickets (Fig. 5-3) is one of the few avitaminoses that can be seen in pure form and can also be seen in affluent countries. In Britain it has been found among Asian immigrants in northern counties where lack of sunlight, a high carbohydrate diet, and possibly also the use of wholemeal flour (containing factors such as phytate, which impair the absorption of calcium) appear to be contributory.

In addition to its role in calcium metabolism, vitamin D also appears to be involved in hemopoiesis and immunologic function. There are reports of impaired hemopoiesis associated with vitamin D deficiency and reversal of the defect on administration of vitamin D. Children with rickets also appear to be abnormally susceptible to infection. Vitamin D may therefore be involved in normal lymphopoiesis or B lymphocyte function. Moreover, monocytes have membrane receptors for dihydroxyvitamin D_3, $1,25$ $(OH_2)D_3$; since monocytes are the precursors of osteoclasts, it is suggested that synthesis of $1,25(OH_2)D_3$ by lymphoid and other tumors may explain the hypercalcemia that is sometimes associated.

Vitamin K deficiency

Vitamin K (phylloquinone) is present in the leaves of most plants, while vitamin K_2 is formed by intestinal bacteria. Vitamin K is needed for the production of clotting factors II, VII, IX, and X (Chapter 13). Vitamin K (from the German, Koagulierung) is therefore essential for normal blood coagulation.

The causes of vitamin K deficiency are as follows:
1. Defective fat absorption, especially obstructive jaundice, celiac, or pancreatic disease (Chapter 14).
2. The newborn lack normal intestinal flora and also have a low intake of vitamin K from human breast milk.
3. Anticoagulants affect vitamin K synthesis rather than absorption.
4. Rarely, prolonged use of broad-spectrum antibiotics in high doses may destroy the intestinal bacteria that synthesize vitamin K.

The effects of vitamin K deficiency are discussed in more detail in Chapter 13.

Thiamine (B₁) deficiency

A disease peculiar to the Far East, where rice is the staple cereal, is characterized by neurologic disturbance and heart disease, which often terminates in sudden death, and has been recognized for approximately 200 years. The disease is termed *beriberi* and was ultimately shown to be caused by lack of thiamine.

Beriberi became severe in the newly formed Japanese navy, in the nineteenth century, when the sailors' diet consisted of little more than polished (white) rice and condensed milk. The disease was eradicated by giving a more varied diet, which included meat and vegetables.

In the United States, thiamine deficiency is virtually only seen in chronic alcoholics.

Pathogenesis. Removal of the outer husk of rice removes thiamine, riboflavin, nicotinic acid, pantothenic acid, and pyridoxine. Lipids and minerals including calcium and iron are also lost.

However, thiamine deficiency appears to be the predominant effect in those who live on a diet mainly of polished rice.

Thiamine appears essential to the normal function of the peripheral nervous system and the myocardium. Although the precise way in which thiamine is involved in these functions is unknown, the improvement in neurologic and cardiac function when thiamine is given to patients with this deficiency has confirmed its importance. The main changes in the peripheral nerves in severe beriberi are myelin degeneration and loss of axoplasm. Beriberi also causes a form of cardiomyopathy with dilatation of the ventricles.

Clinical aspects. Three main types of beriberi have been recognized in the Far East:

1. A chronic, predominantly neurologic form (dry beriberi)
2. An acute form with rapid onset of heart failure and early death
3. A more chronic cardiac form where edema is most prominent (wet beriberi)

The neurologic changes cause alterations in sensation, especially in the legs (peripheral neuropathy). Cardiac disease, including heart failure, may be associated.

When cardiac or neurologic signs develop in any patient where thiamine deficiency appears to be a possibility, the vitamin should be given immediately. Usually deficiencies are multiple, and the other members of this group of water-soluble vitamins should be given at the same time. The response is dramatic in early cases; but where severe damage has already been done, the response is slower and less complete.

Vitamin B₂ deficiency—ariboflavinosis

Ariboflavinosis is still common in underdeveloped countries. In the United States it is only seen among the very poor and in some alcoholics. Ariboflavinosis is never seen when protein intake is adequate; but when the diet is poor, other deficiencies are associated. The main sources of riboflavin are milk, eggs, fish, and meat.

Riboflavin appears to be needed for the formation of pyridoxol 5'-phosphate, an essential coenzyme for tryptophan metabolism. Many riboflavin-dependent enzymes are also present in the brain.

Clinically, ariboflavinosis is characterized by severe oral symptoms. There is inflammation of vermilion border of the lips (cheilitis) and glossitis; the tongue typically acquires a purplish color and a pebbly texture (Fig. 5-4). Sore throat and dermatitis may be associated. Severe itching or burning of the eyes may progress to visual impairment, and mild normochromic, normocytic anemia may be associated.

The disease responds rapidly to riboflavin; but usually other vitamins of this group are needed, and the remainder of the diet must be made adequate.

Vitamin B₆ deficiency

Vitamin B₆ comprises three closely related compounds of which pyridoxine is the most important. Pyridoxal 5'-phosphate is the active form and serves as a coenzyme for many metabolic processes, including transamination and decarboxylation of amino acids.

A specific disease resulting from pyridoxine deficiency has not been clearly defined, but a rare type of microcytic anemia characterized by intramedullary hemolysis appears to respond to large doses of pyridoxine (Chapter 13). Pyridoxine also reduces the incidence of side effects from the antituberculous drug isonicotinic acid hydrazide (Isoniazid), which when given in high doses can cause neurologic symptoms such as neuropathy, mental disturbances and convulsions, and pellagra.

Nicotinamide deficiency—pellagra

Pellagra has been identified since the eighteenth century when it was known as *pelle agro* (literally, rough skin); crusting of the skin, particularly of the hands and neck, painful burning of the mouth, shaking of the body, and mania were described.

Pellagra became epidemic in the southern United States early in this century and remained endemic until the 1940s despite earlier demonstration by Goldberger that it could be treated successfully by improving the diet. Pellagra is still important in parts of Africa and Asia.

Pathogenesis. Pellagra usually results from subsistence on a diet composed mainly of corn (maize) but deficient in protein, particularly meat. Corn lacks two essential amino acids, tryptophan and lysine. Nicotinic acid, although present in appreciable quantities in corn, is biologically unavailable. The main sources of nicotinic acid are liver, yeast, meat, fish, and wheat germ.

As with other avitaminoses, pure nicotinic acid deficiency is little more than a theoretic possibility. In most cases pellagra is probably associated with multivitamin deficiencies, particularly of the B group; nevertheless, the main signs and symptoms respond to nicotinic acid.

Pathology. The skin undergoes both hyperkeratosis and vesiculation. By contrast, there is atrophy of the epithelium of the tongue, loss of papillae, and inflammation; a similar change affects the esophagus. A variety of changes affect the other parts of the gastrointestinal tract, and there may be fatty accumulations in the liver.

The neurologic effects are variable. In severe cases there is atrophy of cerebral neurons and degeneration of peripheral nerves, nerve roots, and spinal tracts.

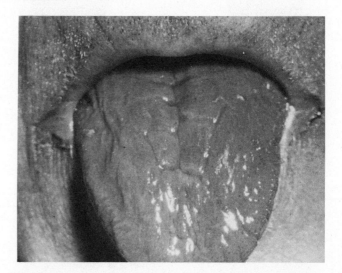

FIG. 5-4. Ariboflavinosis. Typical features are angular stomatitis and the depapillated tongue with a pebbly surface texture. *(Courtesy Curator of the Gordon Museum, Guy's Hospital, London, England.)*

Clinical aspects. Primary pellagra is now exceedingly rare in the United States. Secondary pellagra may occasionally be seen in chronic alcoholics, who more often suffer from thiamine and folic acid deficiencies. Other causes of secondary pellagra are chronic diarrhea or, occasionally, cancer. In its severe form, pellagra causes the four *D*s: dermatitis, diarrhea, dementia, and death.

Early signs and symptoms are weight loss, diarrhea or constipation, indigestion, generalized weakness, and lassitude. The dermal lesions may start as erythema, often with intense burning or itching. Sore mouth is common and may be severe. Changes particularly affect the tongue, and glossitis is probably one of the most reliable early signs. The tongue becomes smooth, dark red, and sore. Small ulcers or more widespread stomatitis and angular cheilitis may also develop. Neurologic disorders tend to appear late in the condition's development when skin and gastrointestinal changes are severe. Typical complaints are vertigo, weakness, headache, disturbances of sensation or complete anesthesia, and often pain in the hands and feet. It is probable that thiamine deficiency may be important in the causation of these neurologic changes. Mental disturbances include confusion, depression, apathy, and delirium. The disease responds well to nicotinamide.

Vitamin B$_{12}$ deficiency

Deficiency of vitamin B$_{12}$ is, in most cases, secondary to gastric atrophy in pernicious anemia (Chapter 13) or less often to diseases causing malabsorption. The deficiency can also be dietary—in those (vegans) who eat no meat or any other animal products—but even in this group it is rare.

Biotin deficiency

It is virtually impossible for a normal person to become biotin deficient, and it was long believed that no clinical syndrome resulted from biotin deficiency. A genetic disorder, multiple carboxylase deficiency, however, causes impaired biotin metabolism which, in neonates, is associated with ketosis, metabolic acidosis and, often, an erythematous rash. In older children total parenteral nutrition may result in an erythematous rash and loss of body hair, and these changes may respond to biotin.

Vitamin C deficiency—scurvy

The signs and symptoms of scurvy were clearly described many hundreds of years ago during the Crusades. The disease became common as a result of lack of fresh food available on sailing ship voyages, which often lasted many months. James Lind, a British naval surgeon, described the disease in detail over 200 years ago and also experimented with diet. He found that giving citrus fruits relieved the characteristic signs and symptoms of "putrid gums, the spots, and lassitude with weakness of their knees."

Later, lime juice became the standard preventive measure, hence the nickname "limey" for a British sailor. At the beginning of this century, infantile scurvy became common in Europe and the United States as the result of increasing substitution of breast milk by canned milk.

Scurvy is rare but is seen occasionally in alcoholics, food faddists, and elderly persons living on grossly unbalanced and inadequate diets. Occasional cases of infantile scurvy are usually the result of bizarre ideas about diet or maternal ignorance or neglect.

Pathology. Ascorbic acid is essential for the synthesis of hydroxyproline and formation of collagen. The essential disturbance in scurvy is therefore failure of various types of connective tissue cells to form their collagen derivatives. Failure of collagen formation by fibroblasts, osteoblasts, and odontoblasts leads to inability to synthesize osteoid and dentin. Therefore there is failure of wound healing and abnormalities in the growing bones of infants. There is loss of integrity of the blood vessel walls, and this appears to be caused by the inadequacy of collagen support.

Ascorbic acid also appears to affect several other metabolic functions, and deficiency may lead to defective synthesis of norepinephrine and serotonin. These, in turn, may cause impaired platelet function, which is also characteristic of scurvy. Vitamin C is also involved in the metabolism of folic acid and, in large doses, promotes the absorption of dietary iron.

Vitamin C has been reported to have a significant anticancer effect, but such reports have not been confirmed in adequately controlled clinical trials.

Neutrophils contain large amounts of vitamin C; macrophages contain lesser amounts. Vitamin C therefore may play some role in defense against infection; however, this has not been confirmed clinically, and megadose vitamin C does not appear to protect against the common cold, as discussed later.

Clinical aspects. Signs and symptoms of scurvy do not develop until after several months of depletion of the vitamin. Fatigue and psychologic disturbances are early symptoms, while the main physical findings are dermatitis (follicular hyperkeratosis) and purpura.

Oral lesions appear late and are a feature only of advanced disease. The characteristic changes are swelling, congestion, and bleeding of the gums (Fig. 5-5). In the past the gingival effects were so severe as to be some of the most troublesome features. Lind described the production of liverlike masses of blood clot from the mouth, and during the Crusades, cutting the gums was carried out to enable the sufferers to eat.

Infantile scurvy has a different clinical picture and is characterized by subcutaneous and subperiosteal hemorrhages, which cause extreme tenderness of the limbs. If subperiosteal

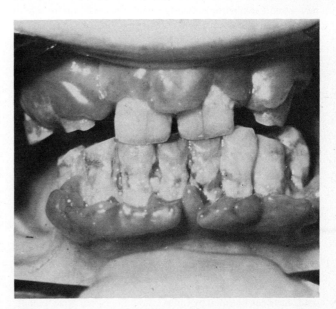

FIG. 5-5. Scurvy. The typical massive overgrowth of the gums is mainly a result of continued bleeding into the tissues (purpura) secondary to gingival infection and inflammation.

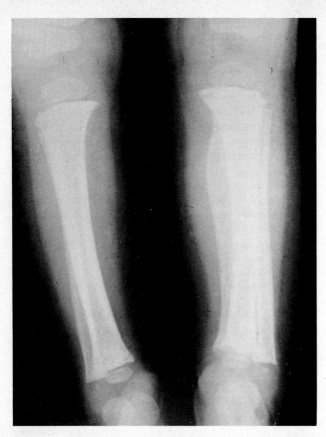

FIG. 5-6. Infantile scurvy. Typical features are the sharply defined epiphyseal ends of the bones as a result of continued calcification but failure of matrix production. Subperiosteal hemorrhage caused by scorbutic purpura has caused an elongated swelling that has become calcified along the length of the left tibia. *(From Cawson RA: Essentials of dental surgery and pathology, ed 4, Edinburgh, Scotland, 1984, Churchill Livingstone.)*

bleeding persists, the raised periosteum can form a shell of new bone (involucrum) clearly visible on radiographs. There may be hemorrhages from other sites, but oral changes or dermatitis are typically absent.

In contrast to rickets, calcification is unimpeded, but because of defective osteoid formation, there is a thick layer of calcified cartilage at the ends of the growing bones.

Diagnosis depends on a dietary history and the presence of purpura. In infants radiographs may show characteristic bony changes (Fig. 5-6). In doubtful cases the ascorbic acid level of the tissues can be measured by assaying its concentration in the buffy coat (white cell layer) of settled blood. However, it is simpler and more convincing to test the response to giving either ascorbic acid or fresh orange juice. The response to treatment can also be monitored in blood and urine samples, but in general it is better to give vitamin C if in doubt, because scurvy can be fatal, apparently as a result of vasomotor instability secondary to defective synthesis of norepinephrine.

Vitamin C and the common cold

The idea that massive doses of ascorbic acid can prevent colds has been extolled by Linus Pauling, a Nobel prize winner. Extensive experimentation has not, however, confirmed this belief, although some trials have suggested that at best, the infection may be mitigated. However, even if there is a marginal

effect of this sort, the continuous consumption of massive doses of vitamin C that has been proposed seems to be out of proportion to any benefits and has possible toxic effects.

Vitamin E

Vitamin E is a group of tocopherols that are antioxidants. It is a fat-soluble vitamin and has long been pushed by unscrupulous or ill-informed entrepreneurs and self-styled nutritionists, for allegedly conferring increased physical endurance, potency, fertility, longevity, and improved cardiac function. Human gullibility is such that these beliefs have been enthusiastically embraced by the lay public. Sadly (or perhaps fortunately) vitamin E is essential for reproductive function only in rats, and the other alleged benefits are also illusory. As a result, the medical profession has long been skeptical of any need for vitamin E in humans.

However, it has become apparent in recent years that vitamin E is essential for normal neurologic function in humans as well as animals. Deficiency is nevertheless rare and likely to develop only as a result of prolonged defects of fat absorption, as in the malabsorption syndromes (Chapter 14) and in association with abetalipoproteinemia in which the neurologic disorders were first observed. In *abetalipoproteinemia*, absence of apoprotein B and malabsorption of fats and fat-soluble vitamins, leads to severe neurologic dysfunction by early adulthood in most of those affected.

Clinically, there is disabling ataxia, impaired proprioception, nystagmus and loss of reflexes. High dosage vitamin E will prevent or sometimes reverse such changes.

Necropsy examination of patients with such spinocerebellar syndromes has shown close correlation with the effects of experimental vitamin E deficiency in animals, namely degeneration and loss of sensory axons in the posterior columns, sensory roots, and peripheral fibers. The pathogenesis is unknown, but one hypothesis is that the antioxidant effect of vitamin E protects against peroxidation of membrane phospholipids rich in polyunsaturated fatty acids.

Vitamin E has also been reported to be beneficial when there is overproduction of or failure to deal with free superoxide radicals (O_2^-). Superoxide radicals are produced within cells but are capable of damaging cell lipids or may even denature deoxyribonucleic acid (DNA) (Chapter 2). Vitamin E may therefore be of benefit, particularly, in counteracting the effects of hereditary deficiency of such enzymes as glucose 6-phosphate dehydrogenase (G6PD) and glutathione synthetase (Chapter 13)—which normally protect cells against free radicals—and in lessening or preventing retrolental fibroplasia or bronchopulmonary dysplasia in infants exposed to oxygen for long periods. Paradoxically however, vitamin E has also been reported to reduce the degree of sickling of erythrocytes in sickle cell anemia (Chapter 13). In view of the fact that sickling is precipitated by hypoxia, an antioxidant seems an unexpected choice of therapeutic agent.

There have therefore been reports of the usefulness of vitamin E in a wide range of conditions, but it cannot be said that its value has been widely confirmed, except for the rare neurologic disorder already mentioned.

Hypervitaminosis

Although an adequate intake of vitamins is essential for health or even life, they are not panaceas. Overdose, particularly of vitamins A and D, can produce severe toxic effects.

Hypervitaminosis A

In infants the effects of acute vitamin A intoxication are drowsiness, vomiting, and raised intracranial pressure. Chronic intoxication causes failure of weight gain, loss of hair, and bone pains. Radiographs show characteristic areas of new bone formation, particularly in the shafts of the long bones.

Toxic effects from vitamin A are seen particularly in tropical countries such as the Philippines, where large amounts are given at 6-month intervals to prevent or treat xerophthalmia.

In adults acute intoxication can develop rapidly. There is severe headache, disturbances of vision, nausea, vomiting, and often drowsiness. Chronic intoxication causes bone pain and skeletal changes similar to those in children. Calcification of ligaments and tendons may also be seen in radiographs. Loss of hair, dermatitis, and angular stomatitis may also develop.

In addition, high doses of vitamin A or its analogs (such as retinoic acid, isoretinoin, etretinate) are teratogenic for humans as well as animals. The effects seen in the offspring of women who have been treated for skin diseases with vitamin A analogs, include hydrocephaly, microtia, with atresia of the external auditory meatus, and microphthalmos.

Vitamin D intoxication

Chronic ingestion of excessive quantities of vitamin D causes hypercalcemia. Many infant foods are already fortified with vitamin D or calcium, but an oversolicitous mother, perhaps influenced by aggressive advertising, may feed the child additional vitamin D concentrates.

Hypercalcemia (Chapter 17) causes loss of appetite, vomiting, and stunting of growth. If persistent, hypercalcemia can cause calcium salts to be deposited in a variety of tissues (*metastatic calcification*) and can severely damage the kidneys.

Vitamin E intoxication

Daily doses of 600 IU daily can cause biochemical disturbances such as raised serum triglyceride and depressed thyroid hormone levels. With larger doses muscle weakness has been reported.

Effects of megadoses of water-soluble vitamins

It had long been thought that overdosage of water-soluble vitamins was prevented by rapid clearance from the body; nevertheless a variety of disorders from this cause have been described.

Nicotinic acid. Large doses of nicotinic acid are sometimes given to treat hypercholesterolemia but can cause flushing, itching, and sometimes, rashes. Jaundice or abnormal liver function with gastrointestinal signs and symptoms such as nausea, diarrhea, abdominal pain, and headache develop in a minority. Other complications include aggravation of peptic ulcers, impaired glucose tolerance, and hyperuricemia.

Thiamine. Thiamine can cause hypersensitivity reactions if given by injection. Such reactions include swelling and itching at the injection site, swelling of the tongue, lips, and eyelids, generalized itching, hay fever, asthmalike symptoms, or anaphylactic shock (Chapter 7), which may be fatal.

Vitamin C. In general, megadosage of vitamin C rarely causes significant ill effects in normal people, but a variety of side effects, including gastrointestinal disturbances and rashes have been reported. "Conditioned deficiency" can sometimes develop when megadosage is stopped. In those with inborn errors of metabolism such as cystinuria, oxalosis, or hyperuricemia, large doses of vitamin C can cause stone formation.

In G6PD deficiency (Chapter 13) hemolysis may be aggravated. Vitamin C can also destroy vitamin B_{12} in food and in very large doses can cause serum cholesterol levels to rise.

Such is the pathetic trust in vitamin megadosage "therapy" that one person received no less than 80 gm of ascorbic acid by the intravenous route and quickly died.

Pyridoxine. Overdosage with pyridoxine has recently been reported to cause sensory neuropathy. This may result from the fact that the family of pyridines, of which pyridoxine is a member, are neurotoxic.

Major minerals

Sodium, chlorine, potassium, and magnesium are essential for life, but dietary deficiencies of these elements do not develop. Iron and calcium deficiencies, however, cause recognizable diseases as discussed in Chapters 13 and 17, respectively.

Iodine

Iodine is essential for the formation of thyroid hormones, and severe iodine deficiency can cause hypothyroidism. In a few parts of the world the iodine content of the soil is low, and compensatory overactivity of the thyroid gland causes enlargement known as *goiter*. Severe maternal iodine deficiency causes cretinism in the newborn (Chapter 18). Dietary or water-borne goitrogens may increase the effects of iodine deficiency. As a result the severity of goiter and hypothyroidism differs in regions that appear to have equally severe iodine deficiencies.

In areas of endemic goiter, iodine is an essential food additive to prevent goiter and cretinism. Excessive iodine intake may cause hyperthyroidism as a result of overproduction of hormones by the goitrous (hyperplastic) gland (Chapter 18).

Trace elements

Many elements, such as cobalt, nickel, manganese, and silicon, are essential in minute amounts for the formation of a wide variety of compounds necessary to life, but the amounts required are so small that deficiency states have not, so far, been detected.

Zinc

Zinc acts as a cofactor for many enzymes such as lactic dehydrogenase and appears to be essential for the growth and development of many animals. Deficiency may lead to failure of growth, hypogonadism, and impaired wound healing.

Zinc deficiency may result from inadequate amounts given during total parenteral nutrition or be secondary to *acrodermatitis enteropathica*. Acrodermatitis enteropathica is a rare disease, particularly of infants; it is characterized by alopecia, diarrhea, dermatitis, and stomatitis. The disease is heritable as an autosomal recessive trait but responds to administration of zinc.

Zinc appears to be essential for the growth and development of many species of animals. It is also an essential component of many enzymes. Experimentally, zinc deficiency in primates causes retarded growth, loss of hair, atrophy of the gonads, and other changes. It is believed that there is a counterpart to animal zinc deficiency in some poverty-stricken populations whose diets are almost devoid of animal protein. It is probable, however, that other deficiencies play a part.

There is also evidence that zinc is essential for repair and that wound healing is delayed by the absence of zinc. Oral administration of zinc restores healing rates to normal.

Copper

Copper is important particularly in blood formation, and deficiency causes a microcytic, hypochromic anemia. Skeletal defects are another effect and include retardation of skeletal development, osteoporosis, increased density of the zone of provisional calcification, and a cuplike defect of the metaphysis. Multiple metaphyseal fractures after minor injuries can result and are typically symmetrical. A variety of other abnormalities have been described in copper-deprived animals.

Copper deficiency is rare in humans but can result from total parenteral nutrition, severe malnutrition, or malabsorption syndromes.

Fluoride

Fluoride is incorporated into the bones and teeth. Fluoride incorporated into the teeth increases resistance to dental caries, but the precise mechanism by which this is achieved remains controversial.

The optimal level of fluoride for this purpose is one part/million (1 ppm) in the drinking water. Higher levels cause discoloration and in more severe cases, defects of dental enamel structure. These defects, known as *mottling* of the teeth, are the most sensitive index of excessive levels of intake of fluorides. The observation of mottled teeth in persons in various communities led to the discovery of the effects of fluoride on the body. However, the belief that fluoride had a protective effect on the teeth was widespread in the nineteenth century, long before its effects had been validated, and pharmaceutical preparations of it were available at the end of the nineteenth century if not earlier.

Incorporation of fluoride into the skeleton increases its density, and in areas where the fluoride content of the water is high (over 6 ppm), osteoporosis (Chapter 17) is less prevalent than in areas of low fluoride intake.

Fluorides are present in excessively high concentrations in the drinking water in some areas, notably in some parts of northern India and in Africa. The main effects of naturally induced fluorosis are, in such areas, mottling of the teeth, hypercalcification of the skeleton, and calcification of ligaments and tendons. Eventually this may severely limit movement. In the worst cases, bony outgrowths from the vertebrae can cause compression of the spinal cord and paraplegia.

Miscellaneous aspects of nutrition
Sugar

Sugar (sucrose) is eaten in enormous quantities in the Western World. Candies eaten at frequent intervals cause increased dental caries and in excessive quantity can contribute to obesity. Compulsive candy eating may sometimes be a symptom of depression.

Some believe that a high dietary sugar intake directly contributes to hyperlipidemia and atherosclerosis, but the evidence that it has any greater effect than other foodstuffs is weak.

Alcohol

Alcohol has a high caloric content but virtually no nutrient value. Chronic alcoholism is therefore an important cause of secondary malnutrition. However, more commonly than overt vitamin deficiencies discussed earlier, alcoholism can cause a great variety of pathologic changes either directly or indirectly. Such disorders include gastritis, hepatitis or cirrhosis of the liver, cardiomyopathy, skeletal myopathy, and later, brain damage.

In some countries, but not all, there is an epidemiologic association between alcohol consumption and cancer of the mouth, pharynx, or esophagus.

Hematologic abnormalities are among the earliest objective effects of excessive alcohol consumption. Macrocytosis is the first change. Later if the diet is defective, megaloblastic anemia resulting from folate deficiency can develop.

Deficiencies of vitamins, particularly thiamine and pyridoxine, are other effects of alcoholism. Such deficiencies are caused by malabsorption, defective metabolism, or neglect of the diet as discussed earlier. Depression of immune function, particularly of cell-mediated immunity, is detectable on in vitro testing.

By contrast there is epidemiologic evidence that modest, regular consumption of wine is associated with a lower mortality rate from myocardial infarction.

More important than the self-inflicted fate of the individual alcoholic is the public health problem. Excessive alcohol consumption is a major factor in violent crime and the epidemic of motor vehicle injuries and deaths; it also accounts for a significant proportion of aircraft accidents and is an important cause of absenteeism from or mismanagement in industry. Alcoholism is also a major cause of the social problems caused by countless broken families.

Food additives

Many are currently obsessed with the idea that food additives are, almost by definition, bad and that only "natural" foods are wholesome. There is no doubt that in the past particularly, some food additives were toxic. Perhaps the most notorious example was butter yellow, a food colorant which proved to be carcinogenic. It is also possible to become allergic to food additives such as the dye, tartrazine.

However, the vast range of highly dangerous toxins produced in nature by plants and molds is conveniently forgotten and many fruits or vegetables can be allergenic. Thus the flavor component of sassafras root and a component of pollen in honey are both potential carcinogens, and there is probably no such thing as a completely safe food, either natural or artificial.

As a result of the widespread concern about food additives, many manufacturers have removed all or most of them from their products, largely as an advertising device. This may in some cases be unfortunate as several additives are beneficial as discussed later.

The definition of food additives by the U.S. Food and Drug Administration (FDA) is "substances added directly to food or substances which may reasonably be expected to become components of food through surface contact with equipment or packaging materials or even substances that may otherwise affect the food without becoming part of it." Some foods are classified by the FDA as additives, but like other safe and acceptable additives are classified as "generally recognized as safe" (GRAS). At the moment, well over 650 substances are on the GRAS list.

Nitrates, nitrites, and nitrosamines. Nitrates are especially abundant in common vegetables and are formed in the soil by bacteria that oxidize ammonia to nitrites. This is followed by oxidation of nitrites to nitrates. Other bacteria can reverse the

process and reduce nitrates to nitrites. Both nitrates and nitrites are used for preserving meats. Beets, celery, lettuce, carrots, and spinach are high in nitrates, and this normally is the main source of intake. Only a small amount of nitrates and nitrites come from cured meats such as bacon.

Nitrites can react in the digestive tract with secondary amines to form nitrosamines. Small amounts of nitrosamines are carcinogenic to animals. Unsmoked tobacco also contains a high level of a carcinogenic nitrosamine.

Although it now appears certain that potentially carcinogenic nitrosamines are produced in the body, tobacco is a far more important source of dangerous nitro compounds than cured meats and other foodstuffs.

Nitrates and human cancer. The epidemiologic evidence of an association between nitrate intake and cancer is controversial as discussed in Chapter 14.

Synthetic antioxidants. Compounds such as ascorbic acid prevent unsaturated fatty acids from becoming rancid and causing spoilage of meat and other fat-containing foods. Antioxidants also inhibit the formation of free radicals in vivo. Moreover, these compounds, when added to the diets of laboratory animals, substantially prolong their lives. Synthetic antioxidants also inhibit the carcinogenic action of polycyclic hydrocarbons, and the recent decrease in the incidence of stomach cancer in the United States has been attributed, at least in part, to the addition of these compounds to foods.

Vitamin E is a natural antioxidant but is less potent than synthetic counterparts and is also readily destroyed by oxidation.

Mold inhibitors. Molds such as *Aspergillus flavus*, which grow on cereals, beans, and nuts (particularly peanuts), are sources of some of the most potent carcinogens known. Mold inhibitors therefore serve a valuable purpose. Examples of mold inhibitors are propionate and sorbate salts. These are used in minute amounts in foodstuffs and are metabolized to carbon dioxide and water. Nevertheless, because of prejudice against so-called chemical additives, many bread manufacturers no longer include propionate in bread, which, as a consequence, becomes moldy more rapidly.

Monosodium glutamate. Monosodium glutamate is the sodium salt of one of the most common amino acids found in proteins, especially those of vegetables. Monosodium glutamate is usually prepared from natural sources and used to enhance the flavor of foods. It is used in the body as a food substance. Excessive quantities of monosodium glutamate can cause toxic effects such as flushing, tachycardia, and nausea as patrons of Chinese restaurants have occasionally found. Doubt has been expressed as to whether there was an organic cause for these symptoms, but, although it is rare, allergy to monosodium glutamate appears to be an entity.

Vitamins and minerals. The use of vitamins as food additives has lessened the incidence of vitamin deficiency diseases such as beriberi and pellagra, while iodine added to salt has caused goiter to disappear from many parts of the world. Vitamins and minerals such as iron, calcium, and iodine should therefore be added to foods in areas where deficiencies are common. Nevertheless, the problem in many areas of the world is that the quantity of food eaten is too small. Notwithstanding the claims of the health food evangelists, synthetic vitamins are identical to their natural counterparts, while some, such as folic acid preparations, are even more effective.

Food-coloring agents. Many synthetic dyes, particularly aniline derivatives, have been used for coloring food. Many of these, such as Red Dye No. 4 and butter yellow have been shown to be toxic or even carcinogenic and have been banned.

Synthetic dyes serve no useful nutritional function, and it is probable that their use will be discontinued. They may be replaced by natural coloring agents such as carotene compounds.

The Delaney Clause. The Delaney Clause, a United States legislation, specifies that "no additive shall be deemed safe if it is found to induce cancer when ingested by man or animals or if it is found after tests which are appropriate for the evaluation of the safety of food additives to induce cancer in man or animals." Supporters of this clause uphold the interpretation that there is no threshold below which carcinogens are ineffective and that lowering the dosage may decrease but does not abolish the risk. Nevertheless, substances such as estrogens and goitrogens have carcinogenic effects at high levels but are naturally present and widely distributed in foods. Estrogens, in particular, are essential for normal bodily function.

Supporters of the Delaney Clause also argue that with the current load of environmental carcinogens of natural or synthetic origin it is essential not to add potentially carcinogenic food additives. On the other hand, it would seem more realistic to attempt to evaluate the carcinogenic hazards of food additives or any other products in quantitative terms.

Dietary fiber

The amount and nature of vegetable fiber has become one of the most emotive subjects in nutrition. The first reference to the importance of fiber in recent years was the hypothesis by Burkitt* in 1969 that a high vegetable fiber intake by Africans was related to their low incidence of cancer and other disorders of the bowel.

Much recent controversy about vegetable fibers stems from their great variety; misunderstandings have arisen as a result of the fact that many of them do not appear fibrous macroscopically, and, paradoxically, some of the important dietary fibers are gums or gelatinous in consistency when hydrated. The essential feature of vegetable fiber in the present context is that they are carbohydrate polysaccharides forming, at molecular level, long chain polymers. Cellulose is the most obviously fibrous food substance and typically forms the husk of wheat and other cereals; however, gums such as karya or guar gum, mucilages from seeds, or even seaweeds form more effective lattices for adsorption of other foods or fluids. Beans are a useful source of dietary fiber, but weight for weight, peas have a higher fiber content. Fiber in the current dietary sense does not refer to the fibrous (collagen) component of meat, since this kind of fiber is largely digestible and has none of the required properties.

Properties of fibers. Properties of fibers include (1) water-holding capacity; (2) adsorptive properties for bile acids, drugs, and other substances; (3) acceleration of bowel transit time; and (4) slowing of glycemia following carbohydrate intake.

The role of fiber in bowel disease. Bulky fibers such as bran appear to be effective in diverticular disease and irritable bowel syndrome. Fiber is an effective laxative because it increases fecal bulk and accelerates fecal transit time. It is widely believed that the postulated ability of fiber to reduce intraluminal pressure makes it valuable for the treatment in diverticular disease. More controversial is the role of a low-fiber diet in colonic cancer. It is suggested that a high-fiber diet can change

---

*Denis P. Burkitt (b. 1907), British surgeon.

the metabolism of the colonic flora, may absorb toxic or carcinogenic compounds, and generally dilute the contents of the colon. By shortening the transit time, it may also reduce the effect of any potential carcinogens present, but the value of fiber in reducing the risk of colonic cancer is difficult to confirm.

Fiber in diabetes and atherosclerosis. Fiber such as guar gum may allow diabetics to consume larger amounts of carbohydrate but at the same time may reduce urinary glucose output to a small degree. The gel-forming polysaccharides also slow glucose absorption, and high-fiber diets may reduce insulin requirements.

There is some evidence that gel-forming polysaccharide types of fiber can also affect lipid metabolism by lowering blood cholesterol and retarding the development of atheroma in animals. Some epidemiologic evidence also suggests that high-fiber diets are associated with a lower incidence of atherosclerosis and its effects. However, it may be just as important that fiber-containing vegetables such as pulses have a high protein content and substitute for meat, which, even when lean, has a high intracellular fat content.

Adverse effects of fiber. Excessive consumption of fiber may cause diarrhea or, if grossly excessive, can possibly cause obstruction particularly if there is a stricture as in Crohn's disease. Fiber also binds to minerals, particularly calcium. Bran in wholemeal wheat flour contains phytates, which also bind to calcium and may contribute to the development of rickets in Asian Indian communities who use coarse wholemeal flour for making chupatties. Iron and zinc may also be lost in the same way.

The effects of fiber therefore are not all beneficial; in particular a high-fiber diet can induce a negative calcium balance, and the more extravagant claims for the benefits of high-fiber diets remain controversial.

Fats

Fats have a high calorific content in relation to their weight and in the form of butter and cream are widely used to enrich and (unfortunately) make food more delicious. Fats are often therefore an important contributory factor in obesity. In addition, animal fats containing saturated fatty acids are believed to be an important factor in the production of atherosclerosis and coronary heart disease (Chapter 10). By contrast, polyunsaturated fatty acids present in vegetable oils (particularly those derived from corn or sunflower seeds) may have a beneficial (though small) effect on blood lipid and cholesterol levels. Some epidemiologic evidence suggests a decreased intake of animal fats and an increased intake of polyunsaturated fatty acids may be associated with a decreased mortality rate from coronary heart disease, but this remains controversial. Increasingly, however, it appears that rather than merely reducing the fat content of the diet, some fats, notably fish oils are beneficial and should be consumed in greater amounts.

Cholesterol transport and metabolism

Dietary fats are absorbed as triglycerides and form chylomicrons in the plasma. Chylomicrons consist of triglyceride and cholesterol bound to apoprotein but lipid metabolism is complex; it is discussed in Chapter 10.

Most of the plasma cholesterol is transported on low density lipoproteins (LDLs), and as a result there is a correlation between plasma LDL levels and ischemic heart disease. High density lipoproteins (HDLs) can also accept cholesterol from various sources, and the levels of HDLs appear to have a negative correlation with ischemic heart disease.

Plasma LDL levels depend partly on diet and the amount of exercise taken but also on the adequacy of LDL and apoprotein membrane receptor function: this is genetically determined with one functional gene for these receptors being inherited from each parent.

The importance of LDL receptors is shown in *familial combined hyperlipidemia* (Chapter 10). In heterozygotes with this disorder only one functional gene is inherited; only half the normal number of LDL receptors are formed and the clearance of LDLs and very low density lipoproteins (VLDLs) is much delayed. In affected patients the plasma LDL levels are approximately double the normal, and the susceptibility to ischemic heart disease is considerably increased. The situation is even worse in homozygotes in whom abnormal LDL receptor genes are inherited from both parents and who have as a consequence plasma LDL levels of approximately four times the normal and a correspondingly increased risk of early ischemic heart disease. Reduction in dietary fat intake and body weight may be effective for mild cases, but cholesterol-lowering drugs may also be necessary.

Diet and hypercholesterolemia

More than 1 in 500 of the population are heterozygous for familial hyperlipidemias of various types, but the contribution of this and other genetic orders to cholesterol levels in the population as a whole is not known.

Eggs are a major source of cholesterol, but total saturated fat (rather than cholesterol) intake has a closer correlation with plasma cholesterol and LDL level. Animal fats are in general highly saturated. Broadly speaking the harder the fat at room temperature, the greater the degree of saturation. Increased intake of polyunsaturated fats by contrast, lowers cholesterol levels, but, although great publicity is given to the benefits of polyunsaturates, their effect on plasma cholesterol is small. Thus if the level of plasma cholesterol is (say) 400 mg/dl, replacement of saturated fats by polyunsaturates in the diet might perhaps lower this level, at best, to 350 mg/dl; this is far from the "ideal" level of below 200 mg/dl.

More recently, monosaturated oils such as olive oil, which were not thought to have the benefits of polyunsaturates, have been reported in several countries, not merely to lower LDL levels; but unlike other fats, to raise HDL levels. This finding has been tentatively related to the longer life span and low incidence of ischemic heart disease in countries bordering the Mediterranean Sea where olive oil is the main fat used.

Fish oils have different effects from animal fats. Fish oils are not merely high in the content of polyunsaturates but also inhibit or even, in large doses, block the synthesis of VLDL triglycerides. Fish oils also interfere with platelet adhesion. It is suggested that the high fish consumption by Arctic Eskimos, is a factor contributing to their low incidence of ischemic heart disease, despite their enormously high intake of animal fats from such sources as seal meat.

A fish oil derivative (MaxEPA) rich in eicospentaenoic acid and other polyunsaturates has also been found to lower blood pressure in persons with mild hypertension.

Alcohol and smoking both tend to raise LDL levels, and both increase the risk of ischemic heart disease by other more obscure mechanisms. Exercise by contrast raises the level of "protective" HDLs.

Racial differences in diet and heart disease

Much has been made of the association between the incidence of heart disease and diet in different countries. Thus in Japan the diet is in general high in carbohydrate and low in fat, and the incidence of ischemic heart disease is very low. By contrast, Asiatic Indians living in Britain have an abnormally high incidence of ischemic heart disease despite a diet with a high vegetable and carbohydrate content and a lower consumption of cigarettes and alcohol than Britons. The incidence of ischemic heart disease is also far higher in Britain than in France even though there are no convincing differences in dietary or smoking habits. However, differences in diagnostic criteria and various other factors may limit the validity of such epidemiologic reports.

Perinatal nutrition—breast-feeding

Cow's milk, particularly when modified by dilution to lower the protein concentration and by the addition of sugar, has long been regarded as providing a convenient and satisfactory substitute for human breast milk. Nevertheless, the advantages of human breast milk include the following:

1. The presence of protective antibodies
2. Absence of bovine antigens capable of causing sensitization
3. Optimal electrolyte concentrations
4. Optimal pH
5. More readily absorbed fats
6. More readily absorbed iron
7. More readily absorbed vitamin D

The antibody in human breast milk is mainly IgA, which acts locally in the infant's intestinal tract. IgA protects against some infections, and gastroenteritis is rare in breast-fed babies. It may also impede absorption of harmful antigens. Other potentially protective components in human milk that may be more active than those from cow's milk, include lysozyme and lactoferrin. Protein, probably β-lactalbumin, in cow's milk (but not in human milk) can cause sensitization and allergy. Cow's milk may also contain traces of antibiotics, which can be sensitizing.

The importance of the nature of the fats in human milk is more controversial. Those in human milk contain more polyunsaturated fatty acids, and it has been claimed, but not proven, that the incidence of coronary arterial disease is less in those who were breast fed. Cow's milk can be a vehicle for infection and in the past served to transmit bovine tuberculosis on a vast scale. Brucellosis can be transmitted in goat's milk in other countries. Infections such as these are a particular hazard to "health food" enthusiasts who insist on consuming unpasteurized milk, and several deaths have resulted. A greater risk, especially in underdeveloped countries, is infection of infant foods prepared from milk powders. The food may be unhygienically prepared or become heavily infected if allowed to stand in a warm environment between feedings.

Human milk fat is more readily absorbed, and it is suggested that this may also improve absorption of fat-soluble vitamins. There is also evidence that vitamin D is better absorbed from breast milk, but this may be because vitamin D in human milk is sulphated and in water-soluble form. Whatever the reason, rickets is exceedingly rare in breast-fed infants.

The electrolyte content of cow and human milk differs considerably; this can occasionally cause electrolyte disturbances because of the infant's more delicate fluid balance and incompletely developed renal mechanisms for dealing with solutes. Unmodified cow's milk can (surprisingly) cause neonatal hypocalcemia and tetany as a consequence of its high phosphate content. Cow's milk can also cause acidosis.

Some of these benefits of breast-feeding are firmly established; others are more controversial. Moreover, there is considerable variation among individuals so that studies are usually based on pooled samples.

Much emotion has been generated in the controversy over the real and postulated benefits of breast-feeding. Nevertheless, it has become apparent that the differences between human and cow's milk are considerably greater than were once thought, and breast-feeding is being increasingly strongly advocated. Breast-feeding does not, however, guarantee infant health, and even breast-fed infants can suffer from malnutrition.

Total parenteral nutrition (intravenous hyperalimentation)

In many conditions, such as inflammatory bowel disease, major intestinal resection, or severe malabsorption, it may not be possible to give the patient adequate nutrition by mouth. Currently, essential nutrients are given, in such cases, exclusively by the intravenous route in the form of concentrated glucose solutions containing protein hydrolysate and electrolyte solutions to which vitamins and minerals may be added. By administration of this fluid by means of a catheter in the subclavian vein, the problem of superficial venous thrombosis caused by hypertonic glucose solutions is avoided.

This method of feeding has greatly improved the management and prognosis of severely burned or comatose patients and many of those with gastrointestinal tract diseases. Various types of cancer, (not necessarily of the gastrointestinal tract) also lead to severe malnutrition (malignant cachexia) for reasons that are not fully understood. The condition of these patients can be improved by intravenous alimentation, which may enable them to withstand treatment better and possibly improve their duration of survival in other ways.

The major hazards of total parenteral nutrition are catheter thrombosis and hematogenous infection, particularly by *Candida albicans*. However, many other opportunistic microbes can enter by this route and cause systemic infections, such as infective endocarditis (Chapter 11), as the patients inevitably also have impaired resistance. Cardiovascular complications can result from fluid overload or hyperchloremia, and other metabolic complications such as copper or zinc deficiency can result from failure to adjust the quantity or composition of the perfusion.

Obesity

Obesity is the single most common nutritional disorder in affluent countries. Obesity is the result of a caloric intake in excess of the energy requirements for physical activity and growth. The disease more frequently affects otherwise healthy persons, but rarely, obesity can be secondary to other disorders, particularly hormonal.

The causes of obesity remain obscure and controversial, and the many varied "slimming diets" that have been proposed testify to the difficulties involved in attempting to lose weight. The severity of the difficulties is illustrated by the more extreme measures that have been used to cause weight loss. These measures include total fasting, gastrointestinal by-pass surgery, insertion of gastric balloons, and jaw wiring. There has been a small but significant number of deaths as a consequence.

Excessive accumulation of fat and increased body weight may be associated with or cause other diseases. In addition, obesity is an obsession of the westernized world as a result of current ideas about how people should look. In the days of the artist, Peter Paul Rubens, for example, the idea of a beautiful woman was one we would today call distinctly fat.

Diseases with which obesity is associated or to which it contributes include the following:

1. *Cardiovascular disease*—There is a significant association between obesity and hypertension; statistically, obesity is associated with a shortened expectation of life.
2. *Diabetes mellitus*—Obesity is the main factor precipitating maturity-onset diabetes mellitus (Chapter 18).
3. *Osteoarthrosis*—Excessive weight throws an increased strain on the weight-bearing joints, particularly those of the hips and knees, and accelerates the progress of osteoarthrosis.

Appetite is the response to many physiologic and emotional stimulatory and inhibitory factors. Researchers have long sought some single central mediator that will switch on or off the feeding center which appears to be in the hypothalamus. The isolation of an overriding mediator of this sort might provide a highly desirable means of controlling obesity. There seems little prospect of finding such a hormone—if indeed it exists—in the foreseeable future.

Selected readings

Alexander JW: Nutrition and infection, Arch Surg 121:966, 1986.

Anonymous (LA): Vitamin E deficiency, Lancet i:423, 1986.

Anonymous (LA): The bran wagon, Lancet i:782, 1987.

Barclay AJG, Foster A, Sommer A: Vitamin A supplements and mortality related to measles: a randomised clinical trial, Br Med J 294:294, 1987.

Ballard-Barbash R and Callaway CW: Marine fish oils: role in prevention of coronary artery disease, Mayo Clin Proc 62:113, 1987.

Bieri JG, Corash L, and Hubbard VS: Medical uses of vitamin E, N Engl J Med 308:1063, 1983.

Bresalier RS and Kim YS: Diet and colon cancer, N Engl J Med 313:1413, 1985.

Council on Scientific Affairs: Vitamin preparations as dietary supplements and as therapeutic agents, JAMA 257(14):1929, 1987.

Flier JS and Underhill LH: New concepts in the biology and biochemistry of ascorbic acid, N Engl J Med 314:892, 1986.

Forman D: Gastric cancer: diet and nitrate exposure, Br Med J 294:528, 1987.

Goodman DWS: Vitamin A and retinoids in health and disease, N Engl J Med 310:1023, 1984.

Health and Public Policy Committee, American College of Physicians, Philadelphia, Pennsylvania, Position paper: Eating disorders: anorexia nervosa and bulimia, Ann Intern Med 105:790, 1986.

Hennekens CH: Micronutrients and cancer prevention, N Engl J Med 315:1288, 1986.

Maher TJ: Natural food constituents and food additives: the pharmacologic connection, J Allergy Clin Immunol 79:413, 1987.

Qizilbash N: Blood pressure and fat intake: a review, J Royal Soc Med 80:225, 1987.

Rifkind BM and Lenfant C: Cholesterol lowering and the reduction of coronary heart disease risk, JAMA 256(20):2872, 1986.

Riis B, Thomsen K, and Christiansen MD: Does calcium supplementation prevent postmenopausal bone loss? N Engl J Med 316:173, 1987.

Rudman D and Williams PJ: Megadose vitamins: use and misuse, N Engl J Med 309:488, 1983.

Sanders TAB: Fish and coronary artery disease, Br Heart J 57:214, 1987.

Sitrin MD, Lieberman F, and Jensen WE et al: Vitamin E deficiency and neurologic disease in adults with cystic fibrosis, Ann Intern Med 107:51, 1987.

Vandongen R: Fish oil and cardiovascular disease, Med J Aust 146:236, 1987.

Weinberger MH: Sodium chloride and blood pressure, N Engl J Med 317:1084, 1987.

Wittes RE: Vitamin C and cancer, N Engl J Med 312:178, 1985.

CHAPTER 6

Inflammation and repair

In the first century AD, Aurelius Celsus in his writings *De re Medicina* described inflamed tissues as being hot, swollen, red, and painful. About a century later, Galen added loss of function to the four *cardinal signs* of inflammation. Although a great deal of knowledge about inflammation has been accumulated since these first simple observations, much remains to be learned.

Inflammation is a reaction of tissues to injury and comprises a complex series of vascular, humoral, and cellular events at or near the site of injury. It is reasonable to regard inflammation as a process which attempts to eliminate offending agents or their effects. Restoration of structure and function of affected tissue is achieved to a varying degree by *reparative processes,* which go hand in hand with inflammation. Inflammation tends to dominate the early events that follow injury, whereas repair begins at an early stage and assumes a major role in the later stages.

Ideally inflammation and repair should restore tissue to its preinjury state. Often, however, this ideal is not achieved. Specialized tissues such as nerve and muscle are replaced by connective tissue. In some inflammatory diseases, such as rheumatoid arthritis or tuberculosis, the inflammatory and reparative processes may be destructive in themselves.

To simplify description, inflammation will be discussed separately from repair. The two processes, in fact, are inseparable.

INFLAMMATION

Inflammation is commonly caused by (1) microorganisms, (2) physical trauma, (3) thermal injury, (4) radiation, (5) foreign bodies including dead tissue, and (6) immune reactions.

It is important to distinguish between the terms *inflammation* and *infection. Infection* is the *presence* and *replication* of microorganisms in the tissues. Infection often leads to inflammation, but this is not invariable. In cholera, for example, large numbers of pathogenic bacteria are present in close contact with intestinal epithelium, but there is no evidence of inflammation or damage to the mucosa. There is, however, severe derangement of intestinal mucosal cell function resulting from the enterotoxin elaborated by *Vibrio cholerae*. It should also be remembered that inflammation can be an immune reaction without the participation of microorganisms, although microorganisms themselves may stimulate immune reactions.

Although previously listed separately as causes of inflammation, infections and immune reactions have much in common. Infections tend to provoke immune reactions. The mediators of inflammation, especially the components of the complement system (see p. 83), are important in the genesis of many immune reactions. Lymphocytes, which are the predominant cells in chronic inflammation, are a major component of the immune response.

The inflammatory processes caused by microorganisms are complex and variable because of the many biologically active substances involved. *Staphylococcus aureus*, for example, a common cause of skin and soft tissue inflammation, produces numerous extracellular enzymes, many of which are capable of modifying the basic inflammatory response, often to the advantage of the organism. *S. aureus* and other bacteria can produce *leukocidins*, which can rapidly kill the leukocytes that arrive on the scene to engulf them.

Our understanding of inflammation is based largely on experimental work with less complex processes, such as thermal and chemical injuries, that have been adjusted in severity to keep tissue necrosis to a minimum.

Inflammation can be classified as (1) acute, (2) chronic, or (3) granulomatous.

Acute inflammation is a short-lived process developing in response to a single episode of injury. The duration of the process is usually measured in hours or days.

Chronic inflammation is prolonged—often lasting weeks or even years—in response to continuous or repeated episodes of injury.

Acute and chronic inflammation can usually also be differentiated microscopically by their different cellular components. *Subacute inflammation* is a vague descriptive term that implies a degree or duration of inflammation somewhere between the acute and chronic types. It has no readily definable pathologic features.

Granulomatous inflammation is a specific form of chronic inflammation that develops in response to certain specific agents such as mycobacteria and many fungi.

Acute inflammation

Acute inflammation is most frequently caused by infectious agents, heat and cold, or physical trauma. It may also be a response to immunologic injury. Despite this diversity of causes, the early phases appear to be the same. The events evolve continuously, but they can be divided into those which are (1) vascular and (2) cellular. Common to both phases are many complex controlling mechanisms or mediators that involve a bewildering network of reactions.

Vascular events

The vascular events of acute inflammation take place in the microvascular circulation, which consists of arterioles, capillaries, and venules. Blood flow into the capillary bed is controlled by the smooth muscle in the arteriolar walls, which can act as a sphincter and adjust the amount of blood entering the capillaries, for example, during exercise.

The order of events as observed in experimental inflammation is as follows:

1. Transient vasoconstriction
2. Arteriolar dilatation

3. Capillary and venule dilatation
4. Increased vascular permeability

Within the first minutes following injury, there is an immediate constrictive reaction in the arterioles proximal to the site of injury. The vasoconstriction is transient and contributes little or nothing to the inflammatory process. It is rapidly followed by dilatation of the arterioles and the beginning of an increased blood flow. Almost simultaneously there is dilatation first of venules, then of capillaries. This reaction, which takes place in the first 30 minutes or so after injury, appears to be caused by chemical mediators such as histamine. The effect of these changes is that previously closed capillaries open up and blood flow to the area increases—*active hyperemia.*

Associated with vasodilatation is an increase in the permeability of the blood vessels, also a chemically mediated process. Under normal conditions, there is loss of fluid from the arterial end of the microcirculation and this fluid is reabsorbed at the venous end. This cyclic process is due to the difference between the hydrostatic pressure (which is high in the arterioles and low in the venules) and the opposing osmotic pressure (Fig. 6-1, *A*). During inflammation hydrostatic pressure increases, preventing reabsorption so that fluid leaves the small vessels at all sites in the microcirculation (Fig. 6-1, *B*). In addition, there is microscopic separation of the vascular endothelial cells, and the interendothelial space becomes wide enough to allow the passage of large protein molecules. The

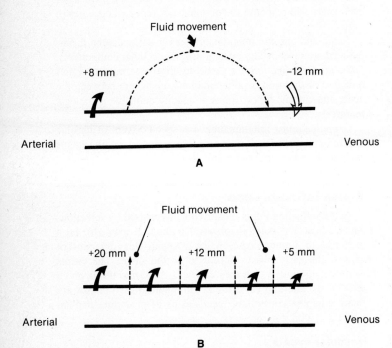

FIG. 6-1. Fluid exchange in capillaries by ultrafiltration under normal conditions (**A**) and in inflammation (**B**). **A,** There is a difference of about +8 mm Hg between hydrostatic and osmotic pressures at the arterial end and −12 mm Hg at the venous end of the capillary system; this results in circulation of fluid into and out of the extravascular space. **B,** In inflammation, mainly because of higher hydrostatic pressure, fluid moves generally from the vessels into the extravascular space.

latter are characteristic of an *inflammatory exudate.* Fibrinogen is the predominant protein that leaves the vessels, but immunoglobulins can also escape in this way. The widespread dilatation of small blood vessels in the inflamed area causes a slowing of the rate of blood flow, a tendency to stasis, and even small areas of thrombosis. These changes account for the *redness, swelling,* and *heat* that typify the inflammatory response. The *pain* of inflammation is probably due to a combination of increased pressure within the inflamed part and the effects of mediators. The vascular changes described previously continue for periods ranging from a few minutes to several hours according to the severity of the injury. Initially, the changes are mediated by vasoactive amines and proteases, but after the first 30 minutes or so they appear to be mediated by a different group of substances as discussed in the section on mediators later in this chapter.

Role of fluid exudate. Inflammatory exudate consists of proteins derived from blood plasma. The high specific gravity (approximately 1.020) is a result of the presence of fibrinogen. Some of the effects of inflammatory exudate are as follows:

1. It contains fibrinogen, which is deposited as fibrin and which may contribute to forming a barrier against further spread of infection.
2. It may help dilute bacterial or other toxins.
3. It contains complement proteins and sometimes specific antibodies that can have a bactericidal effect.
4. It may contain opsonins (p. 81), which enhance phagocytosis by leukocytes.
5. It can act as a vehicle for antimicrobial drugs.

A *transudate,* on the other hand, is a fluid of lower specific gravity (1.010 or less) that escapes from a tissue or membrane. It contains little or no fibrinogen, and thus its composition is very similar to serum. It is usually the result of mild injury to the tissue, which allows fluid and smaller blood protein molecules to escape through smaller gaps in the capillary endothelium.

Cellular events

Leukocytes reach and deal with an infection or other injury as a result of the following sequence of events:

1. Margination and pavementing
2. Emigration
3. Aggregation
4. Phagocytosis

Margination and pavementing. Within the arterioles and venules (though not in the capillaries) when the blood flow is normal, there is a separation of the blood components so that the red and white cells flow in the central axis of the stream. This leaves cell-poor plasma in contact with the endothelial surface. With the slowing of the bloodstream in the early hours of inflammation, the cells move to the periphery. This process, called *margination* brings the white cells into contact with the endothelial surface to which they adhere to form a layer closely applied to the endothelium (Fig. 6-2). This is called *pavementing.* Red cells and platelets may also adhere to the endothelium. This indicates that the phenomenon is not simply a result of an alteration in the surface properties of the white cells but it is also caused by changes in the endothelial cell membrane. The normal, mutually repellant action of leukocytes and endothelial cells is lost in areas of inflammation. The cause is not fully understood at present but pavementing can be abol-

ished experimentally by corticosteroids and prostacyclin (PGI₂). Moreover, recent research indicates that the cytokines, interleukin 1 (IL-1), and tumor necrosis factor (TNF) both promote leukocyte-endothelial attachment; furthermore, a specific molecule, endothelial-leukocyte attachment molecule (E-LAM 1) has been identified on endothelial cell surfaces. This implies that cell membranes of white cells and endothelial cells are both altered in the inflammatory process.

Leukocyte adherence. The adherence of neutrophils and other white cells to endothelial surfaces, other cells and opsonized bacteria, is due, in part, to a group of glycoproteins present on the surface of the neutrophil. One of these for example, known as C3R is the surface receptor for the complement fraction C3b. One of its functions is to act synergistically with the receptor for the Fc fragment of IgG to enhance leukocyte adherence. Lack of this enzyme is associated with severe neutrophil dysfunction and inflammatory disease as discussed later in this chapter.

Emigration. Having applied themselves closely to the endothelium, *emigration* of the white cells into the perivascular tissue begins. The process of emigration appears to be confined to the venules alone. By insinuating themselves between the endothelial cells and then penetrating the basement membrane, leukocytes manage to squeeze their way out of the venules into the surrounding tissues (Fig. 6-3). Once the cells have emerged from the vessels, the basement membrane appears able to reseal itself. Neutrophils are the most active of the emigrating cells, followed closely by monocytes (macrophages), and much later by lymphocytes. Red cells may pass through the vessel wall in small numbers, forced through by hydrostatic pressure. This passive emergence of red cells, which contrasts with the active ameboid movements of the white cells is called *diapedesis* (Fig. 6-4). If larger gaps develop in venule walls, frank hemorrhage into the surrounding tissue can take place.

White cells in inflammation. The white cells that are involved in acute inflammation are (1) neutrophil polymorphs, (2) macrophages (monocytes), (3) eosinophils, and (4) basophils. Lymphocytes and plasma cells appear to play little part in acute inflammation. They are of great importance in chronic inflammation and are described later in this chapter and in Chapter 7. Mast cells can also contribute to the inflammatory response in a similar way to basophils.

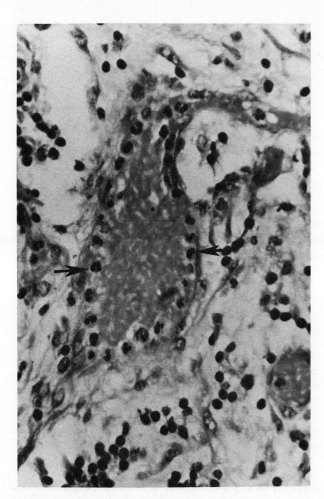

FIG. 6-2. Acute inflammation—margination. A dilated and congested capillary *(arrows)* is shown in which polymorphonuclear leukocytes are arranged around the periphery in contact with the endothelium.

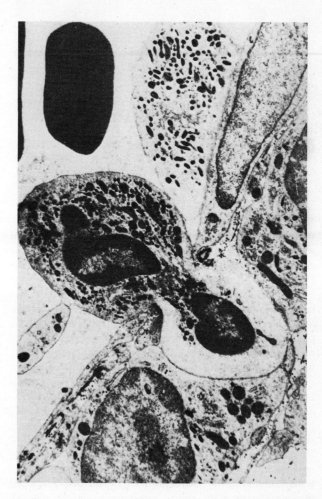

FIG. 6-3. Leukocyte emigration. A neutrophil is squeezing through an endothelial gap. The leading edge is empty of granules. *(From Aspects of acute inflammation, Kalamazoo, Mich., 1969, The Upjohn Co.)*

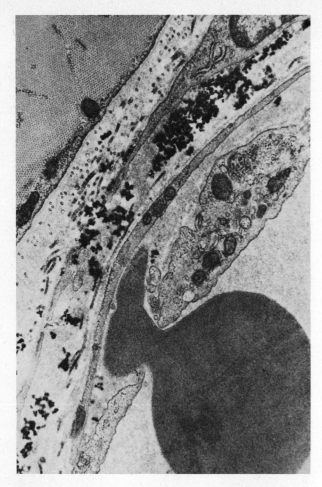

FIG. 6-4. Diapedesis. A red cell is passively squeezed through a preexisting endothelial gap. *(From Aspects of acute inflammation, Kalamazoo, Mich., 1969, The Upjohn Co.)*

Neutrophil polymorph. The mature, segmented neutrophil is about 12 to 14 μm in diameter and has between two and five connected nuclear lobules. With polychromatic stains the nucleus appears deep purple and the cytoplasm pale pink. The cytoplasm contains numerous granules, which are described later in this chapter. The neutrophil polymorph is the predominant cell in acute inflammation, and its main function is the phagocytosis and killing of microorganisms. The killing of many kinds of bacteria by neutrophils and monocytes is mainly the result of the effect of intracellular hydrogen peroxide.

Monocyte. The monocyte or circulating macrophage attains a size of 20 μm. When present in tissues, they are referred to as tissue macrophages or histiocytes. The nucleus is variously oval, kidney-shaped, or convoluted and contains fine chromatin strands. The cytoplasm stains gray-blue and may contain few or many azurophil granules. The monocyte has a phagocytic function in the later phases of the inflammatory process, when it may outnumber the neutrophil. It is possible that monocytes may proliferate at the site of inflammation. Monocytes are capable of secreting a wide variety of substances with a wide range of important biologic activities. These include factors which are involved, not only in inflammation, but in cell-

mediated immunity, reparative processes, and the genesis of fever. These are described elsewhere in the text.

Eosinophil polymorph. The eosinophil is about 16 μm in diameter and has a pale blue bilobed nucleus. Its cytoplasm is rich in large eosinophilic granules. Eosinophils are seen in large numbers in inflammatory conditions where an allergic or hypersensitivity reaction is present or where excessive amounts of certain antigens are found such as those in parasitic worms and their larvae. The basic function of the eosinophil is still not well understood.

Basophil polymorph. The basophil polymorph is about 14 μm in diameter. Its pale blue, bilobed nucleus is almost obscured by many large, deeply rounded basophilic granules. The degranulation of basophils releases, for example, histamine, which acts on venules as one of the mediators of the earlier phases of acute inflammation.

Mast cells. Basophilic cells are present in subcutaneous and other connective tissues, and have a similar function to the circulating basophil polymorph. These tissue cells can release histamine and a variety of other substances that can be involved in the inflammatory process. These include serotonin, eosinophil chemotactic factor (ECF), prostaglandin D2 (PGD_2) and leukotrienes C_4 and D_4 (see pp. 83-84). Small but important differences exist between the mast cells found in the respiratory tract and those present in other sites, since cromolyn, a drug which blocks mast cell degranulation has no effect on the mast cells present in other tissues.

Chemotaxis and leukotaxis. After leukocytes have emigrated from blood vessels, they may be attracted to the site of injury by the process of chemotaxis. *Chemotaxis* is defined as the movement of cells along a gradient of concentration. When the process involves leukocytes, the term *leukotaxis* is applicable; in the context of inflammation, this term is often used synonymously with chemotaxis.

Leukotaxis is a characteristic feature of inflammation. Its mechanisms in vivo are not known and must be largely inferred from in vitro experiments, in which the movement of cells across membrane filters under experimental conditions has been studied by time-lapse photography. The effect of leukotaxis is to cause leukocytes, especially neutrophils, to collect around the site of injury. Several substances appear to be responsible for providing the chemical basis of chemotaxis. These chemotactic factors include certain lymphokines, products of the complement, kallikrein-kinin and coagulation systems, and bacterial enzymes. A specific chemotactic factor for eosinophils (ECF-A), produced by mast cells has been previously noted.

Since chemotaxis is an important mechanism for directing the movement of phagocytic cells, impairment of this mechanism therefore can compromise an individual's defense against microbial disease. Both congenital and acquired defects have been described. Among the former is the *lazy leukocyte syndrome* in which a defective leukotaxic response is associated with gingivitis, stomatitis, and a low white cell count. Affected patients are also subject to severe bacterial infections. Impaired leukotaxis has also been described in some patients with diabetes mellitus or rheumatoid arthritis.

Leukocyte aggregation. Aggregations or collections of leukocytes at or near the site of inflammation are usually greatest in acute bacterial infections caused by pyogenic (pus-producing) bacteria such as *Staphylococcus aureus* and *Neisseria gonorrhoeae*. In most situations the predominant cell is initially the neutrophil, but the macrophage becomes increasingly common as the process progresses. Lymphocytes are usually rare in acute inflammation except in a few bacterial and in many viral infections, where lymphocytes predominate from the beginning. A lymphocytic response is seen, for example, in primary syphilis. Although it is an acute inflammatory process, with respect to the vascular response, it is dominated by the presence of lymphocytes. Small numbers of neutrophils can be found in the very early stages of acute viral meningitis, but the typical cellular reaction is lymphocytic.

Phagocytosis by polymorphonuclear leukocytes. The engulfment of microorganisms, foreign materials, and tissue debris by cells is called *phagocytosis*. It is an important property of neutrophil polymorphs and macrophages (Fig. 6-5, *A* and *B*), but the process is somewhat different in each of these cell types. Phagocytosis consists of three main phases. These include (1) attachment of foreign particles or microorganisms to the surface of the phagocytic cell, (2) their ingestion by the cell, and (3) destruction of particles and killing of bacteria within the cell. An additional requirement is the presence of a suitable surface to act as physical support for the process. This may be a tissue surface, strands of fibrin, or even—in a concentrated cellular exudate—the surface of other phagocytic cells.

Attachment. In the case of bacteria, attachment appears to depend on the coating by materials known as *opsonins* of which there are two main groups. First, there are nonspecific opsonic fragments of the third (C3b) and possibly other components of serum complement. These are capable of opsonizing a wide range of organisms. Second, there are antibodies (particularly IgG), which are directed against the surface components of specific organisms. Opsonic activity has also been ascribed to the glycoprotein, *fibronectin,* which is found in soluble form in blood and body fluids and as an insoluble substance in connective tissues. It appears to act as an opsonin for gram-positive organisms and necrotic tissue debris.

When opsonins have become bound to the bacterial surface, the bacteria stick to the phagocytes because of the receptors on their surface. In the case of opsonization by specific antibodies, the attachment is by means of the Fc component of the antibody, for which polymorphs (and macrophages) have specific surface receptors.

Ingestion and degranulation. After a bacterium or foreign particle has become attached to a phagocyte, it is engulfed. This takes place by means of pseudopodia which extend around the particle until they fuse together. In this way a *phagosome* is formed, and the particle is drawn into the cell. Not all organisms submit to this lethal entrapment. Those, such as *Streptococcus pneumoniae* and *Cryptococcus neoformans*, which have prominent polysaccharide capsules, can resist the phagocytic action of polymorphs. The M protein of *Streptococcus pyogenes* has a similar protective function and serves to enhance the virulence of the bacterium. However, this protective effect can be, in part, neutralized by opsonins. The endotoxin (lipopolysaccharide) component of gram-negative bacterial cell walls in high concentrations can also inhibit phagocytosis. Paradoxically, low concentrations of endotoxin can for unknown reasons, actually enhance the phagocytic process.

While engulfment is taking place, the cell's cytoplasmic granules converge on the phagosomes. These granules, in the neutrophil are of two types. The azurophil (primary) granules, which are large and dense, contain lysosomal hydrolases such as acid phosphatase, myeloperoxidase, lysozyme, and the antimicrobial cationic proteins (1) defensins and (2) bactericidal/permeability increasing protein. Deficiency of these granules and their constituent enzymes can lead to severe infections as discussed later in the chapter.

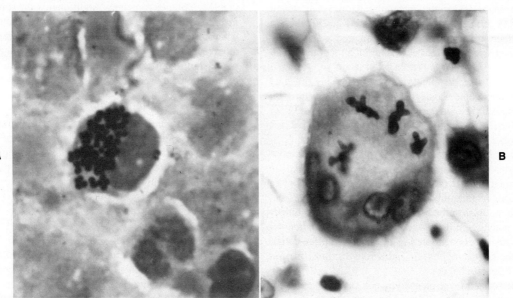

FIG. 6-5. A, Smear of pus from an abscess showing phagocytosis of *Staphylococcus aureus* by a neutrophil. **B,** Section of oral soft tissue showing a multinucleate giant cell with ingested fungal elements in the cytoplasm. *(From McCracken AW and Cawson RA: Clinical and oral microbiology, Washington DC, 1982, Hemisphere Publishing Corp.)*

The specific granules are smaller and less dense. They contain alkaline phosphatase, lysozyme, and lactoferrin (which is an iron-binding antibacterial protein) but no hydrolases or peroxidase.

During engulfment, the cytoplasmic granules, essentially consisting of lysosomes, converge on the phagosomes, fuse with them, and discharge their contents around organisms or particles. This is the process of *degranulation*.

Bacterial killing. The antimicrobial activity within neutrophils appears to result from physicochemical conditions and reactions that include:

1. The acid pH inside the vacuoles containing organisms
2. Cationic proteins from the azurophil granules
3. The lytic action of lysozyme
4. The antibacterial effects of lactoferrin
5. Superoxide anion, a highly reactive radical produced by the removal of one electron from oxygen within the cell
6. Hydrogen peroxide, which is probably the most important

These last two substances are produced in a complex series of reactions. Briefly, superoxide anions are derived from the interaction of molecular oxygen with nicotinamide adenine dinucleotide phosphate (NADPH) in the presence of the enzyme oxidase. The superoxide anions can combine with hydrogen to form hydrogen peroxide or persist as an unstable, highly reactive form of oxygen. It is not surprising therefore that phagocytic activity and intracellular killing is associated with an increased uptake of oxygen by neutrophils. The hydrogen peroxide can enter at least three alternative chemical pathways. First, it can combine with halides (chloride ions, for example) in the presence of myeloperoxidase (present in the primary granules) to form hypochlorite, which has a powerful antibacterial action. Second, hydrogen peroxide can be converted by catalase to water and oxygen. This mechanism is present in certain bacteria, including *S. aureus,* and may contribute to the ability of this bacterium to tolerate intracellular killing mechanisms. Third, hydrogen peroxide may, under the influence of peroxidase, enter the metabolic pathway in which NADPH is regenerated. As discussed later, where hydrogen peroxide production in the neutrophil is impaired as in chronic granulomatous disease, resistance to bacterial infection is much reduced.

After the killing of the phagocytosed organism, the final stage of this microscopic tragedy, is the death of the neutrophil itself at the hands of its own destructive enzyme systems. Other polymorphs (i.e., eosinophils and basophils) take no active part in phagocytosis.

Phagocytosis by macrophages. Macrophages are mononuclear phagocytes that ingest organisms and foreign materials in a manner similar to that described for neutrophils. They are seen in all types of inflammatory reactions. Macrophages develop as promonocytes in the bone marrow and enter the bloodstream as monocytes. In the tissues, they are called *histiocytes* and are particularly concentrated in the liver (Kupffer cells), the lung (alveolar macrophages), and serous cavities (pleural and peritoneal macrophages).

Aschoff* described these phagocytic cells as the *reticuloendothelial system.* This term has been compared to the description of the Holy Roman Empire (which was neither holy, Roman, nor an empire!) since these cells are neither reticular,

---
*Ludwig Aschoff (1866-1942), distinguished German pathologist.

TABLE 6-1. The macrophage-monocyte or mononuclear phagocyte system (reticuloendothelial system)

Site	Cells
Bone marrow	Promonocytes, macrophages
Blood	Monocytes
Tissues/organs	Macrophages
	Connective tissue ("histiocytes")
	Liver (Kupffer cells)
	Lung (pulmonary macrophages)
	Lymphoid tissues (free and fixed macrophages)
	Peritoneum (macrophages)
	Pleura (macrophages)
	Skin (Langerhans' cells)

endothelium, nor a true system! More appropriate terms are the *macrophage-monocyte system* or the *mononuclear phagocyte system* (Table 6-1).

Macrophages contain large numbers of lysosomes, but unlike neutrophils, they do not contain lysosomal myeloperoxidase, cationic proteins, or lactoferrin. They can, however, kill some microorganisms mainly through activated forms of oxygen, including superoxides. The presence of agents such as mycobacteria, histoplasma, and leishmania within the macrophage may be tolerated for considerable periods of time. These organisms may also stimulate proliferation of macrophages.

Unlike neutrophils, macrophages have a long life span and although they may eventually inactivate or kill the ingested organisms, the persistence of intracellular organisms has a great bearing on the natural history of diseases such as tuberculosis or histoplasmosis. Typically these infections may persist for many years without evidence of activity. Eventually, however, active disease may be caused by organisms that have remained viable within macrophages. Additionally, the spread of infected macrophages via the lymphatic system may determine the site where active disease finally develops. This is seen in pulmonary tuberculosis in which early lymphatic spread to the upper lobes of the lungs during primary infection determines the site of reactivation tuberculosis (Chapter 12), if this develops later.

Mediators of inflammation

Numerous humoral substances have been implicated in the stimulation and control of the various phases of inflammation. They are referred to as *chemical mediators of inflammation* and the pathologic results of the activities of these substances include the following:

1. Vasodilatation
2. Increased vascular permeability
3. Leukotaxis
4. Production of pain

Mediators of inflammation arise from two main sources. They are either products of cells stimulated or injured during inflammation, or they are constituents or by-products of biologic cascade reactions. The complement, coagulation, fibrinolytic, and kallikrein-kinin systems are examples of this type of reaction. Most important and fundamental to the inflammatory process are those vasoactive substances that dilate small blood vessels and increase their permeability. Vasoactive substances include the following:

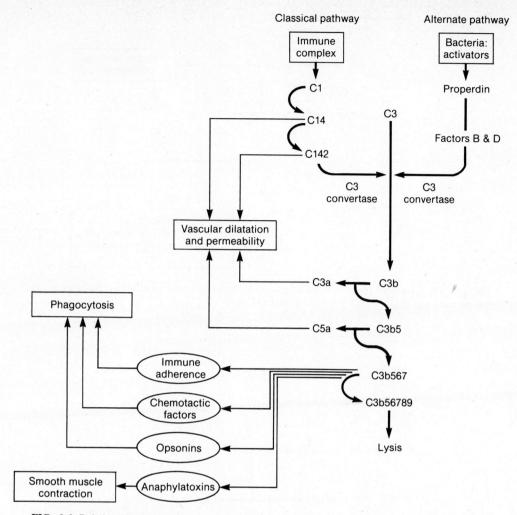

FIG. 6-6. Relationship of complement system to inflammation. The main effects of complement are on vascular permeability and phagocytosis.

1. Histamine is derived from basophils, mast cells, and platelets. Its main action is to cause vasodilatation and vascular permeability in the very early stages of inflammation.
2. Serotonin (5-hydroxytryptamine) has a similar but much less important effect, at least in humans.
3. Many peptides are derived from protein breakdown by proteases.
4. Certain proteolytic enzymes of the complement pathway in particular are vasoactive (Fig. 6-6).

The activity of peptides and proteolytic enzymes is exemplified by the kallikrein-kinin system (Fig. 6-7). This system produces highly vasoactive peptides such as bradykinin and N^2-L-lysylbradykinin. Kinins are highly active compounds and are capable of generating the effects of severe inflammation including the production of pain. Intermediate products of the kallikrein-kinin system include kallikrein and dilute permeability factor (PF/dil), both of which can increase vascular permeability. PF/dil now appears to be a complex of substances rather than a single factor. The end products of the fibrinolytic pathway—i.e., fibrin degradation products (FDPs)—are highly vasoactive. It is important to emphasize that these

two pathways (Figs. 6-7 and 6-8) as well as the coagulation cascade (see Fig. 13-38) are initiated by the conversion of factor XII (Hageman factor) to factor XIIa (Fig. 6-9). This suggests that the activation of factor XII is a fundamental defensive reaction.

Complement components. Components and complexes of the early stages of the complement system are involved in inflammation as a result of immune reactions and appear also to have a role in inflammation that is not of immune origin (see Fig. 6-6). The C3a and C5a fractions are important causes of vasodilatation and increased vascular permeability, both by direct action on blood vessels and indirectly by causing histamine release from basophils and mast cells. C3a and C5a, possibly along with C3b and C3c, can also cause smooth muscle contraction. Collectively, these complement components have been called *anaphylotoxins*. Their participation in the process of *anaphylaxis* (Chapter 7) is confined to animals.

Prostaglandins and leukotrienes. The prostaglandins and leukotrienes, both of which are derivatives of arachidonic acid, have important roles as mediators of inflammation. These substances, which are derived from phospholipid, are widely distributed, especially in vascular endothelium and in blood plate-

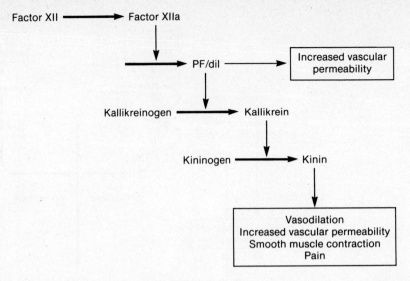

FIG. 6-7. The kallikrein-kinin system and inflammation. This system has a role in vascular permeability and production of pain. *PF/dil*, permeability factor/dilute.

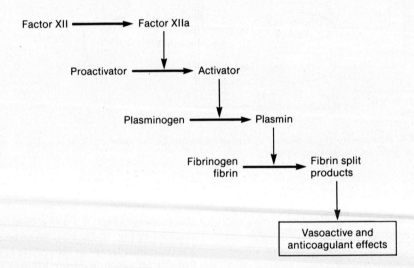

FIG. 6-8. The fibrinolytic system exerts a vasomotor effect mainly through the action of fibrin split products.

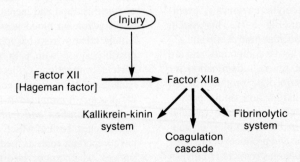

FIG. 6-9. Diagram of interrelationship of kallikrein-kinin, coagulation, and fibrinolytic systems. Note that all three systems are initiated by activation of factor XII.

lets. Briefly, the metabolism of arachidonic acid may follow one of two major pathways:

1. *The prostanoid pathway*—Arachidonic acid is converted by cyclooxygenase to cycloperoxides; these in turn yield prostaglandins (PG) A_2, D_2, E_2, F_2a, and I_2 (prostacyclin) and thromboxane (TXA_2).
2. *The eicosanoid pathway*—Arachidonic acid is converted by lipooxygenase to 5-hydroxyperoxyeicosotetraenoic acid (5HPETE), from which the leukotrienes (LT) A_4 through E_4 are derived. Slow-reacting substance-anaphylactic (SRS-A) consists of LTC_4, LTD_4, and LTE_4.

The precise role of prostaglandins and leukotrienes in inflammation is still unclear, but some of their effects have been determined. For example, PGA_2, PGE_2 and PGI_2 cause vasodilatation, apparently by their direct action on the smooth muscle of the vessel wall, and produce increased blood flow. LTC_4 and LTD_4 derived from mast cells, can also cause vasodilatation and increased vascular permeability. Polymorphonuclear leukocytes can release both PGE_2 and LTB_4, both of which can attract more polymorphs by chemotaxis. Other related actions of prostaglandins include causing pain or increasing sensitivity to it.

The cellular phase of inflammation is also influenced by humoral factors, especially the aggregation of leukocytes and the promotion of phagocytosis. Leukocyte aggregation appears to be enhanced by several chemotactic agents, listed below:

1. Complement fractions
   a. C3a
   b. C5a
2. Fibrin degradation products
3. Kallikrein
4. Leukotriene LTB_4
5. Microbial leucotaxins
6. Prostaglandin PGE_2

The chemotactic substances produced by microorganisms act mainly on neutrophils, but some also act on macrophages, promoting their numbers and activities in the areas of inflammation. Macrophages are also greatly influenced by the products of sensitized lymphocytes. For example, migration inhibition factor (MIF) appears to keep macrophages in the area of the inflammatory response.

In summary it has to be admitted that the precise order, mode of action, and relative importance of mediators of inflammation is not known. At present, it seems likely that the following factors are the most important:

1. *Vascular leakage*—The main mediators are probably vasoactive amines (particularly histamine), kinins (bradykinin) and prostaglandins (A_2, E_2 and I_2).
2. *Leukocyte infiltration*—This is probably caused mainly by the chemotactic components of the complement system, especially the C567 complex. The release of PGE_2 and LTB_4 by damaged neutrophils appears to sustain and augment the leukotactic process.
3. *Tissue damage*—Damage is mainly the result of neutrophil lysosomal products, especially neutral proteases.

In addition to mediators produced by body cells, exogenous factors include vascular damage by chemotactic bacterial products and the direct lethal effect of bacterial toxins on tissue. The events in acute inflammation are summarized in Table 6-2.

TABLE 6-2. Sequence of main events in acute inflammation and their mediators

Events	*Mediated by*
Injury	
Transient arteriolar constriction	Antidromal nerve reflex
Vasodilation, endothelial separation, and increased permeability of venules and capillaries	Amines, kinins, prostaglandins (PGs), leukotrienes (LTs)
Slowing of local circulation	Disturbance of laminar flow
Margination and pavementing of leukocytes	Alteration in leukocyte cell membrane
Leukocyte emigration (±red cell diapedesis) and aggregation	Chemotactic factors including complement fractions, fibrin split products, kallikrein, PGs, and LTs
Phagocytosis	Attachment between leukocytes, bacteria, and foreign materials
Pus formation	Leukocyte proteolytic enzymes

Varieties of acute inflammation

Many terms are used to describe the different varieties of inflammation. Some of these are usefully descriptive; others are relics of the past, and perhaps we should leave them there. Their inclusion is justified only on the grounds that they are still part of the spoken and written language of disease.

Suppurative (purulent) inflammation. Suppurative inflammation is characterized by the formation of pus. Pus is an inflammatory exudate containing white cells, particularly polymorphonuclear leukocytes, in such enormous numbers as to give the fluid a rich, creamy consistency. In addition to leukocytes, pus contains other components of the inflammatory exudate, particularly fibrin, tissue breakdown products, and microorganisms, living or dead.

Suppurative inflammation is most often caused by bacterial infection, particularly by organisms such as *Staphylococcus aureus*, *Streptococcus pyogenes*, and *Neisseria gonorrhoeae*. The appearance and odor of purulent exudates may vary according to the infectious agent and sometimes may provide a clinical clue as to the nature of the causative organism. Pus associated with *Pseudomonas aeruginosa*, for example, is frequently blue-green; anaerobic bacteria, especially of the genera *Bacteroides* and *Clostridium*, commonly produce foul-smelling pus, a consequence of their proteolytic activity.

An *abscess* is a localized area of tissue destruction with the formation of a cavity filled with pus. Staphylococci are important causes, and a common example of an abscess is a boil or furuncle. In this case, entry of staphylococci via a hair follicle leads to septic necrosis of an area of underlying connective tissue. The necrotic tissue becomes separated from the surrounding living tissue and may form an unabsorbed core or be entirely liquefied by leukocytic proteolytic enzymes. A typical acute inflammatory reaction develops at the margins and usually limits the spread of infection. Polymorphonuclear leukocytes attracted to the site of infection gather in such large numbers as to produce a collection of pus. As the lesion progresses, a well-defined abscess wall forms. The innermost layer consists of granulation tissue, consisting of small blood vessels, leukocytes, and fibroblasts (Fig. 6-10). This layer is still sometimes referred to by the archaic name of *pyogenic* (literally, pus-producing) *membrane*. It is called this because of the outpouring of leukocytes from the capillaries of the granulation tissue. More peripherally, proliferating fibroblasts lay down collagen, which, if the abscess becomes chronic, forms a dense fibrous wall. Mononuclear cells, particularly histiocytes and lymphocytes, are present immediately surrounding the area of acute inflammation.

Pus within an abscess is under considerable tension, and this contributes to pain production. The pus also tends to track along a line of least resistance until it reaches a free surface. The abscess can then burst and discharge its contents. The opening formed in this way is known as a *sinus*, but is usually small and drainage of pus is slow. Healing is much accelerated if an abscess is drained by a wide surgical incision. After an abscess has drained, healing is achieved by the formation of granulation tissue, which fills the space. Sometimes the suppurative process results in an abnormal channel forming between two body surfaces, for example, the intestinal tract and the skin. This is known as a *fistula*. It should be noted, however, that the formation of a fistula is not confined to suppurative inflammation. The process can be the result, for example, of chronic inflammation or malignant disease.

Fibrinous inflammation. The characteristic of fibrinous inflammation is the large amount of fibrin present as a result of fibrinogen molecules escaping through damaged vasculature and being converted to fibrin (see Fig. 6-4). Fibrinous inflammation is a frequent reaction observed in membranes lining serous cavities and may follow immunologic or toxin-induced inflammation as well as infection. The pleura that overlies areas of bacterial pneumonitis (Fig. 6-11) is a common site for fibrinous inflammation as is the pericardium in patients with acute rheumatic fever (Fig. 6-12). The replacement of the normally smooth pleural surfaces by rough, irregular deposits of fibrin is usually associated with pain in the chest at the site of inflammation and is the cause of the friction rub heard through a stethoscope as the patient breathes. Chest pain and a friction rub are also typical of fibrinous pericarditis.

If fibrinous inflammation persists, it is replaced by fibrous scar tissue by the process of *organization* described later in this chapter. The scar tissue causes adhesions to develop between the visceral and parietal layers of the pleura or pericardium. This process may be severe enough to obliterate these cavities and impair the function of the lungs or heart.

Catarrhal inflammation. Catarrhal inflammation is an antiquated term which indicates that there is excessive mucus formation as a result of inflammation. The description can best be applied (if used at all) to the common cold, where in addition

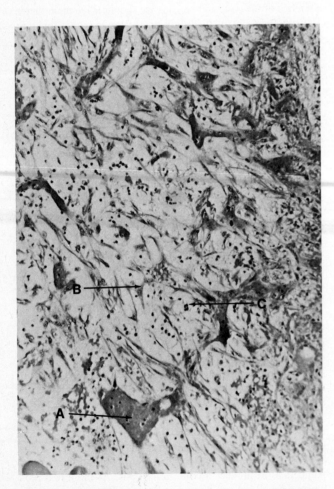

FIG. 6-10. Granulation tissue. The constituents are capillaries *(A)*, fibroblasts *(B)*, and leukocytes *(C)*.

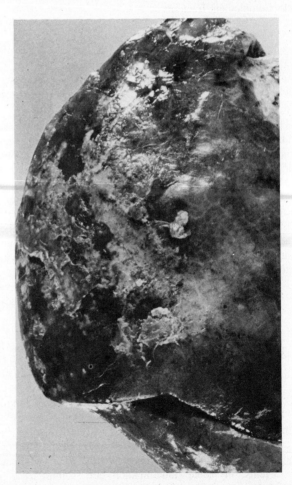

FIG. 6-11. Fibrinous inflammation. The pleural surface of the lung is covered with a shaggy layer of yellowish fibrin, which overlies an area of bronchopneumonia.

to the inflammatory changes in the mucous membranes of the nose, there is a tremendous overactivity of the mucous glands. In the later stages of a cold, mucus contains large numbers of leukocytes. This material is said to be mucopurulent.

Serous inflammation. Serous inflammation implies that the inflammatory exudate resembles serum rather than plasma, that is, it is low or deficient in fibrinogen. Serous exudates are seen when the injury causing the inflammation is slight and the vascular integrity only mildly damaged. This type of inflammation is a common response to mild superficial burns of the skin in which the blister contains a serous exudate.

Pseudomembranous inflammation. Pseudomembranous inflammation is an inflammatory process that takes place on the surface of a mucous membrane. Two factors contribute to pseudomembrane formation. First, there is an inflammatory exudate of fibrin and white cells; second, there is necrosis of the superficial layers of the mucous membrane. This is characteristically seen in diphtheria, where superficial cells, usually of the pharynx, are killed directly by diphtheria exotoxin (Fig. 6-13). It may also be an occasional adverse effect of antimicrobial therapy. In this case, the formation of the pseudomembrane formation is the result of the exotoxin of *Clostridium difficile* (Chapter 14).

Cellulitis. Cellulitis is a term used to describe acute inflammation of loose connective tissues. The organism mainly responsible for cellulitis is the β-hemolytic streptococcus, which has the ability to spread by producing enzymes such as hyaluronidase and fibrinolysins (streptokinase). Specific examples of this type of inflammation are (1) erysipelas, (2) necrotizing fasciitis, and (3) bacterial synergistic gangrene.

Erysipelas is an acute, rapidly spreading inflammation of the subcutaneous tissues, commonly seen in the face. There is little or no pus production, and the spreading edge of the area of acute, vivid red inflammation is clearly demarcated from the adjacent normal skin.

Necrotizing fasciitis is the result of virulent streptococcal infection causing the separation of skin from underlying fascia and reaching relatively avascular fascial planes. The pressure of the inflammatory fluid exudate rapidly opens up the fascial spaces. Necrotizing fasciitis is accompanied by severe systemic toxemia. A severe form of acute cellulitis of dental origin that involves the sublingual and submaxillary spaces and rapidly spreads to the retropharyngeal space is known as *Ludwig's angina*. From there, the inflammatory process may spread to the mediastinum and pleural cavities.

Another severe form of cellulitis, which is occasionally seen as a late complication of surgical wound infection, is *bacterial synergistic gangrene*. This is the result of infection by anaerobic streptococci and either *Staphylococcus aureus* or an enteric bacterium such as *Escherichia coli*. There is intense, spreading inflammation at the margins of the area around the wound, with necrosis of skin in the center of the affected area. Unlike necrotizing fasciitis, there is little associated systemic toxicity, despite the severity of the disease.

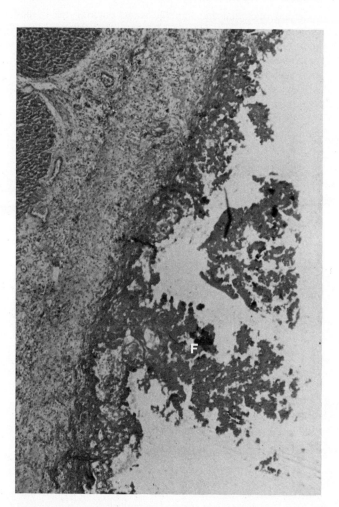

FIG. 6-12. Acute fibrinous inflammation of the pericardium in rheumatic carditis. Fibrin *(F)* appears as an amorphous granular material on the pericardial surface.

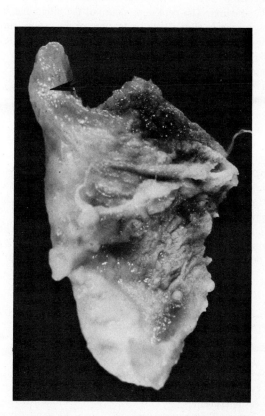

FIG. 6-13. Pseudomembranous inflammation in diphtheria. The pseudomembrane has produced a complete cast of the laryngeal area. The cast of the epiglottis *(arrow)* is clearly shown.

Chronic inflammation

Chronic inflammation implies a process that persists for a long time. It may be a sequel to unresolved acute inflammation, or the process may be chronic from the beginning. The cause may be persistence of the inflammatory stimulus or repeated stimuli. In some instances, as in syphilis and in many viral and rickettsial infections, the nature of the infecting organism initiates a reaction, which histologically has the cellular features of chronic inflammation with lymphocytes as the predominant cells but which, nevertheless, is clinically acute.

Whereas acute inflammation is characterized by an exudative phase and a cellular phase in which the neutrophil is the typical cell, chronic inflammation is largely a cellular response consisting of the following:

1. Lymphocytes
2. Plasma cells
3. Macrophages
4. Fibroblasts

The presence of lymphocytes indicates a response to antigenic stimuli, and often the appearance of plasma cells indicates local production of immunoglobulins.

Plasma cells are derived from B lymphocytes and form antibodies. Characteristically they are oval in shape, 12 by 6 μm, with an eccentric, round nucleus. With hematoxylin and eosin, the cytoplasm stains reddish-blue and the nucleus dark blue. The nuclear chromatin is arranged like the figures on the face of a clock.

Fibroblasts lay down collagen, whereas macrophages consume microbial and necrotic tissue materials in the area of inflammation. Chronic inflammation can be thought of as a "no-decision" contest between the causal stimulus and the protective reaction. The persistent nature of the inflammatory reaction results in slow tissue destruction or distortion from attempts at fibroblastic repair. The gross thickening and distortion of the intestine in Crohn's disease (Chapter 14) is a well-recognized example of chronic inflammation.

Tissue destruction is also a prominent feature of chronic inflammation, one consequence of which is the process of ulceration. An *ulcer*, by definition, is a breach of continuity of an epithelial surface. This process, combined with the other changes typical of chronic inflammation, such as fibroblastic activity and lymphocytic infiltration, is seen in peptic ulceration. Ulceration can also, of course, be an acute process. The formation of fistulas and sinuses (decribed earlier in this chapter) in acute inflammation can also be the result of chronic inflammatory changes.

There is no sharp dividing line between acute and chronic inflammation, but clinically inflammation is regarded as acute if it develops in a matter of hours or days and persists for little longer. Chronic inflammation, by contrast, lasts for weeks, months, or years. Transition from acute to chronic or chronic to acute can also be seen; as a consequence, the histologic picture may be mixed. The essential differences between acute and chronic inflammation are summarized in Table 6-3. Chronic inflammation can develop under the following circumstances:

1. *Chronic inflammation as a sequel to acute*—In cases where the agent that caused acute inflammation is not eradicated, the reaction continues. Possibly the best example is staphylococcal osteomyelitis (Chapter 17). In this disease there is initial acute suppurative inflammation in which bone is killed. The bacteria can then live on in the necrotic bone, inaccessible to the body's defenses.
2. *Chronic inflammation without an acute phase*—Bacteria and other agents, including brucellosis and sterile foreign bodies, do not provoke an acute inflammatory response.
3. *Acute-on-chronic inflammation*—It is not uncommon to find an acute inflammatory reaction superimposed on a chronic one. A common pathologic example is the thickened, chronically inflamed appendix in which evidence of recent acute inflammation in the form of pus formation or fibrinous exudation is readily identified.

Granulomatous inflammation
Cellular components

Certain microbial and mineral agents entering the tissues excite a special form of chronic inflammation called *granulomatous inflammation*. It is characterized by a unique cell called the *epithelioid cell*. The epithelioid cell is probably derived from the macrophage that has been exposed to certain specific antigens, for example, the tuberculoprotein present in *Mycobacterium tuberculosis*.

In histologic sections these cells are pale staining with indistinct cell membranes that merge with those of the surrounding cells to form a network or *syncytium*. Further fusion of cytoplasmic membranes results in the formation of multinucleate giant cells.

A circumscribed collection of epithelioid cells with or without giant cells is called a *granuloma*. This is the characteristic microscopic lesion in tuberculosis, certain fungal infections (histoplasmosis, for example), and sarcoidosis.

In granulomatous inflammation, multinucleate giant cells are frequently present. These are round or oval, up to 50 μm in diameter, and contain numerous nuclei, which are often crowded into a circle or horseshoe arrangement around the periphery of the cell. Such cells are called Langhans' giant cells.* They are formed by the fusion of neighboring epithelioid

---

*Theodor Langhans (1839-1915), German pathologist.

TABLE 6-3. Comparison of features of acute and chronic inflammation

	Acute	*Chronic*
Vascular reaction	Prominent	Less conspicuous
Clinical signs of vascular changes	Warmth, redness, edema	"Cold" swelling
Cellular infiltration	Polymorphs	Mononuclear: lymphocytes, macrophages, plasma cells
Pus formation	Characteristic	Not characteristic
Connective tissue component	Inconspicuous in early stages	Prominent, may produce firm swelling
Pain (effect of mediators)	Often severe	Often absent
Associated immune reactions	Inconspicuous	Often conspicuous and may be contributory

cells, following which the newly formed giant cells lose their phagocytic function.

Langhans' giant cells should be distinguished from *foreign body giant cells* (Fig. 6-14) in which the nuclei are usually scattered indiscriminately throughout the cytoplasm of the cell. Foreign body giant cells are formed in the inflammatory reactions that surround foreign material, for example, surgical silk in tissues. The essential difference between the two forms of giant cells seems to be that sensitization of macrophages precedes the formation of the Langhans' type but does not happen in the case of foreign body reactions.

The causes of granulomatous inflammation are listed below. The pathology of tuberculosis is a classic example of this reaction.

Causes of granulomatous inflammation:
1. Infectious
    a. Mycobacterial infections
        (1) Tuberculosis
        (2) Atypical mycobacteriosis
        (3) Leprosy
    b. Fungal infections
        (1) Blastomycosis
        (2) Cryptococcosis
        (3) Coccidioidomycosis
        (4) Histoplasmosis
    c. Treponemal infection
        (1) Syphilis
        (2) Yaws
    d. Parasitic infestation
        (1) Schistosomiasis
2. Noninfectious
    a. Berylliosis
3. Cause unknown
    a. Sarcoidosis

Histologic structure of the granuloma

The specific feature of the granuloma is a rounded collection of epithelioid cells, which form the bulk of the inflammatory focus. Often Langhans' giant cells are scattered among them (Fig. 6-15). Surrounding the epithelioid cells is a zone of lymphocytes as well as a few plasma cells; finally, there is an outer zone of fibroblasts and strands of collagen. In tuberculosis and some fungal infections the core of the lesion may show caseous necrosis. This is a whitish, cheeselike material (Fig. 6-16) that microscopically stains pink with a bluish tinge. The latter is due to fine particulate remnants of cell nuclei (nuclear dust) (see also Chapter 2).

Variations in the cellular elements of the granuloma are found with different etiologic agents. Neutrophils are often present in mycotic (fungal) granulomas, whereas eosinophils are plentiful

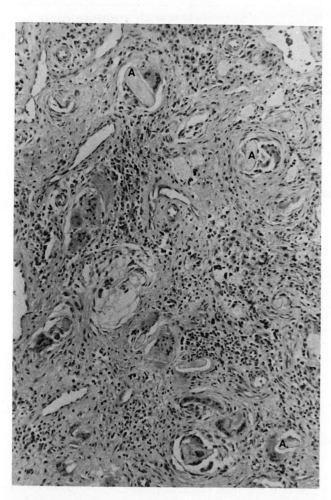

FIG. 6-14. Foreign body reaction. Foreign material *(A)* is surrounded by inflammatory cells, connective tissue, and capillaries. Numerous foreign body giant cells are shown.

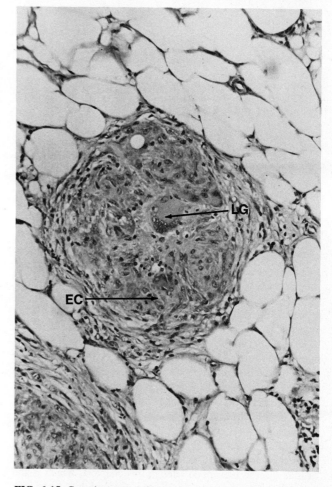

FIG. 6-15. Granulomatous inflammation. The nodule from peritoneal fat consists of pale indistinct epithelioid cells *(EC)* and a typical Langhans' giant cell *(LG)*.

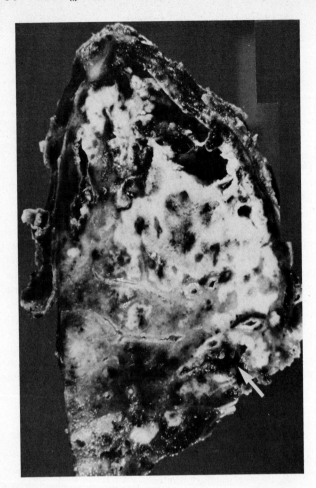

FIG. 6-16. Granulomatous inflammation with caseation and cavitation in advanced tuberculosis of the lung.

in those granulomas that form in response to the eggs of parasites such as schistosomes in the tissues. Plasma cells are prominent in syphilitic granulomas. In sarcoidosis (Chapter 12), a disease of unknown cause, the granuloma does not undergo caseation.

Other "granulomas"

The term *granuloma* is also used in several ways, with less specific meaning than in the descriptions just given, in which the presence of epithelioid cells is the essential feature. The word *granuloma* as it was originally used by Virchow* meant a tumorlike swelling caused by chronic inflammation. It consisted of *granulation tissue*—that is, was composed essentially of new blood vessels, fibroblasts and their products, and inflammatory cells. This broader definition is still widely used today in a clinical setting.

Several other pathologic entities include *granuloma* in their names. Examples are (1) eosinophilic granuloma of bone, which is a localized area of abnormally proliferating histiocytes accompanied by eosinophils (Chapter 13); (2) Wegener's granulomatosis, which is a serious form of vasculitis that affects the respiratory tract (Chapter 10); and (3) chronic granulomatous disease (described later in this chapter), which is the result of defective bacterial killing by neutrophils. The lesions

---

*Rudolph Virchow (1821-1902), distinguished German pathologist.

typically show acute inflammation usually caused by *Staphylococcus aureus* or gram-negative bacteria. Thus the name of the disease is misleading. Nodules of proliferating granulation tissue are also often defined clinically as "granulomas." One of the most common examples is the apical granuloma, which forms at the apex of a dead and infected tooth. Again, *granuloma*, when used in this sense, is a clinical term; these lesions do not have the histologic structure described earlier.

Role of the lymphocyte in chronic inflammation and granuloma formation

Cell-mediated immune responses are discussed more fully in the following chapter, but lymphocytes play an important role in chronic and granulomatous inflammation.

Cell-mediated immune responses to infection are seen, most typically in the tuberculin reaction (Chapter 12). In a patient who has had tuberculosis (even if subclinically), the resulting immunologic response causes an inflammatory reaction in the skin around the injection site. This is the result of a cell-mediated immune response, and histologically the lesions show a predominantly mononuclear cell infiltrate consisting of lymphocytes and epithelioid cells (i.e., a typical granuloma).

Lymphocyte mediators. Lymphocyte mediators appear to play a major role in granuloma formation. These mediators are known as *lymphokines,* which are discussed in Chapter 7.

Reactions associated with inflammation

Several local and general reactions are commonly associated with severe inflammation. Certain characteristic laboratory findings are also associated.

Local reactions are *lymphangitis* and *lymphadenitis*. Generalized or systemic reactions include fever and leukocytosis (see Chapter 8). Laboratory evidence of inflammatory disease is demonstrated by an elevation of the erythrocyte sedimentation rate (ESR) and the appearance in the blood of C-reactive protein. The ESR is particularly influenced by the composition of the plasma proteins especially the α-2-globulins and fibrinogen. In severe inflammation, the relative levels of these proteins are altered, and they are the main cause of the increase in ESR. The ESR returns to normal with resolution of the inflammatory process and can therefore be used to monitor the course of some inflammatory diseases such as rheumatoid arthritis. C-reactive protein is an abnormal "acute-phase" protein that appears in the plasma of patients with major inflammatory disease. C-reactive protein is so-called because it reacts fortuitously, in a precipitin test with the C polysaccharide of *Streptococcus pneumoniae*. Although it is slightly more sensitive than the ESR, the two tests give virtually the same information.

Lymphangitis and lymphadenitis

The main function of the lymphatic system is to return plasma protein lost from the blood vessels to the circulation via the thoracic duct. The lymphatic system is thus extremely important in inflammation, particularly when inflammation is caused by microorganisms and when there is greatly increased loss of plasma protein from inflamed blood vessels. The earliest lymphatic reaction is dilatation of the lymph vessels and increased flow of lymph from the inflamed area to the regional lymph nodes. If the inflammatory process involves the lymphatic vessels, *lymphangitis* is present. This is seen vividly in hemolytic streptococcal infections of the extremities in which the progress of the infection is marked by red lines running up the skin of the arm or leg.

Lymph nodes, which drain areas of inflammation, frequently become enlarged and sometimes painful and tender. This is called *lymphadenitis*. If severe enough, suppuration of the lymph node may result. The characteristic histologic appearance in lymphadenitis is mainly caused by an increase in the activity of cells in the germinal centers. Immature lymphocytes and macrophages increase considerably so that the lymph follicles become enlarged with many pale-staining young cells and with only a rim of mature lymphocytes at the periphery. Inside the follicles cellular debris derived from inflammatory cells undergoes active phagocytosis by histiocytes. This process in the lymph nodes is called *reactive follicular hyperplasia*.

Lymph nodes play an important part in regional defense against infection. Because lymph nodes are in communication with the bloodstream by way of the thoracic duct system, they prevent infections from reaching the systemic circulation and help defend against the many serious complications of septicemia.

Connective tissue reaction in inflammation

Proliferation of fibroblasts is a characteristic and essential feature of the inflammatory response. It starts somewhat inconspicuously in the early stages of acute inflammation and is most prominent in chronic inflammation. The fibrous tissue that forms as a consequence of this activity is partly defensive and partly reparative.

The defensive function of fibrous proliferation is seen by the way in which an abscess becomes walled off, and densely fibrotic lymph nodes can incarcerate live *Mycobacterium tuberculosis*. On the other hand, the importance of this reaction should not be overestimated, since fibrosis can only contain infection if other cellular defense mechanisms are intact. The second function of fibrous proliferation is in healing and repair.

TISSUE REPAIR

The ideal function of the reparative process is to restore dead or disrupted tissue to its normal state. The achievement of this ideal state is limited by the types of cells of which the injured tissue is composed. Three basic cell types are recognized in this context namely *permanent, stable,* and *labile cells.*

Restoration of normal structure and function is absent or rare in the case of permanent cells; it is frequent with stable cells and virtually always takes place with labile cells. Examples of these cell types follow:

Permanent cells	*Stable cells*	*Labile cells*
Neurons	Renal tubules	Epidermis
Cardiac myocytes	Liver	Intestinal mucosa
	Pancreas	Bronchial mucosa
	Adrenal cortex	Bone marrow

Even with some permanent cells, however, there may be attempts at restoration of the damaged tissue. Neuronal axons, if severed, will attempt to restore their continuity if the cell body is intact. Skeletal and cardiac muscle, however, are always repaired by connective tissue. Where restoration of normal architecture fails, there is repair by fibrous scar tissue. This has its most dramatic effect in heart muscle damaged by ischemia.

Tissue repair and organization

A fine distinction is drawn between tissue repair and organization. The term *organization* is reserved for the removal and replacement of *nonviable* substances by macrophage action, vascularization, and fibroblast activity. The nonviable substances include clot, thrombus, and necrotic tissue. Tissue repair, on the other hand, implies restoration of living tissue. Both processes are very similar and frequently can continue side by side.

Repair by fibrous tissue

Fibrous tissue repair has been studied in its purest form in clean, incised surgical wounds of the skin, where the divided edges have been kept in close apposition. This is the situation the surgeon tries to create every time a "clean" surgical operation is performed. This is healing by primary union.

Primary union

The narrow space formed by the surgical incision initially contains a small amount of blood clot. The margins of the wound undergo a mild inflammatory reaction with its typical vascular and cellular components, releasing plasma and polymorphs into the incised space. This reaction lasts 24 to 48 hours. After approximately 24 hours, capillary vessels in the margins begin to bud into the wound, bringing with them macrophages and fibroblasts. The macrophages remove the small amount of cellular debris and hemosiderin derived from hemoglobin breakdown. The fibroblasts begin to lay down extracellular matrix including collagen of both type I and type III structure (Chapter 1). Meanwhile the epidermis begins the restorative process, both by lateral movement of basal cells across the epidermal gap (emigration) and by proliferation of the basal epidermal cells. The small epidermal gap is thus rapidly filled by these two processes, first as a single basal layer, then as these cells proliferate and mature, by the typical multilayered structure of the epidermis.

By the fifth day, the narrow space in the dermis has been filled with fine vascularized connective tissue and ground substance. The macrophages have removed most of the debris from the original hemorrhage and inflammation, and the epidermis has been restored to its normal thickness. At this stage the wound edges will usually maintain apposition without sutures. From then on there is increasing deposition of collagen and decreasing vascularity of the wound. The tensile strength of the collagen gradually increases and there is some degree of remodeling of the scar tissue, partly resulting from the action of collagenases and the effects of local mechanical stress on the wound site. By 2 or 3 weeks, the scar is sound and relatively avascular. This process for many years was also called healing by first intention.

Secondary union

Secondary union is the process in which large gaps in tissue are repaired. There is initially hemorrhage into the wound, with fibrin and blood cells filling the defect. As in primary union, mild, short-lived acute inflammation develops in the margin of the wound. Meanwhile phagocytic activity removes the debris from the surface of the wound, leaving an exposed area of granulation tissue. As collagen is laid down in the deeper layers of the wound, granulation tissue gradually fills in the defect from below. As successive layers of collagen are formed in the

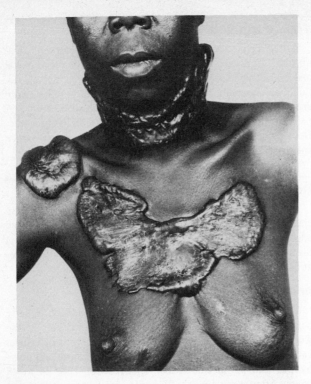

FIG. 6-17. Massive keloid formation in an African woman. *(Courtesy Curator of the Gordon Museum, Guy's Hospital, London, England.)*

granulation tissue, the wound starts to contract as a result of the contractile properties of fibroblasts. These cells are referred to as myofibroblasts because they also have both structural and functional properties of smooth muscle cells. Largely under their influence the wound edges are pulled together, decreasing the size of the wound. Finally, as the gap is closed by a combination of granulation tissue and contraction, the epithelium reunites across the surface of the wound. The connective tissue scar is initially thick and excessive in amount, but normally in time the scar tissue decreases somewhat as a result of lysis of collagen. This process appears to be defective in some people, in particular those of black races. The excessive exuberant connective tissue formed in granulating wounds is called *keloid* (Fig. 6-17). In some African tribes keloid formation as a result of ritual scarification, often of the face, is considered a mark of distinction and beauty.

In primary union (if the injury is slight) skin appendages may regenerate; but with the more severe injuries that are followed by secondary union, there is complete loss of sweat glands, sebaceous glands, and specialized nerve endings and disappearance of hair follicles.

Similar processes to those just described for skin take place in the mucous membranes and solid organs subjected to similar damage. Thus surgical incisions of the bowel wall should repair by primary union with minimal scarring and reunion of the divided mucosa. On the other hand, a large defect such as a peptic ulcer may heal by granulation and, if healing is complete, will be characterized by radial scarring caused by wound contraction. Unfortunately, healing is not always achieved.

Repair of bone

One tissue which has the property of restoring itself completely after injury is bone. However, it must be said that when bones are fractured, their restoration to normal form would rarely be achieved without the application of the basic principles of orthopedics, namely:

1. *Reduction* of the fracture, that is, restoration of the bone to its normal anatomic alignment
2. *Immobilization* of the fracture so that movement between the fracture ends is prevented

The following process, which describes the healing of a fractured long bone, assumes that accurate reduction and adequate immobilization have been achieved.

When a long bone, such as the humerus, is broken at midshaft, the periosteum is partly torn. However, the partially intact periostium is strong enough in most cases to allow the fragments to be externally manipulated into good anatomic alignment and held there, for example, by a plaster cast. In other bones, whether because of peculiarities of the fracture site or the unusual nature of the fracture, open surgical reduction is necessary for good functional results. This usually calls for the insertion of metal plates or pins as a means of internal fixation. For example, fractures of the neck of the femur are mostly treated by inserting a nail to stabilize the fragments and allow the patient to walk within a short time.

At the time of the fracture there is bleeding into the fracture site, clotting of the blood, and formation of a *hematoma*—a tumorlike mass of effused blood. A mild inflammatory reaction takes place in this site, leading to phagocytosis of the breakdown products of the hematoma by macrophages. Capillary vessels grow into the fibrin network, which is predominantly on the external surface of the bone, bringing with them osteoblasts and chondroblasts derived from the inner layers of the periosteum. These cells begin to form extracellular matrix and new cartilage develops at the fracture site. In 7 or 8 days the area in and around the fracture consists of abundant soft vascular connective tissue that contains small islands of cartilage. This tissue is called the *provisional callus*. The process begins on either side of the fracture line, with callus formation progressing axially to seal the gap between the fracture ends. At this stage a little calcification may be seen on a radiograph of the fracture site.

Osteoblasts now begin to lay down firmer osteoid tissue within the provisional callus. This is followed by deposition of calcium salts, and under optimum conditions, the provisional callus is replaced completely by a mass of incompletely organized bone (the *definitive* or *bony* callus) in 4 or 5 weeks.

At this stage the fracture site is stable but surrounded by a large irregular mass of bone. Remodeling of this bone to its normal shape and dimensions now takes place by means of osteoclastic activity. As the limb is used again, the haversian systems reform partly at least because of the effects of physical stress. Finally, the marrow cavity reforms; within 6 to 9 months of the injury, little evidence of the fracture remains. Unlike bone, cartilage is repaired almost exclusively by fibrous tissue.

Factors impairing healing of fractures

Several factors may interfere with the ideal process described. It is worth repeating that alignment and immobilization are essential. If these are not achieved, malunion, that is inadequate or deformed union, is very likely. One undesirable effect that can follow poor fracture alignment is *fibrous union*. In this condition abundant collagen is initially laid down between the bone fragments. This collagen calcifies poorly, if at all, leaving an ineffective, unstable bond at the fracture site. Fibrous union can also be the result of local ischemia or severe periosteal damage. Other factors that predispose to delayed union or nonunion include:

1. The nature of the fracture itself
2. Excessive bleeding at the fracture site
3. Infection
4. Nutritional status of the patient

Nature of the fracture. The anatomic site and degree of bone damage have a bearing on the healing of a fracture. Certain bones, largely because of the peculiarity of their blood supply, heal poorly or slowly when fractured. Thus the scaphoid bone in the wrist frequently heals inadequately following fracture and may undergo avascular necrosis as a result of lack of blood supply to one fragment. Where numerous small bone fragments are produced (a comminuted fracture), the blood supply to some of the fragments is likely to be lost; realignment and immobilization may be difficult, thus creating the conditions for delayed union or malunion. Soft tissue between the ends of the fracture can also prevent normal repair. Fractures of weight-bearing bones often require prolonged immobilization before normal function can be resumed.

Hemorrhage. Excessive bleeding into the fracture site may occur as a result of the severity of the injury and damage to major vessels or as a result of ineffective hemostasis such as in hemophilia. In these circumstances, there is excessive formation of the early provisional callus, which prolongs both the time taken to form the definitive callus and the remodeling process.

Infection. Bacterial infection usually follows a compound fracture, that is, one in which the overlying skin is disrupted permitting entrance of bacteria. Infection is a major, sometimes catastrophic event following a fracture, because the conditions in the tissues are ideal for bacterial proliferation. When open reduction of a fracture is performed, the greatest hazard is the introduction of infectious agents.

Nutritional status. Even when the blood supply to a fractured bone is intact, the general nutritional state of the patient may interfere with proper repair. Deficiencies of vitamins C and D, abnormalities of calcium and phosphorus metabolism and their hormonal control, and severe protein-calorie malnutrition may interfere with normal healing.

Pathologic fractures. A pathologic fracture is one which results from localized or generalized weakening of bone by disease. Fracture of the neck of the femur in elderly persons as a result of osteoporosis (Chapter 14) is a common example of a pathologic fracture caused by generalized bone disease. An example of pathologic fracture resulting from localized bone disease is seen when a fracture is at the site of a bone tumor. In the majority of cases, the injury causing the fracture is trivial; hence the term *spontaneous fracture* is sometimes used synonymously with pathologic fracture. The causes of pathologic fractures are listed below:

Causes of pathologic fractures
1. Congenital
   a. Osteogenesis imperfecta
   b. Osteopetrosis
2. Nutritional and metabolic
   a. Osteoporosis
   b. Osteitis fibrosis cystica
   c. Rickets/osteomalacia
   d. Scurvy
3. Bone cysts
4. Bone tumors
   a. Benign
   b. Malignant
      (1) Primary
      (2) Metastatic
5. Unknown
   a. Paget's disease of bone

Control of reparative processes

The mechanisms that initiate, control, and terminate normal reparative processes are still largely unknown. Mechanisms that may have roles in these functions include:

1. Contact inhibition
2. Humoral inhibitors of cell growth and proliferation
3. Growth factors

Contact inhibition

In artificial monolayer cultures, many types of cells grow actively until they completely cover the available surface area. When this stage is reached, proliferation stops. If neighboring cells are removed, proliferation begins again. The loss of contact between cells caused by injury and its restoration of continuity is a possible mechanism by which repair of epithelium is initiated and then stopped.

Humoral inhibitors

The existence of hormonelike substances that are produced by growing cells and that are capable of stopping cell growth has been postulated. The term *chalone* has been coined for such substances. The existence of such a neat negative feedback system for control of cell proliferation, however, has not been demonstrated.

Growth factors

Several biologic substances have been described in the last 10 years or so that can stimulate cell growth. Such substances have been derived from platelets, macrophages, fibroblasts, and other cells. Platelet-derived growth factors (PDGFs) are among the best characterized of these substances. They are polypeptides, which have been shown to have a variety of effects, especially the stimulation of DNA synthesis and mitotic activity. The role of these and other growth promoting substances, such as somatomedin, which is released from the liver by the action of growth hormone is not known.

Factors that influence soft tissue inflammation and repair

Factors known to alter in some way the outcome of inflammation and repair were mentioned previously on p. 80.

Foreign bodies

Foreign bodies within wounds frequently stimulate inflammation, which, if persistent, impedes the healing of a wound. The presence of foreign bodies causes persistent invasion of phagocytic cells. In some instances, they are polymorphs; in others, especially where insoluble particulate matter is present, macrophages and foreign body giant cells predominate. The inflammatory process tends to continue as long as the foreign material is present. The development of special metals such as Vitallium (Howmedica Inc.) and synthetic polymers such as Dacron (Dupont) that excite little or no inflammatory response has permitted such major advances in surgery as replacement of bones, joints, major vessels, and heart valves. However, if inflammation caused by infection is associated with these prostheses, it will seldom resolve unless the prosthesis is removed.

Infection

Infection, particularly bacterial infection of wounds, is a major obstacle to normal healing because it promotes further inflammation and tissue destruction. Not infrequently infection and foreign bodies cooperate in frustrating primary union.

Age and nutritional status

Elderly people usually heal more slowly than the young, but there is little evidence that the end result of healing is in any way inferior as a result of age alone. However, elderly people have a greater incidence of vascular disease, which can interfere with healing.

The nutritional status of the individual may influence the reparative response. In some situations this too may complicate the effects attributed to age. However, at all ages, major deficiencies of vitamin C (scurvy) and protein can singly or together interfere with collagen synthesis and result in delayed healing and a weakened wound.

Concurrent disease

In addition to scurvy, interference with inflammation and repair is associated with many other disorders. Among these are the following:
1. Diabetes mellitus
2. Vascular disease
3. Uremia
4. Blood diseases and white cell dysfunction

In diabetes mellitus, two major combinations of factors contribute to inflammation and ineffective repair: (1) atherosclerosis and ischemia and (2) increased severity of and possibly increased susceptibility to microbial infections. Vascular disease, which is frequently associated with diabetes, reduces blood supply; this impairs the reparative process. The leg is a frequent site of obstructive arterial disease in diabetics, and minor injuries to the leg often fail to heal and may persist for long periods. Similarly, venous stasis, which accompanies varicose veins, significantly interferes with healing. Those patients who develop varicose ulcers of the leg are usually doomed to suffer the disease until the vascular abnormality has been corrected by surgery.

Whether infections are actually more frequent in diabetics is debatable. Most, however, would agree that infections in diabetics tend to be more severe; among the mechanisms contributing to the severity of infections in diabetes are (1) diminished chemotaxis and (2) impaired phagocytic function of neutrophils.

Patients with elevated blood levels of urea (uremia) have an impaired inflammatory response as a result of at least three different abnormalities: (1) diminished chemotaxis, (2) decreased circulating lymphocytes, and (3) suppression of delayed hypersensitivity. Several blood diseases interfere significantly with inflammation and repair. Hemorrhagic disease from any cause frequently results in excessive bleeding into sites of injury. The resulting large hematomas can physically interfere with healing, as in fractures, and may also predispose to bacterial infection. In aplastic anemia or agranulocytosis there are no white cells to participate in the inflammatory process.

Patients with leukemia, lymphoma, or myeloma do not have sufficient numbers of effective phagocytic white cells because the sites of production of these cells in the bone marrow, spleen, or lymph nodes have been replaced by nonfunctioning malignant cells. Infections that normally stimulate cellular defenses are therefore common complications of these malignancies. Significantly, many of these diseases are caused by organisms that rarely cause infection in the intact host and are therefore known as *opportunistic infections*. Primary defects of white cells, which are the result of abnormalities within the white cells themselves, are uncommon causes of defective inflammation.

Immunosuppressive drugs

Glucocorticoid drugs, which are widely used, have a major inhibitory effect on inflammation and repair. In general, drugs such as hydrocortisone and prednisolone act to suppress inflammation, and appear to do so at several different stages of the inflammatory process. First, they prevent attachment of white cells to vascular endothelium. Second, they have inhibitory effects on vascular permeability and leukocyte migration. Third, because of their ability to stabilize biologic membranes, they interfere with the release of enzymes from lysosomes.

Corticosteroids also interfere with repair by inhibiting protein synthesis, which, in turn, inhibits collagen formation.

Defects of leukocyte function

Susceptibility to infection is greatly increased if neutrophils are too few or if the neutrophils are functionally defective. As shown in Table 6-4, there are a great many of these defects, which may affect microbial killing mechanisms, phagocytosis, or motility.

Disorders of microbial killing mechanisms

Impaired hydrogen peroxide production. Impaired hydrogen peroxide production is the main defect in *chronic granulomatous disease* (CGD), of which several forms are now recognized.

CGD is usually inherited as an X-linked recessive trait; the neutrophils in this disease are defective in cytochrome b-558.

CGD is characterized by multiple recurrent infections of skin, lymph nodes, lungs, and bones. The disease usually starts in childhood and often causes death by the age of 7 years. CGD can also affect adults in whom there is an autosomal mode of inheritance. In this form of the disease cytochrome b-558 is present but does not function. In CGD, the neutrophils are unable to produce sufficient metabolic energy to form hydrogen peroxide. This leads to the following paradoxical situation. Some bacteria produce catalase (which destroys hydrogen peroxide), while others do not. Patients with CGD therefore develop serious infections by catalase-producing bacteria, particularly *Staphylococcus aureus*. On the other hand, affected patients are not susceptible to infection by noncatalase producers such as *Streptococcus pneumoniae* because these bacteria are able to produce enough free hydrogen peroxide as a metabolic product to operate the myeloperoxidase-halide system inside the phagocytes. These organisms therefore contribute to their own destruction. Catalase-positive bacteria, on the other hand, destroy the small amounts of hydrogen peroxide that they themselves produce and therefore survive phagocytosis. Deficiency of glutathione peroxidase, an enzyme that acts earlier in the chain of electron transport than cytochrome also results in defective hydrogen peroxide production and causes CGD. Hydrogen peroxide production is also impaired in glucose 6-phosphate dehydrogenase (G6PD) deficiency (Chapter 13) but only in severe cases where the levels of G6PD are near zero.

A common abnormality that is fortunately only occasionally of clinical significance is *myeloperoxidase deficiency*. The leukocytes in this condition still possess other means of oxidative killing of organisms. Thus the killing process is slow but still effective, and adverse clinical effects are unusual. However, there is an increased association of myeloperoxidase deficiency with fungal infections, especially when the deficiency is secondary to one of the myeloproliferative disorders.

Specific granule deficiency. In this autosomal recessive abnormality, the neutrophil specific granules fail to synthesize. Absence of these granules deprives the neutrophils of antimicrobial properties, such as those of lactoferrin, for example. Similarly, deficiency of primary granules results in the absence of the antimicrobial proteins known as defensins.

Specific granule deficiency is associated with a depressed inflammatory response and recurrent cutaneous and soft tissue infections.

Disorders of phagocytosis

Phagocytosis can be impaired in three main ways:
1. Attachment may be defective as a result of inadequate opsonization of the microorganisms.

2. Engulfment may be impaired.
3. Degranulation may be impaired and the discharge of the granules into the phagosome fails.

Opsonin deficiencies may be caused by defective formation of immune globulins as in hypoagammaglobulinemia or agammaglobulinemia. Alternatively, complement deficiencies may result, especially of C3. Sickle cell disease is probably the most common disease in which an opsonin deficiency is seen. In this condition there is lack of a specific opsonin for pneumococci, resulting in an increased susceptibility to pneumococcal infection.

An important aspect of neutrophil adherence is the role of glycoprotein receptors such as CR3, the receptor for the opsonic fragment (C3b) of complement. Rare cases of *CR3 deficiency* have been described. This is an autosomal recessive abnormality that affects lymphocytes and macrophages as well as neutrophils. Those affected have frequent mucocutaneous infections, recurrent otitis media, severe gingivitis and periodontitis, and often severe pulmonary bacterial or fungal infections.

Other diseases in which defective opsonization is observed include cirrhosis of the liver and lupus erythematosus.

Defective engulfment is mainly caused by drugs, particularly morphine analogs; but these rarely cause sufficiently impaired ingestion of bacteria by phagocytes to have a significant clinical effect. The Chédiak-Higashi syndrome (Fig. 6-18), a rare autosomal recessive disorder, is an example of impaired degranulation. It is characterized by giant lysosomes in the leukocytes and other cells, which include thyroid, renal tubular, and melanin-producing cells. Affected patients are partially albino and have increased susceptibility to infection. The giant lysosomes in the leukocytes fail to fuse with phagosomes with the result that degranulation is defective and discharge of lysosomal contents into the phagocytic vacuole is decreased.

Drugs, particularly, corticosteroids and antimalarial agents, also impair degranulation, but the clinical significance is not known. As mentioned earlier, degranulation fails when normal macrophages engulf tubercle bacilli or the protozoon *Toxoplasma gondii*. The reason for this failure of lysosome-phagosome fusion is not known, but the prolonged intracellular survival of these organisms can have long-term adverse consequences for the host.

TABLE 6-4. Defects of leukocyte function

Defect	Clinical syndromes
Neutropenia	Agranulocytosis; aplastic anemia
	Cyclic neutropenia
	Leukemias
Disorders of microbial killing mechanisms	Chédiak-Higashi syndrome
	Chronic granulomatous disease
	Drugs (e.g., hydrocortisone, sulfonamides)
	G6PD deficiency
	Glutathione peroxidase deficiency
	Impaired hydrogen peroxide production
	Myeloperoxidase deficiency
	Specific granule deficiency
Disorders of phagocytosis	Chédiak-Higashi syndrome
	Complement deficiencies (C3, C5)
	Drugs (e.g., morphine analogs, colchicine corticosteroids, antimalarials)
	Hypogammaglobulinemia
	Hypophosphatemia
	Impaired engulfment
	Impaired degranulation
	Opsonin deficiencies
	Sickle cell disease
Disorders of adherence migration and chemotaxis	Chédiak-Higashi syndrome
	Chemotactic factor inactivators in serum
	Complement deficiencies
	C3R receptor deficiency
	Diabetes mellitus
	Inhibitors of phagocyte locomotion
	Inhibitors in serum
	Intrinsic cellular dysfunctions
	Job's syndrome
	Lazy leukocyte syndrome
	Rheumatoid arthritis
	Uremia

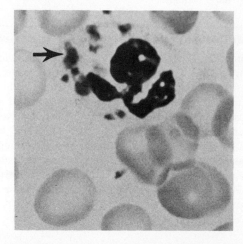

FIG. 6-18. Polymorphonuclear leukocyte in Chédiak-Higashi syndrome. There are prominent large cytoplasmic granules *(arrow)* in the cytoplasm. These are formed by giant lysosomes, which cause defective degranulation.

Disorders of motility and chemotaxis

If the motility of leukocytes is impaired, they are unable to reach sites of infection. These disorders can result from (1) defects in the leukocytes themselves, (2) the presence of inhibitors of motility, and (3) deficiency of chemotactic factors.

Intrinsic cell defects. In the Chédiak-Higashi syndrome, in addition to the defects already described, the motility of the leukocytes is impaired, thus contributing to the susceptibility to infection.

Lazy leukocyte syndrome. The lazy leukocyte syndrome appears to be associated with a primary defect of leukocyte motility. There is neutropenia and increased susceptibility to infection.

In diabetes mellitus, the leukocytes show impaired motility, which can be experimentally rectified by incubating the cells in a medium containing glucose and insulin.

Job's syndrome. Job's syndrome, consisting of hyperimmunoglobulin E, eczema and recurrent staphylococcal infections, is associated with a defect in leukocyte chemotaxis. Demonstration of the chemotactic defect can only be readily achieved at the time the eczema is active.

Inhibitors of leukocyte motility. A few patients apparently possess inhibitory factors in their serum but no other detectable abnormalities. These patients suffer from recurrent infections. In rheumatoid arthritis, leukocyte motility is impaired. This may be the result of the effects of circulating rheumatoid factor complexes on the leukocytes. Leukocyte motility is also impaired when patients have high IgG levels. Certain drugs, particularly corticosteroids and phenylbutazone derivatives, have also been reported to inhibit leukocyte motility.

Deficiencies of chemotactic factors. Complement deficiencies may be the result of a genetic defect or they may be abnormalities of the C3 or C5 components, which generate chemotactic fragments. However, the increased susceptibility to infection associated with these disorders is probably caused by the deficient opsonizing capacity of the serum rather than a lack of chemotactic factors. In sites of infection the bacteria probably release sufficiently strong chemotactic factors to render the complement-derived fragments inessential.

Very high levels of chemotactic factor inhibitors (CFI) have been described in patients with Hodgkin's disease and may contribute to the increased susceptibility to infection experienced by these patients.

Harmful effects of inflammation and repair

Inflammation is justifiably regarded as a valuable defensive reaction, and this is valid in the vast majority of cases. Less often inflammation can do more harm than good, as in rheumatoid arthritis in which severe joint injury is the end result. The reparative process, such as is found in heart valves following rheumatic fever, can also have unfortunate consequences for cardiac function. A more common example of problems caused by the healing reaction is the formation of adhesions, that is, fibrous bands, formed in the peritoneal cavity as a result of infection or foreign body reactions. These adhesions can cause obstruction of the gastrointestinal tract.

Inflammation and cancer

There are two aspects of the relationship between inflammation and cancer. First, it has been argued that chronic inflammation can be precancerous. Second, cancer often provokes an inflammatory reaction, and many now believe that this helps to limit the spread of tumors.

There is little evidence that inflammation alone can cause cancer. Nevertheless, cancer is an occasional complication of long-standing inflammation, particularly of ulceration of the leg secondary to impaired venous drainage or of long-standing chronic osteomyelitis. In these circumstances, the inflammation persists for many years before carcinoma develops. The mechanism of malignant change and its relationship to the inflammatory process are unknown. The postulated role of inflammation in limiting the spread of tumors is highly controversial (Chapter 7).

Selected readings

Amman AJ: Immunodeficiency diseases. In Stites DP, Stobo JD, and Fundenberg HH, editors: Basic and clinical immunology, Los Altos, 1984, Lange Medical Books.

Anderson DC and Springer TA: Leukocyte adhesion dysfunction, Annu Rev Med 38:175, 1987.

Bachner RL: Neutrophil dysfunction associated with states of chronic and recurrent infection, Pediatr Clin N Am 27:377, 1980.

Chambers TJ: Multinucleate giant cells, J Pathol 126:125, 1978.

Cohen S: Role of cell-mediated immunity in the induction of inflammatory response, Am J Pathol 88:502, 1977.

Cotran RS: New roles for the endothelium in inflammation and immunity, Am J Pathol 129:407, 1987.

D'Ardenne AJ and McGee JO'D: Fibronectin in disease, J Pathol 141:201, 1983.

Falloon J and Gallin JI: Neutrophil granules in health and disease, J Allergy Clin Immunol 77:653, 1986.

Ganz T, Selsted ME, and Szklarek D, et al: Defensins: natural peptide antibiotics of human neutrophils, J Clin Invest 76:1427, 1985.

Gospodarowicz D: Growth factors and their action in vivo and in vitro, J Pathol 141:201, 1983.

Honck JC: Inflammation: a quarter century of progress, J Invest Dermatol 67:124, 1976.

Kellermeyer RW and Graham RC: Kinins: possible physiologic and pathologic roles in man, N Engl J Med 279:754, 1968.

Limdak RL, Lewis J, and Granger G: Lymphokines, J Invest Dermatol 67:625, 1976.

Mallech MD and Gallin JI: Neutrophils in human disease, N Engl J Med 317:687, 1987.

Owen DAA: Inflammation and 5-hydroxytryptamine, Br Med Bull 43:256, 1987.

Pearsall NN and Weiser RS: The macrophage, Philadelphia, 1970, Lea & Febiger.

Salmon JA and Higgs GA: Prostaglandins and leukotrienes as inflammatory mediators, Br Med Bull 43:285, 1987.

Sevitt S: Bone repair and fracture healing in man, Edinburgh, 1981, Churchill Livingstone.

White CJ and Gallin JI: Phagocytic defects, Clin Immunol Immunopathol 40:50, 1986.

CHAPTER 7

The immune response and immunologically mediated disease

Immunology is a complex subject, but in essence, the immune system comprises a group of interacting cell types (among which lymphocytes and macrophages play key roles) whose main activity is to defend the body against infection. The immune system has its own internal regulating mechanisms that modulate its responses; however, abnormal immune responses can cause or contribute to many pathologic processes.

Immune responses can also be artificially stimulated or depressed to varying degrees. Historically, the earliest effective exploitation of the powers of the immune response was the introduction of an effective vaccine against smallpox in 1798 by Jenner,* an English country doctor. This discovery ultimately led to the worldwide elimination of this disease, which over the centuries, had killed countless millions of people.

The overwhelming importance of intact immune responses in protecting against infection has, however, been made only too apparent by the *acquired immune deficiency syndrome (AIDS)* epidemic, in which progressive damage to the immune system has (despite the great range of antimicrobrial drugs available) led to tens of thousands of deaths from uncontrollable infections and has spread worldwide. Although this disease can affect virtually any organ, it is only a single example of a means by which disordered immune responses can lead to a great variety of pathologic effects.

By contrast, for patients who require organ transplants, a serious disadvantage of a normally functioning immune system is that it will treat the engrafted organ (unless from an identical twin) as foreign and eliminate it from the body by means of rejection reactions. The discovery of the major histocompatibility complex (MHC) and of the human leukocyte antigen (HLA) system, as discussed later, has contributed greatly to the success of organ transplantation and also to the understanding of immune responses.

In addition to their clinical importance, immune reactions are widely used in the laboratory for diagnostic purposes.

Immunology has, however, become so complex a subject—which expands almost exponentially—that it is no longer possible to summarize its numerous interrelated activities in an understandable fashion in a few pages. In any case the physiology of the immune response is the province of biology or microbiology, and it seems reasonable to assume that the average reader will have an understanding of at least the elements of the subject.

However, some tables and figures have been provided to remind the reader of some salient points.

---

*Edward Jenner (1749-1828), English physician.

TABLE 7-1. Important makers of lymphocytic markers

WHO nomenclature	Function/name	Commercial monoclonal antibody*
CD1	Corticothymocytes	OKT6
CD2	Srbcr† receptor	OKT11
CD3	Mature T cells	OKT3
CD4	Helper/inducer cells	OKT4
CD8	Cytotoxic/suppressor	OKT8

*For simplicity only one commercial type (Ortho) is listed.
†Sheep red blood cell receptor.

Lymphocyte markers

Monoclonal antibodies that bind to surface markers on both B and T lymphocytes are commercially available. They are of considerable value in determining the nature and assessing the activity of lymphocytes in disease processes and for determining the cell types of lymphomas. Antibodies for T lymphocytes are more widely used since there are many subsets with different functions. There has been some lack of uniformity in nomenclature, but it has been common practice simply to refer to these subsets as T1 onwards. The cluster of differentiation (CD) system is increasingly used, and fortunately many of the CD and the earlier OK (Ortho. Kung) numbers correspond. These surface markers change as immature lymphocytes differentiate and mature. Initially they have more markers, and several are lost during maturation. Major T cell specific markers are listed in Table 7-1.

Langerhans' cells

Langerhans' cells are dendritic cells detectable in epithelia of the skin and mucous membranes by their affinity for gold chloride stain. By electron microscopy these cells are recognizable by elongated rod-shaped *Birbeck granules* (see Fig. 13-34) in the cytoplasm.

Langerhans' cells, which carry a T cell marker, are components of the macrophage-monocyte system and are also the dendritic cells of lymph nodes. The Birbeck granules appear to be part of the apparatus by which the cell can take up antigens by a process similar to pinocytosis.

Interleukins and interferons

Hormonelike mediators secreted by immunologically active cells are *lymphokines* and *monokines,* collectively known as cytokines. Particularly important examples are the *interleukins* and *interferons*, which have important activities in various disease processes as mentioned later.

Interleukin 1 (IL 1)

IL 1 is released from macrophages and was formerly known as lymphocyte activating factor (LAF); its properties include the following:

1. Augmentation of IL 2 production by T lymphocytes
2. Mitogenicity for T cells and promotion of their proliferation in response to antigens
3. Induction of mediators of inflammation, acute phase reactants and fever (IL 1 is "endogenous pyrogen" an important mediator of fever.)

Interleukin 2 (IL 2)

IL 2 (formerly known as T cell growth factor, TCGF) is released from T cells in response to the presentation of antigen in association with IL 1. IL 2 interacts with lymphocytes and macrophages in the following ways:

1. Generate certain T effector cells and, in particular, T helper cells and cytotoxic T cells
2. Generate lymphokines such as gamma interferon
3. Influence macrophage activity
4. Enhance natural killer (NK) cell activity as discussed below

IL 2 appears to be particularly important in helping to mediate normal immune responses and its production in AIDS (see below) is greatly depressed. IL 2 has therefore been given experimentally in the treatment of this disease and may ultimately prove to be a useful supplement to antiviral drugs.

Interferons

Interferon was discovered as an antiviral substance over 30 years ago. The interferons (α, β, and γ), however, comprise a family of proteins with a wide variety of activities. α and β (type 1) interferons are produced by leukocytes and fibroblasts, respectively, in response to viruses or double-stranded deoxyribonucleic acid (DNA). γ (type 2; immune) interferon is produced by T lymphocytes in response to antigens and nonspecific mitogens such as lectins.

Activities of the interferons include the following:

1. Antiviral action (Chapter 8)
2. Immunomodulatory actions
3. Possible inhibition of tumor cell proliferation

Immunomodulatory actions of interferons. Immunomodulatory actions of interferons are mainly on macrophages, lymphocytes, and NK cells.

Among other properties, interferons have *macrophage activating factor (MAF)* and *macrophage migration factor (MIF)* activities. Activation of macrophages by interferons also leads to increased expression of receptors for the Fc fragment (FcR) of immunoglobulins. Effects of this include increased ability to phagocytose immune complexes (see below) and to lyse antibody-coated microbes and (possibly) tumor cells.

γ Interferon, in particular, also assists macrophages in the presentation of antigens to T lymphocytes.

Interferons also act on lymphocytes and their humoral or cell-mediated responses, which are enhanced or depressed according to circumstances. In general, administration of interferon, after (but not before) sensitization of lymphocytes by antigen, enhances both humoral and cellular responses; this is probably related to the fact that γ interferon is produced relatively late in the immune response.

Other actions of interferon on lymphocyte activity continue to be demonstrated, but they are complex and their importance in vivo is by no means fully understood.

NK cells (large, granular lymphocytes that lack both T and B cell markers) have cytotoxic activity in vitro against virus-infected cells, certain types of tumor cells, and hematopoietic cells. Interferons enhance NK cell activity by a variety of possible mechanisms but can also make target cells less vulnerable to such activity.

Clinical actions of interferons. α Interferons have become available as pharmaceutical products. As yet they have only been shown to be effective in the control of a rare type of leukemia (hairy cell leukemia) which is associated with the human T cell lymphocytotrophic virus (HTLV II virus) and possibly in some other B cell malignancies such as chronic myelogenous leukemia. There is no evidence of any effect on the common solid tumors, and reports of beneficial effects of interferons on infections such as AIDS remain unconfirmed. The toxic effects of such treatment are unpleasant.

Since most, if not all, cells have interferon receptors, the mechanism of any antitumor effect of these agents is unclear. There is little evidence that interferon acts on tumors in humans via the host immune system, but it may interfere with host support of the tumor by interfering with angiogenesis or host formation of tumor stroma. A stronger possibility seems to be that interferon may act directly on tumor cells by its growth inhibitory properties and may switch off DNA synthesis in certain hemopoietic cells.

Pathologic immune responses

Immune responses, as a broad generalization, may be abnormal in either of two main ways. They may be inadequate (immunodeficiency) or their regulation may be defective. In the case of immunodeficiency, the main consequence is abnormal susceptibility to and inadequate defenses against infection. By contrast, when immunomodulation is defective, immunologic reactions cause varying degrees of damage to host tissues—these are the immunologically mediated diseases. These two categories of disease are not, however, as might be expected, mutually exclusive, and immunologically mediated disorders may complicate immunodeficiency.

IMMUNE DEFICIENCY STATES

In immune deficiency states the activity of one or more components of the immune system is defective. The main consequence is that the ability to combat infections is so impaired that infections are the chief cause of death in the more severe of these disorders. Immune deficiency states have been brought forcibly to public notice by the outbreak of AIDS, which is both transmissible and exceptionally severe.

Immune deficiencies can be primary (Table 7-2) or acquired (see list below) and can affect B or T lymphocytes, or both. However, the role of T lymphocytes in regulating B lymphocyte activity often means that a T cell defect affects antibody production. In addition, there can be failures of production of individual antibodies such as IgA or of complement components.

TABLE 7-2. Major primary immune deficiency diseases

	Etiology or mode of inheritance	Main defect	Cell-mediated responses	Antibody production	Major effects	Associated features and prognosis
Predominantly B cell defects						
X-linked infantile (Bruton) hypogammaglobulinemia	X-linked recessive	Absence of B cells	Usually normal	Absence of all Ig classes	Recurrent bacterial infections	Good responses to antimicrobials and gamma globulin, but increasing lung damage and shortened expectation of life
Predominantly T cell defects						
Congenital thymic aplasia (DiGeorge's syndrome)	Developmental absence of thymus and parathyroids	T cells few or absent	Severely impaired	Normal or impaired	Bacterial, viral, fungal, and protozoal infections	Abnormal facies, congenital heart disease, hypocalcemia, early death
Combined B and T cell defects						
Severe combined immunodeficiency (Swiss type agammaglobulinemia)	X-linked or autosomal recessive; ? stem cell defect	T and B cell deficiency	Severely impaired	Severely impaired	Viral, bacterial, and fungal infections	Early death from infection
Cellular immunodeficiency with abnormal immunoglobulin synthesis (Allibone-Nezelof syndrome)	Unknown	T and B cell defects	Severely impaired	Raised or low	Viral, bacterial, and fungal infections	Chronic pulmonary and fungal infections; death usually in late teens
Immunodeficiency with ataxia-telangiectasia	Autosomal recessive, multisystem abnormality	T and B cell defects	Normal or depressed	Usually depressed; IgA or IgE may be absent	Recurrent infections, especially bacterial	Progressive ataxia and mental defect; recurrent respiratory tract infections or earlier death from infection
Immunodeficiency with thrombocytopenia and eczema (Wiskott-Aldrich syndrome)	X-linked recessive	T and B cell defects	Normal at first but may deteriorate	IgM usually low; IgA and IgE usually raised; normal IgG	Recurrent bacterial infections but increasing susceptibility with age	Early hemorrhage may be fatal; eczema severe; moderate expectation of life

Important causes of secondary immunodeficiencies are as follows:
1. Infections
   a. Parasitic infections (worldwide, a major cause)
   b. Bacterial infections (e.g., tuberculosis)
   c. Viral infections
      (1) AIDS
      (2) Others (e.g., measles) usually transient
      (3) Congenital cytomegalovirus and rubella
2. Malnutrition (worldwide, a major cause)
3. Tumors
   a. Lymphoreticular tumors especially
4. Endocrine and metabolic disorders
   a. Diabetes mellitus
   b. Addison's disease
   c. Chronic renal failure
   d. Hepatic failure
5. Drugs and irradiation
   a. Corticosteroids
   b. Immunosuppressive (cytotoxic) drugs
6. Burns, anesthesia, and surgery

Clinically, any patient who develops recurrent infections—and particularly if the infections respond poorly to treatment or are by otherwise harmless microbes (opportunistic infections)—must be suspected of being immunodeficient.

Primary immunodeficiencies

Most primary immunodeficiencies are genetic, and males are predominantly affected. The severe types are rare, characterized by infections starting in infancy, and frequently fatal.

X-linked (Bruton type*) hypogammaglobulinemia

X-linked hypogammaglobulinemia is a B cell defect probably resulting from a failure of the B cell's development or differentiation. B lymphocytes and plasma cells are scanty or absent, and production of all classes of immunoglobulin (Table 7-3) therefore fails.

Infants are passively protected by maternal antibodies for about 6 months after birth, but thereafter recurrent bacterial

---

*D.C. Bruton (b. 1908), American pediatrician.

infections, particularly of the respiratory tract become frequent and persistent. There is also susceptibility to hepatitis B and echovirus infections although T lymphocytes and cell-mediated immunity are not defective.

The bacterial infections can usually be overcome with the help of antibiotics and immune globulin; however, the recurrent lung infections frequently cause permanent damage, and the expectation of life is reduced.

Congenital thymic aplasia (DiGeorge's syndrome*)

Congenital thymic aplasia is a rare disease resulting from a developmental defect in the formation of the third and fourth pharyngeal pouches. It is characterized by the following:
1. Thymic aplasia, failure of differentiation of T lymphocytes and defective cell-mediated immunity
2. Congenital hypoparathyroidism
3. Cardiovascular defects in many cases

Symptoms, usually of hypocalcemia and tetany, start immediately after birth as a result of hypoparathyroidism. Those who survive the neonatal period suffer recurrent or persistent viral, fungal, or bacterial infections. Although this is a "pure" T cell defect, the latter also leads to impaired B cell activity and antibody production. Pneumonia, chronic diarrhea, and failure to thrive are common consequences.

A thymus graft may restore immune function, but, in addition, replacement treatment for hypoparathyroidism and surgery for any cardiac defects are needed.

Severe combined (Swiss type) immunodeficiency

Severe combined immunodeficiency is the most common, severe primary immunodeficiency disease. There are X-linked and autosomal recessive forms, and the disorder probably results from failure of differentiation of stem cells into T and B lymphocytes. Therefore extreme lymphopenia is seen, and lymphoid tissue is hypoplastic and hard to find.

The severity of the immunodeficiency is such that infants often succumb within the first year of life, although there is partial protection by maternal antibodies for the first 6 months. Infections can thereafter be bacterial, viral, fungal, or protozoal. Typical effects include failure to thrive, chronic diarrhea,

---

*A.M. DiGeorge (b. 1921), American pediatrician.

TABLE 7-3. Some important features of the main immunoglobulin classes

Ig	A	D	E	G	M
Heavy chain	α	δ	ε	γ	μ
Molecular weight	170,000 400,000 (secretory IgA*)	180,000	200,000	150,000	900,000
Ability to activate complement	+ (alternate pathway)	−	−	+ +	+ + +
Functions	Secreted by glands onto mucous surfaces	No proven antibody function	Mediates type I hypersensitivity	Important antibodies to toxins, bacteria, and viruses; late response	Early antibody response to many infections
Approximate average proportion of total Ig's in normal serum	13%	1%	0.002%	80%	6%

*IgA is secreted by glands as a dimer (two molecules) joined by a carrier protein.

persistent candidosis (thrush), pneumonia (including *Pneu-* immunization with live attenuated viral vaccines lead to progressive infections. Furthermore, the absence of T cell function renders affected children vulnerable to graft-versus-host disease as a result of viable lymphocytes present in blood transfusions or given in an attempt to repair immunologic function.

Treatment is by aggressive antimicrobial chemotherapy, and most often isolation in a germ-free environment is necessary. Bone marrow transplantation is the definitive treatment; however, close HLA compatibility is mandatory, and the donor should be a close sibling. Even so, the risks of graft-versus-host disease are high.

Other major, primary immunodeficiencies

Other primary immunodeficiencies are uncommon diseases. But like those described earlier, they are characterized by abnormal susceptibility to infection but most have a variety of other, apparently unrelated manifestations. Their main features are summarized in Table 7-2.

Down's syndrome

Down's syndrome, a common chromosomal disorder causing mental defect and other abnormalities, has been described in Chapter 3. Immunodeficiency, as indicated by decreased T lymphocyte function and impaired primary and secondary antibody responses, leads to increased susceptibility to infection. These infections were, in the past, the main cause of premature death; they are now usually controllable by antimicrobial treatment, and consequently, the expectation of life in Down's syndrome has greatly increased.

Primary monocomponent immunodeficiencies

Very many immunodeficiency states limited to single components of the immune response have now been recognized. The main types are selective immunoglobulin deficiencies, complement component deficiencies, and dysfunctions of phagocytes often caused by enzyme deficiencies. Most of these conditions, apart from selective IgA and C2 deficiency are rare.

Selective IgA deficiency. Selective IgA deficiency is one of the most common primary immunodeficiencies. It may affect about 1 in 600 of the population. Any of three possible clinical effects may be seen in affected individuals. Many remain perfectly healthy, some have increased susceptibility to recurrent respiratory or gastrointestinal infections, whereas some are more susceptible to allergy or less often autoimmune disease.

Since IgA is the only antibody secreted in saliva, it is surprising that deficiency does not lead to any increase in oral infections.

Allergy. Patients with atopic (allergic) disease have an abnormally high incidence of IgA deficiency. The reason is unknown but absence of IgA in secretions may allow intact antigens to be absorbed more readily through mucous membranes. Alternatively lack of IgA may reduce the amount of immunoglobulin for binding to antigens, which may therefore bind with IgE instead.

Complement component deficiencies. A major difficulty in assessing the role of complement activation in human disease is that the individual products appear so transiently in the serum. However, an important source of knowledge about the role of complement comes from genetic deficiencies of individual complement components. These indicate that complement makes contributions that include the following.

Defense against infection. Alternate pathway activation, in particular, plays an essential part in the initial nonspecific defenses by stimulating an inflammatory response and neutrophil activity before the immune system has been able to respond (Chapter 6).

Individual complement components appear to have specific roles in combatting different types of microbes. C1423, for example, appears to be important in viral neutralization, whereas C5 fragment appears to be essential for opsonization of fungi. C8 deficiency causes abnormal susceptibility to gonococcal or meningococcal infections.

Genetic deficiency of many complement components therefore causes increased susceptibility to infection. In particular, C3 and its activation fragments play a key role in the inflammatory response.

Clearance of immune complexes. Antigen-antibody complexes activate complement but are also removed by this process. Therefore deficiencies of several complement components often result in connective tissue diseases such as lupus erythematosus, where immune complex damage is probably the underlying mechanism.

Autoimmune disease. Paradoxically, in view of what has just been stated, complement activation appears to be an important mediator of tissue damage—particularly in the major connective tissue diseases, lupus erythematosus and rheumatoid arthritis, as discussed later. The active (inflammatory) stages of these diseases are marked by *hypocomplementemia* as a result of activation and consumption of complement.

Genetic deficiencies of complement components or complement receptors are mostly rare. Although the expected effects are increased susceptibility to infection, autoimmune disease in other cases as indicated above (particularly lupus erythematosus) can result, whereas others can remain healthy.

C2 deficiency has reportedly been detected in 1% of blood donors. About 60% of those homozygous for C2 deficiency and a small minority of heterozygotes may develop a disease resembling lupus erythematosus.

Complement receptor deficiencies. Complement component receptors are present on the surface of most blood and immunologically active cells in the tissues. They bind to specific components resulting from complement activation. The complement receptor (CR3) for C3 products is present on cytolytic and phagocytic cells. The binding of a C3 fragment to CR3 enhances antibody-dependent phagocytosis of target cells. Genetic deficiency of CR3 therefore confers susceptibility to recurrent, severe infections. The biologic significance of many other complement receptors is unknown.

Secondary (acquired) immunodeficiencies

A great variety of diseases (see Table 7-3) can cause a greater or lesser degree of immunodeficiency. In many cases, such as in the common viral infections the immunodeficiency may only be detectable in vitro and is brief. In others, particularly those caused by neoplastic diseases of the lymphoreticular system such as acute leukemia, infections can form the first signs of the disease and ultimately be the cause of death. Worldwide however, *malnutrition* and *malaria* are major causes of immunodeficiency.

The most common types of severe acquired immunodeficiency are the result of immunosuppressive treatment and, increasingly, AIDS.

Immunosuppressive treatment

Immunosuppression is usually essential for organ transplantation, as discussed later, and also for the treatment of immunologically mediated diseases. The antineoplastic (cytotoxic) drugs are in many cases the same as those used for immunosuppression, but may have an additive effect with the tumor in causing even more severe immunodeficiency.

Immunosuppressive drugs predominantly depress cell-mediated immunity but have various effects on the immune response. Their precise effects, particularly when used in combination, are not fully understood. One end result is, however, the same in that *infection* is the most common cause of death from such treatment. With the advent of newer drugs such as cyclosporine, which have a more selective action, infective complications in organ transplant patients are becoming less common.

The clinical effects of drug immunosuppression therefore have many features in common with AIDS as cell-mediated immunity is mainly affected. Lymphomas are also a complication of either of these conditions, but Kaposi's sarcoma is far more common in AIDS than as a result of immunosuppressive treatment.

The acquired immune deficiency syndrome (AIDS)

So much has been written about this subject that it is possible only to summarize the main features here as follows.

Etiology. AIDS is a transmissible form of severe immunodeficiency caused by retroviruses, the human immunodeficiency viruses (HIV).

Transmission. AIDS is most frequently transmitted by male homosexual intercourse in the West, but in Africa it is mainly transmitted by heterosexual intercourse. Less frequently it is transmitted by blood or blood products. Many intravenous drug abusers and, in the past particularly, recipients of blood trans-

fusions and hemophiliacs have become infected. Intrauterine transmission is also possible.

Antibody formation. Exposure to HIV results in formation of antibodies (which are not, however, protective), and there is some doubt whether the virus is ever eliminated, even from those who remain apparently healthy. HIV antibody positivity is therefore regarded as synonymous with infectivity, but in a few infected persons antibodies are not detectable.

Natural history. Exposure to HIV leads to a variety of possible sequences of events. At the time of writing it appears that a minority of those infected develop full-blown AIDS; however, since the disease was only recognized in 1981, it is not known how many will ultimately develop some form of the disease. As each year passes it becomes evident that fewer and fewer will remain unscathed. Current estimates of the numbers of those infected who will develop the disease range from 10% to 50% as the incubation period in some patients seems occasionally to have been longer than 5 years. The possible effects of HIV infections are summarized diagrammatically in Fig. 7-1.

Immune aspects. The immunologic consequences of HIV infection result from a direct attack on T helper (T4) lymphocytes with reversal of the normal ratio of T helper to T suppressor (T8) cells. As a result there is an increasingly severe defect of cell-mediated immunity and other secondary immunologic abnormalities.

The attack on T4 lymphocytes is made possible by a receptor for HIV on these cells, hence the virus was formerly known as the human T lymphotropic virus type III (HTLV III).

The main secondary immunologic effects of HIV infection are autoimmune phenomena, particularly thrombocytopenic purpura but occasionally lupus erythematosus.

Opportunistic infections. Once the defect of cell-mediated immunity becomes sufficiently severe, infections particularly by opportunistic microbes mark the onset of clinical disease. A sudden increase in the incidence of the protozoal infection *Pneumocystis carinii* pneumonia among previously healthy

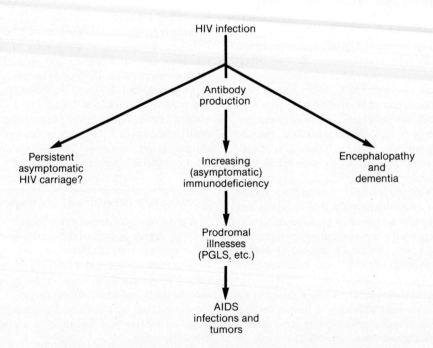

FIG. 7-1. Diagram of possible progression of HIV infection (simplified).

young males led to the recognition of AIDS in 1981. Some of the great variety of infections recognized in AIDS are summarized in the following list:

1. Respiratory
    a. *Pneumocystis carinii*
    b. Aspergillosis
    c. Candidosis
    d. Cryptococcosis
    e. Mucormycosis
    f. Toxoplasmosis
    g. Tuberculosis
    h. Nontuberculous mycobacterioses
    i. Legionellosis
    j. *Pseudomonas aeruginosa*
    k. *Staphylococcus aureus*
    l. *Streptococcus pneumoniae*
    m. *Haemophilus influenzae*
    n. Cytomegalovirus
2. Gastrointestinal
    a. Cryptosporidiosis
    b. Isosporosis
    c. Microsporidiosis
    d. *Mycobacterium avium intracellulare*
    e. Shigellosis
    f. Amebiasis
    g. Giardiasis
    h. Cytomegalovirus
    i. Proctitis (campylobacter, neisseria, chlamydia, herpes simplex)
3. Central nervous system
    a. Herpetic encephalitis
    b. Varicella zoster encephalitis
    c. Toxoplasmosis
    d. Coccidiodomycosis
    e. Cryptococcosis
    f. Aspergillosis
    g. Syphilis
    h. Mycobacterioses
4. Mucocutaneous
    a. Herpes simplex and zoster
    b. Candidosis
    c. *Staphylococcus aureus*
    d. Histoplasmosis
5. Disseminated
    a. Mycobacterioses
    b. Crypotococcosis
    c. Histoplasmosis
    d. Cytomegalovirus

The respiratory and gastrointestinal tract are particularly frequently involved. Persistent diarrhea, often caused by the sporozoan *Cryptosporidium* (formerly thought not to be able to infect humans) or by microsporidia, leads to wasting. In Africa, as a result of this wasting, AIDS is widely known as "slim disease."

Malignant neoplasms. In addition to infections, patients with AIDS are also unusually prone to develop tumors, particularly Kaposi's sarcoma or lymphomas. These tumors are rare in normal persons; in patients with AIDS, the tumors develop in unusual sites, for example, Kaposi's sarcoma of the head and neck region or intracranial lymphoma (Chapters 10 and 20). Although such tumors often respond poorly to treatment, infections remain the most common cause of death in AIDS.

CNS involvement. Brain cells also have receptors for HIV with the result that many of those infected develop a variety of neurologic syndromes (Chapter 20), which can culminate in dementia and death. This can happen even in the absence of the infectious manifestations of AIDS, but intracranial infections are also common in these patients.

Related syndromes. Minor, related, or premonitory diseases can also result from HIV infection. The first sign can be an acute, self-limiting glandular fever-like syndrome that precedes antibody production. More important, however, is persistent generalized lymphadenopathy syndrome (PGLS). The main feature is implied by the name, but in addition there are typically fever, loss of weight, and minor infections such as oral thrush (candidosis) indicative of deteriorating immunologic function. The proportion of patients with this syndrome who progress to AIDS is as yet uncertain, but some appear to recover clinically, at least for a time.

Autoimmunity. A secondary immunologic effect of AIDS is the development of autoimmune disorders and, in particular, autoimmune thrombocytopenic purpura. Such phenomena appear to result from defective modulation of B lymphocyte activity. Major immunologic abnormalities in AIDS are summarized in the following list:

1. Depletion of helper (CD4$^+$) T lymphocytes
2. Depressed responses to soluble antigens
3. Impaired delayed hypersensitivity reactions
4. Decreased γ interferon production
5. Polyclonal B lymphocyte activation
6. Decreased humoral response to immunization
7. Lymphopenia
8. Decreased IL 2 production
9. Decreased cytotoxic response to virally infected cells
10. Increased immune complex formation

Management. The drug zidovudine (azidothymidine, AZT) is the only agent as yet which has any significant effect on HIV and on the clinical manifestations of AIDS. However, the adverse effects, such as marrow depression, can be severe, and the long-term value of this drug is unknown. Currently the value of supplementation of zidovudine with potentially immunopotentiating agents such as α interferon and IL 2, as well as of other antiviral drugs, is being assessed. However, there is little more than a hope that a vaccine can be produced, and a major concern is to limit further spread of the disease, even though it is already worldwide.

Early recognition of infected patients is, as a consequence, of great importance as it is usually neither feasible nor ethical to carry out general testing for HIV positivity, except in the case of blood donors. However, the development of oral thrush, particularly when associated with lymphopenia in a previously healthy young male is strongly suggestive. If such a person, who is not undergoing immunosuppressive treatment, is found to have Kaposi's sarcoma (Chapter 10)—often manifested as a purplish macule or nodule on the skin of the head or neck region or within the mouth—it is virtually pathognomonic of the disease.

Lymph node changes in AIDS. The changes in lymph nodes have been described in cases of persistent generalized lymphadenopathy syndrome (PGLS) and in fully developed AIDS.

Typical findings are decreased numbers of T helper cells in the paracortical region associated with increased numbers of T suppressor cells there and in the follicles. Follicles may initially be hyperplastic but later undergo involution; there is also fragmentation of the follicular dendritic cell network and thinning of the mantle zone.

The effect of AIDS on other individual organs or systems is described in the appropriate chapters later in this text.

Late onset immunodeficiency (syndrome of thymoma, myopathy, hematologic defects, and immunodeficiency)

Thymomas are rare tumors that usually develop late in life. In spite of the role of the thymus in processing T lymphocytes, a thymoma may be associated with either T or B cell defects. In the latter case therefore the first sign may be persistent hypogammaglobulinemia, but defective cell-mediated immunity is more typical.

In addition to abnormal susceptibility to infections, there is frequently myasthenia gravis (Chapter 17) and in some cases hematologic disease, particularly pure red cell aplasia.

Removal of the thymoma improves the neuromuscular and hematologic disorders but has no effect on the immunodeficiency; the outlook for affected patients is poor, especially if the thymoma is malignant. Death may otherwise be due to infection, associated disease such as anemia, or, later, cancer of other organs.

IMMUNOLOGICALLY MEDIATED DISEASE

In contrast to immunodeficiency diseases, the immune response in immunologically mediated diseases appears to be overactive.

Immunologically mediated diseases fall into two main groups. The most frequent type is in response to exogenous (foreign) antigens and form the group of common allergies known as *atopic disease* (see list below) and *contact dermatitis*. In the other less common group there is an abnormal response to endogenous (host) antigens. In the latter case there appears to be partial loss of control of the mechanism of self-tolerance, and such diseases are termed *autoimmune*. Important diseases usually included in this group are also listed as follows:

1. Reactions to foreign antigens.
    a. Type 1 reactions (IgE mediated)
        (1) Allergic rhinitis (hay fever)
        (2) Asthma
        (3) Atopic dermatitis (atopic eczema)
        (4) Angioedema
        (5) Anaphylaxis
    b. Type 4 reactions
        (1) Contact dermatitis
        (2) Some graft rejection reactions
2. Diseases with an autoimmune basis
    a. Connective tissue (collagen vascular) diseases
        (1) Systemic lupus erythematosus
        (2) Rheumatoid arthritis
        (3) Sjögren's syndrome
        (4) Systemic sclerosis
        (5) Polymyositis dermatomyositis
    b. Hematologic disease (Chapter 13)
        (1) Pernicious anemia
        (2) Autoimmune hemolytic anemia
        (3) Idiopathic thrombocytopenic purpura
        (4) Aplastic anemia (some cases)
    c. Gastrointestinal and liver disease (Chapters 14 and 15)
        (1) Chronic atrophic gastritis and pernicious anemia
        (2) Celiac disease
        (3) Chronic autoimmune hepatitis
    d. Renal diseases (Chapter 16)
        (1) Glomerulonephritis (various types)
        (2) Goodpasture's syndrome
    e. Mucocutaneous diseases (Chapter 19)
        (1) Pemphigus
        (2) Pemphigoid
    f. Endocrine diseases (Chapter 18)
        (1) Hypoadrenocorticism (Addison's disease)
        (2) Hashimoto's thyroiditis
        (3) Hyperthyroidism
        (4) Idiopathic hypoparathyroidism
        (5) Diabetes mellitus (some types)
        (6) Polyendocrine deficiency syndromes

In several of these diseases just listed the evidence for an autoimmune basis is slender. Typical features of autoimmune diseases are summarized in the following:

1. More common in women
2. Family history frequently positive
3. Many are HLA D/DR3 or D/DR4 and/or B8
4. Hypergammaglobulinemia
5. Circulating autoantibodies
6. Multiple autoantibodies frequently present but fewer target organs attacked
7. Autoantibodies frequently detectable in unaffected relatives

TABLE 7-4. Summary of important features of hypersensitivity states

Type	Mediators	Mechanism	Effects	Examples of human diseases
I: anaphylactic	IgE	IgE binds to mast cells, releasing histamine, 5 HT, SRS-A	Bronchoconstriction, vasodilatation, increased permeability of vessels	Anaphylactic reactions; atopic allergy
II: cytotoxic	Complement, killer lymphocytes	Lysis of cells having surface antigens	Cell death	Hemolytic anemia; thrombocytopenic purpura
III: immune complex	Antigen/antibody/complement	Formation of immune complexes; release of lysosomal enzymes	Vessel wall damage, especially in the kidney	Serum sickness; various types of glomerulonephritis
IV: cell mediated	Sensitized T cells and lymphokines	Direct cytotoxic action by lymphocytes or effects of lymphokines	Death of target cells	Contact dermatitis; graft rejection

8. Complement activation may be detectable
9. Immunoglobulin deposits or complement may be detectable at sites of tissue damage
10. Active disease usually responds to immunosuppressive treatment.

In an intermediate group, antibodies produced in response to infection, may cross-react with host tissue components. This is the postulated pathogenesis of rheumatic fever (Chapter 11) and post-streptococcal glomerulonephritis (Chapter 16).

The immunologic mechanisms underlying these different diseases are the hypersensitivity reactions summarized in Table 7-4, but more than one may operate in the same disease.

Despite the forbidding complexity of the immune system and its regulation, immunologic disorders apart from the common minor allergies are surprisingly rare. Rheumatoid arthritis is the only type of autoimmune disease that is relatively frequently encountered.

Atopic disease and contact dermatitis

Allergy is a much overused term, frequently misused for diseases with no immunologic basis, but justifiably applied to the atopic diseases, namely asthma and hay fever (Chapter 12), urticaria and eczema (Chapter 19), and some cases of food intolerance in which there is a genetically determined susceptibility to type I hypersensitivity reactions as discussed below. Contact dermatitis is a common Type IV hypersensitivity reaction but appears clinically similar to atopic eczema.

Type 1: immediate type hypersensitivity

Systemic anaphylaxis. In a classic experiment a guinea pig is sensitized by a single injection of 1 mg of egg albumin. This has no visible effect, but if the injection is repeated 2 or 3 weeks later, the sensitized animal reacts almost immediately by severe wheezing due to bronchial constriction and within a few minutes dies from asphyxia. The main findings are intense constriction, particularly of bronchiolar smooth muscle, together with dilatation and increased permeability of capillaries.

In humans, equally acute and, if untreated, fatal anaphylactic reactions can develop, particularly in response to penicillin. Unlike the reaction in the guinea pig, the main effect is a catastrophic fall in blood pressure due to widespread vasodilatation and increased capillary permeability; bronchospasm is usually a minor feature.

The mechanism of anaphylaxis is the result of the reaction of the antigen (allergen) with the specific IgE antibody bound to the surface of mast cells. These then degranulate to release histamine and other mediators such as 5-hydroxytryptamine and leukotrienes.

Clinically, type I reactions are usually less severe but form the basis of the exceedingly common disease known as atopic allergy.

Atopic disease. Susceptibility to atopic disease is genetically determined; it is by far the most common type of immunologically mediated disease, and it is estimated that up to 10% of the population of the United States suffer to some degree from this disorder.

Cell-bound IgE is the mediator and is present in the bronchial tree, nasal mucosa, conjunctival sac, and some other sites. Common extrinsic allergens are grass pollens, mites in house dust, fungal spores, and animal danders (skin scales). These react with cell-bound IgE to release mediators, as described. Sensitivity to foods such as mushrooms or strawberries can

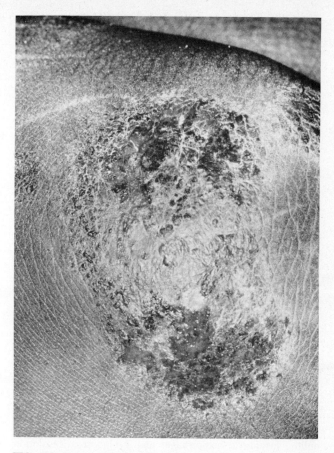

FIG. 7-2. Eczema. The eruption is characterized by inflammation, hyperkeratosis, and desquamation. This type of skin reaction is associated with high serum IgE levels (type I reaction). *(Courtesy Curator of the Gordon Museum, Guy's Hospital, London, England.)*

cause urticaria as a result of material absorbed from the intestinal tract reaching the skin via the bloodstream. IgA deficiency may be present and makes the disease more difficult to manage.

The main types of atopic allergy are asthma, hay fever, urticaria, and eczema (Fig. 7-2). Patients with allergies are also more prone to develop anaphylaxis in response to allergens such as penicillin or intravenous anesthetic agents.

IgE is also formed in normal individuals, but why allergic phenomena develop only in a particular group is unknown.

Type II: cytotoxic type hypersensitivity

Complement-dependent cell lysis. When a cell has surface antigens, combination with antibody can promote adherence by phagocytes, either as a result of opsonic activity or through bound C3. This reaction can kill the cell. Alternatively, the complete complement system up to C8 and C9 can be activated and cause cell destruction by direct membrane damage.

Examples of cytotoxic reactions are autoimmune hemolytic anemia, idiopathic thrombocytopenic purpura, and some graft rejection reactions.

Antibody-dependent cell-mediated cytotoxicity. Experimentally in tissue culture, target cells coated with IgG antibody can be killed in an apparently nonspecific way. They do not undergo phagocytosis, but lymphoid cells bind to the target cell by IgG receptors. These killer lymphocytes (K cells) are nonphagocytic and are neither T or B cells; they may therefore be the same as null cells.

Type III: immune complex hypersensitivity

When soluble antigens react with antibodies, complement may also be activated. As a result, anaphylotoxins and mediators of inflammation can be released.

The outcome of formation of immune complexes in the body depends partly on the absolute amounts of antigen and antibody present. If there is gross antibody excess, complexes are rapidly precipitated and tend to be localized to the site of introduction of the antigen, as in the Arthus reaction.* If there is antigen excess, the complexes are soluble and can cause widespread systemic reactions, as in serum sickness.

Serum sickness. Serum sickness is the classic manifestation of an immune complex reaction in humans. The disease was so termed because it was typically precipitated by administration of animal sera containing antitoxins, such as antitetanic serum.

Serum sickness reactions typically take days or weeks to develop, and the symptoms in specific sites result from the deposition there of antigen-antibody complexes with consequent inflammation. Typical features are joint pains, rashes, enlarged lymph nodes, fever, and malaise. Other hallmarks of immune complex disease, namely vasculitis or glomerulonephritis, can develop but are rare, and usually there is spontaneous recovery after a week or two.

The Arthus phenomenon. The Arthus phenomenon is produced by immunizing an animal until there is a high level of circulating antibodies and then injecting the same antigen locally. At the site of injection an intense inflammatory reaction develops but is mainly localized to the walls of arterioles (vasculitis) leading to hemorrhages and thromboses. Resolution follows phagocytosis and degradation of the antigen-antibody complexes at the site of injection.

Immune complex reactions in general are sometimes loosely referred to as Arthus reactions, but there is considerable doubt as to whether there is a human disease which precisely reproduces this experimental model.

Immune complex lesions. The main effects of immune complex injury are vasculitis and arthritis. Vasculitis with damage to the vessel wall typically leads to hemorrhages or ischemia of the area.

An example of immune complex damage is experimental nephritis induced by the injection of antiglomerular basement membrane into a rabbit. The antibody, followed quickly by complement, binds to glomerular basement membrane. Polymorphonuclear leukocytes, attracted by chemotactic effects of complement components, infiltrate glomeruli and release enzymes that destroy basement membrane.

Different animals vary in their susceptibility to experimental immune complex disorders. It is therefore important to appreciate that results of animal experiments do not exactly reproduce human disease. In humans there seem also to be wide and unexplained variations in susceptibility to immune complex disorders.

Experimentally, foreign serum is one of the most effective causes of immune complex reactions. Other antigens capable of causing similar reactions in humans are a few drugs, such as penicillin and penicillamine. The effects are more severe if antigen is persistently present. Nevertheless, in human immune complex disease the antigen can rarely be identified.

Pathogenesis of tissue damage by immune complexes. Immune complexes cause tissue damage when the complexes are not cleared by phagocytes but are deposited instead in the tissues and are able to activate complement.

Experimentally, deposition of immune complexes appears to depend on the presence of vasoactive amines such as histamine released from mast cells or platelets.

A variety of factors apparently affect the precise sites of deposition of immune complexes. These include their local concentration, their physical size, and the amount of hemodynamic stress on the vessel wall. The latter factor may be the reason for the frequent involvement of the renal glomeruli. The fact that the integrity of the glomeruli is essential for normal renal function also means that damage in such a site is more obvious than when less essential vessels are injured.

A possible sequence of events in immune complex injuries (Fig. 7-3) follows:

1. Formation of immune complexes in the bloodstream
2. Aggregation of platelets and release of vasoactive factors (e.g., histamine) causing increased vascular permeability
3. Permeation of immune complexes into the vessel wall and activation of complement with production of chemotactic factors
4. Emigration of leukocytes into the vessel wall
5. Inflammation and release of neutrophil lysosomal enzymes, causing vessel wall injury
6. Leakage of immune complexes and complement through the vessel wall
7. Local ischemia or hemorrhages resulting from vessel wall damage

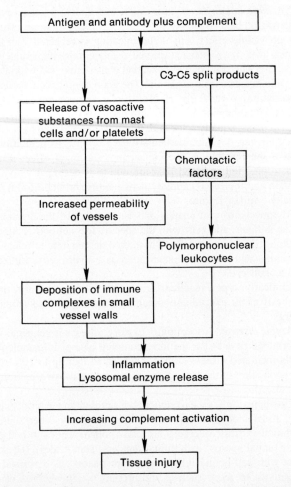

FIG. 7-3. Postulated pathogenesis of immune complex lesions.

---

*N.M. Arthus (b. 1862), French physiologist.

Immune complex disease in humans. Serum sickness is the most typical example of immune complex disease.

The main example of persistent tissue damage associated with immune complex deposition is seen in some types of glomerulonephritis. Other diseases where immune complexes may mediate tissue damage include rheumatoid arthritis or have vasculitis as the prominent feature. The latter include Henoch-Schönlein purpura, lupus erythematosus and polyarteritis nodosa, (also Chapter 10). Examples of diseases associated with immune complex lesions follow:

1. Infective
    a. Infective endocarditis (renal and cerebral lesions)
    b. Poststreptococcal glomerulonephritis
    c. Poststreptococcal Henoch-Schönlein purpura
    d. Chronic hepatitis B
2. Autoimmune disease
    a. Lupus erythematosus
    b. Rheumatoid arthritis
    c. Polyarteritis nodosa
3. Drug reactions
    a. Serum sickness
    b. Penicillamine nephropathy
4. Unknown cause
    a. Many types of glomerulonephritis

Type IV: cell-mediated immune reactions and delayed hypersensitivity

Cell-mediated immune responses have been described earlier.

An intact cell-mediated immune response is shown clinically by a delayed hypersensitivity response to skin testing with potent antigens such as tuberculin or dinitrochlorobenzene (DNCB). Many normal adults are already sensitized to tuberculin as a result of natural exposure to *Mycobacterium tuberculosis*. Sensitivity to DNCB, however, must be induced by

application of this chemical to the skin 7 to 10 days before skin testing.

Anergy (the inability to respond by a delayed hypersensitivity reaction to any antigen) is characteristic of natural and acquired immunodeficiency states where T cells are affected.

Relationships between cell-mediated immunity and delayed hypersensitivity. As mentioned earlier, the delayed hypersensitivity skin test is used as an index of intact cell-mediated responses and one is a manifestation of the other. Nevertheless, many regard cell-mediated immunity as essentially protective and delayed hypersensitivity as a mechanism of tissue damage (type IV reactions). Thus it is postulated, for example, that necrosis (caseation) in tuberculous lesion (Chapter 12) is the result of destruction of bystander cells by the release of macrophage enzymes in an intense cell-mediated reaction. Despite intensive investigation, however, it has not proved possible to determine whether the hypersensitivity component is distinguishable from the protective response. However, both phenomena depend on the same cellular mechanisms, and negative delayed hypersensitivity responses to an infective agent indicates susceptibility to that infection.

Cell-mediated responses, once induced, persist for many years, and the detection of delayed hypersensitivity to a particular antigen cannot be used to infer (as it sometimes is) that this antigen is causing cell-mediated tissue damage. Thus the tuberculin skin test remains positive long after a minimal (subclinical) infection has become quiescent.

The most common example of human disease caused by a type IV reaction is contact dermatitis (Fig. 7-4), which, like a test for delayed hypersensitivity, is a skin reaction.

Summary

The important features of hypersensitivity states are summarized in Table 7-4.

AUTOIMMUNE DISEASE
Self-tolerance and autoimmunity

Survival of the individual depends to a large degree on the ability of the immune system to recognize and eliminate foreign molecules, particularly those of microbes. Host molecules must, however, be recognized as such and protected. This phenomenon is termed *self-tolerance* and is developed early in life; once developed, however, it is so sensitive that implanted human tissue, even from a close relative (other than an identical, monozygotic twin) is treated as foreign and rejected. Immune responses therefore have to be suppressed before organ grafts can be carried out.

The mechanisms of self-tolerance are not fully understood, but the action of T suppressor lymphocytes appears to be important in preventing production of antibodies against host tissues. Impaired T suppressor cell function therefore is possibly an important contributor to loss of self-tolerance, but several other mechanisms, such as the following, have been postulated:

1. Impaired T suppressor cell function
2. Infection by viruses that may (a) contain cross reacting antigens or (b) alter host molecules to make them autoantigenic
3. Binding of foreign haptens, such as drugs, to host tissues to make them autoantigenic
4. Exposure to other foreign antigens that cross-react with host tissue components
5. Nonspecific stimulation of T helper activity (impaired immune modulation)

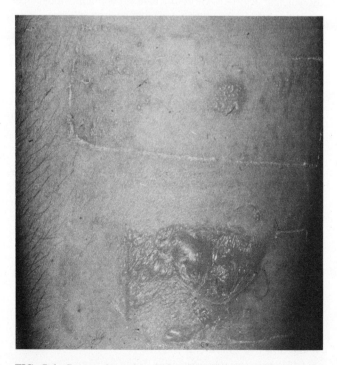

FIG. 7-4. Contact dermatitis. This cell-mediated reaction is due to sensitivity to mercury. A patch test has produced a severe blistering reaction on the skin of the arm.

Whatever the mechanisms by which antigens are allowed to form, many other aspects of autoimmune disease remain unexplained. In particular it is not known why loss of self-tolerance is only partial. As might be expected, when self-tolerance is impaired or lost, multiple autoantibodies may be produced; however, only a limited number of or a single target organ is attacked, and some autoantibodies, once formed, are apparently harmless. It is important to emphasize that the mere presence of autoantibodies therefore is not synonymous with autoimmune disease. For example, relatives of patients with autoimmune diseases, frequently also have circulating autoantibodies but remain healthy. Apparently harmless autoantibodies are also frequently found as age advances.

Types of autoimmune disease

Autoimmune diseases appear to fall into two distinct categories. In one group, mostly endocrine diseases, cell-specific or organ-specific autoantibodies are present and appear to have a direct role in damage to the target organ. In the other, the connective tissue (collagen vascular) diseases, there is a profusion of autoantibodies, but they are not specific to any of the tissues that are attacked.

General features of autoimmune disease

Many diseases of unknown etiology have been postulated as being autoimmune, but it is often impossible to distinguish causative mechanisms from secondary effects or to assess the clinical importance of abnormalities found in the laboratory. The autoimmune diseases, however, share, to a greater or lesser degree, a variety of common features as indicated earlier. None of these features in isolation is likely to be diagnostic; however, the finding of several of them in association with clinical features suggestive of one of the autoimmune diseases is usually informative.

The connective tissue diseases

The connective tissue diseases are discussed here as a "classical" group of immunologically mediated disorders that can affect many body systems and have a variety of common features despite diverse clinical manifestations.

The term *connective tissue disease,* although widely used, is not helpful in understanding the pathogenesis; but alternative terms, namely *collagen vascular* or *rheumatic diseases,* are little better. However, the term *rheumatic disease* is helpful in so far as it serves as a reminder that arthritis or arthralgia is frequently a feature of connective tissue diseases and is the predominant symptom of rheumatoid arthritis, which is the most common type of connective tissue disease.

Typical features of the connective tissue diseases

The connective tissue diseases include the following:
1. Systemic lupus erythematosus
2. Rheumatoid arthritis
3. Sjögren's syndrome
4. Systemic sclerosis
5. Polymyositis and dermatomyositis
6. Mixed connective tissue disease

Other, apparently immunologically mediated diseases such as giant cell arteritis (polymyalgia rheumatica, Chapter 17) or Wegener's granulomatosis (Chapter 10), are often included but with little justification.

Although the connective tissue diseases listed above are often disparate in their clinical manifestations, they tend to share the following common features:
1. Multiple, non-organ-specific autoantibodies are formed.
2. To a variable degree these autoantibodies are shared by different diseases in this group.
3. Sjögren's syndrome can be associated with any of these diseases.
4. Vasculitis is often found and may be the predominant histopathologic feature.
5. Immune complex damage probably underlies the pathogenesis of most of them.
6. Hypocomplementemia is frequently associated with disease activity and may be related to immune complex reactions.
7. These diseases are strongly associated with HLA D/DR3 or D/DR4.
8. Features of any of these disorders can be manifested in mixed connective tissue disease.

The HLA system and autoimmune disease

The HLA system is discussed later in relation to organ transplantation, but there is some association between particular HLA specificities and autoimmune diseases. The main HLA associations between autoimmune and other diseases are listed in Table 7-7.

Autoantibodies in connective tissue diseases

As mentioned earlier, the characteristic features that tend to distinguish the connective tissue diseases from other autoimmune disorders are (1) the autoantibodies are not organ-specific and (2) there is a multitude of them. Antinuclear antibodies are a typical example. These are characteristic of lupus erythematosus but are found more or less frequently in other diseases in this group (Table 7-5). These antinuclear antibodies can include antibodies against single- or double-stranded DNA, ribonucleic acid (RNA), deoxyribonucleoprotein, ribonucleoprotein, and various other extractable nuclear antigens.

Despite speculation extending over many years, the contribution of these autoantibodies to the pathogenesis of these diseases is far from clear. The most readily acceptable hypothesis is that the autoantibodies lead to immune complex formation, complement activation, and inflammation. Release of neutrophil lysosomal enzymes is probably, as a result, the main mediator of tissue damage. The histopathologic effects of such immune complex tissue damage, particularly vasculitis or arthritis is discussed in more detail later.

Systemic lupus erythematosus

Systemic lupus erythematosus (SLE) is a multisystem disease in which arthritis, rashes, fever, and psychiatric disorders are the most common manifestations; neurologic or renal involvement is less common but may be fatal.

The cause of SLE is unknown but genetic factors and possibly viral infection may contribute to the abnormal immunologic reactions. An SLE-like disease can also result from the administration of drugs, particularly the antihypertensive agent, hydralazine, but many others have been implicated.

Immunologic aspects. The main immunologic abnormalities found in active SLE are as follows:
1. Hypergammaglobulinemia

2. Hypocomplementemia
3. Antinuclear antibodies
   a. Anti-DNA antibodies
   b. Anti-RNA antibodies
   c. Antibodies to other nuclear antigens
4. LE cell phenomenon
5. Rheumatoid factor
6. Antierythrocyte antibodies
7. Antiplatelet antibodies
8. False positive VDRL and other serologic tests for syphilis

The most characteristic and constant immunologic finding is the formation of *antinuclear antibodies*, although they are by no means unique to lupus erythematosus. Antinuclear antibodies are the cause of the LE cell phenomenon and probably also responsible for the formation of immune complexes which appear to be the main mechanism of tissue damage.

The LE cell is a polymorphonuclear leucocyte which has ingested altered nuclear material from another white cell (Fig. 7-5). This is due to an IgG antibody which reacts with nuclei from damaged leukocytes in the presence of complement. The result is that nuclear material, immunoglobulin, and complement form a homogeneous mass, which is extruded from the damaged cell and then engulfed by a polymorphonuclear leukocyte.

The LE cell phenomenon is positive in up to 80% of patients with lupus erythematosus at some stage in their disease and rarely positive in other connective tissue diseases. Other antinuclear antibody (ANA) tests are more sensitive (but in most cases less specific) and have in general replaced the LE cell test.

Pathology. The main organs and tissues affected in SLE are shown in Table 7-6.

Necrotizing vasculitis of small arteries is typically present in affected organs; there is fibrinoid change in the vessel walls, in which immunoglobulins, complement (C3), and often DNA are deposited together with fibrin or fibrinogen. There is also leukocytic infiltration of and around the vessel wall.

The late effects of these injuries are fibrous thickening of the vessel walls and narrowing of the lumen. Fibrinoid deposits can also be found in the pleura, pericardium and endocardium (Libman-Sacks endocarditis) (Fig. 7-6).

The joints. The synovia are inflamed and thickened, and there may be foci of fibrinoid change in the underlying connective tissue. The arthritis has features in common with rheumatoid arthritis but differs in that (1) destructive changes are rare, (2) joint pain tends to be less persistent, and (3) tenosynovitis and subcutaneous nodules are rare.

The skin. A distinctive finding is the deposition of immunoglobulin and complement along the dermoepidermal junction in the skin lesions. The IgG and complement deposits have a typical bandlike distribution when examined by immunofluorescence microscopy. These immune complex deposits are also found in the unaffected areas of skin in this disease so that it does not appear that the skin lesions are immune complex mediated.

Oral lesions are associated in 20% of cases and usually consist of white and erythematous areas or shallow ulcers, somewhat similar to lichen planus in appearance.

Similar mucocutanous lesions are the main feature of *discoid lupus erythematosus* (Chapter 19), which lacks the systemic and serologic abnormalities of SLE.

Serous membranes. Inflammation of the pleura or pericardium is common, but the peritoneum is rarely affected.

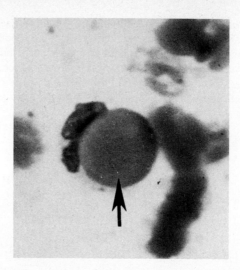

FIG. 7-5. The damaged nuclear mass has been phagocytosed by a polymorphonuclear leukocyte to form a typical LE cell *(arrow)*.

TABLE 7-5. Approximate frequency with which autoantibodies are detectable in collagen disorders

	Rheumatoid factor (%)	Antinuclear factor (%)	LE cells (%)
Systemic lupus erythematosus	20 to 40	100	70 to 80
Sjögren's syndrome	75 to 100	40 to 60	10 to 20
Rheumatoid arthritis	100	10 to 20	5 to 10
Systemic sclerosis	5 to 10	40 to 60	0 to 5
Dermatomyositis	0 to 5	10 to 20	0 to 5

TABLE 7-6. Organs and tissues affected in SLE

Organ system	Frequency of involvement (%)	Typical manifestations
Musculoskeletal	95	Polyarthralgia and arthritis
Mucocutaneous	80	Rashes (various types), oral ulceration
Hematologic	85	Anemia, leukopenia, thrombocytopenia, "lupus anticoagulant"
Nervous system	60	Neuroses and psychoses, strokes, seizures, peripheral neuropathies
Heart and lungs	60	Pericarditis, endocarditis, myocarditis, pleurisy, pneumonitis
Kidneys	50	Proteinuria, nephrotic or nephritic syndromes
Gastrointestinal	45	Sjögren's syndrome, vasculitis (ulceration or perforation), pancreatitis, hepatitis
Eyes	15	Conjunctivitis, retinitis, xerophthalmia
Blood vessels	15	Thromboses
General (nonspecific)	95	Malaise, fever, anorexia, nausea, loss of weight

The heart. When the heart is involved, Libman-Sacks endocarditis* may develop as mentioned earlier. The lesions consist of warty, nonbacterial, vegetations up to 3 mm in diameter, on the valves (see Fig. 7-6). Any valve may be affected, but

---

*E. Libman (1872-1946), American physician; B. Sacks (1873-1939), American physician.

unlike other types of endocarditis, either surface can be affected. Microscopically the vegetations show inflammation and fibrinoid change.

Myocarditis may sometimes develop and is characterized by foci of vasculitis and fibrinoid change in the interstitial connective tissue.

Hematologic changes. Normochromic, normocytic anemia

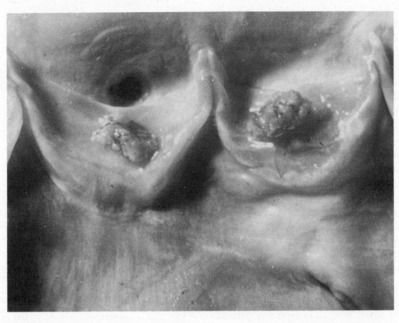

FIG. 7-6. Libman-Sacks endocarditis. These warty vegetations are sterile but are produced by inflammation associated with fibrinoid change initiated in the underlying endocardium.

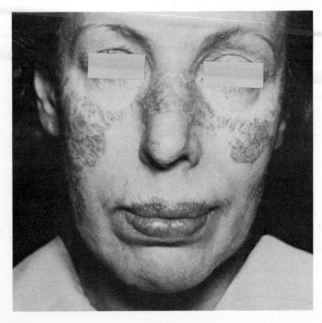

FIG. 7-7. Lupus erythematosus. The facial rash is distributed in typical symmetric fashion across both cheeks and the bridge of the nose, producing a bat's wing–shaped lesion. *(Courtesy Curator Gordon Museum, Guy's Hospital, London, England.)*

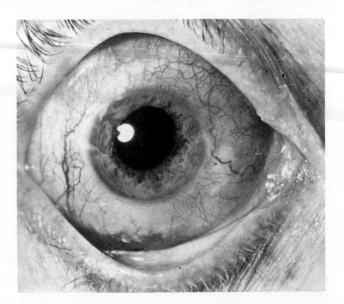

FIG. 7-8. Uveitis in rheumatoid arthritis. Inflammation of the uveal tract (iris, ciliary body, and choroid) can be a prominent feature of autoimmune diseases. The severe inflammation is shown by the leashes of dilated blood vessels spreading on the conjunctiva. Also conspicuous is the irregularity and loss of detail of the iris. *(Courtesy Curator of the Gordon Museum, Guy's Hospital, London, England.)*

is present in up to 80% of patients with active disease. Leukopenia and thrombocytopenia are also common.

The kidneys. The main patterns of glomerulonephritis are (1) focal, (2) diffuse proliferative, or (3) membranous (Chapter 16). These can probably progress from one to another. The diffuse proliferative form is by far the most serious and is characterized by widespread subendothelial deposits of immune complexes.

Clinical aspects. Women are more frequently affected than men in the ratio of up to 9 to 1. The onset is usually between the second and fifth decade.

The main clinical features in approximate order of frequency of SLE are shown in Table 7-6. The "classical" clinical picture is that of a young woman with a butterfly-shaped rash across the face (Fig. 7-7), joint pain, and fever. However, the clinical picture and immunologic findings are so multifarious and variable that detailed criteria for the diagnosis of lupus erythematosus have had to be laid down. In practice, the finding of antibodies to double-stranded DNA and low levels of the complement component, C3, in association with any three of the clinical features described earlier is diagnostic.

Most cases of SLE follow a chronic remittant but benign course, and more than 90% of patients survive for 10 or more years. In those who escape life-threatening complications, the activity of the disease often gradually declines, and after about 5 years anti-DNA titers may fall to low levels.

Many cases are adequately treated with anti-inflammatory drugs, but if the disease is unresponsive, corticosteroids are usually effective. Immunosuppressive drugs, such as azathioprine in addition to corticosteroids, are usually reserved for severe manifestations such as nephritis.

Rheumatoid arthritis

Rheumatoid arthritis is a common and important disease that affects approximately 2% of the population and causes persistent pain and disability. It shares many of the immunologic abnormalities found in lupus erythematosus, but there are also many differences between the two diseases.

Arthritis is the main manifestation of rheumatoid arthritis, and the clinical and pathologic features are described in Chapter 17. Nevertheless, rheumatoid arthritis is a systemic disease and can affect many organs (Fig. 7-8).

Immunopathogenesis. The characteristic abnormality is the formation of a group of immune globulins known as *rheumatoid factors* (RFs). These are usually of the IgM class and directed against autologous IgG and are therefore, in effect, "antiantibodies."

Occasionally RFs are directed against other immunoglobulins. In those patients in whom IgM rheumatoid factors cannot be detected (seronegative rheumatoid arthritis) by the usual methods, RFs may be of the IgG class.

The immunologic reaction to autologous IgG appears to be caused by an abnormality of the immunoglobin, possibly as a result of a viral infection. Thus the IgG combined with a viral antigen may be recognized as "foreign" by the immune system, which responds by antibody production. However, other autoantibodies are also produced in rheumatoid arthritis, as in systemic lupus erythematosus, suggesting that there is also abnormally increased B lymphocyte activity, which probably, in turn, results from defective T suppressor cell control.

Rheumatoid factors are mainly produced in the synovial membranes, and a widely accepted hypothesis for the mechanism of the disease process is as follows:

1. Rheumatoid factors form complexes with IgG, with other RFs, and possibly with other immunoglobulins.
2. The immune complexes activate complement.
3. Complement activation results in chemotaxis of leukocytes, phagocytosis of immune complexes, and release of leukocyte lysosomal enzymes.
4. Lysosomal enzymes, which include collagenases, damage and eventually destroy the synovial membrane. Products of complement activation or activation of T lymphocytes may also contribute to tissue injury.
5. Proliferation of synovial fibroblasts leads to progressive replacement of the synovial membrane by granulation tissue ("pannus").
6. Continued inflammation and loss of the synovial membrane lead to progressive damage to the joint structures and underlying cartilage and bone.

The importance of complement activation in this process is suggested by the low levels (indicating consumption of complement as a result of activation) found in the joint tissues and in the serum in the active stages of the disease.

Other kinds of autoantibodies such as antinuclear factors are also found in rheumatoid arthritis, and in a minority the LE cell phenomenon is also positive.

The finding of rheumatoid factor in the serum is not, incidentally, diagnostic of rheumatoid arthritis, since it is found in other connective tissue diseases, in other unrelated diseases where there is no joint damage, and even in normal persons.

The precise pathogenesis of rheumatoid arthritis, it must be admitted, remains far from clear, and there are many unexplained features.

Sjögren's syndrome*

Sjögren's syndrome is characterized by *xerostomia* and *xerophthalmia* (dry mouth and dry eyes) as a result of destruction of salivary and lacrimal tissue. Another connective tissue disease is often associated. Sjögren's syndrome develops in 10% to 15% of patients with rheumatoid arthritis. It is reported to be found in up to 30% of patients with SLE and in approximately 70% of patients with chronic biliary cirrhosis. It is also a common feature of graft-versus-host disease. The same glandular changes can also develop in the absence of connective tissue disease, and the condition is then known as sicca (dry) syndrome.

Immunologic findings. Antibodies to extractable nuclear antigens, anti SS-A and anti SS-B, are virtually specific to Sjögren's syndrome. There is typically also a raised titer of rheumatoid factor. Antisalivary duct antibodies, antinuclear antibodies, antithyroid autoantibodies, and other autoantibodies may also be detected.

In spite of the histopathologic similarities of the glandular changes to those in Hashimoto's thyroiditis (Chapter 18), there are no antibodies to acinar cell components, and the antiduct antibody found in Sjögren's syndrome appears to have no role in the pathogenesis of the disease. In spite of the presence of these antibodies, duct tissue survives and even proliferates in Sjögren's syndrome. The immunopathogenesis of this disease is therefore obscure.

Pathology. Despite the difficulty of correlating the immu-

---

*Henrick Sjögren (b. 1899), Swedish ophthalmologist.

nologic findings in Sjögren's syndrome with the pathologic process, the histologic picture is strongly suggestive of immunologically mediated tissue destruction. The glandular tissue is progressively more widely infiltrated by T and B lymphocytes, starting periductally but eventually replacing all the acinar tissue. The final picture is of a sheet of lymphocytes, scattered among which are islands of proliferating ductal tissue (Fig. 7-9).

Sjögren's syndrome is discussed further in Chapter 14.

Systemic sclerosis (scleroderma)

Systemic sclerosis is characterized by progressive fibrosis of skin and subcutaneous muscle (Fig. 7-10) and visceral connective tissue. The result is inexorable loss of mobility of the affected parts and usually a fatal outcome as a result of heart disease secondary to pulmonary fibrosis or renal involvement. As with the other connective tissue diseases, Sjögren's syndrome may be associated.

Immunologic findings. Antinuclear antibodies are detectable in up to 95%. In addition to other autoantibodies anti-Scl 70 appears to be specific to systemic sclerosis and may be predictive of pulmonary involvement.

The immunopathogenesis of systemic sclerosis is obscure. Lymphocytic infiltrates in the tissues are scanty but may be seen in a perivascular distribution. Inflammation and vasculitis are not, however, apparent, although it is postulated that the disease is mediated by damage to blood vessels as the progressive fibrous replacement of tissues is certainly suggestive of chronic ischemia.

Unlike other connective tissue diseases, systemic sclerosis shows no response to immunosuppressive treatment. The disease is discussed further in Chapter 19.

Polymyositis and dermatomyositis

Polymyositis and dermatomyositis can be regarded as variants of one another; they are inflammatory diseases of skin and muscle (the name is chosen according to which system is predominantly affected) and are sometimes associated with other connective diseases or possibly in some cases with cancer.

Myositis is characterized by muscle pain and weakness, insidious in onset, and typically spreading upward from the lower to the upper limbs and sometimes to the face. Biopsy shows monocytic infiltration and degeneration of muscle and perivascular inflammatory infiltrates.

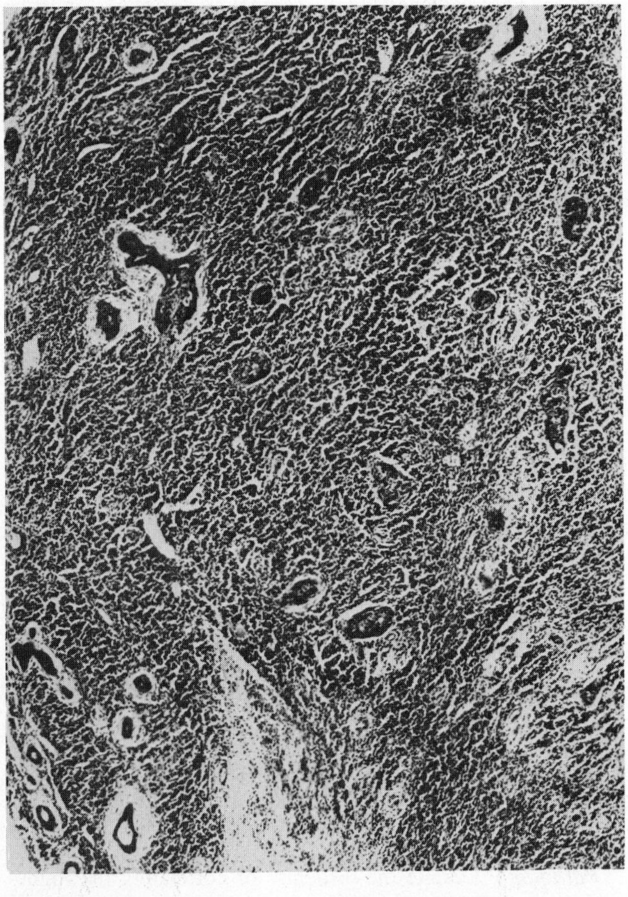

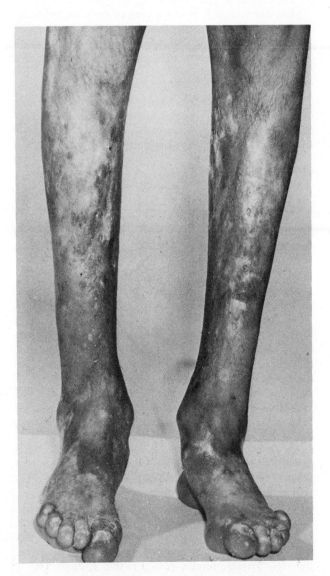

FIG. 7-9. Sjögren's syndrome (salivary gland section). This is the typical appearance of the late stage. All the secretory tissue has been destroyed, and only islands of proliferated duct tissue remain, surrounded by the dense infiltrate of lymphocytes.

FIG. 7-10. Systemic sclerosis. The fibrosis has caused contracture of the skin, and over a wide area dermal appendages have been destroyed, producing a scarred appearance (see also Fig. 19-3). *(Courtesy Curator of the Gordon Museum, Guy's Hospital, London, England.)*

Severe muscle disease may be associated with pulmonary or myocardial involvement. Muscle enzymes (creatine phosphokinase, CPK) are released into the blood to levels corresponding to the severity of the muscle damage.

Dermatitis takes the form of characteristic rashes; a purplish suffusion of the upper eyelids is pathognomonic but uncommon.

Raynaud's phenomenon (Chapter 10) is relatively common, and Sjögren's syndrome develops in a minority.

Antibodies such as rheumatoid factor or antinuclear antibodies may be found, but there is no diagnostic immunologic test. Diagnosis is largely dependent on muscle biopsy and serum CPK levels.

Mixed connective tissue disease

Mixed connective tissue disease (MCTD) is a more uncommon form of connective tissue disease but illustrates the links between these disorders.

MCTD is characterized by the following clinicopathologic features in varying combinations:
1. Raynaud's phenomenon or arthralgia is often seen at onset.
2. Arthralgia or arthritis is the most common feature, but joint disease is rarely destructive.
3. Lupus erythematosus-like skin lesions are common.
4. Pulmonary involvement resembles that in systemic sclerosis.
5. Painful myositis resembles polymyositis, but it is generally milder.
6. Renal disease is increasingly frequently reported, but unlike SLE appears to be an immune complex nephropathy.
7. The central nervous system is involved in more than 50% of patients, but the consequences are rarely fatal.
8. The pathologic findings with the exceptions of those mentioned are similar to related connective tissue diseases.

Immunologic aspects. The most characteristic abnormality in MCTD is the formation of antibodies to ribonucleoprotein (anti-RNP), and antibodies to extractable nuclear antigens (anti-ENA) are almost invariably also found. Other findings are more variable, and there are probably no absolutely specific criteria of diagnosis.

TRANSPLANT IMMUNOLOGY AND GRAFT REJECTION

Destroyed or diseased organs can sometimes be replaced by organs from several possible sources. These sources differ mainly in the extent to which the new organ or tissue will be tolerated by the recipient. The following terms are used:
1. *Autograft*—An autograft is tissue taken from one site on the donor and grafted back onto another. This is frequently done with skin, for example, after a disfiguring injury when skin from the thigh can be used to replace facial skin loss.
2. *Isograft*—An isograft is a graft from a donor who is syngeneic, that is, of identical genetic constitution to the recipient, usually an identical (monozygotic) twin.
3. *Allograft (homograft)*—An allograft is a graft from a donor to a recipient who is allogeneic, that is, a member of the same species but of different genetic constitution. This is the most common type of transplant.
4. *Xenograft (heterograft)*—A xenograft is a graft between different species of animals.

Blood transfusion is an allograft and is tolerated by the recipient when the ABO and major blood groups of donor and recipient are matched. In some ways tissue grafts are treated in a similar fashion to transfused blood by a recipient, but the tissue antigens are different from and much more complex than the blood group systems. Tissue antigens are present on the white blood cells and are known as human lymphocyte antigens (HLA).

THE HUMAN HISTOCOMPATIBILITY SYSTEM

The search for a histocompatibility system (comparable to the ABO blood groups) to enable the prediction of the acceptability of transplanted organs has led to the discovery of the major histocompatibility complex—the HLA (*h*uman *l*eukocyte *a*ntigen) system—and the mapping of many of the genes that determine the system.

The antigens by which HLA specificities are recognized are determined by genes that occupy a large region of the short arm of the *sixth chromosome*. The main loci that have been identified so far have been designated A though D and DR (D related). Specificities that have been incompletely defined have the suffix *w*.

Individual antigens of the A, B, and C loci (class I antigens) are identified by means of antisera, whereas those of the D and DR loci (class II antigens) are identified by mixed lymphocyte culture.

Class I (A, B, and C) antigens are expressed on all nucleated cells, whereas class II (D and DR) are normally only expressed on some cells and, in particular, B lymphocytes of the immune system.

Clinical relevance of the HLA system

The following are important aspects of the HLA system:
1. *Organ transplantation*—Histocompatibility is critical in determining the level of tolerance with which an organ and, in particular, bone marrow is accepted. Tissue typing is usually an essential measure in selecting a donor organ as discussed later. Matching at the D and DR loci appears to be particularly important.
2. *Immune responses*—As discussed earlier, activation by an antigen, especially of B lymphocytes, usually depends on presentation of the antigen in association with a host HLA-D or -DR antigen.
3. *Host defense against infection*—Class II HLA antigens are (as mentioned earlier) involved in antigen presentation to cytotoxic T lymphocytes, which may be important in defense against viral infections.
4. *Associations with disease*—Various HLA specificities are significantly more frequently found in association with certain diseases than in normal persons. In the latter, these specificities may sometimes indicate susceptibility to that disease. However, in most cases the associations are not so strong as to be of diagnostic value (Table 7-7).
5. *Autoimmunity*—The involvement of HLA-D and -DR specificities in normal antigen handling and immune responses together with the association between various D and DR specificities with autoimmune diseases such as rheumatoid arthritis has led to widespread assumptions that such specificities are directly related to autoimmune activity. There is no evidence as yet that this is the case, but it is possible that viruses can induce the expression of D or DR specificities on human cells and thus render them recognizable as antigens.

TABLE 7-7. Examples of associations of HLA with some diseases

Diseases	HLA
Connective tissue diseases	
SLE	D/DR3
Rheumatoid arthritis	D/DR4
Sjögren's syndrome	D/DR3 or DR4
Endocrine diseases	
Addison's disease	D/DR3
Hashimoto's thyroiditis	D/DR5
Diabetes mellitus (some types)	D/DR3 or DR4
Renal diseases	
Goodpasture's syndrome	D/DR2
IgA nephropathy	D/DR4
Membranous nephropathy	D/DR3
Hematologic disease	
Pernicious anemia	D/DR5
Others	
Pemphigus vulgaris	D/DR4
Ankylosing spondylitis	B27
Narcolepsy	D/DR2

NOTE: With the exception of ankylosing spondylitis and narcolepsy, where the association with the HLA types indicated is between 90% and 100%, most of the diseases listed have a frequency of association of approximately 50%. Many of the autoimmune diseases are frequently also associated with HLA-B8.

Although there are significant associations of different HLA specificities with autoimmune diseases (as discussed earlier), the strongest associations are with diseases where no autoimmune mechanism has been demonstrated. The best known of the latter is that of *ankylosing spondylitis* (Chapter 17) in which 95% of patients are HLA-B27. Over 20% of apparently normal persons found to be HLA-B27 have unrecognized signs of or later develop ankylosing spondylitis. More remarkably it has been found that 100% of patients with *narcolepsy* (uncontrollable attacks of sleep) are HLA-DR2. With these exceptions, determination of HLA specificities has not proved useful in the diagnosis of disease.

Despite a variety of hypotheses, the significance of any association of a particular HLA specificity with a particular disease is unknown. A possible mechanism is that particular HLA specificities may be linked with genes that are responsible for the disorder.

HLA compatibility and organ transplantation

The degree of toleration of an organ graft depends closely on the degree of HLA compatibility. It is clearly not possible to test for all antigens in this system, which shows intense polymorphism. Furthermore, in the case of kidneys, for example, a match for only 6 antigens at the A, B, and DR loci can be found in no more than 1 in 1,000 of the population. Also suggestive of the problems of HLA polymorphism is the fact that organs donated from close relatives have a far better prognosis than equally well-matched organs from unrelated (cadaveric) donors. These considerations aside, matching for the HLA-DR and the HLA-B loci appears to give the best success rates. As discussed later ABO (blood group) compatibility is also essential to prevent acute rejection.

Although the closest possible HLA matching is desirable, modern supportive and, particularly, immunosuppressive treatment can often, to a great extent, make up for less than perfect matching. Cyclosporine, with its more selective action on T lymphocytes, has had a major effect on transplant success rates.

In practice, different organs vary widely in the immune responses they provoke in the recipient; livers are more readily tolerated than kidneys, for example. Furthermore, a major determining factor is often the availability of organs; in a patient near to death, transplantation with a poorly matched organ may be preferable to waiting for a better match. By contrast, bone marrow transplantation where many immunologically active cells are implanted requires, as nearly as possible, perfect matching.

First and second set graft reactions

That graft rejection is immunologically mediated is indicated by *first* and *second set* graft reactions. If an incompatible tissue is transplanted from one animal to another, it is rejected after a time (first set reaction). If, however, a second graft is given to the same recipient from the same donor, then rejection is more rapid and violent. The great rapidity and specificity of the second set reaction suggests that it is an immunologic reaction. This is further illustrated by the fact that if the original recipient is given another graft, but from a *different* donor, the graft is rejected by a first set reaction.

Animals can, however, be made tolerant of allografts if either (1) the transplant is made early in life before the immune system has developed or (2) if the thymus is removed before T lymphocytes can differentiate.

The immunologic nature of graft reactions has been abundantly confirmed in recent years, and the importance of T lymphocytes in graft rejection has been confirmed by the value of cyclosporine and monoclonal anti-T cell sera for controlling rejection reactions.

Rejection mechanisms

The process of organ rejection can, for simplicity, be regarded as developing in the following stages:
1. Antigens released from the graft enter the host via the efferent lymphatics. The most important of these antigens appear to be on donor leukocytes expressing large numbers of class II (DR) antigens.
2. The donor antigens activate host cellular and humoral immune responses and, in particular, cytotoxic T lymphocytes.
3. Activated host cells and antibodies travel by the bloodstream to the graft and attack it. The chief target cells are those bearing class II (D and DR) antigens; such antigens can be present on cells not normally carrying them as they can be induced by lymphokines, produced by activated host T lymphocytes.

Rejection mechanisms are both humoral and cell mediated and can be hyperacute, acute, or chronic.

Hyperacute rejection. Humoral factors play the predominant role in these reactions, which typically develop in a patient already sensitized as a result of such factors as ABO incompatibility, previous blood transfusion, or earlier attempts at engraftment.

An *immediate hyperacute reaction* is characterized by sludging of white cells, platelet microthrombi, and thrombosis of glomeruli of the donated kidney. The result is failure of revascularization and ischemic necrosis ("white kidney").

Hyperacute rejection may, however, be less immediate and characterized by gross infiltration by neutrophils and deposition of antibody and complement in the graft.

Hyperacute rejection can usually be prevented by appropriate

immunosuppressive preparation, but once it develops, it is irreversible.

Acute rejection. A graft may be rejected after 1 or 2 weeks. The process is characterized by infiltration of the graft by host T lymphocytes and macrophages. The reaction has features suggestive of delayed-type hypersensitivity, but there is also evidence of cytotoxic T cell activity. The variation in reported findings may be due to the difficulties (particularly in the past) of identifying subsets of mononuclear cells in biopsies and partly by the effects of different immunosuppressive regimens.

Histologically, acute cellular rejection in the kidney manifests as tubular injury by lymphoid cells; acute humoral rejection involves vascular occlusion (mainly by activation of the clotting process), producing ischemic graft injury, at worst renal infarction. This is discussed more fully in Chapter 16.

General features of acute rejection include loss of function of the graft associated with local pain and swelling, fever, malaise, leukocytosis, and thrombocytopenia.

Late acute reactions are less violent and characterized by relatively mild lymphocytic infiltration of the graft with depositions of immunoglobulins in vascular endothelium and immune complex-type reactions. This is suggested by the adherence of leukocytes, platelets, and fibrin to the endothelium. Connective tissue proliferation in the inflamed area causes progressive vascular obstruction.

Acute rejection should be controllable by appropriate immunosuppressive treatment.

Late rejection. The characteristic feature of late rejection is gradual loss of function of the grafted organ after a period of 6 or more months. The precise immunopathogenesis remains controversial, and the reaction may represent the late effects of humoral and cellular immunologic damage.

The histopathologic features are progressive narrowing of arteries caused by intimal proliferation as well as deposition of platelets and fibrin. There is often also subendothelial accumulation of immunoglobulins and complement, which may represent immune complex reactions to the graft or to a continuation of the original disease process. These deposits become covered by intimal proliferation with the result that, ultimately, the combination of these processes leads to such severe intimal thickening that the lumen of the vessels becomes obliterated and there is progressive ischemic damage to the engrafted organ.

Late rejection is generally resistant to immunosuppression.

Control of graft rejection

The main measures taken to reduce the chances of rejection of an organ graft include the following:

1. Blood group compatibility between donor and recipient and multiple preoperative transfusions of compatible blood—the latter appears to have an immunosuppressive effect, although the mechanism involved is controversial
2. Matching of tissue (HLA) antigens particularly at the DR locus
3. Use of immunosuppressive drugs

Immunosuppressive drugs include relatively nonspecific drugs such as azathioprine and more selective agents such as cyclosporine and monoclonal anti-T cell antibodies. Cyclosporine's main modes of action appear to be on activated lymphocytes to block the production of lymphokines necessary for immune responses and to depress IL 2 production by macrophages. T cell–dependent proliferative reactions and some other functions, such as T cell cytotoxicity, are inhibited. Overall, the main immunosuppressive action of cyclosporine appears

to be by depression of T4 (helper) lymphocyte function. Unfortunately, cyclosporine is nephrotoxic; however, it significantly improves graft survival rates, and its adverse effects are considerably less than those of earlier agents.

To monitor the requirements for immunosuppressive treatment, needle biopsies or aspirates from the engrafted organ are examined for signs of rejection reactions, and treatment is modified accordingly.

GRAFT-VERSUS-HOST DISEASE

As already discussed, the normal reaction of the host's immune system is to attack incompatible transplanted tissue. If, however, the host is severely immunodeficient, immunologically active cells in the donor tissue can attack the host. This phenomenon, known as graft-versus-host disease (GVHD) can be regarded as a rejection reaction in reverse and can develop only in the following circumstances:

1. There is incomplete histocompatibility between donor and host tissues.
2. The engrafted tissue or blood cells are immunocompetent.
3. The host cells are immunodeficient.

GVHD is most common after bone marrow transplantation because more intense immunosuppression is required or because the transplant is being given for an immunodeficiency disease such as severe combined (Swiss type) immunodeficiency. GVHD develops in approximately 50% of patients who have had bone marrow transplants. It must also be added that although the incidence of GVHD is related to the degree of donor-host incompatibility, it has also occasionally been reported after syngeneic grafts.

Although it is clear that T cells are the main mediators of the reaction, the immunologic basis of GVHD is unclear, and conflicting findings have been reported. Suppressor (CD8) T lymphocytes are numerous in tissues under attack, and the cells of these tissues are rich in surface DR antigens, which appear to render them liable to attack. Infection also appears to be a factor precipitating GVHD, but GVHD also increases susceptibility to infection.

The main target organs attacked in GVHD are the skin and oral mucosa, the gastrointestinal tract (including the liver and salivary glands), and lymphoid tissue.

GVHD can be acute (usually starting 1 to 2 months after transplantation) or chronic (usually starting 6 months to 2 years afterward). Acute GVHD mainly affects the skin, gastrointestinal tract, and liver, whereas chronic GVHD causes more widespread multisystem effects.

Acute GVHD. A rash is often the first sign of acute GVHD. Pruritus (itching) and erythema may be followed by bulla formation and exfoliation. In the mouth there is frequently a lichenoid reaction (Chapter 19) and loss of salivation as a result of a Sjögren-like syndrome. Hepatitis and enteritis are frequently associated with severe skin reactions.

Hepatitis is characterized by cholestasis, bile duct necrosis, and inflammation of the portal triads.

In the gut there is necrosis of basal cells of the crypts, abscess formation, and crypt destruction in severe cases. Malabsorption and diarrhea result and may progress to hemorrhage and ileus.

Depletion of lymphoid tissue, lymphopenia, and hypogammaglobulinemia result in immunodeficiency. Infection, as a result, is an important cause of death.

Chronic GVHD. Chronic GVHD causes a scleroderma-like skin reaction in most patients; there is subcutaneous fibrosis and, in severe cases, joint contractures. A lichenoid reaction of the skin and oral cavity and a Sjögren-like syndrome with dryness of the mouth and eyes are usually associated. Gastrointestinal involvement causes dysphagia, regurgitation, diarrhea, abdominal cramps, and malabsorption, but severe liver damage is rare.

Bone marrow involvement causes anemia, leukopenia, and thrombocytopenia, but there is usually eosinophilia. Infection secondary to immunodeficiency is the chief cause of death.

Other possible effects are respiratory disease with cough, asthma, or chronic obstructive disease caused by pulmonary fibrosis, and arthralgia or arthritis, and muscle weakness.

After bone marrow transplantation, GVHD is an important factor affecting survival, which falls to 20% when GVHD is moderate or severe, since treatment is rarely successful. Various combinations of drugs have been used in the attempt to prevent GVHD; of these the combination of cyclosporine with methotrexate appears currently to be most effective. Experimentally T cell depletion by means of monoclonal antibodies acting against specific subsets appears to be an even more promising approach, and recent results suggest that it is effective in humans.

TUMOR IMMUNOLOGY

Tumor cells arise from host tissues but nevertheless harm and frequently kill the host. The behavior of tumor cells is in some ways like that of invading microbes; like them, it might be expected that tumor cells would be recognized as foreign by the host immune system and be antigenic.

The belief that there might be an immune reaction to tumors is founded on observations such as the following:

1. Most cancers, particularly carcinomas, evoke a lymphocytic reaction in the surrounding tissues.
2. Immunodeficient patients have an increased susceptibility to certain types of tumors.
3. Very rarely, malignant tumors appear to undergo spontaneous remission.

As a consequence, it has been postulated that the immune system exerts a monitoring function to recognize and destroy tumor cells as they develop. Though this *immune surveillance* theory has been widely espoused and great expectations have been held out for treatment of cancer by immunostimulation, early optimism has not been justified so far.

Animal and human tumors

Inevitably, most of the work on tumor immunology has been carried out in animals. Artificially induced tumors, however, differ in very many ways from the common, "spontaneous" human tumors, which have no identifiable cause. In particular, and unlike the latter, experimentally induced tumors are highly antigenic. The immunogenicity of artificially induced tumors is also directly related to the nature and dose of the inducing agent. Moreover, histologically similar tumors may have distinct and different antigenic structures, specific to the inducing agent rather than to the tumor cell type.

Human tumor cell antigens

The only antigens from human tumors that have been identified are fetal proteins and tumor products, such as hormones, which are not specific to the tumor cell. Immunization against such antigens also does not protect the host and may even promote tumor growth. After many years work, no truly specific human tumor antigens have yet been identified.

Cancer in immune deficiency states

Animal studies. In animals severe depression of T cell activity is followed by increased susceptibility to tumors. This increased susceptibility is, however, mainly to virus-induced tumors and much less to chemically induced or spontaneous tumors. More remarkable is the observation that in several thousand congenitally athymic (nude) mice, which lack T cell activity, no spontaneous tumors were found during their life span. These animals also showed no increased susceptibility to chemical carcinogens but were highly susceptible to oncogenic viruses.

These findings therefore indicate that immunodeficiency of this type does not increase susceptibility to tumors per se but only to oncogenic viruses.

Cancer in human immune deficiency states. In these disorders, especially in children with immunodeficiency diseases, the incidence of cancer is greatly increased. On the basis of the "immune surveillance" hypothesis, a great excess of the common types of cancer (such as neuroblastoma or nephroblastoma in children and cancer of the bronchus, breast, prostate, and bowel in adults) would be expected. This, however, is not the case, and there is an overall excess of otherwise uncommon lymphoreticular tumors. There appear to be several mechanisms to account for this observation.

First, lymphomatous change can apparently follow persistent bombardment of the lymphoreticular tissues by antigens. When the immune system is unable to respond, there is no antibody production to exert feedback control. Antigens therefore continually stimulate the lymphoid tissues, and the process is self-perpetuating.

Second, in the natural immunodeficiency diseases there is evidence that chromosomal abnormalities may underlie both the immune defect and increased susceptibility to cancer. Some chromosomal disorders are known to be associated with an increased cancer risk, as with the Philadelphia chromosome and in xeroderma pigmentosum. A chromosomal abnormality has been identified in ataxia telangiectasia, and even first-degree relatives who are immunologically normal have an increased susceptibility to cancer.

The increased susceptibility to cancer may therefore be due to an underlying defect of DNA, which could be both potentially premalignant and also cause impaired lymphocyte function.

Third, in renal transplant patients most of the excess of cancers are lymphoreticular tumors and skin cancers. The susceptibility to cancer, however, is not related to the depth of immunosuppression, and patients who have repeatedly rejected grafts have also developed cancer.

Several immunosuppressive drugs are mutagenic and are probably also carcinogenic. This is suggested by the fact that the use of these drugs for the treatment of cancer in otherwise normal patients has been followed by the development of new tumors.

Skin cancer in transplant patients is related to the amount of exposure to sunlight, and the process may be accelerated by the cocarcinogenic action of immunosuppressive drugs.

Fourth, in the connective tissue disorders, which are often treated with immunosuppressive drugs, there is also an increased incidence of cancer. This, however, happens even in the absence of immunosuppressive treatment.

Fifth, removal of the thymus in humans is not associated with any increased susceptibility to tumors.

The findings in immune deficiency states do not therefore appear to support the "immune surveillance" hypothesis and may be summarized as follows:

1. Malignancies in immunodeficiency diseases are not the common tumors of childhood or adult life. There is a great excess of the otherwise uncommon lymphoreticular tumors.
2. The risk of malignancy is not directly related to the degree of depression of the immune response.
3. In congenital immune deficiency states chromosomal abnormalities may both predispose to malignancy and also cause defective lymphocyte function.
4. Several immunosuppressive/cytotoxic drugs are known to be mutagenic and may be carcinogenic for humans.
5. Severely immunodeficient animals, particularly congenitally athymic mice, show no increase in spontaneous tumors.
6. Thymectomy in humans is not associated with any increase in tumors.

In addition, there is increasing evidence of the activity of oncogenic viruses, whose activity may be released in immunodeficiency states.

Increasingly, however, it has become apparent that the common solid tumors do not produce specific antigens recognizable by the host immune system, and little evidence exists for a significant defensive host response. Alternatively such tumors may have effective mechanisms of escape from immune defenses.

Immunotherapy of cancer

Early attempts to control tumors by nonspecific immunostimulation with BCG vaccine or suspensions of *Corynebacterium parvum* have failed. More specific approaches, such as injection of irradiated allogeneic leukemia cells, have also proved ineffective.

Optimism yet remains about the potential value of *monoclonal antibodies* targetted against tumor cells, but formidable problems persist. As yet the treatment of tumors in humans with these agents has had little success.

Interferons have been discussed earlier, but α interferons have proved highly successful in the treatment of a rare disease, hairy cell leukemia (Chapter 13), which is associated with the retrovirus, HTLV-II. It is possible therefore that the antitumor effect of α interferon in this disease may be due to its antiviral as much as to any immunomodulatory effect. The response to α interferon of other tumors, such as chronic myelogenous leukemia, Kaposi's sarcoma in AIDS, and lymphomas, has been less encouraging.

Paradoxically therefore, despite decades of promise that some form of immunostimulation would conquer cancer, cytotoxic drugs, which are essentially immunosuppressive, have not been displaced as the mainstay of medical treatment of this group of diseases. However, in view of the technical problems of producing sufficiently specific, immunologically active tumoricidal reagents, hope of future success by this means should not be abandoned.

Selected readings

Baldwin WM III and Sanfilippo F: Antibody-mediated graft versus host reactions in renal transplantation, Immunology Today 8(78):219, 1987.

Balkwill FR and Smyth JF: Interferons in cancer therapy: a reappraisal, Lancet ii:317, 1987.

Barbour SD: Acquired immunodeficiency syndrome of childhood, Pediatr Clin N Am 34(1):247, 1987.

Biggar RJ: The clinical features of HIV infection in Africa, Br Med J 293:1453, 1986.

Boylston AW, and Cook HT et al: Biopsy pathology of acquired immune deficiency syndrome (AIDS), J Clin Pathol 40:1, 1987.

Colten HR: Hereditary angioneurotic edema, 1887 to 1987, N Engl J Med 317(1):43, 1987.

Dinarello CA and Mier JW: Current concepts: lymphokines, N Engl J Med 317(15):940, 1987.

Durant JR: Immunotherapy of cancer, N Engl J Med 316(15):939, 1987.

Edwards L: Interferon, Arch Dermatol 123:743, 1987.

Emlen W, Pisetsky DS, and Taylor RP: Antibodies to DNA, Arthritis Rheum 29(12):1417, 1986.

Gale RP: Graft-versus-host disease, Immunol Rev 88:193, 1985.

Garcia CF and Lifson JD et al: The immunohistology of the persistent generalized lymphadenopathy syndrome (PGL), Am J Clin Pathol 86(6):706, 1986.

Gluckman JC and Klatzmann D: Lymphadenopathy-associated-virus infection and acquired immunodeficiency syndrome, Ann Rev Immunol 4:97, 1986.

Guinan ME and Hardy A: Epidemiology of AIDS in women in the United States 1981 through 1986, JAMA 257(15):2039, 1987.

Ho DD and Pomerantz RJ et al: Pathogenesis of infection with human immunodeficiency virus, N Engl J Med 317(5):278, 1987.

Hoxie JA: Current concepts in the virology of infection with human immunodeficiency virus (HIV), Ann Intern Med 107(3):406, 1987.

Keown PA and Stiller CR: Kidney transplantation, Surg Clin North Am 66(3):517, 1986.

Kessler HA and Blaauw B et al: Diagnosis of human immunodeficiency virus infection in seronegative homosexuals presenting with an acute viral syndrome, JAMA 289(9):1196, 1987.

The Lancet: AIDS in Africa, Lancet ii:192, 1987.

Lauder I and Campbell AC: The lymphadenopathy of human immunodeficiency virus infection, Histopathology 10:1203, 1986.

Maury CPJ: Interleukin 1 and the pathogenesis of inflammatory diseases, Acta Med Scand 220:291, 1986.

Leads from the MMWR. Revision of the CDC surveillance case definition for acquired immunodeficiency syndrome, JAMA 258(9):1143, 1987.

Mock DJ and Roberts NJ: Proposed immunopathogenic factors associated with progression from human immunodeficiency virus seropositivity to clinical disease, J Clin Microb 25(10):1817, 1987.

Muggia FM and Lonberg M: Kaposi's sarcoma and AIDS, Med Clin North Am 70(1):139, 1986.

Newmark P: AIDS in an African context, Nature 324:611, 1986.

O'Reilly RJ: New promise for autologous marrow transplants in leukemia, N Engl J Med 315(3):186, 1986.

Pahwa S, Kaplan M, and Fikrig S et al: Spectrum of human T-cell lymphotropic virus type III infection in children, JAMA 255(17):2299, 1986.

Pedersen C, Nielsen CM, and Vestergaard et al: Temporal relation of antigenaemia and loss of antibodies to core antigens to development of clinical disease in HIV infection, Br Med J 295:567, 1987.

Schroeder JS and Hunt SA: Cardiac transplantation: where are we? N Engl J Med 315(15):961, 1986.

Seligman M, Pinching AJ, and Rosen FS et al: Immunology of human immunodeficiency virus infection and the acquired immunodeficiency syndrome, Ann Intern Med 107:234, 1987.

Serafin WE and Austen KF: Mediators of immediate hypersensitivity reactions, N Engl J Med 317(1):30, 1987.

Sterioff S, Engen DE, and Zincke H: Current status of renal transplantation, Mayo Clin Proc 61:573, 1986.

Van Buren CT: Cyclosporine: progress, problems, and perspectives, Surg Clin North Am 66(3):435, 1986.

Witt DJ, Craven DE, and McCabe WR: Bacterial infections in adult patients with the acquired immune deficiency syndrome (AIDS) and AIDS-related complex, Am J Med 82:900, 1987.

CHAPTER 8

Pathogenic mechanisms in infectious diseases

Infection is defined as the presence and replication of microorganisms in the tissues of a host. *Infectious disease* is present when the biologic activities of the microorganisms injure the host severely enough to cause clinical signs and symptoms. When infection does not result in signs and symptoms of disease in the host, inapparent or *subclinical* infection is said to be present. For example, during an influenza epidemic, nonimmune persons may be infected by influenza virus but do not become ill. They do, however, develop specific antibodies in response to the replicating influenza virus. In sharp contrast, other individuals infected by the same virus can develop fulminating respiratory disease, which can be fatal. The factors that determine whether inapparent infection or severe infectious disease develop are usually not known. However, in general terms the outcome of infection depends on (1) the quantity and virulence of the organism, (2) the integrity of the host defenses, and (3) in the modern era of antimicrobial agents, the interaction of specific antibiotics with both the causative organisms and their host.

Infectious diseases are thus the result of temporary or permanent failure of the many protective mechanisms of the body to ward off infectious agents. In this chapter the means by which microorganisms are able to cause disease as well as the various reactions of the body to these invaders will be considered. Specific infections will also be described, but because many are dealt with in detail in the chapters on systemic disease, only brief summaries of most will be given here. A few infectious diseases which are multisystemic will, however, be dealt with more fully here.

Nonspecific protective mechanisms

There are many nonspecific mechanisms that protect the body against attack by infectious agents. These mechanisms are found on the external and internal surfaces of the body including the lumina of the alimentary, respiratory, and urinary tracts.

Skin

The intact skin forms a formidable barrier to infectious agents. It is unlikely that any microorganism can penetrate the intact skin, although it is probable that some bacteria such as leptospira, *Treponema pallidum,* and *Francisella tularensis,* can gain access to the body through microscopic breaches of the epidermis. Although keratin is absent from mucous surfaces, it is also likely that intact mucous membranes resist penetration by microorganisms. Some parasites, however, such as schistosomal cercaria and hookworm larvae can penetrate intact skin, while the larval stages of several nematodes, including hookworm, ascaris, and trichinella, can invade the body through intact intestinal mucous membranes. The ability

of schistosomes and probably other parasitic larvae to penetrate the skin is due to the enzymic action of glandular secretions of the larvae.

Skin that is kept continually moist can provide a suitable condition for infection by dermatophytic fungi, a situation that is seen in the external auditory canal in swimmer's ear and between the toes in athlete's foot. Other protective mechanisms in the skin are its acid pH and the bactericidal effect of the long chain fatty acids present in the sebaceous secretions.

Mouth

The general defense mechanisms of the oral cavity are no better understood than those of other body surfaces. The free flow of saliva is important in carrying away great numbers of microorganisms, which are ultimately swallowed and killed by gastric acid. In conditions that cause xerostomia (dry mouth) this mechanism breaks down, and diseases, especially caries and periodontal disease, can become rampant, as the oral flora changes.

Unlike the skin where hair follicles provide a protective environment for staphylococci, corynebacteria, and other bacteria, the oral mucosa has no such hiding places. The teeth and gingival margins, however, provide a protective environment as a result of their complex morphology and retain bacterial plaque. This layer of bacteria and polysaccharides is so adhesive that it can only be removed by toothbrushing. The consequence is that gingivitis is almost inevitable.

In contrast to the teeth and gums, the oral mucosa is infected relatively rarely. Bacterial infections are exceedingly uncommon. Syphilis and tuberculosis are almost the only examples, and even these require special circumstances to become established. The main infections of the oral mucosa are caused by viruses (especially *Herpesvirus hominis*) and fungi (especially *Candida albicans*). The reasons for freedom from infections of the oral mucosa are unknown. Saliva contains IgA and lysozyme, but these appear to have little effect against caries or periodontal disease. Two possibilities are that the profuse natural oral flora may compete with potential bacterial pathogens, or more probably, that such potential pathogens may lack the necessary attachment mechanisms for the cells of the oral mucous membranes and as a result may be unable to initiate infection.

Stomach

The gastric secretion of hydrochloric acid is a very important mechanism especially against bacterial pathogens. In cholera, ingestion of 10^9 organisms/ml is necessary to overcome the killing effect of gastric pH and cause infection. Persons who are achlorhydric are therefore more susceptible to intestinal bacterial infections, including salmonella infections and intestinal tuberculosis.

Intestines

Intestinal motility appears to protect against enteric infections. Two factors are thought to be involved. First, with normal motility the chances of bacterial pathogens attaching to the surface of intestinal mucosal cells are lessened; second, reduction of intestinal motility increases the density of the bacterial population with an increased risk of infection. It has been shown in bacillary dysentery that the use of drugs that inhibit intestinal motility can prolong the duration of symptoms.

The normal gastrointestinal tract flora is mainly anaerobic and is present in high concentration (about 10^{12} organisms/g of feces). End products of anaerobic bacterial metabolism include organic acids, which have an inhibitory effect on bacterial pathogens. Interference with the normal flora of the bowel, for example, by antibiotics may suppress this mechanism. This may result in promotion of growth of pathogenic bacteria and opportunistic organisms such as *C. albicans*, or select out minority species from the normal flora, which may then become pathogenic. This latter mechanism is thought to be responsible for the pathogenesis of antibiotic-associated colitis. Antibiotics, such as clindamycin, tetracycline, and penicillin, inhibit or kill the common anaerobic species in the bowel. However, *Clostridium difficile*, a minority strain among the intestinal anaerobes, is unaffected by these antibiotics and multiplies freely. This bacterium is then capable of producing sufficient exotoxin to cause necrosis of the intestinal mucosa (see also Chapter 14).

Respiratory tract

Lysozyme is an enzyme present in high concentration in the tears. It is capable of causing lysis of some bacteria by acting on their cell wall, and as such, may be an important defense mechanism for the eye and the upper respiratory tract. The configuration of the upper respiratory tract creates turbulence in air flow which leads to larger particles impinging on the mucosal surfaces. The ciliated epithelium lining the respiratory tract and its associated layer of mucus form an important protective mechanism. The constant upward movement of mucus caused by ciliary movement is able to clear almost all inhaled particles from the respiratory tract. The few particles reaching the alveoli are ingested by alveolar macrophages. Injury to this mechanism during measles, for example, can create conditions for secondary bacterial infection of the bronchi, which in turn can lead to bronchopneumonia.

The respiratory secretions contain nonspecific viral inhibitors, which are mucoid substances capable of saturating the attachment mechanisms of several respiratory viruses, including influenza virus, and in this way may prevent many viral infections.

Urinary tract

The urinary tract is normally sterile throughout its length with the exception of the lower urethra. The mechanisms contributing to its sterility include (1) the hypertonic urine present in the renal medulla, (2) the possible antimicrobial effect of urea and other urinary constituents, (3) the pH of the urine, and (4) the flushing effect of the urinary flow.

Female genital tract

The main protective mechanism in the female genital tract is the normally low pH. This is the result of acid production from the metabolism of glycogen by lactobacilli. Glycogen synthesis is, in turn, promoted by the action of estrogens.

PATHOGENIC MECHANISMS OF MICROORGANISMS

Each major group of microorganisms—viruses, bacteria, fungi, and protozoa—together with helminths, have unique properties which confer on them the ability to cause disease. Some important examples of these, together with the typical human host responses, will be discussed briefly. As already mentioned the larger the dose and the greater the virulence of an infectious agent to which the host is exposed, the more likely disease is to develop.

Pathogenic mechanisms in viral diseases

Viruses are small, obligate intracellular parasites. They consist of a core of either DNA or RNA surrounded by a protein coat or capsid; in some instances they possess an outer envelope, which is derived from the host cell (Fig. 8-1). This structure provides a basis for virus classification (Table 8-1), which can be modified by the physical type of the nucleic acid (single or double stranded) and the molecular weight of the virus. The presence or absence of an envelope and the type of nucleic acid also determine the way in which the virus interacts with its host cell.

Viruses must gain access to the interior of the host cell because they require many of the cell's biosynthetic processes

TABLE 8-1. Simplified viral classification based on morphology and nucleic acid

Nucleic acid	Viral symmetry	Envelope	Size (nm)	Virus
DNA	Icosahedral	No	70	Adenovirus
	Icosahedral	Yes	150	Herpesvirus
	Complex	Yes	160	Poxvirus
RNA	Icosahedral	No	20	Picornavirus
	Icosahedral	Yes	60	Rubella virus
	Helical	Yes	100	Influenza virus

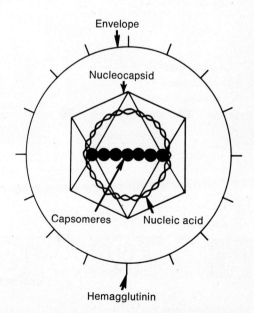

FIG. 8-1. General structure of an icosahedral virus particle.

for replication. In doing so they alter the cell function and frequently the cell morphology. These latter changes can often permit a pathologic diagnosis of viral infection.

The steps in viral infection of a host cell are as follows:

1. Attachment of the virus to the cytoplasmic membrane of the host cell
2. Penetration of the cytoplasmic membrane by the virus (Fig. 8-2)
3. Uncoating of the virus particle, that is removal of the protein coat
4. Synthesis of viral nucleic acid and protein
5. Assembly of structurally mature viruses
6. Release of viruses from the host cell (Fig. 8-3)

Viral latency

Certain viruses, especially the herpesvirus family, can remain dormant within the host cell for long periods. They remain integrated with the host cell genome until triggered by a variety of stimuli to undergo a period of replication. This is the property of *viral latency*.

Infections of *Herpesvirus hominis* are excellent examples of latent infection. Initial oral infection by *H. hominis* type 1 is usually asymptomatic although occasionally it may cause herpetic stomatitis. Thereafter, apparently for the lifetime of the host, the virus resides in the ganglion of the trigeminal nerve, from which it may be reactivated at intervals and cause characteristic faciolabial herpes (fever blisters). The mechanisms for reactivation are obscure, but precipitating factors include ultraviolet light, fever, and menstruation.

Alterations in cellular morphology caused by viral replication vary from little or none to total dissolution of the cell. Some morphologic changes are readily seen in histologic or cytologic preparations of virus-infected tissues, and these may be typical or highly suggestive of the causal agent. The morphologic features that are very suggestive of viral infection are (1) the presence of *inclusion bodies* and (2) the formation of *giant cells* in infected tissues.

A viral inclusion body is an intracellular structure formed in the course of viral synthesis. Viral inclusions are readily seen by microscopy when stained by acid dyes such as acid fuchsin. They are found in the nucleus or in the cytoplasm, a feature which may further assist in recognition of the causative virus. Inclusions can consist of masses of virus particles, viral components especially nucleic acids, or remnants of viral synthesis with few or no viral particles present. Some examples of viral inclusions are listed in Table 8-2. Members of the genus *Chlamydia*, which are obligate intracellular bacteria, also produce inclusions that are typically basophilic and present in the cytoplasm (Fig. 8-4). It was this property which for many years resulted in their classification as "basophilic viruses."

Giant cells formed in viral-infected tissues are thought to develop in one of two ways. First, the cell nucleus may divide without division of the cytoplasm. Second, the cytoplasmic membranes of neighboring cells may fuse to form a large syncytial mass. A typical viral giant cell from a case of chickenpox is shown in Fig. 8-5. The common viruses that can cause giant cell formation are listed as follows:

1. Paramyxoviruses
   a. Measles virus
   b. Mumps virus
   c. Parainfluenza viruses
   d. Respiratory syncytial virus
2. Herpesviruses
   a. Cytomegalovirus
   b. Herpesvirus hominis type 1
   c. Herpesvirus hominis type 2
   d. Varicella-zoster virus

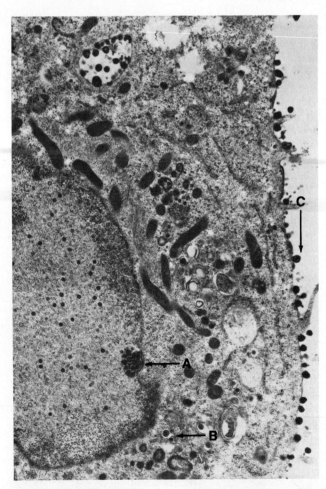

FIG. 8-3. Electron micrograph of a virus-infected cell. Virus particles are present in the nucleus *(A)* and the cytoplasm *(B)* and are budding at the cell surface *(C)*.

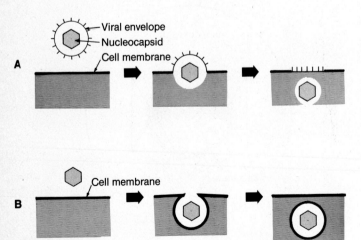

FIG. 8-2. Cell penetration by virus particles. **A,** Enveloped virus. **B,** Nonenveloped virus.

Cell lysis by viruses

The lytic destruction of cells by viruses is a common result of many virus infections. The final event in enterovirus infection, for example, is the lysis of the host cell upon release of new viral progeny. When epithelial surfaces are involved, replication of uninfected cells usually replaces the necrotic cells fairly rapidly. However, destruction of ciliated respiratory epithelium, which is a common feature of some viral infections (influenza, for example), damages the normal mucociliary defense mechanism and predisposes the affected person to secondary bacterial invasion. Some cells, however, especially neurons, are destroyed without replacement. This is seen most vividly in poliomyelitis where motoneurons are destroyed by viral replication and motor paralysis results (Chapter 17).

Host response to viral infection

The main pathologic and immune responses to viral infections are (1) inflammation, (2) antibody formation, (3) interferon formation, and (4) cellular immunity.

Inflammation. Inflammation is considered in detail in Chapter 6. It is worth emphasizing again, however, that although most viral infections are acute in nature, the typical cellular response in viral-induced acute inflammation is *lymphocytic*. Occasionally, neutrophils are present in the inflammatory ex-

TABLE 8-2. Common inclusion bodies caused by viruses and chlamydiae

Agent	Site of inclusion	Staining characteristic	Remarks

Herpesvirus group
  H. hominis
  H. varicella-zoster
  Cytomegalovirus
	Nucleus + + +
	Cytoplasm +
		Eosinophilic	Nuclear inclusions usually surrounded by a halo

Rabiesvirus	Cytoplasm	Eosinophilic	Negri body

Poxvirus group
  Vaccinia virus
  Smallpox virus
	Cytoplasm	Eosinophilic	Guarnieri body

Measles virus	Nucleus + + Cytoplasm +	Eosinophilic	Measleslike inclusions seen in subacute sclerosing panencephalitis
Adenovirus	Nucleus	Amphophilic	

Chlamydia group
  Psittacosis
  Inclusion conjunctivitis
  Trachoma
  Lymphogranuloma venereum
	Cytoplasm	Basophilic	Fastidious obligate intracellular bacteria

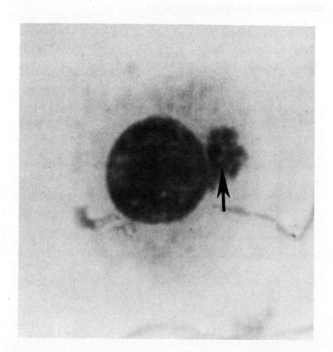

FIG. 8-4. Cytoplasmic inclusion body *(arrow)* in a smear from the eye of a patient with trachoma. These inclusions are typically basophilic.

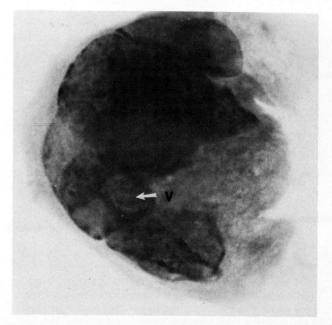

FIG. 8-5. Smear from skin lesion in chickenpox, showing a multinucleate giant cell with nuclear inclusions *(V)*.

udate, even in the absence of secondary bacterial invaders. Neutrophils are seen, for example, in the cerebrospinal fluid in the early stages of viral infections of the central nervous system, and commonly in the inflammatory exudate of infections caused by *Herpesvirus hominis.* In the peripheral blood, it is not uncommon to find a mild polymorph leukocytosis, for example, in enteroviral infections. A lymphocytosis, however, is characteristic of infectious mononucleosis, viral hepatitis, and cytomegalovirus infections.

Antibody formation. A variety of antibodies is formed in response to viral infections. These antibodies include the three main classes of immunoglobulins: IgG, IgM, and IgA. As in other infections, IgM antibodies are detected early in the disease

TABLE 8-3. Types of interferons

Type	Source	Induced by
I α	Leukocytes	Virus or RNA
I β	Fibroblasts	Virus or RNA
II γ	T lymphocytes	Antigens or lectins

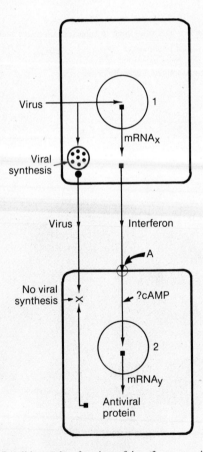

FIG. 8-6. Possible mode of action of interferon on viruses. Viral infection of *cell 1* results in (a) new viral synthesis and (b) production of mRNA$_x$ which codes for interferon. Interferon reaches *cell 2* where it first interacts with a surface receptor *(A)*, then possibly as a result of cyclic AMP activity, stimulates production of mRNA$_y$. This RNA codes for a specific protein, which, in turn, inhibits viral synthesis in cell B. *(From McCracken AW and Cawson RA: Clinical and oral microbiology, Washington DC, 1982, Hemisphere Publishing Corp.)*

and are good evidence of current or very recent infection. With one agent, cytomegalovirus (CMV), IgM antibodies appear not only in the early stages of the initial infection, but can reappear if there is recrudescence of the disease months or even years later. Secretory IgA antibodies are an extremely important immune response in viral infections, whether they are naturally acquired or artificially induced by live attenuated viral vaccines. Their presence in the nasopharyngeal and intestinal secretions is an important defense against respiratory or enteric viruses.

Autoantibodies are thought to play a part in the pathogenesis of some viral infections. Mumps virus appears to augment its pathogenicity by releasing cellular antigens that stimulate antibodies against the patient's own cells.

Interferon production. The production of interferons is an important mechanism that appears to be partly responsible for termination of viral infections. The classification of interferons is shown in Table 8-3. Interferons are proteins that have many effects on cell functions (Chapter 7), including enhancement of antibody production and macrophage activity as well as protecting cells against the effects of invading viruses.

The main sources of interferons are leukocytes, fibroblasts, and T lymphocytes. Leukocyte and fibroblastic interferons (type I) are produced not only in response to viral infection but their production can be stimulated by other microbial agents and inducer substances containing double-stranded RNA, such as synthetic polynucleotides. T lymphocytes can produce type II (immune) interferons during immune reactions. Unlike antibodies, interferons are not specific for the agent that induced them. They are, however, specific for the species in which they were induced. Thus interferons that are induced in chick embryos by influenza virus can block infection of chicken tissues by several different viruses. These interferons, however, do not block infection of human tissue, for example, by influenza virus. The mode of action of interferon at cellular level is shown in Fig. 8-6.

Cellular immunity. Although more is known of humoral immunity in viral infections, cellular immunity appears to play an important part along with interferon in bringing viral infections to an end.

The responsible cell is the T lymphocyte, which in this context has two main functions:

1. A cytotoxic effect that destroys virus-infected cells
2. Recruitment of macrophages, which are responsible for phagocytosis of viral particles and cell debris

Macrophages appear to be capable of ingesting viral particles. Some, called *permissive macrophages,* will allow further replication of viruses rather than cause their destruction following ingestion. The property of permissiveness in macrophages appears to be determined by genetic factors. Thus it is possible that genetic abnormalities that affect macrophages may determine the severity and outcome of viral infections.

Range of host-virus interactions

The outcome of host-virus interaction varies considerably according to the properties of the virus and the host. On the one hand there are infections in which the virus is eradicated during or within a finite time following the illness. This is seen in many respiratory tract infections in which the virus can only be isolated in the early stages of the illness and at no other time thereafter. Only specific viral antibodies remain as evidence of infection. Influenza and mumps are examples of diseases in which the virus is totally eliminated from the body following recovery. Usually the recovered host is left with permanent immunity to the causative viruses. On the other hand, several viruses, once they have established infection, will persist in the host cells for long periods, which may last for the lifetime of the host. These viral infections are of three types—latent, slow and chronic.

Latent viral infections. Latent viral infections begin either with an acute illness, during which the virus can be isolated from the host, or an asymptomatic infection. Thereafter, for the life of the host, the virus remains dormant in host cells, from which it may periodically emerge causing a recrudescent illness during which the virus may again be isolated. Although antibodies to the virus are present in the host, they are not protective and fail to eliminate the virus. The best known example of a latent virus is *Herpesvirus hominis*. Indeed, viral latency is a characteristic of the family of herpesviruses.

Slow virus infections. In the last 20 years, it has been recognized that certain chronic diseases of the nervous system are caused by viruses or by unique viruslike agents called *prions*. Prions are composed of protein; as yet, no nucleic acids have been demonstrated in their composition. Slow virus diseases are characterized by very long incubation periods that may last up to several years, followed by progressive deterioration in nervous system function that leads inevitably to death. The term *slow* applies to the prolonged nature of the illness. There is no evidence that viral synthesis, for example, proceeds at anything but a normal rate. Human immunodeficiency virus (HIV), the cause of acquired immunodeficiency syndrome (AIDS), is also a slow virus. In this instance the virus attacks the T lymphocytes, particularly those helper T cells which possess OKT4 or Leu 3 antigens.

The reason for the slow progression of these infections is not known. *In subacute sclerosing panencephalitis (SSPE),* which is caused by a measleslike virus, it is possible that, having entered and replicated within the host cell, the viruses are prevented by host antibody from leaving the cell and can only infect neighboring cells in some restricted way. Slow cell-to-cell transfer of viruses is the result. Thus it may take many months for measles virus to enter and destroy sufficient neurons for the disease to become clinically apparent.

Progressive multifocal leukoencephalopathy (PML), which is caused by simian virus (SV) 40, becomes clinically apparent when the patient is immunosuppressed. This suggests that the virus is normally rendered harmless by host defense mechanisms, only becoming pathogenic when immune mechanisms fail.

Creutzfeldt-Jakob disease and *kuru* are two similar nervous system demyelinating diseases caused by prions. The former has been transmitted, with fatal results by corneal transplant and injections of growth hormone preparations made from human pituitary glands. The route of infection in most cases, however, is not known.

Kuru is also a demyelinating disease that is confined to tribes in eastern New Guinea. The infection is spread by the consumption of human remains. With the proscription of cannibalism the disease appears to be dying out.

Diseases caused by prions are also seen in animals. The best studied is scrapie, a demyelinating disease affecting the central nervous system of sheep. There are striking similarities between the pathologic changes in scrapie and Creutzfeldt-Jakob disease. The spongelike appearance of the brain and the presence of plaques of amyloid are common to both diseases. Purified extracts of brain tissue from both diseases contain the same specific protein (PrP). This protein is closely associated with infectivity, although no nucleic acids have as yet been detected in infectious preparations of brain. This has led to the conclusion that prions may possibly be a unique, new class of agents consisting of infective, self-replicating proteins. Much remains to be learned about these agents and slow virus diseases. Their study is likely to lead to a better understanding of degenerative diseases of the nervous system such as multiple sclerosis and amyotrophic lateral sclerosis (Chapter 20).

Chronic virus infections. There are a few viral infections that can give rise to persistent diseases of fluctuating severity, during the course of which viruses are continually being shed even in the presence of specific antibodies. Three important examples of this type of virus disease are hepatitis B (Chapter 15), chronic Epstein-Barr virus infection (Chapter 12), and congenital rubella syndrome (discussed later in this chapter). Patients with persistent hepatitis B and children with congenital rubella syndrome are important sources of epidemic spread of the infections. The continued presence of viruses in the body fluids of patients with hepatitis B is related to failure of the patient's immune system to develop antibodies to hepatitis B surface antigen, despite the formation of antibodies to other components of the virus. The reason for failure or delay in formation of this antibody is not known.

HIV is yet another important example of a virus that continues to be shed by its host despite the presence of circulating antibodies.

Infections caused by specific viruses

The important common viruses and the diseases that they cause are listed in Table 8-4.

Adenoviruses

Adenoviruses are 70 nm, nonenveloped DNA viruses; over 40 serotypes have been identified. This group of viruses causes respiratory tract infections that range in severity from the common cold to viral pneumonia. Adenoviruses also cause epidemics of conjunctivitis, and ocular infection frequently accompanies adenoviral upper respiratory disease. Types 11 and 21 have been described as causes of acute hemorrhagic inflammation of the bladder, a self-limiting disease of young children. Recently described serotypes 40 and 41 are believed to cause infantile gastroenteritis.

Diseases associated with adenoviruses are generally mild with few complications. The viruses replicate in the mucosal cells of the respiratory and intestinal tracts. Their pathologic effects in the respiratory tract range from mild acute inflammation to, on rare occasions, fatal viral pneumonitis. In these cases there is interstitial inflammation of the lung and necrotizing bronchitis. Cells with intranuclear inclusions have been described in the pulmonary lesions. This severe form of adenoviral disease is now recognized as a life-threatening complication in immunosuppressed patients, particularly those who have undergone renal transplantation.

Arboviruses

The arboviruses (*arthropod-borne* viruses) comprise a large, heterogeneous group; characteristically, they are transmitted by and multiply within blood-sucking arthropods, especially mosquitoes and ticks. Arboviruses are normally spread among animals and birds by arthropods. Humans can become occasional and accidental hosts when they intrude into this pathway of infection.

TABLE 8-4. Important viral groups and their diseases

Virus group	Virus	Associated diseases	Also refer to chapter
Adenovirus	Many serotypes	Respiratory, ocular, and bladder infections	12 and 16
Arbovirus	Several hundred species	Central nervous system infections; hemorrhagic fevers	20
Hepatitis	Hepatitis A	Viral hepatitis	15
	Hepatitis B		
	Hepatitis non-A, non-B		
	Possibly others		
Herpesvirus	Herpesvirus hominis 1 and 2	Mucocutaneous eruptions; encephalitis	14, 19, and 20
	Varicella-zoster	Chickenpox; shingles; encephalitis; pneumonitis	12 and 19
	Cytomegalovirus	Congenital and acquired diseases, which can affect all organ systems	
	Epstein-Barr	Infectious mononucleosis	13
Myxovirus	Influenza	Influenza	12
	Parainfluenza	Bronchiolitis and pneumonia	12
	Respiratory syncytial virus	Bronchiolitis and pneumonia	12
	Measles	Measles	
	Mumps	Mumps	
Papillomavirus	Types 6, 11, 16, 18	Associated with genital and other carcinomas	19, 21
Picornavirus	Poliovirus	Poliomyelitis	14
	Coxsackievirus A and B	Infection of central nervous system, heart, respiratory tract, skin, and mucous membranes	11, 12, 19, and 20
	Echovirus	Infection of central nervous system, skin, and mucous membranes	19 and 20
	Rhinovirus	Common cold	12
Poxvirus	Vaccinia	Vaccinia	19
Retrovirus (HTLV* series)	HTLV 1	Human T cell leukemia: tropical spastic paraplegia	
	HTLV 2	Hairy cell leukemia	
	HTLV 3 (HIV 1)†	Acquired immunodeficiency syndrome	
	HTLV 4 (HIV 2)†	Acquired immunodeficiency syndrome	
	HTLV 5	?Human leukemia/lymphoma	
Rhabdovirus	Rabies	Encephalomyelitis	20
Togavirus	Rubella	Rubella	19

HTLV, human T cell lymphotropic virus.
†*HIV*, human immunodeficiency virus.

Arboviruses frequently cause only mild illness or asymptomatic infection, but they may also cause one of the following:

1. Hemorrhagic fever
2. Hemorrhagic fever with hepatitis and nephritis (i.e., yellow fever)
3. Dengue syndrome of fever, rash, severe headache and arthralgia, and lymphadenopathy.
4. Meningoencephalitis

Examples of arboviruses and their associated diseases are listed in Table 8-5.

Hemorrhagic fevers. Hemorrhagic fevers are caused by several viruses of which dengue virus is the most common. The pathologic effects of this infection are thought to be a result of immunologic reactions that activate complement and the process of disseminated intravascular coagulation (Chapter 12). These in turn can lead to shock, thrombosis, hemorrhage, and renal failure.

Yellow fever. Yellow fever has similar pathogenic mechanisms, but in addition, there are major pathologic changes in the liver and kidneys in severe cases. The liver lobules show partial (midzonal) or complete necrosis, and the cytoplasm of the hepatocytes contains large hyaline apoptotic masses called

Councilman bodies. Intranuclear viral inclusions may also be present. There is fatty degeneration and necrosis of the proximal renal tubules. As a result of liver damage, jaundice (hence yellow fever) usually accompanies the clinical picture of hemorrhagic fever described earlier, and renal failure develops in severe cases. The overall death rate is about 5%. As a result of the use of a highly effective vaccine and mosquito control, yellow fever, at least for the present, is an uncommon disease.

Dengue fever. The pathogenesis of dengue fever, caused by dengue viruses, is a peripheral vasculitis. This appears to be mediated by immunologic reactions similar to those in hemorrhagic fevers, which, as already mentioned, can be caused by the same viruses. Although it is symptomatically dramatic with very severe headache and joint pains, dengue fever has a low mortality rate in the absence of hemorrhagic manifestations.

Hepatitis viruses

Many viruses are capable of causing inflammatory liver disease. They include hepatitis A and B viruses, non-A, non-B agents, δ agent, coxsackieviruses, rubella, and members of the herpesvirus family (Chapter 15).

TABLE 8-5. Some important arbovirus diseases and their vectors

Virus group	Disease	Vector
Alphavirus	Eastern equine encephalitis	Aedes mosquito
	Western equine encephalitis	Culex mosquito
	Venezuelan equine encephalitis	Culex, Aedes and other species
Bunyavirus	California encephalitis	Not determined
Flavivirus	Dengue fever	Aedes mosquito
	St. Louis encephalitis	Culex mosquito
	Yellow fever	Aedes mosquito
Reovirus	Colorado tick fever	Dermacentor tick

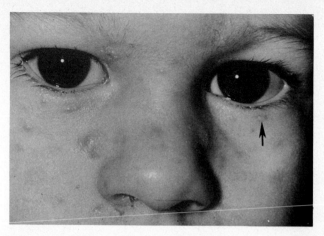

FIG. 8-7. Cutaneous lesions of chickenpox *(arrow).* The lesions are oval, superficial, and surrounded by a narrow zone of erythema.

Herpesviruses

The members of the large herpesvirus family that affect humans are listed in Table 8-4. Herpesviruses are enveloped DNA viruses, which average about 150 nm in diameter. They are unique in their relationship with humans in that all have the ability to integrate with the genome of certain host cells and remain latent for long periods, possibly for life.

The factors that control latency and reactivation are poorly understood. However, immunodeficiency, whether caused by disease, treatment or both, is commonly associated with reactivation of this group of infections. Many recurrences of infection as a result of *Herpesvirus hominis* or varicella-zoster virus are also seen in otherwise healthy people.

Pathologic characteristics of herpesvirus infections include the following:

1. Formation of vesicular mucocutaneous lesions seen with *Herpesvirus hominis* type 1 (HSV 1), *Herpesvirus hominis* type 2 (HSV 2) and varicella-zoster virus (VZV)
2. Formation of giant cells with eosinophilic, intranuclear, and intracytoplasmic inclusions seen with HSV 1, HSV 2, VZV, and CMV.

The clinicopathologic features of *Herpesvirus hominis* infections are described in Chapters 19, 20, and 23.

Varicella-zoster virus. Chickenpox (varicella) is the result of primary infection of a nonimmune person with VZV. Reactivation of a latent VZV infection results in herpes zoster (shingles).

Chickenpox is contracted by inhalation of virus-infected droplets. From the respiratory tract the virus reaches the lymphatic system and enters the blood stream to be carried to the skin and mucous membranes (Fig. 8-7) including the epithelial lining of the respiratory tract.

The pathologic features of chickenpox are very similar to those described in mucocutaneous herpetic infections. Vesicles form in the skin and mucous membranes and typically contain inflammatory cells and multinucleate giant cells (Fig. 8-5). Occasionally, especially in adults, varicella virus causes a severe interstitial pneumonitis (Chapter 12) and rarely, a viral encephalitis (Chapter 20).

In childhood, chickenpox is a mild illness, characterized by fever, a vesicular rash particularly on the trunk, and often vesicles in the mouth. The skin lesions characteristically appear in small crops at different times so that both early and late lesions can be seen simultaneously. Complications are rare in children; however, in adults the disease is more severe, and the risk of complications, especially varicella pneumonitis, is higher. Infants born of mothers with active chickenpox are liable to develop the disease in severe form immediately before or shortly after birth. Atypical rashes, especially with hemorrhagic lesions, are seen in immunodeficient children and adults. The hemorrhagic nature of these lesions is usually due to thrombocytopenia.

Shingles (zoster). Shingles is caused by reactivation of VZV, which is thought to remain latent in the cells of nerve root ganglia following an initial attack of chickenpox. It is described in Chapter 19.

Cytomegalovirus. Most human infections by CMV are asymptomatic. Clinically significant infections can take place as follows:

1. In the developing fetus (congenital infection)
2. As a primary infection of nonimmune persons
3. By reactivation of latent infection in immunosuppressed patients

Congenital CMV infections are generally most serious when transmission to the fetus takes place in the first trimester of pregnancy. However, transmission resulting in disease in the infant can take place in the later months of gestation. The results of intrauterine infection on the fetus vary, but stillbirth or neonatal death are relatively common. In those infants who survive, there may be little overt evidence of the disease. In others the following may be present at birth:

1. An acute necrotizing encephalomyelitis, particularly involving the periventricular brain tissue and resulting in calcification in and around the ventricular system, which, in turn, frequently leads to hydrocephalus
2. Multiple organ involvement, including the liver, lungs, and kidneys, as well as the central nervous system by cell destruction and inflammation (Fig. 8-8, *A* and *B*)

In some children defects, especially mental retardation, may not be detected until later in childhood. Children with congenital CMV infection excrete the virus in saliva and urine for many months or years and are a major source of the disease.

In some congenitally infected infants, the salivary glands are involved, hence the earlier name of salivary gland inclusion disease.

Primary infection of nonimmune persons is usually asymptomatic or results in a mild illness. It is thought to be transmitted by droplet infection or by contact with secretions of congenitally infected infants. The clinical features of the illness are

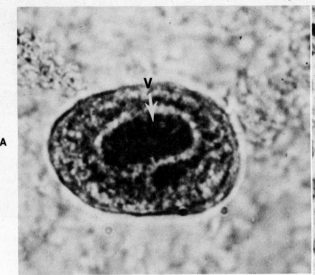

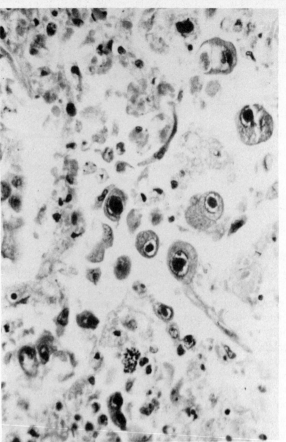

FIG. 8-8. A, Congenital cytomegalovirus infection. Micrograph of urinary sediment shows a renal tubular cell containing a large intranuclear viral inclusion body *(V).* **B,** Generalized cytomegalovirus infection in an immunosuppressed patient. Lung section shows typical enlarged, inclusion-bearing cells. *(From McCracken AW and Cawson RA: Clinical and oral microbiology, Washington DC, 1982, Hemisphere Publishing Corp.)*

fever, malaise, pharyngitis, and lymphadenopathy. Atypical lymphocytes are present in the peripheral blood. In all these respects, the disease closely simulates infectious mononucleosis. CMV disease can also be sexually transmitted. A similar syndrome (postperfusion syndrome) sometimes follows open heart surgery or blood transfusion. The apparent source of virus is the donor blood.

CMV infection is extremely common following kidney, liver, heart, and bone marrow transplantation. The donor organ is thought to be the source of CMV in most of these cases.

The CMV genome has been detected in the cells of Kaposi's sarcoma, suggesting a possible etiologic relationship between the virus and this malignancy, especially in the context of AIDS.

Reactivation of latent CMV infection is a common sequel to immunosuppressive treatment of disease in which the immune system is compromised. CMV infection is, for example, extremely common in patients with AIDS and can involve the adrenal glands (causing adrenal insufficiency) and the nervous system as well as the lungs, kidneys and other organs.

Postmortem evidence of reactivated CMV is common in patients who have died of leukemia or lymphoma. The CMV-infected cells are demonstrable in almost every organ of the body in these cases (Fig. 8-8). The lungs, liver, kidney, pancreas, and the retina of the eye are the organs most frequently involved. The typical histologic appearances are those of enlarged parenchymatous cells (i.e., cytomegaly) with intranuclear, eosinophilic inclusion bodies associated with a variable amount of chronic inflammatory cell infiltration.

Effective preventive and therapeutic measures have not yet been developed for CMV infections, although CMV retinitis in patients with AIDS has been successfully treated with an analog of acyclovir.

Epstein-Barr virus. Epstein-Barr virus (EBV) is the etiologic agent of infectious mononucleosis (Chapter 12) and has also been associated with two forms of cancer, Burkitt's lymphoma and nasopharyngeal carcinoma of Chinese males. Its etiologic role in these two malignancies remains uncertain.

Orthomyxoviruses and paramyxoviruses

Orthomyxoviruses are large enveloped RNA viruses that have an affinity for mucoid substances as a result of the presence of neuraminidase on the viral envelope. Paramyxoviruses have a similar structure and composition but do not possess neuraminidase. Orthomyxoviruses and paramyxoviruses together comprise the myxoviruses.

Infections by myxoviruses fall into three broad categories:
1. Primarily respiratory infections: influenza, parainfluenza, respiratory syncytial virus (RSV)
2. Systemic infection with involvement of skin and mucous membranes: measles
3. Systemic infection localizing mainly to the parotid glands: mumps

Influenza. Influenza is an acute respiratory infection caused by *influenza A* or *B* viruses. Pathologically, it is characterized by inflammatory changes in the bronchial and bronchiolar mucosa. There is loss of the ciliated epithelial cells and infiltration of the submucosa with lymphocytes and macrophages. Frequently, secondary bacterial infection, by *S. pneumoniae* or *S. aureus,* for example, leads to further acute inflammation with a neutrophil polymorph infiltrate. From the bronchi, bacterial infection can spread readily to the alveoli, giving rise to bronchopneumonia. Rarely, influenza virus involves the alveoli, giving rise to a severe, sometimes fatal primary viral pneumonitis (Chapter 12).

Clinically, uncomplicated influenza is characterized by fever, myalgia, and cough. Complications are mainly caused by secondary bacterial infections or serious impairment of respiratory function. One rare and serious complication of influenza (as well as several other viral diseases) is *Reye's syndrome* of encephalopathy and hepatic failure. The syndrome is seen mainly in children and death results in about one third of cases. The cause of Reye's syndrome is not known. Aspirin has been postulated as a risk factor, but this has not been firmly established. Pathologically, there is severe fatty change involving the liver lobules and cerebral edema. Avoidance of aspirin in treating children with acute viral infections seems a prudent precaution but no specific preventive or therapeutic measures are available.

Prevention of influenza A and B by vaccination against strains of the two viruses prevalent in the community is highly advisable for patients with chronic heart, lung, and kidney disease. If such patients contract influenza they run a high risk of fatal illness.

Respiratory syncytial virus (RSV) and parainfluenza. These paramyxoviruses are common causes of severe respiratory disease in infants. RSV, in particular, can cause fatal infection. In RSV disease, the pathologic changes are mainly in the bronchioles, which become infiltrated with inflammatory cells. The lining epithelium becomes necrotic. Multinucleate giant cells can be detected in the bronchiolar lumen. Parainfluenza viruses (types 1, 2, and 3) cause acute inflammation of the larynx, trachea, and bronchi in young children, giving rise to the laborious breathing and pronounced cough that typify the old clinically descriptive term *croup*. Occasionally viral pneumonia may develop. RSV and parainfluenza viruses usually cause only mild, coldlike illnesses in adults. Preventive vaccines against both of these viruses have been singularly unsuccessful.

Measles. Measles is the most important and potentially the most severe of all the common childhood fevers. Transmission is by droplet infection. After a period of proliferation first in the upper respiratory tract, then in the cells of the reticuloendothelial system, the virus reaches the mucous membranes (including the conjunctivae) and the skin by way of the blood stream. In a few instances the lung parenchyma or the meninges and brain may be involved at this stage.

The pathologic changes in the skin are found in the vicinity of small blood vessels where small aggregates of lymphocytes and monocytes are present. Measles virus antigens can also be demonstrated in these sites.

In the oral mucous membranes, similar lesions are present and develop a bluish-white necrotic center. These are *Koplik's spots,* which precede the appearance of the skin lesions. There is lymphoid hyperplasia throughout the body, and multinucleate giant cells may be seen in sections of lymphoid tissue. Occasionally, primary measles pneumonitis develops, characterized by a giant cell reaction and interstitial inflammation.

In the typical cases of measles, following an incubation period of 10 to 14 days, fever, Koplik's spots, conjunctivitis, and a maculopapular rash develop; the rash begins on the face and spreads down the body. The main complications of measles are the following:

1. Bacterial infections of the lung, bronchi, paranasal sinuses, and middle ear
2. Viral penumonia
3. Acute meningoencephalitis
4. Rarely, subacute sclerosing encephalitis, a slow virus disease of the central nervous system, a possible development months or years after the measles attack

Atypical measles is seen in persons who have received killed measles vaccine in the past. In this form of measles, the clinicopathologic picture appears to be mainly a result of hypersensitivity reactions. Koplik's spots are absent and the rash is urticarial in many cases. Other features of atypical measles include edema of the hands and feet, interstitial pneumonia, and pleural effusion.

The use of live attenuated vaccines has resulted in a 95% decline in measles in the United States and other countries. Care must be taken, however, to avoid vaccination of infants with immunodeficiency diseases, since this is likely to result in fatal illness caused by the attenuated measles virus.

Enteroviruses

The enteroviruses—poliovirus, coxsackieviruses A and B, and echoviruses—are commonly present in the intestinal tracts of normal individuals. In a minority of those infected with enteroviruses, overt disease develops (Table 8-6).

The pathologic effects of enteroviruses are a result of invasion and destruction of the cells in the target organs and associated inflammatory changes (Fig. 8-9). Examples are the destruction of motoneurons in poliomyelitis and cardiac myocytes in coxsackievirus myocarditis, respectively, following invasion of these cells by lytic viruses. The pathogenesis of enterovirus infections is shown in Fig. 8-10.

Clinically, enteroviral infections are characterized by fever, sometimes accompanied by rashes: depending on the virus and target organ, there are a variety of signs and symptoms referable to the nervous, cardiovascular, respiratory, and integumentary systems (Table 8-6).

Newly discovered enteroviruses are now assigned sequential numbers and have been associated with a variety of illnesses.

TABLE 8-6. Spectrum of diseases caused by enteroviruses

Disease	*Virus and serotype*
Bronchitis, pneumonia	Enterovirus 68
Epidemic myalgia (Bornholm disease; pleurodynia)	Coxsackie B1 to B5, echovirus 1
Hand-foot-and-mouth disease	Coxsackie A16, A4, A5, A7, A9, A10
Hemorrhagic conjunctivitis	Coxsackie A24, enterovirus 70
Herpangina	Coxsackie A1 to A6, A8, A10
Myopericarditis	Coxsackie B1 to B5, coxsackie A4, A14, echovirus 9 and 22
Meningitis	Many serotypes of coxsackieviruses and echoviruses; enterovirus 71
Poliomyelitis	Polioviruses 1, 2, and 3
Upper respiratory tract infection	Coxsackie A10, A21, A24

For example, enterovirus type 70 has been responsible for major outbreaks of hemorrhagic conjunctivitis throughout the world: type 71 has caused outbreaks of hand-foot-and-mouth disease or poliomyelitis-like illness in several countries.

Most enteroviral infections resolve without sequelae. In a few patients infected by coxsackievirus and other enteroviruses, there are permanent effects or even death caused by neuronal or cardiac damage, respectively. In the United States, the few cases of poliomyelitis reported each year are almost invariably associated with exposure to live attenuated poliovirus vaccine.

Vaccine strains can regain neurovirulence during passage in a human host. Despite this rare complication, live attenuated trivalent poliovaccine has been highly successful in eliminating or controlling poliomyelitis in many countries. Inactivated vaccines have also been highly successful in reducing or eliminating the disease.

Rabies

Rabiesvirus is a bullet-shaped, enveloped RNA virus belonging to the Rhabdoviridae family. It causes destructive, in-

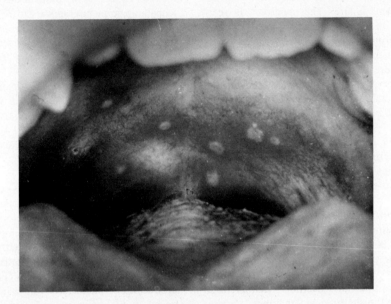

FIG. 8-9. Palatal lesions in herpangina caused by coxsackievirus A. The yellow necrotic patches are surrounded by a zone of erythema. The lesions are extremely painful.

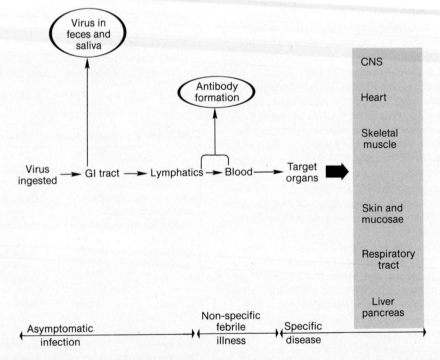

FIG. 8-10. Pathogenesis of enteroviral infections. *(From McCracken AW and Cawson RA: Clinical and oral microbiology, Washington DC, 1982, Hemisphere Publishing Corp.)*

flammatory disease affecting the central nervous system and occasionally the myocardium. The pathologic and clinical effects of rabies are discussed in Chapter 20.

Rubella

Rubella virus is a 60 nm enveloped member of the Togavirus family. It causes two types of infection in humans, congenital and postnatal.

Congenital rubella is by far the most important form of the disease. When a nonimmune mother is infected during the first trimester of pregnancy, there is at least a 50% chance that the fetus will develop abnormalities. Numerous defects have been described, and virtually every organ may be damaged in some way (Table 8-7). The most common abnormalities are heart disease and eye and hearing defects. Growth retardation is frequent. Follow-up studies have shown a high incidence of insulin-dependent diabetes following congenital rubella.

The pathologic processes that contribute to these multiple defects are caused by the following effects of the virus:

1. Inhibition of cell mitosis
2. Cell necrosis followed by focal fibrosis and calcification mainly in the central nervous system and its appendages
3. Vasculopathy caused by proliferation of vascular endothelial cells
4. Chromosome damage

Postnatal rubella is a mild, self-limiting febrile illness of childhood, characterized by cervical lymphadenopathy followed by a maculopapular rash. The incubation period is between 2 and 3 weeks. During this time the virus can be detected in circulating leukocytes. The pathogenesis of the rash is not understood although it is a consequence of a viremia and the virus has been isolated from the skin. The current view is that the rash is the result of antigen-antibody complexes acting on the vascular endothelium rather than viral invasion of endothelial cells.

Rubella in adults is a more severe illness, and especially in women, arthritis is a painful sequel that can persist for several weeks. The presence of virus and viral antigens in the affected joints suggests that the arthritis too may have an immunologic basis.

Other diseases of viral or presumed viral etiology

Diseases included in this category and not described elsewhere are:

1. Parvovirus disease
2. Roseola (exanthem subitum)
3. Kawasaki disease (mucocutaneous lymph node syndome)

Parvoviruses. Parvoviruses are very small (20 nm), nonenveloped DNA viruses. They are known to cause diseases in animals but recently have been shown to be associated with outbreaks of erythema infectiosum ("fifth" disease). Evidence of infection by human parvoviruses (HPV) can be demonstrated in patients who have received multiple transfusions. It is particularly high in young hemophiliacs receiving factor VIII concentrates; 97% of this group of patients have antibodies to parvoviruses.

The usual clinical consequence of HPV infection is erythema infectiosum. Parvovirus 19 is thought to be the etiologic agent and has been implicated in several epidemics. The pathogenesis of erythema infectiosum is not known. Clinically, the disease is a mild, febrile illness associated with a vivid rash on the cheeks in the earlier stages of the disease. A variety of nonspecific symptoms may accompany the disease. As with rubella, with which it can be easily confused, the disease is more severe in adults than in children.

Parvoviruses are also reported as causing (1) episodes of marrow aplasia in patients who have pre-existing hemolytic anemias or myalgic illnesses and (2) arthralgia, particularly in young women (Chapter 17).

Roseola. Roseola is an acute febrile disease of young children. The epidemiology of the disease and its ability to be transmitted to humans by ultrafiltrates of serum from cases of roseola are good evidence that a virus is the responsible agent.

The characteristics of the disease are high fever lasting several days associated with cervical lymphadenopathy, followed by a return of temperature to normal and the simultaneous appearance of a maculopapular rash. The disease has few complications, and there is no specific treatment.

Kawasaki disease. Kawasaki disease is a disease of unknown cause of young children that is particularly prevalent in Japan. It is characterized by persistent fever; ocular, skin, and mucous membrane inflammatory changes; and acute enlargement of cervical lymph nodes. Although many causes have been proposed, the epidemiologic features of the disease are consistent with an infectious agent possibly a virus.

The most significant pathologic features are in the heart, where there are inflammatory changes throughout the coronary arteries and the development of microaneurysms. Acute inflammatory changes similar to those seen in viral myocarditis have been demonstrated in almost all cases subjected to myocardial biopsy. The death rate in Kawasaki disease is 2% mainly from cardiac complications. The current recommended treatment is with aspirin.

TABLE 8-7. Clinical spectrum in the congenital rubella syndrome*

System	Abnormalities
Alimentary	Esophagitis Hepatosplenomegaly Pancreatitis
Cardiovascular	Myocarditis Patent ductus arteriosus Pulmonary stenosis Ventricular septal defect
Bone	Metaphyseal abnormalities
Ear	Deafness
Endocrine	Diabetes mellitus
Eye	Coloboma Corneal clouding Chorioretinitis Microphthalmia
Hemolymphatic	Thymic aplasia Thrombocytopenia
Renal	Glomerulonephritis Kidney anomalies
Respiratory	Pneumonitis
Skin and connective tissues	Dermal hematopoiesis Hyperelastosis

*Low birth weight and failure to thrive are also common effects.

Pathogenic mechanisms in bacterial diseases

Bacteria are much more biologically complex than viruses. It is not then surprising that the mechanisms bacteria use to infect humans are much more diverse than those described for viral infections. Among the mechanisms that will be considered are the following:

1. Attachment of bacteria to host cells
2. Intracellular and extracellular growth of bacteria
3. Tissue penetration by bacteria
4. Elaboration of toxins

Bacterial attachment

In order to gain access to tissues when epithelial surfaces are intact, bacteria must attach themselves to superficial cells. If it were not so, bacteria such as *Neisseria gonorrhoeae* in the urethra and *Vibrio cholerae* in the intestine would be swept on by the flow of urine or the intestinal contents and prevented from establishing disease in their respective sites. These two bacteria, along with *Escherichia coli* and other gram-negative organisms, possess structures called either *pili* (hairs) or *fimbriae* (fringes). These short, fine, hairlike structures composed of protein arise from the bacterial cytoplasmic membrane. They enable bacteria to attach to other cells including other bacteria. It is by means of a special class of pilus that bacterial genetic materials may be transmitted from one bacterium to another. The other class of pili are important in the initial stages of gonococcal infection and a variety of intestinal infections including cholera, gastroenteritis of infants and of travellers caused by *Escherichia coli* and possibly other enteric bacteria.

Another mechanism of attachment that has been described for group A β hemolytic streptococci is an affinity between M protein of the cell wall of the streptococcus and the cytoplasmic membrane of pharyngeal cells. *Bordetella pertussis*, the cause of whooping cough, possesses two hemagglutinins that promote its attachment to ciliated respiratory epithelium.

The ability of certain bacteria to attach to heart valves may be an important factor in the pathogenesis of infective endocarditis (Chapter 10). The attachment of *Streptococcus mutans* to enamel is an important aspect of dental caries. The bacterium forms glucans by which means it readily attaches to tooth enamel. Glucans are glucose polymers, which *S. mutans* can synthesize from sucrose.

Organisms of the genus *Mycoplasma*, which are cell wall deficient bacteria, are unique because their plastic physical structure enables them to apply themselves very closely to cell membranes. In cell cultures such attachment can intefere with host cell function in a variety of ways including causing death of the host cell. It is likely that in mycoplasmal infection this mechanism plays a role in cell damage, as for example, in primary atypical pneumonia (Chapter 12).

Bacteria which do not possess specific attachment mechanisms probably require some previous injury, albeit microscopic, to skin or epithelial surfaces in order to initiate infection. *Treponema pallidum*, the cause of syphilis, probably gains entry to the body in this way.

Intracellular growth of bacteria

Bacteria can be found both inside and outside cells (Table 8-8). Some are obligate intracellular parasites; some are capable of an intracellular or extracellular existence, while others are found only within phagocytic cells often in the process of being

TABLE 8-8. Cell relationships of some common bacteria

Bacterium	Intra-cellular	Extra-cellular	Type of cell involved
Rickettsiae	+	−	Endothelial
Chlamydiae	+	−	Epithelial
Mycobacterium leprae	+	−	Macrophage
M. tuberculosis	+	+	Macrophage
L. monocytogenes	+	+	Macrophage
Brucella species	+	+	Macrophage
Treponema pallidum	−	+	None
Corynebacterium diphtheriae	−	+	None
Bordetella pertussis	−	+	None

destroyed. Obligate intracellular parasites, such as rickettsiae, appear to damage their host cells by using certain biosynthetic pathways or products to further their own ends. In the case of rickettsiae, the cells mainly affected are vascular endothelial cells. In view of the enormous numbers of these cells and their universal distribution in the body, it is not surprising that rickettsial infections such as typhus are both serious and frequently can involve all parts of the body.

Mycobacteria (including *M. tuberculosis*), the nontuberculous mycobacteria, and Brucella are capable of survival and growth within and outside macrophages. Thus although phagocytosed, they can resist the killing effects of their phagocytic host cell, probably because of the chemical nature of their surface. The intracellular persistence of these organisms has several implications. First, such infections tend to persist for lengthy periods because the intracellular bacteria are protected from the effects of antibodies and complement. Second, because macrophages may be carried to other sites in the body, dissemination of infection may be facilitated. Third, the ability of antimicrobial drugs to kill such organisms may be seriously impaired by their intracellular habitat. Consequently, such infections require prolonged treatment to eradicate the infectious agent.

Tissue penetration by bacteria

Some bacteria remain on the surface of an epithelial layer; others invade that layer to varying degrees.

Bordetella pertussis multiplies in the mucous layer, which is normally present overlying the respiratory epithelium. The organism is attached to, but does not invade the epithelium. In this site, however, it elaborates a variety of virulence factors which appear to account for its pathogenicity. *Corynebacterium diphtheriae* behaves in a similar way in the pharynx. *Vibrio cholerae* and *Escherichia coli* in the bowel, can both cause diarrheal illness of varying severity. Both of these bacteria remain on the surface of the intestinal mucosa, where they elaborate toxins. *Salmonella enteritidis* and most other Salmonella species, which are common causes of bacterial enteritis, have been shown by immunofluorescence studies to penetrate just below the intestinal mucosa, while *Shigella sonnei*, which causes bacillary dysentery, penetrates into the colonic submucosa.

The consequence of different capacities of enteric bacteria to penetrate intestinal mucosa is a difference in the degree of host inflammatory response. Thus *V. cholerae* produces no inflammatory response at all despite the severity of the disease. Salmonella infections are associated with the mildest of in-

TABLE 8-9. Important bacterial exotoxins

Toxinogenic organism	Main action of toxin	Pathologic effects
Corynebacterium diphtheriae	Interferes with polypeptide synthesis of enzymes concerned with fatty acid metabolism	Necrosis of pharyngeal and laryngeal epithelium; fatty change in heart muscle; peripheral neuritis
Clostridium tetani	Binds to central nervous system gangliosides	Tetanic muscle spasm
Clostridium perfringens	Lecithinase	Red cell lysis; tissue necrosis
Clostridium botulinum	Inhibition of acetylcholine release at cholinergic synapses	Descending paralysis
Staphylococcus aureus	Central nervous system effect; specific action not known	Nausea; vomiting; diarrhea
Vibrio cholerae	Augments adenylcyclase activity in intestinal mucosa	Active transport of water and electrolytes from mucosal cells to intestinal lumen

flammatory responses only and the mucosa remains intact. Shigella organisms deep in the mucosa cause a severe acute inflammatory response with considerable tissue destruction and consequent mucosal ulceration.

Toxin production by bacteria

The best understood mechanism by which bacteria cause disease is toxin production. Toxins are of two main types; exotoxins, which are secreted by the bacteria, and endotoxins, which are components of the bacterial cell wall.

Exotoxins. Bacteria of many species produce soluble toxic substances in great variety. The role of most of these in disease is unclear, but in some infections, the production of exotoxins is the main determinant of the organism's pathogenicity or can cause all the essential features of the disease. Examples of exotoxins and their activities are shown in Table 8-9.

The mode of action of the toxins of *V. cholerae* and *E. coli* have greatly contributed to the understanding of bacterial diarrheas. Cholera toxin is a protein that attaches to a specific receptor—GM1 ganglioside—on the mucosal cell. This is followed by an increase in adenyl cyclase activity and increased production of intracellular cAMP from ATP. The result of this reaction is a greatly increased transfer of water and electrolytes from mucosal cells to the intestinal lumen (Fig. 8-11). Some enterotoxigenic strains of *E. coli* possess a heat-labile toxin (LT), which has very similar effects to cholera toxin; others produce a heat-stable toxin (ST), which causes increased fluid secretion from intestinal cells by stimulating guanyl cyclase activity. Some ST-producing strains also secrete LT resulting in a more severe diarrheal illness. It is likely that other intestinal bacteria can behave in a similar way to *V. cholerae* and *E. coli*. In the early stages of shigellosis (bacillary dysentery), especially in young children, the initial watery diarrhea, which may precede the true dysenteric stage of the disease, is thought to be caused by a cholera-like enterotoxin.

Pore formers. Some bacterial toxins cause lysis of red blood cells. Examples are α toxin of *S. aureus*, streptolysin O from *S. pyogenes*, and *E. coli* hemolysin. The lytic mechanism is the result of formation of a porous molecule in the red cell envelope, similar to that formed by perforin 1, a product of T and NK lymphocytes or by C9 in complement mediated cell lysis (Chapter 2). This mechanism is also thought to explain the cytolytic effects of *Pseudomonas aeruginosa* and the pathogenic protozoon *Entamoeba histolytica*.

Endotoxin. The cell wall of gram-negative bacteria contains lipopolysaccharides. These substances when released in significant amounts from lysed organisms can have serious patho-

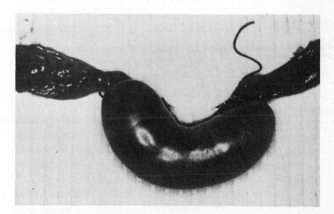

FIG. 8-11. Effects of *Escherichia coli* exotoxin on a loop of rabbit ileum. Eighteen hours after instilling a filtrate of toxinogenic *E. coli*, the segment of bowel, isolated by ligature is grossly distended due to excessive exudation of fluid. *(From Dupont HL: Enteropathogenic organisms, Med Clin N Am 62:945, 1978.)*

logic effects. The active substance that appears to account for these effects is a lipoidal acylated glucosamine dissacharide, called lipid A. Lipid A has the following effects:

1. It activates the (a) complement system, (b) kallikrein-kinin system, and/or (c) fibrinolytic system.
2. It can generate a generalized Shwartzman reaction with disseminated platelet thrombi.

The clinical effect of these processes is *endotoxin shock,* a very serious and complex condition characterized by fever, major disturbances of the circulation especially hypotension (Chapter 10) and disseminated intravascular coagulation (Chapter 13). It is a complication of severe sepsis, especially when caused by gram-negative enteric bacteria, and frequently has a fatal outcome. The presence of circulating endotoxin can be detected in serum by its ability to cause gelation of amebocytes derived from the horseshoe crab *(Limulus polyphemus).* Horseshoe crab amebocytes have a function similar to platelets in man and are exquisitely sensitive to the presence of endotoxin.

Host response to bacterial infection

Host responses to bacterial infections are highly variable. For example, the pathologic effects of exotoxins (see Table 8-9) are very diverse. However, there are responses that are common to most bacterial diseases. These are (1) inflammation and associated phenomena and (2) immune responses by antibodies and cellular immunity.

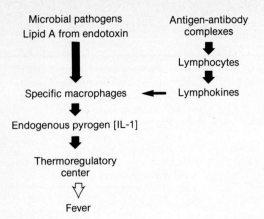

FIG. 8-12. The pathogenesis of fever. *IL-1*, interleukin 1.

TABLE 8-10. Some non-infective causes of fever

Cause	Example
Collagen-vascular disease	Polyarteritis nodosa
Drugs	Drug fever
Granulomatous disease	Sarcoidosis
Neoplasms	
Primary	Certain hepatic and renal tumors
Metastatic	Many metastatic tumors
Lymphoma	Hodgkin's disease
Others	Cyclic neutropenia
	Erythema nodosum
	Familial Mediterranean fever

Inflammation. Bacterial infection is among the most common causes of inflammation. The type of inflammation is often conditioned by the species of bacterium causing the infection. Thus infections caused by *Staphylococcus aureus* and *Streptococcus pyogenes* are typically acute inflammatory processes with polymorphonuclear leukocytes predominating. Typhoid fever, on the other hand, is characterized by a macrophage response and a tendency to tissue necrosis, while *Mycobacterium tuberculosis* produces typical granulomatous inflammation and caseous necrosis. Inflammatory changes are often seen in regional lymph nodes that drain a focus of bacterial infection. These can vary from reactive hyperplasia (Chapter 6) to frank inflammation within the lymph nodes themselves *(lymphadenitis),* sometimes leading to suppuration and abscess formation.

The systemic effects of inflammation frequently seen with a wide range of bacterial disease are fever and leukocytosis.

Fever. Fever (pyrexia) for practical purposes can be defined as an oral temperature greater than 37.2° C (99.0° F) in an individual at rest. Fever is caused by the action of endogenous pyrogen (EP) on the hypothalamus (Fig. 8-12). Recent studies have shown that, contrary to previous speculation, EP is an exclusive product of bone marrow-derived macrophages and not of polymorphs or macrophages in general. These studies have also shown that EP is indistinguishable from interleukin 1 (IL 1). Thus EP (IL 1) is released by specific macrophages in response to a variety of stimuli, which include bacterial endotoxin, immune complexes, some viruses, and the process of phagocytosis itself. The effect of EP on the thermoregulatory center is similar to that produced by cold; it causes vasoconstriction of the skin and shivering (chills). These result in an elevation of central temperature, which is usually followed by vasodilatation, sweating, and subsidence of fever. EP is thought to exert its effect on the hypothalamic center by stimulating the production of prostaglandins. Another action of EP, unrelated to its temperature effects is to cause the level of plasma iron to fall. This has an inhibitory effect on microorganisms, many of which depend on critical iron levels for toxin formation and replication. It has recently been observed experimentally that the ability of EP to cause T cell proliferation is greatly enhanced with increase of temperature in the range of human fever. If such a mechanism is present in vivo it will be the first instance of fever being directly beneficial to the immunologic protection of the human host.

Causes of fever. Although fever is most commonly the result of infection, it must not be forgotten that there are other non-infectious causes of fever, with radically different forms of treatment. The main causes of fever other than infections are listed in Table 8-10.

Fever of unknown origin. Patients who have daily fevers of 101.5° F or higher for 21 days, during which the cause has not been determined by clinical investigation, are said to have "fever of unknown origin" (FUO). Resolving the cause of an FUO is one of the more difficult and sometimes frustrating endeavors of diagnostic medicine. However, in expert hands, about one third of cases are found to be the result of infections; neoplastic and granulomatous diseases each account for about 20%, connective tissue diseases for 10% to 15%. The remainder are rare diseases or are undiagnosed despite intensive and repetitive investigations.

Leukocytosis. Leukocytosis, the elevation of the white blood cell count above 10,000/μL, is a frequent accompaniment of infection. Acute inflammatory foci in the body are usually associated with increased numbers of circulating white cells, particularly neutrophils in the blood (neutrophilia). The sources of these neutrophils are:

1. A mitotic pool of neutrophil precursors in the bone marrow
2. A marginal pool of mature neutrophils, which are stationary, attached to the walls of small blood vessels, particularly in the lungs

Neutrophilia is the result of release of neutrophils from both pools. The mechanisms controlling the production and release of neutrophils are as yet ill defined. Possible neutrophil regulators include a colony-stimulating factor present in blood and urine and a neutrophila-inducing factor present in bone marrow. The neutrophils present in acute infections frequently contain dense granules in their cytoplasm ("toxin" granulation).

The circulating neutrophils in infectious diseases are often seen to be young cells with few lobes. Even younger metamyelocytes or myelocytes may be present. When a graph of numbers of lobes in neutrophils in infection is compared to that in a normal population, the curve is shifted to the left. Thus the increased number of young and immature cells is termed "a left shift" and is an indicator of infection (Fig. 8-13).

Eosinophilia. Eosinophilia is the presence in the peripheral blood of more than 500 eosinophils per μL. There are many causes of eosinophilia but in the context of infection, parasitic infestations are the main etiologic agents. The presence in blood or tissues of larval stages of various parasitic worms, such as

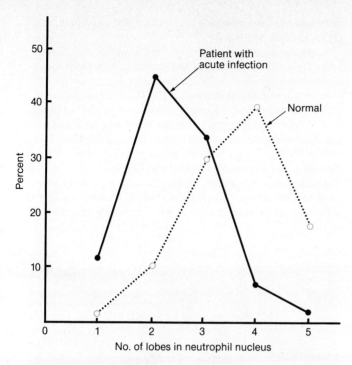

FIG. 8-13. "Left shift" in neutrophils. In acute infection younger neutrophils, with fewer lobes in their nuclei, enter the circulation. Their distribution, compared with normal *(dotted line)*, is shifted to the left.

is seen in filariasis or trichinellosis, is usually accompanied by a high circulating eosinophil count.

Lymphocytosis. Some infectious diseases are associated with a lymphocytosis—an increase in circulating lymphocytes above 4000 per µL. Among the causes are viral infections—such as infectious mononucleosis (Chapter 13) and viral hepatitis (Chapter 15)—and bacterial infections—including pertussis (whooping cough), tuberculosis and brucellosis. The factors that affect the behavior of lymphocytes are discussed in detail in Chapter 7. Among other important causes of increased circulating lymphocytes is chronic lymphocytic leukemia, most commonly found in older adults.

Immune response to bacterial infection

Immune responses are dealt with in Chapter 7, but a few points are worth further emphasis.

Opsonins. Opsonins are substances that promote phagocytosis. They may be nonspecific components of the complement system or specific antibodies of IgM or IgG classes. They facilitate the attachment of bacteria to the cytoplasmic membranes of phagocytic cells.

Antitoxins. The exotoxins produced by bacteria (see Table 8-9) are usually highly antigenic as a result of their protein composition and readily stimulate antibodies that are capable of neutralizing the effects of toxin. Such antitoxins may also be artificially stimulated in vivo by formalin-treated toxins (toxoids). Toxoids, although highly antigenic, are without toxic effects. They are extensively used for immunization against diphtheria and tetanus.

Effects of complement. Among the many biologic effects of complement is the lysis of bacteria. This lytic property can readily be demonstrated in vitro, but the role of com-

plement in the destruction of bacteria in vivo is unclear. The final process in complement-mediated lysis is the activation of an enzyme that perforates the bacterial cell membrane, allowing the entrance of excess water and resulting in rupture of the cell.

Prevention of bacterial attachment. The importance of bacterial attachment in the initial phases of infection has already been emphasized. This mechanism may be inhibited by secretory antibodies of the IgA class. In the case of some enteric pathogens these antibodies may be stimulated by a vaccine prepared against bacterial pili.

Another aspect of this protective mechanism has been elucidated in gonococcal urethritis. Repeated exposure to gonorrhea does not confer resistance to further gonococcal infection despite the fact that local antigonococcal IgA is present in the urethral mucosa. However, *Neisseria gonorrhoeae* has been shown to produce a protease that cleaves IgA. This strongly suggests that this process accounts for its ability to cause frequent reinfection.

Cell-mediated immunity. With certain bacteria, notably the mycobacteria, the immune response is largely cell mediated; humoral antibodies, although they are present, play little or no part in the host defenses.

Autoimmunity. Bacteria may stimulate autoantibodies in the following ways:

1. Releasing sequestered host antigens during tissue inflammation and destruction—The host antigens are normally sheltered within cells from antibody-forming cells, but, when released from damaged cells, stimulate antibodies to the host's own tissues. The Wassermann antibody (Chapter 23), which is demonstrable in syphilis and other infectious diseases, is thought to be of this type.

2. Stimulating cross-reacting antibodies—In pulmonary infection caused by *Mycoplasma pneumoniae* (Chapter 12) antibodies are formed that have specificity for the universal red cell I antigen. The resultant interaction between the antigen and the autoantibody may be severe enough to cause hemolytic anemia. In the pathogenesis of rheumatic carditis (Chapter 11) antibodies formed in response to group A β-hemolytic streptococci, which may cross-react with the sarcolemma of cardiac myocytes, have been implicated as a possible etiologic mechanism.

Infections caused by specific bacteria
Staphylococcus aureus

Staphylococcus aureus is a gram-positive coccus, frequently present in the nose and on the skin of healthy people, which is capable of infecting almost any tissue of the body and causing disease which can range from a trivial cutaneous infection to fatal generalized disease. The diseases caused by *S. aureus* are summarized in Table 8-11. The pathologic basis of staphylococcal disease rests on the ability of the organism to cause suppurative inflammation (Fig. 8-14) and to produce a wide range of enzymes and toxins, some of which have profound pathologic effects.

Among the many enzymes produced is fibrinolysin which along with hyaluronidase appears to facilitate the spread of the organism in soft tissues. The production of leukocidins affords the organism some protection against the predatory activities of phagocytic leukocytes.

Among the many exotoxins produced by *S. aureus* are those

TABLE 8-11. Staphylococcal diseases

Site of infection	Disease	Pathogenic mechanism
Blood	Bacteremia	Blood-borne infection leading to abscess formation in many organs
Bone and periosteum	Osteomyelitis	Suppurative inflammation
Central nervous system	Meningitis, brain abscess	Suppurative inflammation
Heart valves and cardiovascular prostheses	Endocarditis	Vegetation formation with septic emboli
Intestinal tract	Staphylococcal food poisoning	Toxin acting mainly on nervous system
Lung	Pneumonia	Suppurative inflammation
	Empyema	Suppurative inflammation
Skin and soft tissues	Furuncle, impetigo, carbuncle	Suppurative inflammation
	Wound infection	Suppurative inflammation
	Epidermal necrolysis	Toxin acting on skin
Various sites but especially female genital tract	Toxic shock syndrome	Toxin which ?activates kinins

that cause (1) food poisoning, (2) scalded skin syndrome, and (3) toxic shock syndrome.

Staphylococcal food poisoning. Certain strains of *S. aureus* under favorable environmental and nutritional conditions found in improperly cooked or stored foodstuffs can evolve potent exotoxins (enterotoxins A through F). These toxins appear to act in two ways: first, by central stimulation of the vomiting centers, after absorption; second, by interfering with sodium and water reabsorption from the intestine causing diarrhea. This form of food poisoning typically develops in four hours or less following consumption of the contaminated food.

Scalded skin syndrome. Staphylococcal dermatonecrotic toxin acts on cells of the epidermis, where it causes splitting at the level of the stratum granulosum. This results in a clinical

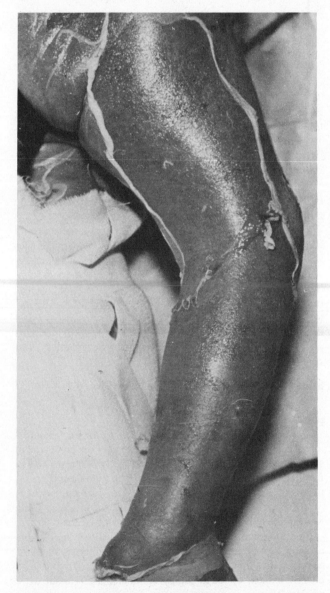

FIG. 8-15. Epidermal necrolysis (scalded skin syndrome). There is extensive desquamation of the epidermis caused by the effects of a specific dermatonecrotic toxin produced by some strains of *Staphylococcus aureus*. *(Courtesy Curator of the Gordon Museum, Guy's Hospital, London, England.)*

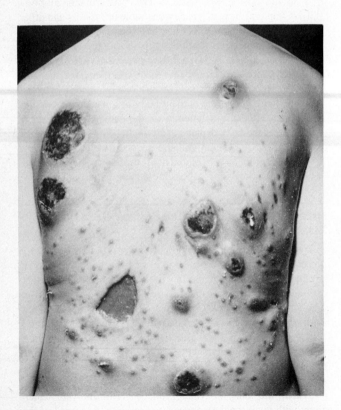

FIG. 8-14. Severe staphylococcal skin sepsis causing numerous carbuncles on the back. The patient died from generalized staphylococcal infection. A large abscess was found in the liver at autopsy. *(Courtesy Curator of the Gordon Museum, Guy's Hospital, London, England.)*

appearance resembling scalded skin (Fig. 8-15) usually in young children. Scalded skin syndrome is also called epidermal necrolysis and Ritter's disease.*

Toxic shock syndrome. Toxic shock syndrome (TSS) is characterized by fever, hypotension, desquamating rash, and serious dysfunction of most organ systems. The evidence is overwhelmingly in favor of a staphylococcal exotoxin—exotoxin C—as the cause of this disease. Exotoxin C is identical to enterotoxin F, one of the toxins associated with food poisoning. TSS can develop during any infection with toxin-producing *S. aureus* or *S. epidermidis*. Most cases have been associated with the use of vaginal tampons and are caused by *S. aureus*. This reached epidemic proportions in the early 1980s when hyperabsorbent tampons were widely used, apparently providing suitable conditions for vaginal staphylococcal colonization and toxin production. Approximately 50% of the cases that are not associated with the use of tampons are caused by *S. epidermidis*. Recently, TSS has been seen as a result of *S. aureus* infections of the respiratory tract complicating epidemic influenza. The case fatality rate for toxic shock syndrome is 3% to 4%. Death is due mainly to renal failure and hyaline membrane disease of the lung. Treatment is directed at managing the hypotension and eliminating *S. aureus* with an appropriate antibiotic.

Other staphylococci. In recent years, other species of staphylococci *S. epidermidis* and *S. saprophyticus* in particular, have been recognized as important causes of human disease. *S. epidermidis* is a frequent cause of infection of vascular prostheses used in heart valve and arterial surgery. The source of infection is the patient's own skin where *S. epidermidis* is frequently

---

*Gottfried Ritter von Rittershain (1820-1883), German physician.

found as part of the normal bacterial flora. *S. saprophyticus* is a fairly common cause of urinary tract infection in women. It is occasionally found as a constituent of the normal vulvovaginal flora, which is the likely source of infection.

Streptococci

Streptococci comprise a large group of gram-positive cocci capable of causing a wide range of human diseases. Streptococcal disease appears to be the result of one or more of the following:

1. Acute suppurative inflammation
2. The effects of toxins
3. Hypersensitivity to streptococci or their products

About 90% of streptococcal infections of humans are caused by β hemolytic streptococci of Lancefield group A *(S. pyogenes)*. Other β-hemolytic streptococci, grouped on the basis of their cell wall polysaccharide, that are important causes of human disease are groups B, C, D, and G. Other streptococci that are important causes of human disease are *S. pneumoniae* (pneumococcus), the viridans group of streptococci and anaerobic streptococci. The main infections caused by streptococci are listed in Table 8-12.

Like staphylococci, streptococci elaborate a variety of enzymes and toxins that contribute to their pathogenicity. Fibrinolysins and hyaluronidase are examples. The latter may be an important factor in the rapid spread of infection in tissue, which is a characteristic of many streptococcal diseases.

Another product of some group A streptococci is erythrogenic toxin. This toxin is the product of lysogenic (prophage-containing) strains and is responsible for the typical punctate erythematous rash and "strawberry tongue" of scarlet fever. Scarlet fever may be caused by group A streptococcal infections

---

TABLE 8-12. Types of streptococcal disease

Site	Organism	Disease	Pathogenic mechanisms
Central nervous system	*S. agalactiae* (group B)	Neonatal meningitis	Acute inflammation
Heart	*S. pyogenes*	Rheumatic fever	?Hypersensitivity to streptococci
			Also involving joints, connective tissue, and central nervous system
	S. viridans	Bacterial endocarditis	Vegetation formation with septic emboli
	S. pneumoniae		
	S. faecalis		
	S. bovis		
Lungs	*S. pneumoniae*	Lobar pneumonia	Suppurative inflammation
		Bronchopneumonia	
		Empyema	
Oropharynx and tonsils	*S. pyogenes*	Acute pharyngitis	Suppurative inflammation
		Tonsillitis	
	S. pyogenes	Scarlet fever	Suppurative inflammation of the pharynx plus erythrogenic toxin production
Teeth and gingivae	*S. mutans*	Dental caries	Complex
	Anaerobic streptococci	Dental abscess	Suppurative inflammation often with gas production
Skin and soft tissues	*S. pyogenes*	Erysipelas	Suppurative inflammation
		Impetigo	
		Wound infection	
Uterus and adnexa	*S. pyogenes*	Puerperal sepsis	Suppurative inflammation
	Anaerobic streptococci		
Urinary tract	*S. faecalis*	Cystitis	Ascending infection and suppurative inflammation
	S. bovis	Pyelonephritis	
	S. pyogenes	Glomerulonephritis	Hypersensitivity to streptococci

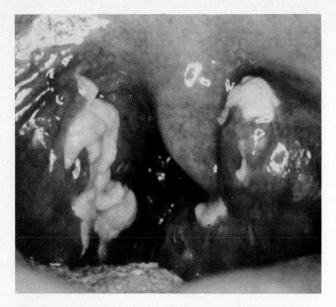

FIG. 8-16. Streptococcal pharyngitis. Typical redness and swelling of pharynx and tonsils with a thick, purulent exudate on both tonsils. *(From McCracken AW and Cawson RA: Clinical and oral microbiology, Washington DC, 1982, Hemisphere Publishing Corp.)*

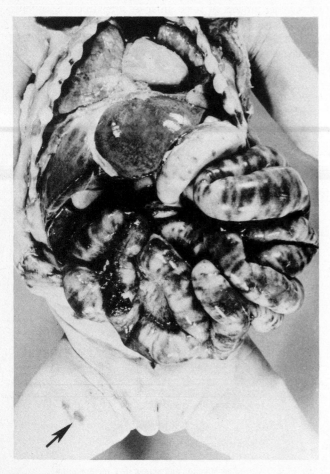

FIG. 8-17. *Pseudomonas aeruginosa* bacteremia. There are areas of severe hemorrhagic necrosis throughout the intestinal tract. Similar lesions in the skin *(arrow)* are present and are called *ecthyma gangrenosum.*

in any site but the tonsils or pharynx are the usual sources (Fig. 8-16).

Infections by group B streptococci *(S. agalactiae)* are a major cause of neonatal sepsis and meningitis. The main source of these organisms is the genital tract of the mother.

Group D streptococci are important causes of urinary tract infections and infective endocarditis. Their main significance is that many are resistant to multiple antibiotics, and for this reason successful treatment of these infections is often difficult.

The most common infections caused by *S. pneumoniae* are those of the lungs, the paranasal sinuses and the middle ear. From these sites, local spread to the meninges or, via the blood-stream, to the meninges and heart valves is a very serious complication. The capsule of *S. pneumoniae* allows the organism to resist phagocytosis and is an important virulence factor. One aspect of pneumococcal disease that remains a serious and unexplained problem is the high death rate especially in persons over 50, despite adequate and early administration of appropriate antibiotics.

The role of viridans streptococci, especially, *S. mutans* in dental caries is discussed elsewhere. Viridans streptococci are important agents of infective endocarditis. One species, *S. milleri,* in addition to causing some cases of endocarditis, has now been associated with a wide range of serious suppurative infections including empyema.

Enteric gram-negative bacteria. The main gram-negative enteric bacteria causing human diseases are *Escherichia coli, Klebsiella* and Enterobacter species, Proteus species, Salmonella and Shigella species. Of these, *E. coli* is most commonly isolated from clinical sources. It causes disease by at least four mechanisms:

1. Acute suppurative inflammation as in urinary tract or wound infection
2. Release of bacterial endotoxin, which can cause serious hypotension (endotoxin shock)
3. Production of exotoxin in the intestine by some strains of the organism, which causes profuse watery diarrhea
4. Invasion of the intestinal mucosa by other strains of the bacterium causing a dysentery-like illness.

The main sites of *E. coli* infection are the following:

1. The urinary tract
2. Postoperative wound sites
3. Meninges especially in neonates
4. Intestinal tract

The pathogenic mechanisms of diseases caused by Klebsiella, Enterobacter, and Proteus species are similar to those caused by *E. coli. Klebsiella pneumoniae* causes a severe cavitating form of pneumonitis (Friedländer's pneumonia). Infections by these gram-negative organisms are very frequently acquired by patients in hospital (nosocomial infections).

Salmonella and Shigella infections are described fully in Chapter 13.

Several enteric and nonenteric gram-negative bacilli including *Serratia marcescens* and Pseudomonas species mostly cause nosocomial infections. Pseudomonas infections (Fig. 8-17) are particularly important in patients with burns or hemolymphatic malignancies.

Spirochetes. Three genera of spirochetes, *Treponema, Borrelia,* and *Leptospira,* cause disease in humans. The most important spirochetal infection is syphilis, which is caused by *Treponema pallidum* (Chapter 23). The pathologic and clinical features of other spirochetal diseases are tabulated in Table 8-13. The table includes the newly recognized Lyme disease

TABLE 8-13. Pathologic and clinical features of spirochetal diseases other than syphilis

Organism	Disease	Pathogenesis and pathology	Main clinical features
Borrelia recurrentis (and other species)	Borreliosis (relapsing fever)	Transmitted by ticks or lice; organisms spread from skin to bloodstream, causing inflammatory changes and infarcts in liver, kidney, spleen, and meninges	Fever, rash, jaundice, and hemorrhagic tendencies
Borrelia burgdorferi	Lyme disease	Transmitted by tick saliva or tick feces; infection spreads from skin to lymphatics, then via bloodstream to brain, liver, and spleen, causing inflammatory lesions; neuronal degeneration found in chronic form	Fever, headache, expanding macular rash, lymphadenopathy, cardiac complications; arthritis, both acute and chronic; neuropathy in chronic cases
Leptospira interrogans	Leptospirosis	Transmission via abraded skin from water contaminated with animal urine; pathogenesis unknown; fatal cases show hepatic and renal tubular necrosis	Highly variable from mild transient illness to fever, severe malaise, conjunctivitis, hepatitis, meningitis, and hemorrhagic tendencies
Treponema pertenue	Yaws (frambesia)	Person-to-person transmission by direct contact; primary cutaneous lesion followed by multiple secondary mucocutaneous lesions; later tertiary lesions in bone and skin; basic pathologic changes are in small vessels, which show periarteritis and endarteritis; tissue necrosis (gumma) is characteristic	Papular skin lesions in early stages with later multiple necrotizing lesion of skin and bone

(Chapter 17), named for the Connecticut town where the disease was first recognized in its epidemic form in 1975.

Corynebacteria. The most important human corynebacterial infection is diphtheria. It is caused by *Corynebacterium diphtheriae,* a gram-positive rod with club-shaped ends. Virtually all of the pathologic effects of *C. diphtheriae* are the result of the action of its exotoxin, which can be lethal to all human cells. The action of the toxin causes the following:

1. Localized superficial tissue necrosis in the pharynx or larynx (pseudomembrane formation)—The skin is also a possible site of initial inoculation (cutaneous diphtheria). Superficial necrosis of the skin develops at the site.
2. Severe fatty change and necrosis of cardiac muscle by interference with protein synthesis at the stage of interaction of tRNA with the ribosomes
3. Myelin degradation in peripheral nerves

Death from diphtheria is due to either myocardial failure or airway obstruction by diphtheritic membrane.

Haemophilus influenzae. Haemophilus influenzae is a small gram-negative coccobacillus. It is capsulated, and most human infections are caused by organisms with type B polysaccharide capsule. It is an important pathogen in children, particularly in those aged 1 to 5, although infections in adults appear to be increasing.

Important infections caused by *H. influenzae* are as follows:

1. Meningitis
2. Acute epiglottitis
3. Bronchopneumonia

The organism causes an acute inflammatory reaction, often with considerable fibrinous exudate. In acute epiglottitis, inflammatory edema is the prominent process, which may occlude the airway.

Bordetella pertussis is morphologically similar to *H. influenzae* and is the cause of whooping cough (pertussis). The exact pathogenesis of the characteristic inspiratory whoop is not known. Possible explanations include increased sensitivity to histamine and serotonin, induced by products of the organism, which results in paroxysms of coughing. A characteristic feature of the disease is the high lymphocyte count in the peripheral blood in most children over 6 months old.

Brucella. The four species of *Brucella* which can cause human disease are primarily animal pathogens, as seen in the following columnar material:

Species	Animal host
B. abortus	Cattle
B. canis	Dog
B. melitensis	Goat
B. suis	Pigs

Most human cases of brucellosis are caused by *B. melitensis* and *B. abortus,* and many affected persons are dairymen, farmers, and veterinarians. Others occasionally acquire the disease usually by consuming unpasteurized dairy products.

The organisms enter via the respiratory or alimentary tracts, reach the bloodstream via the lymphatic system and are widely distributed throughout the body within the cytoplasm of macrophages. They can excite a granulomatous inflammatory response in the liver, spleen, bone marrow, and lymph nodes. The granulomas are frequently necrotic in the center, and the areas of necrosis may coalesce to form "abscesses" in any of the affected organs. Healing takes place by means of fibrosis.

The clinical effects of brucella infection are variable. They range from subclinical infection to serious systemic illness with many complications. Acute and chronic forms of the disease are observed. High fever, rising and falling in a wavelike (undulant) manner, is typical of the acute disease; there is weight loss, profound malaise and enlargement of liver, spleen, and lymph nodes. Frequently, the patient improves symptomatically only to relapse 2 to 3 months later. Chronic forms of the disease are much less dramatic. There is only a low-grade fever, localizing signs are usually absent, and personality changes resulting from central nervous system involvement can be mistaken for psychiatric illness. The diagnosis is made by blood culture or the demonstration of specific antibodies. Treatment is usually with tetracycline and an aminoglycoside antibiotic, but relapses are common even after adequate treatment.

Francisella tularensis. Francisella tularensis is the cause of tularemia, a disease usually characterized by inflammatory skin or ocular lesions and regional lymphadenitis. If untreated, the infection can spread by the bloodstream to the lungs. The organism is a highly infectious animal pathogen. Human infections are due to tick bites, inhalation, or accidental skin or mucous membrane inoculation of infected animal body fluids. The organism causes granulomatous inflammation and necrosis in lymph nodes and lung. The diagnosis is made by demonstration of specific antibodies to *F. tularensis*. Treatment is with aminoglycosides or tetracycline.

Yersinia. Members of the *Yersinia* genus are small, gram-negative coccobacilli. *Y. pestis* is the most notorious species and is the cause of bubonic and pneumonic plague—the "Black Death" of the Middle Ages. Sporadic cases of plague are still seen in many Asian and African countries, and occasional cases are seen in the southwestern United States. The organism is a pathogen of rodents and is transmitted to man by the bite of the rat flea. The pathogenesis of plague is similar to that of tularemia, except that the inflammatory process is acute and hemorrhagic. Lymph node enlargement ("bubo") is prominent in the early stages. With rapid multiplication of the organism, hypotension, possibly resulting from endotoxemia, and severe disturbances of hemostasis develop. Pulmonary involvement is usually a late and terminal event. Streptomycin is the drug of choice.

Mycobacteria. The mycobacteria (acid-fast bacilli) are a group of gram-negative rods that possess a cell wall rich in mycolic acids. The mycobacteria of importance in human disease are (1) *M. tuberculosis,* (2) the nontuberculous mycobacteria, and (3) *M. leprae*. Tuberculosis and pulmonary infection by the nontuberculous mycobacteria are described in Chapter 11. Other infections caused by the latter are summarized in Table 8-14.

M. leprae is the cause of leprosy, but it has not been grown in artificial culture. However, the disease has been propagated in the nine-banded armadillo. Pathologically, leprosy in humans is characterized by the following:

1. Granulomatous inflammation in nerve fibers, skin, and mucous membranes
2. A variable histopathologic picture that depends on whether or not there is a well-developed immune response to *M. leprae*

When the cell-mediated immune response is well developed, the disease is called *tuberculoid* leprosy; when it is poor or absent, *lepromatous* leprosy develops.

Histopathologically, in tuberculoid leprosy the lesions in the skin, cutaneous nerves, and dermal appendages resemble those of tuberculosis but without caseation: that is, epithelioid cells, Langhans' giant cells, and lymphocytes are present. Nerve destruction is a prominent feature. Bacilli may be seen close to nerve fibers, but generally they are extremely difficult to find in stained sections. Clinically, in this form of leprosy the disease is localized to one or two areas of the skin, especially in the legs and feet (Fig. 8-18). Such areas are anesthetic, rough, and red. In dark-skinned persons, loss of pigment (vitiligo) is typical.

In lepromatous leprosy, the lesions consist of histiocytes and a few scattered lymphocytes. Some of these histiocytes have foamy cytoplasm and contain mycobacteria (Fig. 8-19). Numerous bacilli can be seen in stained sections: spherical collections called *globi* are prominent. Nerve destruction is minimal.

Clinically, lepromatous leprosy is most prominent in the face, although the skin of the whole body may be involved. Thickening of the skin, especially of the forehead and ears, is common. Tumorlike swellings (lepromas) may be seen, and eyebrow hair is lost. The face may take on a leonine (lionlike) appearance.

TABLE 8-14. Diseases associated with nontuberculous mycobacteria

Disease	Mycobacterial species
Skin ulcers and soft tissue infections	*M. chelonei*
	M. fortuitum
	M. marinum
	M. ulcerans
Lymphadenitis (especially cervical)	*M. avium-intracellulare*
	M. scrofulaceum
Pulmonary infection (including patients with AIDS)	*M. avium-intracellulare*
	M. kansasii
	M. szulgae
	M. simiae
	M. scrofulaceum
Tendon sheaths, bone, and joint	*M. kansasii*
	M. avium-intracellulare
	M. fortuitum
	M. chelonei
Disseminated disease (including patients with AIDS)	*M. avium-intracellulare*
	M. kansasii
	M. fortuitum

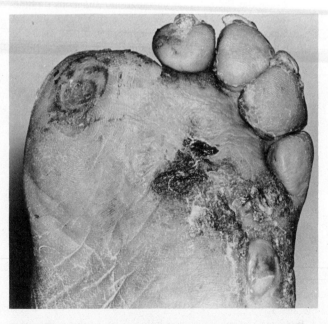

FIG. 8-18. Leprosy. Destruction of nerves by granulomatous inflammation has led to trophic changes in the skin, and loss of sensation has resulted in unheeded injury. As a consequence there is extensive ulceration and loss of the great toe. *(Courtesy Curator of the Gordon Museum, Guy's Hospital, London, England.)*

Nasal congestion and discharge caused by bacterial invasion of the mucous membranes are frequent. This may result in destruction of nasal cartilage. Scrapings of the nasal mucosa in such cases contain large numbers of mycobacteria. If untreated, the disease can spread to internal organs, especially the liver and spleen.

Tuberculoid and lepromatous leprosy are two extremes of reaction to this infection. The lepromin test, in which killed *M. leprae* are injected into the skin, is a means of differentiating the two forms of leprosy. A positive test indicates tuberculoid leprosy, and a negative test indicates lepromatous leprosy. However, the majority of cases of leprosy are dimorphic; that is they have clinical, pathologic, and immunologic features somewhere between tuberculoid and lepromatous disease. Dapsone has long been the drug of choice; more recently it has been given in combination with other drugs, notably rifampicin and clofazimine. Treatment extends over many years and may have to be continued for life. Endemic leprosy still exists in the United States especially in southern Texas.

Anaerobes

Many bacterial species are strictly anaerobic; that is, they are intolerant of oxygen and die rapidly in its presence. An-

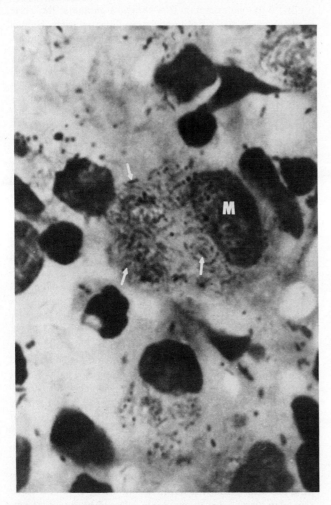

FIG. 8-19. Acid-fast stain of skin biopsy of patient with lepromatous leprosy. The cytoplasm of a macrophage *(M)* contains many acid-fast bacilli. *(From McCracken AW and Cawson RA: Clinical and oral microbiology, Washington DC, 1982, Hemisphere Publishing Corp.)*

aerobic organisms form the majority of the normal bacterial populations of the mouth, the intestine, and the vagina. Other anaerobes that can cause human disease are normal inhabitants of the soil.

The classic anaerobic organisms are *Clostridium tetani, C. perfringens,* and *C. botulinum,* which cause, respectively, tetanus, gas gangrene, and botulism. However, many other anaerobic species, mainly those listed in the following, can cause a variety of serious infections.

1. *Actinomyces israelii*
2. *Bacteroides fragilis*
3. *Bacteroides melaninogenicus*
4. *Clostridium perfringens*
5. *Clostridium ramosum*
6. *Fusobacterium nucleatum*
7. *Peptostreptococcus anaerobius*
8. *Peptostreptococcus intermedius*
9. *Peptococcus magnus*
10. *Propionibacterium acnes*

Anaerobic bacteria are found in mixed culture in about one third of these infections. Frequently, several anaerobes are present in the same lesion.

Clinical conditions associated with anaerobic bacteria follow:

1. *Abdominal*
   a. Actinomycosis
   b. Appendicitis
   c. Clostridial enterocolitis
   d. Peritonitis
   e. Subphrenic and intraabdominal abscesses
2. *Female genital tract*
   a. Endometritis
   b. Pelvic abscesses
   c. Puerperal sepsis
3. *Nervous system*
   a. Botulism
   b. Brain abscess
   c. Tetanus
4. *Oral and dental*
   a. Actinomycosis
   b. Acute necrotizing ulcerative gingivitis
   c. Fascial space infection
   d. Osteomyelitis of the jaw
   e. Periodontal disease
5. *Respiratory tract*
   a. Actinomycosis
   b. Aspiration pneumonia
   c. Bronchiectasis
   d. Empyema
   e. Lung abscess
6. *Soft tissue*
   a. Abscess
   b. Gas gangrene

Tetanus, gas gangrene, and botulism are the result of the elaboration of highly potent bacterial toxins and are described elsewhere (Chapters 16 and 19). The mechanisms by which most other anaerobes cause disease is less well-understood. However, certain properties of the organisms and the host are worth noting:

1. Many anaerobes produce a variety of extracellular enzymes, including lipases, proteases, ribonucleases and deoxyribonucleases, and lecithinases, all of which can contribute to tissue necrosis. Suppurative necrotizing in-

flammation with the production of foul-smelling pus is characteristic of many anaerobic infections.

2. Some, such as *Bacteroides fragilis,* a common cause of anaerobic infection have a capsule, which is an important determinant of virulence.
3. The anaerobic conditions that favor the growth of anaerobes prevent the process of phagocytosis, for which the presence of oxygen is required. The activity of some antimicrobial drugs (e.g., aminoglycosides) is also impaired by anaerobic conditions.

Anaerobic infections are favored by several predisposing factors:

1. The presence of necrotic tissue or foreign material
2. Tissue ischemia
3. The presence of other bacteria that can produce the necessary redox potential that favors anaerobes

From a clinical standpoint, there are certain features that should arouse suspicion that an anaerobic infection may be present. These are as follows:

1. Infections near sources of endogenous anaerobes—These are usually near mucosal surfaces such as the mouth or anus.
2. Infections contaminated with excreta or soil
3. Infections of ischemic tissue
4. Infections associated with extensive tissue damage and necrosis
5. Infections that have a foul-smelling discharge or gas production

Anaerobic infections are usually treated with antibiotics combined with surgical drainage.

Chlamydiae

Chlamydiae are highly specialized bacteria that are obligate intracellular parasites. They cause at least five important diseases (Table 8-15).

A characteristic microscopic feature common to all types of chlamydiae is the formation of basophilic cytoplasmic inclusion bodies, which are an aid to histologic diagnosis.

Properties of chlamydiae that appear to account for their pathogenicity include:

1. A heat-labile toxic factor, which can be neutralized by specific antibodies
2. Ability to prevent the formation of phagolysosomes and thus interfere with the lethal phase of phagocytosis

Antibody production is a feature of chlamydial infections, but there is also experimental evidence that cell-mediated immunity has a role in protection of the host.

Chlamydial infections are characterized by acute inflammation in which polymorphs, macrophages, and lymphocytes are seen, together with characteristic inclusion-bearing cells. Sometimes, however, these are few in number, and culture of inflammatory exudates may be required to demonstrate the inclusion-producing properties of the organism. Chlamydial infections generally respond to treatment with tetracyclines (see also Chapter 23).

Mycoplasmas

The mycoplasmas are small, free-living bacteria that lack a cell wall. Two species, *Mycoplasma pneumoniae* (Eaton agent) and *Ureaplasma urealyticum* (T strain mycoplasma) cause disease in man. Evidence is accumulating that a third species *(M. hominis)* may also be pathogenic for man. *M. pneumoniae* is

an important cause of respiratory tract disease; *U. urealyticum* appears to account for a significant proportion of cases of nongonococcal urethritis (Chapter 22). *M. hominis* has recently been strongly implicated as a cause of pyelonephritis, pelvic inflammatory disease, and postpartum fever.

Mycoplasmas, having no cell wall, are very plastic organisms and frequently apply themselves very closely to cell membranes. Little is known of their pathogenic mechanisms in humans, but it is possible that their affinity for cell membranes is important.

In animals, tissues infected with mycoplasmas contain infiltrates of lymphocytes and plasma cells, and inflammatory changes are present in small blood vessels. Similar findings have been reported in a few fatal human cases of *M. pneumoniae* infection. *M. pneumoniae* infection is associated in about half the cases with an antibody directed against the I antigen of the patient's own red cells. These antibodies act best at 4C and are called *cold agglutinins.* One possible explanation is antigenic similarity between the surface of the organism and the red cell envelope.

Mycoplasmal infections respond to erythromycin or tetracycline, but the response is seldom dramatic.

Rickettsiae

Rickettsiae are small, gram-negative pleomorphic coccobacilli. With one exception (*Rochalimaea quintana,* the cause of trench fever) they are obligate intracellular parasites. Human rickettsioses are mainly acquired as the result of infection transmitted by insects (Table 8-16).

In the United States, Rocky Mountain Spotted Fever (RMSF), which is transmitted by ticks, is the most important rickettsial disease. Similar tick-borne diseases are seen in many other areas of the world; Indian and South African tick bite fevers, for example. The pathogenesis and pathology of RMSF exemplifies the processes seen in the more severe, systemic rickettsioses.

Rocky Mountain spotted fever. Despite its name, RMSF is predominantly a disease of the eastern seaboard of the United States and is caused by *R. rickettsii.* Following inoculation of this highly infectious agent into the skin, it gains entrance to endothelial cells. The severity of rickettsial diseases in general is largely the result of their affinity for vascular endothelial cells so that infection is usually widely disseminated and can involve every organ in the body.

Rickettsiae multiply in and are released from endothelial cells, then spread to and infect other endothelial cells. This results in widespread endothelial damage, increased vascular permeability, and inflammation at the sites of endothelial injury. In these areas, inflammatory cells, lymphocytes, with a few polymorphs and macrophages infiltrate around the small blood vessels. Inflammatory edema may develop, especially around small pulmonary vessels. Microthrombi, which lead to hemorrhagic infarction, can affect any organ, especially the liver, spleen, and adrenal glands. In fatal cases, there is widespread organ damage; myocarditis, renal tubular necrosis, and cerebral, cutaneous, and other infarcts are common. Patients who have glucose 6-phosphate dehydrogenase deficiency are, for unknown reasons, much more likely to die from RMSF. Apart from the widespread vascular invasion, the severity of the disease may also be due to endotoxin released by the organism. This, however, has not been confirmed.

Clinically, RMSF begins as an influenza-like illness, which

TABLE 8-15. Disease caused by chlamydiae

Organism	Disease	Pathogenesis and pathology	Clinical features
C. psittaci	Psittacosis	Disease of psittacine birds transmitted to humans by inhalation of dried bird feces: interstitial pneumonitis, which may spread to spleen and meninges	Fever, pneumonitis, spleno-megaly, delirium
C. trachomatis (types L1, L2, L3)	Lymphogranuloma venereum	Sexually transmitted; minor genital lesion followed by extensive regional lymph node suppuration	Painful inguinal and pelvic lymphadenopathy
C. trachomatis (types A, B, Ba, C)	Trachoma	Spread by direct contact or by flies: acute inflammation of conjunctiva may involve the cornea and progress to blindness	Conjunctivitis: keratitis; leading cause of blindness in the world
C. trachomatis (types D through K)	Inclusion conjunctivitis	Acute conjunctivitis	As for trachoma but the cornea is not involved
C. trachomatis (types D through K)	Nongonococcal urethritis, bartholinitis, Fitz-Hugh-Curtis syndrome, Reiter's syndrome	Sexually transmitted suppurative inflammation: (1) urethral mucosa, (2) Bartholin's glands, (3) perihepatic inflammation, (4) ?hypersensitivity reaction to chlamydia	Purulent urethral discharge; vulvar pain and swelling; fever, upper abdominal pain; urethritis, arthritis, conjunctivitis, rash

TABLE 8-16. The rickettsioses

Group	Rickettsia species	Disease	Vector	Clinicopathologic features
Typhus	R. prowazekii	Epidemic typhus	Louse	Fever, rash, prostration, multisystem infection; many complications including shock and hemorrhage
	R. prowazekii	Recrudescent typhus	None	Milder form of typhus; recrudescence of latent infection
	R. mooseri	Endemic	Flea	Similar to epidemic typhus
Spotted fever group	R. rickettsii and other species	Rocky Mountain spotted fever and other locally named diseases	Tick	Similar to typhus
	R. akari	Rickettsialpox	Mite	Fever, papulovesicular rash; self-limiting disease
Scrub typhus	R. tsutsugamushi	Scrub typhus	Mite	Crusting, necrotic lesion on skin at site of infection; fever, rash, lymphadenopathy; complications and relapses common in untreated cases
	Coxiella burnetii	Q fever	Ticks, but vector not necessary	Fever, headache, interstitial pneumonitis
	R. quintana	Trench fever	Louse	Fever, prostration, rash

is dominated by intense headache. This is followed by a macular rash especially on the arms, hands, legs, and feet and a wide range of effects of multiorgan dysfunction. Death in untreated cases is usually the result of pulmonary, cardiac, or renal complications.

The diagnosis of RMSF is made by the demonstration of specific antibodies to *R. rickettsii*. The traditional Weil-Felix test, which used X strains of *Proteus* species as antigens, is for diagnostic purposes useless and should no longer be used. Treatment for RMSF is by tetracycline or chloramphenicol and should be begun as early as possible.

Nocardia and actinomycetes

Nocardia and *Actinomyces* species are morphologically similar; they are generally gram-positive, branching bacteria. The essential difference between them is that the former is aerobic and acid-fast, the latter is anaerobic and not acid-fast.

Nocardiosis is the disease caused by one of the species of *Nocardia*, usually *N. asteroides* or *N. brasiliensis*. These are saprophytic, predominantly soil bacteria that cause opportunistic infections in humans; i.e., they cause disease only in persons debilitated by other illnesses, especially those who have malignancies or are immunosuppressed.

The initial site of infection is either the lung as a result of inhalation of the organisms or the skin when a wound is contaminated by soil. The former route can give rise to pulmonary and disseminated disease, the latter may cause a *mycetoma*—a suppurating subcutaneous swelling.

The pathologic process associated with nocardiosis is suppurative, necrotic inflammation with abscess formation. This is most striking in the lungs, but the process frequently spreads to involve the pleural cavity (causing empyema) and the brain (by way of the bloodstream), although virtually any organ may be affected. Tangled masses of organisms—"sulfur gran-

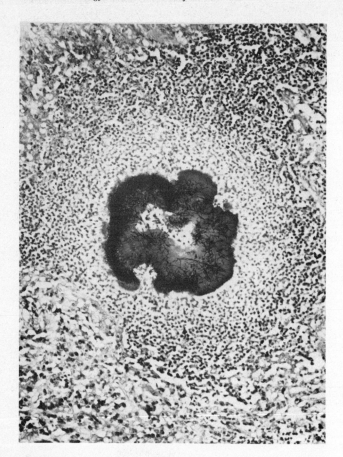

FIG. 8-20. Actinomycosis. Closely packed actinomycetes *(A)* are surrounded by an inflammatory reaction, which mainly consists of polymorphonuclear leukocytes.

ules"—are only seen in superficial tissues. The drug of choice for nocardiosis is sulfadiazine. Treatment is often unsuccessful because of the seriousness of the underlying disease.

Actinomycosis. Actinomycosis is caused by *Actinomyces israelii* or in a few instances by members of the genus *Arachnia,* which are commensals of the oral cavity. The infection originates most commonly in the mouth, but occasionally it begins in the intestine or the lung, giving rise to cervicofacial, abdominal, and thoracic actinomycosis, respectively. The characteristic features of actinomycotic lesions are (1) granulomatous inflammation with suppuration and cavitation and (2) the presence of "sulfur granules" (Fig. 8-20). There is slow expansion of the lesions, which results in tissue destruction and the formation of sinuses and fistulae. In cervicofacial disease these sinuses communicate with the skin of the face and neck. In abdominal and thoracic actinomycosis, fistulous tracts develop between organs and communicate with the skin and mucosal and serosal surfaces. The systemic effects of actinomycosis are surprisingly mild or even absent until late in the disease. The treatment of actinomycosis is with penicillin, augmented where necessary with surgical drainage or excision of necrotic tissue.

Pathogenic mechanisms in fungal diseases

Knowledge of the pathogenic mechanisms of fungi is limited. The following mechanisms appear to be involved: (1) tissue invasion by fungal elements often associated with variable inflammatory responses and (2) hypersensitivity to fungal antigens.

Tissue invasion

Fungal spores enter the body mainly by inhalation; they may also gain access to skin that is macerated or to mucous membranes, if local conditions are favorable. In susceptible individuals, those who have defective cellular immunity or those who have received massive doses of spores, tissue invasion develops. Typically, this is associated with a granulomatous inflammatory response. Examples of invasive fungi are *Histoplasma capsulatum* and *Coccidioides immitis.* In the absence of effective cell-mediated immunity, disseminated disease caused by these fungi is very likely to develop (Chapter 12).

Dermatophytic fungi (which invade skin, hair, and nails) produced keratinase, which enable them to penetrate these structures (Chapter 19).

Hypersensitivity

Allergic reactions in the lung may be caused by inhalation of spores. This is seen, for example, in some individuals exposed to the spores of *Aspergillus fumigatus.* There is interaction in the lung between the fungus and specific IgE antibodies with the development of an immediate hypersensitivity pneumonitis and eosinophilia. Patients with this disease develop asthmatic attacks associated with fever and chills.

An allergic component is present in infections by the common dermatophytic fungi such as those that cause ringworm or athlete's foot. The "Id" reaction, in which desquamation of the epidermis of the hands develops in dermatophytic infections, is an example of this allergic component.

Pathogenic mechanisms in protozoal disease

In comparison to bacteria, protozoa are highly complex. Consequently, their pathogenic mechanisms, such as are known, are as numerous as their species. Because these mechanisms are so diverse, a summary of the salient pathogenic mechanisms, the pathology, and clinical aspects of protozoal infections is shown in Table 8-17.

Pathogenic mechanisms in helminthic disease

Helminths that infest humans (Table 8-18) are even more numerous and complex than the protozoa. Many of them are uniquely successful in their relationships with humans. Frequently, they produce neither disease nor symptoms unless their numbers are great. Again, much more is known about the host reactions to the presence of worms than the pathogenic properties of the worms themselves. Some properties worthy of note are as follows:

1. Simple mechanical effects, such as obstruction of the lumen of a viscus—In infestation by *Ascaris lumbricoides* (giant intestinal roundworm) intestinal obstruction can be caused by a mass of worms, especially in children. Sometimes a single worm can enter the bile duct, leading to biliary obstruction and jaundice.
2. Tissue penetration by worms or their larvae leading to eosinophilic inflammatory reactions—An example of this can be seen in early infestation by ascaris, during which the larval worms enter the lungs via the circulation and give rise to an eosinophilic pneumonitis.

TABLE 8-17. Summary of pathologic and clinical aspects of protozoal infections

Disease	Parasite	Pathogenesis and pathology	Clinical aspects
Amebiasis	*Entamoeba histolytica*	1. Humans infected by swallowing cystic form of protozoon	Asymptomatic infection ("cyst passer"); present in about 10% of population of United States
		2. Cysts develop into amebae, which can invade the lower intestinal mucosa and lead to ulceration; ulceration may heal spontaneously or progress	Abdominal pain, diarrhea, blood in stools
		3. Amebae can spread to liver via portal vein causing amebic liver abscess	Fever, abdominal pain, liver enlargement; fatal if untreated
		4. Further spread to other organs by contiguity or bloodstream may take place	Destructive lesions of skin, lung, peritoneum, etc.; usually fatal
Giardiasis	*Giardia lamblia*	1. Infection by swallowing cystic form of protozoon	Asymptomatic infection very common
		2. Heavy infection leads to interference with intestinal absorption of nutrients including fat; mechanisms of interference unknown	Abdominal pain, diarrhea with excess fat in stools (mild steatorrhea)
Malaria	*Plasmodium falciparum* *P. vivax* *P. malariae* *P. ovale*	1. Infection by bite of female anopheline mosquito	Incubation period of malaria
		2. Parasite enters liver cells and undergoes division (schizogony)	
		3. a. Parasite leaves liver to enter red blood cells; replicates in red cells and destroys them before infecting more red cells	Period of malarial attack; high fever, malaise, headache
		b. Parasite stimulates phagocytic activity in monocyte-macrophage system increasing red cell and platelet destruction	Anemia and thrombocytopenia
		c. *P. vivax* and *P. ovale* return to liver where they remain for weeks or months reemerging to red cell phase (Fig. 8-5)	Relapsing malaria
		4. *P. falciparum* can rapidly invade central nervous system blood vessels and can also cause a wide variety of serious derangements of microcirculation in kidney and other organs	Major complications almost exclusively *P. falciparum* Cerebral malaria Blackwater fever and renal failure Hyperpyrexia
Leishmaniasis Visceral	*Leishmania donovani*	1. Small unicellular protozoon transmitted to human by bite of sandfly	Minor skin lesion
		2. Protozoon phagocytosed by macrophages and spread of infection throughout monocyte-macrophage system via macrophages	Fever with enlargement of lymph nodes, liver, and spleen
		3. Depression of protein synthesis in liver and normal red and white cell production in marrow leading to depressed immunity and hemorrhagic tendencies	Progressive weight loss, anemia, bleeding, susceptibility to infections; death in 1 or 2 years if untreated
Cutaneous	*Leishmania tropica* and other species	Protozoon transmitted to human by sandfly; macrophage response confined to skin (cutaneous), mucous membranes, and associated cartilage (mucocutaneous)	Subacute spreading inflammatory lesions on exposed areas of skin; in mucocutaneous form, destructive lesions of face can develop
Trypanosomiasis African (sleeping sickness)	*Trypanosoma gambiense* and *T. rhodesiense*	1. Leaf-shaped protozoon transmitted to human by bite of tsetse fly with local multiplication in skin	Incubation period ± minor skin lesions
		2. Spread to blood and lymphatics with enlargement of lymph nodes	Fever, lymphadenitis, parasitemia
		3. After 12 to 18 months protozoon penetrates central nervous system leading to encephalitis	Lethargy, apathy, coma (sleeping sickness), death from dehydration, starvation, intercurrent infection
South American (Chagas' disease)	*Trypanosoma cruzi*	1. Humans infected by scratching feces of reduviid bugs containing *T. cruzi* into skin	Incubation period with minor skin lesions; some asymptomatic infections
		2. Spread to blood and lymphatic system	Fever, facial edema, lymphadenitis
		3. Spread to heart muscle and intrinsic autonomic nerve plexuses of colon	Myocarditis, heart failure, megacolon

Continued.

TABLE 8-17. Summary of pathologic and clinical aspects of protozoal infections—cont'd

Disease	Parasite	Pathogenesis and pathology	Clinical aspects
Toxoplasmosis	*Toxoplasma gondii*	1. Small leaf-shaped protozoon; humans infected by ingesting oocysts; main source is domestic cat; majority of persons have no overt evidence of infection	Asymptomatic infections
		2. Infection of nonimmune pregnant mother can lead to congenital toxoplasmosis in which there are: a. Microcysts of *T. gondii* with lymphocytic reaction and necrosis and calcification in brain b. Retinochoroiditis in the eyes	Stillbirth; hydrocephalus; severe mental retardation; visual defects
		3. Infection of nonimmune young adults mainly involves monocyte-macrophage system but may spread to the eyes	Fever; malaise; lymphadenitis; mononuclear blood picture
		4. Reactivation of latent infections in immunosuppressed patients leads to cerebral and pulmonary inflammation	Pneumonitis; encephalitis
Pneumocystosis	*Pneumocystis carinii*	1. Small spherical or leaf-shaped protozoon infects human by unknown route	Asymptomatic infections common
		2. In neonates and immunosuppressed persons, especially patients with AIDS, the organism causes progressive pulmonary alveolar infiltrates in which plasma cells are prominent with occasional spread to other organs	Fever; pneumonia; progressive dyspnea

3. Consumption of essential nutrients by worms, for example, the sucking of blood by hookworms leading to anemia and hypoproteinemia

Again, the preferential absorption of vitamin B_{12} by the fish tapeworm *(Diphyllobothrium latum)* can lead to the development of megaloblastic anemia in susceptible individuals (Chapter 13).

Host response to helminthic infestation

As mentioned earlier, host response to many intestinal or blood-dwelling worms may be completely absent. Nowhere is this more dramatically seen than in schistosomiasis. In this disease, the adult worms lie permanently within the venous plexuses of the abdominal viscera, apparently totally immune to any attack by humoral or cellular immune mechanisms. The worm achieves this by incorporating host antigens, including those of the ABO blood group, into its surface, and thus disguised—a wolf in sheep's clothing as it were—is able to avoid the effects of immune attack. The worms meanwhile, continue to lay thousands of eggs, which can cause severe inflammatory changes in the bowel, bladder, lung, or liver depending on the species of worm (Table 8-18).

Eosinophilia. One very common reaction to helminthic infestation particularly when larval forms invade the tissues, is eosinophilia, which may be localized or generalized. Increased numbers of circulating eosinophils are a common finding in many worm diseases. When inflammatory reactions are associated with worms, eosinophils are usually a prominent feature of the inflammatory exudate. The function of eosinophils in worm infestation is largely unknown; however, they are able to discharge their cytoplasmic granules around worms in tissues. This may contribute to the demise of the worm or in the dissolution of dead worms, around which eosinophilic infiltration can be intense.

Inflammation. In parasitic diseases inflammatory reactions are seldom associated with adult worms unless they die while still in the tissues, but they are commonly related to worm larvae or eggs that are deposited in tissue. The anatomic site of such inflammation is of great importance, particularly if the central nervous system, the eye, or another major organ is involved.

The eggs of blood flukes or schistosomes, unlike adult worms, evoke a severe granulomatous inflammatory response in which eosinophils again are common. Indeed the whole pathogenesis of schistosomiasis is the result of a host response to the eggs and, depending on the site of egg deposition, can cause severe inflammatory disease in the bowel, liver, bladder, or lung. In onchocerciasis, in which larvae migrate from the site occupied by the adult worm in the subcutaneous tissue of the head, the inflammatory response frequently takes place around the eye. If untreated, it commonly leads to blindness. Deposition of larvae (cysticerci) of the pork tapeworm *(Taenia solium)* in the soft tissues of the body and in the brain can result from hematogenous dissemination of the larvae following intraintestinal rupture of a gravid worm segment. This results in tumorlike inflammatory masses in muscle, subcutaneous tissues, eye, brain, and spinal cord; these masses are the main pathologic feature of *cysticercosis.*

Immune responses to helminthic infestations

Antibodies. The most noteworthy immune response to helminthic infestation is the production of IgE antibody. One function of IgE is to attack the worms, possibly by combining with their surface antigens to stimulate mast cell degranulation and release inflammatory amines. Again, IgE may possibly act as an opsonin, which allows macrophages to attack the worm.

Cell-mediated immunity. Although it seems certain that cell-mediated immunity plays a part in defense against helminths,

TABLE 8-18. Helminths: pathogenesis and clinical manifestations

Worm	Pathogenic mechanisms	Clinical manifestations	Worm	Pathogenic mechanisms	Clinical manifestatins
Enterobius vermicularis (pinworm)	Worm produces irritant secretion	Local irritation only	*Fasciola hepatica* (liver fluke)	Obstruction of biliary tract	Jaundice Hepatic fibrosis
Ascaris lumbricoides (giant roundworm)	Mechanical obstruction by adult worms	Intestinal obstruction Biliary obstruction Airway obstruction	*Schistosomes* (blood flukes)	Eggs produce granulomatous inflammation in bladder, bowel, liver, and lungs	Hematuria, hepatic fibrosis, portal hypertension, pulmonary fibrosis, and hypertension
	Migration of larvae through lungs	Eosinophilic pneumonitis	*Taenia solium* (pork tapeworm)	Worm segment ruptures in human intestine allowing larvae to penetrate tissues	Cysticercosis of muscles, eye, and central nervous system
Trichocephalus trichiurus (whipworm)	Irritation	Rectal prolapse ? in predisposed patients	*Diphyllobothrium latum* (fish worm)	Worm absorbs vitamin B_{12}	Megaloblastic anemia in predisposed individuals
Necator americanus (hookworm)	Worm sucks blood from intestinal wall	Anemia Hypoproteinemia Wasting Edema	*Echinococcus granulosus* (dog tapeworm)	Human swallows egg and acts as intermediate host; larvae develop as growing cysts in liver, lung, kidney, etc.	Hydatid disease
Trichinella spiralis	Larvae invade intestinal tract, blood, and muscle	Diarrhea, vasculitis, myositis Severe allergic reactions Eosinophilia			
Wuchereria bancrofti (filarial worm)	Adult worms occupy lymph nodes leading to lymphatic obstruction	Elephantiasis			

the precise means by which it takes place are unclear. With some parasitic infections (for example, schistosomiasis) the inflammatory response to the presence of schistosome ova in the tissues is of the delayed hypersensitivity type.

SPREAD OF INFECTION

Infection, like cancer, can spread in several ways: (1) local contiguous spread, (2) spread along natural passageways, (3) lymphatic spread, and (4) spread via the blood stream (bacteremia, viremia, fungemia).

Local contiguous spread

Local spread of infection largely depends on the outcome of the contest between the host response and the infecting organism. Thus local extension of the infective process is favored by the following:

1. Products of the organisms—For example, hyaluronidase, which hydrolyzes hyaluronic acid in extracellular matrix is produced by many bacteria, especially streptococci and staphylococci. The production of abundant gas, especially by anaerobic bacteria such as *Clostridium perfringens* can assist the spread of infection by physical separation of cell and tissue layers, as seen in gas gangrene.
2. Presence of necrotic tissue and/or foreign materials
3. Lack of effective local inflammatory and immune responses—This may be due to many causes, as discussed in Chapter 6, particularly diabetes mellitus and immunodeficiency states.
4. Site of infection located in certain tissue planes or spaces, where there are no anatomic barriers—for example, in the retropharyngeal space
5. Effect of antimicrobial drugs, which can greatly modify

the spread of infection by killing or inhibiting the growth of microorganisms

Conversely, infection tends to be contained by fibrinous exudates, a prompt effective leukocyte response, connective tissue barriers, and early treatment with a suitable antibiotic.

Spread along natural pathways

The following lists the natural pathways along which infection can spread:

1. Any of the hollow viscera of the body, especially in the upper and lower airways, the intestinal tract, and the urinary tract
2. Along blood vessels especially the veins
3. Within the central nervous system

Descending infection from the nasopharynx to the trachea and bronchi and from there to the alveoli is a common sequence of events in the pathogenesis of bacterial bronchopneumonia particularly when this disease is preceded by a viral infection such as measles or influenza. Many enteric infections (bacillary dysentery, for example) can begin in one part of the intestine and spread by means of the intestinal contents to lower regions of the alimentary tract. By contrast, bacteria can spread upward within the urinary tract giving rise to inflammatory disease in the bladder and occasionally the ureters and kidneys. This mechanism is almost exclusively seen in women, in whom it is attributed to the shortness of the urethra and the colonization of the lower urethra by rectal bacteria.

Infection within the central nervous system (as for example, in bacterial meningitis) can be disseminated by the circulating cerebrospinal fluid to other areas of the brain and spinal cord.

Lymphatic spread

Infection commonly spreads via lymphatic channels to the regional lymph nodes, in which intense cellular proliferation and phagocytic activity develops. This is associated with tender, often painful enlargement of the lymph nodes (lymphadenitis), which frequently accompanies acute infections. The phagocytic activity within lymph nodes is an important defense mechanism. Its failure to contain infection can lead to invasion of the blood stream by the infective agent by way of the thoracic duct. This route of spread is important in the pathogenesis of several major infectious diseases: typhoid fever and poliomyelitis are two important examples.

Spread by the bloodstream

It seems likely that at least some species of bacteria, viruses, and fungi can enter the bloodstream with no adverse consequences to the patient. Certainly bacteremia is a common event in healthy people in whom small numbers of bacteria enter the blood following toothbrushing, vigorous chewing, and defecation. These bacteria are part of the normal flora of the gingivae and the colon. The number of bacteria is small and they are cleared from the blood in 10 to 20 minutes by the macrophage-monocyte system. Bacteria frequently enter the bloodstream during surgical procedures. The main sources are the skin, oral and genital mucous membranes and the gastrointestinal tract. Bacteremia is an important process in the pathogenesis of many infections (as is viremia). Bacteremia should, however, be distinguished from *septicemia* and *pyemia,* which are sometimes used (often incorrectly) as synonyms for bacteremia.

Septicemia is the presence of bacterial toxins in the blood, whereas *pyemia* is septicemia with the formation of multiple foci of suppuration (abscesses). Both terms are often used rather loosely to describe illnesses in which blood-borne infection has taken place. Bacteremia, however, is detectable in the laboratory by blood culture. There are no practical diagnostic methods to confirm septicemia and pyemia.

Bacteremia may be (1) an obligatory event in the pathogenesis of certain infections or (2) a complication arising in the course of an infection.

In meningococcal meningitis the circulation of *N. meningitidis* in the bloodstream precedes bacterial invasion of the meninges in all cases. By contrast, during the course of pneumococcal pneumonia, *S. pneumoniae* invades the bloodstream in about one third of patients and may give rise to serious infective complications in the heart valves and meninges.

Bacteremia can arise from many sources. The most direct is the introduction of bacteria into the circulation by contaminated needles, as seen in drug addicts, or as a consequence of poorly managed intravenous therapy.

Foci of infection in any part of the body can give rise to bacteremia. Abscesses in the kidney and the lung are particularly likely to spread infection in this way. Entry into the bloodstream from these foci may be direct, as for example, when a pulmonary tuberculous lesion erodes a blood vessel, or as already mentioned, entry may be indirect via the lymphatic system.

The consequences of the entry of bacteria into the bloodstream are often very serious. Metastatic (pyemic) abscesses may arise in any organ, but the kidney is affected most often. Other sites that are particularly vulnerable to infection by circulating organisms are the (1) meninges, (2) heart valves (infective endocarditis), and (3) cardiovascular prostheses, such as synthetic vascular grafts or plastic and metal valves. Infec-

tion of human heart valves is more likely if the patient has had previous valvular disease. Infective endocarditis is a severe disease when it affects either natural or artificial valves. Once infected, they are a source of further continuous shedding of bacteria into the bloodstream, resulting in widespread infective complications.

The clinical effects of bacteremia are variable, but with certain bacteria (such as *N. meningitiditis, S. aureus,* and *P. aeruginosa,* for example) a fatal outcome is not uncommon despite antibiotic treatment. The most consistent clinical findings are episodes of high fever, with chills and leukocytosis. The diagnosis is confirmed by aerobic and anaerobic cultures of the blood which allow the antimicrobial susceptibility of the offending bacterium to be ascertained as a guide to treatment.

Viremia. The presence of viruses in the bloodstream is common in many virus diseases. Most viruses reach the blood via the lymphatics either from the respiratory or the gastrointestinal tracts. Arthropod-borne viruses are unique in that they are injected directly into the skin by the biting insect.

The circulation of viruses in the blood accounts for both the generalized and localized manifestations of many viral diseases. Rashes that are frequently prominent in viral illnesses, such as measles and rubella, are caused by bloodborne spread of the viruses to the skin and mucous membranes.

Viremia is an essential process that precedes invasion of the central nervous system in viral meningoencephalitis, the heart muscle in viral myocarditis, or the liver in viral hepatitis. The presence of viruses in the blood has been confirmed by culture in many viral diseases; usually the viruses have been found to be associated with leukocytes particularly with polymorphs.

It appears very likely that viremia can take place without the development of signs or symptoms; this is inferred from those frequent instances in which specific viral antibodies can be demonstrated in individuals who can give no history of any illness related to infection by that virus. Clinically, viremia is usually associated with fever and chills.

Other methods of spread

Infections can spread along nerves. This, however, is probably seen only in three viral diseases, rabies, herpes simplex and zoster. In these diseases, the viruses spread along nerve trunks; in the case of rabies the virus appears to enter the central nervous system via the peripheral nerve axoplasm. In the latter two diseases, the viruses spread peripherally along nerve trunks to reach mucocutaneous sites.

Relationships among host, parasite, and antimicrobial agents

With the introduction of many antimicrobial agents in the last fifty years, a third party has intruded into the almost venerable relationship between host and parasite. These drugs have highly specific antimicrobial activity, particularly against bacteria. There are currently few bacteria for which a specific bacteriocidal or bacteriostatic drug is not available. Thus the simple contest of organism versus host has now been greatly complicated by therapy. Although antimicrobial drugs have successfully altered many infectious diseases in favor of the host, other interactions of the triumvirate of host, organism, and drug must be taken into account. These interactions include the following:

1. The effect of the drug on the host—An understanding of the absorption, distribution, and excretion of antimicrobial agents together with their potential toxic effects is essential, especially in patients with renal failure.
2. The effect of the organism on the drug—The ability of the organism to inactivate antibiotics or to develop resistance to or tolerance of these drugs is an important consideration in the management of infectious diseases. It is, for example, unwise particularly in a hospital to treat staphylococcal infections with penicillin G, because the majority of such infections are caused by organisms which inactivate penicillin by producing β-lactamase (penicillinase).
3. Infections in immunocompromised patients—In immunocompromised patients who have infections, the beneficial effects of humoral and cellular defense mechanisms are diminished or lost. Thus the patient is almost totally dependent on the antimicrobial drug to treat his infection. In these circumstances, only bactericidal drugs are likely to be effective.

Herxheimer reaction (Jarisch-Herxheimer reaction)

The Herxheimer reaction, named for a German dermatologist who described it in patients being treated for syphilis, is an acute systemic reaction that develops in 2 to 48 hours after antimicrobial therapy is begun. Characteristically, it begins with nausea, headache, malaise, and fever. Later there is intensification of the patient's inflammatory lesions. In some patients there may be severe shock. The diseases in which the Herxheimer reaction is a serious risk of injudicious treatment are as follows:
1. Brucellosis
2. Leprosy
3. Syphilis
4. Typhoid

The reaction is a response to a rapid massive killing of organisms. At least two substances, bacterial endotoxin and a heat-stable pyrogen have been implicated in this reaction.

Selected readings

Andresen BD, Alexander MS, and Ng KJ et al: Aspirin and Reye's disease: a reinterpretation, Lancet 1:903, 1982.

Atkins E: Fever: its history, cause and function, Yale J Biol Med 55:283, 1982.

Deiner TO, McKinley MP, and Prusiner SB: Viroids and prions, Proc Natl Acad Sci 79:5220, 1982.

Dinarello CA: Interleukin-1, Rev Infect Dis 6:51, 1984.

Jackson GG, Thomas H, editors: Bayer Symposium VIII: the pathogenesis of bacterial infections, Berlin, 1985, Springer-Verlag.

Morris JG Jr and Black RE: Cholera and other vibrioses in the United States, N Engl J Med 312:343, 1985.

Melnick JL: Enteroviruses: polioviruses, coxsackieviruses, echoviruses and newer enteroviruses. In Fields BN, editor: Virology, New York, 1985, Raven Press.

Myerhoff J: Lyme disease, Am J Med 75:663, 1983.

Nunove T: Human parvovirus (B 19) and erythema infectiosum, J Pediatr 107:38, 1985.

Prusiner SB: Prions: novel infectious pathogens, Adv Virus Res 29:1, 1984.

Rapp F: The biology of cytomegalovirus. In Roizman B, editor: The herpesviruses, vol 2, New York, 1983, Plenum Publishing Corp.

Steere AC, Schoen RT, and Taylor BA: The clinical evolution of Lyme arthritis, Ann Intern Med 107:725, 1987.

Stroop WG and Baringer JR: Persistent, slow and latent virus infections, Prog Med Virol 28:1, 1982.

Wolff SM: Biological effects of bacterial endotoxins in man, J Infect Dis (Suppl.) 128:259, 1973.

Youmans GP, Paterson PY, and Sommers HM: The biologic and clinical basis of infectious diseases, Philadelphia, 1985, W.B. Saunders Co.

CHAPTER 9

Disorders of tissue growth

The main categories of disorders of tissue growth include the following:
1. Hyperplasia and hypertrophy
2. Hypoplasia, aplasia, and agenesis
3. Heterotopia (choristoma)
4. Hamartoma
5. Metaplasia
6. Dysplasia
7. Neoplasia

HYPERPLASIA AND HYPERTROPHY

Hyperplasia (*-plasias;* Gr., development, formation) is an absolute increase in the *number* of cells in a tissue. The individual cells usually maintain their normal morphologic and functional features. Hyperplasia is seen in both physiologic and pathologic conditions. In women, a common example of hyperplasia is breast enlargement in puberty, during pregnancy, and at lactation. In elderly men, obstruction of the urinary tract is frequently due to prostatic enlargement, a manifestation of glandular and stromal hyperplasia of the prostate gland.

In contrast to hyperplasia, *hypertrophy* indicates an increase in the cell *size*. Such a phenomenon is commonly observed in cardiac and skeletal muscles, where cells respond to increased stress or work by enlarging rather than by cell division.

Because hyperplasia, by definition, is an excessive proliferation of cells, it may be thought to be a stage of neoplastic change. This may happen in some sites, such as the breast or endometrium, but in most situations hyperplasia shows no tendency to subsequent neoplastic change. In simple terms, a neoplastic process is hyperplastic, but a hyperplastic process is not necessarily neoplastic.

HYPOPLASIA, APLASIA, AND AGENESIS
Hypoplasia

Hypoplasia is a reduction in the number of cells in an organ. It can be developmental or acquired. Examples of developmental hypoplasias are those of the kidneys, lungs, or liver (Fig. 9-1). The defective organs may be nonfunctional, which is incompatible with life. On the other hand, only one of the paired organs such as the kidneys may be affected, and the other may then show compensatory hyperplasia. With aging, acquired hypoplasia is seen in most organs.

Aplasia

Aplasia is usually an acquired condition where there is total loss of a particular cell population within tissue or organ. It is the extreme of hypoplasia. The most common example is aplasia of the bone marrow, in which production of normal marrow hematopoeitic cells ceases. This condition is clinically known as aplastic anemia (Chapter 13). Marrow aplasia (or hypoplasia) is not uncommonly a side effect of drugs, of which the most publicized example is the antibiotic chloramphenicol.

Agenesis

Agenesis is a developmental failure of formation of an organ. Agenesis of an organ may be unilateral or bilateral, partial, or total. When a vital organ fails to develop, life cannot be sustained.

HETEROTOPIA

Heterotopia is a term that describes the presence of morphologically normal tissue at a site where it is normally not present. It usually reflects an aberrant developmental disorder during embryogenesis. Examples of heterotopia in man are numerous, such as the presence of thyroid tissue in the anterior mediastinum or adrenal tissue in the testis (Fig. 9-2). This heterotopic tissue is often referred to as ectopic. *Choristoma* or *aberrant rest* are synonyms for heterotopic tissue.

HAMARTOMA

The term *hamartoma* was first used by Albrecht* to describe ". . . tumor-like malformations in which occur only abnormal

---

*Karl Albrecht (1851-1894), German anatomist.

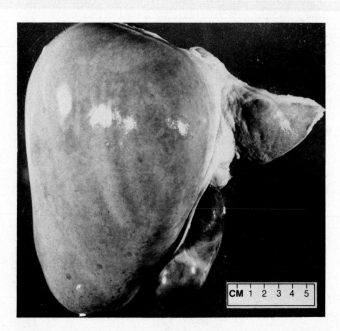

FIG. 9-1. Hypoplasia of the left lobe of the liver. This was an incidental finding at autopsy; the defect caused no apparent ill effects.

mixing of the normal components of the organ." This description of hamartoma as a growth malformation remains the conventional definition of this lesion, but in recent years, some authors consider these masses as complex neoplasms. They may be congenital or acquired. The lung is one site where hamartomas are commonly encountered in adults. They consist of a closely intermixed epithelial and mesenchymal elements, that include bronchial-like cells, myxoid fibrous tissue, cartilage, and fat.

METAPLASIA

Metaplasia (meta-; Gr., change) is a change in the development of a tissue from one type of functional differentiation to another. It usually arises as an adaptive mechanism to an abnormal local environment, as in chronic irritation or inflammation. The metaplastic tissue is more protective but often loses the function of the tissue it has replaced. Metaplasia is more commonly encountered in epithelial tissue than in connective tissue. A common example of metaplasia is the change of the ciliated columnar epithelium of the respiratory tract to a stratified squamous type as a response to excessive smoking (Fig. 9-3). In general, metaplasia is a reversible process if the exogenous irritant is removed from the environment. If exposure

persists, it may act sometimes as a prelude to a neoplastic process. In this regard it is important to emphasize that metaplasia per se does *not* represent a neoplastic change.

DYSPLASIA

The word *dysplasia* (dys-; Gr., ill, difficult, abnormal) denotes an abnormality of development, but it is used in pathology to describe a disordered proliferation of tissue cells, commonly epithelial. It is characterized by a loss of a well-defined pattern of maturation, alteration in size and shape of cells, and disorganization of the tissue as a whole (Fig. 9-4).

Dysplastic cellular changes can be induced by chemicals, viruses, chronic inflammation, or irritation. However, in man, the precipitating cause is not known in the majority of cases.

Under certain rare circumstances it appears that dysplasia can be reversible when the precipitating cause is removed. However, there seems to be no way in which dysplastic lesions can be made to revert completely to normal.

There is undoubtedly a relationship between dysplasia and neoplasia, but this can only be expressed in statistical terms. It is not possible, because of the difficulties of objective assessment, to quantify the premalignant potential of an individual dysplastic lesion. Because the risk is there and it cannot be precisely evaluated, the tendency is usually to regard dysplastic lesions as premalignant although malignant change is not invariable.

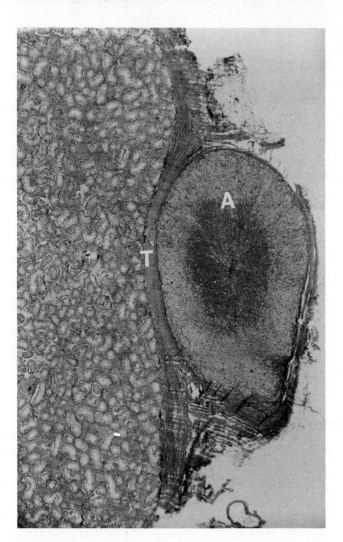

FIG. 9-2. Ectopic adrenal gland tissue *(A)* is located outside the tunica of the testis *(T)*.

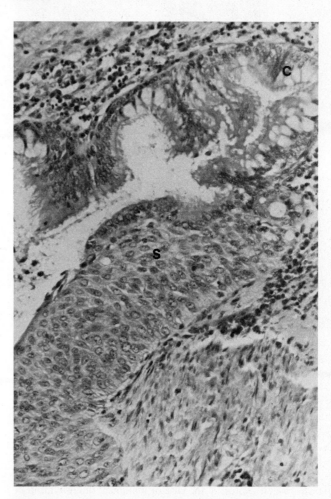

FIG. 9-3. Squamous metaplasia in bronchial epithelium. Note the transition from columnar *(C)* to squamous *(S)* epithelium.

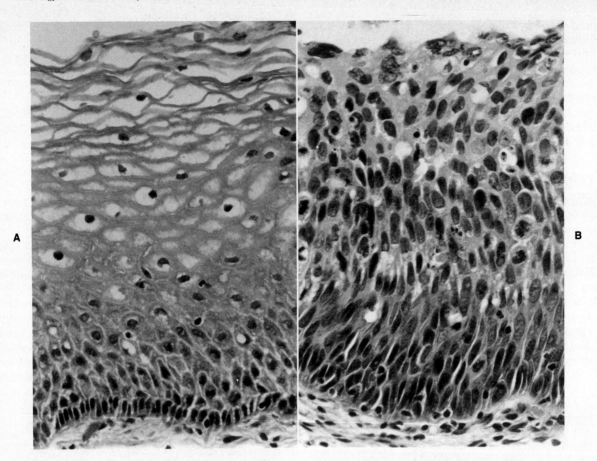

FIG. 9-4. A, Normal ectocervical mucosa showing stratified squamous epithelium. With maturation, the nuclei become smaller, round, and flattened. The cytoplasm is abundant. **B,** Dysplasia of the cervical squamous mucosa showing loss of maturation, disorganization, and nuclear enlargement with variation in size and shape.

NEOPLASIA

Neoplasms (neo-; Gr., new) are usually conveniently referred to as *tumors,* and the two terms are used synonymously. Nevertheless, the term *tumor* literally means no more than a swelling. The latter is characteristic of, but not exclusive to, neoplasms. It may be the result of many other processes such as inflammation or the accumulation of fluid in a cyst. The study of neoplasms and the clinical specialty of managing them is called *oncology* (oncos; Gr., tumor).

It is almost impossible to define a neoplasm in all-embracing terms because exceptions can be found to many of the accepted features of neoplasms. Their essential characteristics can, however, be summarized as follows:

1. New growth—This is the literal meaning of the term neoplasia and describes a process of unexpected proliferation of cells in the parent tissue.
2. Abnormality—It is self-evident that the growth of this new tissue is not part of the normal growth process. Most tumors in adults appear long after normal growth has been reached.
3. Excessive growth—This is one of the most obvious features of neoplasms. They produce swelling that at the very least can press on adjacent structures, obstruct passageways, or, in the case of malignant tumors, infiltrate and destroy surrounding tissue.
4. Lack of useful function—Neoplasms are never of benefit to the host. They may in some cases be functional and

secrete hormones, but these have pathologic effects. Even in the case of benign tumors, proliferation of tissue (such as muscle in a myoma) typically impairs the function of the organ from which it arises.

5. Autonomy—The growth of tumors is uncontrolled, and they are uncoordinated with their local environment.
6. Self-perpetuating—In a few cases the stimulus that provoked the initiation of neoplastic growth can be identified. Nevertheless, once the neoplastic process has started, removal of this stimulus has no effect, and the tumor continues to grow of its own accord.
7. Parasitic—Neoplasms acquire a blood supply from the host tissues and compete with host cells for nutrients. This is done so successfully that neoplasms can continue to flourish while the patient is dying.

To summarize, the main properties of a neoplasm are that it is an abnormal and excessive growth of new cells; it is uncoordinated with the host tissues, autonomous, persistent, and parasitic.

Classification

Several classification schemes have been proposed in the study of neoplasms, but the most widely used classification *combines the differentiation of the tumor and its biologic behavior.* The name of a tumor is usually based on the type of normal differentiation which it mostly resembles. This commonly correlates with the tissue of origin, but the two are not

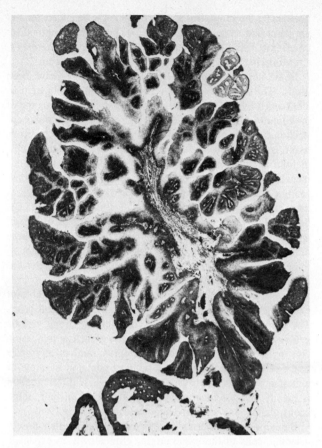

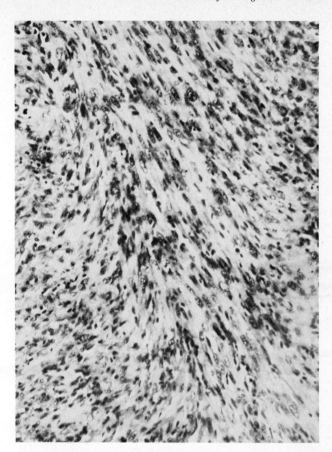

FIG. 9-5. Squamous cell papilloma. This benign tumor consists of fine fingerlike processes of squamous epithelium growing out from vascular connective tissue core.

FIG. 9-6. Fibrosarcoma. The spindle-shaped cells have an obvious resemblance to fibroblasts and form interlacing bands and a little reticulin. The highly cellular picture and the variation in size and staining of the nuclei are typical of malignancy.

TABLE 9-1. Classification of nomenclature of neoplasms

Tissue of origin or line of differentiation	Benign	Malignant
Epithelium		
Surface epithelium		
Squamous	Squamous papilloma	Squamous cell carcinoma
Transitional	Transitional cell papilloma	Transitional cell carcinoma
Glandular epithelium	Adenoma	Adenocarcinoma
Mesenchyme		
Fibrous tissue	Fibroma	Fibrosarcoma
Fatty tissue	Lipoma	Liposarcoma
Bone	Osteoma	Osteogenic sarcoma
Cartilage	Chondroma	Chondrosarcoma
Muscle		
Smooth muscle	Leiomyoma	Leiomyosarcoma
Skeletal muscle	Rhabdomyoma	Rhabdomyosarcoma
Neural tissue		
Nerve sheath	Neurofibroma, neurilemoma	Neurogenic sarcoma
		Malignant schwannoma
Nerve cell	Ganglioneuroma	Neuroblastoma
Glial tissue		Astrocytoma
Endothelium		
Blood vessels	Hemangioma	Angiosarcoma
Lymph vessels	Lymphangioma	Lymphangiosarcoma
Blood cells (lymphoreticular)		
Hematopoietic cells		Leukemia
Lymphoid cells		Lymphoma, myeloma
Germ cell	Mature cystic teratoma (dermoid cyst)	Teratoma

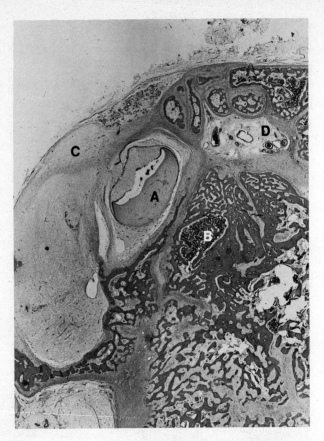

FIG. 9-7. Teratoma. The small area of the tumor shows a few of the many structures present. These include a tooth germ *(A)*; a focus of hemopoietic marrow in a large mass of irregular bone *(B)*; some poorly formed glandular tissue consisting mainly of ducts *(C)*; and a group of thin walled vessels in a loose connective tissue stroma *(D)*.

necessarily the same. Based on their biologic behavior, tumors are described as *benign* or *malignant*, but a few intermediate types exist. Malignant tumors are often referred to as *cancer,* a term derived from the Latin word *cancrum*—a "crab."

In the nomenclature of tumors, several suffixes have been useful. The suffix *-oma* denotes tumor. Benign tumors are usually named by adding the suffix -oma to the histogenic type of the tumor cell. For example, a benign tumor of glandular epithelium is called an *adenoma* and a benign tumor of fibrous tissue is called *fibroma*. A papillary tumor of squamous epithelium is called *papilloma* (Fig. 9-5). Malignant tumor nomenclature follows a similar scheme, but with a few additions. Malignant tumors of epithelium are called *carcinomas,* whereas those of mesenchymal tissues are called *sarcomas* (sarc; Gr, fleshy) (Fig. 9-6). Table 9-1 lists several examples of benign and malignant tumors of various lines of differentiation. These tumors can be categorized into four major groups: epithelial, mesenchymal, lymphoreticular, and germ cell. The latter encompasses a unique group of neoplasms referred to as *teratomas*. Teratomas are exceptional in that they are capable of exhibiting differentiation into more than one germ cell layer. The totipotential tumor cells may differentiate along various germ cell lines, producing specialized tissue such as skin, muscle, thyroid, brain tissue, intestinal epithelium, or any other tissue of the body (Fig. 9-7). The most common example of teratoma is the dermoid cyst of the ovary, where differentiation is mainly along ectodermal lines producing skin, hair, sebaceous glands, and sometimes tooth structures (Fig. 9-8).

Benign tumors are usually composed of cells which closely resemble cells of the tissue origin, grow slowly in expansile fashion, and most important, are confined to the organ in which they arise and will not disseminate through the body (*metastasize*). In contrast, malignant neoplasms consist of cells with significant abnormal morphologic features, grow rapidly and invade adjacent tissues. Most critically they are capable of spreading through the body and establishing growths at remote

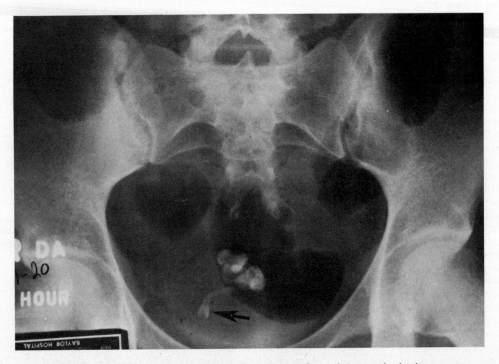

FIG. 9-8. Radiograph of an ovarian teratoma. The presence of a tooth *(arrow)* is clearly apparent.

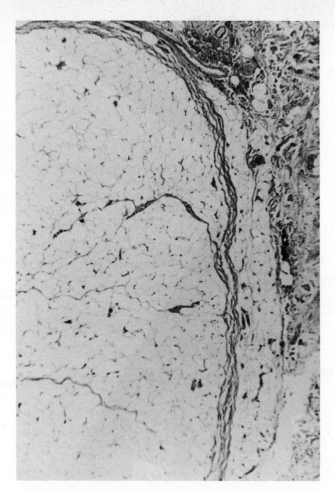

FIG. 9-9. Tumor showing distinct differentiation into mature adipose tissue, thus classifying it as lipoma. Note the capsule of fine fibrovascular connective tissue.

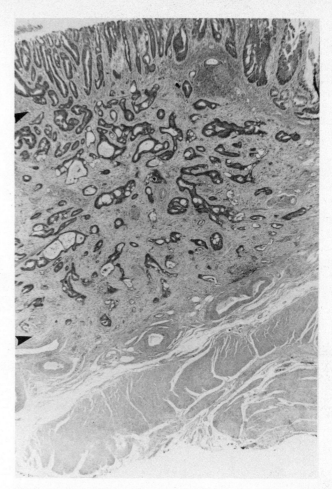

FIG. 9-10. Loss of differentiation in an adenocarcinoma of the colon. At the top, adenomatous hyperplastic glands are seen. The invasive component *(between arrowheads)* shows disorganization with formation of abnormal irregular and complex glands.

sites. For better understanding of the differentiating features between these two groups, it is imperative to review the general biologic, morphologic, and functional characteristics of neoplasms.

Differentiation and anaplasia

Neoplasms consist of two components: the *parenchyma* and the *stroma*. The tumor cells themselves represent the parenchyma; their supportive matrix is referred to as stroma.

Differentiation describes the extent to which the parenchymal cells of a neoplasm resemble those of the parent tissue. In well-differentiated tumors, the resemblance to the parent tissue may be such as to make the origin obvious (Figs. 9-9 and 9-10). Generally speaking, all benign tumors are well differentiated and the better differentiated the tumor, the slower is its growth. Although loss of differentiation is one of the most characteristic features of malignant tumors, well-differentiated tumors can also be highly malignant.

Anaplasia is more characteristic of malignant cells and indicates their cytologic lack of differentiation. Anaplastic tumors bear little or no resemblance to the parent tissue. The tumor cells typically have an increased amount of chromosomal material resulting in disproportionately enlarged nuclei, which appear *hyperchromatic* (i.e., dark staining with hematoxylin) (Fig. 9-11). Nucleoli and increased mitoses are commonly

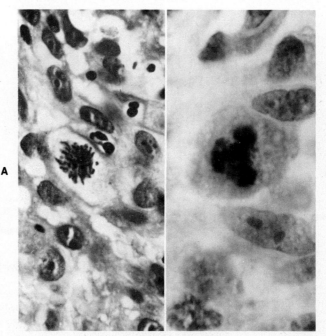

FIG. 9-11. A and **B,** Anaplastic neoplasm showing nuclear hyperchromasia, pleomorphism, asymmetry, and increased mitotic activity **(A)** with abnormal forms **(B).**

prominent and reflect the high proliferative activity of the tumor cells. The increase in chromosomal material may not affect all the chromosomes in the individual cell uniformly, with certain chromosomes, or parts of chromosomes, being replicated, and others being unaffected, or even deleted (Fig. 9-12). This de-

viation from the normal diploid chromosomal complement of the cell *(aneuploidy)* is reflected in *asymmetry* in the structure of the nucleus and in the distribution of the chromatin in the nucleus. It results in the appearance of nuclei with bizarre shapes and chromatin aggregates that vary in size and staining

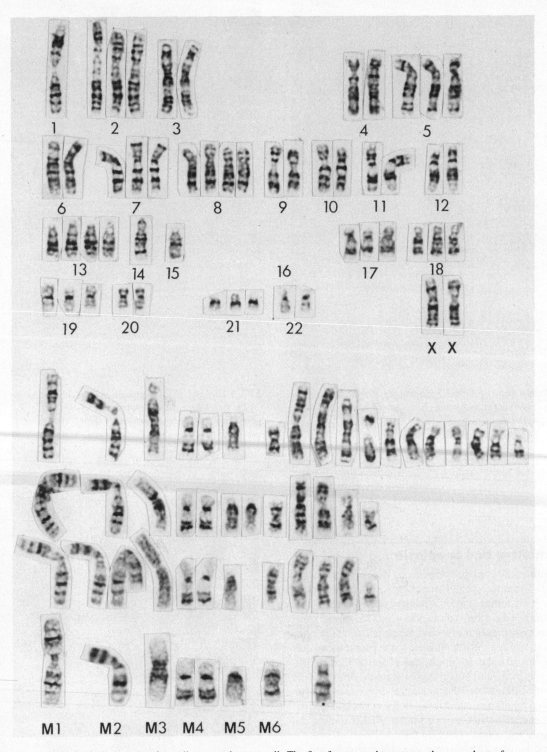

FIG. 9-12. Karyotype of a malignant melanoma cell. The first four rows demonstrate the normal set of chromosomes; however, the fifth row shows an additional set of chromosomes in the same cell. The last three rows represent similar abnormal chromosomes recovered from three additional cells within the same tumor. Note the consistent banding pattern within these individual abnormal chromosomes. *(Courtesy Dr. Sen Pathak.)*

intensity from one portion of the nucleus to the next. Moreover, the number of chromosomes may not be uniform from one cell to another in the same neoplasm; this lack of uniformity results in *nuclear pleomorphism* (i.e., striking variability in nuclear morphology from one cell to the next) (Fig. 9-11).

In the classification of the anaplastic and undifferentiated tumors, pathologists may apply several techniques in an attempt to characterize the nature of the tumor cells. These include histochemistry, immunocytochemistry, cytogenetic probing and chromosomal analysis, electron microscopy, and tissue culture.

Functional activity by tumors

In general, functional activity of a tumor correlates well with the degree of differentiation of its parenchymal cells. Well-differentiated neoplasms continue to produce substances characteristic of the tissue from which they originated. Thus keratin may be produced by squamous cell carcinoma (Fig. 9-13), melanin pigment by malignant melanoma (Fig. 9-14), and osteoid by osteogenic sarcoma (Fig. 9-15). Other neoplasms elaborate hormones or enzymes. Insulin may be produced by carcinoma of the pancreatic islets and acid phosphatase by carcinoma of the prostate.

The production of hormones or other substances is no indication that the tumor is benign, and the functional activity of these products may also have pathologic effects. Thus excessive parathormone production by a parathyroid adenoma can lead to bone resorption and deposition of calcium in the kidney (renal calcinosis). Furthermore, the production of detectable substances such as these can lead to the diagnosis of the tumor.

Unlike the previous examples where the neoplastic product is similar to that formed by the parent tissue, some tumors give rise to abnormal substances, most commonly polypeptide hormones. These products are not known to be synthesized by that particular tissue under normal or physiologic conditions. This heterotopic production of a protein probably represents an abnormal regulation of the gene expression (see later). In the case of hormone production, the phenomenon is referred to as *ectopic hormone production* (Table 9-2). An undifferentiated carcinoma of the lung can produce adrenocorticotrophic hormone (ACTH), while peritoneal fibrosarcoma can produce an insulin-like hormone. Other tumors are capable of producing proteins which are normally expressed during fetal life only. *Carcinoembryonic antigen* (CEA) is produced by various gastrointestinal malignancies and *α-fetoprotein* is produced by hepatocellular carcinoma. These proteins function as extremely useful markers in the diagnosis and in monitoring the effectiveness of treatment of these neoplasms.

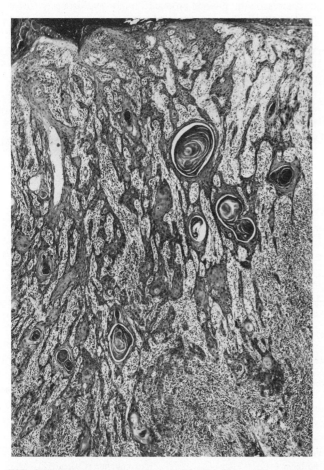

FIG. 9-13. Squamous cell carcinoma of the lip. This malignant tumor is invading the deeper tissues. The whorls of keratin produced in the depths of the lesion is a typical feature.

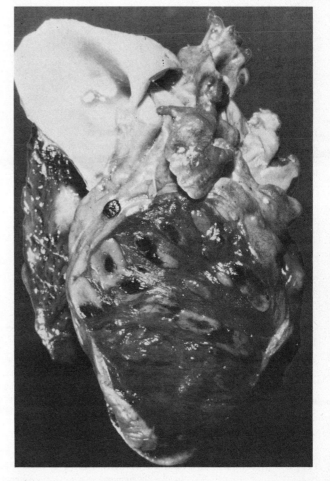

FIG. 9-14. Metastatic melanoma in the heart. The tumor has continued to produce melanin, and the metastases are almost black. This is an uncommon site for metastases. *(Courtesy Curator of the Gordon Museum, Guy's Hospital, London, England.)*

The immunocytochemical detection of intermediate filaments as well as several other cytoplasmic proteins is widely used to determine the functional differentiation of a variety of neoplasms. This technique contributes significantly to a better classification of tumors, understanding their nature, and in certain situations monitoring their biologic behavior. For example, a poorly differentiated tumor may be shown to be epithelial if keratin intermediate filaments can be identified by antibodies to keratin (Fig. 9-16).

Stroma of tumors

The stroma is the connective tissue in which the tumor grows and on which the tumor depends for its blood supply. In epithelial tumors the stroma is produced by the host tissue. In these neoplasms, the fibrous connective tissue component of the stroma varies considerably in amount. At one extreme, it is minimal and the epithelial component is described as *encephaloid* or *medullary*. At the other extreme, the stroma is excessive and is called *desmoplastic* or *scirrhous*.

The stroma of connective tissue neoplasms (sarcomas) is formed in part by the tumor itself. This is not surprising considering the fact that the production of stroma is one of the differentiating functions of mesenchymal cells. For this reason, sarcomas tend to be highly vascular and can spread early and widely by the bloodstream.

In order to maintain an adequate blood supply, which is vital to their growth, tumors produce "tumor-angiogenesis factor (TAF)." This substance is capable of inducing proliferation of new vascular channels from existing vessels of the host in the vicinity of the tumor (Fig. 9-17). Angiogenesis is not unique to neoplasms, and may be observed in other pathologic processes, such as chronic inflammatory conditions. A variety of normal tissues and tumors, both benign and malignant, secrete angiogenic factors. As angiogenesis is promoted, a cascade of events involving a variety of soluble polypeptides and other factors is stimulated. The outcome is the migration of endothelial cells followed by changes in the adjacent basement membrane components. It is suggested that the latter may carry specific growth promoting sequences that facilitate and sustain the endothelial cell growth.

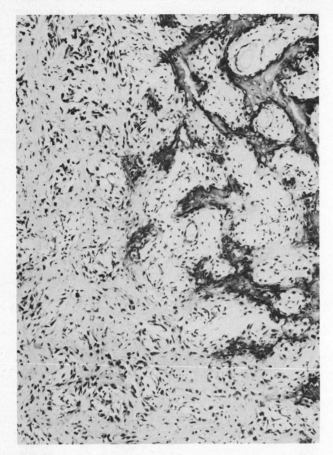

FIG. 9-15. Osteogenic sarcoma. The malignant cells are dark and angular. They produce osteoid, the unmineralized matrix of bone. To the right, calcification of the osteoid is seen with the formation of irregular trabeculae.

TABLE 9-2. Production of hormones by tumors

Tissue	Tumor	Hormone	Clinical features
Hormones appropriate to (normally secreted by) tissue of origin			
Adrenal cortex	Adenoma, carcinoma	Cortisol	Cushing syndrome (Chapter 18)
Islet cells (pancreas)	Adenoma	Insulin	Hyperinsulinism (Chapter 18)
Parathyroid gland	Adenoma, carcinoma	Parathormone (PTH)	Hyperparathyroidism (Chapter 18)
Placental tissue	Choriocarcinoma	Gonadotrophic hormone (HCG)	(Chapter 21)
Thyroid	Adenoma	Thyroxin	Hyperthyroidism (Chapter 18)
Hormones inappropriate to (ectopically produced by) tumors			
Liver	Hepatoblastoma	Gonadoptrophic hormone (HCG)	Precocious puberty (Chapter 15)
Lung	Squamous cell carcinoma	Parathormone (PTH)	Hypercalcemia (Chapter 12)
	Small cell carcinoma	Adrenal corticotrophic hormone (ACTH)	Cushing syndrome (Chapter 12)
		Antidiuretic hormone	Hyponatremia (Chapter 12)
Soft tissues	Fibrosarcoma	Insulin-like	Hypoglycemia (Chapter 17)

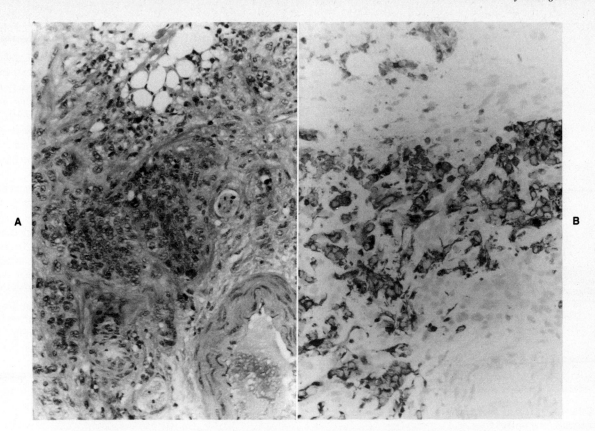

FIG. 9-16. A, Poorly differentiated infiltrating neoplasm lacks distinctive features upon examination with hematoxylin and eosin and routine histochemical stains. **B,** Immunostaining with antibodies to keratin demonstrates the positive dark cytoplasmic staining thus indicating the epithelial differentiation of this neoplasm.

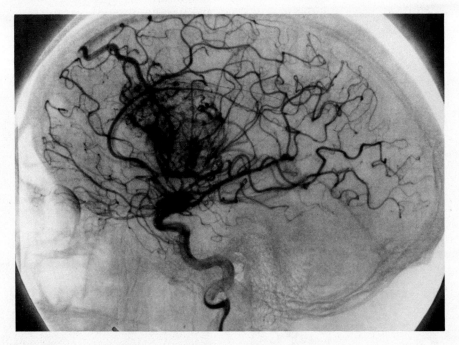

FIG. 9-17. Cerebral angiogram shows the formation of numerous new vessels in a glioblastoma multiforme, a highly malignant neoplasm of glial tissue.

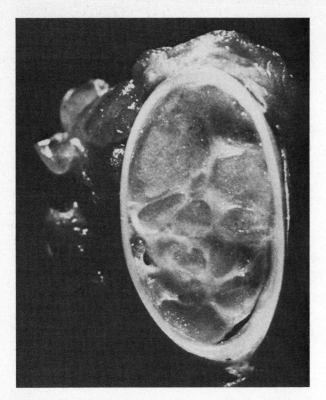

FIG. 9-18. Lipoma. Note the smooth, well-defined capsule and the lobular arrangement of the tumor.

Spread of malignant tumors (metastasis)

Benign tumors, by definition, remain localized and many are surrounded by a fibrous capsule (Fig. 9-9, 9-18). In contrast, malignant tumors are almost never encapsulated, typically invasive and extend into adjacent tissues. They may invade lymphatic and vascular channels and nerves (Fig. 9-19). Even more characteristically, they are capable of *metastasis,* which means the transfer of neoplastic disease from one part of the body to a distant anatomic site, thus creating a *secondary deposit.*

Pathways of metastasis. Dissemination of malignant tumors takes place by four major routes:

1. Lymphatic spread—Spread by the lymphatic system is particularly characteristic of carcinomas which invade and grow along lymphatic channels (Fig. 9-20). Spread to lymph nodes usually follows the anatomic lymphatic drainage of a particular tissue or organ. For example, metastatic carcinoma of the outer quadrants of the breast usually involves the axillary lymph nodes on the same side. Adenocarcinoma of the colon commonly metastasizes to regional pericolonic lymph nodes (Fig. 9-21). Exceptionally, lymphatic spread may be paradoxical and may be observed in opposite sides or may skip some of the more proximal lymph node groups (Fig. 9-22). Because the lymphatic system ultimately drains into the

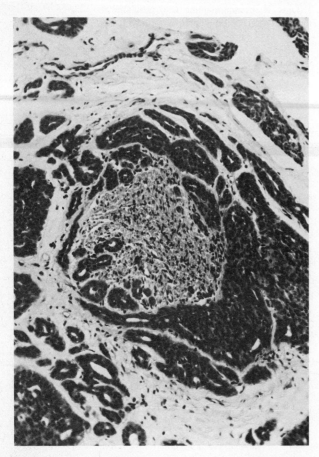

FIG. 9-19. Adenoid cystic carcinoma—perineural invasion. Invasion around and along the nerve sheath and, to a lesser extent, among the axons is typical of this tumor. In spite of the malignant nature of the tumor, the cells are remarkably uniform.

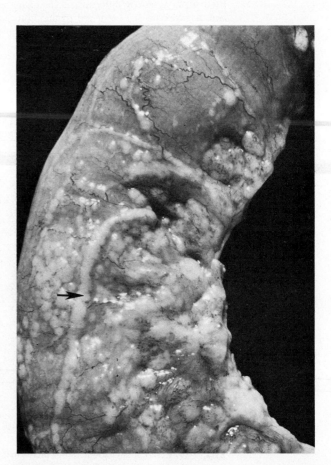

FIG. 9-20. Lymphatic spread of carcinoma. Tumor cells from a gastric adenocarcinoma have permeated the subserosal lymphatic vessels. The lymph vessel arrowed is particularly striking. *(Courtesy Curator of the Gordon Museum, Guy's Hospital, London, England.)*

bloodstream, carcinoma cells can reach the blood by the thoracic duct.

2. Hematogenous spread—Early spread via the bloodstream is characteristic of sarcoma. It would be misleading, however, to leave the reader with the notion that sarcomas and carcinomas have exclusive and selective pathways of metastasis. Sarcomas can also metastasize to lymph nodes, whereas carcinomas can invade blood vessels and, within the lumen, form a tumor "thrombus," which can subsequently embolize to distant sites. Generally, venous spread is more common than arterial spread. Thus it is not surprising that the lung and liver, which are the major drainage sites for vena cava and portal venous flow, are two of the most common sites of hematogenous dissemination (Fig. 9-23).

3. Seeding through body cavities (transcoelomic spread)— The peritoneal cavity is the most common site of this mode of spread. It is typically seen in association with ovarian carcinoma, where widespread seeding of all peritoneal surfaces may take place. Tumors may also seed across other body cavities, such as the pleural cavity, the pericardial cavity, the subarachnoid and joint spaces. An example of transcoelomic spread is extension of a carcinoma of the stomach through its wall into the peritoneal cavity to produce secondary deposits in the ovaries. This is known as *Krukenburg tumor* (Fig. 9-24).

4. Transplantation—Transplantation refers to the mechanical carriage of fragments of tumor cells by surgical instruments during operation or needles during diagnostic procedures. Although there are well-documented instances where this has happened, transplantation is rare.

Biologic phenomena in tumor growth and metastasis

Both experimental and human studies indicate that tumor growth is a very slow process that evolves over many years (Fig. 9-25). Tumors appear to grow exponentially. In experimental tumors, the doubling time increases as the tumor grows. In most situations, a tumor is the outcome of a monoclonal proliferation of a single cell that has selective growth advantage over the normal cells from which it arose. Supportive evidence for this contention is provided by multiple myeloma, a plasma cell neoplasm. In this tumor, a single idiotypic immunoglobulin, or a fragment thereof, is produced and secreted by the tumor cells. This indicates an identical genetic program in each of these malignant plasma cells for the synthesis of this protein. This phenomenon is only conceivable if the cells are derived from one precursor cell (i.e., are monoclonal). In exceptional examples, neoplasms appear to arise from polyclonal populations. In other instances, tumors of similar differentiation may arise multifocally in either synchronous or metachronous

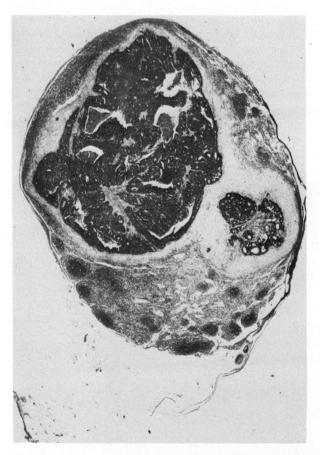

FIG. 9-21. Metastases of adenocarcinoma in a lymph node. The two deposits are surrounded by a fibrous reaction. The remaining lymphoid tissue has been displaced to the periphery. The intense darkly staining malignant cells and the suggestion of a glandular pattern are apparent.

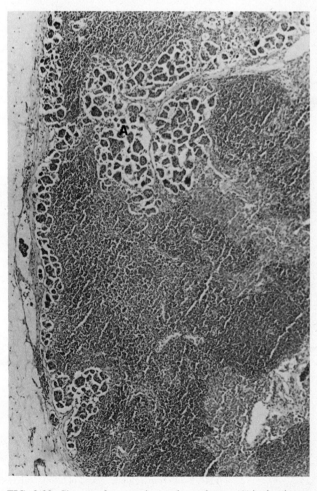

FIG. 9-22. Clusters of metastatic gastric carcinoma *(A)* in the sinuses of a lymph node in the neck.

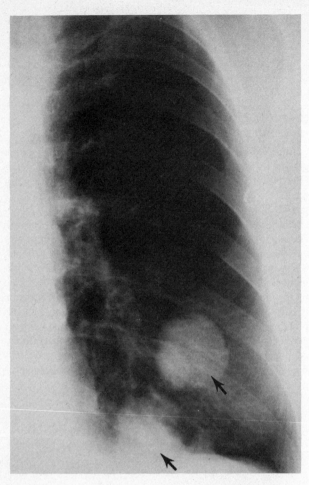

FIG. 9-23. Radiograph of the chest showing two large round metastatic tumors *(arrows)*. The primary carcinoma in the kidney was much smaller than the pulmonary metastasis.

fashion. This is exemplified by multifocal colonic adenocarcinoma and lobular mammary carcinoma.

All tumors acquire a state of growth that is at least initially confined to an anatomical structure. Benign tumors maintain their confined pattern, whereas malignant tumors go on to disseminate and be a major cause of morbidity and mortality. In carcinomas, there is a stage in their growth where the anaplastic cellular changes are limited by a basement membrane to a mucosal surface (Fig. 9-26). This is referred to as *carcinoma in situ* (CIS). The latter usually becomes invasive carcinoma, but in some situations, such as the uterine cervix, this may take many years. If untreated, CIS does not necessarily develop into invasive cancer and in some cases may even appear reversible. Because of the unpredictability of the biologic behavior of CIS, every attempt should be made to remove that lesion, since it is potentially curable at this stage.

Growth factors and receptors

Proliferation of most cells, including malignant variants, is controlled to a large extent by the interactions between specific growth factors and their receptors. Under ordinary physiologic conditions, such an interaction is expressed by the exogenous release by one cell type of peptide proteins which bind to specific receptors on the cell surface of other cell types at a distant site (endocrine function) or at a nearby location (paracrine function) (Fig. 9-27). Many polypeptide growth factors have been characterized recently in different physiologic systems. Some relate specifically to proliferation, differentiation and transformation of cells. Most notable in this group are the *insulin family, epidermal growth factor family, platelet-derived growth factor family, type B transforming growth factor,* and *colony stimulating factors.* Malignant cells escape these normal growth controls through several mechanisms. First, tumor cells are capable of endogenous synthesis of their own growth factors which bind to the functional receptors on the surface of the

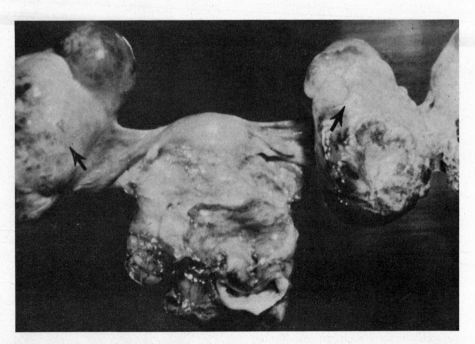

FIG. 9-24. Transcelomic spread of tumor. A Krukenberg tumor of the ovaries *(arrows)*, which originated from a primary gastric carcinoma, is shown.

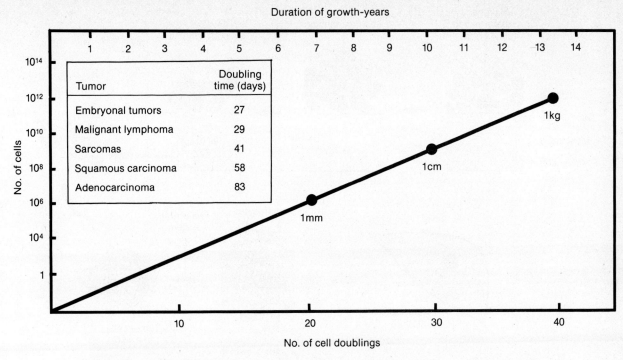

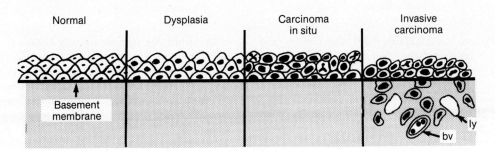

FIG. 9-25. Graphic illustration of tumor growth assuming a consistent 100-day doubling time. This clearly shows the long time it takes for a tumor to grow before it is clinically detected. The table lists the doubling time for a variety of tumors.

FIG. 9-26. An illustration showing the progression of carcinoma. In carcinoma in situ, the dysplastic changes are advanced and involve the entire thickness of the mucosal surface, defined by a basement membrane. In invasive carcinoma, the tumor cells break through the basement membrane into adjacent stroma and may gain access into lymphatic channels *(ly)* or blood vessels *(bv)*.

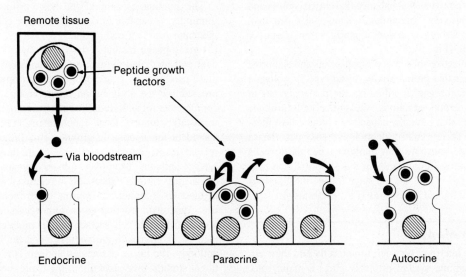

FIG. 9-27. Possible modes of peptide secretion and sites of action.

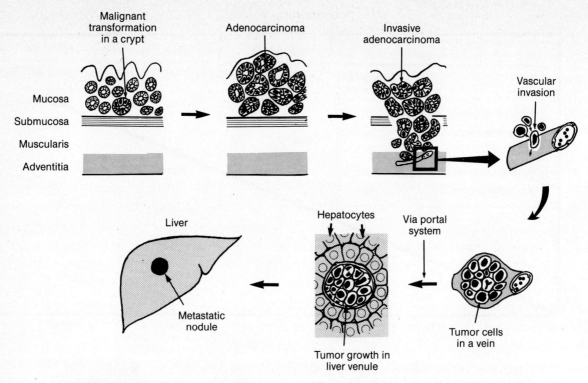

FIG. 9-28. An illustration of the different stages of an infiltrating and metastatic adenocarcinoma of the colon. The tumor has invaded blood vessels, formed tumor emboli, and metastasized to the liver.

tumor cells (autocrine function) (Fig. 9-27). This reduces their dependence on exogenous factors and renders them autonomous. Second, tumor cells exhibit increased receptiveness to stimulation by these peptides. This may be accomplished through increased numbers of receptors on their surface, increased affinity of the receptors, or increased sensitivity of the cell to the signal generated by the peptide-receptor complex. The genetic control of some of these mechanisms will be discussed in a subsequent section.

Unfortunately, the majority of malignant tumors are not clinically detected at the *in situ* stage. Invasive cells typically lose their cohesiveness and contact inhibition, alter their cell junctions and cytoskeleton, change their surface glycoproteins, and release proteolytic enzymes that enhance their invasiveness and penetration into basement membranes. Thus, they can gain access to adjacent stroma, and subsequently vascular and/or lymphatic channels (Fig. 9-28).

Tumor cells synthesize abnormal proteoglycans and elaborate proteolytic enzymes that preferentially digest type IV collagen of the basement membrane or solubilize the proteoglycans in basal lamina. In certain situations, the tumor cells produce soluble metabolites that have the capacity to induce host mesenchymal cells to secrete matrix degradative enzymes. These functions clearly demonstrate that malignant neoplastic cells are capable of creating an environment that supports their proliferation and migration and sets the stage for the most serious complication of malignant neoplasms (i.e., metastasis).

Tumor immunology

In the complex interplay between tumor cells and their environment, the immune system probably plays a major role. Tumors express new antigens, called *tumor-associated antigens*

(TAA), which are immunologically distinct from histocompatibility antigens and are responsible for their interaction with the host immune system. These *neoantigens* exist extracellularly and intracellularly, but the majority are located at the outer cell surface, in the form of glycoproteins, glycolipids or mucins. They are detected in spontaneous tumors in man and animals as well as in virally, chemically, or radiation-induced tumors in experimental animals. Their expression is the result of processes that transform normal cells into neoplastic cells. Actually, most TAA consist of normal cell components that are expressed in aberrant amounts or at inappropriate times or locations. Their production probably reflects a failure of the control system of cellular gene transcription.

The immune system of the host, primarily cell-mediated immunity, is capable of destroying tumor cells through several mechanisms: (1) T cell mediated cytoxicity, (2) natural killing, (3) macrophage mediated cytoxicity, and (4) antibody dependent cell mediated cytoxicity. The activation of any or all of these mechanisms is dependent on environmental factors, expressed surface antigens on tumor cells, and availability of components for individual immune responses. In invasive and metastatic tumors, these mechanisms may fail to limit the spread of the neoplastic growth. This failure may in part be related to the known heterogeneity of tumors in expressing surface antigens. Moreover, tumors are capable of modulating the surface antigen expression in relationship to the antibodies in their environment. In murine experimental models, it has been demonstrated that some tumor-associated antigens disappear from the cell surface within minutes to hours during their incubation with antibodies. Upon the removal of excess antibody, the tumor-associated antigen is re-expressed. Additional studies have shown that the expression of class I histocompatibility antigens is anomalous, thus allowing the cells to evade the immune system and progress to metastasis. Therefore it appears that a variety of means exist by which tumors can avoid destruction by the host's immune system. A combination of mechanisms are probably required to enable the neoplasm to establish itself.

Biology of metastatic tumor cells

As discussed earlier, invasion of blood or lymphatic vessels is the usual route of distant dissemination (Fig. 9-28). As expected, this is accomplished by the breakage of the matrix and wall of vessels including the endothelial basement membrane. Gaining access to the circulation is not by itself sufficient for the tumor cells to successfully establish metastatic growth. Several interdependent factors are involved in the outcome. Experimental studies have demonstrated that there is a critical minimal number, estimated to be several thousand to a million tumor cells, necessary to initiate distant growth. Other significant variables include the type of tumor cell and the defensive mechanisms of the various organs of the host.

By the time they are diagnosed, most tumors are heterogeneous and comprise several subpopulations of cells with varying biologic behavior. This is true irrespective of the monoclonal or polyclonal origin of a particular neoplasm. This diversity exhibits itself in regard to numerous cellular functions, including (1) metastatic potential, (2) growth rate, (3) surface receptors, (4) cytoplasmic markers, (5) antigenicity, (6) response to treatment, and others. Studies on animal and human neoplasms indicate that this heterogeneity is a phenomenon acquired during the progressive growth of a tumor and is attributed primarily to chromosomal instability and subsequent genetic changes (see later).

When mechanically trapped within a host blood vessel, the tumor cells must attach to the endothelium, interact with exposed subendothelial basement membrane, penetrate the vascular wall, and finally enter the organ parenchyma. This is accomplished by specific surface glycoproteins, such as laminin and fibronectin, plasma membrane receptors, secretion of proteolytic enzymes, and by modifying the matrix to enhance

tumor cell locomotion. For example, in animal models, intravenously injected tumor cells selected for their ability to attach via laminin, produced metastasis ten times more frequently than cells lacking this property.

In summary, tumor invasion, both at local and distant sites, is a complex multistep process that culminates in the initiation of metastasis and progressive tumor growth and subsequently contributes to the host's death.

Sites of metastasis

As previously discussed, biologic phenomena may, in part, explain some clinical observations. For example, the sites of secondary deposits are not generally dictated by simple factors such as the richness of the blood supply: for example, secondary deposits rarely form in skeletal muscles or myocardium. Similarly the spleen, although it is an effective filter and contains large amounts of lymphoid tissue, is also a rare site of metastatic tumors. The most common site for metastasis is the liver, particularly for tumors of the gastrointestinal tract, pancreas, breast, and malignant melanoma of the skin (Fig. 9-29). The lung is the typical site for metastasis of sarcomas and also of carcinomas, especially from the breast, thyroid, and kidney (see Fig. 9-23). Carcinomas frequently metastasize to bone (Figs. 9-30 and 9-31), but paradoxically sarcomas that originate in bone rarely form metastases in other bones.

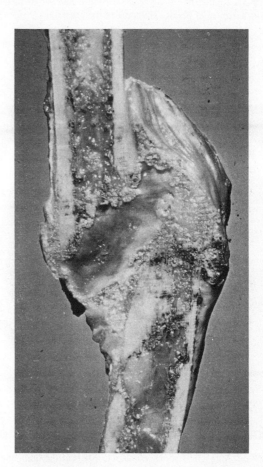

FIG. 9-30. Pathologic fracture of the humerus at the site of a metastatic bronchial carcinoma. *(Courtesy Curator of the Gordon Museum, Guy's Hospital, London, England.)*

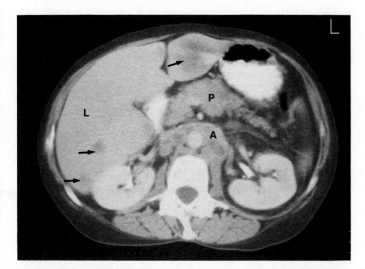

FIG. 9-29. Computerized tomogram (CT) of the abdomen showing a tumor of the pancreas *(P)* with metastasis to para-aortic lymph node *(A)* and liver *(L)*. In the latter, multiple radiolucent areas are seen *(arrows)*.

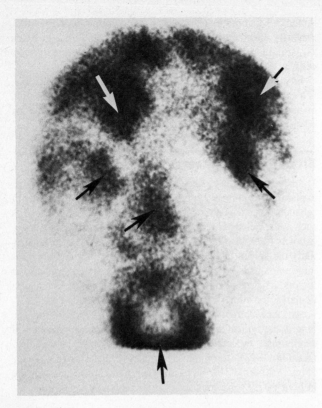

FIG. 9-31. Radioactive bone scan showing a number of metastatic deposits *(arrows)* of breast carcinoma in the chest.

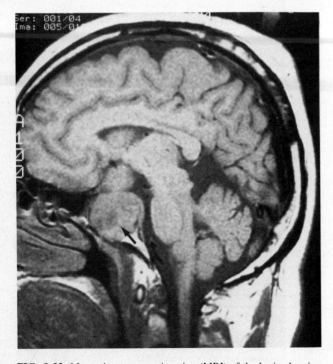

FIG. 9-32. Magnetic resonance imaging (MRI) of the brain showing a large pituitary adenoma distending the sella turcica *(arrow)* and showing suprasellar extension.

Clinical behavior and effects of neoplasms

Having discussed the major characteristics of neoplasms, tabulating the distinguishing features between benign and malignant tumors becomes a much easier task (Table 9-3). However, it is important to emphasize the following points:

1. In certain instances, the anatomic location of the neoplasm, and not its usual biologic behavior, dictates its clinical course. For example, a benign tumor of the brain may prove to be fatal because it is in a part of the brain, such as the brainstem, which does not lend itself to easy surgical removal (Fig. 9-32).
2. The spectrum of benign and malignant neoplasms encompasses a group of tumors of intermediate malignant potential (i.e., they are locally invasive but do not metastasize). An example is basal cell carcinoma of the skin (Chapter 19) (Figs. 9-33 and 9-34).
3. In general, malignant change in benign tumors is exceedingly rare. There are, however, few exceptions. An example is carcinoma arising in pleomorphic adenoma of the salivary glands.
4. The major clinical manifestation of a neoplasm, benign or malignant, may be the consequence of products of the tumor cells. For example, a thyroid adenoma can produce an excessive amount of thyroxin, thus leading to thyroid overactivity (hyperthyroidism) (Chapter 18).

Systemic effects of tumors

Like benign tumors, malignant tumors are capable of causing local pathologic effects. However, in view of their invasive character and metastatic potential, clinical features in addition to their mass effect are frequently seen (Fig. 9-35). These include loss of function, ulceration, pain, and hemorrhage (Figs. 9-36 and 9-37). In addition, malignant tumors may cause systemic effects. One important example is *cachexia,* a description given to the emaciated debilitated state of patients with advanced cancer. Evidence that cachexia is mediated by a circulating substance comes from experiments with parabiotic pairs of rats (two rats joined by a common circulation). The tumor is grown only in one partner and the partner without tumor also experiences anorexia and weight loss. A peptide,

TABLE 9-3. A comparison of benign and malignant tumors

	Benign	*Malignant*
Behavior		
	Expansive	Invasive
	Remain localized	Spread to distant sites (metastasize)
	Encapsulated	No capsule
	Slow growth	Rapid growth
	Closely resembles parent tissue	Varying degrees of loss of differentiation
	Cell reproduction apparently normal	Disordered reproduction
	Normal mitotic figures	Abnormal mitoses
Effects on patient		
	Pain rare	Can cause severe pain
	Little effect on host nutrition	Cachexia

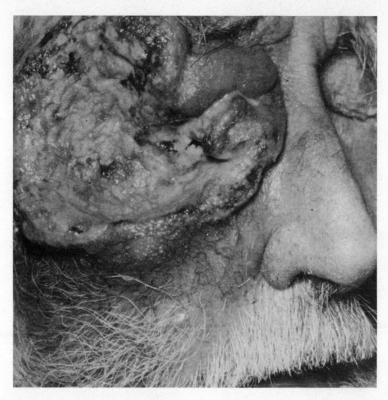

FIG. 9-33. A gross example of neglected basal cell carcinoma of the skin that has destroyed the orbit and part of the face. In spite of the extreme severity of the local effects, there are no metastases.

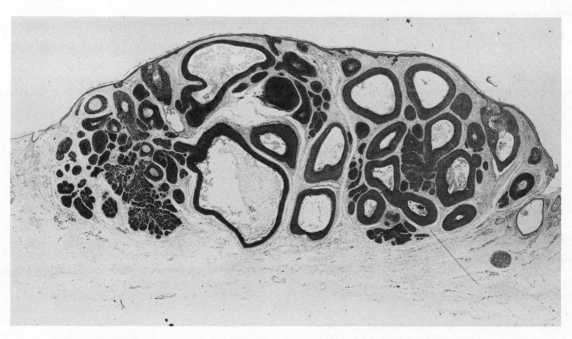

FIG. 9-34. Basal cell carcinoma. This specimen shows the uniform, small, darkly staining tumor cells forming rounded processes extending into the deeper tissues. In some of these there has been cystic change, which is a fairly common feature.

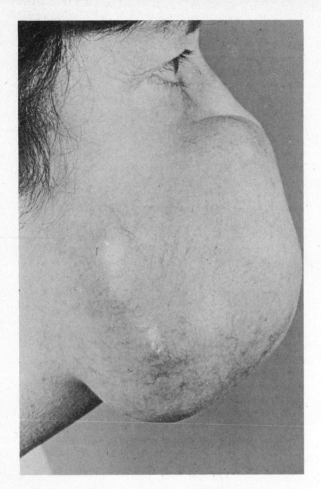

FIG. 9-35. Pleomorphic adenoma. This neglected but benign tumor of a minor intraoral salivary gland has produced an enormous, disfiguring swelling but has not affected the general health of the patient nor given rise to any distant effects.

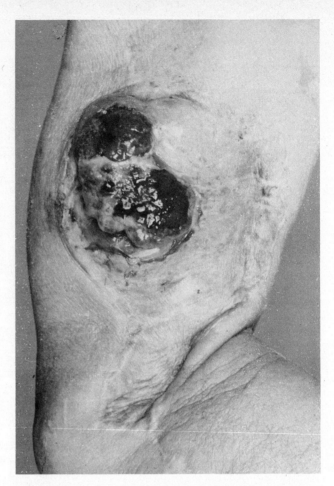

FIG. 9-36. Ulcerating rhabdomyosarcoma of the biceps. *(Courtesy Curator of the Gordon Museum, Guy's Hospital, London, England.)*

named *cachectin,* has been identified as the mediator of this phenomenon. Earlier experiments have demonstrated its secretion by macrophages as a prohormone (propeptide) in response to endotoxin or other bacterial and protozoal products. This prohormone is subsequently cleaved to form the mature polypeptide. The close similarity or identity of cachectin to tumor necrosis factor (TNF) has been recently demonstrated. For example, the administration of cachectin/TNF, a well-characterized tumor cell product, to animals causes diarrhea, weight loss, fever, and lethal shock. The catabolic actions are partly mediated by suppression of synthesis of several adipocyte-specific messenger ribonucleic acid (mRNA) molecules and prevention of differentiation of adipocytes. Lipoprotein lipase is specifically suppressed.

Another unique feature of malignant tumors, usually carcinomas, is to cause unusual clinical syndromes, such as *migratory thrombophlebitis* and *nonbacterial thrombotic endocarditis* (Fig. 9-38). Other examples include rashes as in *acanthosis nigricans* and *dermatomyositis.* The mechanisms of these biologic phenomena are not completely understood, but factors secreted by tumors appear to induce or indirectly mediate these effects.

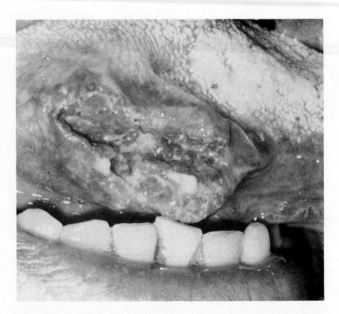

FIG. 9-37. Squamous cell carcinoma of the tongue. The formation of an ulcer with a thickened, rolled edge is typical. *(Courtesy Curator of the Gordon Museum, Guy's Hospital, London, England.)*

Principles of treatment of tumors

The treatment of malignant neoplasms usually depends on two major factors: the *grade* and the *stage* of the tumor in question. The scoring of the former depends on the cytologic differentiation of the neoplastic cells, whereas the stage reflects the size of the tumor, its local extension, and evidence of distant metastasis. There is more than one conventional system for grading and staging tumors. These vary from one organ to another, but the general principles are similar. The higher the grade and/or stage of a particular tumor, the worse its prognosis will be. For example, the "unfavorable histology" group of nephroblastoma (Wilms' tumor), which characteristically shows cytologic anaplasia, has a much worse prognosis than the "favorable histology" group of this renal neoplasm. Furthermore, children with tumors of higher stage, irrespective of their grade, are treated more aggressively.

Etiology and pathogenesis (carcinogenesis)

Most biologic phenomena are a product of an interplay of several factors. Throughout the life of a subject, there is an ongoing interaction between the host and the environment, and

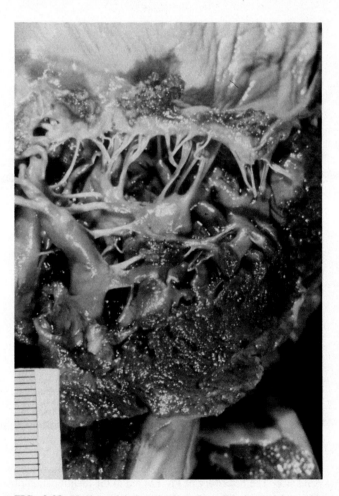

FIG. 9-38. Nonbacterial thrombotic endocarditis in a patient with adenocarcinoma of the pancreas. Note the vegetations along the leaflets of the mitral valve.

this interaction determines the outcome of most pathologic processes, including neoplasia. The major carcinogenic influences that have been identified are as follows:

1. Genetic factors
2. Chemical carcinogens
3. Physical agents, particularly radiation
4. Microbial carcinogens, particularly viruses
5. Immunologic factors

Genetic factors and oncogenes

The advances in molecular biology indicate that normal cell growth is the outcome of a harmonious interaction between unique segments of DNA, constant in location and conserved in evolution. This finding has revolutionized the study of neoplasia in recent years and prompted several authors to consider cancer as a genetic disease. About 40 genes, referred to as *oncogenes* are widely distributed throughout the genome. They are expressed in a temporally related and tissue specific manner and are involved in the control of cellular proliferation, differentiation, and carcinogenesis. They are probably active during embryogenesis, wound healing, tissue repair, and normal cell replacement. The cellular genome also includes genes that are responsible for suppressing the development of a tumor cell phenotype. Both oncogenes and suppressor genes *(antioncogenes, emerogenes)* are in continuous interaction with the influences exerted by their environment.

Oncogenes were first identified in retroviruses (oncogenic RNA viruses). Subsequent studies proved that oncogenes are not unique to viruses and demonstrated their presence in a wide range of living cells, including those of the fruit fly *(Drosophila)* and man. In view of this wide distribution, it is more likely that retroviruses acquired their oncogenes from host cells and *not* vice versa. For viruses to replicate, they usually integrate their genome into the host's deoxyribonucleic acid (DNA) through a specific sequence of events (see later). Hybridization between the two genomes will contribute to the acquisition of oncogenes by viruses. Because of this feature, most cellular oncogenes (or proto-oncogenes) are designated, largely for historic reasons, by abbreviations of their homologues in the corresponding viruses (Table 9-4).

In normal cells, the expression of cellular oncogenes (proto-oncogenes) is tightly regulated. They encode directly or indirectly for nuclear and cytoplasmic proteins. In the nucleus, the function of these proteins is not completely understood, but it is thought that they regulate gene expression. The cytoplasmic proteins function as growth factors, protein kinases (some of which are growth factor receptors), and proteins homologous to transducing proteins, which play a role in membrane signaling (Table 9-4). The enhancement of these functions by activating oncogenes will contribute to the phenotypic expression and growth of a particular cell.

In animal and experimental models of neoplasia and in examples of human cancer, several qualitative and quantitative abnormalities that involve oncogenes have been identified (Table 9-5). These may be present within the gene itself or in close proximity to it. Recognizable abnormalities include (1) *point mutations,* (2) *chromosomal rearrangements,* (3) *deletions (truncation),* and (4) *gene amplification* (Fig. 9-39).

Amplification refers to the duplication of regions of DNA to form linear arrays containing a variable number of copies

TABLE 9-4. Cellular proto-oncogenes (oncogenes) and retroviral oncogenes

Oncogene	Retrovirus	Location of gene products	Function of gene products
Ha-*ras*	Harvey murine sarcoma virus	Plasma membrane	Signal transduction
Ki-*ras*	Kirsten murine sarcoma virus	Plasma membrane	Signal transduction
erb-B	Avian erythoblastosis virus	Plasma membrane	Growth factor receptor
fms	Feline sarcoma virus	Plasma membrane	Growth factor receptor
erb-A	Avian erythroblastosis virus	Cytoplasm	Glucocorticoid receptor
src	Rous avian sarcoma virus	Membranes, cytoplasm	Protein-tyrosine kinase
abl	Abelson murine leukemia virus	Membranes, cytoplasm	Protein-tyrosine kinase
mos	Moloney murine leukemia virus	Cytoplasm	Protein-serine/threonine kinase
sis	Simian sarcoma virus	Cytoplasm	Platelet-derived growth factor
myc	Avian myelocytomatosis virus	Nuclear	Unknown
fos	FBJ murine sarcoma virus	Nuclear	Activation of cell division ? cellular memory

TABLE 9-5. Examples of oncogenes and associated neoplasms

Oncogene	Method of identification	Neoplasm
N-*myc*	Amplification	Neuroblastoma
L-*myc*	Amplification	Lung carcinoma
N-*ras*	Transfection	Neuroblastoma
bcl-1,2	Chromosomal translocation	B-cell lymphoma
bcr	Chromosomal translocation	Chronic myelogenous leukemia
int-1,2	Insertional mutagenesis	Breast carcinoma

of the original region. Through a poorly understood mechanism, these alterations lead to the "activation" of an oncogene. Its protein product will in turn contribute to a state of uncontrolled proliferation. A single oncogene may be activated by more than one mechanism. A group of cellular oncogenes is not associated with recognizable chromosomal abnormalities; however, their existence has been identified through DNA transfection. In this assay, DNA from certain tumor cells, but not normal cells, induces immortalized mouse fibroblast cell lines (NIH3T3) to exhibit biologic features of neoplastic cells. This follows the entry of exogenous DNA into the host cells and its integration with their genome. One additional mechanism by which an oncogene is thought to be activated is *insertional mutagenesis*. This applies primarily to certain models of viral oncogenesis. The introduction of an enhancer sequence by the proviral genome into the host's genome will lead to the activation of adjacent base pairs which may include an oncogene (Fig. 9-40).

The altered expression of an oncogene is *not by itself sufficient to cause neoplasia*. Carcinogenesis is a complex process arising from either a structural change in the DNA or by modification of regulatory genes responsible for the repression of autonomous growth. It is very likely that human cancer is the outcome of multiple steps involving multiple genes. The distinctive and differentiating features of a neoplasm, including the previously described heterogeneity, are a reflection of a selective group of genes that the cell is capable of transcribing. The order of these events may not be as significant as the cumulative effect of all these mutations in conferring a selective growth advantage on the tumor cell. Although the evidence for an association between chromosomal aberrations and cancer is clear, the nature of the relationship remains elusive.

Several questions pertaining to these chromosomal changes remain unresolved. For example, are they a causative factor in neoplasia, the result of neoplasia or a manifestation of a fundamental factor causing neoplasia?

Chromosomal and pedigree studies

Evidence of an association between genes and cancer comes from chromosomal studies on individual tumors and pedigree studies of families showing increased risk of developing neoplasms. The first specific chromosomal abnormality to be associated with malignancy was the demonstration that 90% of patients with chronic myelogenous leukemia have the Philadelphia (Ph') chromosome. This often represents a reciprocal translocation between chromosomes 9 and 22 (Fig. 9-41). This finding is not, however, limited to myeloid cells, but may be seen in erythroid and megakaryocytic elements as well. It has been demonstrated that this abnormality includes an oncogene, c-*abl*, which is translocated from its locus on chromosome 9 and fused to a "breakpoint cluster region" *(bcr)* on the long arm of chromosome 22. In hematopoietic cells of mice, an activated oncogene of this kind leads to growth factor independence. The discovery of Ph' has led to the identification of numerous consistent karyotypic abnormalities in other types of leukemia, lymphoma, and solid tumors. These include chromosomal gain, deletion, inversion, and translocation (Table 9-6). Karyotyping studies have significantly contributed to the recognition of morphologic subsets of leukemia and lymphoma

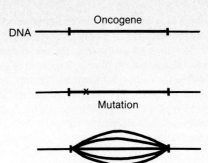

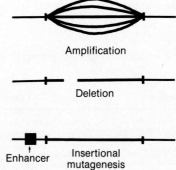

FIG. 9-39. Possible mechanisms by which oncogenes are activated: (a) mutation—a limited qualitative alteration of the base sequence; (b) amplification—duplication of genetic material forming linear arrays of gene; (c) deletion—loss of part of the normal base sequence of the gene; (d) insertional mutagenesis (see text and Fig. 9-40).

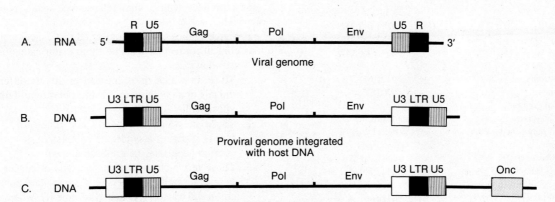

FIG. 9-40. Schematic illustration of "insertional mutagenesis" model of viral carcinogenesis, depicting the RNA genome of avian leukosis virus *(A)*. When its RNA is transcribed into DNA and integrated into the host's genome, the end sequences are flanked by long terminal repeat (LTR) sequences *(B)*. LTR contains an enhancer that increases the rate of expression of most nearby DNA sequences, including those of an oncogene *(C)*.

FIG. 9-41. Philadelphia chromosome. Karyotype showing 9-22 translocation typically seen in patients with chronic myelogenous leukemia. *(Courtesy Dr. Sen Pathak.)*

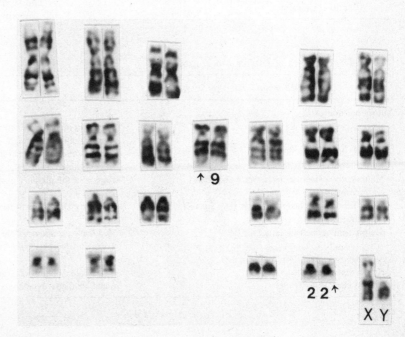

characterized not only by specific chromosomal abnormalities, but also by median survival, and unique morphologic and clinical features. In lymphoid neoplasms, the use of cloned gene probes permits the assessment of *rearrangement of genes* normally responsible for coding for immunoglobulins, their components, or their receptors. The presence of specific rearrangements is indicative of a clonal proliferation of the lymphocytes and thus determines their neoplastic nature.

Similar observations have been made in several kinds of solid tumors (see Fig. 9-12, Tables 9-5 and 9-6). For example, retinoblastoma, an embryonal tumor of the retina, is strongly associated with homozygosity of a mutant allele on chromosome 13, band q14. Most germ cell tumors, irrespective of histologic type, demonstrate a specific chromosomal change, an isochromosome of the short arm of chromosome 12.

Abnormal expression of oncogenes has been demonstrated in many hematopoietic and solid tumors. It has been examined by three different methods: (1) transfection assays, (2) DNA, RNA blots and in situ hybridization, and (3) immunohistochemical demonstration of oncogene products, such as p21 of the *ras* oncogene. The most commonly described alterations involve the following genes: *myc, erb*-B, H-*ras,* Ki-*ras,* and *ebl*. In certain situations, the detection of an abnormal expression of an oncogene is helpful for diagnostic and prognostic purposes. In neuroblastoma, another example of embryonal tumor of neural tissue, the presence of amplified N-*myc* gene (many copies) correlates with the stage of the disease and the overall survival. Moreover, the greater the N-*myc* copy number, the worse the patient's prognosis irrespective of the stage. Similarly, in breast carcinoma, an amplified c-*erb* B-2 (or *neu*) gene correlates with a high relapse rate and a poor overall survival.

Pedigree studies have demonstrated that cancer exhibits various clinical forms that fall into three major categories (Table 9-7) as follows:

1. Those in which the same cancer affects different individuals in a pedigree (e.g., retinoblastoma, familial polyposis coli)
2. Those in which a cancer—not necessarily the same type—is part of a syndrome complex (e.g., multiple endocrine neoplasia, neurofibromatosis)
3. Those in which more than one type of cancer develops in several family members (e.g., hereditary nonpolyposis colorectal cancer—Lynch syndrome II), where cancer of the colon is associated with other forms of cancer, particularly carcinoma of the endometrium, ovary, and pancreas.

With the exceptions of a few autosomal recessive syndromes, the predisposition to tumor development in all these forms of heritable cancer is dominantly inherited.

The study of sporadic and familial forms of retinoblastoma has contributed to Knudson's ingenious "two-hit" hypothesis

TABLE 9-6. Neoplasms with specific (primary) chromosomal changes

Neoplasm	Chromosomal change
Benign neoplasms	
Meningioma	− 22, 22q −
Mixed tumor (salivary glands)	t(3;8), t(9;12)
Colonic adenoma	12q, +8
Malignant neoplasms	
Carcinoma	
Urinary bladder	i(5p), +7, −9/9q −
Prostate	del(10) (q24)
Kidney	del(3) (p21)
Ovary	6q −, t(6;14)
Sarcoma	
Liposarcoma	t(12;16)
Synovial	t(X;18)
Embryonal tumors	
Retinoblastoma	del(13) (q14)
Wilms' tumor (nephroblastoma)	del(11) (p13)
Neuroblastoma	del(1) (p32 p36)
Ewing's sarcoma and peripheral neuroepithelioma	t(11;22) (q24; q12)
Germ cell tumors	i(12p)
Leukemia and lymphoma	
Chronic myelogenous leukemia	t(9;22)
Acute nonlymphocytic leukemia	t(9;22), t(8;21), t(15;17)
Acute lymphocytic leukemia	t(9;22), t(8;14)
Small noncleaved lymphoma (Burkitt's lymphoma)	t(8;14)

TABLE 9-7. Examples of familial cancer syndromes

Syndrome	Associated neoplasms
Autosomal dominant	
Familial polyposis coli	Adenocarcinoma of colon, adenomatous polyps
Gardner syndrome	Adenocarcinoma of colon, desmoid tumor
Peutz-Jeghers syndrome	Adenocarcinoma of small intestine and colon, tumors of ovary
Neurofibromatosis	Neurofibroma, neurogenic sarcoma, pheochromocytoma
Multiple endocrine neoplasia type I (Wermer syndrome)	Tumors of the pituitary gland, pancreatic islet cells, and parathyroid gland
Multiple endocrine neoplasia, type IIA (Sipple's syndrome)	Medullary carcinoma of the thyroid, pheochromocytoma, parathyroid tumors
Multiple endocrine neoplasia type IIB	Medullary carcinoma of the thyroid, pheochromocytoma, parathyroid tumors, mucosal ganglioneuromas
Autosomal recessive	
Xeroderma pigmentosum	Basal and squamous cell carcinoma of skin and malignant melanoma
Ataxia-telangiectasia	Acute leukemia, lymphoma, and possibly gastric cancer

of carcinogenesis. He has proposed that at least two independent mutations are necessary for the expression of a malignancy. These events result in the loss of both alleles at the same locus. In the familial form, the first mutation ("first hit") is inherited in the germ line, and thus is present in every cell of the body. Tumor development requires only one additional mutation ("second hit") in any single cell of the appropriate tissue. In the sporadic form, the two events are restricted to the somatic target cell (i.e., the retinoblast). In both forms of retinoblastoma, the outcome is identical and is usually expressed as a deletion of band 14 of the long arm of chromosome 13. The retinoblastoma model supports the existence of *suppressor genes*. The loss of both alleles of a particular gene removes the suppression of the continuous expression of transforming genes and oncogenes, resulting in tumor development. Similar mechanisms have been identified in several tumors, such as Wilms tumor, osteogenic sarcoma, and familial polyposis coli.

The list of tumors associated with chromosomal abnormalities continues to grow. The use of recombinant DNA probes which recognize individual chromosome specific markers, known as restriction-fragment-length polymorphisms (RFLP), have revolutionized the clinical studies in neoplasia. As the loci of genes responsible for individual heritable cancers are mapped, patients who are predisposed to these tumors will become amenable to genetic counseling (carrier detection and prenatal diagnosis) as is now the case with other genetic disorders. This has been successfully implemented in the early detection of cases of familial retinoblastoma. The identification of putative cancer genes increases the likelihood of cloning such genes and subsequent characterization of their biochemical composition. This may provide additional insight into the mechanisms that underlie the development of cancer as well as help in designing new approaches to the treatment of cancer that would primarily target these genetic abnormalities.

Chemical carcinogens

In 1775, a London surgeon, Sir Percival Pott, related carcinoma of the scrotal skin to exposure to soot among chimney sweeps. In 1914, Yamagiwa and Ichikawa were successful in inducing carcinoma in rabbits' ears by repeated applications of coal tar. Since that time, a wide variety of chemical compounds have been analyzed for their carcinogenic potential. Based on human studies and experimental animal models, it seems that chemical carcinogens exert their effect by three major modes of action as follows:

1. Direct action—The carcinogen, without preceding conversion or biochemical alteration, is capable of exerting its effect by irreversible interaction with DNA or in certain situations, by binding to RNA or proteins.
2. Procarcinogenic action—The chemical carcinogen requires metabolic or enzymic conversion to exert its carcinogenic effect.
3. Promotor action—The chemical lacks intrinsic carcinogenic potential, but exerts its action by enhancing the effect of direct-acting carcinogens or procarcinogens.

Numerous chemical carcinogens have been identified (Table 9-8). Examples of these include the following:

1. Alkylating agents—These are direct-acting, but generally weak carcinogens. They are used clinically in the treatment of cancer (e.g., cyclophosphamide, chlorambucil, busulfan, nitrogen mustard and analogs). Women treated for disseminated ovarian carcinoma with alkylating agents are at increased risk of developing leukemia.
2. Polycyclic aromatic hydrocarbons—The first recognized examples of carcinogens belong to this category which includes soot (coal tar), dimethylbenzanthracene, benzpyrene, and cholanthrene. Potent carcinogens of this type do not merely induce neoplasms when painted on the skin, but also cause malignant change in deep organs when injected. Most of these chemicals are procarcinogens. Their ultimate carcinogenic metabolites are dihydrodiol epoxides which are strongly electrophilic and bind to nucleophilic sites, including DNA, RNA and protein. Exposure to coal tar and many of its products remains an industrial hazard, and it is believed that compounds similar to coal tar hydrocarbons may be the cause of lung cancer in cigarette smokers.
3. Aromatic amines and azo dyes—These are also procarcinogenic and are mostly metabolized in the liver. Examples of this group include acetaminofluorene and benzidine. β-Naphthylamine, widely used in the aniline dye industry, is associated with urinary bladder carcinoma. The dye butter yellow was at one time used as a coloring for margarine until its potent carcinogenicity was appreciated.
4. Other carcinogens—The list of chemical carcinogens is extensive. These encompass some natural products (e.g., aflatoxin B), drugs and hormones (e.g., diethylstilbestrol), metals and inorganic compounds (e.g., arsenic compounds, asbestos), industrial products (e.g., vinyl chloride) and food additives and sweeteners (e.g., saccharin for animals).

TABLE 9-8. Examples of chemical carcinogens

Chemical	*Tumor site*
Alkylating agents	
Nitrogen mustard, melphalan cyclophosphamide, chlorambucil and others	Leukemia, urinary bladder
Vinyl chloride	Angiosarcoma of liver
Polycyclic hydrocarbons	
Tars, soots and oils	Skin, lung
Aromatic amines and azo dyes	
β-Naphthylamine	Urinary bladder
Benzidine	Urinary bladder
Natural products (food, plant or beverage components)	
Aflatoxin (from mold on peanuts)	Liver
Betel nuts	Buccal mucosa
Saccharin	Urinary bladder
Medications	
Androgenic anabolic steroids	Liver
Diethylstilbestrol	Vagina
Phenacetin	Renal pelvis
Inorganic compounds	
Chromium	Lung
Nickel	Lung, nasal sinuses
Asbestos	Serosal membranes, lung
Arsenic	Skin

Chemical carcinogenesis and human cancer

In the United States any substance for human consumption that has been shown experimentally to be carcinogenic for animals is either banned or carries a warning label. It must be appreciated, however, that animals differ widely in their susceptibility to cancer. Rats, which are widely used as experimental animals, develop cancers of some types very readily. It is obviously also difficult, if not impossible, to compare the degree of experimental exposure to the agent with what is happening naturally in humans. It is not feasible to confirm the experimental findings by setting up comparable experiments on humans. Although it is a justifiable assumption that a substance which is carcinogenic for animals is also carcinogenic for humans, this is unproven. Alternatively, the risk may not be significant for humans because exposure to the putative carcinogen may not be great enough to induce tumors under natural circumstances. Thus, in the case of saccharin, vast quantities have been used as a noncaloric sweetener for dieting purposes and by diabetics. There is also no good evidence that diabetics who have used saccharin habitually for many years show any increased incidence of bladder cancer nor that victims of bladder cancer had an increased consumption of saccharin.

There is *no* test which will reliably predict whether a chemical agent is carcinogenic for humans. However, it is usual to resort to certain tests to detect the mutagenicity of the chemical in question. In general, carcinogenicity correlates well with mutagenicity but it is equally important to keep in mind that not all carcinogens are mutagens and conversely some mutagens are noncarcinogenic. A widely used test for screening for mutagenicity is the Ames test which uses a specific mutant strain of the bacterium, *Salmonella typhimurium* which is unable to synthesize histidine. The bacterium, the test chemical, and a mammalian tissue extract (commonly rodent liver) are incubated in soft agar containing a trace of histidine, to allow limited growth and expression of mutations. If mutagenic, the chemical or its metabolite (a product of the action of the liver extract on the chemical) reacts with the bacterial DNA. It may induce a second mutation, which allows the bacterium to resume histidine biosynthesis and consequently to form visible bacterial colonies.

Mechanisms of chemical carcinogenesis

Several models have been proposed for chemical carcinogenesis. Nevertheless, there is general acceptance in all these models that the expression of malignancy in a transformed cell population is the outcome of a sequence of events that follow a critical interaction between a carcinogen and a single cell or a group of cells. Other commonly shared features are as follows:

1. The effect of carcinogens is dose dependent. A critical level of dosage, or threshold is necessary.
2. There is a latent period. Carcinogenesis is a slow, complex process that evolves over an extended period of time. The agent has to be applied for a long period before any change becomes apparent. The effect of individual short exposures may be additive.
3. Cellular changes are transmitted to daughter cells, and the process once initiated is often irreversible.

4. Carcinogenesis may be influenced by noncarcinogens.
5. Carcinogenesis depends on cell proliferation. This may be a requirement of certain models of experimental carcinogenesis, but as noted earlier, hyperplasia is not necessarily a precursor of carcinomatous change in humans and malignant change can take place in hypoplastic or atrophic epithelial cells.

One of the most widely accepted stepwise models of chemical carcinogenesis is the *initiation-promotion-progression model:*

1. The initiator, which is a carcinogen, must be applied first. It is most effective at certain stages of the cell cycle, usually at the beginning of DNA synthesis.
2. The initiated cell is usually permanently altered and rendered capable of giving rise to tumor. This process is often, but not always, associated with DNA changes. In specific models of chemically induced tumors, point mutations of oncogenes have been demonstrated (see Table 9-9).
3. The *promotor,* commonly a noncarcinogen, enhances the expression of the phenotypic characteristics of the *transformed* or "initiated" cell. The effect is typically reversible and nonadditive.
4. Promotion is usually expressed by a focal proliferation within a tissue or organ.
5. *Progression* is the process whereby the focal proliferation evolves into a malignant process.

It is important to emphasize that this sequence remains speculative and applies mostly to experimental carcinogenesis. Whether any human cancers are the result of this strict three stage process of initiation-promotion-progression, remains unresolved. It is very possible that some carcinogens act as both initiators and promoters, but in others, promoting substances are needed. Examples include croton oil, phenol, teleocidin, aplysiatoxin and palytoxin. Phorobol esters are normally present in plants, while teleocidin, aplysiatoxin and palytoxin have been isolated from fungi, algae and plants. These chemicals exhibit a wide range of effects, most notably increased cell proliferation, induction of enzymes in the polyamine synthetic pathway, and alterations in surface proteins. These effects may be mediated through their activation of protein kinase, a function controlled by oncogenes. For example, phorbol ester can activate the *fos* gene which is capable of detecting incoming signals at the cell membrane and converting them to lasting responses that require gene activity, such as cell division and possibly memory formation.

Cocarcinogenesis is a term used to describe the interaction

TABLE 9-9. Carcinogen-activated oncogenes in experimental carcinogenesis

Oncogene	Tumor	Carcinogen
Ha-*ras*	Mammary carcinoma	Nitrosomethylurea
	Skin papilloma/carcinoma	Dimethylbenzanthralene
Ki-*ras*	Renal carcinoma	Methyl (methoxymethyl) nitrosamine
erb-B (*neu*)	Neuroblastoma	Ethylnitrourea
	Schwannoma	Nitrosomethylurea

of several factors in the production of cancers. A possible example of cocarcinogenesis in humans is cancer of the lung found in asbestos workers who are also heavy cigarette smokers.

Radiation carcinogenesis

Both experimental studies and epidemiologic data have demonstrated the carcinogenic effect of solar and ionizing radiation in humans.

Ionizing radiation. The various forms of ionizing radiation—electromagnetic (x rays, gamma rays) or particulate (alpha particles, beta particles, protons, neutrons)—are proven carcinogens, but have varying degrees of potency (Chapter 5). Possible theoretical mechanisms of radiation carcinogenesis include chromosomal damage or induction of somatic mutations. The genetic defects are thought to be introduced directly into the genome by linear energy transfer or by chemical modification due to by-products produced by free radical interaction with DNA. Recent studies point to a possible role of oncogene activation in radiation induced cancer. In the neoplastic transformation of embryo fibroblasts, at least two cooperating oncogenes on different chromosomes are activated. In experimental thymic lymphoma, *Ki-ras* oncogene is activated by gamma rays.

Since the discovery of x-rays in the late 19th century, considerable information has been obtained about the physical properties of radiation and its biologic effects, including cancer. Some of these known facts about radiation-induced cancers have been summarized by the Committee on the Biological Effects of Ionizing Radiation:

1. Radiation-induced cancers are morphologically indistinguishable from similar natural cancers.
2. Radiation can induce cancer in almost every tissue in the body.
3. The sensitivity to radiation carcinogenesis varies considerably for various tissue and organs. Examples of tissue with high sensitivity include female breast, thyroid gland, hematopoietic cells especially myeloid elements.
4. Cancer induction by radiation has a characteristically long latent period. The length of this period is dependent on the type of cancer and may extend from years to decades.
5. Age and sex are major risk factors of cancer from exposure to radiation. Other host and environmental factors may also play a role.
6. Dose-response relationships may not be the same for all radiation-induced cancers.
7. Risk estimates of radiation-induced cancers are based primarily on high dose data. The risk estimate for low-dose exposure remains undetermined. The prevailing view is that the risk of cancer is directly proportional to the dose.

In humans, a wealth of information on the relationship between ionizing radiation and cancer comes from epidemiologic studies on occupational, therapeutic and military exposures.

Occupational exposure. Miners in certain parts of central Europe were recognized several centuries ago to have a high risk for a peculiar type of lung disease. It was eventually discovered that there was exposure to radioactive dust or gas (radon) and that the lung disease was bronchial carcinoma, at that time a rare disease. A similar hazard has existed in some mines in the United States (see Chapter 4).

Cancer was also a serious hazard in the early days of radiology. In ignorance of these dangers early workers, including Roentgen* himself, often placed their hands in the x-ray beams and developed skin cancers. Before the use of modern equipment and protective measures, radiologists had a disproportionately higher incidence of leukemia and skin cancer compared with other medical specialties.

In the early part of this century, luminous watch dials were handpainted with light-emitting, radioactive materials. To achieve the necessary fine detail, the workers wetted the tips of their brushes with their tongue or lips. Ingestion of this radioactive material was followed by a high incidence of bone sarcomas and leukemias in these young women.

Therapeutic irradiation. Neoplastic change is a rare hazard of therapeutic irradiation. Radiation treatment of the skin for benign conditions, such as removal of excessive hair, has led to skin cancers. Radiation of cancer of the mouth has occasionally led to development of otherwise rare sarcomas of the jaws or oral soft tissues. In the past the fashion for irradiating the thymus in children for "thymic asthma" was followed by a high incidence of thyroid cancer many years later. Radiation of the head and neck region in general is also associated with an increased incidence of thyroid and salivary gland cancers, which are also otherwise rare.

The strongest evidence for the carcinogenic effect of therapeutic irradiation is the high incidence of leukemia after radiation of the spine for ankylosing spondylitis. In these patients the incidence of leukemia is approximately 10 times that in the normal population.

Atomic explosions. As if to prove once and for all the carcinogenic effect of ionizing radiation, the effects of the atomic bombs dropped in Hiroshima and Nagasaki should have erased any doubts. Among survivors the incidence of acute leukemia has been approximately 15 times higher than that of controls, and there has been also a considerable excess of other cancers. The carcinogenic effect of this exposure is still being seen by new cases developing more than 30 years afterward. Among these, the majority are solid tumors, such as neoplasms of the thyroid, breast, and lung.

Ultraviolet radiation. The ultraviolet component of sunlight is carcinogenic. The ozone layer of the atmosphere provides a natural protection to humans against this form of radiation. The preservation of this layer is a source of great concern to the international community since the discovery that certain chemicals such as fluorocarbons can compromise the ozone layer and render the population at increased risk of developing radiation-induced cancer. Radiation of approximately 300-nm wavelength is responsible for such injuries. It has little power of penetration, and as a consequence the tumors induced are superficial. Frequent sites are the skins of the face and the vermilion border of the lower lip. The mechanism of the carcinogenic effect of ultraviolet radiation is not totally understood, but it is attributed to alterations in the DNA structure through the formation of pyrimidine dimers (e.g., thymine dimers).

---

*Wilhelm Conrad von Roentgen (1845-1923), German physicist.

Tumors induced by excessive exposure to sunlight are basal cell carcinoma, squamous cell carcinoma and malignant melanoma of the skin. The risk of skin cancer is related to the amount of exposure; consequently those engaged in outdoor occupations, particularly farmers, are at greatest risk.

Skin cancer related to sunlight is most prevalent in countries where there is both strong sunlight and a large fair-skinned population, such as the southern United States and northern Australia. In the United States it is calculated that the incidence of cancer of the lower lip doubles for every 250 miles nearer the equator. The Texan 10-gallon hat has probably also acted as an effective cancer preventive for many.

An example of an interaction between more than one factor in the induction of cancer is *xeroderma pigmentosum*. In this autosomal recessive disorder, in which DNA repair is defective, there is increased vulnerability to skin cancer, particularly in those parts of the body exposed to the sun.

Microbial carcinogenesis

For decades, a causal relationship between microbial organisms and cancer has been suspected. In 1911, Peyton Rous* successfully induced a sarcoma in fowls by using a cell free filtrate. Since that time, viruses, more so than other microorganisms, have been strongly associated with cancer. Several DNA and RNA viruses have proven carcinogenic potential in particular species of animals (Table 9-10). In man, a cause-and-effect relationship between viruses and cancer has been more difficult to establish. However, in rare situations, there is strong evidence that such a relationship exists (Table 9-11). The association of cancer to bacteria and parasites is less well understood, but there is growing evidence that they may act as cofactors in the pathogenesis of some cancers.

The role of microorganisms in neoplasia is a complex one and it is impossible to apply Koch's postulates to the study of carcinogenesis in the same manner as they are applied to bacterial infections. However, the studies on viruses and cancer have dramatically contributed to our understanding and knowledge of oncogenes.

Viruses and cancer

Tumor viruses are specific both for the type of tumor they produce and the animals in which the tumors develop (species specific). One problem, therefore, in comparing human and animal tumor viruses is that the common human cancers (breast, lungs, and digestive organs) are uncommon sites of cancer in animals.

It is worth noting, for example, that despite the inoculation of avian leukemia virus into thousands of recipients of yellow fever vaccine and ingestion of oncogenic simian viruses in early polio vaccines (before the presence of these viruses was suspected) there has been no evidence of any increase in malignant disease attributed to these agents.

The role of oncogenic viruses in humans comes from epidemiologic and serologic studies. In addition, electron microscopy, biochemical, and immunologic techniques have been

---

*Francis Peyton Rous (1879-1970), American pathologist and Nobel Laureate.

TABLE 9-10. Virus-cancer relationships in animals

Virus (family)	Host	Neoplasm
Marek's disease virus (herpesvirus)	Chicken	Lymphoma
Lucké's tumor virus (herpesvirus)	Frog	Renal adenocarcinoma
Mammary tumor virus (retrovirus B)	Mouse	Mammary adenocarcinoma
Feline leukemia virus (retrovirus C)	Cat	Leukemia
Rous sarcoma virus (retrovirus C)	Fowl	Sarcoma
Simian sarcoma virus (retrovirus C)	Woolly monkey	Sarcoma

TABLE 9-11. Virus-cancer relationships in humans

Virus (family)	Neoplasm
Papilloma (papova)	Squamous papilloma and squamous cell carcinoma
Epstein-Barr (herpesvirus)	Burkitt lymphoma, nasopharyngeal carcinoma
Cytomegalovirus (herpesvirus)	Kaposi sarcoma
Herpes simplex—type 2 (herpesvirus)	Uterine cervical carcinoma
Hepatitis B virus	Hepatocellular carcinoma
Human T-cell lymphotropic virus-I (retrovirus C)	T-cell leukemia/lymphoma

used to detect viruses in human tumors. Nevertheless, the demonstration of a virus in a tumor by any of these techniques is not necessarily irrefutable evidence of its etiologic role in the pathogenesis of that particular neoplasm and it may be a mere passenger.

Both DNA and RNA viruses have been associated with neoplasms in humans and animals. There are four families of DNA viruses associated with cancer: papillomaviruses, herpes viruses, adenoviruses, and poxviruses. The latter two are known to cause tumors in animals, but not in humans. Hepatitis B virus infection in humans is linked to hepatocellular carcinoma.

Papillomaviruses. Although originally included in the *papovavirus* family, it is now considered a distinct group. Individual types of papilloma viruses are known for their selective effects on the squamous epithelium. They are the cause of common viral warts of the skin, condyloma acuminatum of genitalia, and squamous papilloma of the larynx. Condyloma acuminatum is strongly linked to dysplasia of the uterine cervix and subsequent squamous cell carcinoma. Similarly in the skin, certain subtypes give rise to *epidermodysplasia verruciformis** which often evolves into squamous cell carcinoma.

---

*A rare familial disease characterized by flat, wartlike skin lesions and associated with papillomavirus types 5,8,14.

Herpes viruses. There is epidemiologic evidence and experimental data to indicate a relationship between human cancer and (1) Epstein-Barr virus (EBV), (2) herpes simplex virus type 2, and (3) cytomegalovirus. This relationship is not completely understood, but it seems to be dependent on a variety of biochemical and physical cofactors. This is best exemplified by EBV.

EBV is associated with Burkitt's lymphoma, a malignant neoplasm of lymphoid tissue commonly seen in children (Chapter 13). The original descriptions were from Central Africa and New Guinea, where the disease is prevalent. However, this tumor is not confined to Africa and has been described in all parts of the world. In Africa, the tumor is frequent in areas where the altitude and humidity are favorable to anopheline mosquitoes. This geographic distribution corresponds to an endemic area of malaria, which may be a predisposing factor. Patients with Burkitt's lymphoma commonly have high titers of antibodies to EBV. Moreover, the viral genome has been identified in the tumor cells by nucleic acid hybridization techniques. In recent years mainly due to the epidemic of acquired immunodeficiency syndrome (AIDS) and the prevalence of other immunosuppressed states, there has been a disproportionate increase in the incidence of Burkitt's-like lymphoma and other less frequent types of lymphoma, such as immunoblastic sarcoma. Some of these patients too, have high titers of EBV antibodies. Identification of EBV particles in lymphoma cells of a child with primary immunodeficiency disease, has been reported.

Exposure of tissue cultures of normal human fetal lymphoid B cells to EBV induces *lymphoblastic transformation*. These transformed cells are capable of maintaining continuous proliferation in culture, an effect that is characteristic of a transforming virus. Other features characteristic of fully evolved cancer cells are also present. Although this may suggest that EBV is the "cause" of Burkitt's lymphoma, the in vitro changes in the lymphoid cells only partly resemble those of true malignant transformation, and their behavior in vivo is another matter. Of interest are the descriptions in Burkitt's lymphoma of chromosomal translocation between chromosome 8 and other chromosomes, commonly chromosome 14. The breakpoint appears in close proximity to an oncogene, c-*myc*. It is tempting to speculate that viral infection, such as that of EBV, may enhance the emergence of chromosomal abnormalities in the lymphoid cells and consequently the expression of an oncogene.

There is convincing evidence that EBV is the cause of infectious mononucleosis, a self-limiting condition in which lymph nodes are typically enlarged. Moreover, there is a rapid rise in the titer of antibodies to EBV. The morphologic changes in the lymph node in this disease resemble those of malignant lymphoproliferative disorders, making the microscopic distinction between them very difficult.

Nasopharyngeal carcinoma, which is particularly common in China is also associated with high titers of antibodies to EBV. It is possible that this EBV-induced malignant transformation depends on cofactors produced by tung oil trees that grow in those parts of the world.

Herpes simplex virus type 2. Some association exists between infection of the female genitalia by herpes simplex virus type 2 (HSV2) and cancer of the uterine cervix. The evidence is based on seroepidemiologic studies and the demonstration of the viral genome in some tumor cells. The epidemiologic data on the carcinogenic potential of HSV2 parallels that of human papilloma virus, suggesting that there may be a synergistic interaction between the two viruses.

Hepatitis B virus (HBV). In Southeast Asia and Africa, where the HBV carrier state is very common, the relative incidence of hepatocellular carcinoma is significantly higher than in other parts of the world.

RNA viruses (oncornavirus, retroviruses). The RNA viruses were the first proven to be oncogenic in animals. These viruses possess RNA-dependent DNA polymerase and are also called retroviruses. It was not until recently that one retrovirus, human T-cell lymphotrophic virus-I (HTLV-I), had been incriminated as the cause of a rare form of leukemia in humans (see later). Retroviruses are capable of inducing leukemias and sarcomas in birds, and mammary tumors, leukemias, and sarcomas in mice and other animals. They can be grouped into four distinct types—A, B, C, and D—based on their morphology. Type C has proved to be the most important in humans, both in relation to malignancies and certain immune deficiency states.

Transmission of retroviruses varies with the particular agent. Some are transmitted from one host to another as infectious agents *(horizontal spread)*. These are often oncogenic and exhibit a consistent pattern of induction of malignant lymphoproliferative disorders. Other retroviruses are acquired genetically as a congenital infection (i.e., *vertical transmission*). Here, viral replication in the parent cells is not efficient, is dependent on activation by halogenated pyrimidines or other agents, and cells from distant species are required for complete replication.

For a long time, there have been great doubts about the existence of human retroviruses. However in 1980, a type C retrovirus (HTLV-I) was isolated from fresh and cultured lymphocytes of a patient with cutaneous T cell lymphoma. Subsequent seroepidemiologic studies identified several regions of the world where HTLV-I is endemic, such as the Caribbean, southwestern Japan, and Africa. In those areas, the virus is linked to lymphoma and leukemia and has been isolated on numerous occasions. As in natural animal leukemia viruses, only a proportion of HTLV-I infected individuals develop cancer. It is possible that other factors such as the host immune response, age at exposure, and viral doses are important in oncogenesis. In *in vitro* experiments, HTLV-I is capable of infecting T lymphocytes. The infected cells closely resemble leukemia cells in many features such as their altered morphology, increased growth rate, tendency to grow in clumps, reduced dependence on T cell growth factor, and immortality in culture.

The identification of HTLV-I has paved the way for the identification of a family of human retroviruses that include HTLV-II and the notorious human immunodeficiency virus (HIV; formerly HTLV-III), the virus associated with the AIDS epidemic. These viruses exhibit selective infectivity of the helper population of T lymphocytes (lymphotropic). HTLV-II was originally isolated from a patient with hairy cell leukemia and subsequently from an intravenous drug addict. Patients with HIV infection are also at a significantly increased risk of developing malignant neoplasms, such as lymphoma, leukemia, and Kaposi sarcoma. The exact relationship between the HIV and these various neoplasms is a subject of extensive on-going research.

Mechanism of viral oncogenesis

Most of the information on viral oncogenesis relates to work on RNA viruses or retroviruses. Upon infecting a cell, a virus first uncoats its envelope and capsid. Then its RNA is copied by reverse transcriptase into DNA, which in turn becomes integrated into the host cell genome. This integration allows the virus to replicate by using the host cell's mechanisms for protein synthesis.

The induction of malignancy by a retrovirus may be slow or rapid. Slow-induction viruses contain three genes, called Gag, Pol, and Env. They carry information for the synthesis of capsid proteins, reverse transcriptase, and envelope proteins, respectively. These viruses characteristically lack genetic information for transforming cells or oncogenes. In contrast, the rapid transforming virus, such as the Rous sarcoma virus, carries one additional gene, an oncogene (v-onc) that enhances its replication. A family of transforming genes has been characterized and each is typical of a particular retrovirus. A v-onc is unnecessary for virus growth, but is required for the oncogenic state. Mutations affecting any or all of the other genes, but sparing v-onc, do not necessarily prevent transformation.

Viral oncogenes have been identified in the DNA of a wide range of species. This indicates the following: (1) the viral oncogenes must have been rigorously conserved during evolution to allow hybridization with other species' DNAs, (2) contrary to earlier beliefs, it would seem much more likely that the v-onc genes are derived from normal cellular proto-oncogenes than the other way round. The incorporation into the retroviral genome (transduction) took place during recombinational events between viral DNA and cellular DNA in retrovirus infected cells.

Despite the similarities of v-onc to proto-oncogenes, the two are not identical for the following reasons: (1) their localization on different chromosomes, (2) the expression of proto-oncogenes is unrelated to the expression of endogenous proviruses, (3) proto-oncogenes are more complex entities in which protein-coding sequences (exons) are interrupted by introns.

The mechanism, or mechanisms, of viral oncogenesis is (are) not totally understood for all retroviruses. However, in specific situations, as in avian leukosis virus, the provirus with its long terminal repeat units (LTR) integrates into the host's DNA at a site very near to the proto-oncogene (insertional mutagenesis) (see Fig. 9-39). LTR contains an enhancer sequence that increases the expression of most DNA sequences within a few thousand base pairs in either direction. Consequently, the proto-oncogene is activated and contributes to oncogenesis. In certain situations, it is very possible that a viral infection may become dormant and that activation takes place upon the exposure of the host to other environmental factors, such as chemicals, radiation, or other viral agents. The story of viruses and cancer is far from complete and the future will bring us more enlightening information on this very intriguing subject.

Selected readings

Barbacid M: Mutagens, oncogenes and cancer, Trends Genet 2:188, 1986.

Baylin SB, and Mendelsohn G: Ectopic (inappropriate) hormone production by tumors: mechanisms involved and the biological and clinical implications, Endocr Rev 1:45, 1980.

Becker FF: Recent concepts of initiation and promotion in carcinogenesis, Am J Pathol 105:3, 1981.

BEIR: Committee on the Biological Effects of Ionizing Radiation: The effects on populations of exposure to low levels of ionizing radiation, Washington, DC, 1980, National Academy of Science.

Beutler B and Cerami A: Cachectin: more than a tumor necrosis factor, N Engl J Med 316:379, 1987.

Boice JD Jr and Fraumeni JF Jr, editors: Radiation carcinogenesis: epidemiology and biological significance, New York, 1984, Raven Press.

Cavenee WK, Murphree AL, Shull MM, et al: Prediction of familial predisposition to retinoblastoma, N Engl J Med 314:1201, 1986.

Farber E: Chemical, evolution, and cancer development, Am J Pathol 108:270, 1982.

Farber E and Sarma DSR: Hepatocarcinogenesis: a dynamic cellular perspective, Lab Invest 56:4, 1987.

Frost JK: The cell in health and disease, ed 2, Basel, 1986, S Karger, 16-28, 126-144.

Furcht LT: Critical factors controlling angiogenesis: cell products, cell matrix, and growth factors, Lab Invest 55:505, 1986.

Gallo RC: Human T-cell leukemia (lymphotropic) retroviruses and their causative role in T-cell malignancies and acquired immune deficiency syndrome, Cancer 55:2317, 1985.

Goodenow RS, Vogel JM, and Linsk RL: Histocompatibility antigens on murine tumors, Science 230:777, 1985.

Gould VE: Histogenesis and differentiation: a re-evaluation of these concepts as criteria for the classification of tumors, Human Pathol 17:212, 1986.

Iozzo RV: Proteoglycans and neoplastic-mesenchymal cell interactions, Human Pathol 15:2, 1984.

Iozzo RV: Proteoglycans and structure, function, and role in neoplasia, Lab Invest 53:373, 1985.

Knudson AG: Hereditary cancer, oncogenes and anti-oncogenes, Cancer Res 45:1437, 1985.

Krokowski E: The prevention of metastases as the central problem of future cancer therapy. In Kaiser HE, editor: Neoplasms-comparative pathology of growth in animals, plants, and man, Baltimore, 1981, Williams and Wilkins.

Lebovitz RM: Oncogenes as mediators of cell growth and differentiation, Lab Invest 55:249, 1986.

Liotta LA: Tumor invasion and metastasis: role of the basement membrane, Am J Pathol 117:339, 1984.

Liotta LA and Hart IR: Tumor invasion and metastasis, vol 7, Developments in oncology, The Hague, 1982, Martinus Nijhoff Publishers.

Machowiak PA: Microbial oncogenesis, Am J Med 82:79, 1987.

Mossman KL: Ionizing radiation and cancer, Cancer Invest 2:301, 1984.

Paul J: Oncogenes, J Pathol 143:1, 1984.

Poiesz BJ, Ruscetti FW, and Gazdar AF, et al: Detection and isolation of type C retrovirus particles from fresh and cultured lymphocytes of a patient with cutaneous T-cell lymphoma, Proc Natl Acad Sci USA 77:7415, 1980.

Reddy BS, Cohen LA, McCoy GD, et al: Nutrition and its relationship to cancer, Adv Cancer Res 32:237, 1980.

Sandberg AA: Application of cytogenetics in neoplastic diseases, CRC Critical Reviews in Clinical Laboratory Sciences 22:219, 1985.

Sandberg AA and Turc-Carel C: The cytogenetics of solid tumors—relation to diagnosis, classification and pathology, Cancer 59:387, 1987.

Sklar JL, Weiss LM, and Cleary ML: Diagnostic molecular biology of non-Hodgkin's lymphoma. In Berard C, Dorfman RF, and Kaufman N, editors: Malignant lymphoma, International Academy of Pathology Monograph, Baltimore, 1987, Williams & Wilkins.

Slamon DJ, de Kernion JB, and Verma IM, et al: Expression of cellular oncogenes in human malignancies, Science 224:256, 1984.

Taylor CR: Immunomicroscopy: A diagnostic tool for the surgical pathologist, vol 19, Major problems in pathology, Philadelphia, 1986, W.B. Saunders Co.

Theologides A: Anorexins, asthenins, and cachectins in cancer, Am J Med 81:696, 1986.

Todara GJ and Huebner RJ: The viral oncogene hypothesis: new evidence, Proc Natl Acad Sci USA 69:1009, 1972.

Tucker MA, D'Angio GJ, and Boice JD: Bone sarcomas linked to radiotherapy and chemotherapy in children, N Engl J Med 317:588, 1987.

Varmus HE: Viruses, genes, and cancer: the discovery of cellular oncogenes and their role in neoplasia, Cancer 55:2324, 1985.

Weinberg RA: A molecular basis of cancer, Sci Am 249:126, 1983.

Weinberg RA: The action of oncogenes in the cytoplasm and nucleus, Science 230:770, 1985.

Weisburger JH, Wynder EL, and Horn C: Nutritional factors and etiologic mechanisms in the causation of gastrointestinal cancers, Cancer 50: 2541, 1982.

Wheelock EF and Robinson MK: Endogenous control of the neoplastic process, Lab Invest 48:120, 1983.

Willman CL and Fenoglio-Preiser CM: Oncogenes, suppressor genes, and carcinogenesis, Human Pathol 18:895, 1987.

CHAPTER 10

Cardiovascular disease: diseases of blood vessels

The most significant effect of blood vessel disease is obstruction and reduced blood supply to an organ (ischemia). *Atherosclerosis* is by far the most medically (and economically) important disease of arteries.

Hypertension is the result of abnormal vessel function, that is, increased arteriolar tone, but it is also a major contributory cause of atherosclerosis and therefore ischemia.

Heart disease is considered separately in Chapter 11, but it must be emphasized that diseases of the heart and of the blood vessels interact closely and frequently. In many cases, therefore, circulatory disturbances result from the combined effects of blood vessel and heart disease. The most common examples are hypertension and cardiac ischemia resulting from atherosclerosis of the coronary arteries. The effects of the latter vary from gradually developing congestive heart failure to myocardial infarction, acute circulatory failure, and sudden death. Thrombotic and ischemic lesions in other parts of the body can also be associated when vascular disease is widespread.

Cardiovascular disease is common and is also the most frequent cause of death in the United States and other countries whose people have a similar life-style. It is therefore necessary that health care workers understand these diseases.

Examination of the cardiovascular system

Traditional clinical methods of examining the heart and circulatory function include palpation of the pulse and use of the stethoscope. Valve and other defects disturb blood flow and cause murmurs. The valve affected and the type of defect (stenosis or regurgitation) can be recognized by the character and timing of the murmur heard with the stethoscope. Measurement of blood pressure with a sphygmomanometer allows exact quantitation of hypertension or hypotension.

Ophthalmoscopy allows the blood vessels of the retina to be visualized directly. Hypertension causes constrictions at points where arteries cross veins.

Clinical methods such as these are by no means obsolete but are now supplemented with other highly sophisticated techniques.

Electrocardiography (ECG) measures the electrical activity of the heart. More precise assessment may mean placing intraesophageal or intracardiac electrodes. An ECG also gives an objective picture of heart rate and the character of any rhythm disorders (such as conduction disturbances) and areas of inactivity, usually due to myocardial infarction.

The effect of stressing the heart can be shown by ECG monitoring during exercise or even long term, with portable equipment (Holter monitoring). Ambulatory monitoring of blood pressure can also be carried out.

Radiography shows any enlargement of the heart and the state of the pulmonary vessels. The latter are prominent when there is a left-to-right shunt. *Angiography* is a refinement of radiography, in which radiopaque material is injected into the arteries to show their degree of patency. Biplane angiography and cineangiography are further refinements.

Echocardiography uses a beam of ultrasound that reflects differentially from soft tissue surfaces and provides a detailed picture of abnormalities not detectable by radiography, such as vegetations on heart valves in infective endocarditis.

Cardiac catheterization shows the patency of coronary arteries, valvular or other cardiac lesions (such as a congenital defect), or the efficiency of a prosthetic heart valve.

Cardiac catheterization is used to enable selective angiography to be carried out and to measure intracardiac pressures and blood gas levels. Valve function or localization of valve and other lesions can thus be more precisely determined. This is particularly important in the preoperative assessment of congenital defects.

Radioisotope scanning will reliably detect myocardial infarcts and can be used to assess their progress. Thallium and nuclear imaging can demonstrate the quality of regional myocardial perfusion and any abnormalities of wall motion.

Computed tomography (CT scanning), Doppler electrocardiography, digital subtraction angiography, and magnetic resonance imaging (MRI) are increasingly also used.

Cardiac biopsy is used to monitor rejection reactions after heart transplants.

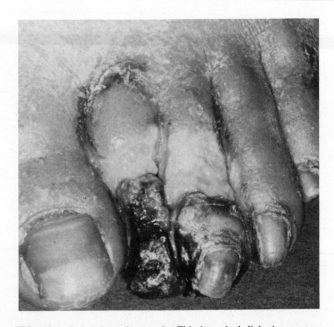

FIG. 10-1. Ischemia and necrosis. This is typical diabetic gangrene of the foot secondary to severe atherosclerotic changes in the arteries. *(Courtesy Curator of the Gordon Museum, Guy's Hospital, London, England.)*

DISTURBANCES OF THE CIRCULATION

Ischemia

Ischemia is the term used when blood vessel obstructions restrict the supply of blood to the tissues. It is one of the most serious effects of vascular disease, although not all vascular diseases cause ischemia. Mönckeberg's sclerosis, for example, produces severe changes in the arterial wall, but since the lumen is not reduced, there is no interference with blood flow.

Causes of ischemia

The most common cause of ischemia is arterial obstruction. This in turn is usually the result of thrombosis, embolism, spasm, atherosclerosis (or less often other arterial diseases) (Fig. 10-1), or occlusion by external pressure. Important causes and effects of ischemia are summarized in Table 10-1.

Less frequently, ischemia can result from venous obstruction, which can cause sufficiently increased venous pressure to impede the blood flow. Increased venous pressure after cardiac failure also impairs the blood supply to the tissues.

Effects of ischemia

The effects of ischemia vary widely. Acute ischemia can cause death of part of an organ *(infarction)* or even of the whole body if the heart or brain is affected. Less severe, chronic ischemia can cause symptomless cell death, particularly in the heart or brain, or temporary pain in the chest or legs when the oxygen needs of the tissues are increased.

Hypoxia. The reduced oxygen supply is the main contributor to tissue damage. Some tissues, such as neurons and cardiac muscle, are particularly vulnerable and can quickly die.

Accumulation of metabolites. The failure to remove metabolic waste products is a major cause of pain in ischemic muscles. Hypoxia forces tissues to use the glycolytic pathway for respiration. Lactic acid then accumulates, causing metabolic acidosis, which further damages the tissues.

The effects of ischemia on tissues depend on the degree of blood flow restriction, the rapidity with which ischemia develops, tissue sensitivity to hypoxia, and the activity and oxygen needs of the tissue.

Hypoxia

Hypoxia is a state of inadequate tissue oxygenation. As mentioned earlier, ischemia always causes hypoxia. Hypoxia, however, is not only caused by a reduced blood supply, but also by any factor that impairs oxygenation of the blood or reduces its availability to the tissues. It can affect the whole body.

Hypoxia can be categorized as follows (Table 10-1):

1. *Hypoxic hypoxia* results when oxygenation of the blood is reduced. This in turn can be caused by inadequate oxygen exchange, which is frequently secondary to lung disease; inadequate oxygen intake because of respiratory obstruction or failure of the oxygen supply during anesthesia; or congenital heart disease with a left-to-right shunt, which causes the blood to bypass the lungs.
2. *Anemic hypoxia* is the result of abnormally low levels of hemoglobin. The oxygen-carrying capacity of the blood is reduced accordingly.
3. *Stagnant (ischemic) hypoxia* may be localized as a result of vessel obstruction or generalized as in cardiac failure.
4. *Toxic hypoxia* is caused by cell poisons, such as carbon monoxide or cyanide, that prevent oxygen uptake by red blood cells or tissues, respectively.

Unless it is caused by ischemia, hypoxia affects all tissues, but the brain and heart are particularly sensitive. If more than one disease affects the oxygen supply to the tissue, then the effects of hypoxia are aggravated. Thus, when there is atherosclerotic coronary artery disease, anemia further endangers the myocardium.

As with ischemia, the effects of hypoxia depend on its severity, rapidity of onset, and duration. In the case of strangulation, for example, hypoxia can cause death in a few minutes. At the other extreme, in a fainting attack there is only transient cerebral anoxia and loss of consciousness.

Clinical aspects

Acute hypoxia can cause sudden loss of consciousness or even death. Chronic hypoxia, by contrast, usually causes breathlessness (dyspnea) and often, cyanosis. Common causes of chronic hypoxia are lung disease, particularly emphysema (Chapter 12) and cardiac failure. Hypoxia of the heart muscle (usually due to coronary artery disease) can affect heart rhythm, which in extreme cases can culminate in ventricular fibrillation or cardiac arrest, and death.

Hypoxic hypoxia is one of the most common and dangerous complications of general anesthesia. For example, the patient may have a degree of respiratory obstruction, but many anesthetic agents, particularly the intravenous barbiturates, such as thiopental, are potent respiratory depressants. Such factors can cause hypoxia of the respiratory center, which further depresses respiration and possibly the cardiovascular center, leading to worsened (stagnant) hypoxia or total respiratory failure.

Thrombosis

A *thrombus* is a solid, adherent mass formed within a blood vessel by deposition of elements from the circulating blood. Unlike a clot, a thrombus may be formed from platelets alone, particularly in fast-flowing arterial blood, but in veins especially, fibrin is usually deposited. In essence, a thrombus is an aggregation of platelets (Fig. 10-2), fibrin, and red and white blood cells. Once formed, fibrin is usually deposited on the initial platelet thrombus, particularly in veins, to produce a friable mass filling part of the vessel. This process of platelet thrombus formation followed by deposition of fibrin can be

TABLE 10-1. Hypoxia and its causes

Respiratory causes (hypoxic)	*Anemic*	*Stagnant (ischemic)*	*Toxic*
Blockage of airway	Low oxygen-carrying capacity of blood	Poor circulation (heart failure)	Cellular poisons (e.g., cyanide)
Shortage of oxygen (e.g., anesthesia)		Local obstruction	block oxygen uptake
Impaired gas exchange in lungs			

repeated several times, until a layered structure is built up (Fig. 10-3).

The mass is also adherent. If it breaks off to be carried away by the bloodstream, it becomes an *embolus*. Although emboli often originate as detached fragments of thrombus, they can also form from other material such as tumor cells, as discussed later.

Arterial thrombi are a direct cause of obstruction and ischemia of the organ supplied. The best known example is thrombosis of the coronary arteries, although the role of thrombotic obstruction in producing the syndrome of myocardial infarction is controversial (Chapter 11).

Effects of venous thrombosis are mainly indirect. The most disastrous consequence is when a venous thrombus detaches to form a massive embolus, which can block the pulmonary arteries.

Thrombosis can affect the arteries but is much more common in veins, where the sluggish blood flow favors thrombosis. The widely different conditions prevailing in arteries, as compared with veins, suggest that the mechanisms of venous thrombosis probably differ in many respects from those of arterial thrombosis.

At the risk of oversimplification, arterial thrombosis depends on severe damage to the endothelium, which leads to platelet adherence and aggregation. Venous thrombosis, by contrast, can develop in the absence of obvious vascular damage, and a sluggish blood flow is often the main contributory factor.

Antemortem and postmortem thrombi

Arterial thrombi consist predominantly of platelets interspersed with fibrin, which may form clearly defined layers. Relatively few red blood cells are incorporated, and arterial thrombi are paler and firmer than venous thrombi. The latter typically consist of strands of fibrin entangling large numbers of red blood cells, forming a soft red cast of the blood vessel lumen.

After death, the clotting process continues slowly. The result is a clot forming a cast of (but not adherent to) the vessel lumen and having a gelatinous consistency. The slow coagulation of the blood allows the red blood cells to settle into the dependent part of the clot. As a result, the upper zone is pale, with a translucent "fatty" appearance. It is important to distinguish these postmortem clots from true, antemortem, thrombi.

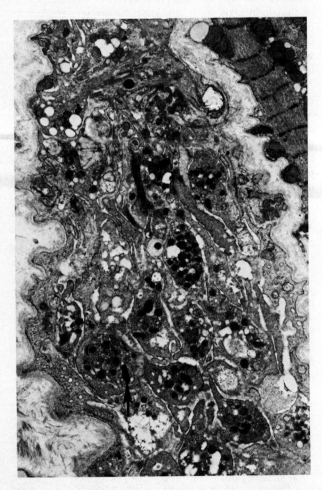

FIG. 10-2. A platelet thrombus in a capillary blood vessel. The electron-dense granules in the platelets contain serotonin *(arrow)*.

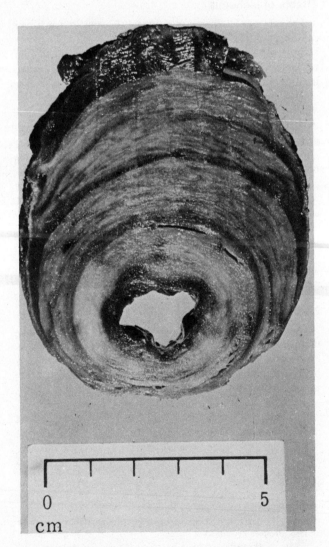

FIG. 10-3. Thrombosis. The formation of the thrombus, layer on layer, of platelets alternating with fibrin and red blood cells has progressed until the lumen of the vein has been almost occluded. *(Courtesy Curator of the Gordon Museum, Guy's Hospital, London, England.)*

Pathogenesis

The hemostatic mechanism is delicately balanced. First, hemostasis, which prevents excessive blood loss after an injury, depends on platelet adhesion and aggregation as well as coagulation. This process is initiated by damage to the vessel wall, particularly the endothelium. Second, a fibrinolytic mechanism prevents extensive intravascular coagulation. Despite the fibrinolytic mechanism, platelet aggregation and intravascular clotting can, under appropriate circumstances, go on to produce extensive thromboses.

Mechanisms of thrombosis

Three main factors are commonly involved in thrombosis; however, their relative importance in contributing to arterial rather than venous thrombosis differs. The three main factors include the following:

1. Changes in the vessel wall. Atherosclerosis is the most important cause of endothelial damage.
2. Stasis or turbulence of blood flow. This also can be caused by atheromatous plaques.
3. Changes in blood coagulability.

Vessel injury. In the initial phase of hemostasis, platelets adhere to the damaged area of the vessel and aggregate to a platelet plug if the vessel is small enough. Injury to the vessel wall, however microscopic, is probably the precipitating factor in the formation of most thrombi. Arterial thrombosis depends on adhesion of platelets to areas of atherosclerotic damage or inflammatory injuries to the endothelium or endocardium. Thus a myocardial infarct can cause a thrombus to form even within a ventricle.

Platelet adhesion and clotting. As discussed in more detail in Chapter 13, this is a complex process initiated by damage to the vessel wall, but mediated by adenosine triphosphate, thromboxane, and other factors. Platelets thus build up a nidus and form an irreversibly coherent platelet mass (Fig. 10-2). Release of clotting factors from the damaged platelets in turn causes blood to coagulate and to form a clot that adheres to the platelet mass.

Stasis and turbulence. Arterial thrombosis depends on severe disturbance of blood flow; this is often also caused by atherosclerosis. Gross damage to vessel walls or the endocardium creates areas of turbulence within which there are minute zones of relative stasis, and these bring plasma-clotting factors into effective relationships with platelets adhering to the damaged area.

By contrast, the fast laminar flow of blood in normal arteries sweeps these plasma-clotting factors away and may also sweep away aggregating platelets before irreversible adhesion can develop.

For these reasons thrombosis is far more common in the slowly flowing blood in the veins. Any factor that slows venous blood flow further is a potent cause of thrombosis.

Nevertheless, evidence suggests that mere stasis does not trigger thrombus formation and that some damage to the vessel wall, however minute, is necessary to activate the process.

Altered blood coagulability. Venous thrombosis is a common complication of postoperative and posttraumatic states. It also seems that under these circumstances the coagulability of the blood increases. Increased coagulability is obviously protective if further blood loss is to be prevented. Diseases characterized by increased platelet production or decreased platelet destruction are also characterized by thrombotic tendencies.

Increased coagulability cannot be demonstrated in the test tube in such cases. It has been suggested that the state of hypercoagulability is due to the release of activated clotting factors, which are normally absent from the circulating blood but which are released either from the tissues directly or are formed within the vessels. Thus increased coagulability may develop in localized areas of stasis and as a consequence may be undetectable in the systemic circulation.

As might be expected, thrombosis is rare among patients with severe congenital deficiency of clotting factors. Nevertheless, such patients are by no means insusceptible to thrombosis, which can happen even in patients with hemophilia.

Anticoagulant drugs, particularly heparin, have been used for many years to prevent venous thrombosis, but they are by no means completely reliable or effective. Aspirin or prostacyclin analogs are valuable in the prevention of arterial thrombosis after, for example, heart operations.

In view of these considerations, it is hardly surprising that there is as yet no single hematologic test that reliably predicts thrombotic tendencies.

Pregnancy. In the early postpartum period, thromboses are a major complication, and during pregnancy raised levels of plasma coagulation factors can be found. Nevertheless, the incidence of leg vein thrombosis is five or six times higher after delivery than before. This is another example of the disparity between the circulating levels of clotting factors and thrombotic disease.

Oral contraceptive agents. Extensive studies have shown that the risks of deep vein thrombosis and strokes are five or six times higher in users of oral contraceptives than in comparable nonusers. The estrogen component of oral contraceptives is related to the complication of venous and arterial thromboembolism. However, pregnancy (or more precisely, the postpartum state) also contributes to thrombosis, and by preventing pregnancy, contraceptives reduce this risk.

Diseases associated with thrombotic tendencies

The risk of thrombosis is increased in the following conditions:

1. Heart disease, especially congestive heart failure and arrhythmias
2. Increased platelet production or decreased destruction
3. Cancer, especially of the lung, gastrointestinal tract, and genitourinary tract
4. Ulcerative colitis
5. Obesity
6. Impaired mobility because of old age, injuries to the legs or pelvis, and paralytic states

Apart from impaired mobility, the way by which many of these conditions contribute is unknown.

Fate of thrombi

The possibilities include the following four examples.

Lysis. A thrombus can sometimes be dissolved, largely by the action of the fibrinolytic mechanism (Chapter 13), and the patency of the vessel's lumen is restored.

Retraction and recanalization. Retraction of the clot leaves space within the original vessel lumen to allow the blood flow to be partially reestablished (Fig. 10-4).

Organization and scarring. The thrombus is invaded by fibroblasts and capillary buds to form granulation tissue. Ultimately, the vessel is completely obliterated by fibrous scar-

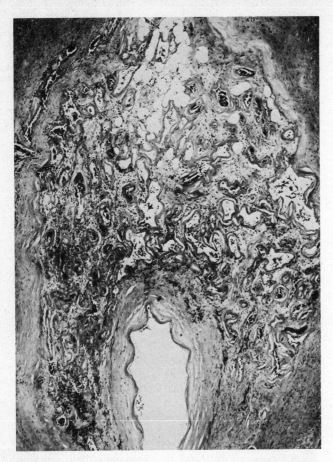

FIG. 10-4. Recanalized thrombus. The walls of the artery are visible at the edges of the photo. Its lumen has been obliterated by a thrombus that has organized and is now perforated by many small and large vessels.

ring. A variation of this picture is organization of a thrombus within a vein followed by calcification to form a *phlebolith*.

Detachment. Detachments can range from small fragments of thrombotic vegetation breaking away from a damaged heart valve in infective endocarditis to the sudden separation of a massive thrombus from the wall of a vein. The resulting embolus can reach, and sometimes block, pulmonary arteries, with disastrous consequences.

Clinical aspects

Thrombi can obstruct vessels (infarction is the main complication when arteries are blocked) and can give rise to emboli. The most massive emboli are the result of the detachment of major venous thrombi. The effects depend on the site and structure of the thrombus.

Arterial and cardiac thrombosis

Thrombosis in this part of the circulation is always a result of severe damage to the vascular or cardiac endothelium, gross disturbance of blood flow, or both. Arterial thrombosis is usually a direct or indirect consequence of atherosclerosis.

The main causes of intraarterial and intracardiac thrombosis can be summarized as follows:

1. Severe atherosclerosis
2. Aneurysms
3. Myocardial infarction

4. Endocarditis, particularly rheumatic fever and infective endocarditis
5. Atrial fibrillation
6. Damage to the endocardium during cardiovascular surgery

An arterial thrombus consists of a platelet nidus on which an adherent mass has formed by a repeated sequence of clotting and platelet aggregation to form a series of more or less well-defined zones of aggregated platelets interspersed with layers of coagulated fibrin.

Effects of arterial thrombosis. The effects inevitably depend on the extent of the collateral circulation and the completeness with which the artery is obstructed. The possibilities follow:

1. *No effect.* This is the consequence of thrombosis of a minor artery in an organ that has an abundant collateral blood supply.

2. *Relative ischemia.* Partial obstruction of an artery, such as may be caused by an atherosclerotic plaque in a coronary artery, can allow the tissue to perform without trouble until the demands on it are increased. Thus partial occlusion of a coronary artery can cause angina (pain) on exertion.

3. *Degenerative changes.* Gradual reduction of the blood supply to a specialized tissue, such as the myocardium, leads to progressive fibrosis. This is a common consequence of long-standing atherosclerosis.

4. *Infarction.* Infarction is the consequence of sudden, complete obstruction of an artery supplying a tissue that has no collateral blood supply. This sequence of events is often most disastrous in the heart or brain.

5. *Remote effects.* Arterial thrombi can also give rise to emboli.

Thrombosis in specific arteries

Coronary thrombosis. Atherosclerosis can cause coronary occlusion leading to myocardial infarction, but the relationship between coronary thrombosis and the clinical syndrome known as myocardial infarction is complex.

Thrombosis in aneurysms. Aneurysmal dilatation can be a complication of atherosclerosis of the aorta or, less commonly, of tertiary syphilis. Thrombosis is a complication particularly of atherosclerotic aneurysms. Such a thrombus can occlude branches of the aorta arising nearby, such as the iliac, renal, or mesenteric arteries. In addition, the thrombus can give rise to systemic emboli.

Cerebral thrombosis. Atherosclerosis and thrombosis have been estimated to account for up to 35% of all strokes. Occlusion of a cerebral vessel leads to cerebral infarction, causing major disturbances of function, particularly unilateral paralysis (Chapter 20).

Intracardiac thrombosis

Valvular thrombosis. This is a complication of damage to the endocardium of the heart valves, particularly as a consequence of infective endocarditis. The vegetations formed in this disease are friable, so fragments break off relatively readily. Embolic phenomena are therefore a well-recognized feature of infective endocarditis. Thrombus formation associated with insertion of prosthetic heart valves is also a source of emboli.

Mural thrombosis. Mural thrombosis is a consequence of damage to the endocardium resulting from myocardial infarction. Thrombi in this site can release systemic emboli that can complicate myocardial infarction.

Atrial thrombosis. Atrial thrombosis is a common complication of atrial fibrillation, in which there is both turbulence and relative stasis in various parts of the atria (Fig. 10-5).

Atrial fibrillation commonly accompanies cardiac failure, particularly that associated with mitral valve disease. Thrombosis in a fibrillating atrium can release emboli into the systemic circulation. Alternatively, the thrombus can occasionally build up within the atrium to form a spherical mass, which can act as a ball valve.

Venous thrombosis

Unlike arterial thrombosis, venous thrombi can form even in a fit, young person. Although uncommon, it is a well-recognized misfortune in persons who sit for long periods, leading to venous stasis in the lower legs.

About 95% of venous thrombi develop in the leg veins, especially those of the calf. Contributory factors follow:

1. Age
2. Prolonged immobilization
3. Local pressure
4. Trauma (either accidental or surgical), particularly to the legs or pelvis
5. The postpartum state
6. Cardiac failure
7. Cancer and other diseases

Those most at risk are elderly patients with a fractured femur, patients who have had surgical operations, and patients who are in cardiac failure. The young and healthy, even athletes, are not immune, however. Stasis in the leg veins is by far the most important single factor, but hypercoagulable blood is also a factor in venous thrombosis.

Pathology. Once thrombosis has been initiated, coagulation in the slow-moving venous blood can readily extend as a long tail, forming a cast of the vein lumen. The thrombus itself further slows the bloodstream until there is complete occlusion and further extension of the thrombus.

These thrombi, therefore, consist largely of clot, a tangled mass of fibrin threads enmeshing red blood cells. Venous thrombi are red and friable as a consequence.

Thrombophlebitis is an inflammation adjacent to and involving the wall of the vein causing localized thrombosis (Figs. 10-6 and 10-7). Thrombosis itself gives rise to inflammatory changes, so that the distinction between phlebothrombosis and thrombophlebitis is often academic. An infection can involve a vein and the thrombus. The release of infected emboli can produce metastatic abscesses (pyemia).

Migratory thrombosis is a phenomenon of unknown cause. It is characterized by thrombus formation in many veins at different times and is an uncommon but significant manifestation of cancer.

Effects of venous thrombosis

Local effects. These may be absent, but there is sometimes local tenderness, as in thrombosis of leg veins, and edema of the ankles. The local effects are unimportant in most cases because of the abundant collateral venous circulation.

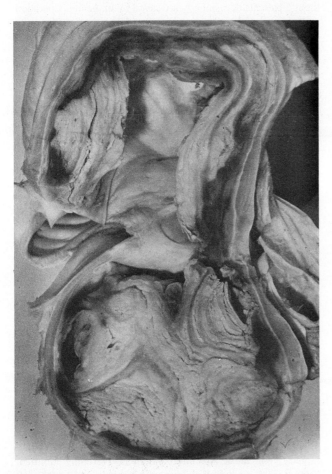

FIG. 10-5. Atrial thrombosis. The patient had long-standing mitral stenosis and atrial fibrillation, which caused successive layers of thrombus to form in the dilated atrium. *(Courtesy Curator of the Gordon Museum, Guy's Hospital, London, England.)*

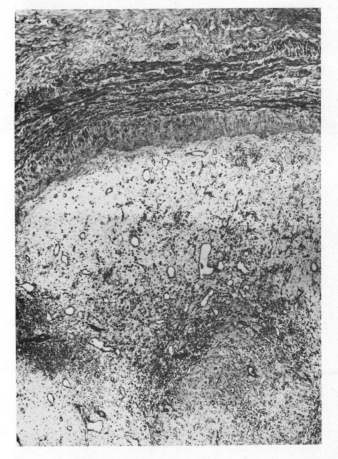

FIG. 10-6. Organizing thrombus in a vein. In contrast to thrombosis in an artery, a thrombus has formed on normal vein wall. Most of the thrombus has been replaced by delicate granulation tissue in which many thin-walled blood vessels can be seen.

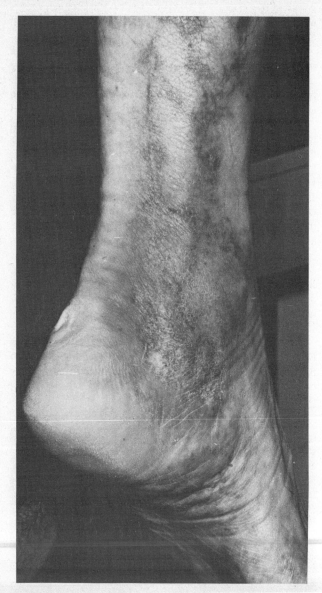

FIG. 10-7. Thrombophlebitis. Typical darkening of the skin over an inflamed and thrombotic vein in a patient with Behçet's syndrome (Chapter 19).

Remote effects. The most serious aspect of venous thrombi is as a source of emboli. Pulmonary embolism is probably the cause of 10% to 20% of all hospital deaths. The source of these pulmonary emboli is the deep veins of the leg or pelvis in 95% of cases.

Clinical aspects. Deep vein thrombosis, particularly in the calf, was believed at one time to be detectable by tenderness on pressure (Homans' sign*). This sign is not reliable, however, and recent studies using isotope-labeled fibrinogen show that only a few patients have detectable signs or symptoms of thrombosis. More than 60% of elderly patients may have phlebo-thrombosis after surgery.

Historically, *cavernous sinus thrombosis* was one of the most dreaded complications of dentistry because it was uniformly fatal. It is secondary to suppurative infections in the nasal

---

*J. Homans (1877-1950), American surgeon.

sinuses or the upper half of the face, including the teeth. The infection is initially unilateral but rapidly spreads to the opposite side via the circular sinus. Patients are acutely ill and febrile and have severe retroorbital pain. The eyes protrude, there is edema of the conjunctivae and eyelids, and there may be paralysis of the third, fourth, and sixth cranial nerves and paresthesia of the fifth cranial nerve. Complications include blindness, cerebral abscess or edema, and death. On the rare occasions when cavernous sinus thrombosis develops, it usually responds well to antibiotics if treated early and aggressively.

Embolism

Embolism (Fig. 10-8) is the term used to describe occlusion of a vessel by the impaction of an embolus. Most emboli are detached fragments of a thrombus, but can be categorized into five main types: detached thrombi, gas, fat, tumor cells, and miscellaneous, such as foreign bodies.

Thrombotic emboli

Pulmonary embolism. Pulmonary emboli almost invariably arise from the leg veins.

Massive pulmonary embolism (Figs. 10-9 to 10-11) results when an extensive venous thrombus detaches and passes through the right side of the heart and then curls up and blocks the pulmonary artery. The consequences are sudden severe dyspnea, chest pain, loss of consciousness, and often death. Although patients occasionally are saved by immediate operation and removal of the embolus, this is rarely successful. The most important factor in lowering mortality is prevention of leg vein thrombosis in patients at risk.

Minor pulmonary emboli have little detectable effect in healthy lungs. In unfit patients, particularly those confined to bed or those who have heart failure and in whom the general circulation is impaired, pulmonary emboli cause edema and hypoxia of a segment of the lung and infarction.

Minor pulmonary emboli can give rise to a septic infarct if they block an end artery, such as in the kidney. Alternatively, they can cause multiple metastatic (pyemic) abscesses. For example, the liver can become infected as a consequence of severe infection of the appendix.

Gas emboli

Air emboli. Although oxygen readily dissolves in the blood, a large air bubble admitted into a vessel does not dissolve quickly and can cause obstruction. Air emboli can form in the following circumstances:

1. *Head and neck surgery.* If the jugular vein is opened, air can be sucked in and is immediately transported to the right ventricle. If the air bubble is large enough, the pumping action of the heart causes severe foaming, loss of output from the right ventricle, and death. Fortunately, this is rare.

2. *Open heart surgery.* The risk of air being sucked into the veins is high in open heart surgery. Although the technical difficulties are considerable, it is possible to prevent this complication.

3. *Aspiration of fluid from the pleural cavity.* One hazard of introducing a needle into the pleural cavity is that a pulmonary vein can be punctured and air inadvertently admitted. Even a small air bubble is immediately transported to the left ventricle and from there to a pulmonary or cerebral vessel. Immediate death can result.

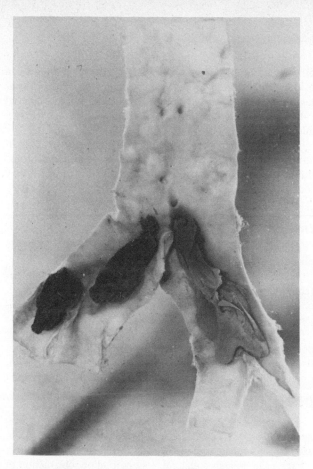

FIG. 10-8. Embolism. Thrombotic emboli have been arrested at the bifurcations of the common iliac arteries. Raised, pale, and smooth atheromatous plaques are present in the aorta above. *(Courtesy Curator of the Gordon Museum, Guy's Hospital, London, England.)*

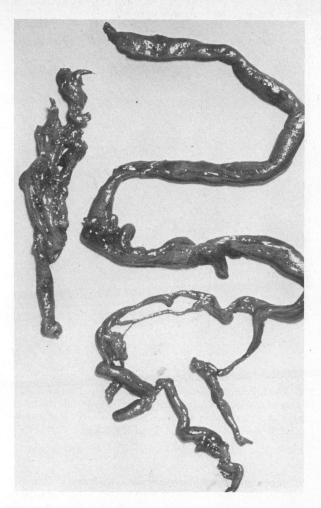

FIG. 10-9. Pulmonary embolism. The large thrombi that arose in the deep veins of the leg were found at autopsy, occluding the pulmonary artery. The patient died suddenly a week after an abdominal operation. *(Courtesy Curator of the Gordon Museum, Guy's Hospital, London, England.)*

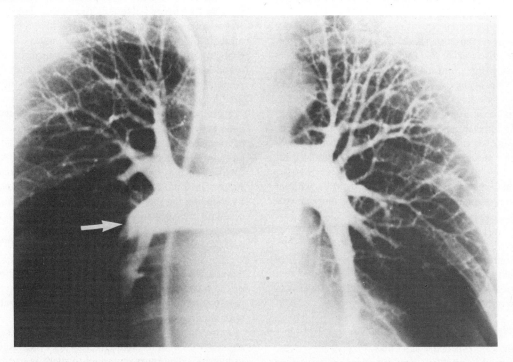

FIG. 10-10. Pulmonary embolism. The pulmonary arteriogram shows the abrupt interruption *(arrow)* of the arterial blood flow to the right lower lobe.

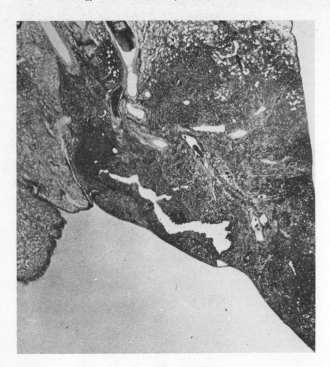

FIG. 10-11. Pulmonary infarction due to embolus. The embolus can be seen in a branch of a pulmonary artery *(arrow)*, and the infarct appears as a dark area in the lower lobe. *(Courtesy Curator of the Gordon Museum, Guy's Hospital, London, England.)*

Nitrogen embolism (decompression syndrome). This is a hazard for divers or workers in deep tunnels subjected to high atmospheric pressures. Sudden decompression causes nitrogen to come out of solution and form bubbles in the blood. Nitrogen at high pressure is also soluble in lipids and thus can produce bubbles in the central nervous system when the pressure falls. This can damage the spinal cord.

Clinically, the most common symptom is severe pain in the joints or muscles ("the bends").

Neurologic complications are usually in the legs and vary from disturbances of sensation *(paresthesia)* to total paralysis.

Bubbles can also reach the pulmonary capillaries. This causes difficulty in breathing and can lead to sudden loss of consciousness from asphyxia. Rapid collapse and sudden death follow in the worst cases.

The industrial hazard is well recognized, and strict precautions are taken to prevent rapid decompression. If this happens accidentally, however, the victim is put into a pressure chamber to redissolve the nitrogen. The pressure is then gradually reduced.

Many persons who deep-sea dive for sport do so without adequate training or understanding of the risks of nitrogen embolism.

Fat emboli

The main source of fat emboli is the bone marrow after fractures. Usually no more than minute globules escape, but occasionally greater amounts of fat escape and can cause cerebral embolism.

Tumor emboli

Malignant tumors, especially sarcomas, involve blood vessels and can spread to produce secondary deposits in various sites.

Miscellaneous emboli

One of the less common types of embolus is a fragment of atherosclerotic plaque. A wide variety of foreign bodies can also enter the bloodstream. These include fragments of disintegrating prosthetic heart valves, plastic tubing from arterial catheters, and insoluble material contaminating drugs used by addicts.

Parasites, especially schistosome eggs, can enter the bloodstream and reach the liver or lungs, where they cause a chronic inflammatory reaction and fibrosis of the vessel in which they lodge.

Infarction

Infarction is a localized area of ischemic necrosis caused by obstruction of the blood supply to an organ.

The main causes of acute ischemia are complications affecting atheromatous plaque, that is, thrombosis, hemorrhage, or rupture; embolism; twisting of the mesentery and strangulated hernias; and injuries to an artery.

With few exceptions, infarcts are the consequence of thromboembolic events, but are often the combined effects of a reduced blood supply and a decrease in the functional activity of the tissue.

Determinants of infarction

The vascular anatomy. Infarction is an inevitable consequence of complete occlusion of an end artery. The heart, brain, and kidneys are therefore especially vulnerable. Most other organs have enough collateral vessels to allow obstruction of a small artery without damage to the part. Nevertheless, even in the lungs, infarction can follow obstruction of a small vessel if other disease is present.

Rapidity of occlusion. Usually an infarct is the result of sudden occlusion. Gradual narrowing allows a collateral circulation to develop. However, in the heart, there is a limit to the extent to which this can be achieved.

Vulnerability of the affected tissue. The more specialized the cells, the more vulnerable they are to damage by hypoxia. Nerve cells of the brain suffer irreversible damage if deprived of their blood supply for 3 to 4 minutes. Myocardial cells probably die within 5 minutes of complete obstruction of the blood supply; parenchymal cells of the kidneys are also vulnerable. Connective tissue cells, particularly fibroblasts, survive hypoxia for long periods.

Functional activity of the tissue. Tissues are more readily damaged when functionally active, especially in the heart. Myocardial infarction probably results, in most cases, from partial obstruction of a coronary artery together with a demand for oxygen that is beyond the ability of coronary arteries to supply. In some cases, it may be possible to prevent infarction by reducing the metabolic needs of a tissue. Thus, in the case of a limb, when a major artery has become obstructed, complete rest and cooling may lower the metabolic needs sufficiently to permit the tissues to survive.

The heart cannot be rested so completely, but damage after a myocardial infarct may be minimized by reducing the activity of the heart by such means as controlling arrhythmias or hypertension (as appropriate), and reducing sympathetic activity with suitable drugs.

Efficiency of the general circulation and oxygen-carrying capacity. Infarction is more likely when other factors contribute to hypoxia. The most important of these is cardiac failure but another is anemia. Obstruction of the pulmonary artery has

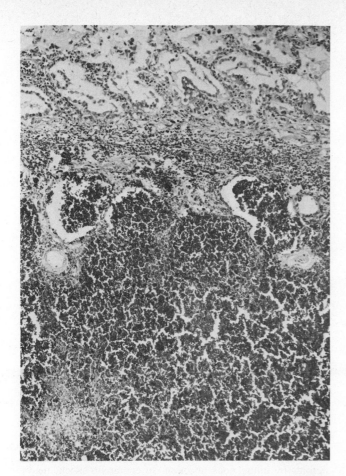

FIG. 10-12. Infarct of the lung. Above are relatively normal alveoli, which are sharply demarcated from the infarcted area stuffed with red blood cells below.

little effect in a healthy person, but in the patient in cardiac failure it can cause a pulmonary infarct.

Pathology

A typical infarct is conical, with its apex close to the point of obstruction. In the early stages, infarcts are usually red because red blood cells are trapped in the ischemic tissues and leak into the area from the periphery.

The appearance depends mainly on the amount and texture of blood normally in the tissue. The distinction between red and white infarcts is of little practical significance. In compact organs infarcts become almost white and bloodless as the blood leaches or is squeezed out. In spongy organs, such as the lungs, infarcts remain filled with red blood cells, which are only slowly absorbed.

The cells in an infarcted area undergo necrosis and autolysis (Fig. 10-12). Any blood cells remaining in the area break down and are eventually absorbed, but hemosiderin (a blood pigment) often persists. Eventually, the area undergoes fibrosis until no more than a scar is left. In the central nervous system the infarcted area is repaired by gliosis. Occasionally, an infarct may become infected, leading to abscess formation.

Shock syndrome

Shock is the term given to a variety of syndromes characterized by overall inadequacy of tissue perfusion. Inadequate supplies of oxygen and nutrients result in deterioration of cel-

lular function and, if untreated, death. An obvious example is massive blood loss leading to an inadequate circulating volume and severe hypotension; however, shock can develop in the absence of hypotension.

Whatever the cause, metabolites (particularly lactic acid) accumulate. This condition, known as metabolic lactic acidosis, is characteristic of all forms of shock. These syndromes present an acute threat to life.

On rare occasions, shock is due not so much to circulatory failure but to the inability of vital organs to make use of the blood supply.

At the risk of oversimplification, most forms of shock can be regarded as being either central or peripheral in origin. In peripheral circulatory failure, the essential change is loss of circulating volume. In central failure the heart fails as a pump; hence, this type of failure is often called *cardiogenic shock*.

There are three main types of shock:
1. Hypovolemic shock
2. Vascular shock, including endotoxemic shock
3. Cardiogenic shock

Clinical features

The effects of shock are shown in the skin, brain, respiration, renal function, and blood. Typical features are pale, cold, sweaty skin that becomes cyanotic; restlessness and disorientation progressing to coma; a thin rapid pulse; arrhythmias that may progress to ischemic ECG changes and heart failure; rapid, shallow respiration with impaired gas exchange; a low output of urine; hemoconcentration and sludging of blood cells, together with acidosis and hypoglycemia.

Hypovolemic shock

Hypovolemic shock is characterized by acute loss of so much of the plasma volume that an adequate blood pressure can no longer be maintained.

The main causes of hypovolemic shock include hemorrhage, extensive burns causing plasma loss, and loss of fluid and electrolytes by severe diarrhea or vomiting.

The chief effect of acute loss of circulating blood volume is a greatly diminished venous return and, as a consequence, an equally rapid fall in cardiac output and blood pressure. The effects of hemorrhage on the circulation depend on a variety of factors, particularly the amount and rate of loss. Thus, a rapid loss of 20% of the blood volume has much more severe effects than gradual leakage of even 40% of the blood volume. In this latter case, compensatory mechanisms partly make up for the deficiency. In addition, the hemoglobin level of the blood and the state of the cardiovascular and respiratory systems of the patient before the accident inevitably affect the outcome.

Compensatory mechanisms. The fall in circulating volume and in blood pressure stimulate the mobilization of fluid from the extravascular compartment. Up to 1 L of fluid per hour may reenter the circulation in this way. Increased sympathetic activity causes an increased heart rate and force of contraction. Arterioles and veins are contracted, increasing the peripheral resistance. In addition to catecholamines, antidiuretic hormone and aldosterone are secreted in increased amounts, and the combined effect is to reduce the blood flow to the skin, kidneys, muscles, and viscera, allowing a better blood supply to the heart and brain.

The kidney is severely affected; glomerular filtration and urine output are reduced. These immediate changes, by making best use of the reduced plasma volume to support the heart and brain, may be life saving in the short term. In the long term, however, the early reflex vasoconstriction cannot be maintained and is followed by vasodilatation. This is made worse by metabolic acidosis and the accumulation of vasodilator substances, such as histamine and the kinins. The veins are less sensitive to metabolic acidosis. This decreased sensitivity tends to cause stagnation of blood in the venous and capillary beds, allowing transudation of plasma into the tissues and further depletion of the blood volume.

Metabolic acidosis, one of the critical factors in the deterioration of the patient in shock, is due to impaired perfusion of the peripheral tissues. Here the shortage of oxygen forces the cell to depend on glycolytic pathways, which have lactic acid as the end product. The increasing acidosis stimulates increased release of carbon dioxide from the lungs in an attempt to compensate. In addition, the hypoxic state of the cells impairs their metabolism further, and the deleterious changes become progressively more complex and severe.

Shock due to fluid and electrolyte loss. Persistent severe vomiting or diarrhea, as in cholera and severe dysentery, can cause sufficiently massive loss of fluid and electrolytes to deplete the extracellular fluids and in turn lead to critical reduction in circulating volume. In countries with high temperatures the patient may be dehydrated even before the start of the disease, thus worsening its effects.

Vascular shock

In vascular shock, fluid is diverted to peripheral vessels or into the extracellular compartment. Neurogenic factors, bacterial endotoxin, acute anaphylaxis, and acute adrenocortical insufficiency are causes of vascular shock.

Neurogenic shock. Shock can follow general anesthesia, spinal or epidural anesthetics, or result from severe pain. It is postulated that shock under these circumstances is due to an effect on central neural control mechanisms, with widespread peripheral vasodilatation and pooling of blood. Nevertheless, with general anesthesia there are so many other possibilities, such as effects of the anesthetic agent itself, the condition of the patient, and the effects of surgery, that the underlying mechanisms and sequence of events in a rapid reaction of this sort are rarely clear.

Endotoxin shock. Endotoxin shock is common but poorly understood and has a variable presentation. It is usually due to severe gram-negative bacillary infections characterized by massive release of endotoxin. Experimentally, endotoxin (lipopolysaccharide) stimulates the release of anaphylatoxins, histamines, kinins, and probably other substances that can cause widespread vasodilatation, peripheral stagnation, and anoxia. It is also possible that endotoxins can directly damage cells and thus interfere with their oxidative processes. The cells may then be unable to use even an adequate blood supply. Damaged cells may include those of the vasomotor center, with consequent deterioration of vascular control and peripheral circulatory failure.

Anaphylaxis and acute adrenocortical insufficiency

Widespread vasodilatation and increased capillary permeability are the main features of anaphylactic shock. A somewhat similar reaction, although due to a different basic mechanism, is that seen in patients with impaired adrenocortical function.

Probably the main cause of anaphylactic shock is penicillin,

but some intravenous anesthetic agents and a few other drugs can have the same effect. Shock in patients receiving corticosteroids can be a result of surgical operations, particularly under general anesthesia, and can be fatal unless adequate additional doses of corticosteroids are given preoperatively.

Although the basic mechanisms may be somewhat different, the essential changes are loss of circulating volume, venous return, and cardiac output. In addition, because plasma rather than whole blood is lost, there is hemoconcentration with increased viscosity of the blood and sludging of red blood cells. This further impedes blood flow through and perfusion of the tissues.

An addisonian crisis (Chapter 18) is a severe form of shock caused by adrenocortical insufficiency, hypotension, and fluid and electrolyte loss.

Cardiogenic shock

Cardiogenic shock is due primarily to a severe fall in cardiac output, most commonly as a result of myocardial infarction. Other causes are severe arrhythmias, massive pulmonary embolism, the end stage of congestive cardiac failure, severe myocarditis, or cardiac tamponade.

Measures to counteract shock

The underlying factor in hypovolemic and vascular shock is the fall in circulating volume and blood pressure. The most important immediate measure, therefore, is rapid infusion of fluid, either blood, plasma, or plasma substitutes.

In anaphylaxis or operative shock in patients receiving corticosteroids, it is also essential to give large doses of corticosteroids by intravenous injection. In endotoxin shock, heavy doses of antibiotics should be given, but corticosteroids, although they have been widely used, are of no proven benefit in reducing mortality.

Vasoconstrictors, used to reduce vasodilatation and capillary permeability, may be dangerous in shock because they also reduce renal perfusion. Dopamine, however, increases both blood flow to the essential organs and also cardiac output. In view of the different causes of shock, each needs to be treated appropriately.

Hypervolemia

The main cause of increased blood volume is administration of excessive quantities of parenteral fluids; hypervolemia is therefore an important complication of transfusion.

The effect is to progressively increase the circulating volume and the venous return. This has two effects. First, there is increased transudation of fluid into the tissues and edema, especially of the lungs. Second, the increased venous return can overload the heart and can lead to cardiac failure.

Edema

Edema is the name given to excessive accumulation of fluid in the interstitial tissue spaces. Edema can be localized, particularly as a result of inflammation, or generalized, as in cardiac failure.

Edema results from escape of excessive amounts of fluid or from its inability to return to the blood as a result of the following:

1. Generalized edema

a. Increased hydrostatic (venous) pressure
b. Decreased osmotic pressure of plasma proteins
c. Increased osmotic pressure of tissue fluid due to sodium retention
d. Increased vascular permeability
2. Localized edema
a. Increased vascular permeability
b. Increased hydrostatic (venous) pressure
c. Lymphatic obstruction

An important additional factor that determines both the readiness with which edema develops and its distribution is tissue tension. In some cases more than one mechanism operates; in others the cause is unknown. Specific pathologic conditions associated with edema are discussed individually and are summarized as follows:

1. Generalized
a. Cardiac failure
b. Nephrotic syndrome
c. Hepatic cirrhosis and failure
d. Starvation, malabsorption syndromes, and protein-losing enteropathy
e. Cushing's syndrome
2. Localized
a. Inflammation
b. Hypersensitivity (type I) reactions (urticaria and acute angioedema)
c. Venous obstruction
d. Lymphatic obstruction

Generalized edema

Cardiac failure. Cardiac failure leads to retention of sodium and water as a result of impaired renal perfusion and complex hormonal changes (Chapter 11). The results are increased blood volume and raised venous pressure (Fig. 10-13).

The fluid retained in the tissues has a low protein content and is known as a transudate. Hydrostatic pressure seems to be the main factor in the production of cardiac edema.

In left ventricular failure the pulmonary venous pressure is raised. Pulmonary edema is therefore the main feature and is facilitated by the loose texture of the lungs. In right-sided heart failure the systemic circulation is affected, causing edema of the rest of the body, but especially in the ankles and areas of low tissue tension, such as the peritoneal cavity. Gravity also affects pulmonary edema, which is made so much worse by recumbency that the patient may be unable to breathe when lying down.

Some aspects of cardiac edema remain obscure. Sodium and water retention and edema often precede the rise in venous pressure. Nevertheless, the latter greatly worsens the condition. Thus cardiac edema can be improved by reducing salt intake, improving the pumping efficiency of the heart by giving cardiac glycosides, and increasing fluid excretion by giving diuretics. As cardiac failure becomes more severe, ridding the body of excess fluid may become insurmountable.

Nephrotic syndrome and other hypoproteinemic states. The nephrotic syndrome (Chapter 16) is characterized by gross proteinemia and hypoalbuminemia. The resulting fall in the osmotic tension of the blood is the basic cause of edema in this and other hypoproteinemic states (Fig. 10-14). Starvation, severe malabsorption, and many other diseases of the gastrointestinal tract that impair protein absorption (protein-losing enteropathy) are associated with edema.

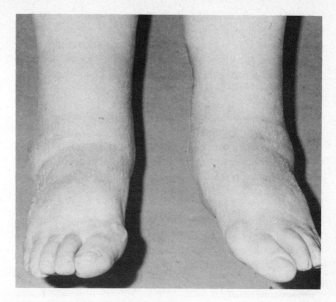

FIG. 10-13. Edema of right-sided cardiac failure. Edema of the ankles, where venous return is most severely impaired, is typical. *(Courtesy Curator of the Gordon Museum, Guy's Hospital, London, England.)*

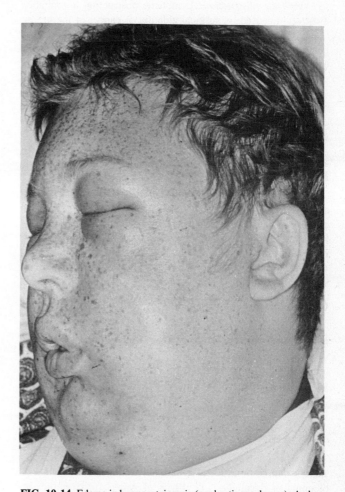

FIG. 10-14. Edema in hypoproteinemia (nephrotic syndrome). A characteristic clinical feature is the involvement of the face and eyelids as severely as more dependent parts. *(Courtesy Curator of the Gordon Museum, Guy's Hospital, London, England.)*

Hepatic cirrhosis and failure. Advanced hepatic cirrhosis is accompanied by lymphatic obstruction, portal hypertension, and impaired protein synthesis. These lead to accumulation of transudate in the peritoneal cavity (ascites). The ascitic fluid may impede the venous return from the legs and increase the tendency to edema of the ankles.

Localized edema

Inflammatory edema. Inflammatory edema is the result of increased capillary permeability caused by chemical mediators, mainly vasoactive amines such as histamine and kinins. The escaped plasma protein and tissue breakdown products increase the osmotic tension of the extracellular fluid and enhance the edema.

Hypersensitivity reactions. These reactions result from the release of chemical mediators when IgE reacts with sensitized mast cells. Edema is superficial in urticaria or may involve deeper tissues, such as the glottis, causing respiratory obstruction.

Venous obstruction and edema. Venous obstruction and edema are typically caused by thrombosis, particularly of leg or pelvic veins. Leg edema is common in late pregnancy and is possibly partly due to pressure on the pelvic veins by the gravid uterus. Other factors, such as fluid retention, also contribute.

Lymphatic obstruction. Lymphatic obstruction is probably most often caused by surgical ablation of cancer of the breast (Fig. 10-15). In radical mastectomy the lymph nodes and lymphatics of the axilla are removed. Edema of the arm and hand can be troublesome and persistent as a consequence.

Massive edema causing *elephantiasis* of the legs and scrotum is the result of infestation of the lymphatics by the parasitic nematode *Wuchereria bancrofti* and similar nematodes. Lymphangitis and eventually fibrous obstruction develop when the worms die.

Fluid, electrolyte, and acid-base balance

Disturbances of fluid, electrolyte, or acid-base balance can develop in isolation or in various combinations. In practical clinical terms the subject is beset with difficulties, particularly because of movements of electrolytes from one compartment in response to changes in another. Moreover, many of the variables cannot be measured directly. Only the basic principles are discussed here.

Water balance

Fluid intake is mostly from drinks, but food also contains water; more water is formed by oxidation of food (*metabolic water*).

Fluid is lost in the urine, feces, and perspiration, and under normal circumstances fluid intake and loss are balanced. Fluid restriction leads to decreased secretion in urine (*oliguria*) and feces, but loss in insensible perspiration cannot be controlled.

Water deficiency (dehydration)

Pure water deficiency is relatively uncommon, but causes include deprivation (due to the inability to ingest water because of coma or dysphagia), or a lack of water, for example, in shipwrecked sailors. Excessive excretion is also a problem. Failure to consume enough water to compensate for excessive loss in diabetes insipidus (Chapter 18) is a rare cause.

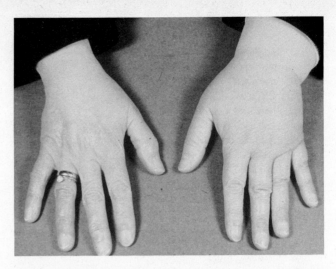

FIG. 10-15. Edema due to lymphatic obstruction. Following radical mastectomy the lymphoid tissue of the axilla has been removed and has led to typical unilateral edema.

Under desert conditions especially, there can be both inadequate intake and excessive loss by sweating. The predominant effect is then loss of salt in the sweat, as discussed later.

Effects. Water deprivation primarily affects the extracellular fluid, causing it to become hypertonic. Intracellular water moves out, so that the water deficiency is shared between the two compartments. Sodium and protein concentrations in the plasma are raised, however. In the attempt to reduce water loss, the body increases secretion of antidiuretic hormone (except in diabetes insipidus) and reduces output of urine. Clinically, water deprivation causes thirst, oliguria, hypotension, and eventually coma.

The essentials of treatment are to give water by mouth or, if the patient cannot swallow, a 5% glucose solution intravenously.

Salt (sodium) depletion

Salt depletion is usually associated with excessive fluid loss, but salt depletion alone can develop as a result of excessive sweating and drinking large amounts of water. Causes of sodium depletion include the following:

1. Renal disease ("salt-losing nephritis") and uremia
2. Diarrhea and vomiting
3. Addison's disease (Chapter 18)
4. Severe diabetes with polyuria

In some of these conditions acid-base balance is disturbed at the same time.

Effects. Sodium is mostly extracellular, and sodium loss causes the extracellular fluid to become hypotonic. Two consequences are oliguria and osmotic movement of extracellular fluid into the intracellular compartment. This further decreases extracellular fluid volume.

Clinically, the effects are similar to those caused by pure dehydration, except that thirst is not a feature; but the fall in blood pressure is more severe and may lead to renal failure. The reduced plasma sodium is an important diagnostic feature.

The essential treatment is to give salt by mouth, but in more severe cases it is preferable to give intravenous isotonic saline until signs of dehydration disappear and blood pressure and pulse rate become normal. It is dangerous, however, to give water alone, since this further dilutes the extracellular fluid and perpetuates the movement of water into the cells.

Potassium depletion

One cause of excessive potassium loss is severe diarrhea. Vomiting or other causes of loss of intestinal secretions are usually less important causes. Another factor is excessive renal loss. The mechanisms are usually complex but include use of thiazide diuretics and increased production of urine *(osmotic diuresis)* in response to the hyperglycemia of diabetes mellitus. Potassium-losing nephritis and hyperaldosteronism are additional causes.

Effects. Potassium is mainly intracellular, but when depleted it tends to move into the extracellular fluid. The plasma potassium level therefore tends to remain within normal limits and conceal the level of potassium depletion until it is very severe. There may, however, be depressed plasma sodium and bicarbonate levels as a result (it is believed) of compensatory migration of sodium and hydrogen ions into the cells. This can lead to alkalosis and sodium depletion.

In severe potassium-losing nephritis, by contrast, the kidneys cannot secrete an acid urine, and acidosis develops.

Potassium depletion severely affects cellular function, most obviously in muscle, brain, and kidneys.

Clinically, the effects of potassium depletion include the following:
1. Muscle weakness
2. Cardiac irregularities
3. Mental changes, including apathy and confusion, which may progress to coma
4. Impaired renal function

Among other effects, excretion of hydrogen ions in place of potassium can cause aciduria and a paradoxic alkalosis. The inability of the kidneys to concentrate the urine can lead to polyuria, dehydration, and thirst.

The main principles of treatment are to give potassium salts, preferably orally. Secondary salt and water depletion should also be treated.

Potassium excess

The causes of potassium excess include the following:
1. Renal disease or anuria
2. Overdosage of potassium salts or of potassium-conserving diuretics
3. Addison's disease, if unusually severe

The effects of potassium excess are difficult to recognize and confusingly similar to those of *hypokalemia*. The effects include lethargy progressing to confusion or stupor, muscle weakness, and irregularity, particularly slowing of the heart rate, which may lead to cardiac arrest. The diagnosis is based on the history and a raised serum potassium level.

Treatment is complex, but important principles include the following:
1. Reduced potassium intake in drugs and food, such as protein and fruit juices
2. Ion exchange resins to absorb potassium from the gastrointestinal tract
3. Glucose and insulin administration to promote the migration of potassium; this effect is enhanced if an infusion of isotonic sodium bicarbonate is also given
4. Water and salt administration if these are depleted and correction of any acidosis to enable a normal circulation and, as far as possible, normal renal function
5. Calcium gluconate intravenously to reduce the toxic effect of potassium on the heart
6. In severe acute cases, removal of potassium by hemodialysis

Disturbances of acid-base balance

Precise regulation of the pH of the blood between 7.37 and 7.45 is essential for normal body function. The main base is bicarbonate, but the phosphates and proteins of the blood, including hemoglobin, are also bases and powerful buffers. The pH of the blood mainly depends on the ratio between its main acidic component, carbonic acid, and bicarbonate. The carbonic acid concentration, in turn, is determined by the carbon dioxide levels (PCO_2) in the pulmonary alveoli. Under normal circumstances carbon dioxide, produced by metabolic processes in the tissues, is excreted by ventilation from the lungs, since carbon dioxide directly stimulates the respiratory center.

The kidneys also play an essential role in acid-base balance by excreting bicarbonate and acid anions.

Carbonic acid is quantitatively by far the most important acid produced in the body, but an excessive amount is normally excreted readily via the lungs. Acids that cannot be excreted by this route are normally buffered in the blood, mainly by the bicarbonate–carbonic acid system, and the acidic anion is ultimately excreted by the kidney.

Acid-base balance can be disturbed if the body produces too much acid or if the respiratory or renal excretion mechanisms are disturbed. Acid-base disturbances are therefore either respiratory or metabolic (nonrespiratory).

Respiratory alkalosis. Overbreathing causing excess loss of carbon dioxide can be neurotic *(hyperventilation syndrome)* or, more rarely, the result of damage to the respiratory center or the result of overventilation with a mechanical respirator.

The direct effects of the low PCO_2 are a fall in plasma carbonic acid and also in plasma ionized calcium, which can cause tetany.

Respiratory acidosis. Respiratory acidosis may be acute or chronic and can result from the following:
1. Carbon dioxide retention (hypercapnia)
   a. Respiratory obstruction (especially during anesthesia)
   b. Excess carbon dioxide in respired air (anesthetic mismanagement)
   c. Respiratory depression due to drugs and other causes
   d. Chronic obstructive pulmonary disease
2. Hypoxia that induces anaerobic glycolysis. This may give rise to lactic acidosis (secondary metabolic acidosis), which can worsen the effects of carbon dioxide accumulation due to impaired respiratory exchange.

The compensatory responses are:
1. Hyperventilation. Usually the patient cannot hyperventilate unless any underlying respiratory disorder is relieved.
2. Buffering of excess carbonic acid by plasma proteins, especially hemoglobin.
3. Renal excretion of hydrogen ions, but retention of bicarbonate. If carbon dioxide levels continue to rise, however, renal compensation eventually fails.

The effects of hypercapnia include peripheral vasodilatation, increased heart rate, headache, drowsiness, and finally coma.

Metabolic alkalosis. The main causes of metabolic alkalosis are as follows:

1. Excessive loss of gastric acid by vomiting or other means
2. Overindulgence in alkalis, particularly sodium bicarbonate, by patients with peptic ulcer or indigestion
3. Severe potassium depletion

Alkalosis is a secondary effect of the compensatory movement of hydrogen and sodium ions into the intracellular fluid, as discussed earlier. The kidney's ability to excrete hydrogen ions may also be impaired.

Effects. The main compensatory mechanism is respiratory retention of carbon dioxide. Aciduria is a frequent and paradoxic response and is partly the result of carbon dioxide retention, which causes increased reabsorption of bicarbonate. In addition, metabolic alkalosis is frequently associated with loss of chloride (as a result of vomiting, for example), which prevents the kidneys from producing an alkaline urine.

The clinical effects of metabolic alkalosis depend on the causes. They may include tetany and also disturbances of cerebral function, which may lead to stupor. This may be mainly the result of associated potassium and water loss.

The main principles of treatment are to give isotonic sodium chloride intravenously in patients with normal renal function. This enables excess bicarbonate to be excreted in the urine; the chloride is retained. In more severe cases an ammonium chloride infusion is given in addition to sodium chloride and, if necessary, potassium chloride.

Metabolic acidosis. The main causes of metabolic acidosis include the following:

1. Excessive production of acids, particularly in diabetic ketoacidosis; hypoxia (due to shock, for instance) can also cause acidosis by inducing anaerobic glycolysis
2. Impaired excretion of hydrogen ions in renal failure
3. Excessive loss of base in intestinal contents, as a result of persistent diarrhea, fistulae, or prolonged aspiration

Effects. The main compensatory changes include stimulation of respiration to excrete carbon dioxide, and excretion of hydrogen ions and a more acid urine by the kidneys.

Clinically, the most obvious feature of metabolic acidosis is the increasingly deep and rapid respiration (air hunger). In diabetic ketoacidosis (Chapter 18) there tends also to be water and salt depletion, whereas in chronic diarrhea there is water and potassium loss and their attendant effects.

Hypertension

Hypertension is the term given to a sustained elevation of blood pressure. There is no sharp dividing line between "normal" blood pressure and hypertension. In practice, hypertension is diagnosed at an arbitrary point when the blood pressure at rest exceeds 160/90. By this criterion, approximately 34 million Americans may be affected.

The main immediate cause of hypertension appears to be a sustained increase in arterial tone and, as a consequence, increased peripheral resistance.

In 90% of the cases the basic cause of persistently elevated blood pressure is unknown, and the disorder is therefore called *essential hypertension.* In about 10% of the cases hypertension is caused by renal or endocrine disease or vascular anomalies (secondary hypertension).

Epidemiology

The main epidemiologic aspects follow:

1. Hypertension is twice as common in women as men, but the latter suffer its effects more severely.
2. The incidence of hypertension among American blacks is about twice as high as among whites, and the death rate is correspondingly greater.
3. If both parents are hypertensive, then 50% of their offspring are also affected. But inheritance is polygenic, and the rate of rise of blood pressure with increasing age also appears to be largely determined by external (nongenetic) factors.
4. Environmental factors appear to play a part but are difficult to assess. Hypertension appears, for instance, to be much less common in Chinese living in China than in those living in the United States.
5. The complications of hypertension—atherosclerosis and coronary artery disease—are undoubtedly more common in affluent westernized society than in poor countries.
6. Hypertension and its complications increase in severity with age.
7. Excessive salt intake is associated with hypertension.
8. Obesity and hypertension are associated, and reduction in body weight leads to a fall in blood pressure.
9. It is widely believed that an important factor in the production of hypertension is "stress," whatever that may be. Acute emotional disturbance, such as fear, anger, or anxiety, produces a rapid rise in blood pressure, and this reaction is mediated through the autonomic nervous system. It has been suggested that those who are susceptible to this form of labile hypertension ultimately develop progressive, essential hypertension. This is unproven, and no definable pattern has yet emerged from studies attempting to relate hypertension with psychosocial factors. Nevertheless, the increasing evidence that sympathetic activity may play a role in the production of hypertension in some patients suggests that emotional factors may be involved.

Pathogenesis

Paradoxically, there have been greater advances in the development of new drugs to control hypertension than in understanding the underlying mechanisms. Such drugs include the angiotensin-converting enzyme inhibitors that block the conversion of angiotensin I to angiotensin II (as discussed below) and the calcium channel blocking drugs (calcium ion antagonists). Of the multiple mechanisms responsible for chronic essential hypertension, three contribute and interact with each other, but the relative importance of each is uncertain:

1. The renin-angiotensin pathway
2. Sympathetic activity
3. Calcium (and possibly sodium) ion movement

Goldblatt* showed experimentally that restriction of the blood supply to a kidney, short of complete obstruction, caused hypertension. It is now widely believed that this effect is mediated by a complex sequence of interactions by the renin-angiotensin-aldosterone (RAA) system (Fig. 10-16).

Renin is a proteolytic enzyme released from the kidney in response to various stimuli, including ischemia. Angiotensin II exerts a complex negative feedback control of renin release. In simple terms, a rise in blood pressure normally stimulates an increased urinary output of sodium and water. This in turn lowers blood pressure by diminishing plasma volume. On the other hand, a severe reduction in salt intake activates the renin-angiotensin system to raise the blood pressure by vasoconstric-

---

*H. Goldblatt (1891-1976), American physician.

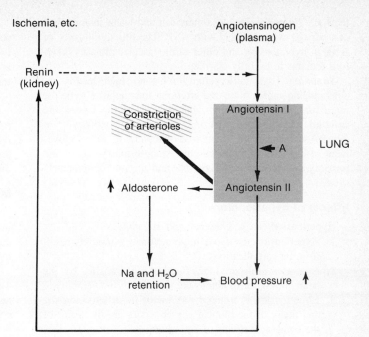

FIG. 10-16. The renin-angiotensin mechanism in the genesis of hypertension. *A* indicates the site of action of angiotensin-converting enzyme.

tion. In this way a delicate balance exists between sodium retention and renin release to maintain the blood pressure.

In humans, unilateral renal ischemia causes hypertension and greatly raised levels of renin in the vein leaving the ischemic kidney. Restoration of the blood supply or nephrectomy abolishes the hypertension.

In more than 50% of hypertensive patients, however, plasma renin levels are within normal limits, and in 25% renin levels are not only subnormal but also do not rise in response to salt depletion. Raised plasma renin levels are found in fewer than 20% of hypertensives. The mechanism by which the RAA system may operate in the pathogenesis of human essential hypertension remains controversial.

Aldosterone, a mineralocorticoid, affects the blood pressure by controlling sodium and water retention and thus blood volume. Hypersecretion of aldosterone, as in primary aldosteronism (Conn's syndrome*) is characterized by sodium and water retention and hypertension. This is a rare cause of hypertension, but illustrates the negative feedback mechanism, in that renin secretion is depressed.

Plasma catecholamine levels in hypertension. In up to 40% of patients with essential hypertension, plasma catecholamine levels are abnormally high. These high levels may indicate increased sympathetic activity contributing to the development of hypertension, but this has not yet been proven.

Calcium mediation of vascular tone. Contraction of vascular smooth muscle depends on calcium binding to calmodulin, a small binding protein. The calcium-calmodulin complex sets in train a course of events that causes myosin to react with actin and the muscle to contract. Unlike skeletal muscle, the intracellular stores of calcium are minimal in smooth muscle, so that contraction depends on the availability of calcium in the cytosol. Arterial smooth muscle is particularly

sensitive to drugs that block this entry of calcium, and it is increasingly believed that calcium may be the final common path by which vascular tone is increased in hypertension.

Recently considerable attention has been given to calcium intake and metabolism in the pathogenesis of hypertension. Despite the role of intracellular calcium in raising vascular tone, some evidence has been found to suggest that hypertension (in some patients at least) is associated with calcium deficiency and that in some hypertensives, calcium supplementation lowers blood pressure to a small degree. The calcium deficiency hypothesis for hypertension is not widely accepted but increasing attention is being paid to the interactions between sodium and calcium ions both as dietary components and at the cellular level in hypertension. The ability of dietary salt to raise blood pressure may, for example, be related to its ability to affect calcium metabolism; evidence also suggests that calcium-regulating hormones interact with the renin-angiotensin system and that such interactions may regulate intracellular and extracellular calcium levels.

Atrial natriuretic peptide. Although the importance of calcium ions in mediating contraction of vascular smooth muscle is accepted, the significance of other modifying substances is more difficult to assess. These substances include several peptides, in particular, atrial natriuretic peptide (ANP). ANP was originally isolated from atrial wall but has since been found in other tissues. Some evidence suggests that although ANP enhanced sodium secretion by the kidneys, it allowed accumulation of sodium in vascular smooth muscle. The entry of sodium into vascular smooth muscle cells triggers the entry of calcium into the cytosol and hence muscular contraction (vasoconstriction). However, current work has confirmed that atrial natriuretic peptide also causes vasodilatation, rather than vasoconstriction and blocks the action of angiotensin II. Moreover, the renal effects of ANP may vary according to electrolyte and hormone levels. If circulating levels of angiotensin II are high, its actions may be significantly blocked by ANP. Fur-

---

*J.W. Conn (b. 1907), American physician.

thermore, hypertensives lose more salt and water than do normal persons when infused with ANP. The full significance of ANP in hypertension and other cardiovascular diseases therefore remains to be fully clarified.

Summary. Essential hypertension has no single readily understandable cause. Increased arteriolar tone appears to be the main immediate mechanism, but the underlying causes are complex and the mediators may include an abnormality of the RAA mechanism, increased sympathetic tone, movement of calcium ions into vascular smooth muscle cells, and possibly interactions between ANP and the renin-angiotensin system.

Effects of hypertension

Hypertension can be characterized as follows:
1. Hypertension itself has no symptoms; symptoms result from its complications
2. No organs are spared the effects of hypertension, but the heart, brain, and kidneys are particularly vulnerable.
3. Hypertension is a major risk factor for atherosclerosis, and many of the clinical consequences are the result of the combined effects of both diseases.
4. The complications of hypertension can be catastrophic, and it is one of the most important factors contributing to coronary artery disease, congestive heart failure, and cerebrovascular accidents.
5. The degree of damage to affected organs is directly related to the blood pressure level.

Cardiac effects. Hypertension alone, by imposing a persistent overload on the left ventricle, causes progressive hypertrophy until the increased bulk of the myocardium outstrips its blood supply. Hypertension leads to left-sided heart failure or ischemic heart disease. Hypertension also plays an important role in coronary artery disease, but mainly because it contributes to atherosclerosis.

The blood vessels. The three main effects of hypertension on blood vessels are atherosclerosis, arteriolosclerosis, and rupture of weakened vessels causing hemorrhage.

Arteriolosclerosis. Arteriolosclerosis is a direct effect of hypertension on the arterioles in which the intima thickens and the muscle layer hypertrophies, especially in the renal vessels. The kidney undergoes gradual atrophy and glomeruli and tubules become fibrotic, a condition known as *nephrosclerosis.* Elsewhere, arteriolosclerosis has little significant effect.

Hemorrhage. Excessive strain on blood vessels may cause them to rupture, but usually only when there is disease of the vessel walls. Rupture of a berry aneurysm of the circle of Willis, cerebral hemorrhage, or aortic dissection can be consequences of severe hypertension.

Control of hypertension

It seems that the effectiveness of drugs in controlling hypertension would be related to the pathogenesis. In practice, blood pressure can be lowered by drugs that act centrally to reduce cardiac output, sympathetic antagonists that also reduce cardiac output, drugs that cause vasodilatation by a variety of means (including blocking calcium entry), and drugs that block the conversion of angiotensin I to angiotensin II. By contrast, studies on the effects of dietary salt and of calcium on blood pressure produce conflicting results, but reducing salt intake (and in some people, increasing calcium intake) is beneficial even if the effect is small.

Clinical aspects. Although hypertension and its effects cause no symptoms until complications develop, severe hypertension is readily detected during a medical checkup. If hypertension is found, the current consensus is that the patient should be treated even though symptoms may be absent. It is less certain, however, whether such treatment prolongs life.

Even severe hypertension can be asymptomatic and unsuspected. Vague complaints such as headache or dizziness are relatively common once the patient has been made aware of the disease. Otherwise, the first overt sign of hypertension is often a heart attack or stroke.

Malignant (accelerated) hypertension

This is a less common form of hypertension that can develop in a person with previously normal blood pressure, or it may complicate essential and secondary hypertension. About 5% of hypertensives have the malignant form.

Malignant hypertension is associated with malignant nephrosclerosis. Microscopically, the main features of malignant nephrosclerosis are thickening of the intima and media of the renal arterioles with fibrinoid change and, even more striking, hyperplasia of the intima, which progressively obliterates the vessel lumens. In addition, microthrombi sometimes form within the vessels.

The glomeruli themselves are not primarily attacked. Nevertheless, they suffer severe secondary ischemic changes. The proximal tubules are particularly sensitive to ischemia and undergo degenerative changes.

Clinical aspects. Patients are usually relatively young adults. Severe hypertension often causes no symptoms, and the first manifestation of the disease is one of its complications.

Clinical examination shows papilledema (swelling of the optic disc) with retinal hemorrhages and exudates. Cardiac failure and rapidly deteriorating renal function are also common.

In the absence of treatment, many patients die within a year, usually from renal failure or, less often, as a result of a cerebrovascular accident or cardiac failure. The condition must be regarded as a medical emergency, and vigorous antihypertensive treatment has significantly increased the expectation of life. About 50% now survive for at least 5 years. If the disease is not detected before renal damage is advanced, however, the expectation of life is poor.

Hypertensive encephalopathy

Hypertensive encephalopathy is an acute neurologic syndrome caused by severe (malignant) hypertension.

Pathology. Cerebral edema and hemorrhages, ranging from petechiae to gross bleeding, are the usual features. The intracranial pressure is raised. Microscopically, the main features are small hemorrhages, necrotic changes in arteriole walls, minute infarcts, and glial cell clusters.

Clinically, this syndrome is characterized by headache, nausea and vomiting, convulsions, confusion, stupor, and coma.

The blood pressure should be lowered as quickly as possible. If this cannot be done, the patient may die.

Secondary hypertension

A few cases of hypertension are due to identifiable underlying disease. Although the clinical term "treatable hypertension" is sometimes used, this is only true in some cases. Essential hypertension is also treatable. The main causes of secondary hypertension are renal, including renovascular and renal parenchymal disease; hyperaldosteronism (Conn's syndrome); Cushing's syndrome; and pheochromocytoma. Patients with secondary hypertension may also progress to malignant hypertension.

Renovascular and renal parenchymal hypertension are described more fully in Chapter 16. Renovascular hypertension is associated with high circulating renin levels, whereas in renal parenchymal hypertension the renin levels are variable and not necessarily raised. The basic lesion in renovascular disease is ischemia, and, if the lesion is unilateral, removal of the affected kidney should restore the blood pressure to normal. The picture in renal parenchymal hypertension is more variable, and the disease is often bilateral and untreatable.

The following endocrine disorders cause hypertension and are discussed in more detail in Chapter 18.

Primary aldosteronism. Primary aldosteronism is due to hypersecretion of aldosterone, usually by an adenoma of the adrenal cortex. The basic mechanism of hypertension in this case is severe sodium retention. Plasma renin is depressed because of the feedback mechanism.

Cushing's syndrome. Cushing's syndrome is also a disease of the adrenal cortex. It is characterized by hypersecretion of glucocorticoids, which also have some mineralocorticoid effect, and the basic mechanism is again sodium retention. Some patients with Cushing's syndrome may also overproduce mineralocorticoids.

Pheochromocytoma. Pheochromocytoma is a tumor of the adrenal medulla, which actively secretes epinephrine and norepinephrine. Norepinephrine excessively stimulates adrenergic receptors and causes severe peripheral vasoconstriction. The increased peripheral resistance causes a rise in blood pressure. This is made worse by the stimulant effect of epinephrine on the heart, causing increased cardiac output.

Oral contraceptives. The estrogen component of these agents can cause secondary hypertension, apparently by stimulating hepatic synthesis of angiotensinogen. This leads to increased production of angiotensin and also of aldosterone.

In most women this effect is slight, but, if it becomes severe, the blood pressure can be restored to normal by discontinuing the oral contraceptive agent.

DISEASES OF BLOOD VESSELS

Arteriosclerosis is not a specific pathologic entity but is a general term that literally means "hardening of the arteries." This term is not merely vague but also inaccurate in many cases. The diseases comprised by arteriosclerosis include atherosclerosis and Mönckeberg's sclerosis. Arteriolosclerosis affects small arteries and is a consequence of hypertension, as discussed earlier.

Atherosclerosis

Atherosclerosis is characterized by the formation of thickened fatty plaques in arterial walls, particularly medium-size and large arteries. The most important arteries affected are therefore the coronary and cerebral arteries and the aorta (Fig. 10-17). Atherosclerosis produces gradual or, if there are secondary changes, sudden occlusion of the vessel. It can also weaken the walls, particularly of cerebral arteries. Atherosclerosis plays a crucial role in the production of coronary artery disease and cerebrovascular disease.

Atherosclerosis, like hypertension (with which it is closely associated), produces no symptoms until complications develop. In humans the initiation and progression of atherosclerosis therefore must be based on inferences drawn from information about its main complication, coronary artery disease. Statistics relating to the mortality from myocardial infarction are frequently used as an index of the incidence of severe atherosclerosis.

Although coronary artery disease and atherosclerosis are closely associated, they are different diseases, and their pathogenesis is not necessarily identical, since other risk factors are involved. Theories about atherosclerosis are inevitably also based on experiments on animals, which may not respond in the same way as humans.

Epidemiology

Atherosclerosis as a cause of cardiovascular complications is a disease of the affluent, especially in the United States,

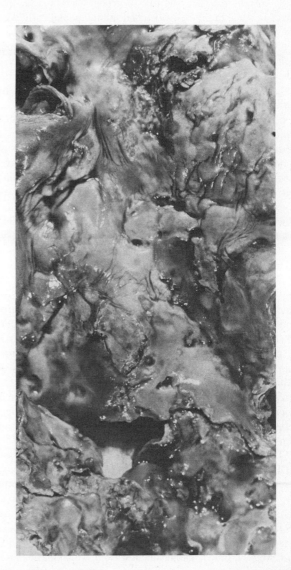

FIG. 10-17. Atherosclerosis of the aorta. Close-up of the endothelial surface shows the gross irregularity and areas of ulceration in the aortic intima.

Great Britain, Australia, New Zealand, Finland, and other Scandinavian countries. In countries where the standard of living is low, such as India, parts of Africa, and South America, atherosclerosis is a much less severe problem.

The incidence of complications increases with age. Certain risk factors can be identified:

1. *Serum lipoprotein and cholesterol levels.* A raised level of low-density serum lipoprotein is a major risk factor. Hypothyroidism, for instance, is associated with high plasma cholesterol levels and unusually early coronary artery disease in women.

2. *Blood pressure.* The higher the blood pressure, the greater the risk, especially in patients over 45.

3. *Cigarette smoking.* It is not known precisely how this affects atherosclerosis, but epidemiologic evidence makes it clear that heavy cigarette smoking is an important contributory factor.

4. *Diabetes mellitus.* Diabetes also is a high-risk factor. The role of a high blood glucose level rather than hyperlipidemia, which is commonly also present, is not clear.

5. *Genetic aspects.* The role of genetic factors is far from clear. In some families, myocardial infarction and early death are frequent, whereas other families apparently living under similar conditions reach a great age without complications. Genetic factors may also affect the incidence or severity of atherosclerosis through other mechanisms. For example, diabetes mellitus is partly genetically determined. Familial hyperlipidemia is also a high-risk disease.

6. *Hormonal factors.* Until they undergo the menopause, women are much less severely affected by complications of atherosclerosis than are men. By about age 70, the sexes are almost equally affected. Evidence suggests that this effect is mediated by estrogens. Combinations of risk factors are not so much additive as synergistic. High serum lipoprotein levels, high blood pressure, cigarette smoking, and a raised blood glucose level increase the risk of complications from atherosclerosis about thirteen times.

7. *Diet.* Serum lipoprotein and cholesterol levels are affected by diet in a complex fashion. The high animal fat content of Westernized diets is widely believed to be a factor in atherosclerosis and its complications. In several countries a lowered mortality from myocardial infarction has been reported, and this has been associated with a generally lower consumption of animal fats. The relationship between the quantity and types of fats eaten and the incidence or severity of atherosclerosis may be important, but this relationship, although widely accepted, remains controversial in humans.

Lipid metabolism and ischemic heart disease. Serum lipoproteins are of three main types: very low-density lipoproteins (VLDLs), low-density lipoproteins (LDLs), and high-density lipoproteins (HDLs).

The importance of the different lipoproteins is that increased LDL levels are characterized by a higher incidence of coronary artery disease. Accelerated disease is characteristic of homozygous familial hyperlipoproteinemia (Table 10-2) in which serum LDL levels are at a high level. By contrast, increased HDL levels carry with them a lower expectation of coronary artery disease and related mortality.

Currently, little is known about ways in which plasma levels of HDL can be increased or ways in which high LDL levels might be converted into raised HDL levels. Apart from genetic factors affecting blood lipids, LDL levels may be controlled to

some extent by diet, and HDL levels are apparently increased by exercise, which explains why exercise helps prevent coronary artery disease.

Lipoproteins consist of cholesterol together with triglyceride or phospholipid, and an *apoprotein.* The numerous apoproteins determine the conformation, receptor binding, and metabolism of lipoproteins and can exchange between the lipoproteins.

Lipoprotein metabolism. Fats are absorbed from the gut as triglycerides and form chylomicrons in the plasma. Chylomicrons consist of a triglyceride and cholesterol bound to apoprotein. In the plasma, chylomicrons are converted to a small amount of LDL (cholesterol bound to apoprotein) and a larger amount of *remnant lipoprotein* (differing in its composition from chylomicrons only in the attached apoprotein), which is taken up by the liver via its apoprotein receptors. The remainder is taken up by fat and muscle where it is hydrolyzed to fatty acids, for use as an energy source, or to triglyceride for storage.

Within the liver the lipoprotein is converted into VLDL, which contains a high proportion of triglyceride. In the plasma, VLDL is converted into intermediate density lipoprotein (IDL) and into LDL, which is taken up by peripheral cells. Part, however, is also broken down by plasma lipases and taken up by fat and muscle as triglyceride.

Apoproteins. Apoproteins determine the composition, receptor binding, and metabolism of lipoproteins. Eight major apoproteins have been identified. Since apoproteins, particularly apo A1 and apo B are major determinants of HDL and LDL levels, measurement of individual apoproteins may possibly be better predictors of ischemic heart disease risk than measurement of lipoprotein levels.

Important apoproteins include the following:

1. *Apo A1* forms about 40% of the HDLs. Genetic variants or the absence of apo A1 are associated with low HDL levels and increased susceptibility to ischemic heart disease.

2. *Apo B100* is synthesized by the liver, secreted in VLDLs, and is also a major component of LDLs. Hyperlipoproteinemia and abetalipoproteinemia are genetic diseases characterized by fat malabsorption and low levels of apo B100. The resulting low levels of LDL and VLDL are associated with a decreased risk of ischemic heart disease. High levels of apo B are associated with hypoalbuminuria or with prolonged estrogen therapy, which may explain the increased risk of ischemic heart disease in such conditions. This also applies to familial hypercholesterolemia in which, as a result of the genetic defect of apo B receptors, there are very high levels of apo B and

TABLE 10-2. Important familial hyperlipoproteinemias*

Disease	*Lipoproteins†*		*Risks†*	*Prevalence*
Familial hypercholesterolemia	LDL	↑ ↑	CHD + +	Common
			CVD +	(1/500)
Familial hypertriglyceridemia	VLDL	↑	CHD ±	Common
	HDL ?	↓	CVD ±	(1/600)
Familial combined hyperlipidemia	LDL	↑	CHD + +	Very common
	VLDL	↑ ↑	CVD + +	(1/300)
Remnant hyperlipidemia	VLDL	↑	CHD +	Rare
	CRs	↑ ↑	CVD +	(1/10,000)

*Modified Goldstein classification; other, rare varieties omitted.
†*LDL,* Low-density lipoproteins; *VLDL,* very low-density lipoproteins; *HDL,* high-density lipoproteins; *CRs,* chylomicron remnants; *CHD,* coronary artery disease; *CVD,* cerebrovascular disease.

LDL, and premature coronary artery disease. High levels of apo B and VLDL are also features of familial combined hypercholesterolemia. Interaction of apo B−containing lipoproteins with components of arterial walls appears to be important in the accumulation of lipids there.

3. *Apo C11* acts as a cofactor for lipoprotein lipase. Inherited apo C11 deficiency therefore results in hypertriglyceridemia, and these levels may be so high in homozygotes as to confer a risk of pancreatitis and sometimes of vascular disease. Inherited variants of apo C111 (a major protein of VLDL) may also result in hypertriglyceridemia.

4. *Apo E* is synthesized in several organs but particularly in the liver. Apo E is an important component of VLDL and of remnant lipoproteins, but there are several apo E phenotypes that vary in their capacity to bind to receptors and affect the catabolism of their lipoproteins accordingly.

5. *Remnant hyperlipidemia,* a rare disorder of lipoprotein metabolism, is associated with the apo E2/E2 phenotype. Apo E2 binds weakly to lipoprotein receptors, delaying remnant lipoprotein clearance. Because less VLDL is converted to LDL, triglyceride and cholesterol levels increase. This accelerates atherosclerosis both of coronary and peripheral arteries and leads to premature death. However, only a minority of those expressing the apo E2/E2 phenotype have hyperlipidemia, and another factor, either genetic or environmental, appears to be needed for remnant hyperlipidemia to develop.

Apoproteins and ischemic heart disease. Several genetic apoprotein defects have been identified by family studies. Some of these, as mentioned earlier, are associated with low HDL or high triglyceride levels and premature death from ischemic heart disease. Other polymorphisms at the apoprotein gene locus result in a variety of other disorders with hypercholesterolemia or hypertriglyceridemia and accelerated atherosclerosis, establishing a broad correlation between particular apoprotein disorders and premature ischemic heart disease. However, the contribution of genetic lipoprotein metabolism defects to atherosclerosis in the general population is unknown.

In summary, the chief identifiable (and potentially treatable) risk factors for atherosclerosis appear to be:
1. Serum cholesterol (LDL) levels
2. Hypertension
3. Cigarette smoking

Pathogenesis

The main theories put forward to explain the development of atherosclerosis are hemodynamic stress, lipid infiltration and platelet adherence, and myointimal proliferation. These theories are by no means mutually exclusive, but their relative importance cannot as yet be determined.

Hemodynamic stress. The relationship between hypertension and atherosclerosis is close. Epidemiologically, the complications of hypertension and atherosclerosis are intimately associated. More direct evidence shows that atherosclerosis only develops in highly stressed vessels, namely arteries, not veins, and does not affect the pulmonary arteries unless pulmonary hypertension develops. Atherosclerotic lesions tend also to be more common at sites such as bifurcations of arteries in which hemodynamic stress appears to be greater.

Despite these findings, the mechanisms by which hypertension may contribute to atherosclerosis remain obscure. Although acute hypertension leads to breakdown of the intermembranous complexes of endothelial cells, there is no hard evidence that chronic hypertension either damages the endothelium or makes it more permeable to substances that induce myointimal proliferation. Earlier theories that denudation of endothelium (an injury that is readily produced experimentally) is the initiating event in atherosclerosis have not been confirmed in studies of the disease in humans.

Atherosclerosis-like changes, notably fatty streaks, also form in the walls of coronary and other arteries in children. These fatty streaks may regress, but subsequent development of fibrous plaques may precede the development of hypertension. The mechanism by which these childhood fatty streaks form is unknown, but it is possible that the process may be initiated by active vesicular lipoprotein transport through intact endothelial cells. The adverse effects of hypertension may therefore act on already diseased areas of the arterial walls.

Lipid infiltration. Hypercholesterolemia is associated with atherosclerosis both epidemiologically and experimentally. In monkeys, high-fat and high-cholesterol diets lead to the attachment of leukocytes to arterial endothelium. Macrophages also migrate beneath the endothelium and become foam cells by taking up local accumulations of lipid. Fatty streaks, which are histologically similar to those in humans, expand by migration of smooth muscle cells into the area from the media. When high plasma lipid and cholesterol levels persist for months, endothelial cells overlying the fatty streaks separate, initially at arterial branches or bifurcations. The underlying connective tissue with its content of lipid-laden macrophages, may thus become exposed; conditions then favor the adhesion of platelets and secondary changes. It is also possible that changes in surface components of endothelial cells may permit platelet adhesion, but this has not been confirmed.

Despite the close association between hypercholesterolemia and atherosclerotic disease in humans, any mechanism for hypercholesterolemic vascular damage remains controversial.

Platelet adherence. Platelets release a variety of mediators and in particular, platelet-derived growth factor (PDGF). The latter is both chemotactic and mitogenic. Platelets also secrete a variety of chemotactic factors and a substance apparently identical with PDGF is also produced by macrophages. In addition, macrophages secrete fibroblast growth factor, as well as the potent chemotactic factor, leukotriene B$_4$.

The plasma half-life of PDGF is only a few minutes, but various plasma proteins appear able to promote its local mitogenic activity. PDGF is the growth factor that has been most fully investigated, and although it is likely that other growth factors are also involved, the fact that, in animal experiments, platelet depletion prevents the formation of proliferative lesions, even when the endothelium is damaged, suggests that platelet-derived factors are particularly important in atherogenesis.

Many cells transformed by retroviruses and other viruses secrete molecules similar to if not identical with PDGF, but the role of viruses in the pathogenesis of atherosclerosis is, as yet, speculative.

Myointimal proliferation. Fatty streaks, particularly at arterial branches and bifurcations, become infiltrated by macrophages and also expand as a result of increasing numbers of smooth muscle cells that have migrated from the media into the intima. Electron microscopy has also shown that the so-called fibrous cap of uncomplicated atherosclerotic lesions is formed from smooth muscle cells rather than fibroblasts. Nevertheless collagen accumulates in association with the muscle cells. The migration of the latter appears to result from the formation, in the initima, of chemotactic factors to which smooth muscle cells respond. Many of these smooth muscle cells proliferate in response to mitogens, particularly PDGF, and also accumulate lipids (Fig. 10-18) (for which they have receptors) and thus increase the mass of the plaque. It has been suggested, however, that macrophage infiltration is an early if not an initiating event, that precedes loss of endothelial continuity and that macrophages may be the prime source of mediators of myointimal migration and proliferation.

Another aspect of this complex story is the evidence that myointimal proliferation is monoclonal and arises from a single

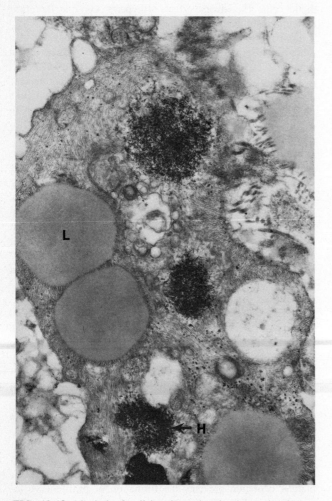

FIG. 10-18. Myointimal cell in atherosclerotic plaque showing cytoplasmic accumulations of lipid droplets *(L)* and hydroxyapatite crystals *(H)*.

myointimal cell, probably as a response to mutagens. The latter could include tobacco products or oxidized lipids. However, not all investigators have confirmed this finding. It has also been found that endothelial cells and even smooth muscle cells secrete mitogenic peptides, but it is difficult to reconcile findings that suggest an endogenous origin for myointimal proliferation with those described earlier.

Cigarette smoking, a major risk factor for atherosclerosis, may contribute by its known mutagenic properties to myointimal proliferation and can also affect blood lipids, but the sum total of its effects is unclear.

In addition to all the findings, of which only a few have been described, it has become apparent that endothelial cells have a far greater range of functions and secrete or process many more substances than was previously suspected. However, the contribution of endothelial dysfunction to the pathogenesis of atherosclerosis is far from clear.

Ultimately, it must be admitted that the many findings as a result of investigation of early human lesions, as well as experimental atherosclerosis, have failed to clarify the nature of the initiating processes or to allow the formulation of a unifying theory. Currently, it appears possible only to state that in the pathogenesis of the uncomplicated lesions of atherosclerosis:

1. Lipid infiltration of the intima to produce fatty streaks is a very early event and can precede any factors, such as hypertension or hyperlipidemia. Macrophages (foam cells) predominate in fatty streaks.

2. Some fatty streaks progress when myoepithelial cells, which proliferate in the plaque, migrate into them and form the so-called fibrous cap. Others may regress.

3. There is no evidence that injury (in its ordinary sense) to the endothelium is an initiating event but hyperlipidemia may cause endothelial cell changes that promote adherence of platelets and monocytes and lead to increased macrophage infiltration and lipid accumulation. Endothelial dysfunction, rather than denudation of an area of arterial wall, may be a critical early event.

4. A variety of cells, such as platelets and macrophages, secrete growth factors, particularly PDGF (or apparently identical substances), as well as chemotactic factors.

5. The different risk factors for atherosclerosis may act by separate pathways. Thus hypercholesterolemia may lead to monocyte and platelet interactions, resulting in release of growth and chemotactic factors. Hypertension and possibly other etiologic factors such as smoking and diabetes mellitus may, by contrast, act by direct stimulation of endothelial cells to promote the secretion of mediators of intimal infiltration and proliferation.

6. The findings in experimental atherosclerosis produced by such means as introduction of catheters to damage the endo-

TABLE 10-3. Pathogenesis of atherosclerosis

Risk factors	Complications in plaques	Main effects
High serum lipids Hypertension Cigarette smoking High blood glucose level Genetic factors Oral contraceptives	Atherosclerosis Fibrosis Ulceration Thrombosis Hemorrhage Medial damage	Coronary artery disease Cerebrovascular disease Intermittent claudication Atherosclerotic aneurysms of aorta Renal ischemia

thelium, are of uncertain relevance to human disease. Clearly, however, the difficulties involved in elucidating the initiating events in human atherosclerosis are formidable. Important factors in the pathogenesis of atherosclerosis and its main effects are briefly summarized in Table 10-3.

Pathology

Atherosclerosis predominantly affects the intima. The media is involved secondarily and usually to a much lesser degree.

Three types of lesions are recognizable. These represent increasing degrees of severity and are generally regarded as stages in the progress of this disease.

Fatty streaks. These can be found (particularly in the aorta) in children, as mentioned earlier. The streaks are virtually always present by the time the tenth year has been reached, and their extent increases with age.

Fatty streaks consist of yellowish plaques, slightly raised above the surrounding arterial lining but not sufficient to cause obstruction. These plaques consist essentially of smooth muscle cells with lipid (mainly cholesterol) (Fig. 10-19) in and around them and in macrophages. Fatty streaks are ubiquitous and even affect nutritionally deprived infants in parts of the world where the complications of advanced atherosclerosis are relatively rare. Moreover, fatty streaks not uncommonly develop in different sites from those of more severe lesions. The relationship

of these lesions to those of adult atherosclerosis is therefore problematic, but in some cases it appears that they form the basis for atherosclerosis in later life.

Fibrous (atheromatous) plaques. These plaques (Fig. 10-20) are whitish and thick, but at normal arterial pressure they apparently do not significantly reduce blood flow.

In mildly affected areas normal intima separates the plaques, but in severely affected areas they become confluent. Their striking feature is the heavy accumulation of lipid in and around smooth muscle cells (Fig. 10-21). The latter are also surrounded by collagen, elastic fibers, and proteoglycans. This complex of cells, lipid, and matrix forms a cap overlying more extensive deposits of lipid and cell debris (Fig. 10-22).

The complicated lesion. Fibrous plaques can increase in size as a result of further lipid accumulation and fibrosis until the

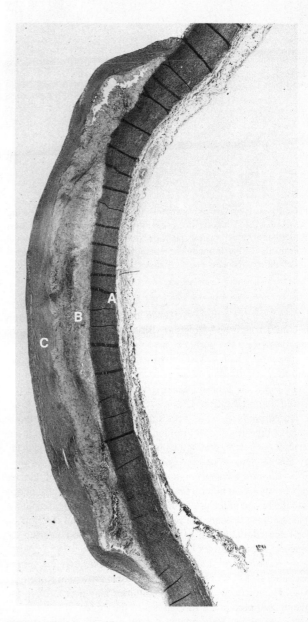

FIG. 10-20. Atheromatous plaque in the aorta. The media *(A)* shows as a dark zone, whereas the plaque shows a deeper zone *(B)* mainly of fatty material and a cellular cap *(C)* of proliferated myointimal cells, which give a smooth surface to the plaque.

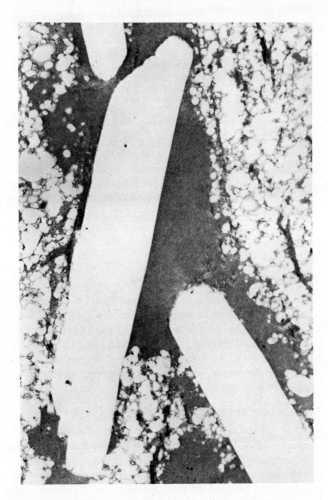

FIG. 10-19. Electron micrograph showing typical rhomboidal clear spaces left by cholesterol crystals.

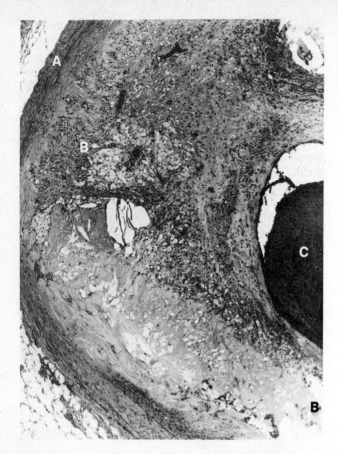

FIG. 10-21. Coronary artery atherosclerosis and thrombosis. The media *(A)* has been reduced to a thin rim; the arterial lumen has been obliterated by atheromatous plaque (extending from *B* to *B*) on which a thrombus *(C)* has formed. The atheromatous plaque shows a mixture of cellular components and fatty material.

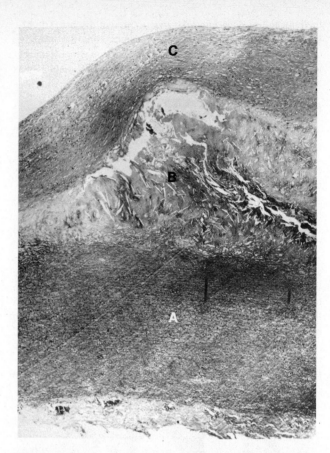

FIG. 10-22. Higher power view of part of Fig. 10-19. There is fatty atheromatous deposit *(B)* above the media *(A)* but overlain by the cellular cap *(C)*.

intima becomes grossly thickened and the surface of the plaque becomes rough and irregular. Blood vessels from the media also grow into the normally avascular intima.

The progress of the lesions from this stage onward is variable, and they may undergo one or more of the following changes:

1. *Fibrosis.* Fibrous scarring is common and may be followed by calcification.

2. *Thrombosis.* A thrombus usually forms gradually and in stages (Fig. 10-23). A thrombus is only likely to occlude arteries if the greater part of the lumen has already been obstructed by atherosclerosis.

3. *Rupture of atheromatous plaque.* Rupture of the fibrous cap overlying an atheromatous deposit can release fatty debris into the lumen of the artery. Blood can also penetrate the plaque and infiltrate beneath the intima. A thrombus can develop on the released material or as a consequence of blood entering the plaque. These changes can occlude arteries.

4. *Hemorrhage into atheromatous plaques.* As the intima becomes grossly thickened, blood vessels grow into it from its base. Hemorrhage from these capillaries may leak through the plaque and precipitate thrombosis in the lumen.

5. *Embolism.* Detachment of fatty material or development of a thrombus after the rupture of plaque are uncommon complications. The effects vary with the size of the embolus, but serious effects follow only if a relatively large vessel is blocked.

6. *Calcification.* Calcification tends mainly to affect severe lesions (especially in elderly patients), particularly at the edges of the fatty deposits and in the depths of the intima.

7. *Damage to the media.* Progress of the plaque leads to weakening of the arterial wall, damage to the media, and in some cases to aneurysm formation or rupture. This is important in the brain and aorta.

Regression of atherosclerosis

In animals, starvation or dietary modification causes only atheromatous plaques to regress. In humans, prolonged starvation may also have the same effect. The possibility of regression of advanced plaques, which are much more important, is more problematic. All that can be hoped at the moment is that dietary modifications may possibly prevent atheromatous plaques from progressing.

Distribution of atherosclerosis

As a general rule, atherosclerosis affects the more highly stressed vessels, but the distribution is erratic. The distribution of complicated lesions can also differ from that of fatty streaks. Severe, advanced lesions are found, especially in the aorta and coronary and cerebral arteries; nevertheless, the distribution seems also to be quite arbitrary. There may be severe aortic lesions but little in the coronary arteries or vice versa. The determinants of the distribution of atheroma are unclear.

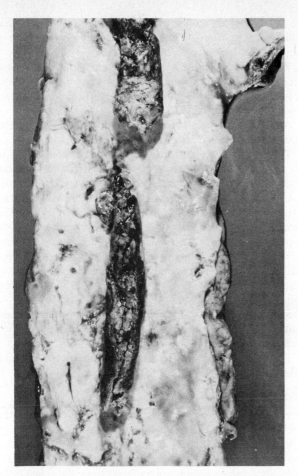

FIG. 10-23. Thrombus formation. Two large antemortem thrombi are shown lying in an atheromatous aorta. Note the pale, compact, and rather dry appearance of the thrombi.

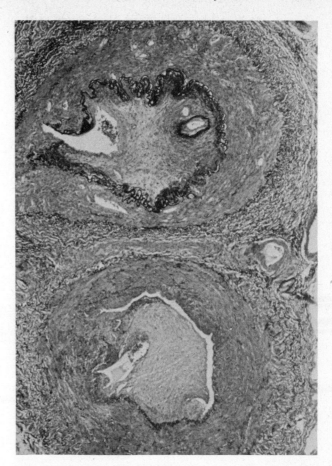

FIG. 10-24. Thromboangiitis obliterans (Buerger's disease). Inflammatory changes have involved the whole of the neurovascular bundle and caused almost complete obstruction of both vessels.

Effects of atherosclerosis in specific sites

Atherosclerosis is a major contributory factor to heart attacks and strokes. On the other hand, the majority of people reach old age with moderate or severe atherosclerosis and yet have no symptoms. The results of atherosclerosis are unpredictable, but when it causes disease, the main sites are as follows:

1. *The coronary arteries.* Occlusion causes ischemic heart disease.

2. *Cerebral arteries.* Effects are gradual narrowing, causing slow impairment of mental function; acute obstruction and cerebral infarction; or rupture, causing cerebral hemorrhage.

3. *Vertebral arteries.* Obstruction is an important cause of cerebral ischemia.

4. *The aorta.* Atherosclerosis in the aorta progresses in severity from its proximal to its distal segments. Plaques are frequently confluent below the renal arteries and tend to be particularly severe around the orifices of the lower aortic branches, causing ischemia. Aneurysm formation is a recognized but uncommon complication. The arch of the aorta, where hemodynamic stresses are greatest, is frequently unaffected; the lower end, where the stresses are presumably much less, is the main site. This is one of the unpredictable aspects of this disease.

5. *Leg arteries.* These are more frequently affected with advancing age. Increasing obstruction causes ischemic muscle pain on exercise and limping *(intermittent claudication)*. More severe disease can cause gangrene of the foot and lower leg.

Other arterial diseases
Mönckeberg's medial calcific sclerosis

Mönckeberg's sclerosis* produces dramatic appearances on radiographs. It is not, however, an important arterial disease because the lesions do not encroach on the vessel lumen or impede blood flow. This disease is seen only in the elderly and is characterized by calcification within the media of medium-sized arteries. In extreme cases a length of the vessel, such as the radial artery, is converted into a hard, calcified tube.

Thromboangiitis obliterans

Thromboangiitis obliterans, also known as Buerger's disease,† is a hazard of cigarette smoking, especially in men between ages 20 and 40. It is characterized by inflammation and thrombosis of medium-sized arteries, especially of the legs and to a lesser extent the arms. The inflammatory changes often involve adjacent veins or even nerves (Fig. 10-24).

The arterial walls show a nonspecific inflammatory reaction, together with thrombosis and varying degrees of organization and partial recanalization. The changes vary in severity, but the common and characteristic result is fibrous occlusion and

---

*J.G. Mönckeberg (1877-1925), German pathologist.
†L. Buerger (1879-1943), American urologist.

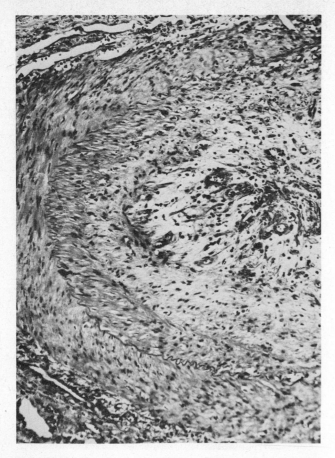

FIG. 10-25. Thromboangiitis obliterans (Buerger's disease). This high-power view shows complete occlusion of an artery as a result of thrombosis and organization.

periarterial scarring, which usually encircles an entire neurovascular bundle (Fig. 10-25).

The inflammatory changes produce red tender areas over superficial affected arteries. The course of the disease is unpredictable but in general is remittent and relapsing. In the mildest cases the development of collateral vessels may keep pace with obstruction of the arteries, and symptoms are slight. But the arterial changes frequently cause ischemia and coldness with pain, especially of the feet. There may also be intermittent claudication. The most severe cases can progress to gangrene of the extremities.

The most important measure in the management of Buerger's disease seems to be to stop the patient from using any form of tobacco.

Syphilitic arteritis and aortitis

Arteritis is a feature of all stages of syphilis, but tertiary disease can have severe effects. Syphilis is a common disease, but as a result of early effective treatment, tertiary stage disease has become rare.

Pathology. Syphilitic endarteritis is characterized by concentric intimal thickening of small vessels. There is a mononuclear infiltrate around their periphery (perivascular cuffing) extending into the adjacent connective tissue.

Syphilitic arteritis has its most severe effects on the vasa vasorum of the aorta. The consequences of the narrowing of these nutrient arteries are ischemic destruction of the elastic tissue and smooth muscle of the media and intima and their replacement by fibrous tissue. The changes are most severe in the region of the aortic arch.

Weakening of the media allows the aorta to dilate under the stress of the blood pressure and can produce a syphilitic aneurysm or cause dilatation of the aortic valve ring and incompetence.

A further effect of fibrosis resulting from syphilitic aortitis is stenosis of the orifices of the coronary arteries.

Typical syphilitic arteritis can affect the cerebral arteries in the tertiary stage. The lumen of smaller arteries can become obliterated, causing areas of cerebral ischemia and dysfunction.

Clinical aspects. The main consequence of syphilitic aortitis is cardiac disease, in particular, left ventricular failure. The incompetence of the aortic valve, together with great ventricular hypertrophy, leads to the characteristic collapsing (water hammer) pulse due to enormously powerful ejection of blood from the left ventricle. This is followed by immediate regurgitation during diastole. Thus a wide difference exists between systolic and diastolic pressures, that is, an elevated pulse pressure.

Stenosis of the coronary orifices, together with the low diastolic pressure, contributes to angina and occasionally to myocardial infarction.

The ultimate consequence is usually death from congestive heart failure. The most dramatic complication, however, is rupture of a syphilitic aneurysm and fatal hemorrhage.

Vasculitis

Vasculitis is inflammation of and damage to vessel walls, especially those of arteries (arteritis). Overall, vasculitis is a relatively common complication of infections, but is less often the predominant feature of a disease. Although rare, polyarteritis nodosa is a "classic" form of vasculitis in which all the features are secondary to the arterial damage.

Vasculitis is commonly assumed to be immune complex mediated (type 3 hypersensitivity reaction), and leakage of immunoglobulins and complement components through the damaged arterial wall may be detectable, but antigens can rarely be identified. Moreover, in at least one such disease, the predominantly cutaneous reaction known as bullous erythema multiforme, the immunologic findings are stated to be those of vasculitis, but histologic evidence of the latter is lacking.

Classification of different types of vasculitis is difficult and controversial. Classic polyarteritis nodosa, for example, is typically of unknown cause but is generally distinguished from hypersensitivity-mediated vasculitis. Nevertheless, an identical disease can be related to the hepatitis B antigen or result from the administration of a variety of drugs. Moreover, "hypersensitivity" vasculitis is usually, but confusingly, distinguished from "allergic" vasculitis.

As a further indication of the complexities involved in this group of diseases, lymphoid granulomatosis is commonly included, but mounting evidence (helped by the use of T-lymphocyte markers) has indicated that it is a T-cell lymphoma with strong angiocentric and angiodestructive propensities.

Since the cause of the majority of cases is unknown, the following classification is suggested:

I. Primary forms of vasculitis (of unknown cause but some with features suggestive of hypersensitivity reactions)
  A. Polyarteritis nodosa
  B. Churg-Strauss syndrome, hypersensitivity variant
  C. Vasculitis associated with giant cells

1. Giant cell (cranial) arteritis
2. Takayasu's (pulseless) disease
3. Wegener's granulomatosis
   D. Kawasaki disease
II. Vasculitis associated with connective tissue diseases*
III. Vasculitis associated with infections or drugs
   A. Viral infections, including hepatitis B and infectious mononucleosis
   B. Bacterial infections, including streptococci (Henoch-Schönlein purpura), infective endocarditis, and syphilis
   C. Rickettsial infections
   D. Serum sickness
   E. Drug reactions (usually serum sickness–type reactions, but sometimes polyarteritis nodosa)

Polyarteritis nodosa

Polyarteritis nodosa is characterized by foci of necrotizing inflammation of medium-sized arteries with a random distribution of lesions and an episodic course producing highly variable clinical effects.

Polyarteritis nodosa is probably immunologically mediated. It may be a complication of the use of various drugs. Some patients have circulating antibodies to hepatitis B, and in such patients HB immune complexes may be detected in the walls of affected arteries.

Lesions can affect any medium-sized or small artery, particularly those of the kidneys, heart, skeletal muscles, liver, gastrointestinal tract, or, less often, subcutaneous tissues.

The inflammatory changes are patchy in localized segments of an artery, typically producing discrete nodules.

Microscopically, acute inflammation begins in the intima and media but extends to involve ultimately the entire thickness of the arterial wall and immediately surrounding tissues (Fig. 10-26). The characteristic picture is damage to the arterial wall associated with fibrinoid change (necrotizing vasculitis). The inflammatory infiltrate is mixed but eosinophils are occasionally present in great numbers. Thrombosis, aneurysm formation, and hemorrhage are possible effects of damage to the arterial wall.

Healing is by fibrosis, sometimes obliterating the lumen. The main effects of the arterial lesions are ischemia and infarction of the tissues supplied.

Clinical aspects. Fever, malaise, weakness, and loss of weight are often features of the acute phase, but the clinical picture is highly variable. Possible manifestations follow:

1. Renal involvement with pain, hematuria, and albuminuria, sometimes progressing to hypertension
2. Gastrointestinal tract lesions that can produce abdominal pain, diarrhea, and melena
3. Peripheral neuritis or spinal cord involvement
4. Subcutaneous or submucosal lesions that produce inflamed tender swellings readily mistaken for a local infection; diagnosis can be confirmed by biopsy

The course is completely unpredictable. Often the disease persists, with acute recurrences for years until a vital organ, particularly the kidney, is irreversibly damaged. The progress can be modified by giving corticosteroids or other immunosuppressive drugs. In a few cases it appears that the disease

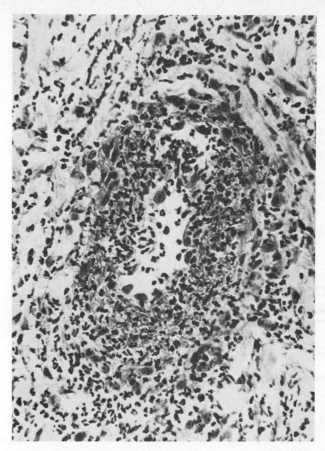

FIG. 10-26. Polyarteritis nodosa. This arteriole is surrounded, and its fine structure is obliterated by inflammatory cellular infiltrate. A few swollen endothelial cells are protruding into the arteriolar lumen. This biopsy specimen is from a girl of 19 with small submucosal oral swellings. She also had peripheral neuritis and evidence of mild renal involvement.

can be acute, but self-limiting and after a few weeks or months does not recur.

Churg-Strauss syndrome

In Churg-Strauss syndrome* the vasculitic lesions are indistinguishable microscopically from polyarteritis nodosa, but pulmonary disease (asthma) is typical. Eosinophilia and extravascular granuloma formation are also features (hence the alternative name, allergic granulomatosis and angiitis), and lesions may also involve the skin or nerves. The cause and any immunologic basis for this condition are unknown.

Giant cell arteritis

Giant cell arteritis, also known as cranial or temporal arteritis, is characterized by patchy granulomatous inflammatory lesions of large- and medium-sized arteries but is most conspicuous when the temporal arteries are affected.

Etiology. The cause is unknown. Abnormalities in serum proteins, including high γ-globulin levels and a greatly raised erythrocyte sedimentation rate, have led to the belief that this is an immunologic disorder. However, no characteristic im-

---

*Vasculitis is a major feature of systemic lupus erythematosus but can also be associated with any of the connective tissue diseases (Chapter 7).

*J. Churg (b. 1910), American clinical pathologist; L. Strauss (b. 1913), American pathologist.

munologic abnormalities are found, and the disease is unrelated to connective tissue diseases (Chapter 7).

Pathology. In addition to the temporal and other cranial arteries, the aorta and its branches can be affected (Fig. 10-27). The disease produces nodular swellings. The temporal artery is most conspicuous and becomes firm, swollen, and tortuous, often with inflammation of the overlying skin.

Histologically, inflammation involves both the media and intima. There is infiltration of mononuclear cells typically associated with multinucleate giant cells. The intimal damage leads to formation of thrombi, which usually become organized. Severe changes in the internal elastic lamina, sometimes going on to complete destruction, are also characteristic. Healing is by fibrosis, particularly of the media, thickening of the intima, and partial recanalization of the thrombus.

Clinical aspects. Giant cell arteritis is rare in persons under age 55. It is a relatively common cause of sudden onset of severe headache after middle age.

The disease may start as an influenza-like illness with malaise, weakness, low-grade fever, and weight loss. More specific symptoms depend on the vessels involved. The best known is involvement of the cranial arteries, with severe throbbing headache and tenderness over affected vessels (Fig. 10-28). Involvement of the ophthalmic artery causes disturbances of vision or sudden blindness.

More widespread systemic involvement causes diffuse ische-mic muscle pain on exercise; a condition known as *polymyalgia rheumatica* (Chapter 17).

In about 20% of cases giant cell arteritis can also cause ischemia of the masticatory muscles and pain during mastication. Investigation for cranial arteritis is essential when this symptom suddenly develops in an older person, because damage to sight may follow.

Diagnosis can be confirmed by biopsy when an affected artery is accessible but, in typical cases the clinical features are so distinctive as to be virtually diagnostic.

Giant cell arteritis in most cases follows a fairly benign course and eventually undergoes spontaneous remission. The onset of complications, particularly visual disturbances, makes it essential to establish the diagnosis and to give systemic corticosteroids immediately. These are usually quickly effective and should be continued until the erythrocyte sedimentation rate falls to normal.

Takayasu's disease

The chief clinical features of this uncommon disease,* also called pulseless disease, are complete or almost complete absence of pulses at the wrists, visual disturbances, and often cerebrovascular complications. Most patients are young women, frequently of Asian origin.

Takayasu's disease is an arteritis of the aortic arch or its branches with effects corresponding to the branches affected.

---

*M. Takayasu (1860-1938), Japanese ophthalmologist.

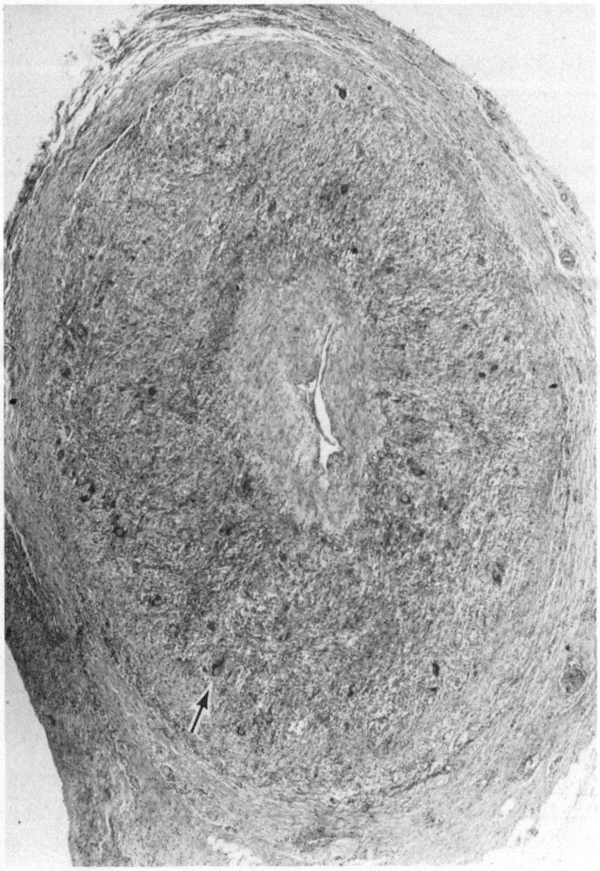

FIG. 10-27. Giant cell (cranial) arteritis. The lumen is almost obliterated by inflammation and fibrous proliferation. Giant cells are difficult to see at this low magnification *(arrow).*

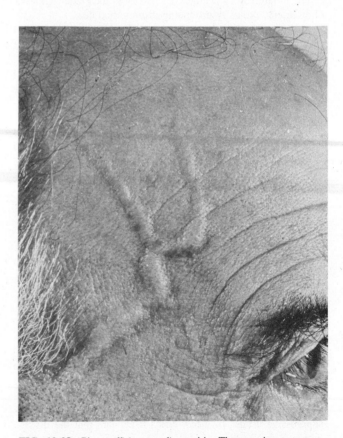

FIG. 10-28. Giant cell (temporal) arteritis. The prominent, tortuous appearance of the temporal artery is typical. *(Courtesy Curator of the Gordon Museum, Guy's Hospital, London, England.)*

Microscopically, mononuclear cells infiltrate the media and adventitia, often associated with giant cells and sometimes granuloma formation. Obstruction to arteries in the arms can lead to raised blood pressure in the lower extremities.

Because of the risk of blindness or strokes, treatment with bypass grafts is necessary to restore an adequate blood flow beyond the obstructed vessels.

Wegener's granulomatosis

Wegener's granulomatosis,* like polyarteritis nodosa, is rare and also thought to be immunologically mediated, although the immunologic findings are variable and of no value in diagnosis. The disease is characterized by acute necrotizing vasculitis and granulomatous lesions, particularly of the upper respiratory tract, where it can destroy the nasal septum and is a recognized cause of midline granuloma syndrome (Chapter 12). The lower respiratory tract is frequently also involved, but the most severe effects are on the kidneys.

Pathology. The main feature is an acute focal necrotizing arteritis resembling polyarteritis nodosa. However, giant cells near the affected arteries are typical of Wegener's granulomatosis. Necrotizing focal or diffuse proliferative glomerulonephritis is often fatal.

Clinical aspects. The onset of the disease is highly variable, but a characteristic presentation resembles acute sinusitis with suppurative discharge and bleeding (epistaxis) from the nose. Alternatively, Wegener's granulomatosis can occasionally produce characteristic gingival lesions ("strawberry gums") as the first sign. Death in renal failure is the usual outcome. Immunosuppressive treatment can cause remission.

Kawasaki's disease

Kawasaki's disease† is a cause of vasculitis in children but is somewhat similar to polyarteritis nodosa. It is seen frequently in Japan and less frequently in the United States and Europe. It is described in Chapter 8.

Peripheral vascular disease
Raynaud's disease and phenomenon

Raynaud's disease* is a common peripheral vascular disorder in which digital arteries become spastic as an exaggerated physiologic response to exposure to cold. The vascular spasm can also be precipitated by emotional or other factors and is common in otherwise healthy young women. In an attack, the fingers become pale or cyanotic and often painful. Warming is followed by erythema and recovery.

Raynaud's phenomenon, by contrast, is associated with connective tissue diseases, in which it tends to be more severe and persistent. Ischemic damage to the nails and peripheral skin, or even gangrene can result.

Raynaud's phenomenon can also result from other conditions such as occlusive vascular disease or occupations involving vibratory trauma to the hands.

Intermittent claudication

Claudication literally means limping; it is due to ischemic pain in the calves during exercise. The ischemia in most cases is due to atherosclerosis but can be caused by thromboangiitis obliterans.

Intermittent claudication itself is benign, and spontaneous improvement is common. About 40% of patients improve and 40% remain unchanged; only 20% need surgery, but about half of these require amputation. By contrast, the underlying disease is more dangerous, and there is a mortality of 20%, mainly from myocardial infarction, up to 12 years from the onset of claudication. The management of claudication is therefore the same as that for ischemic heart disease.

The less common arterial diseases are summarized in Table 10-4.

*M. Raynaud (1834-1881), French physician.

*F. Wegener (b. 1907), German pathologist.
†T. Kawasaki, Japanese pediatrician.

TABLE 10-4. Summary of the less common arterial diseases

Disease	Vessels involved	Age and sex	Pathologic vascular changes	Main symptoms
Medial calcific stenosis (Mönckeberg)	Medium-sized arteries	>50	Calcification of media; no obstruction	None; artery is hard; no impedance of blood flow
Thromboangiitis obliterans (Buerger)	Medium-sized vessels (e.g., tibial arteries and veins)	Young males who smoke	Acute inflammation of arterial and venous walls; involves adjacent structures (e.g., nerve trunks)	Thrombophlebitis; ischemic changes in extremities (e.g., gangrene of toes)
Giant cell arteritis	Large and medium arteries (e.g., temporal)	Elderly	Granulomatous inflammation with giant cells in arterial wall; vascular obstruction	Temporal pain, tenderness, sudden blindness (cranial arteries) Polymyalgia rheumatica
Syphilitic arteritis	Small arteries, especially of aortic wall	M > F; >40	Chronic inflammation and fibrosis of small arteries	Aortic aneurysm
Radiation arteritis	Arteries in irradiated areas	Any	Intimal and medial fibrosis and obliteration	Ischemia; aseptic necrosis of, for example, jaw bone; susceptibility to infection
Polyarteritis nodosa	Muscular arteries	Adults	Necrotizing inflammation of vessel walls	Renal, cardiac; hepatic or gastrointestinal ischemia
Wegener's granulomatosis	Arteries; arterioles	Adults of either sex	Local necrotizing arteritis and granulomas with giant cells	Respiratory tract, kidneys, spleen
Raynaud's disease	Small arteries (e.g., digital)	Young females	Virtually none	Pallor cyanosis of extremities

Aneurysms

An aneurysm is a localized dilatation of a blood vessel caused by an area of weakness of the wall. In large arteries this results from defects of or damage to the media. Increased stress on the arterial wall by hypertension is an important contributory factor.

Aneurysms are usually spindle shaped (fusiform) or saccular (Fig. 10-29). Their chief danger is that of rupture, which often kills the patient. The main types of aneurysms follow:

1. Syphilitic
2. Atherosclerotic
3. Dissecting
4. Congenital
5. Ventricular
6. Mycotic
7. Traumatic

Syphilis, atherosclerosis, and medial necrosis are the main causes of aortic aneurysm. The most common and important site of congenital aneurysms is the circle of Willis; they are a major cause of subarachnoid hemorrhage (Chapter 20).

Syphilitic aneurysms

Syphilitic aneurysms are mainly of historical interest and are now the least common cause of aortic aneurysm. The mechanism of production of the syphilitic aneurysm has been described earlier.

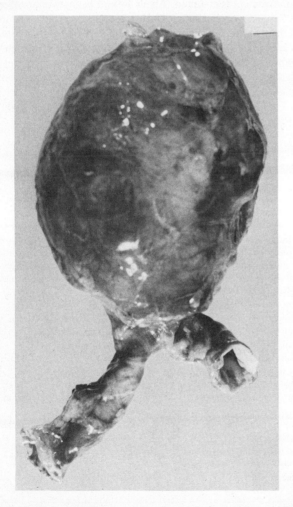

FIG. 10-29. A large saccular aneurysm arising from the internal iliac artery, which was severely atherosclerotic.

Syphilitic aneurysms affect the ascending aorta and arch, which are otherwise rarely affected. These aneurysms can reach an enormous size.

Clinically, in addition to the cardiovascular effects of aortitis, a syphilitic aneurysm produces effects by pressure on adjacent structures, such as the esophagus, trachea or bronchi, nerves, and great veins. Erosion of the chest wall is also characteristic, causes severe pain, and allows the pulsatile swelling to reach the surface.

The result, death, is most often from left ventricular failure. Rarely, this type of aneurysm was the cause of one of the most dramatic terminations of this, or any other, disease, when it burst and projected a fountain of blood through the eroded chest wall.

Atherosclerotic aneurysms

Atherosclerosis affects the abdominal aorta most severely and, although it is an uncommon complication of this disease, it is probably the most frequent cause of aortic aneurysms. They are usually fusiform. Thrombus formation on the large area of atheromatous plaque can sometimes fill the aneurysm.

Clinically, most patients are men over 50 and in at least 50% of cases are hypertensive. Atherosclerotic aortic aneurysms typically produce a pulsatile swelling in the middle of the upper abdomen and often abdominal or back pain.

Surgical repair is possible in selected cases and may be needed to relieve symptoms; large or rapidly expanding aneurysms have a high risk of rupture. Patients whose aneurysms rupture, if treated by skilled surgery without delay, have a survival rate of 50%.

The essential problem, however, is that atherosclerotic aneurysm of the aorta is usually only one aspect of widespread disease, and at least half these patients have ischemic heart disease.

Acute aortic dissection

This is a common disease, also known as dissecting aneurysm, that is frequently confused clinically with myocardial infarction because it causes similar symptoms and effects.

The older term, dissecting aneurysm, is misleading because there is little significant dilatation of the aorta. Instead, there is splitting of the media, allowing blood to extravasate between the layers of the aortic wall. Blood enters this zone through a tear in the intima and such a tear can usually (but not invariably) be found. Dissection can spread along branches of the aorta or burst into the surrounding tissues or body cavities. Spread of the dissection or blockage of their lumens by clot can cause fatal ischemia of the brain, heart, or kidneys according to how far the process spreads.

Aortic dissection results from weakening of the aortic wall (Fig. 10-30) from a variety of possible causes. An important example is medial cystic necrosis in which there is loss of muscle and elastic fibers in the media, associated with accumulations of proteoglycans ("mucoid"). The cause of medial cystic necrosis is unknown, and it is a common postmortem finding even in the absence of aortic dissection. Aortic dissection can also be a complication of Marfan's syndrome (Chapter 7) in which there is a heritable defect of collagen formation. The main feature, however, common to most cases of aortic dissecting aneurysms is hypertension.

Clinically, the majority of patients are men of middle age or older except when dissection is associated with Marfan's syndrome or pregnancy. Because the typical symptom is acute,

agonizingly severe chest pain, aortic dissection is frequently mistaken for myocardial infarction. Also, like the latter, sudden death can follow, particularly if the aneurysm ruptures. In other cases, death may follow later from ischemia of a vital organ, but in a few cases there is spontaneous healing or recanalization.

The diagnosis of aortic dissection can usually be made antemortem, by the clinical features, lack of ECG and other changes typical of myocardial infarction and, definitively, by angiography. Many cases can be successfully treated (depending on the extent of spread of the dissection) by surgery or by vigorous antihypertensive therapy.

Congenital aneurysms

Congenital aneurysms are often called berry aneurysms because of their shape and color. They form in cerebral arteries of the circle of Willis. They are the main cause of subarachnoid hemorrhage (Chapter 20), since the aneurysmal wall consists of little more than intima and readily ruptures.

Ventricular aneurysms

Aneurysm of the ventricular wall is a complication of myocardial infarction. These aneurysms result from replacement of

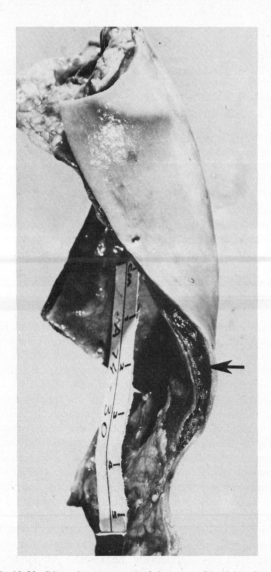

FIG. 10-30. Dissecting aneurysm of the aorta. Blood has forced a false channel *(arrow)* between the layers of the aorta.

the necrotic areas of muscle by a relatively thin fibrous tissue. The latter not only fails to contract but also bulges during systole and so reduces the heart's efficiency.

These aneurysms rarely burst but contribute to congestive heart failure and are also a site of thrombus formation. Systemic emboli can therefore be released.

Mycotic aneurysms

Mycotic aneurysm is a misleading name for damage to the wall of an artery by bacterial infection of a thrombus. Cerebral arteries are most often affected, usually as a complication of infective endocarditis.

Damage to the arterial wall is usually so severe that these aneurysms rupture while still minute in size.

Traumatic aneurysms

These are rare complications of physical injuries, such as stab or gunshot wounds. Trauma causes false aneurysms in most cases, because the vessel wall is usually perforated by the injury, and the outer wall of the aneurysm is formed by the adjacent tissues and organizing hematoma.

An abnormal communication between arteries and veins is another possible consequence of trauma and is termed an *arteriovenous aneurysm (AV fistula)*.

Diseases of veins
Varicose veins

Varicose veins are abnormally dilated and tortuous veins, caused by increased venous pressure or disease of the venous wall. Virtually any veins can be affected but the superficial leg veins are most frequently involved because of the increased venous pressure there. Venous pressure in the legs, when standing, is approximately five times that during recumbency. Pregnancy is an important precipitating or exacerbating factor as a result of pressure of the gravid uterus on the iliac veins. In addition, any condition that contributes to weakening of the connective tissue support of the veins increases susceptibility to this disorder, but there also appears to be a genetic element.

Microscopically there is irregular thinning of the vein wall, as well as areas of compensatory thickening and thromboses. In addition, there are deformities of the valves; these are predominantly secondary to the dilatation of and thromboses in the veins but also worsen the varicosities.

The most important secondary effects of varicose veins are varicose ulcers and thromboses. Bleeding is not a significant complication.

Varicose ulcers are persistent trophic ulcers of the leg that result in part at least, from the impaired circulation. Bacterial colonization of these ulcers is almost invariable but their etiology is complex and the management is difficult. Clinically similar ulcers can also result from arterial disease.

Esophageal varices are dilated esophageal veins. They are a typical complication of portal hypertension, resulting from cirrhosis of the liver (Chapter 15). Bleeding from esophageal varices can be fatal.

Hemorrhoids are dilated rectal and anal veins. Constipation and pregnancy are important predisposing factors but occasionally they are secondary to venous obstruction by a tumor. Bleeding during defecation is almost invariable but can be so persistent as to cause iron deficiency anemia. In severe cases the veins can prolapse through the anus and become strangulated and infected.

Tumors of blood vessels
Pyogenic granuloma

This is a common vascular tumorlike hyperplastic lesion affecting the skin or oral mucous membranes. It is thought to be a reaction to minor injury.

Clinically, pyogenic granuloma forms a rapidly growing nodule that may reach a centimeter in diameter. It is red because of the prominent vascular component and bleeds readily.

Microscopically, the main feature is the presence of wide vascular spaces in a loose edematous connective tissue stroma, together with a widespread and often dense acute inflammatory infiltrate in most cases. Despite the name, pus production is not a feature and the older name, granuloma telangiectaticum, is more appropriate but less convenient.

A histologically identical lesion sometimes develops on the gum margins during pregnancy (pregnancy epulis).

Pyogenic granuloma responds to excision, which also allows the diagnosis to be confirmed, but it is probably a self-limiting condition.

Hemangioma

A hemangioma is not a true tumor, but a malformation (hamartoma) consisting either of a mass of fine capillaries (capillary hemangioma) or large thin-walled sinusoids (cavernous hemangioma) (Fig. 10-31). Hemangiomas are typically congenital, developmental anomalies affecting the skin (nevi, birthmarks). When located on the face, they sometimes extend to involve the underlying oral mucous membrane and gingival tissues, (mucocutaneous angiomatosis) and a particularly severe form is the Sturge-Weber syndrome in which the meninges of the same side are also affected (Chapter 20).

Clinically, superficial hemangiomas appear as bluish or red areas on the skin or as raised lesions of varying extent. Prominent cavernous hemangiomas in the mouth can be traumatized and bleed severely.

Rare intraosseous hemangiomas produce loculated areas of radiolucency, the nature of which may not become apparent until operation or biopsy is attempted.

Hemangiomas can undergo neoplastic change, as discussed in Chapter 14.

Leiomyoma

Vascular leiomyoma is a benign tumor that can arise from the smooth muscle of blood vessel walls. It consists of interlacing strands of smooth muscle cells of small blood vessels.

Other vascular tumors

Hemangioendotheliomas arise from endothelial cells, whereas hemangiopericytomas arise from the pericytes that proliferate outside the reticulin sheath of capillaries. The glomus tumor is a painful subcutaneous variant of hemangiopericytoma. Malignant variants (angiosarcomas) of these benign tumors also exist. All are rare.

Kaposi's sarcoma

From having been one of the least frequently seen tumors in the United States, Kaposi's sarcoma* has become common as a result of the spread of acquired immunodeficiency syndrome (AIDS).

---

*M.K. Kaposi (1837-1902), Hungarian dermatologist.

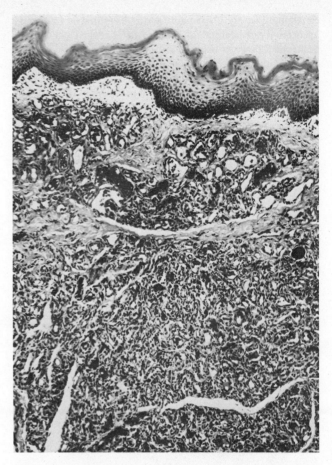

FIG. 10-31. Capillary hemangioma. The lesion consists of vast numbers of fine capillaries, many of which (more deeply) are imperforate and consist of rosettes of endothelial cells.

As originally described in 1872, Kaposi's sarcoma was a rare entity, affecting elderly persons of central European or Mediterranean origin. Later it was found to be common in Central Africa where, in some areas, it formed up to 12% of all malignant tumors. At this time Kaposi's sarcoma affected the lower extremities and usually had an indolent course, with late involvement of viscera. In AIDS-related cases, by contrast, Kaposi's sarcoma is often seen in young adults and typically affects the upper part of the body. The head and neck area, including the mouth, are frequently involved, but the tumor has been reported in many sites. Kaposi's sarcoma can be a complication of immunosuppressive treatment, with a similar site distribution as that seen in persons with AIDS.

Pathology. Kaposi's sarcoma (Fig. 10-32) appears to be of endothelial origin, as indicated by the presence of the factor VIII marker in the cells. The microscopic features depend largely on the stage of development of the tumor. Early, in the "presarcomatous" stage, angiomatous proliferation resembles granulation tissue, with formation of irregular capillary-like channels with perivascular cuffing by lymphocytes and plasma cells. If cutaneous or mucosal, trauma may be superadded and make diagnosis at this stage difficult. In the intermediate stages, the angiomatoid proliferation becomes widespread with formation of vast numbers of fine vascular channels that appear slitlike when cut longitudinally. Perivascular proliferation of spindle-shaped and angular cells is associated. Ultimately, these

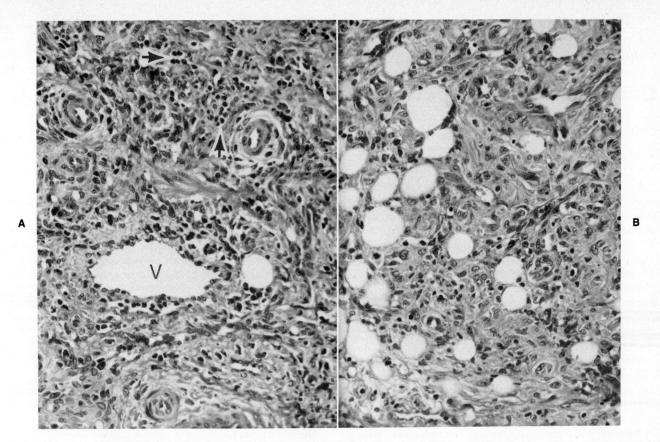

FIG. 10-32. Kaposi's sarcoma. **A,** Soft tissue invasion by oval and spindle-shaped cells. Many small, cleftlike vascular spaces *(arrows)* are filled with red blood cells. Note typical lymphocytic infiltration around vessel *(V)*. **B,** Section from same patient shows infiltration of fatty tissue by tumor cells.

latter cells dominate the picture, mitotic activity becomes conspicuous, and there is frequently extravasation of erythrocytes leading to deposition of hemosiderin. Central necrosis may develop.

The etiology of Kaposi's sarcoma is unknown. A seroepidemiologic association with cytomegalovirus (an infection commonly associated with AIDS) has been reported but also disputed. It is frequently assumed, however, that the immunodeficiency of AIDS releases the oncogenic potential of some virus, which remains unidentified. A genetic component may also exist in that in both AIDS-associated and African Kaposi's sarcoma have a strong association with HLA-DR5.

For unknown reasons, Kaposi's sarcoma is common in male homosexuals with AIDS, but rare among hemophiliacs who have acquired the disease from contaminated blood products.

Clinically, Kaposi's sarcoma in AIDS typically appears as purplish-red macular areas in the skin or mucous membranes of the head and neck region of at least 50% of patients. Lesions in viscera and other sites frequently develop early in the course of the disease.

The response to chemotherapy is poor, and most AIDS patients with this tumor die from infections secondary to the immunodeficiency.

Selected readings

Kaplan NM and Meese RB: The calcium deficiency hypothesis of hypertension: a critique, Ann Intern Med 105:947, 1986.

Kent KM: Coronary angioplasty, N Engl J Med 316:1148, 1987.

Hypertension: Is there a place for calcium? Lancet i:359, 1986.

McCluskey RT and Fienberg R: Vasculitis in primary vasculitides, granulomatoses, and connective tissue diseases, Hum Pathol 14:305, 1983.

Miller NE: Associations of high-density lipoprotein subclasses and apolipoproteins with ischemic heart disease and coronary atherosclerosis, Am Heart J 113:589, 1987.

Paulin S: Assessing the severity of coronary lesions with angiography, N Engl J Med 316:1405, 1987.

Pietinen P and Huttunen JK: Dietary determinants of plasma high-density lipoprotein cholesterol, Am Heart J 113:620, 1987.

Resnick LM, Miller FB, and Laragh JH: Calcium-regulating hormones in essential hypertension, Ann Intern Med 105:649, 1986.

Ross R: The pathogenesis of atherosclerosis—an update, N Engl J Med 314:488, 1986.

Schwartz SM and Reidy MA: Common mechanisms of proliferation of smooth muscle in atherosclerosis and hypertension, Hum Pathol 18:240, 1987.

Shiels RA: A history of Kaposi's sarcoma, J R Soc Med 79:532, 1986.

Steinberg D: Lipoproteins and atherosclerosis: some unanswered questions, Am Heart J 113:626, 1987.

Yanagawa H, et al: Nationwide epidemic of Kawasaki disease in Japan during winter of 1985-86, Lancet ii:1138, 1986.

CHAPTER 11

Cardiovascular disease: diseases of the heart

Diseases of the heart are very common and are usually serious. Ischemic heart disease and hypertension are the leading causes of death today. The heart may sometimes be primarily affected, as in congenital heart disease, but it is more frequently damaged as a result of disease that initially involves blood vessels, lungs, or other organs. Whatever the cause of heart disease, the result in many instances is *heart failure*.

Methods of examining the cardiovascular system have been discussed at the beginning of Chapter 10.

Types of heart disease

The main types of heart disease are as follows:

1. Valvular disease. Abnormal function of the heart valves can greatly reduce the efficiency of the heart and overstress it. Valvular disease can be congenital or acquired.

2. Disorders of the conducting system. Serious disturbances of heart rhythm or excessively slow or fast beating can greatly affect cardiac output and have severe consequences.

3. Disease of the heart muscle. Disease of the heart muscle can be intrinsic, as in the cardiomyopathies, or a result of infection, but more commonly it results from ischemic damage due to coronary artery occlusion.

4. Disease of the pericardium. Fibrosis of the pericardium or accumulation of fluid in the pericardial sac can severely restrict the movement of the heart.

Heart failure

Heart failure is present when the cardiac output becomes insufficient for the metabolic needs of the tissues. Failure is a relative term and results from the heart's inability to respond to the load imposed on it.

Heart failure can be acute but is more often chronic. *Acute failure* is present when cardiac output is grossly reduced, such as after a massive myocardial infarct. *Chronic failure* develops when the heart can no longer compensate for a defect that has been present for some time. Defects of cardiac valves as a result of rheumatic fever can cause failure of this type.

The main causes of heart failure are as follows:
1. Myocardial diseases
2. Excessive outflow resistance (e.g., hypertension and aortic or pulmonary stenosis)
3. Excessive afterload (incomplete emptying of the heart) (e.g., aortic or mitral regurgitation)
4. Increased metabolic demands, as in thyrotoxicosis and anemia

The most important causes are *hypertension*, which places a persistent and excessive load on the heart, and *coronary artery disease*, which, by causing myocardial ischemia, can greatly reduce pumping efficiency.

High- and low-output failure

Cardiac failure that is mainly the result of inadequate output is called *low-output failure*. Less frequently, extracardiac diseases such as anemia, pulmonary disease, or thyrotoxicosis can also lead to cardiac failure. The cardiac output is increased in such conditions, but it cannot provide adequate oxygenation for the demands of the tissues. This is known as *high-output failure*. Sooner or later, however, in high-output failure the heart succumbs to the excessive load or impaired oxygenation; output declines and low-output failure develops.

Pathophysiologic aspects

The functional aspects of heart failure in many cases are more important than morphologic cardiac changes. The normal heart can pump out all the venous blood returned to it. Because cardiac output depends on the venous return (Frank-Starling principle*), the ventricles empty more fully during exercise. The heart beats faster and ejects a larger volume of blood at each contraction (increased stroke volume). The normal heart therefore has great functional reserves and during violent exercise can increase its output to about five or six times its resting level.

The first clinical manifestation of failure is diminution of cardiac reserve, evidenced by a decreasing ability to perform exercise. Before this happens, however, the following compensatory mechanisms develop:
1. Hypertrophy of the myocardium
2. Increased blood volume
3. Increased adrenergic activity
4. Peripheral vasoconstriction

Hypertrophy of the myocardium. The heart enlarges as a consequence of an increase in muscle bulk. This enables the heart to pump more powerfully, but the extent of this improvement is limited.

Increased blood volume. The kidneys retain sodium and water by mechanisms discussed later. Sodium and water retention increases the blood volume and in turn the venous return and cardiac output.

Increased adrenergic activity. Increased levels of circulating catecholamines also contribute to the increased cardiac output and can cause widespread vasoconstriction.

Peripheral vasoconstriction. Peripheral vasoconstriction develops as heart failure advances, and blood is thus diverted from the skin and extremities to the heart, lungs, viscera, and muscles. At the same time, peripheral resistance imposes a greater load on the heart.

---

*A.E. Frank (1884-1957), German physician; E.H. Starling (1866-1927), English physiologist.

Systemic effects of heart failure

When the heart is failing, the ventricles gradually fail to empty completely, and venous pressure rises. Two main effects of cardiac failure account for most of the symptoms: reduced blood flow to and oxygenation of all tissues and congestion, that is, accumulation of blood in the tissues as a result of impaired venous drainage. The organs most severely affected are the kidneys, lungs, liver, spleen, and brain.

Kidneys. Because of inadequate cardiac output, the circulating volume decreases. The response to this is vasoconstriction and sodium retention by the kidney. Angiotensin II, norepinephrine, and vasopressin are also released in an apparent attempt to maintain adequate tissue perfusion, while the vasoconstrictor action of angiotensin II on the glomerular efferent arterioles (Chapter 10) maintains glomerular filtration. In addition to increasing perfusion pressure, norepinephrine may also increase sodium retention to some extent. Vasopressin acting on a renal receptor increases water reabsorption, as well as augmenting vasoconstriction. Although these findings have been confirmed in established heart failure, they appear to be anteceded by sodium and water retention triggered by mechanisms that are not yet fully understood but appear to be in part neurohumoral. Eventually the blood flow to the kidneys may become so inadequate that excretion is impaired and azotemia (increased nitrogenous compounds in the blood) develops.

Lungs. The main effects of left ventricular failure are pulmonary congestion and edema. When pressure rises in the pulmonary veins, fluid escapes from the thin-walled, congested alveolar capillaries, and edema develops readily.

Pulmonary edema has the immediate effect of impeding gaseous exchange. In the most extreme cases the patient can literally drown in his or her own secretions. This can happen when a patient has a myocardial infarct (causing acute left ventricular failure) and is then laid flat on the back with the idea of improving blood supply to the brain.

Eventually, persistent distention of the pulmonary capillaries leads to fibrous thickening of their walls, impairs gaseous exchange, and causes the lungs to become stiffer and less compliant. Leakage of blood from the congested capillaries often causes the sputum to be blood stained *(hemoptysis).* Damaged red blood cells accumulate in the alveoli and are engulfed by macrophages. These become laden with hemosiderin and are known as *heart failure cells* (Fig. 11-1).

Brain. In advanced cardiac failure, inadequate oxygenation of the brain can cause such symptoms as anxiety, loss of concentration, restlessness, and irritability. The effects are more severe in the elderly in whom the cerebral circulation is often already reduced by atherosclerosis.

Liver. Congestion and enlargement of the liver *(chronic passive venous congestion)* is characteristic of right ventricular failure. As the circulation fails, zone 3 of the acinus (the area

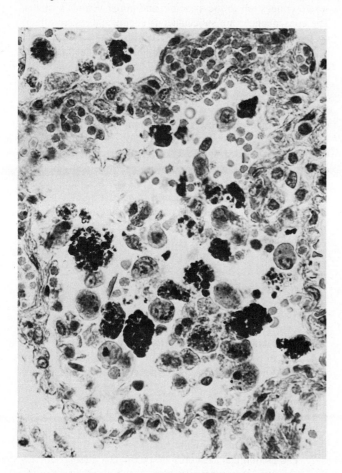

FIG. 11-1. Chronic passive congestion of the lung caused by left-sided heart failure. The pulmonary vessels are engorged; many alveoli are filled with red blood cells, and numerous hemosiderin-laden macrophages (heart failure cells) are seen.

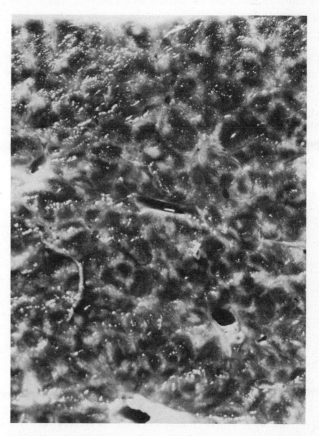

FIG. 11-2. Liver in chronic venous congestion. This close-up of the cut surface of the liver shows the pattern formed by alternating areas of vascular congestion surrounded by pale areas of liver cell necrosis. The appearance resembles the cut surface of a nutmeg. *(Courtesy Curator of the Gordon Museum, Guy's Hospital, London, England.)*

close to the hepatic vein) suffers most severely from hypoxia and may degenerate or die. Zone 1, close to the hepatic artery and portal vein, becomes dark red because of congestion, whereas the peripheral area (zone 3) becomes yellow as a result of fatty change (Chapter 14). The resulting mottled appearance of the liver resembles the cut surface of a nutmeg (nutmeg liver) (Fig. 11-2).

In severe but prolonged failure, the liver can become fibrotic (cardiac cirrhosis), but significant disturbance of liver function is an uncommon, late development.

Spleen. Venous congestion causes the spleen to become enlarged and mildly fibrotic.

Cyanosis

Cyanosis is the name given to the bluish color of mucous membranes (particularly the lips) and the skin. It is a sign of hypoxia and appears when the capillary blood contains more than 5 g of reduced hemoglobin per deciliter.

In heart failure, the blood moves sluggishly through the tissues and becomes excessively deoxygenated; this phenomenon is called *central cyanosis* (i.e., it is central in origin). A contributory factor to the cyanosis of heart failure is hypoxia of the marrow, which stimulates increased production of red blood cells *(secondary polycythemia)*. The inability to oxygenate this increased amount of hemoglobin causes cyanosis to deepen.

Central cyanosis, seen in the lips or within the mouth, is usually an indication of severely impaired cardiovascular or respiratory function, which can make general anesthesia hazardous.

By contrast, *peripheral cyanosis* is seen in the ears, nose, and fingertips of people exposed to extreme cold; the local circulation shuts down, causing excessive deoxygenation in the exposed areas.

Left-sided and right-sided heart failure

Cardiac failure can predominantly affect either the left or right ventricle. The causes and effects of left-sided failure differ from those of right-sided failure. However, failure of one side of the heart eventually leads to failure of the other, since the cardiovascular system is a closed circuit.

Left ventricular failure. The most common causes of left-sided heart failure are:
1. Coronary artery disease (atherosclerosis)
2. Hypertension
3. Aortic and mitral valvular disease

The cardinal features of left ventricular failure are:
1. Pulmonary venous congestion
2. Pulmonary edema
3. Left ventricular hypertrophy
4. Impaired blood supply to the brain and kidneys

Clinically, typical consequences of pulmonary edema are cough and difficulty in breathing (dyspnea) during exercise as early complaints; later, shortness of breath at rest becomes particularly distressing and characteristic. The sputum is frothy and pink with blood in severe cases.

When the patient is lying down, fluid can accumulate in the lungs in even greater quantities, and one of the most unpleasant consequences of left-sided failure is *paroxysmal nocturnal dyspnea (cardiac asthma)*, a sudden, terrifying attack of severe breathlessness that wakes the patient with a sensation of suffocation. As left-sided failure worsens, the patient cannot

TABLE 11-1. Main causes and effects of heart failure

	Left-sided heart failure	*Right-sided heart failure*
Main causes	Coronary artery disease	Cor pulmonale
	Hypertension	Sequel of left-sided failure
	Aortic and/or mitral disease	
Main effects	Pulmonary edema	Systemic edema
		Portal congestion
	Severe dyspnea	Hepatomegaly and splenomegaly
	Renal insufficiency	More severe renal insufficiency

breathe at all when lying down (orthopnea) and has to be propped up with pillows or must sleep sitting upright.

Right ventricular failure. Pure right-sided heart failure is uncommon. The main cause is *cor pulmonale*, which is heart disease secondary to pulmonary disorders that persistently overload the right ventricle.

Other causes of right-sided heart failure are left-sided failure, particularly when there is mitral valve stenosis; uncommon causes are tricuspid or pulmonary valve lesions and infarction of the right ventricle.

Right ventricular failure causes increased back pressure and severe congestion in the systemic and portal venous systems. The consequences are subcutaneous edema and severe effects on the liver, spleen, and kidneys, as already described.

Venous congestion also affects the gastrointestinal tract, causing loss of appetite, indigestion, nausea, and impaired absorption of food.

Another consequence of increased portal venous pressure is the escape of large amounts of fluid into the peritoneal cavity (ascites), which can cause gross abdominal distension.

Edema of the most dependent parts of the body is characteristic of right-sided heart failure. If the disease is severe or of very long standing, edema of the legs, abdomen, and even chest wall can be so massive that the body becomes grossly distended with fluid. This is termed *anasarca*.

The principles of treatment of heart failure are determined by the underlying pathology and comprise the following:
1. Relief of any underlying cause, such as hyperthyroidism or anemia or, in some cases, surgical replacement of a damaged valve.
2. Improving myocardial function by giving a cardiac glycoside such as digoxin.
3. Reducing fluid retention with diuretics, which can have a strikingly beneficial effect by reducing congestion and improving function of all affected tissues.
4. Use of vasodilators when there is widespread vasoconstriction may be helpful by reducing peripheral resistance and the load on the heart.

Summary (Table 11-1)
Left-sided heart failure
1. Coronary artery disease, hypertension, and aortic or mitral disease are the main causes.
2. The predominant features are pulmonary edema and progressive respiratory difficulty.

Right-sided heart failure
1. Cor pulmonale is the main cause.
2. The predominant effects are chronic venous congestion

and edema of dependent parts, particularly of the legs and abdomen.

Common features of heart failure

1. Failure of one side usually leads to failure of the other, producing the full-blown picture of congestive cardiac failure.
2. Both left-sided and right-sided heart failure reduce cerebral and renal blood flow, causing increasingly impaired function of the brain and kidneys.

Disorders of cardiac control

Disturbance of the regular heartbeat (arrhythmia) or gross changes in heart rate are usually the result of lesions of the sinoatrial or atrioventricular nodes or the conducting tissues. The chief effect of these disturbances is usually reduced cardiac output and sometimes increased oxygen demands by the myocardium.

Tachycardia is an increase in the heart rate. The rate of beating of the whole heart may be increased (sinus tachycardia) or the atria or ventricles alone may be affected.

Sinus tachycardia is a normal response to exercise or fear. It can also be the result of hyperthyroidism or a feature of acute cardiac failure when the myocardium may become overstressed and its oxygen demands outstrip the coronary blood supply.

Atrial tachycardia is often paroxysmal and of unknown cause. In an otherwise normal patient, this may cause no more than the sensation of palpitation. Filling of the ventricle can be reduced, however, causing faintness or breathlessness; if there is heart disease, ischemic pain or cardiac failure can result.

Paroxysmal atrial tachycardia can be accompanied by conduction defects causing varying degrees of heart block, but the ventricular rate may also be very rapid, and cardiac failure results. Alternatively, the ventricle may contract at a fraction of the atrial rate, and function is affected accordingly.

Atrial fibrillation is the name given to totally uncoordinated and ineffective atrial contraction and is the most common type of chronic arrhythmia. Common causes are rheumatic valve disease, ischemic heart disease, or thyrotoxicosis. The effects are impaired ventricular filling, and irregular but usually rapid ventricular rate, and often thrombus formation in the atrium. Untreated atrial fibrillation can therefore aggravate heart failure or cause embolic disease and is an important cause of strokes in the elderly.

Ventricular tachycardia, a persistently increased ventricular rate above about 140 beats per minute, is usually the result of serious disease, such as ischemic heart disease or digitalis overdose. Myocardial pain and heart failure or cardiac arrest are typical consequences.

Ventricular fibrillation, as discussed earlier, is the most serious type of arrhythmia. It is usually the result of acute myocardial ischemia and is the most common cause of sudden death. Other possible causes of ventricular fibrillation include sympathetic overactivity associated with halothane anesthesia or thyrotoxicosis or an overdose of epinephrine, cocaine, or digitalis.

Ventricular fibrillation may be terminated by applying a strong direct current (DC cardioversion) across the heart with an electrical defibrillator.

Cardiac arrest results from similar causes to those of fibrillation, of which it is often a consequence and from which it cannot be distinguished clinically. Cardiopulmonary resuscitation should be started immediately.

Sinus bradycardia, a heart rate below 60 beats per minute, is unimportant in a healthy young person. In the elderly, especially those with heart disease, bradycardia may cause sudden loss of consciousness *(syncope).*

In *sick sinus syndrome* the pacemaker function of the sinoatrial node is disordered. This can cause bradycardia, sinoatrial block, or atrial tachycardia or fibrillation. Bradycardia may be severe enough to cause circulatory failure and loss of consciousness. Alternatively, overrapid atrial contraction or fibrillation can have any of the effects described earlier.

In *sinoatrial block* the initial pacemaker impulse fails or comes at longer or irregular intervals. If many beats are lost, consciousness may be disturbed or lost.

Disorders of conduction (heart block)

Conduction can be blocked anywhere between the atrioventricular node to points on the branches of the bundle of His. The causes include ischemic heart disease, acute rheumatic fever, myocarditis, or drugs, particularly digitalis.

Minor degrees of heart block can only be detected on an electrocardiogram or as a slow pulse (beating at half the atrial rate, for example).

Complete heart block causes a regular pulse, usually of 30 to 40 beats a minute (idioventricular rhythm). The cardiac output is then so reduced as to cause pallor, loss of consciousness, and cyanosis. Recovery follows when the heart rate increases.

Conduction disturbances such as these can often be effectively treated by implanting an artificial pacemaker.

Congenital heart disease

Congenital heart disease includes developmental anomalies of the valves, of the heart itself, and of the adjacent great vessels. Congenital heart disease is probably present in about 1% of live births and is often associated with other developmental anomalies. The prognosis has been greatly improved by cardiac surgery; without such treatment, it is estimated that at least 40% of affected infants would die during the first 5 years of life. The early recognition of the precise nature of developmental cardiac anomalies is therefore of great practical importance because of the possibility of repair or at least amelioration of many of these defects.

Among school-age children congenital heart disease is now far more frequent than rheumatic heart disease, the incidence of which has steadily declined. Congenital malformations are the most common form of heart disease in children up to the age of 4 years.

The causes of developmental anomalies of the heart are not known, but both genetic and environmental factors may play a part. For example, genetic factors appear to be important in atrial septal defects, whereas the best-known environmental hazard is rubella during the first trimester of pregnancy. The role of other infections and drugs is more problematic. Congenital heart disease, especially atrial septal defect, is common in persons with Down's syndrome (Chapter 3).

General effects

There are too many congenital anomalies of the heart to discuss them in detail, but they have certain common features. Most interfere with the normal laminar flow of blood through the heart and great vessels. The resulting turbulence produces cardiac murmurs, which are sometimes dramatically loud. These anomalies also bring with them the risk of infective endocarditis.

Another common feature of many of these anomalies is that the blood can be short circuited through a defect in the heart or between the great vessels. These shunts can divert the blood from the right ventricle into the systemic circulation, bypassing the lungs (right-to-left shunt). The shunted blood is therefore not oxygenated, and cyanosis is obvious, often from birth (blue babies). If blood flows from left to right, part of the output of the right ventricle is recirculated through the lungs (left-to-right shunt). There is no cyanosis at first; however, this type of shunt tends to cause pulmonary hypertension, and eventually right ventricular hypertrophy becomes sufficient to reverse the shunt and cause *late-onset cyanosis* (cyanose tardive). The presence or absence of cyanosis forms the basis for classifying congenital heart disease (Table 11-2).

Ventricular septal defect

The site of ventricular septal defects (VSDs) is high, near the atrioventricular septum; their size varies from a minute pinhole to failure of formation of the whole septum. Very large VSDs usually cause death in infancy unless the defect is corrected, but survival into middle age is possible with smaller defects.

Blood initially flows from the stronger left ventricle to the right, causing enlargement of the latter. Where the jet of blood from the left ventricle hits the lining of the right ventricle, an area of endocardial thickening (jet lesion) can develop. Later pulmonary hypertension may develop and, if severe enough, can cause reversal of the direction of blood flow through the defect and late-onset cyanosis.

In the early stages, the main clinical sign is a loud systolic murmur synchronous with contraction of the ventricles; this sign is sometimes called a *machinery murmur*.

Surgical correction of the defect is usually successful, but in persons with uncorrected defects the most common cause of death is right-sided heart failure. Less often, infective endocarditis involves the margins of the defect or the jet lesion in the right ventricle.

Atrial septal defect

Females are affected more frequently than males by atrial septal defect (ASD) (Fig. 11-3). Survival into middle age is usual because the defect has relatively little effect on cardiac function. The main cause of death in ASD is right-sided heart failure. Infective endocarditis is rare. Occasionally, emboli pass through the septal defect from the right into the left side of the heart and the systemic circulation. This is known as *paradoxical embolism*. Surgical correction is usually successful.

Patent ductus arteriosus

The ductus arteriosus that joins the pulmonary artery to the aorta usually closes by the third month of life, but is sometimes delayed for up to a year. Patent ductus arteriosus may be an isolated lesion but is more often associated with other, adjacent malformations. The ductus may vary from a mere opening between the apposed pulmonary and aortic trunks to a distinct vessel about 1 cm in diameter. A patent ductus shunts blood from the aorta into the pulmonary artery.

Females are more often affected than males, and the most

TABLE 11-2. Classification of congenital heart disease

Disease	Percentage
Acyanotic congenital heart disease	
Ventricular septal defects	20 to 30
Atrial septal defects	10
Patent ductus arteriosus	13
Coarctation of the aorta	10
Isolated pulmonary stenosis	10
Cyanotic congenital heart disease	
Transposition of great vessels	10
Tetralogy of Fallot	10

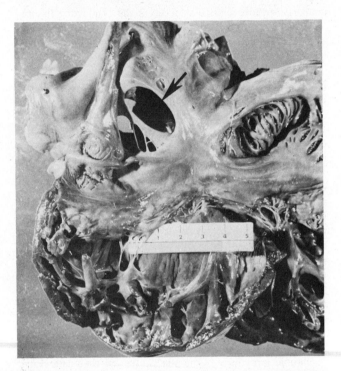

FIG. 11-3. The heart has been opened to show a large patent foramen ovale (atrial septal defect) *(arrow).*

striking feature is a loud, continuous, sawing, systolic-diastolic murmur.

Patent ductus is compatible with survival into middle age, but if uncorrected, the usual cause of death is right-sided heart failure; infective endocarditis is also a hazard. A patent ductus is, however, readily correctable by surgery.

A patent ductus can be beneficial when associated with other congenital defects, particularly when there is obstruction to the outflow from the right ventricle as in the case of transposition of the great vessels. Under these circumstances a patent ductus can provide sufficient collateral pulmonary blood flow to maintain life. This collateral flow is usually only for a limited time because the ductus progressively constricts in most cases.

Normal closure of the ductus arteriosus appears to be determined by certain prostaglandins, whereas other prostaglandins maintain its patency. In preterm infants, a patent ductus can often be closed by giving indomethacin, an inhibitor of prostaglandin synthesis. For patients in whom continued pa-

TABLE 11-3. Hemodynamic features of congenital heart disease

Defect	Direction of shunt	Cyanosis	Effects and complications*
Ventricular septal defect	L →→ R Later R →→ L (sometimes)	None unless R →→ L shunt develops	RVF IE
Atrial septal defect	Little effect	Absent	RVF Paradoxical emboli IE
Patent ductus arteriosus (aorta opens into pulmonary artery)		Absent	RVF IE
Coarctation of aorta	None	Absent	"Upper half" hypertension Aortic aneurysm IE Cerebral hemorrhage
Transposition of great vessels (origins of aorta and pulmonary artery reversed)	R →→ L	Severe	Rapid congestive heart failure

Tetralogy of Fallot
  Pulmonary stenosis
  Ventricular septal defect
  Straddling of interventricular septum by aorta
  Right ventricle hypertrophy
	R →→ L	Severe	Syncope
			Heart failure
			Respiratory tract infection
			IE

*RVF, Right ventricular failure; IE, infective endocarditis.

tency of the ductus is essential, prostaglandin E_1 is administered. This overcomes the problem of progressive hypoxia and often death before elective surgery can be carried out.

Coarctation of the aorta

Coarctation is a narrowing of the aorta, usually distal to the subclavian arteries. As a result, blood reaches the upper half of the body normally, but the blood supply to the lower half of the body is restricted or depends on collateral vessels. The condition is detectable by stronger than normal pulses at the wrist but weak or absent femoral pulses. More than 50% of these patients also have a bicuspid aortic valve.

Unlike other developmental anomalies, males are predominantly affected. Two main varieties can be distinguished. The *infantile type* is characterized by gross narrowing of the aorta proximal to the ductus arteriosus, which remains patent. Most infants with this defect die soon after birth unless it is surgically repaired.

The *second type* of coarctation is usually asymptomatic until it produces complications in adult life. The narrowing of the aorta is much less severe and is distal to the ductus arteriosus. Symptoms are usually a consequence of severe hypertension, proximal to the narrowing, and, typically, in the upper part of the body with a low blood pressure distally. Collateral vessels, particularly the intercostal arteries, become enlarged and cause notching of the ribs, visible on radiographs.

The severe hypertension affecting the proximal part of the aorta leads to aortic medionecrosis and dissection (Chapter 10), which is often fatal before middle age. Other complications are infective endocarditis, cerebral hemorrhage, or left-sided congestive heart failure from the local hypertension. Surgical correction can be carried out, but is difficult.

Pulmonary stenosis

The truncus arteriosus may divide unequally, resulting in a small pulmonary artery and valve; the severity of this stenosis inevitably affects the outcome. The main symptoms are undue breathlessness on exertion and fatigability. Death in childhood

is usually from right-sided heart failure, but surgical correction is increasingly successful.

Transposition of the great vessels

This severe defect affects males more often than females and is characterized by reversal of the origins of the aorta and pulmonary artery. Cyanosis and breathlessness are present from birth, congestive heart failure develops rapidly, and death follows within the first year. Coexistent anomalies such as septal defects or a patent ductus allow a slightly longer survival time by providing communication between the pulmonary and systemic circuits. Surgical correction is difficult but, as with other congenital defects, is increasingly more successful.

Tetralogy of Fallot

The tetralogy of Fallot* is the most common form of cyanotic heart disease compatible with survival into early adult life. The components of the tetralogy are:
1. Pulmonary stenosis
2. Ventricular septal defect
3. Straddling of the interventricular septum by the aorta; blood from both ventricles can thereby enter the aorta
4. Compensatory hypertrophy of the right ventricle

The course of this disease depends on the degree of pulmonary stenosis. If stenosis is severe, survival depends on persistence of a patent ductus to allow blood to enter the pulmonary vessels.

The clinical effects of tetralogy of Fallot are many, but the two most obvious early features are severe cyanosis and loud murmurs heard over the precordium. Later clubbing† of the fingers and toes develops. Physical development is poor as a

---

*E.L.A. Fallot (1850-1911), French physician.
†Finger clubbing is the name given to bulbous swelling of the fingertips and increased convexity of the nails. It is associated with a variety of chronic pulmonary diseases and rarely with other disorders, but its cause is unknown.

result of an inadequate systemic blood supply. Compensatory polycythemia results from hypoxia of the bone marrow.

Children with tetralogy of Fallot tend to squat after exertion because this gives some relief from breathlessness. They often have paroxysms of cyanosis and breathlessness for no obvious reason. These characteristically cause cerebral anoxia and syncope.

The prognosis is poor if untreated, but surgical correction, although formidably difficult, is usually successful. Causes of death are heart failure, intercurrent respiratory tract infection, and sometimes infective endocarditis.

Hemodynamic features of congenital heart disease are summarized in Table 11-3.

Ischemic heart disease

Ischemic heart disease is the result of an inadequate coronary blood flow caused, in the vast majority of cases, by atherosclerosis.

Epidemiology and etiology

Ischemic heart disease is now the main cause of death in westernized countries, accounting for more than 35% of deaths in affluent countries apart from Japan. In all types of ischemic heart disease, males are affected more than females in a ratio of four to one, but after age 70 the prevalence becomes equal.

Because atherosclerosis is the main cause of coronary narrowing, the etiologic determinants of ischemic heart disease are mostly similar to those of atherosclerosis. However, other factors also appear to affect the vulnerability of the myocardium.

Types of ischemic heart disease

An inadequate blood supply can affect the heart with varying degrees of severity, but there is usually an initial period, often lasting many years, without symptoms. The main types of heart disease caused by ischemia are:

1. Chronic atherosclerotic (ischemic) heart disease
2. Angina pectoris
3. Myocardial infarction

The factors that determine the effects of ischemia on the heart include the following:

1. The speed of narrowing of the coronary arteries. If this is slow, anastomotic channels may have time to develop.
2. The severity of the narrowing of the arteries.
3. The size and number of the vessels most severely affected and the presence or adequacy of intercoronary anastomoses.
4. The oxygen requirements of the heart. Hypertension, myocardial hypertrophy, or any factor impairing cardiac efficiency increases the oxygen demand. Any factor causing hypoxia aggravates the effects of ischemia.

Chronic atherosclerotic heart disease. Atherosclerosis is an almost inevitable feature of advancing years and causes slow, patchy narrowing of the coronary and other arteries. However, severe lesions are seen even in individuals in their twenties, as shown by autopsy studies during the Korean and Vietnam Wars. Atherosclerosis does not necessarily impede the blood flow, and ischemic heart disease develops only when the coronary arteries have narrowed enough to cause damage to the myocardium.

Pathology. The pathologic features are atherosclerotic narrowing of the coronary arteries and patchy myocardial fibrosis.

The left ventricle, particularly near the apex, is most severely affected. Ischemia causes necrosis of muscle fibers, which undergo autolysis. There is a minor inflammatory cellular infiltrate, the necrotic tissue is removed, and proliferation of fibroblasts leads to replacement of the dead muscle by fibrous tissue. In severe cases pale streaks of fibrosis in the myocardium can be seen when the heart is cut across (Fig. 11-4).

Chronic ischemia reduces the efficiency of the heart to such a degree that failure may eventually follow. Conduction defects are common and arrhythmias often develop.

Clinical aspects. Chronic ischemic heart disease typically progresses slowly over the course of years without symptoms and is often therefore found by chance at autopsy. Alternatively, the degenerative changes can produce symptoms during periods of stress, particularly intercurrent infections. If the patient lives long enough, there is a good chance of heart failure developing. In some cases damage to the conduction tissues can cause arrhythmias, which can contribute to severe symptoms or cause sudden death. In other cases angina pectoris or myocardial infarction supervene, and these may be the first overt indications of vascular disease.

Angina pectoris. Angina pectoris is the name given to acute attacks of severe chest pain, which are usually brought on by exercise and relieved by rest. In most cases there is underlying atherosclerotic heart disease, but the acute episode does not appear to cause irreversible myocardial damage.

Pathogenesis and pathology. The main contributory causes of angina are as follows:

1. Coronary artery narrowing by atherosclerosis
2. Coronary spasm
3. Reduced coronary artery filling
4. Increased oxygen demands by the myocardium

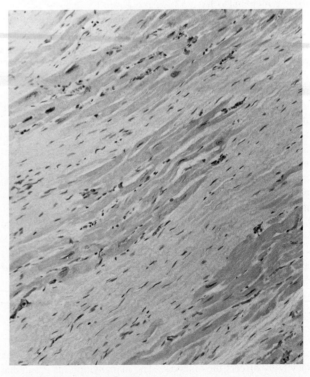

FIG. 11-4. As a result of chronic ischemia bands of fibrous tissue are present, separating darker cardiac myocytes.

Severe coronary atherosclerosis is usually found at autopsy in patients with a history of angina. In other patients spasm of the coronary arteries has been demonstrated by means of cineangiography.

Reduced coronary artery filling can be caused by stenosis of their origins in the aorta. This is typically but rarely caused by syphilitic aortitis.

Clinical aspects. The most common precipitating causes of anginal chest pain are physical exertion (particularly in cold weather) and emotion, but pain is relieved by rest.

The pain of angina pectoris is retrosternal and often described as a sense of strangling, choking, or tightness of the chest. The sensation is rarely, however, the unbearable, crushing, intense pain of myocardial infarction. Angina often radiates to the left side, sometimes to the left upper arm, and occasionally to the left jaw. Electrocardiographic changes are characteristic either at rest or after exercise.

Pain usually persists only for a few minutes or at most for a quarter of an hour. It is, however, more quickly relieved by giving nitrates, which cause widespread vasodilatation. Pain relief from nitrates helps confirm the diagnosis. Patients may have repeated attacks of angina for years; others, after one or two attacks, have a myocardial infarct. Management is based on controlling aggravating factors such as obesity, hypertension, or smoking. When pain is severe and unresponsive to drugs, coronary bypass surgery may be considered.

Myocardial infarction. Myocardial infarction is the most severe form of ischemic heart disease. The most typical symptom is intense and persistent chest pain that is unrelieved by rest. It is by far the most common cause of sudden death.

Ischemia leading to myocardial infarction can result from sudden occlusion of the coronary arteries or from a rapid increase in the demand of the myocardium for oxygen beyond the capacity of the coronary arteries to supply it.

The term myocardial infarction is, however, widely used for two distinct entities: a clinical syndrome and a pathologic lesion. Although usually associated, these are separate conditions. To simplify matters, the clinical syndrome of intense, substernal, crushing pain, unrelieved by rest and often terminating early or later in death, will be referred to here as a *heart attack.* The term *myocardial infarction,* on the other hand, will be restricted to the specific lesion found at autopsy or demonstrated objectively in life by release of cardiac muscle enzymes and characteristic electrocardiographic changes.

The need to distinguish heart attacks from myocardial infarctions is important because an infarct does not necessarily follow a heart attack and vice versa. Even when there is the typical sequence of heart attack followed by myocardial infarction, symptoms precede irreversible damage, and objective signs of infarction appear only several hours after the onset of the clinical attack.

Pathogenesis. Severe and widespread coronary atherosclerosis is found in about 90% of persons who have had a myocardial infarction. The main risk factors are essentially the same as those for the development of atherosclerosis, namely, hypertension, smoking, and hyperlipidemia. Angina or myocardial infarction may in fact be the first manifestation of severe atherosclerosis. It is also widely accepted that the precipitating cause of the heart attack is thrombus formation (or other complication) affecting the atheromatous plaque and occluding the vessel. Nevertheless, an occluding thrombus is rarely found at autopsy, and in up to 10% of cases there may be no significant arterial disease.

Evidence also suggests that the frequency with which thrombosis in coronary arteries is found at autopsy depends on the duration of survival. A thrombus is present in only a small minority of those who die less than an hour after a heart attack. In many cases, therefore, thrombosis superimposed on atheromatous plaque is probably secondary deterioration of the circulation as a result of the heart attack rather than the cause.

The importance of thrombosis in the pathogenesis of myocardial infarction is controversial. Thrombus formation has been found in only a small minority of those who die within an hour of the onset of the attack. It has been argued in many cases that thrombosis involving an atheromatous plaque could be secondary to the deterioration of the circulation as the result rather than the cause of the heart attack. The counterargument is that failure to find a thrombus at autopsy is the result of intense fibrinolytic activity during a severe heart attack. Supporting the belief of thrombosis as the main cause of acute obstruction is the effectiveness of thrombolytic treatment in restoring patency of the coronary vessels if given within 2 to 3 hours.

The role of coronary artery spasm in precipitating acute heart attacks is uncertain. Arterial spasms have been observed by cineangiography, but spasmolytic drugs, unlike thrombolytic drugs, do not appear to be of significant benefit.

About 25% of patients with coronary artery disease die very suddenly. Autopsy examination has confirmed the presence of severe and widespread coronary artery disease, but more than 40% of these patients have no acute lesions. In those in whom acute lesions have been found, thrombosis is much less common than rupture of an atheromatous plaque.

Arrhythmias play an important part in heart attacks: first, by contributing to the cause; second, as a consequence of the ischemic episode. Arrhythmias as a result of a damaged conduction system reduce cardiac efficiency and increase oxygen demands of the heart. These effects may culminate in myocardial infarction if coronary artery disease is present.

Arrhythmias are a common sequel to heart attacks, and the most severe arrhythmia, ventricular fibrillation, is the main cause of death in the early stages. In ventricular fibrillation, effective cardiac pumping stops, causing total ischemia of the myocardium and the brain. Sudden death is inevitable in a matter of minutes unless effective treatment (such as electrical defibrillation) is immediately given.

Other contributory factors. Any factor that impairs oxygenation of the heart muscle may also precipitate infarction when the coronary blood flow is marginal. Risk factors include the following:

1. *Smoking.* The mortality from ischemic heart disease is twice as high among smokers (20 or more cigarettes a day) as among nonsmokers. Smokers are also more susceptible to sudden cardiac death. The reasons are unknown but may be the result of increased carbon monoxide levels in the blood (depressing oxygenation), platelet aggregation, or the effects of nicotine on the autonomic nervous system. In addition, as discussed earlier, smoking is a major risk factor for the development of atherosclerosis.

2. *Anemia.* When the body is at rest, the oxygen content of hemoglobin is reduced by 20% to 30% in most tissues. In the myocardium, by contrast, reduction may be up to 70% even under normal conditions. Therefore, the heart muscle is particularly susceptible to reduced oxygenation of the blood.

3. *Physical activity.* The risk of myocardial infarction is greater among the sedentary than among those who are phys-

ically active. On the other hand, violent exertion, in joggers for example, can precipitate a heart attack when the coronary blood supply is marginal.

4. *Emotional stress.* Emotion, such as violent anger or fear, produces increased sympathetic activity, leading to increased oxygen demands by the heart, and is a well-recognized factor precipitating angina. The majority of sudden deaths, however, happen when the patient is relaxing or asleep. If angina develops during general anesthesia, it may be precipitated by hypoxia or arrhythmia.

5. *Hypotension.* The blood pressure can be depressed by a variety of causes such as hemorrhage, drugs, or anesthesia. Coronary filling is reduced as a result.

6. *Hypoxia.* Reduced oxygenation of the blood obviously aggravates the effects of reduced coronary blood flow. Important potential causes of hypoxia are anesthetics, especially intravenous barbiturates.

Pathology. Information about the acute changes of myocardial infarction comes from autopsy studies on those who have survived long enough for an infarct to develop. Relatively little is known about the acute changes in those who survive an attack.

Sites affected. Disease of the right coronary artery (supplying the posterior wall of the left ventricle and the posterior part of the interventricular septum) and of the left anterior descending artery (supplying the anterior wall of the left ventricle and the anterior part of the interventricular septum) account for ap-

proximately 80% of the cases. Disease of the left circumflex coronary artery, which supplies the lateral wall of the left ventricle, accounts for the remaining 20%. Infarcts therefore affect the left ventricle in the great majority of cases.

Macroscopic features. A myocardial infarct is characterized by necrosis of the muscle and often damage to the endocardium or pericardium. The changes are typical of ischemic necrosis. Descriptions of the early features of infarction vary because it is rarely possible to know precisely when the process started and thus the age of the lesion.

Macroscopic changes probably do not become visible until at least a day after the attack begins. The first sign is that the area of damage becomes paler than the surrounding normal muscle. The border becomes hyperemic after about 48 hours, whereas the central dead area becomes yellowish and progressively softer (Fig. 11-5). These changes spread through the infarct after about 10 days. Areas of hemorrhage into or around the infarct are common. If the patient survives long enough, the necrotic area eventually is replaced by a fibrous scar.

Large infarcts extend through the full thickness of the muscle, but smaller infarcts are enclosed within normal muscle, usually near the endocardial surface. When the endocardium is involved, it becomes rough; there is a fibrinous exudate, and thrombus formation (mural thrombus) may be superimposed.

Fibrinous or serofibrinous pericarditis is less common and is usually localized to the area overlying the infarct. Alternatively, there may be generalized pericarditis. Pericarditis usually resolves with healing of the infarct, but occasionally healing is followed by organization and permanent fibrous adhesions.

Microscopic features. The escape of enzymes from the damaged muscle can be detected histochemically about 8 hours after the start of the clinical attack. Histologic changes develop

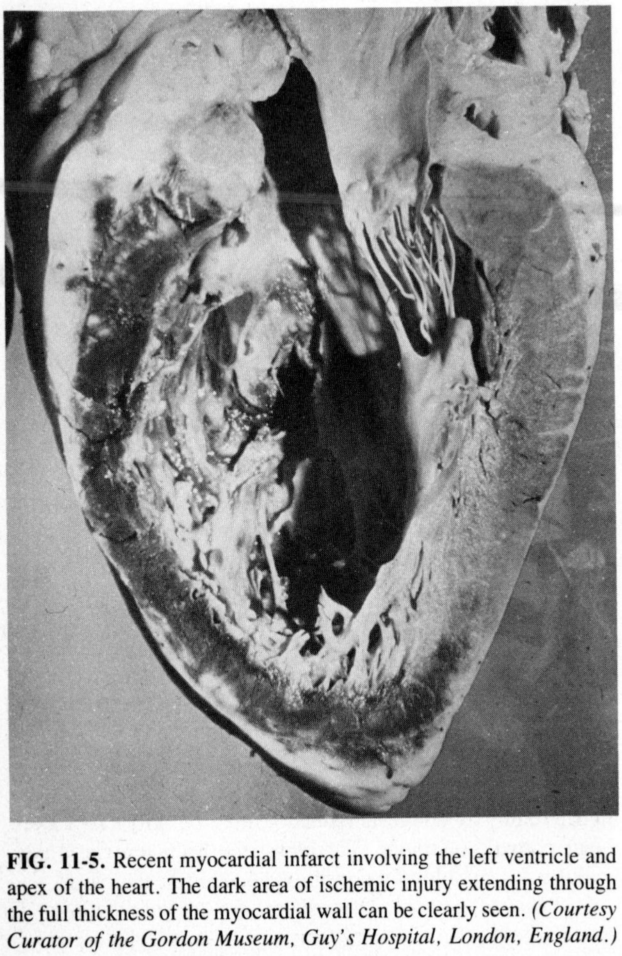

FIG. 11-5. Recent myocardial infarct involving the left ventricle and apex of the heart. The dark area of ischemic injury extending through the full thickness of the myocardial wall can be clearly seen. *(Courtesy Curator of the Gordon Museum, Guy's Hospital, London, England.)*

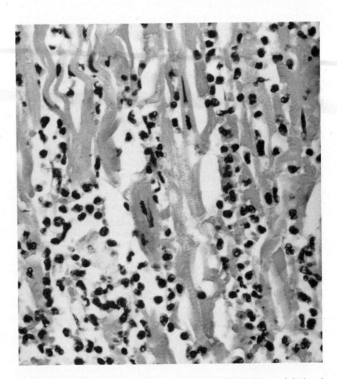

FIG. 11-6. Photomicrograph of acute myocardial infarct of 3 days' duration. Note the abundant neutrophils and fragmented necrotic cardiac myocytes.

about 24 hours after a heart attack and are essentially the same as in any other infarct (Figs. 11-6 and 11-7). Death of muscle cells is shown by swelling, loss of striations, and disappearance of the nuclei. The infarcted area becomes infiltrated by leukocytes, which emigrate from the surrounding living tissue. There is autolysis and phagocytosis of the dead cells by macrophages. After about a week, granulation tissue proliferates at the periphery and gradually replaces the necrotic tissue. Collagen fibers begin to form in the third week, and the damaged area is progressively replaced by fibrous tissue, which matures during the following weeks.

Abnormalities of serum enzyme levels. Several enzymes are released when cardiac muscle cells die. Creatine phosphokinase (CPK) determination is the most sensitive enzymatic test for myocardial infarction, and the most specific isoenzyme is CPK-MB. Serum levels of CPK-MB start to rise 3 to 6 hours after the onset of chest pain and peak at 7 to 17 times the upper limit of normal in 18 to 24 hours. The enzyme then rapidly disappears from the circulation unless the patient has a second infarct or the original infarct extends.

Raised serum CPK-MB* levels therefore provide objective evidence of myocardial infarction after a heart attack and serial measurements also indicate the severity of the lesion. Serum levels of other enzymes, such as aspartate aminotransferase and

---

*Electrophoretic separation methods have shown that there are two CPK isoenzymes—M, derived from muscle, and B, derived mainly from brain. Normally only a small MM fraction is present in serum. In myocardial infarction, the MM fraction is usually increased, but a second MB fraction (CPK-MB) appears, which is virtually diagnostic of myocardial injury. A BB fraction can be seen following brain and other tissue injury.

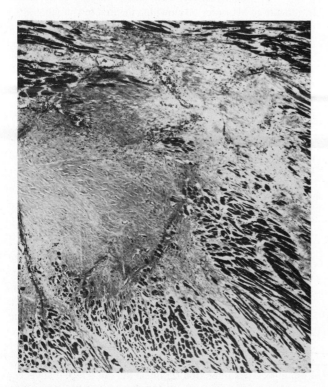

FIG. 11-7. Healed myocardial infarct. The fibrous scar replaces an extensive area of dead muscle and also extends between surviving muscle fibers where there has been patchy ischemic damage.

lactate dehydrogenase (LDH), also increase at different times and rates, but an increase in the ratio of LDH1 isoenzyme to LDH2 to 1 or greater is a typical finding.

Electrocardiographic changes. Contraction of the heart causes electrical activity, which is recorded on an electrocardiogram. Ischemia of the heart muscle gives rise to characteristic changes: elevation of the ST segment and abnormal Q waves. The raised ST segment gradually falls back to the baseline, but the T waves remain symmetrically inverted. The development of this series of changes confirms the diagnosis of myocardial infarction.

Effects and complications

PUMP FAILURE AND SHOCK. A reduction in the amount of contracting muscle affects cardiac function. Arterial pressure tends to fall, which can reduce coronary flow. Myocardial function is even further weakened, and the size of the infarct may increase. Further deterioration of cardiac function is caused by arrhythmias and metabolic acidosis as a result of inadequate blood supply. A vicious circle of myocardial damage, arterial hypotension, reduced coronary blood flow, and deteriorating cardiac function is established. As a result, this syndrome has a high mortality rate.

CONGESTIVE CARDIAC FAILURE. Some degree of left ventricular failure usually results from myocardial infarction. A high proportion of those who survive the early complications develop congestive heart failure, which may be fatal in the short or long term.

ANGINA PECTORIS. Acute changes in atheromatous plaques in the coronary arteries are frequently associated. In those who survive, some narrowing of the coronary lumen is common. This is shown by the frequent development of angina pectoris in the months after an acute attack.

MYOCARDIAL RUPTURE. Rupture of the myocardium (Fig. 11-8) is uncommon but usually happens within the first week, and the incidence increases with the age of the patient. The myocardium continues to contract, but blood bursting through the necrotic area fills the pericardial sac and prevents the heart from filling (tamponade). Acute hypotension and death are almost inevitable.

CARDIAC ANEURYSM. Aneurysm (Fig. 11-9) is a later complication. It results from dilatation of the fibrous scar during systole and causes further deterioration of pumping efficiency of the heart.

THROMBOEMBOLISM. Clinical signs of thromboembolism complicating myocardial infarction are relatively uncommon, but thrombi are found in at least 45% of the cases at autopsy. Embolism may cause or contribute to death in about 25% of the fatal cases. Because the vast majority of infarcts affect the left ventricle, the emboli are released into the systemic circulation and can block the coronary arteries or cerebral vessels.

Clinical aspects. The cardinal clinical feature of a heart attack (myocardial infarction) is acute and increasingly intense, crushing substernal pain. It is probably the most severe and terrifying kind of pain that can be experienced and is inevitably associated with severe anxiety and a justified sense of doom. The pain and anxiety contribute to further deterioration by stimulating intense sympathetic activity. The pain often radiates to the left arm and neck and, occasionally, as with angina, is not felt in the usual substernal site but in the left jaw for example.

Tachycardia, arrhythmias, breathlessness, and often vomiting or sudden loss of consciousness as a result of shock are common. Some patients die very suddenly, and about 30% die

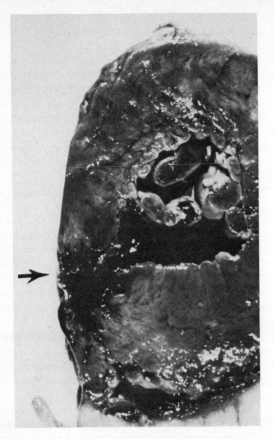

FIG. 11-8. Myocardial rupture. As a result of myocardial infarction, the left ventricular wall has become soft and weakened (myomalacia cordis) resulting in rupture and sudden death.

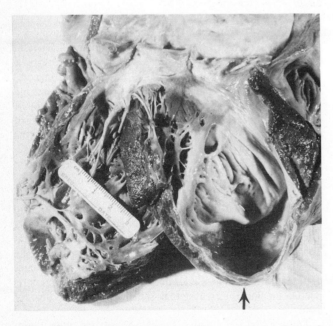

FIG. 11-9. Left ventricular aneurysm. The myocardium of the left ventricle has been replaced by fibrous tissue as a result of a previous infarction. As a result of intracardiac pressure, the ventricular wall has stretched outward and formed an aneurysm *(arrow).*

before reaching the hospital, especially if emergency care is inadequate or delayed.

Arrhythmias can be detected in at least 90% of patients, particularly at the onset of the attack. Arrhythmias are responsible for death in the early stages, but many of them are preventable.

Some degree of left ventricular failure is almost invariable and produces clinically evident effects in over 60% of patients. In the most severe cases, acute pulmonary edema and severe breathlessness result.

The loss of contractile tissue as a result of damage to the myocardium usually causes a fall in blood pressure. This may be slight, but in 10% to 12% of patients the fall in blood pressure is severe, and cardiogenic shock develops. About 80% of those in cardiogenic shock do not survive.

In a minority of cases, infarction is painless but may be detected by electrocardiography in a patient who develops acute heart failure. Old, healed lesions are also found at autopsy in persons who have had no history of acute pain. The reason for these painless infarcts is unknown.

Characteristic electrocardiographic changes (particularly elevation of the ST segment, as already described) develop within 24 hours. Raised serum enzyme levels from the damaged heart muscle (CPK-MB) are detectable 4 to 8 hours after the onset of the attack. A delay in raised serum enzyme levels and of electrocardiographic changes indicates that extensive myocardial damage is not immediate; the implications of this are discussed later.

Pathophysiologic basis of management. Experimentally, mitochondrial changes can be seen by electron microscopy about 20 minutes after the onset of ischemia. Increasing evidence has shown that there is a short interim period when effects on the myocardium may be reversible. A heart attack that is treated immediately and effectively may not necessarily be followed by infarction. Measures taken within the first few minutes after the start of the attack are major determinants of the patient's fate.

Immediate resuscitative measures initiated by trained personnel are often effective. In one series, for example, 40 patients who suffered cardiac arrest or developed ventricular fibrillation outside the hospital were resuscitated by ambulance personnel. Thirty-two of these patients were alive when followed up at periods between 6 months and 3½ years later.

The essential measures for the initial management of a heart attack are based on the pathophysiology of the condition and include the following:
1. Relief of pain
2. Relief of anxiety
3. Maintenance of adequate oxygenation
4. Control of arrhythmias
5. Cardiopulmonary resuscitation if necessary

Relief of pain and anxiety are particularly important because they cause sympathetic overactivity, and the consequent outpouring of epinephrine contributes to the severity of the arrhythmias. Morphine is effective and nitrous oxide and oxygen are also valuable for this purpose. In addition, antiarrhythmic drugs are usually needed, but their choice depends on electrocardiographic identification of the type of disturbance. β-Blocking drugs, however, have been shown to reduce the mortality from myocardial infarction significantly, but a recent advance, related to the pathogenesis of the disease, has been the introduction of thrombolytic therapy. If a thrombolytic drug is administered within 4 hours of the onset of the attack, recanalization frequently follows, the size of the infarct is limited, and

mortality and morbidity are reduced. Although thrombolytic therapy may cause hemorrhage, the risk appears to be small and should be even less with newer agents such as tissue plasminogen activators.

Survival from myocardial infarction. Survival depends on many interacting factors, which fall into two main groups: intrinsic (patient) and extrinsic. Intrinsic factors include the following:

1. Size of the infarct
2. Preexisting disease
   a. Ischemic heart disease
   b. Hypertension
   c. Other cardiovascular disease
   d. Diabetes mellitus
3. Age

Other contributory factors have been discussed earlier, but the main extrinsic factor affecting survival is the rapidity with which skilled medical care is given. The critical period is within 2½ hours after the onset of the attack; 50% of all deaths come in this period, mostly because of delay in getting medical care. Even if facilities and medical skill are available, many factors may prevent them from reaching the patient in time.

The second factor affecting mortality, as mentioned earlier, is the introduction of drugs such as β-blocking and thrombolytic agents.

About 50% of patients die within a year of the attack, the great majority within the first 3 months. About one third of the deaths take place within an hour of the attack, and more than 70% of these patients die before they can get medical aid.

Of those who survive, the most common complication in the first year is angina pectoris (about 50%), and more than 20% develop congestive heart failure. Only about 5% have a second infarct in this period, and clinically significant thromboembolic phenomena are rare. If there is complete clinical and electrocardiographic recovery, however, survival for 10 to 20 years is possible. The outcome of myocardial infarction is diagramed in Fig. 11-10.

RECENT CHANGES IN MORTALITY. Although mortality from myocardial infarction rose progressively until the mid-1950s,

it has subsequently declined. In the United States and some other countries this change has been attributed to a decreased consumption of animal fats, an increased consumption of polyunsaturated fats, and a decrease in cigarette smoking by men. However, the degree of correlation is inconsistent between the rates of myocardial infarction deaths and, for example, smoking habits and serum cholesterol levels; between men and women; and between older and younger age groups. Furthermore, it is hard to explain why the decline in mortality became evident at different times in different American states, especially because mortality from a variety of other unrelated diseases has declined significantly.

The decline in mortality from myocardial infarction underlines the uncertainty about the etiology of this disease. However, some account must be taken of improvements in treatment and in particular the introduction of such drugs as the β-blocking agents, which have been shown in an extensive multinational controlled trial to have reduced the immediate mortality from myocardial infarction by 30%. It is also likely that the greatly increased attention to immediate care after heart attacks and newer treatments outlined earlier, have played a significant part in this trend.

Aortocoronary bypass surgery. The replacement of atheromatous and partly occluded coronary arteries by healthy vessels seems a logical, although technically difficult, means of overcoming coronary artery disease. In little more than a decade coronary bypass surgery has become an almost commonplace operation. Since the first report in 1969, of surgical bypassing of an obstructed coronary artery by means of a reversed segment of autologous saphenous vein, the number of such operations has progressively increased to a current estimated level of more than 200,000 a year in the United States alone. In expert hands the operative mortality may now be less than 1.5% and the long-term outcome has also improved.

Although bypass operations seem an obvious means of overcoming the effects of coronary artery obstruction, it has been difficult to confirm their effectiveness. Several large surveys involving thousands of patients have compared the survival rates for surgical as opposed to medical treatment. Unexpectedly, the survival rates for both groups show little difference except for those patients with significant left ventricular dysfunction.

Patients most likely to benefit from coronary bypass surgery are those with otherwise uncontrollable angina, with significant left main branch obstruction, or with significant left ventricular dysfunction.

Major problems that affect the long-term success of bypass surgery are obstruction of the graft by recurring atherosclerosis and the inability of many patients to change a life-style that contributed significantly to the development of the disease.

Percutaneous transluminal coronary angioplasty. In this procedure a balloon catheter is inserted into the coronary artery and dilated to reduce the obstruction caused by atheroma. The success rate in terms of improvement in symptoms and exercise tolerance is currently about 75%, but the duration of the benefit is less easy to assess because the procedure has only been used on any scale in the last decade.

Summary. The events that precipitate myocardial infarction are rarely clear. There are many conflicting findings, and inevitably much less is known about those who recover from heart attacks than about those who die. The main findings are as follows:

1. The majority of myocardial infarcts are associated with severe atherosclerosis of the coronary arteries.

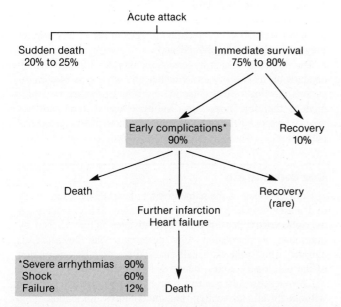

FIG. 11-10. Outcome of myocardial infarction. The column at lower left shows the relative incidence of the main causes of death. (Figures are approximate.)

2. Acute ischemia sufficient to cause death of an area of myocardium is the basic mechanism involved, but the precise cause of the ischemic episode is less clear, and several mechanisms may be involved.

3. Only those who die at least 24 hours after a heart attack can be shown to have objective evidence, either grossly or microscopically, of an infarct. In those who do not die immediately, objective evidence of infarction is shown by release of cardiac muscle enzymes and by electrocardiography.

4. In those who die immediately after a heart attack, infarction is not found because it has not had time to develop.

5. Early control of severe arrhythmias is an important factor in reducing mortality from heart attacks.

Mechanisms that *may* be involved in fatal acute myocardial ischemia include the following:

1. Occlusion of coronary vessels by thrombosis or hemorrhage relating to atheromatous plaque.

2. Severe dysrhythmias or spasms of coronary vessels contribute to subsequent development of thrombosis secondary to deterioration of cardiac function and blood flow.

3. Lethal dysrhythmias (sudden cardiac death) without pathologic changes apart from preexisting chronic ischemic heart disease; however, if successful cardiopulmonary resuscitation is given, the patient may have no subsequent objective evidence of cardiac damage.

Sudden cardiac death. A significant proportion (estimated at approximately 50%) of patients with ischemic heart disease, die suddenly and unexpectedly. The cause in most cases, as confirmed by continuous electrocardiographic monitoring, is ventricular tachycardia rather than fibrillation, as was earlier believed, although the one readily progresses to the other.

The importance of the distinction is that ventricular tachycardia is entirely "electrical" in origin and is not the result of damaged myocardial cellular membranes, the usual cause of ventricular fibrillation.

Immediate cardiopulmonary resuscitation can abort sudden cardiac death without showing signs of myocardial damage. In the hospital, diagnosis of the precise cause (ventricular tachycardia or fibrillation) of sudden collapse of a patient with ischemic heart disease should enable the appropriate treatment to be given.

Hypertensive heart disease

Hypertension (Chapter 10) may be defined as a persistently raised blood pressure of more than 160/90 mm Hg at rest. In about 90% of the cases the cause is unknown, and the disease is referred to as *essential hypertension*. The effect of hypertension on the heart is a sustained increase in its work load.

Pathogenesis and pathology

Systemic hypertension leads to progressive hypertrophy of the left ventricle. The heart, therefore, becomes larger and heavier. These changes are frequently accompanied by coronary atherosclerosis. The combination of limited ability of the coronary blood supply to expand and the increased oxygen demands of the hypertrophic myocardium is a common cause of left ventricular failure (Fig. 11-11). In effect, the hypertrophied heart muscle outstrips its blood supply. Atherosclerosis, particularly of the coronary vessels, is accelerated by hyper-

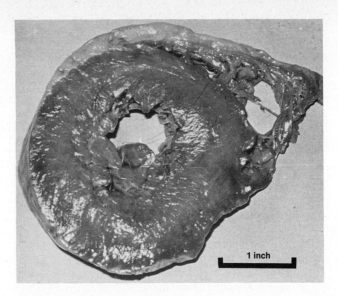

FIG. 11-11. Myocardial hypertrophy. The myocardium of the left ventricle is almost four times its normal thickness as a result of long-standing essential hypertension. It is obvious that the coronary arteries, even if unobstructed by atheroma, would have increasing difficulty in maintaining an adequate blood supply to this bulk of muscle. *(Courtesy Curator of the Gordon Museum, Guy's Hospital, London, England.)*

tension so that atherosclerotic heart disease is superimposed on the changes caused by the hypertension itself. Cardiac failure is accelerated, and often the patient develops angina or myocardial infarction. Other organs that are often severely affected are the kidneys and the brain.

Clinical aspects

Hypertensive heart disease is symptomless until failure or other complications develop. Cardiac arrhythmias and left ventricular failure progressing to congestive cardiac failure, angina, or myocardial infarction are the most common complications, but severe hypertension is sometimes first manifested by its effects on other organs. The first sign may be a stroke or, less often, renal failure.

Investigation may show cardiac enlargement and changes in the heart sounds. Characteristic changes in the retinal arteries may be visible by ophthalmoscopy.

The degree to which hypertension shortens life expectancy depends on its severity and whether and what type of complications develop. Early detection by blood pressure measurement is therefore important. Antihypertensive treatment has greatly improved the prognosis, particularly of malignant hypertension.

Cor pulmonale

Cor pulmonale is the name given to heart disease secondary to disease of the lungs or pulmonary vessels. It is characterized by right ventricular hypertrophy and later failure caused by pulmonary hypertension. Cor pulmonale can be acute or chronic. The former is usually caused by embolic obstruction of the pulmonary artery, which is frequently fatal.

Chronic cor pulmonale is caused by emphysema (with or without chronic bronchitis), pneumoconioses, idiopathic interstitial fibrosis, bronchiectasis (Chapter 12), and pulmonary vascular abnormalities (e.g., pulmonic valve stenosis).

Pathologic and clinical features

The changes characteristic of cor pulmonale resemble those of hypertensive heart disease, except that the right ventricle instead of the left ventricle is primarily affected. Therefore, right ventricular hypertrophy is followed by right-sided heart failure and systemic venous congestion. The clinical effects are the result of both the lung disease and impaired cardiac function, which together limit oxygenation of the tissues.

Clinically, in the earlier stages, the patient has a cough, breathlessness on exertion or wheezing, and other signs of underlying lung disease. Later, right-sided heart failure develops, and cyanosis may be especially prominent. Intercurrent respiratory tract infections aggravate the symptoms or can precipitate heart failure.

The management of cor pulmonale is to stop the patient from smoking and to improve respiratory function by physiatrics and appropriate drugs (Chapter 12). When heart failure develops, it must be treated along conventional lines, but largely because of the irreversible nature of the underlying disease, response to treatment is often poor.

Thyroid (hyperthyroid) heart disease

Excessive thyroid hormone production raises the metabolic rate and activity of the myocardium and also sensitizes the myocardium to sympathetic activity (Chapter 18). In addition, the heart has to meet the increased metabolic demands of the rest of the body. If untreated, the persistent overload on the heart, together with tachycardia and a tendency to arrhythmias, can lead to cardiac failure or myocardial infarction. This is especially likely in the older patient who may have other preexisting heart disease.

Severe tachycardia, with or without arrhythmias, is the main clinical feature and is made worse by emotional or other stresses. High-output cardiac failure may develop later.

Myxedematous heart disease

In myxedema (Chapter 18), the metabolic rate is slowed, and the activity of the heart is also depressed. Another feature of myxedema is hypercholesterolemia, which is associated with a high incidence of atherosclerosis. Patients with myxedema are therefore prone to ischemic heart disease (angina or myocardial infarction). The latter is unusual in its sex distribution because myxedema is more common among females.

Cardiomyopathies
Alcoholic heart muscle disease

Chronic heavy alcohol intake damages muscle, both cardiac and skeletal. Experiments suggest that alcohol itself, rather than other constituents of alcoholic beverages, has a direct toxic effect on muscle. Patients with sickle cell trait appear to have a greater susceptibility to alcoholic heart disease.

Pathology. In the myocardium lysis of muscle cells can be seen. In addition, glycogen-like material or glycoprotein accumulates between the muscle fibers; interstitial fibrosis may also be found.

Cardiac damage is usually a result of both prolonged and excessive alcohol intake. Nevertheless, in an experiment on a healthy and eager volunteer who was given 12 to 16 ounces of Scotch whisky a day for 5½ weeks, the resting heart rate began to increase, the circulation time was prolonged, and venous pressure started to rise. After 4 months on this "treatment," a cardiac arrhythmia developed. When the alcohol was stopped, there was spontaneous reversion to normal.

In the chronic alcoholic a variety of cardiac signs and symptoms may develop. Pulmonary hypertension and right-sided heart failure, mild enlargement of the heart, and episodes of atypical precordial pain are not uncommon. Palpitations are sometimes a major complaint and are presumably caused by arrhythmias. There is also a relatively high incidence of sudden unexpected death in young alcoholics, which is believed to be a result of ventricular fibrillation.

Clinical aspects. Chronic alcoholism is often unsuspected, particularly if the person is a respected member of the community. Alcoholics are also notoriously unreliable about the amount of alcohol they admit to consuming. In view of the high and increasing prevalence of alcoholism, alcoholic heart disease, like other complications of this type of addiction, is a serious problem. Alcoholism should be suspected in any patient with any of the cardiac disorders mentioned earlier and in whom no other cause is apparent. In known alcoholics, the possibility of heart disease or liver damage should always be investigated before a general anesthetic is given.

Infective myocarditis

In addition to toxic cardiomyopathy, which may be a cause of sudden death in acute diphtheria, the heart may be directly involved in some viral infections, particularly in children. Myocarditis is a recognized but rare complication of measles and mumps but is more commonly caused by coxsackievirus B types 1 through 5 (Fig. 11-12).

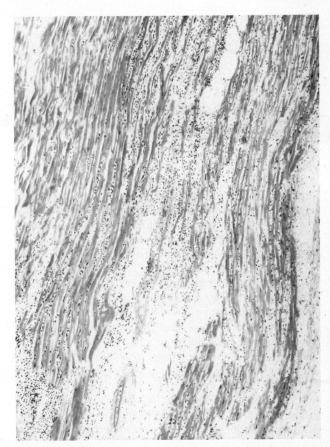

FIG. 11-12. Viral myocarditis. The cardiac myocytes are necrotic, and many have lost their nuclei. There is an interstitial inflammatory infiltrate of lymphocytes.

The different infective agents cause essentially similar pathologic changes and, unlike other forms of cardiomyopathy, are characterized by inflammatory cell infiltration, edema, and sometimes necrosis of the myocardium, which often becomes dilated and flabby. Fibrinous pericarditis is commonly associated.

Clinically, in many individuals myocarditis causes no symptoms and is overshadowed by the systemic features of the infection. If severe, myocarditis may become apparent as tachycardia and rhythm disorders, sometimes with anterior chest pain. Severe cases can progress rapidly to heart failure and death. In young children the rapid onset of pulmonary edema as a result of cardiac failure can be mistaken for pneumonia. Inappropriate and ineffective treatment may therefore be given. In other cases, especially in adults, there appears to be complete or almost complete recovery.

AIDS-related cardiac disease

Although cardiovascular disease is not a major feature of acquired immunodeficiency syndrome (AIDS), the heart does not escape damage. Autopsies confirm that in approximately 50% of those dying from this disease, lymphocytic myocarditis is the most common finding and in most cases is of presumed viral etiology; in a small group, however, *Toxoplasma gondii* has been found in the myocardium, and one such case was fatal. Otherwise, AIDS-related myocarditis does not seem to have significant clinical effects.

Kaposi's sarcoma can involve the heart and tuberculous pericarditis has also been reported.

Idiopathic cardiomyopathies

Several varieties of idiopathic cardiomyopathy, defined as primary heart muscle disease of unknown origin, are recognized. They are rare, although it is probable that many cases escape diagnosis. The main examples are congestive and hypertrophic cardiomyopathy, characterized by myocardial degeneration and hypertrophy, respectively. Some cases appear to be familial and others may be viral.

Congestive dilated cardiomyopathy. Congestive (idiopathic) dilated cardiomyopathy is of unknown cause, although viral infection is suspected. The disease is not distinguishable from known causes of myocardial diseases such as alcoholism and like them leads ultimately to heart failure. Congestive cardiomyopathy is characterized by decreased force of contraction of the left ventricle with slow and inadequate emptying. There is progressive enlargement of the heart mainly because of dilatation of the left ventricle, leading to pulmonary hypertension and, later, right ventricular failure. The underlying pathologic changes appear to be myocardial degeneration and fibrosis. The main clinical manifestation of congestive cardiomyopathy is heart failure.

Hypertrophic cardiomyopathy. Hypertrophic cardiomyopathy (idiopathic hypertrophic subaortic stenosis) is often familial and transmitted as an autosomal dominant trait but is otherwise of unknown cause.

Grossly, there is massive hypertrophy of the left ventricular wall in the absence of systemic or myocardial disease capable of having this effect. The hypertrophy is typically asymmetrical; the posterior free wall is the least affected in most cases, and the ventricular cavity is normal or reduced in size. Hypertrophy may be severe enough to obstruct filling of and outflow from the ventricle.

Microscopically the main features are disorganization of myocardial cells, myocardial fibrosis, and abnormalities of the small intramural arteries.

The myocardial cells are enlarged and disarrayed, often in bundles at irregular angles to each other or presenting an interwoven appearance. Fibrosis develops even in the absence of coronary artery obstruction and ranges from patchy interstitial fibrosis to gross scarring. The intramural arteries show medial and intimal thickening, and narrowed lumens. These abnormal vessels are more numerous at the margins of areas of fibrosis and the latter may therefore be the result of ischemia.

The clinical consequences of the myocardial abnormalities are most commonly dyspnea on exertion, angina-like pain and, later, left ventricular failure. Hypertrophic cardiomyopathy is possibly the main cause of sudden death in young athletes.

Cardiac transplantation

After the first heart transplants in South Africa in 1967, initial enthusiasm was followed by such disappointing results that the operation was abandoned by virtually all but Shumway at Stanford University. A particular problem with heart transplants is that the organ must start pumping immediately after the patient is removed from the heart-lung machine. Improvements in such aspects of management as selection of patients and organs, immunosuppressive treatment, and aftercare have been such that more than 50% survive for at least a year and at the time of writing one patient is still alive after 18 years.

For conditions such as cardiomyopathies causing uncontrollable heart failure, heart transplantation can dramatically improve the quality and expectation of life. The technical difficulties of the operation and controlling rejection have largely been overcome. However, important obstacles to cardiac transplantation are the shortage of donor hearts and the cost of the operation.

Rheumatic fever

Rheumatic fever is an inflammatory disease characterized by fever, malaise, widespread transient arthritis, carditis, chorea, and lesser effects on other organs. The joint pains are usually the most troublesome symptom but are harmless.

The most important effect of rheumatic fever is damage to the heart valves. Usually no symptoms occur at the time of the disease, but after some years symptoms of chronic rheumatic heart disease emerge.

Rheumatic fever has become rare in such countries as Great Britain and the United States (although there are signs of its reemergence) but is common in Africa, Asia, and South America where it has a high death rate.

Etiology and pathogenesis

Rheumatic fever is generally believed to be an immunologically mediated disease in which susceptible patients have an abnormal response to streptococcal infection with antibodies that cross-react with cardiac tissue. The evidence for the relationship between streptococcal infection and rheumatic fever is largely epidemiologic, however. The main points are as follows:

1. Rheumatic fever develops in susceptible patients 1 to 4 weeks after streptococcal pharyngitis or scarlet fever caused by group A β-hemolytic streptococci.

2. More than 95% of patients who develop rheumatic fever have serologic evidence of recent streptococcal infection even when it was not clinically evident.

3. Recurrences of streptococcal infection in susceptible persons cause recurrences of rheumatic fever and progressively more severe cardiac damage.

4. Prevention of streptococcal infections by long-term antibiotic prophylaxis prevents recurrences of rheumatic fever.

5. Effective antibiotic treatment for streptococcal infections and improvements in social conditions have been associated with the great decline in the incidence of rheumatic fever in the Western world.

6. Although rheumatic fever follows streptococcal infection, the lesions are sterile.

7. Antibodies against heart tissues can be detected in the sera of up to 60% of patients with acute rheumatic fever. Other studies have shown that in about 50% of patients with active or inactive rheumatic disease, antibodies against β-hemolytic streptococci are cross-reactive with cardiac muscle.

8. Streptococcal components that share common antigenic determinants with joint and brain tissues that are attacked in acute rheumatic fever have been identified.

9. Some persons who develop rheumatic fever produce higher and more sustained titers of streptococcal antibodies than those who have uncomplicated streptococcal infection.

10. Susceptibility to rheumatic fever is believed to be genetically determined, and one or more B-cell alloantigens have been found in the great majority of rheumatic fever patients but rarely in controls. As yet, however, no specific HLA-associated phenotypes have been identified.

Immunologic aspects

The M protein of the cell walls of streptococci has been shown to have cross-reactivity with myocardial sarcolemma. Cross-reactivity between group-specific cell wall polysaccharide and cardiac valve glycoprotein and between a streptococcal protoplasmic antigen and neuronal tissue of the caudate and subthalamic nuclei have also been reported.

Although it seems likely that immunologic reactions triggered by streptococcal infection are responsible for tissue damage in rheumatic fever, no specific immunologic mechanism has been identified. Thus streptococcal antibodies can be shown to bind to cardiac tissues, but it has not been possible to demonstrate them at the sites of tissue damage or prove that they are cytotoxic. Attention has therefore turned to the possibility of cell-mediated tissue injury, but this has proved difficult to confirm in humans.

Pathology

The *Aschoff body** is the characteristic lesion of rheumatic fever (Fig. 11-13). Aschoff bodies are fusiform in shape and are found most often in the heart, joints, and other connective tissues.

Microscopically, the Aschoff body begins as a focus of swollen, weakly staining collagen fibers. This so-called fibrinoid change is caused by the presence of glycoprotein. The area of degeneration becomes infiltrated by neutrophils and lymphocytes, but macrophages ultimately become predominant.

Large undifferentiated mesenchymal cells known as *Anitschkow myocytes*† and multinucleate cells, probably formed by fusion of macrophages, also appear. Digestion of the damaged collagen and proliferation of connective tissue follow, and the

---

*K.A.L. Aschoff (1866-1942), German pathologist.
†N.H. Anitschkow (1885-1964), Russian pathologist.

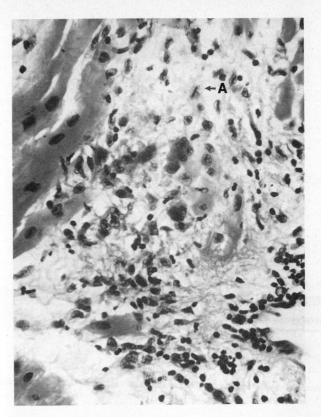

FIG. 11-13. Aschoff node in rheumatic carditis. A high-power view of the subendocardial connective tissue shows a focus of fibrinoid change surrounded by Anitschkow myocytes *(A)*.

lesion heals to leave a microscopic focus of scarring. Perversely, immunofluorescence studies do not show the antibodies against heart tissue in the Aschoff bodies.

Heart. There is inflammation of all three layers (pancarditis) of the heart to varying degrees.

Myocardium. Aschoff bodies are mainly present just beneath the endocardium and around the small arteries. The rare deaths during the acute phase are a result of myocardial failure, but the myocardium shows no specific changes. Aschoff bodies are few or undetectable, and the only obvious gross features are edema and flabbiness of the muscle and dilatation of the heart.

Endocardium. The valves are the site of the most important changes. Inflammation and formation of Aschoff bodies just beneath the surface lead to loss of endothelial cells, particularly along the lines of contact of the cusps. Platelet thrombi form on these denuded areas, and fibrin deposition follows. In this way, warty vegetations (Fig. 11-14) form along the lines of closure of affected valves. The mitral and aortic valves are particularly affected. These vegetations are small and firm and do not detach to release emboli. Inflammation and organization, however, cause the malformations to become permanent, and fibrosis causes distortion of the valves. Inflammatory changes in the heart valves start in this way, but at this stage in acute rheumatic fever their immediate effect on cardiac function is minimal.

During recurrences of the disease, damage is increased, but even so the effects on the valves (stenosis or regurgitation) do not become clinically apparent for some years. This delayed development of chronic rheumatic heart disease is partly a result of the slowly progressive distortion of the valves, but mainly it is a result of the ability of the heart to compensate for their inefficiency for a considerable period.

Pericardium. Pericarditis (Figs. 11-15 and 11-16) is common and varies in severity, but it is usually of little clinical importance. Inflammation and formation of Aschoff bodies in the subserosa may lead either to a serofibrinous effusion, or in severe heavy deposits of fibrin cause the surface of the heart to become shaggy.

Joints. Arthritis is the most common and conspicuous feature of the acute phase of rheumatic fever. Aschoff bodies are present in the synovial membranes; nevertheless, inflammation is transient, and healing follows without permanent damage.

Chorea. Chorea is a highly characteristic but uncommon manifestation of rheumatic fever. It consists of spasmodic, involuntary muscular movements, which in the past were called *St. Vitus' dance.*

Skin. Only a minority of patients with rheumatic fever have dermal lesions. The best known are subcutaneous nodules produced by large areas of fibrinoid change and inflammation or a rash called *erythema marginatum,* consisting of red rings mainly on the trunk.

Clinical and epidemiologic aspects

The incidence of rheumatic fever after epidemics of untreated streptococcal pharyngitis was about 3% a few decades ago. Over the past 30 years, however, both the incidence of and mortality from rheumatic fever have declined in developed countries until in many of them it has become a rare and mild disease. The cause of this decline is not entirely clear, but it is likely that better socioeconomic conditions have diminished the spread of streptococcal infection. Prompt antibiotic treatment of streptococcal infections in susceptible patients and

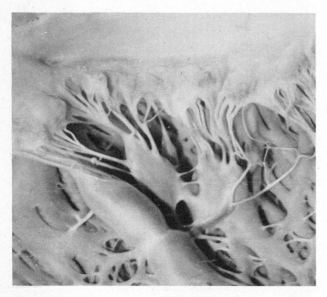

FIG. 11-14. Rheumatic endocarditis. The vegetations on this mitral valve are warty but pale and relatively insignificant compared with infective endocarditis in Fig. 11-21. *(Courtesy Curator of the Gordon Museum, Guy's Hospital, London, England.)*

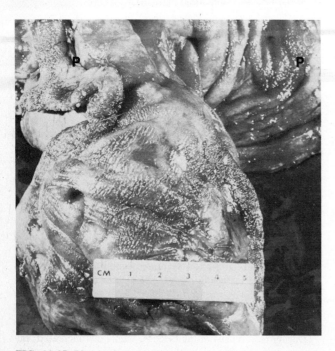

FIG. 11-15. Rheumatic pericarditis. The parietal pericardium *(P)* has been reflected to show fibrinous inflammation in both visceral and parietal layers of the pericardium. This pale shaggy appearance is sometimes described as "bread-and-butter" heart.

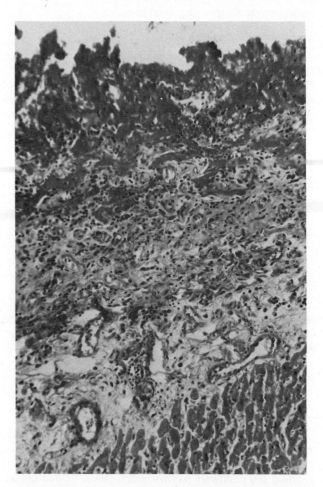

FIG. 11-16. Rheumatic pericarditis. The pericardium is swollen and infiltrated with inflammatory cells. A prominent fibrinous exudate is present on the pericardial surface.

prevention of recurrent infections may have played a part, but it also seems likely (although impossible to confirm) that there has been a decline in streptococcal virulence, as suggested by the falling incidence of carditis even among those who develop rheumatic fever and the decrease in the frequency of other complications of streptococcal infections. A lesser prevalence of rheumatogenic strains of streptococci is another possibility. That this picture may change again is suggested by the recent eightfold increase in rheumatic fever (associated with the M protein type 18) among children in Utah. The disease remains common among poverty-stricken communities, probably because overcrowding promotes spread of streptococci.

Clinically, the majority of patients have their first attack between the ages of 5 and 15.

Streptococcal infection may cause a sore throat or may be asymptomatic. In either case infection has subsided before the onset of rheumatic fever. The onset and manifestations of rheumatic fever are highly variable. Joint pains are the most common symptom and may be associated with an acute febrile illness. In others chorea may occur alone, or chronic rheumatic heart disease may be found in later years in a patient with no history of rheumatic fever.

Arthritis causes joint pain and swelling and characteristically flits from joint to joint but leaves no permanent effects.

Cardiac involvement can be detected by tachycardia and the onset of characteristic murmurs. These are usually caused by such factors as dilatation of the valve rings secondary to general dilatation of the heart rather than inflammation of the valves. There is usually also clinical or radiologic evidence of heart enlargement. Myocarditis is often shown by arrhythmias and can lead to cardiac failure. The acute phase of the disease subsides in 6 to 12 weeks.

The diagnosis depends both on the clinical picture and on laboratory findings. The major criteria are polyarthritis and pancarditis, but serologic evidence of earlier streptococcal infection, particularly antistreptolysin A, or less frequently antibodies to other streptococcal antigens, can usually be demonstrated. Other findings are leukocytosis and a raised erythrocyte sedimentation rate. Individually none of these findings is specific. The diagnosis must therefore be made on the presence of at least two of the major clinical criteria, together with serologic findings.

The prognosis depends on the severity of cardiac damage. Even when rheumatic fever was more common and severe, only about 1% of patients died in the acute phase, usually from fulminating myocarditis. The long-term prognosis, in terms of the likelihood of developing chronic rheumatic heart disease, also depends on whether carditis develops in the acute attack, its severity, and whether or not rheumatic fever is allowed to recur. However, in recent years rheumatic fever has not merely become uncommon, but it rarely causes permanent cardiac damage.

In those who suffer valve damage, there is usually a period of many years when the only detectable abnormality is a cardiac murmur before chronic rheumatic heart disease becomes apparent. Alternatively, in a few persons infective endocarditis can supervene.

Salicylates are the most effective drugs for controlling fever and joint pains. It is even more important to prevent recurrences by prescribing continuous penicillin treatment, if necessary, for many years. Complications such as congestive heart failure have to be treated by conventional means as they arise.

TABLE 11-4. Clinicopathologic spectrum of rheumatic fever

Affected organ	Effects in acute stage	Late effects
Joints	Acute, transient arthritis	None
Skin	Subcutaneous nodules Erythema marginatum	None
Central nervous system	Chorea	Chorea may appear months after acute rheumatic attack; may last several years
Heart		
Pericardium	Acute pericarditis	Usually minor
Myocardium	Acute myocarditis; may lead to heart failure	Usually none
Endocardium	Endocarditis with rheumatic vegetations	Distortion and functional defects of heart valves, especially mitral and aortic; infective endocarditis may complicate

Summary

1. Rheumatic fever develops in susceptible patients 1 to 4 weeks after infection by group A β-hemolytic streptococci.
2. The characteristic lesion is the Aschoff body, consisting of a minute focus of fibrinoid change and inflammatory cells.
3. The main symptom of rheumatic fever is joint pain, but there is no permanent damage.
4. Carditis is the main and most severe effect. Its most important feature is the formation of minute vegetations on the valves and underlying inflammatory changes.
5. Death (from acute myocarditis and failure) in the acute stage is now exceedingly rare.
6. Subsequent streptococcal infections lead to recurrences of rheumatic fever and increasing cardiac damage.
7. Recurrences can be prevented by long-term antibiotic treatment.
8. If recurrences are avoided, rheumatic fever can be followed by apparent recovery and an asymptomatic period, usually of many years.
9. The clinicopathologic spectrum of rheumatic fever and its consequences are summarized in Table 11-4.

Chronic rheumatic heart disease

Chronic rheumatic heart disease as a result of acute rheumatic fever many years previously is still prevalent and, despite the decline in the incidence of rheumatic fever, is the most common cause of acquired valvular disease in adults. However, as causes of heart (as opposed to valvular) disease, hypertension and occlusive coronary artery disease are considerably more common in older adults.

Pathogenesis and pathology

The inflammatory changes affecting the valves in the acute phase are followed by organization and fibrosis. Contraction of this scar tissue causes gradual distortion that can lead to valve stenosis or incompetence. A stenotic valve orifice has a

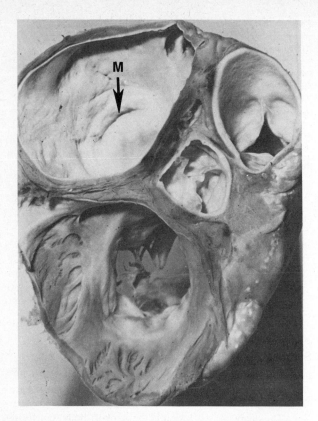

FIG. 11-17. Mitral stenosis. The mitral valve *(M)* viewed from the left atrium has been reduced to a mere slit. The left atrial muscle is hypertrophic, and the atrial chamber is dilated. *(Courtesy Curator of the Gordon Museum, Guy's Hospital, London, England.)*

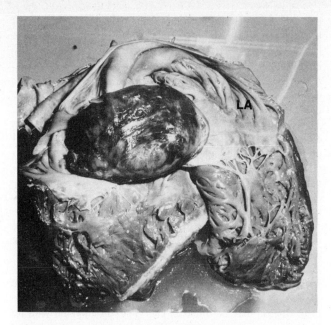

FIG. 11-18. Mitral stenosis with ball-valve thrombus. A large oval thrombus completely fills the left atrium.

narrowed opening, and the heart has to beat more forcibly to maintain an adequate output. The distorted leaflets of an incompetent valve fail to shut so that the blood regurgitates immediately after systole. The ventricle becomes overloaded during diastole by this backflow, in addition to the normal venous filling. Moreover, to maintain a normal output, the ventricles have to continually reeject the regurgitated blood and are in a situation not unlike a person desperately trying to bale water out of a rapidly leaking boat.

Stenosis and regurgitation are often combined so that the heart has to force the blood through a narrowed valve orifice, as well as deal with excessive diastolic filling, but usually one type of dysfunction predominates. The most common valvular abnormality in chronic rheumatic heart disease is mitral stenosis (Figs. 11-17 to 11-19). Aortic regurgitation is also common and may be combined with mitral stenosis. Isolated aortic valve disease is uncommon, and the tricuspid and pulmonic valves are rarely involved.

Chronic rheumatic heart disease is essentially a consequence of mechanical, hemodynamic effects caused by the distorted valves. Typically it develops many years after rheumatic fever has become inactive. As mentioned earlier, the latter may have been so mild or inconspicuous that only 60% of patients with chronic rheumatic heart disease are aware of having had rheumatic fever in the past.

Clinical aspects

Women are more frequently affected than men. Chronic rheumatic heart disease becomes apparent first as a heart mur-

mur without symptoms. These characteristic murmurs are caused by the disturbance of blood flow over the distorted valves. Cardiac failure gradually develops usually in early adult life. Mitral stenosis mainly causes right ventricular failure but may be combined with aortic regurgitation, causing left-sided heart failure.

In the past, death from cardiac failure before middle age was the usual outcome, but the prognosis has been greatly improved by surgical replacement of the damaged valve. Infective endocarditis, however, remains a hazard of artificial valves, as well as of untreated rheumatic heart disease.

Summary

1. Chronic rheumatic heart disease is the long-term consequence of carditis, which started during the course of acute rheumatic fever.
2. During the long latent period the only detectable signs are cardiac murmurs caused by progressive distortion of the heart valves.
3. The mitral and aortic valves are chiefly affected. Stenosis and regurgitation develop to varying degrees.
4. Cardiac function is progressively impaired by the malfunctioning of the valves, which ultimately progresses to cardiac failure.
5. Surgical correction of the valve defects has greatly improved the prognosis.
6. Infective endocarditis is a well-recognized but uncommon complication of damage to the valves, whether or not the damage has been corrected surgically.

Mitral valve prolapse

Prolapsed or "floppy" mitral valves are common and are believed to be present in some degree in up to 5% of the population. The defect is common in generalized disorders of collagen formation such as Marfan's syndrome, but similar valve defects, in the great majority of cases, are unassociated

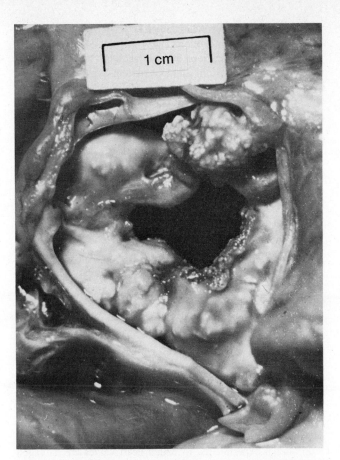

1 cm

FIG. 11-19. Rheumatic valve disease—late stages. The valve has been grossly distorted by progressive inflammation and fibrosis; there has also been extensive calcification of the fibrotic areas. The valve is now rigid and unable to open fully or close completely. Functionally there was both stenosis and regurgitation. *(Courtesy Curator of the Gordon Museum, Guy's Hospital, London, England.)*

with any systemic disorder. There are also several subtypes of mitral valve prolapse, in terms of morphologic changes and hemodynamic effects, so that they may represent the effect of a variety of genetic and other disorders. Mitral valve prolapse can be a feature of rheumatic heart disease.

Clinically, mitral valve prolapse has a familial tendency and is more common in women. The defect is typically found between the ages of 14 and 30 and is usually asymptomatic but detected as one or more clicklike murmurs just after the first heart sound. Such clicks may be followed by a high-pitched late systolic murmur that may be described as a "whooping" or "honking" sound. In a small minority of cases, mitral regurgitation develops and may progress to cardiac failure, particularly if the chordae tendineae rupture. Prolapsed mitral valves are occasionally also the site of origin of infective endocarditis but do not in general appear to confer a high risk of this infection.

Microscopically, there is considerable variation between the subtypes of prolapsed mitral valves. Typical features include extensive myxomatous change, particularly in the posterior leaflet, together with enlargement of the mitral annulus and elongation of the chordae tendineae. The sudden tensing of these elongated chordae is the cause of the characteristic click.

Calcific aortic valve stenosis

Stenosis (usually mild) and calcification of the aortic valve are relatively common autopsy findings in the elderly. These characteristics are believed to result from senile degenerative changes, but there is sometimes an underlying congenital, bicuspid defect.

Clinically, the lesion only rarely causes critical aortic obstruction leading to heart failure, and it is usually asymptomatic. However, stenosis may confer susceptibility to infective endocarditis and may be a cause of the increased incidence of this disease in the elderly.

Calcification of the mitral valve annulus is another possible finding in the elderly. It may be associated with ischemic heart disease, but although it may occasionally restrict the mitral orifice, it rarely affects function.

Infective endocarditis

Infective endocarditis is a severe, potentially lethal disease resulting from colonization of the endocardium by bacteria or other microbes. Progressive damage to the heart, particularly the valves, and usually, lesions in the kidneys, brain and other sites are the results.

Previously this disease was known as *subacute bacterial endocarditis,* but it is usually either acute or chronic and can be caused by bacteria, fungi, or rickettsiae. The course of the disease depends on a variety of factors, including the virulence of the infecting organisms, the state of the host's defenses, and the effects of treatment (Fig. 11-20). The clinical picture of the disease has changed in recent years and from being a disease of young adults with congenital or rheumatic heart disease, infective endocarditis now has its peak incidence in those over 60.

Etiology

Two prerequisites are usually necessary for the development of infective endocarditis. The first is a preexisting lesion, either a valve defect or a vascular anomaly such as coarctation of the aorta. The second factor and precipitating event is bacteremia.

Dental extractions happen to have been the first procedures that were recognized as causing bacteremias in healthy persons and that in susceptible persons could lead to infective endocarditis. For purely historical reasons dental operations are given prominence as a precipitating cause of infective endocarditis, but currently they are implicated in less than 15% of the cases. Other factors, such as cardiovascular surgery, now provide a portal of entry for organisms either in large numbers or of unusual virulence, and prosthetic valve or vascular replacements provide a site that is particularly vulnerable to infection. In addition, the more virulent bacteria can also attack normal valves.

Microbiology

Streptococci, particularly viridans streptococci, are the single most frequent group of causative bacteria, but the frequency of isolation of particular bacteria varies according to the circumstances. In the case of intravenous drug addicts, for example, and patients with prosthetic valves that are frequently infected at operation, *Staphylococcus aureus* and *Staphylococcus epidermidis* are particularly important because the bacteria are then likely to have come from the patient's skin or other external source.

Viridans streptococci probably most often come from the oral cavity and account for 45% to 54% of natural valve infections. The importance of viridans streptococci may depend on their attachment mechanisms; these may enable them to adhere to the valvular endocardium, but the plastic or metal of prosthetic valves may present less favorable surfaces.

Less frequent but still important are *Streptococcus faecalis* and, in alcoholics especially, *Streptococcus pneumoniae*. *Candida albicans*, which may be introduced by an intravenous catheter, accounts for a small but increasing number of cases and is difficult to treat.

The organisms that infect prosthetic heart valves differ from those which infect natural valves. Immunosuppression and drug addiction also affect the picture. Thus any figures quoted for the frequency of isolation of different bacteria in series of cases of infective endocarditis are meaningless unless the circumstances are defined.

Portals of entry

In very many, probably the majority of patients, the portal of entry of the bacteria is unidentifiable. However, enormous numbers of bacteria colonize the gum margins in most mouths, and it can readily be shown that dental extractions release showers of bacteria into the bloodstream. Even toothbrushing frequently causes minor bacteremias, as may chewing candies, but such minor bacteremias usually appear to be of no significance even in patients with heart lesions. However, as mentioned earlier, a dental operation precedes the onset of infective endocarditis in only a small minority of patients.

Currently, other medical procedures provide many more portals of entry. The most important of these is cardiac surgery. Portals of entry for organisms include:

1. Dental extractions and occasionally other dental procedures
2. Cardiovascular surgery
3. Indwelling intravenous catheters
4. Instrumentation of the urinary tract
5. Intravenous injections by drug addicts

In addition, prepartum and postpartum sepsis, respiratory tract and skin infections, and burns are possible sources, but it is estimated that up to 50% of cases of infective endocarditis are now a direct consequence of cardiac surgery.

Host factors

Although potential sources of bacteremias can be identified, bacteremia is not synonymous with infective endocarditis. Even in persons with heart lesions, bacteremias only rarely lead to infection, probably because only a few bacteria enter the circulation or other unknown factors do not favor colonization of a valve.

Distorted valves, cardiovascular prostheses, or congenital defects can produce localized turbulence of blood flow in which there are areas of relative stasis. The damaged endocardium favors platelet and fibrin deposition. This in turn provides a "sticky" surface to which bacteria can readily adhere and colonize the endocardium. In nearly half the cases, however, in some recent series, no preexisting cardiac lesion has been detected.

Systemic factors also affect susceptibility to this disease. One of the most important is immunosuppressive treatment, which greatly depresses the patient's resistance to infection. Another debilitating condition is chronic alcoholism, and cocaine addiction appears to confer an increased risk of infective endocarditis among intravenous drug abusers.

In animal experiments, in which heart valves are damaged and bacteria are injected into the bloodstream, infective endocarditis can be made to develop in virtually 100% of cases, probably as a result of the large bacterial inoculum and the active unhealed cardiac lesion. Such models do not therefore accurately reproduce human infective endocarditis in which

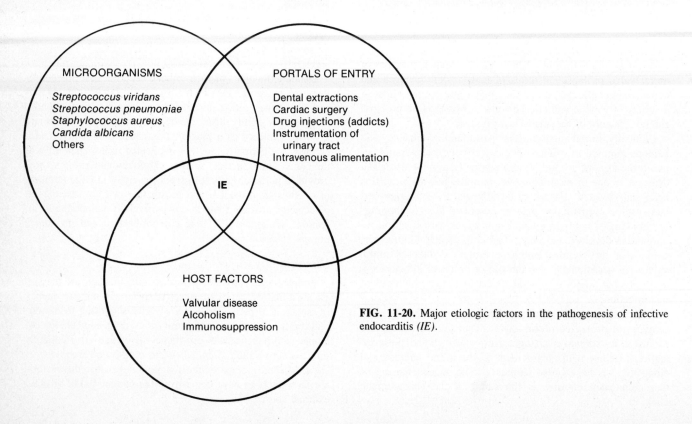

FIG. 11-20. Major etiologic factors in the pathogenesis of infective endocarditis *(IE)*.

there are mysterious aspects. Thus infective endocarditis is uncommon in Down's syndrome despite the fact that there is a natural immunodeficiency and congenital valve lesions are frequently present. In acute leukemia also, despite the frequency of septicemias, infective endocarditis appears to be rare. The reason why infective endocarditis has become a disease of the elderly is also obscure.

These clinical aspects of susceptibility to infective endocarditis must be borne in mind when evaluating any experimental (animal) model of endocarditis or when trying to assess the effectiveness of prophylactic measures.

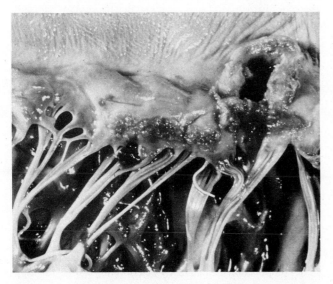

FIG. 11-21. Infective endocarditis. The vegetations are massive, crumbly, and hemorrhagic. Top and to the right, the valve has been perforated by the infective process. *(Courtesy Curator of the Gordon Museum, Guy's Hospital, London, England.)*

Pathology

The characteristic lesions are friable, warty masses *(vegetations)* on the leaflets of the affected valves (Fig. 11-21) and their consequences. Vegetations may be up to several centimeters in diameter and form at the free margins of the valve leaflet (Fig. 11-22). This is in contrast to the vegetations of rheumatic heart disease, which are small and firm, form in a relatively orderly fashion along the lines of valve closure, and contain no organisms.

Histologically, vegetations consist of irregular, tangled masses of fibrin strands, platelets, and blood cells. The valve to which the vegetation is attached shows vascularization, inflammatory changes, and proliferation of granulation tissue into the vegetation.

The vegetations can have a variety of effects. Locally, because of the proliferative and fibrotic changes they provoke, they cause distortion of and severe loss of efficiency of the affected valve. The valve may become perforated, or one of the attached chordae tendineae may rupture, with the disastrous consequences of hyperacute cardiac failure (Fig. 11-23).

The consequence of infective endocarditis is therefore progressively more severe cardiac damage, which is often the cause of death if treatment is delayed or inadequate.

Kidneys. The kidneys (Fig. 11-24) are involved in 30% to 50% of all patients, as indicated by such signs as hematuria or progressively impaired renal function. It is probable, however, that the kidneys are involved in all cases, but renal function is often unaffected. Lesions may sometimes result from multiple infected emboli, but those of glomerulonephritis secondary to infective endocarditis have histologic appearances suggestive of immune complex disease.

Brain. Cerebral involvement is relatively common and may produce a misleading clinical state of psychosis or neurosis that is likely to be misdiagnosed. The cerebral lesions, like those in the kidneys, have an appearance suggestive of immune complex disease rather than direct embolization.

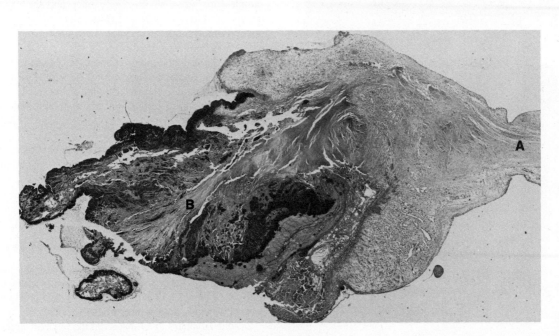

FIG. 11-22. Infective endocarditis. The enormous size and irregular shape of the vegetation can be compared with the relatively normal part of the valve *(A)*. A large part of the vegetation consists of fibrin and great masses of darkly staining bacteria (around *B*).

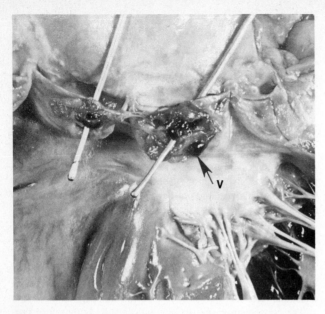

FIG. 11-23. Infective endocarditis. The aortic valve cusps are distorted and perforated. Vegetations *(V)* are present on the ventricular aspect of the valve.

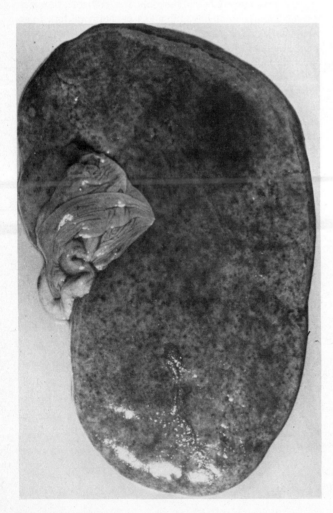

FIG. 11-24. The kidney in infective endocarditis. The capsule has been stripped off to show numerous small subcapsular hemorrhages. *(Courtesy Curator of the Gordon Museum, Guy's Hospital, London, England.)*

Embolic phenomena. Emboli readily break off the friable vegetations and can land in unpredictable fashion in any part of the systemic circulation. The effects are most dramatic when emboli block coronary, cerebral, or retinal vessels.

Clinical aspects

The peak incidence of infective endocarditis is now in the sixth and seventh decades, and the source of the infection is often obscure. The insidious onset of the disease can make early diagnosis difficult, but two characteristic features are low intermittent fever and changing cardiac murmurs. The changing character of the murmurs is a result of the progressive growth of the vegetations and damage to the valves. There is usually (but not always) mild leukocytosis, but the erythrocyte sedimentation rate is always raised and anemia develops.

A common feature is finger clubbing and brownish (café au lait) spots on the skin, but linear (splinter) hemorrhages under the fingernails are seen less often than in the past. Tender nodules in the ends of the fingers (Osler's nodes*) are characteristic and almost diagnostic. Other symptoms are variable and include appetite loss, weight loss, arthralgias in some patients, and weakness.

In many patients the indefinite clinical picture is punctuated by more dramatic embolic events. These particularly affect the spleen, kidneys, brain, or joints, and their arrival is usually indicated by sudden local pain or, if in the brain, by sudden deterioration of cerebral function. Hematuria is an important sign of renal involvement, whereas any type of cerebral disturbance can result from foci of damage in the brain.

Acute endocarditis caused by *Staphylococcus aureus* is a rapidly prostrating illness with high fever, multiple septic embolic complications, and quickly deteriorating cardiac function.

Early confirmation of the diagnosis and identification of the infecting organism are essential and depend on the blood culture. The chances of isolating organisms in a single random sample are about 80%, despite a constant bacteremia. In an adult, 5 to 10 ml of blood should be taken; if three blood samples are taken at 30-minute intervals, the chances of a positive culture are increased to at least 95%. Failure to get a positive blood culture in infective endocarditis is usually a result of previous antibiotic treatment.

If a positive blood culture cannot be obtained, despite conscientious attempts, treatment must be started on the basis of the clinical picture, particularly that of low-grade intermittent fever and changing cardiac murmurs. Intermittent fever in a patient known to have valve disease is almost diagnostic of infective endocarditis.

In the past, deaths from infective endocarditis were a result of overwhelming infection or severe renal damage causing azotemia. Currently the main cause of death is cardiac failure, but embolic infarction of the brain, for example, may cause sudden death.

The treatment of infective endocarditis depends on giving adequate doses of bactericidal antibiotics, selected on the bacteriologic findings. For viridans streptococci infection, penicillin alone or combined with gentamicin is widely and effectively used. Another effective measure is early surgical excision of affected valves and their replacement by a prosthetic valve, especially when there is severe insufficiency.

Despite advances in antibacterial therapy and cardiovascular surgery, treatment not infrequently fails. The mortality from

---

*W. Osler (1849-1919), Canadian physician.

infective endocarditis remains at approximately 30%, usually from cardiac failure. This persistently high mortality is the result of infection by particularly virulent bacteria or other organisms such as *Candida albicans,* for which treatment is unsatisfactory. In some cases, because of the insidious onset of the disease, the diagnosis is made too late for effective treatment as the cardiac damage is advanced and severe. Chronic alcoholics, those receiving immunosuppressive treatment, and drug addicts also have a poor prognosis.

Prevention

Despite the changing picture of infective endocarditis, viridans streptococci still account for many cases, and dental and other operations that cause bacteremia are a threat to susceptible patients. It is mandatory, therefore, to give such patients antibiotics prophylactically. Patients at risk are those with rheumatic valve disease or a congenital defect or those who have had prosthetic heart valves inserted. The severity of the defect is not an indication of the level of risk because mild valvular lesions are more susceptible to infective endocarditis than severe ones.

Penicillin is generally the first choice for prophylaxis, because viridans streptococci are usually sensitive and the toxicity of the drug is low. In the United States penicillin G or V is recommended for most patients. In Great Britain and most of the rest of Europe, however, amoxicillin is now the first choice because of the high blood levels produced by oral administration and because the slower excretion allows bactericidal blood levels to persist for 6 to 9 hours. These have been shown in human experiments effectively to clear bacteremias after dental extractions.

If the patient is allergic to penicillin, the choice of drug is more difficult and in some cases, vancomycin has to be used, despite the difficulties of administration and its potential toxicity.

The American Heart Association has recommended more vigorous antibiotic prophylaxis with the use of streptomycin with penicillin or vancomycin in some circumstances. These recommendations were based largely on the results of animal experiments and are currently controversial.

Infective endocarditis is a relatively common complication of the insertion of prosthetic heart valves, particularly in the immediate postoperative period. Prosthetic valve endocarditis has a high mortality rate. Even the most vigorous antibiotic prophylaxis is frequently unsuccessful and may also be followed by antibiotic-resistant infections.

Diseases of the pericardium

The pericardium is often involved in diseases of the myocardium. This is usually of minor importance. Nevertheless, disease of the pericardium can on rare occasions lead to cardiac failure.

Pericarditis

The causes of pericarditis are summarized in the box at right. Pathologically, pericarditis is either fibrinous or associated with effusion of fluid into the pericardial sac or both. In most cases the pericarditis resolves with little residual damage, but rarely there is inflammation with fibrosis of the pericardium severe enough to cause constriction (constrictive pericarditis). This can prevent the heart from expanding fully during diastole and can lead to heart failure.

Clinically, the chief symptom of pericarditis is chest pain when fibrinous inflammation is present. This is often associated with a grating sound (pericardial friction rub) when the heart is auscultated. The pain and rub disappear with resolution or the development of a fluid effusion.

Hydropericardium and hemopericardium

Accumulation of fluid in the pericardial sac *(hydropericardium)* can be caused by either an inflammatory exudate as a complication of pericarditis or, much more commonly, by a transudate complicating cardiac failure. It is uncommon for hydropericardium to cause any significant ill effects. *Hemopericardium,* the accumulation of blood in the pericardial sac, can be caused by a penetrating chest wound or rupture of a myocardial infarct or aortic aneurysm. Sudden accumulation of blood in the pericardial sac is often sufficient to prevent the heart from dilating during diastole and can cause acute and fatal cardiac failure *(cardiac tamponade).*

Tumors of the heart

Tumors of the heart are exceptionally rare. The main examples of primary tumors are the myxoma and rhabdomyoma.

Cardiac myxoma

This is the most common cardiac tumor. It usually arises from the left atrial septal wall and forms a rounded or cauliflower-like mass. If it is large enough, it can obstruct the mitral orifice and, rarely, cause sudden death by impaction there. The more common effects are emboli formed by small fragments of the friable mass breaking off.

Microscopically, cardiac myxomas consist of loose connective tissue containing stellate cells surrounded by a mucoid matrix. This matrix typically contains deposits of hemosiderin as a result of minute internal hemorrhages. The surface is covered by endothelium on which small organizing thrombi frequently form.

Congenital rhabdomyoma

Cardiac rhabdomyomas are generally believed to be hamartomas rather than true tumors, because they are almost exclusively found in infants and, although benign, lack encapsulation. The tend also to be associated with some other congenital defects such as tuberous sclerosis.

Microscopically, cardiac rhabdomyomas form multiple nodular masses of large glycogen-filled cells that may show cross-striations.

Other cardiac tumors

Primary malignant tumors such as rhabdomyosarcomas are even more rare than benign tumors. Secondary deposits are more common, although overall the heart is an unusual site for metastases.

CAUSES OF PERICARDITIS

Infection (e.g., coxsackievirus pericarditis)
Immunologically mediated (e.g., rheumatic fever, systemic lupus erythematosus)
Myocardial infarction
Trauma to the chest
Miscellaneous: uremia, neoplasia, and unknown causes

Selected readings

Ball M and Mann JI: Apoproteins: predictors of coronary heart disease? Br Med J 293:769, 1986.

Bisno AL: Acute rheumatic fever: forgotten but not gone, N Engl J Med 316:476, 1987.

Buxton FE: Sudden cardiac death—1986, Ann Intern Med 104:716, 1986.

Coumel P, Leclercq J-F, and Leenhardt A: Arrhythmias as predictors of sudden death, Am Heart J 114:929, 1987.

Edwards WD: Cardiomyopathies, Hum Pathol 18:625, 1987.

Francis GS: Sodium and water excretion in heart failure: efficacy of treatment has surpassed knowledge of pathophysiology, Ann Intern Med 105:272, 1986.

Kannel WB: Hypertension and other risk factors in coronary heart disease: part 2, Am Heart J 114:918, 1987.

Ledford DK and Espinoza LR: Immunologic aspects of cardiovascular disease, JAMA 258:2974, 1987.

Lee TH and Goldman L: Serum enzyme assays in the diagnosis of acute myocardial infarction, Ann Intern Med 105:221, 1986.

Levett JM and Karp RB: Heart transplantation, Surg Clin North Am 65:613, 1985.

Mancini DM et al: Central and peripheral components of cardiac failure, Am J Med 80(suppl 2B):2, 1986.

Maron BJ et al: Hypertrophic cardiomyopathy: part 1, N Engl J Med 316:780, 1987.

Maron BJ et al: Hypertrophic cardiomyopathy: part 2, N Engl J Med 316:844, 1987.

Nadas AS: Update on congenital heart disease, Pediatr Clin North Am 31:153, 1984.

Rose AG: Etiology of acquired valvular heart disease in adults, Arch Pathol Lab Med 110:385, 1986.

Ruffolo RR and Kopia GA: Importance of receptor regulation in the pathophysiology and therapy of congestive heart failure, Am J Med 80(suppl 2B):67, 1986.

Schroeder JS and Hunt S: Cardiac transplantation: Update 1987, JAMA 258:3142, 1987.

Terpenning MS, Buggy BP, and Kauffman CA: Infective endocarditis: clinical features in young and elderly patients, Am J Med 83:626, 1987.

Veasy LG et al: Resurgence of acute rheumatic fever in the intermountain area of the United States, N Engl J Med 316:421, 1987.

Weinstein C and Fenoglio JJ: Myocarditis, Hum Pathol 18:613, 1987.

CHAPTER 12

Diseases of the respiratory system

Anatomic considerations

The anatomy and physiology of the lungs are complex and beyond the scope of this text. However, it is necessary to review briefly some structural aspects of the respiratory tract before beginning a discussion of pulmonary diseases.

The respiratory tract includes the nasopharynx and paranasal sinuses, larynx, trachea, bronchi and their subdivisions, and lungs. The airways of the respiratory tract are lined with tall, columnar, ciliated epithelium intermixed with mucus-secreting goblet cells. Ciliary activity is constant in health and moves the overlying blanket of mucus upward. This important cleansing mechanism has been called the *mucociliary elevator;* its activity can be impaired by drugs, especially anesthetic agents.

The alveoli of the lungs are lined with a continuous layer of epithelium in which two types of cells are found: pneumocytes types 1 and 2. Type 1 pneumocytes are thin, flattened cells that are only seen clearly by electron microscopy. Type 2 pneumocytes are plumper, rounder cells containing granules and appear to produce a phospholipid called *surfactant*. Surfactant lowers surface tension within the alveoli, which keeps them patent, and is a major factor in maintaining the elastic properties of the lungs. Surfactant-like secretions are also produced by Clara cells scattered among the bronchiolar respiratory epithelial cells.

The airways, beginning with the trachea and mainstem bronchi, undergo successive divisions and subdivisions. The areas where small bronchi lack cartilage in their walls and the lining epithelium changes to a cuboidal type are called *terminal bronchioles*. These lead in turn to respiratory bronchioles, alveolar ducts, and finally to the alveoli. The pulmonary tissue served by one terminal bronchiole is called an *acinus* and can be considered as the fundamental respiratory unit of the lung.

The true weight of each lung is about 250 g. The greater weights observed at autopsy reflect varying degrees of postmortem fluid retention.

The lungs are divided by major fissures into three lobes on the right side and two on the left. Further subdivision of each lobe and segments into lobules is important to the radiologist and surgeon for localization of lesions and pulmonary surgery.

The lungs are covered by the visceral pleura, which is lined by flat mesothelial cells. The visceral pleura over each lung is reflected as the parietal pleura onto the inner chest wall and mediastinum. This creates a right and left pleural cavity, each of which is under slight negative pressure, thus maintaining the lungs closely applied to the chest wall.

The lungs have a dual blood supply from the bronchial arteries and the pulmonary arteries. The bronchial arteries arise from the aorta and supply the bronchi and pleura. The pulmonary arteries, in addition to conveying venous blood to the lungs, supply the alveoli. There are rich anastomoses between the bronchial and pulmonary arteries. Under some pathologic conditions the bronchial arteries may be the main source of arterial blood supply to the lungs. In the alveoli, the pulmonary capillaries are separated from the alveolar air by (1) an endothelial basement membrane, (2) a thin layer of elastic and collagenous tissue, (3) an epithelial basement membrane, and (4) the alveolar pneumocytes. These layers form the alveolar septae.

Investigation of pulmonary disease

The main techniques used to investigate pathologic changes in the lungs and their consequences are:
1. Radiography, tomography, angiography, bronchography, and radioactive scanning techniques
2. Pulmonary function studies
3. Blood gas measurements
4. Bronchoscopy
5. Pulmonary and pleural biopsy and cytology
6. Culture of microorganisms
7. Skin testing

Chest radiographs are essential in the diagnosis of pulmonary disease, and have virtually succeeded the stethoscope as the main method of investigating the lungs. The bronchial tree can be outlined by a bronchogram in which radiopaque material is instilled into the airways and a radiograph taken. Pulmonary lesions seen on plain x-ray films can be examined in more detail by focusing on the lesion while placing the rest of the lung field out of focus. This is the process of tomography. A highly sophisticated form of computed tomography (CT scan) can be used to investigate virtually any organ of the body by viewing it radiographically in transverse planes. It is particularly useful for localizing pulmonary lesions.

Valuable information about the pulmonary circulation can be obtained by angiography. After injection of radiopaque material, the appearance of the pulmonary vasculature is recorded by still or cineangiography. Scintiphotography (radioactive scanning) has been used mainly to detect tumors or areas of inflammation. Radionuclides, such as ^{67}Ga, are injected intravenously. The radioactive material is concentrated in sites of inflammation or tumors and is detectable by a scanning device, which records the location on film. The value of magnetic resonance imaging, a highly sophisticated, noninvasive technique for visualizing cross sections of the body in many different planes, has still to be assessed for pulmonary disease.

Pulmonary function studies are measurements of pulmonary ventilation, diffusion of gases across the alveoli, perfusion of the lung by the pulmonary circulation, and distensibility (compliance) of the lung.

Partial pressures of oxygen and carbon dioxide (Po_2 and Pco_2) in the arterial blood measure pulmonary efficiency and are essential for the proper management of patients with severe respiratory tract disease and respiratory failure.

Almost every air passage of the lung can be visualized by means of the fiberoptic bronchoscope. In addition to directly viewing the lesions, the operator can obtain fluid, lung, or bronchial biopsy specimens or brushings of the bronchial surface for laboratory examination.

Biopsies of the lung and bronchi are usually obtained via the bronchoscope, although in some conditions, it may be necessary to perform a thoracotomy to obtain satisfactory lung tissue. Needle biopsies of the pleurae sometimes yield diagnostic information, whereas cytologic examination of pleural fluid, bronchial washings or even sputum may reveal malignant cells.

Cultures of sputum, bronchial washings, or transtracheal aspirated fluid are frequently used to determine the identity of an infecting microorganism.

Skin tests, particularly for tuberculosis, are commonly used as part of the investigation of pulmonary disease. Similar tests are less frequently used for suspected nontuberculous mycobacterial infection and histoplasmosis.

Infections of the respiratory tract

Respiratory tract infections are among the most common afflictions of humans. Most frequent are those which affect the upper respiratory tract and which are often included in the common cold syndrome (acute coryza). In the United States they account for at least half of the time lost at work and at school due to illness.

Common cold syndrome

The common cold is a mild, self-limiting disease in which nasal irritation, mucus production, and very mild systemic symptoms are the most prominent features. It is a viral infection, but at least 150 serotypes from at least 11 viral groups can be responsible for the same clinical and pathologic state. (See box below.)

Viruses that virtually always cause colds (but rarely anything more) should be distinguished from those which sometimes produce colds but also more serious respiratory disease and

from others that cause diseases in which a coldlike prodrome precedes the major illness.

The viruses invade the nasal epithelium and cause two main effects: (1) inflammation of the nasal mucous membrane with the excessive production of mucus (catarrh) and (2) loss of superficial ciliated epithelial cells. During the 5 to 7 days of the infection, the nasal discharge, which initially is clear and mucoid, becomes opaque, yellowish, and tenacious as the inflammation subsides and polymorphonuclear leukocytes emigrate into the mucus. Complications are usually caused by obstruction of the eustachian tubes or ostia of the paranasal sinuses, leading to otitis media and sinusitis, respectively.

Contrary to long-held beliefs, cold viruses can often be transmitted to the nose of the host by touch and not exclusively by the inhalation of aerosolized droplets as previously believed. Patients with colds contaminate their hands with virus-infected secretions. These are then transmitted to the nose of the new host directly by touch or indirectly (e.g., door handles or taps).

Clinically, the common cold syndrome is a mild, self-limiting infection with a worldwide distribution. The continuing failure of medical science to "cure" the common cold, long a cliché with professional entertainers and the public, can be attributed to the enormous number of virus types (see previous box) and the viral nature of most colds. The former makes vaccine development unlikely; antiviral drugs are impractical for such a relatively minor illness. At present, with nonspecific remedies, the common cold lasts about 7 days; without treatment it lasts about a week!

Sinusitis

Sinusitis is inflammation of one or more of the paranasal sinuses. It may be acute or chronic.

The following can initiate acute sinusitis:
1. Direct extension of a viral cold to the paranasal sinuses
2. Involvement of the sinus mucosa in allergic rhinitis
3. Extraction of upper teeth, which can cause an oroantral fistula, or when a root is forced into the maxillary antrum
4. Forcible entry of infected or irritant materials, which can be caused by pressure changes during diving in an aircraft or by vomiting against a closed nose and mouth usually to avoid social embarrassment

Chronic sinusitis for unknown reasons frequently accompanies bronchiectasis (discussed later in this chapter).

The bacteria most commonly isolated from patients with acute sinusitis are *Haemophilus influenzae*, *Staphylococcus aureus*, and *Streptococcus pneumoniae*. In addition, anaerobic bacteria are commonly present in the antral secretions of patients with chronic sinusitis. Obstruction of the outlets (ostia) of the sinuses, usually as a result of inflammatory edema, initiates the attack. Deviation of the nasal septum, commonly associated with sinusitis, predisposes to such obstruction.

Pathology. In acute sinusitis there is acute inflammation of the sinus mucosa with destruction of the superficial epithelium and production of mucopurulent secretions. In most instances this process will resolve with restoration of the epithelium. In some instances, as a result of persistent or recurrent infection, chronic sinusitis develops. It is characterized by mucosal thickening and the formation of rounded or elongated masses of thickened mucous membrane called *polyps*.

Although uncommon, the complications of sinusitis can be very serious. They include brain abscess, cavernous sinus thrombosis, and meningitis.

> ### VIRUSES ASSOCIATED WITH COMMON COLD SYNDROME
>
> **Group 1—Viruses causing only common cold syndrome**
> Rhinoviruses (100 + serotypes)
> Coronaviruses (20 + serotypes)
>
> **Group 2—Viruses causing common cold syndrome and more severe respiratory tract infections**
> Adenoviruses (especially types 1 to 7, 14, and 21)
> Influenza viruses (A, B, and C)
> Parainfluenza viruses (4 serotypes)
> Respiratory syncytial virus
>
> **Group 3—Viruses causing common cold syndrome and infections of other systems**
> Coxsackievirus A (especially type 21)
> Coxsackievirus B (especially types 4 and 5)
> Echoviruses (especially types 11, 20, and 25)
>
> **Group 4—Viruses causing common cold as prodromal stage of more serious illness**
> Measles virus
> Mumps virus

Mild upper respiratory tract infections have been associated with the nonviral agents *Mycoplasma pneumoniae*, *Coxiella burnetii*, and *Chlamydia psittaci*.

Clinical aspects. Acute sinusitis is characterized by pain and tenderness over the affected sinus. Pain in sphenoidal or ethmoidal sinusitis is referred to the back or side of the head. In chronic sinusitis the main complaint is of persistent mucopurulent nasal discharge. Most cases of acute sinusitis resolve after treatment with analgesics and decongestants. In more severe infections, antibiotics may be necessary. Surgery is usually reserved for chronic cases.

Other conditions of the nose and sinuses

Zygomycosis (mucormycosis, phycomycosis). Invasion of the paranasal sinuses by fungi, especially *Mucor* and *Rhizopus* species, is a serious complication of poorly controlled diabetes mellitus, hemolymphatic malignancies, and immunosuppression. Fungal hyphae proliferating in the sinuses invade blood vessels, causing hemorrhagic inflammation and tissue necrosis. The disease may spread to involve the orbit or the brain. Treatment is that of the underlying cause, together with antifungal therapy and sometimes surgery. Only half of the cases successfully respond to treatment; those who do are almost exclusively diabetics.

Rhinoscleroma. Rhinoscleroma is a rare granulomatous infection of the nose due to *Klebsiella rhinoscleromatis*. On microscopic examination, nodular masses consisting of chronic inflammatory cells and large foamy macrophages containing the gram-negative bacteria are found.

Midline lethal granuloma. Also called malignant granuloma of the nose, this disease of unknown cause behaves like a destructive, malignant process. It begins in the nose or the sinuses as an area of necrosis that spreads and can destroy wide areas of orofacial tissue. Many cases are now believed to be T-cell lymphomas, which on pathologic examination, are pleomorphic and show strong angiocentric and angiodestructive changes. A high proportion of the remaining cases are Wegener's granulomatosis, in which there is an infiltrate of normal lymphocytes and macrophages and a necrotizing vasculitis. The disease may be controlled by radiation or cytotoxic therapy, followed by reconstructive surgery.

Laryngotracheobronchitis

Inflammation of the main air passages is most commonly caused by infectious agents, but it may also be produced by noninfectious causes such as irritant vapors and allergic reactions. Primary infectious causes are:

1. Influenza viruses
2. Parainfluenza viruses
3. Respiratory syncytial virus

Bacterial infections by *S. pneumoniae* and staphylococci are usually secondary to virus infections, but primary bacterial laryngotracheobronchitis is sometimes caused by *H. influenzae* and diphtheria. In the former, the larynx and epiglottis are especially prone to severe inflammation, and there is danger of acute obstruction of the airway by inflammatory edema. In diphtheria, airway obstruction is caused by blockage by the pseudomembrane, which sometimes forms in the larynx, trachea, or bronchi.

Pathology. In laryngotracheobronchitis, the mucosa is acutely inflamed, often with loss of ciliated epithelium (Fig. 12-1). Secondary invasion by bacteria such as staphylococci and pneumococci can lead to suppuration.

Clinically, the most important complication is laryngeal obstruction, which may require emergency tracheostomy to save the patient's life. This is most likely in young children because of the small size of their airway.

CAUSES OF LARYNGEAL OBSTRUCTION	
Acute	**Chronic**
Allergy	External pressure from:
Diphtheria	Aneurysms
Foreign bodies	Tumors of adjacent structures
H. influenzae laryngitis	Laryngeal tumors

Laryngeal obstruction. Laryngeal obstruction can be acute or chronic. Some of the important causes are listed in the box. Among the acute causes, angioedema (Figs. 12-2 and 12-3) is perhaps the most dramatic (Chapter 19).

Whooping cough (pertussis). An infectious disease of children, whooping cough is characterized by a paroxysmal cough and thick mucopurulent sputum. It is usually caused by *Bordetella pertussis* but some cases are due to *B. parapertussis*. A similar syndrome has been attributed to adenoviruses.

Pathogenesis. The pathogenesis of whooping cough is still unclear. The organism remains on the respiratory mucosal surface, where it incites an inflammatory response and the production of tenacious sputum. Two features of the disease—the altered reactivity of the bronchial smooth muscle and the extraordinary lymphocytosis—are attributed to the effects of bacterial endotoxin release.

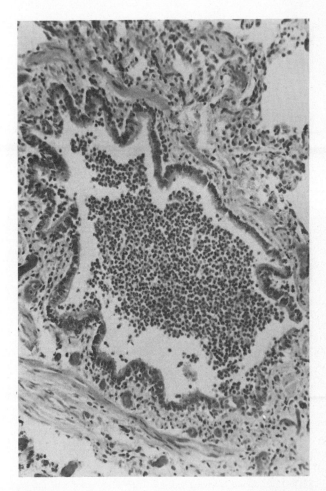

FIG. 12-1. Acute bronchitis. There is some loss of the bronchial epithelium and the bronchial lumen contains many pus cells.

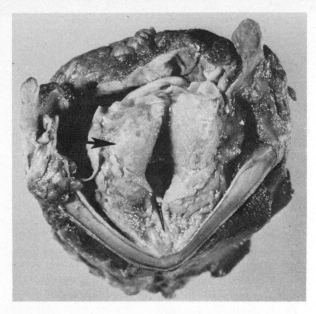

FIG. 12-2. Acute laryngeal edema. Note intense swelling of laryngeal tissues and vocal cords *(arrow)*. The patient died of acute asphyxiation.

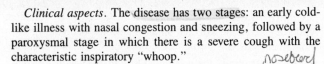

Clinical aspects. The disease has two stages: an early cold-like illness with nasal congestion and sneezing, followed by a paroxysmal stage in which there is a severe cough with the characteristic inspiratory "whoop."

Complications are frequent and range from epistaxis and ocular hemorrhages, resulting from very high venous pressure caused by coughing, to occlusion of bronchi by bronchial secretions, leading to pneumonia and later to bronchiectasis. The clinical picture is very typical, especially in the presence of pronounced lymphocytosis; white blood cells may number $200,000/\mu m$ (normal is 1500 to $4000/\mu m$).

The epidemic spread of whooping cough can be greatly reduced by killed vaccines. However, reports of serious adverse reactions to the vaccines have prompted efforts to improve their safety and efficacy. Treatment is by erythromycin, which has little effect on the course of the disease, but prevents bacteriologic relapse and may reduce transmission of infection.

The pneumonias (pneumonitis)

Pneumonia can be defined as inflammation of the lung parenchyma, characterized by an inflammatory exudate within the interstitium and/or the alveoli. Pneumonia can be caused by infectious or noninfectious agents. The former are considered here; noninfectious pneumonias are discussed later in the chapter.

Classification based on anatomic distribution and pathologic changes or etiologic agents is not completely satisfactory. An-

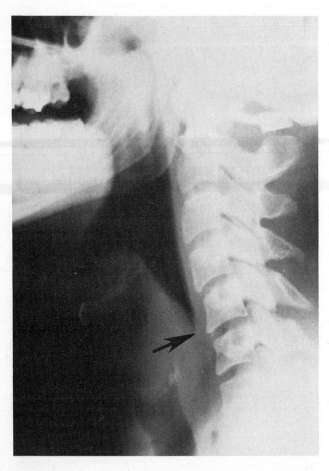

FIG. 12-3. Acute laryngeal edema. Lateral radiograph of the neck shows that the normal dark shadow of the airway is occluded *(arrow)* by acute laryngeal edema.

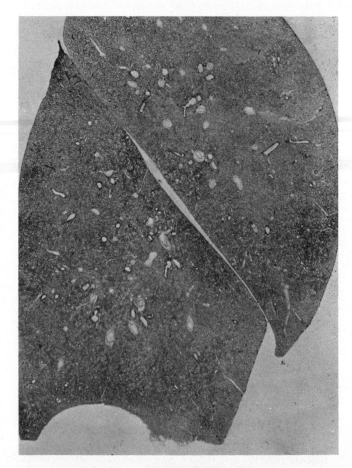

FIG. 12-4. A normal whole lung section. *(Courtesy Curator of the Gordon Museum, Guy's Hospital, London, England.)*

atomically, pneumonias may be considered to be lobar, lobular, or interstitial.

Lobar pneumonia describes an inflammatory process that involves the alveoli of an entire lobe, without involvement of the bronchi. *Lobular pneumonia* (more traditionally known as *bronchopneumonia*) describes a process of pulmonary inflammation in which both the bronchi and the lobules they supply are involved in the inflammatory process.

Interstitial pneumonia means that the inflammation is primarily in the interstitium of the lung rather than within the alveoli. Interstitial pneumonias are commonly caused by viruses.

Lobar pneumonia

Etiology. The term lobar pneumonia is virtually synonymous with pneumococcal pneumonia, since 90% of the cases in which the pneumonic process involves an entire lobe are caused by *S. pneumoniae*. The serotypes isolated from adults differ from those in children. Types 1, 3, 4, and 8 are the main causes in adults; types 6, 14, 19, and 23 are the main causes in children. It is noteworthy that with one exception, type 3, these organisms are not the serotypes that are normally part of the resident flora of the oropharynx and nasopharynx. The causative organisms in the remaining 10% of cases are mainly *S. aureus* and *Klebsiella pneumoniae*. In patients with acquired immunodeficiency syndrome (AIDS), primary pneumonias caused by *S. aureus* and *Branhamella catarrhalis* (a bacterium for-

merly believed to be a harmless commensal organism) are now fairly common.

Pathogenesis and pathology. The pathologic processes described here are those seen in untreated pneumococcal pneumonia. When adequate antibiotic treatment is given early in the illness, few patients develop the full range of pathologic changes. Despite antibiotics, deaths from pneumococcal disease, especially in the very young and those over 55, are still common.

S. pneumoniae reaches the alveoli through the airways and initiates an inflammatory response, which spreads rapidly to involve a complete lobe. More than one lobe may be affected at the same time. Initially, the alveolar capillaries become congested. This is followed by the appearance in the alveoli of a fibrin-rich exudate containing a few polymorphonuclear leukocytes and red blood cells. On gross examination, the lung (Fig. 12-4) takes on a solid, deep red appearance, which pathologists in the past compared to liver *(red hepatization)*.

By this time the inflammatory process has reached the pleura and acute fibrinous pleurisy (pleuritis) develops over the surface of the affected lobe. The cellular stage of the acute inflammatory process is characterized by the appearance of numerous polymorphonuclear leukocytes (Fig. 12-5) within the alveoli, changing the gross appearance of the lung from red to *gray hepatization* (Fig. 12-6). At this stage, tremendous phagocytic

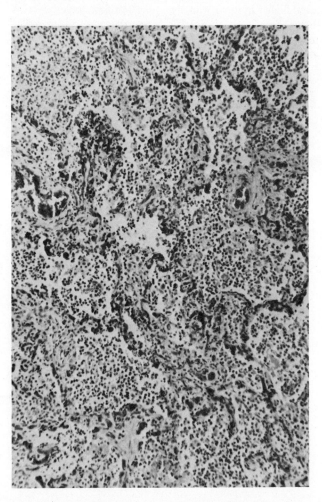

FIG. 12-5. Lobar pneumonia. The alveoli are filled with polymorphonuclear leukocytes. This produces the gross appearance of gray hepatization.

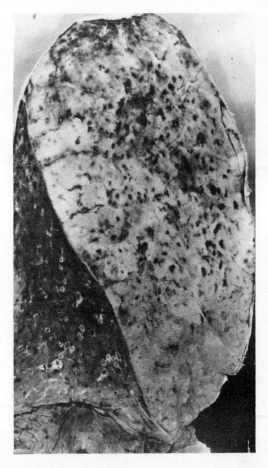

FIG. 12-6. Lobar pneumonia; gray hepatization. Note complete consolidation of the upper lobe. The lung is gray-white as a result of the large numbers of polymorphonuclear leukocytes filling the alveoli. Compare with Fig. 12-4. *(Courtesy Curator of the Gordon Museum, Guy's Hospital, London, England.)*

activity and lysis of leukocytes begins. During these stages of active inflammation, perhaps 30% or more of patients have positive blood cultures for *S. pneumoniae*.

In the most favorable circumstances, resolution is finally achieved by means of enzymatic and macrophage activity so that the inflammatory exudate is completely removed without suppuration. The fibrinous pleural exudate resolves by fibrovascular repair. Unlike the lung parenchyma, which returns to normal, the pleural surface is permanently scarred and thickened, sometimes with adhesions between the visceral and parietal pleural layers. Without antibiotic therapy, progressive toxemia with failure of the pulmonary consolidation to resolve led to the deaths of about one third of the patients in the past. In others a variety of complications developed, some of which were also fatal.

The main complications of lobar pneumonia, with the possible exception of bacteremia, are more common and severe with *S. aureus* and *K. pneumoniae* than with *S. pneumoniae*. The main complications include the following:
1. Lung abscess
2. Empyema (pus in the pleural cavity) caused by extension of suppuration to the pleura
3. Distal effects of bacteremia
   a. Purulent meningitis
   b. Acute endocarditis

4. Pulmonary fibrosis of the affected lobe as a result of failure of resolution and organization of the inflammatory alveolar exudate (Fig. 12-7)

Clinical aspects. Early inflammatory changes in the lung are associated with sudden onset of high fever and chills, malaise, and frequently inspiratory pain in the chest caused by pleurisy. Patients often cough up small amounts of blood-stained sputum. Many develop herpetic lesions on the lips. If untreated, there is progressive dullness to percussion on the affected side, continuing fever, and worsening of the patient's clinical state. The most favorable outcome in untreated patients is a sudden improvement in the patient's condition and subsidence of fever (defervescence) around the end of the first week of the illness (the crisis) that corresponds to the resolution phase described earlier.

Deaths are the result of cardiorespiratory failure or the effects of major complications such as meningitis or endocarditis. The administration of antibiotics, particularly penicillin G or erythromycin, usually changes the clinical picture dramatically. Fever and pleuritic pain subside in 1 to 3 days. Signs of pulmonary consolidation also subside, usually within a week.

The diagnosis rests on radiographic demonstration (Fig. 12-8) of pulmonary consolidation and the presence of polymorphonuclear leukocytes in the sputum. Despite the use of antibiotics, the death rate in bacteremic pneumococcal pneumonia is about 20% in the 12- to 50-year-old age group and even higher in those who are over 50 or have underlying systemic disease. For this reason, a pneumococcal vaccine, originally containing 14 but now consisting of 23 types of pneumococci, has been developed. The vaccine confers effective

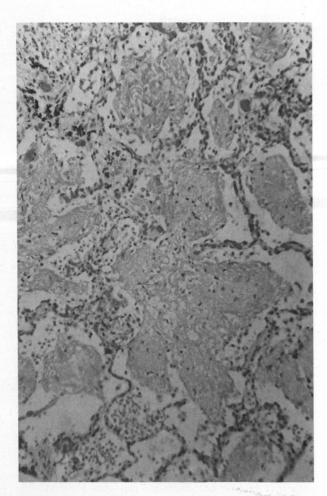

FIG. 12-7. Nonresolution of lobar pneumonia. Residual fibrin plugs, seen in the alveolar spaces, will eventually be replaced by fibrous tissue.

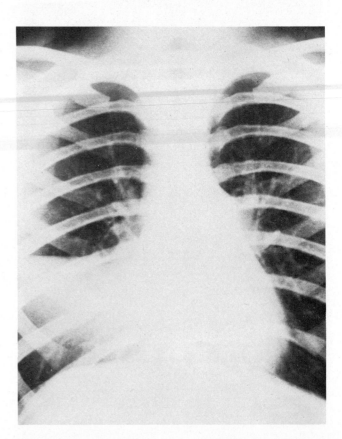

FIG. 12-8. Lobar pneumonia. In this radiograph the consolidation zone in the right lower lobe is sharply delineated by the line of the horizontal fissure.

immunity on most patient groups except children under 2 years and patients with lymphomas. It is recommended especially for those who have sickle cell anemia or who have undergone splenectomy.

Lobular pneumonia

Etiology. Lobular pneumonia (bronchopneumonia) is caused by extension of inflammation of the bronchi and bronchioles into the alveoli. In this respect, the disease differs from lobar pneumonia, in which the bronchi and bronchioles are normal. The main predisposing conditions in lobular pneumonia are:

1. Acute viral or bacterial bronchitis or bronchiolitis such as influenza and whooping cough
2. Chronic bronchitis and bronchiectasis
3. Cardiac failure
4. Cancer
5. Immunosuppression

In addition, any condition that is likely to cause aspiration of upper respiratory tract secretions or gastric content commonly results in pulmonary infection. Such conditions include anesthesia, alcoholism, and coma from any cause. The inhalation of irritant fumes and gases can also predispose to bronchopneumonia.

The microorganisms causing lobular pneumonia are much more varied than those causing lobar pneumonia, and very often more than one organism is involved. Generally they are derived from the normal flora of the upper respiratory tract. Common bacteria isolated from patients with lobular pneumonia are:

1. Streptococci, especially *S. pneumoniae,* but different types from those causing lobar pneumonia.
2. *S. aureus*
3. *H. influenzae*
4. Anaerobic bacteria of the genera *Bacteroides* and *Fusobacterium*
5. Gram-negative aerobic bacilli, especially *Klebsiella, Pseudomonas,* and *Proteus* species and *Escherichia coli*
6. Various fungi (e.g., *Candida albicans, Aspergillus*), which are especially common in patients with AIDS

The gram-negative aerobic bacteria are especially common as a cause of lobular pneumonia in hospitalized patients or those receiving immunosuppressive therapy. *Legionella pneumophila,* the cause of Legionnaire's disease, also causes lobular pneumonia.

Pathogenesis and pathology. The inflammatory changes begin in the bronchi and spread down into the related areas of the lung parenchyma, especially to the lower lobes, by gravitational drainage. The resultant inflammatory process is patchy and lobular in distribution with relatively normal lung tissue lying between the pneumonic areas. The affected areas become consolidated with large numbers of polymorphonuclear leukocytes, with milder degrees of inflammation at the margins (Fig. 12-9). With some bacteria, such as *S. aureus* and *K. pneumoniae,* necrosis and abscess formation may be prominent. Spread of infection to the periphery of the lungs results in fibrinous pleurisy.

Immunosuppressed patients are often unable to mount an adequate white blood cell response to the infecting organisms, and overwhelming infection develops rapidly. In these circumstances the lungs contain a fibrinous exudate with many bacteria but few polymorphonuclear leukocytes.

Clinical aspects. Bronchopneumonia, or lobular pneumonia, is almost always a complication of underlying illness. The clinical manifestations, unlike those of lobar pneumonia, are variable and sometimes minimal despite the severity of the pathologic process. Fever is common. A cough, especially one that produces purulent sputum, during the course of another infection that predisposes to pneumonia, is very suggestive of the disease. If the disease is untreated, resolution is unlikely, and complications such as lung abscess, empyema, and bronchiectasis are almost inevitable.

The diagnosis again rests on radiography and on the identification of the causative organisms by bacteriologic examination of lower respiratory tract secretions. Selection of the correct treatment is based on antimicrobial susceptibility studies because of the diversity of organisms and their patterns of sensitivity to antimicrobial agents.

The outlook in lobular pneumonia depends on many factors. Severe disease or death is most likely in the very old and the very young, in those with severe underlying disease, especially the immunosuppressed, and when treatment is delayed or inappropriate. Lobar and lobular pneumonias are compared in Table 12-1. The clinicopathologic effects of bronchopneumonia due to specific organisms are compared in Table 12-2.

Community-acquired and hospital-acquired pneumonias.

The epidemiologic and clinical features of various pneumonias caused by infectious agents allow the pneumonias to be classified as hospital acquired (nosocomial) or community acquired.

Hospital-acquired pneumonias comprise those that are generally of the lobular type. They affect patients with underlying illnesses and are caused by a wide range of bacteria, especially

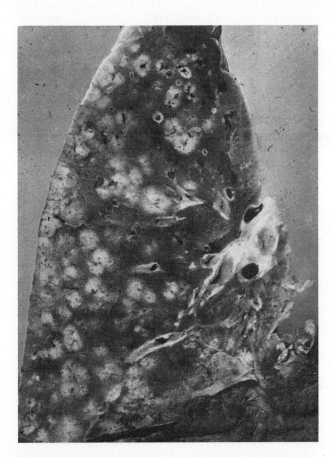

FIG. 12-9. Bronchopneumonia. Many round white areas of pneumonic consolidation appear throughout the lung. Each pneumonic area surrounds a small bronchus. *(Courtesy Curator of the Gordon Museum, Guy's Hospital, London, England.)*

TABLE 12-1. Comparison of lobar and lobular pneumonia

	Lobar	Lobular
Etiology	90% *S. pneumoniae*, 10% *S. aureus* and *K. pneumoniae*	*S. pneumoniae*, *S. aureus*, *H. influenzae*; anaerobes; enteric gram-negative rods
Predisposing diseases	Usually none	Measles, influenza, neoplasms
Age group	Mainly adult	Very young and older adults
Pathology	Alveolar consolidation, pleurisy; bronchi normal; can resolve without treatment	Bronchial inflammation, alveolar consolidation, pleurisy; rarely resolves without treatment
Complications	Uncommon in treated patients	Frequent
Local	Lung abscess, empyema	Lung abscess, empyema
Distant	Hematogenous spread, especially to meninges, heart valves	Hematogenous spread to brain

TABLE 12-2. Associated clinical conditions and pathology of other bacterial pneumonias

Organism	Associated conditions	Main pathologic features
S. aureus	Influenza, measles, pertussis, AIDS	Acute hemorrhagic inflammation; abscess formation
K. pneumoniae	Chronic liver disease, diabetes mellitus	Pulmonary consolidation; cavity formation
L. pneumophila (occasionally other species)	Air-conditioning and humidifying equipment	Pulmonary consolidation; alveoli contain fibrin macrophages, polymorphonuclear leukocytes; cyst formation
Pseudomonas aeruginosa	Immunosuppression; mechanical respiratory support	Hemorrhagic inflammation; vascular invasion by bacteria

gram-negative bacilli, and fungi, as previously mentioned. These organisms are usually derived from patients' resident bacterial flora or occasionally from the hospital environment.

Community-acquired pneumonias frequently affect patients who are otherwise healthy and are almost exclusively caused by one of three microorganisms:

1. *S. pneumoniae*
2. *Mycoplasma pneumoniae*, the cause of primary atypical pneumonia
3. *L. pneumophila* and related species, the cause of legionellosis (Legionnaire's disease)

Mycoplasma (primary atypical) pneumonia

Etiology. Mycoplasmas are unusual bacteria that do not possess a cell wall. *M. pneumoniae* (formerly known as the Eaton agent) is the most important pathogenic member of this curious group.

M. pneumoniae causes a form of pneumonitis called *primary atypical pneumonia*. This is an unsatisfactory term because it

may be applied to pneumonias caused by other infectious agents, such as viruses or rickettsias.

Mycoplasma pneumonia has also been called *cold agglutinin–positive pneumonia* because cold agglutinins to the I antigen of red blood cells appear in some patients. However, about 50% do not develop cold agglutinins, and these antibodies are demonstrable in some patients with viral pneumonia.

Pathogenesis and pathology. *M. pneumoniae* multiplies extracellularly and has a strong affinity for the cytoplasmic membranes of epithelial cells. By this means the organism appears able to damage or interfere with the cell membrane. Knowledge of the pathology of mycoplasma pneumonia is limited because it is rarely fatal. In those few fatal cases, the findings have been mild bronchial hyperemia with intact respiratory epithelium and fibrinous pleurisy. Patchy areas of interstitial pneumonitis, in which plasma cells are prominent, and collections of mononuclear cells in the alveoli have been described, particularly in the upper lobes.

Clinical aspects. Mycoplasma pneumonia is a very common disease. Only pneumonia caused by *S. pneumoniae* is more common. By contrast, in military populations and possibly in young adults in the general population, *M. pneumoniae* may be the most common cause of pneumonia. The disease is curious in that signs and symptoms are often mild despite radiographic evidence of widespread disease. Fever, malaise, chest pain, and coldlike symptoms are common; hemorrhagic inflammation of the eardrum has been described in some patients. A chronic nonproductive cough is typical. A few patients develop hemolytic anemia as a result of cold antibodies. Most patients develop complement-fixing antibodies that are diagnostically useful. Mycoplasmas can be isolated from throat swabs or sputum. Complete recovery is the rule even without treatment with erythromycin or tetracycline, the two drugs of choice. In some outbreaks, patients have complained of persistent lethargy, weakness, and malaise long after the radiographs are normal. The reason for this is not known. After *M. pneumonia* infection, a few patients develop a severe inflammatory disease involving the mucous membranes of the eye, mouth, and genital tract (Stevens-Johnson syndrome).*

Legionellosis. Legionellosis is a term used to describe pulmonary disease caused by bacteria of the genus *Legionella*. The most notorious outbreak caused by these organisms was among those who attended an American Legion conference in Philadelphia in 1976, when the term "Legionnaire's disease" was coined. However, several outbreaks of the same disease had been reported in the previous 10 years but no etiologic agent was identified.

Etiology. The etiologic agent was isolated and identified in 1978 and has been named *L. pneumophila*. Since then it has been established that at least one other similar bacterium, *L. micdadei*, can occasionally cause Legionnaire's disease.

Pathogenesis and pathology. *L. pneumophila* appears to be a water bacterium but can also be found in dry soil. Infection is by airborne spread, such as from contaminated air-conditioning cooling towers.

The role of the many extracellular products of *L. pneumophila* in the pathogenesis of pulmonary disease has not yet been established. It is postulated that the organism can enter macrophages and in effect paralyze their phagocytic activity.

The main pathologic findings in the lung in fatal cases of le-

---

*A.M. Stevens (1884-1945), American pediatrician; F.C. Johnson (1894-1934), American pediatrician.

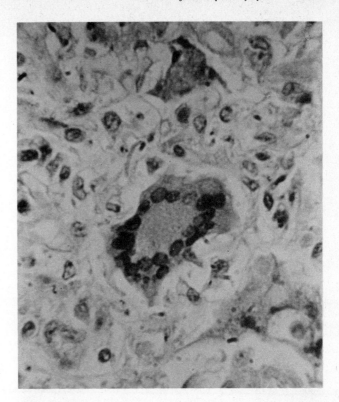

gionellosis are those of a lobular type of pneumonia, varying from discrete patches of inflammation and consolidation to involvement of whole lobes and the presence of small abscesses. Pleural inflammation with effusion is common but seldom severe. The alveolar exudate consists of polymorphonuclear leukocytes, macrophages, and fibrin; similar inflammatory cells are present in the interstitium where the alveolar septae are thickened and edematous. Numerous bacteria can be demonstrated in sections stained by Dieterle's silver impregnation method and specifically identified by immunofluorescence. In several cases, infection has spread to the pericardium and myocardium.

The death rate can be as high as 10%; causes of death range from cardiorespiratory failure to endotoxin shock.

Clinical aspects. Asymptomatic infections in young persons are probably common, but the disease affects mainly the elderly. Apart from a high incidence of diarrhea, there are no specific clinical findings to distinguish legionellosis from other pneumonias. The antimicrobial treatment of choice is erythromycin.

Viral pneumonia

Etiology. Following are the viruses that can cause pneumonia:

1. Influenza viruses, especially influenza A
2. Parainfluenza viruses
3. Respiratory syncytial viruses
4. Adenoviruses
5. Varicella (chickenpox)
6. *Herpesvirus hominis*
7. Cytomegalovirus
8. Measles virus

The first four of these viruses can cause primary pulmonary infection, whereas the remainder usually cause pneumonia as a complication of a generalized illness. Cytomegalovirus (CMV) is now a frequent cause of pneumonia in immunosuppressed patients, including those with AIDS. This is usually the result of reactivation of latent infection, often in association with other latent agents, such as the protozoa *Pneumocystis carinii* or *Toxoplasma gondii*, on which CMV may have a growth-promoting effect.

Among the viruses listed, respiratory syncytial, parainfluenza, and measles cause viral pneumonia almost exclusively in children. Fatal viral pneumonia may result from the vaccination of an immunodeficient child with live attenuated measles vaccine (Fig. 12-10).

Influenza virus pneumonia can affect all age groups. A most devastating form of this disease was particularly common in young, previously healthy adults during the world influenza pandemic in 1918 to 1920 and contributed to 20 million deaths.

Varicella pneumonia is almost exclusively a disease of adults. Only 10% of the patients are less than 19 years old.

Pathogenesis and pathology. Virtually all viral pneumonias are characterized by interstitial inflammation, with microscopic appearances similar to that previously described for mycoplasma pneumonia (Figs. 12-11 and 12-12). Some of the distinguishing features of the different viral pneumonias are listed in Table 12-3.

Clinical aspects. Common to most viral pneumonias are fever, chills, and a nonproductive cough. Because no specific treatment is currently available, the management is essentially to maintain respiratory function (by mechanical ventilation if necessary) and prevent or treat secondary bacterial infection. Hyperimmune globulin has been used to ameliorate varicella pneumonia. Deaths as a result of influenza, measles, and re-

FIG. 12-10. Lung in measles pneumonia. The microscopic appearances are of an intense interstitial pneumonitis with a multinucleate (Warthin-Finkeldey) giant cell. The patient was an immunodeficient infant who received live attenuated vaccine. (*From McCracken AW and Cawson RA: Clinical and oral microbiology, Washington DC, 1982, Hemisphere Publishing Corp.*)

spiratory syncytial virus pneumonia are common. Persistent or even permanent impairment of gaseous diffusion is common after varicella pneumonia.

Chlamydia *and* Coxiella *pneumonias*. Pneumonia is a complication of several infamous infectious diseases such as plague and typhus, which are now, fortunately, much more rare than in the past. Two agents that are unusual but true bacteria can cause primary pneumonia in humans: (1) *Chlamydia psittaci*, the cause of psittacosis in humans, and (2) *Coxiella burnetii*, the cause of Q (for query) fever. Both of these organisms are primarily pathogens of animals or birds, but occasionally these organisms spread from animals to humans (zoonosis).

Psittacosis. *C. psittaci* is an obligate, intracellular bacterium that mainly parasitizes parakeets, parrots, or budgerigars (psittacine birds), but the disease has been described in many other bird species, including turkeys, pigeons, and finches. In birds the disease is called *ornithosis*. Humans are infected by inhalation of particles containing the organisms, which are derived from the droppings or respiratory secretions of birds.

The pathologic changes in the lung consist of an interstitial pneumonia with lymphocytes and macrophages present both in the interstitium and the alveoli. Basophilic intracytoplasmic inclusions are present in the alveolar macrophages.

Clinically, psittacosis is an atypical pneumonia, very often accompanied by splenomegaly. Severe headache is consistently present; progressive delirium is seen in untreated cases. A few cases have been complicated by *C. psittaci* endocarditis. Tetracyclines are considered the most effective drugs for treatment; however, even in treated cases, the mortality is 5%.

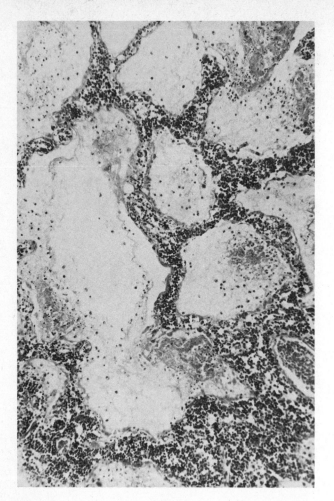

FIG. 12-11. Lung in viral pneumonia demonstrating the characteristically interstitial lymphocytic infiltrate.

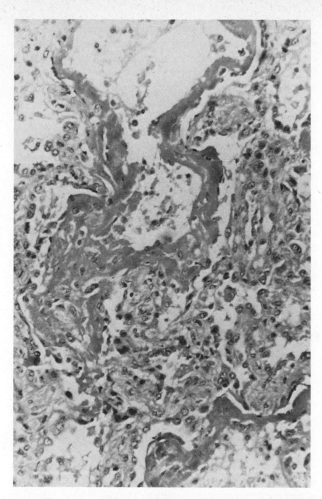

FIG. 12-12. Influenzal pneumonia. Hyaline material lines the terminal air spaces of the lung.

TABLE 12-3. Pathologic features of viral pneumonias

Virus	Pathologic findings	Inclusions	Remarks	Outcome
Influenza	Bronchitis, bronchiolitis, interstitial pneumonia, mononuclear infiltrates of alveolar septae, hyaline membrane, pulmonary edema	Absent	Almost always caused by influenza A	High fatality rate
Measles	Bronchitis, bronchiolitis, hyperplasia of bronchiolar epithelium, interstitial pneumonia, multinucleate giant cells	Present in giant cells, nuclei, cytoplasm	Only found in children from 6 months to 2 years	Always fatal
Adenovirus	Bronchial ulceration and necrosis, submucous lymphocytic infiltration, interstitial pneumonitis, alveolar cell desquamation, hyaline membranes	Present; nuclear in bronchi, alveolar cells	Usually caused by types 3 and 7	Usually resolves
Parainfluenza and respiratory syncytial virus	Bronchiolitis, peribronchiolar lymphocytic infiltrates, multinucleate giant cells	Present; nuclear and cytoplasmic occasionally seen	Serious infection in infants; mild in adults	Mortality rate about 5% in infants for RSV
Varicella	Interstitial pneumonia, mononuclear infiltrate in alveolar septae, pulmonary edema, giant cells	Present; nuclear in giant cells	Mainly in adults or immunosuppressed patients	Commonly fatal in adults; gaseous exchange impairment also common
CMV	As for varicella	As for varicella	Affects immunosuppressed patients	Often fatal

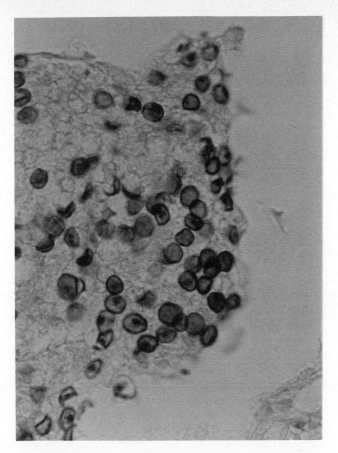

FIG. 12-13. Lung in pneumocystis infection. Many oval or collapsed cystic parasites are seen, staining darkly with silver stain, against a background of amorphous foamy material.

An interstitial pneumonitis with similar pathologic features has been recognized in neonates in recent years. This disease is caused by *Chlamydia trachomatis,* an organism closely related to *C. psittaci.* Infection is transmitted from mother to infant during delivery. The source of infection is the maternal cervix, which is the site of asymptomatic or undiagnosed chlamydial cervicitis (Chapter 23).

Q fever. The causative organism, *Coxiella burnetii,* is a pathogen of livestock and wild animals, among which it is spread by ticks. Human infection is caused by inhalation of infected particles. Little information is available regarding the pulmonary pathology, since the infection is often asymptomatic or causes an acute interstitial pneumonia that is usually self-limiting and very rarely fatal. Hepatitis with hepatosplenomegaly is present in many cases. Fatalities in Q fever are rare and are due to endocarditis, which can develop months or even years after the initial infection. Although tetracycline and chloramphenicol are effective drugs in other rickettsial diseases, it is not known whether they are effective in Q fever, since most cases are undiagnosed or treated empirically.

Pneumocystis pneumonia. Pneumonia caused by *Pneumocystis carinii* is the most important cause of protozoal pneumonia, a disease that is seen almost exclusively in immunocompromised patients, especially those with AIDS. The organism, a round or oval parasite, often forms a small cyst or rosette of six to eight parasites. Its life cycle and the source of infection for humans are not known, but rodents are a likely source. Strong epidemiologic evidence suggests airborne human-to-human spread of infection in outbreaks in institutions. A majority of the population has antibodies to *P. carinii,* indicating that asymptomatic infection is very common.

Pulmonary infection can affect the following:
1. Infants with immune deficiency diseases
2. Patients of all ages with disseminated malignancies
3. Patients who are immunosuppressed from any cause, particularly those with AIDS

The pathologic features of *Pneumocystis* infection of the lung, which begins at the hilum and spreads peripherally, include:
1. An interstitial inflammatory reaction
2. A mononuclear cell infiltrate with moderate numbers of plasma cells
3. Intraalveolar, eosinophilic, foamy material
4. Intraalveolar fibrosis, granulomas, and calcification as the disease progresses and becomes chronic
5. The presence of organisms that stain brown-black with silver stains within the alveoli (Fig. 12-13)

The clinical features, as would be suggested by the gradual development of the pathologic changes, consist of insidious onset of slowly increasing dyspnea and fever. The diagnosis is confirmed by chest radiography and the demonstration of the protozoan in a lung biopsy or bronchial brushings. The current effective treatment of pneumocystosis is cotrimoxazole or pentamidine. However, the outcome is greatly affected by the underlying immunosuppressed state.

Pulmonary tuberculosis

Tuberculosis is defined as an infectious disease caused by *Mycobacterium tuberculosis* (tubercle bacillus) or rarely by *M. bovis.* This definition is necessary to distinguish tuberculosis from infections by the nontuberculous ("atypical") mycobacteria, some of which can cause pulmonary disease resembling tuberculosis (Table 12-4).

Etiology. *M. tuberculosis* is a slender, acid-fast bacillus between 1 and 4 μm in length. Important cellular components of *M. tuberculosis* include a number of complex lipids, such as mycolic acids, which appear to have a role in the pathogenesis, especially in the process of caseation. Protein antigens derived from *M. tuberculosis* (tuberculoproteins) have a major role in the hypersensitivity reactions associated with the infection.

Infection by tubercle bacilli is usually by droplets entering the respiratory tract. Because pasteurization of milk is almost universal in advanced countries, infection by *M. bovis* via the intestinal tract is rare.

Pathogenesis. About 95% of nonimmune persons exposed to *M. tuberculosis* for the first time become infected but have no clinical evidence of disease; that is, they have an asymptomatic primary infection. Five percent of those infected develop disease localized to the lungs, whereas in a few persons, progressive disease spreads to other organs. This is called *primary tuberculosis.* All of these nonimmune individuals, within a short period of time, develop a cell-mediated immune response to mycobacterial antigens (i.e., they have become sensitized to *M. tuberculosis*). Many months or years after the primary infection, some of these sensitized persons develop tuberculous lesions in the lungs. This is called *reactivation,* or *recrudescent, tuberculosis.*

Whether persons infected with *M. tuberculosis* develop active disease or not depends on the properties of both the host and the bacterium. Host resistance depends on, among other things, age and race. Infections in young children are more

TABLE 12-4. Nontuberculous mycobacteria that cause diseases of the lungs and other systems

Mycobacterium	Lungs	Tendons, bones, joints	Cervical nodes	Skin	Disseminated disease
M. avium-intracellulare	C	UC	UC	—	UC
M. chelonei	U	C	UC	C	UC
M. fortuitum	U	UC	UC	C	UC
M. kansasii	C	C	UC	UC	C
M. marinum	—	UC	—	C	—
M. scrofulaceum	UC	UC	C	—	UC
M. simiae, M. szulgi, M. xenopi	UC	—	—	—	—

C, Common; *UC*, uncommon; —, not described.

likely to progress to serious disease than in adults. For unknown reasons, fair-skinned persons are less likely to develop progressive disease than dark-skinned (African, American Indian, or Eskimo) persons. Black males with tissue type Bw15 are particularly susceptible. The infecting organisms may vary in their numbers and virulence. Clearly a large inoculum of virulent *M. tuberculosis* is most likely to cause active disease than a small dose of an attenuated strain.

Tuberculin test. The procedure for demonstration of cell-mediated immunity to *M. tuberculosis* in vivo is the *tuberculin* test. The antigen used in the test is a protein extracted from tubercle bacilli (tuberculoprotein). Seibert's purified protein derivative (PPD-S), which was originally prepared from cultures of *M. tuberculosis,* is used in the United States. A positive reaction is a zone of inflammatory induration of 10 mm or more in diameter at the injection site of a dose of 5 tuberculin units. The implications of a positive test are (1) that live tubercle bacilli are present somewhere in the body, mainly in lymph nodes (i.e., infection is present), and (2) that the greater the size and severity of the skin reaction, the greater are the chances of active disease being present. Negative tuberculin reactions usually mean that the person has not been infected by *M. tuberculosis.* Rarely, patients with severe disseminated tuberculosis fail to respond to the tuberculin test and are said to be *anergic.*

Reactions of 5 to 9 mm of induration are believed to be caused by either weak hypersensitivity to *M. tuberculosis* or hypersensitivity to mycobacteria other than *M. tuberculosis.* Currently, in the United States, 0.3% of children entering school are tuberculin positive. Five percent of adults under 30 and 17% of adults in the 30 to 40 age group also react positively.

The tuberculin test is thus an important method in the following circumstances:
1. In the clinical diagnosis of tuberculosis
2. In the epidemiologic study of tuberculosis at the community level
3. To detect nonimmune persons who are at risk if exposed to the disease, for example, nurses; this application is important in those countries, such as Great Britain, where bacille Calmette-Guérin (BCG) vaccine is given to nonimmune persons

In clinical medicine it is rare for a diagnosis of tuberculosis to be considered when the tuberculin test is negative. In addition to providing important information about the incidence and prevalence of tuberculosis in a community, the tuberculin test performed at annual intervals can be used to detect changes in skin reactivity, for example, among schoolchildren. A child in the United States who has converted from tuberculin negative

to positive can be detected and treated with isoniazid (INH). Such chemoprophylaxis is estimated to reduce the expected incidence of reactivation tuberculosis by 93%. When a child has converted from tuberculin negative to positive, the source of infection, invariably a close household contact with active pulmonary tuberculosis, can also be identified and treated.

Pathology. The two forms of tuberculosis found in humans are primary tuberculosis, which is seen in nonimmune persons, and reactivation tuberculosis, which develops in patients with a considerable degree of immunity.

Primary tuberculosis. The first interaction between *M. tuberculosis* and the lung was studied in the guinea pig, which responds to the organism in a very similar way to humans. Within the alveoli, where the bacteria alight, there is a mild fibrinous inflammatory exudate in which a few polymorphonuclear leukocytes and macrophages collect. Usually this inflammatory focus remains microscopic. Occasionally bacteria may spread via the lymphatics to the hilar nodes and then to the systemic and pulmonary circulation. Once the organisms spread to the circulation, they are disseminated to many tissues and all parts of the lungs. This is *miliary* (literally, like a millet seed) tuberculosis. The tuberculin test is negative during this phase.

During the 4 to 6 weeks after initial entry of *M. tuberculosis* into the lungs, the cell-mediated immune response develops. T lymphocytes, sensitized by exposure to tuberculoprotein, and histiocytes (macrophages) begin to appear in the early acute inflammatory focus. The histiocytes phagocytose tubercle bacilli, but the bacteria continue to multiply intracellularly, disrupting their host cells and attracting more histiocytes. The ensuing process is a classic example of granulomatous inflammation.

Microscopically, the histiocytes form focal collections of pale-staining cells, which lose their definitive outlines. The name *epithelioid cells* has been given to these cells purely because of their morphology. They are, of course, not of epithelial origin but are altered macrophages and are the characteristic features of true granulomatous inflammation. Among them, multinucleate giant cells can often be seen. The giant cells in which the numerous nuclei are arranged peripherally, often in the shape of a horseshoe, are known as Langhans' giant cells. The rounded, focal collections of epithelioid cells and Langhans' giant cells are called *tubercles* or *tuberculous follicles* or *granulomas.* During this time, the small subset of lymphocytes that naturally recognize tuberculous antigens processed by the histiocytes is activated and proliferates. Four to 6 weeks after initial exposure to the organism, the tuberculin skin test converts from negative to positive because the activated lymphocytes can now respond to the inoculum of tuberculoprotein in the skin.

Concurrent with development of skin hypersensitivity, the center of the tubercle may undergo caseation or caseous necrosis (Fig. 12-14). Both epithelioid cells and bacteria undergo degeneration and form a yellowish-white mass, which reminded the earlier gourmet pathologists of cheese (Latin, *caseum*). Caseous material contains lipids derived from the tubercle bacilli. Microscopically, it is an amorphous, eosinophilic substance in which basophilic remnants of nuclear material are seen. The exact cause of caseation is not known, but it may be caused by toxic lymphokines released by the sensitized T-lymphocytes that have now begun to infiltrate the tuberculous focus. Thus the characteristic granuloma of tuberculosis is a focus consisting of the following:

1. A central zone of caseation
2. A zone of histiocytes (epithelioid cells) in which Langhans' giant cells may be seen (Fig. 12-15)
3. A peripheral zone of T-lymphocytes
4. Variable numbers of tubercle bacilli

The components of tuberculous lesions vary according to the concentration of tuberculous antigens and the degree of intensity of the cell-mediated immune response to these antigens. With a small infecting dose of organisms and a vigorous cellular immune response, a well-organized granuloma with no central caseation and a periphery containing abundant lymphocytes and fibroblasts develops. This lesion is sometimes referred to as a "hard tubercle." With increasing size of the infecting dose of organisms but still in the presence of a high cellular immunity, there is an increasing tendency to caseation and the lesions tend to be less well organized. Lack of cellular immunity is associated with an acute fibrinous and granulocytic exudate and an abundance of bacteria.

Thus the outcome of primary tuberculous infection is conditioned by host and bacterial factors. In most cases the initial tuberculous focus is small; infection does not spread, and as host resistance develops, the focus heals spontaneously by fibrosis with no clinical evidence of disease. In less favorable circumstances, the site of the primary infection, which is commonly just under the pleura in one of the lower lobes of the lung, enlarges and undergoes caseous necrosis. This is called the *Ghon** or *primary focus* and together with the hilar lymph nodes, which are enlarged by the tuberculous process, comprise the Ghon or primary complex.

In the majority of cases of primary tuberculosis, the caseous foci in the lungs and hilar nodes undergo healing by fibrosis and eventually calcification. In some, however, the disease may progress in the following ways:

1. Via the bronchi
2. Via the bloodstream
3. To the pleura

SPREAD VIA THE BRONCHI. A progressively enlarging and caseating Ghon focus can erode and discharge its contents into a bronchus. The effects are to produce a small cavity in the original focus and sometimes to initiate tuberculous broncho-

---

*A. Ghon (1866-1936), Czechoslovakian physician.

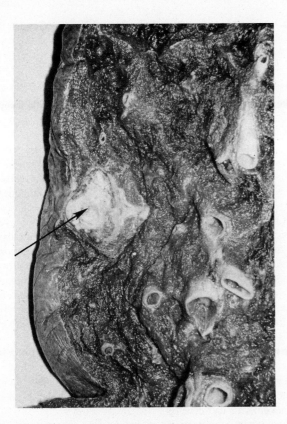

FIG. 12-14. Primary pulmonary tuberculosis. Arrow indicates a small caseating subpleural tuberculous lesion. This is a typical primary (Ghon) focus. *(Courtesy Curator of the Gordon Museum, Guy's Hospital, London, England.)*

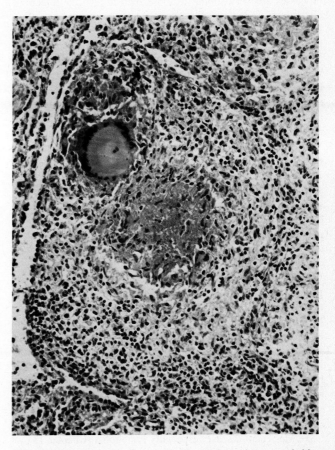

FIG. 12-15. Pulmonary tuberculosis. Caseated area is surrounded by epithelioid cells, Langhans' giant cells, and lymphocytes.

pneumonia by the spread of infected material into the area of lung supplied by that bronchus. This is particularly likely in young children.

SPREAD VIA THE BLOODSTREAM. Tubercle bacilli can enter the blood in one of two ways. First, in the early stages of primary infection tubercle bacilli, transported to the hilar lymph nodes by the lymphatic vessels, may reach the thoracic duct and from there the systemic circulation. Second, erosion of a blood vessel in an area of caseation can discharge bacteria directly into the bloodstream.

The result of hematogenous spread of large numbers of organisms is miliary tuberculosis, in which numerous, small tubercles are established in the lungs, liver, meninges, kidneys, adrenal glands, and spleen. The most serious effect is tuberculous meningitis (Chapter 20). Before antituberculous treatment was available, miliary tuberculosis was 100% fatal. If only a few organisms enter the bloodstream, they may alight, for example, in the kidney and produce a localized infection.

SPREAD TO THE PLEURA. Spread of a tuberculous focus to the pleura is associated with an inflammatory response, usually in the form of a profuse fluid exudate that forms a pleural effusion. This complication is more frequent in young adults. The fluid that collects in the pleural space is clear and yellow, has a high protein content, and contains a moderate number of lymphocytes. Mycobacteria are very scarce in the fluid of a tuberculous pleural effusion. Only 20% of cases yield positive cultures. Because of this, the tuberculin test is very important in establishing the tuberculous nature of a pleural effusion.

Other forms of primary tuberculosis. Primary infection can also take place in the eye and in the intestine. The pathologic processes are very similar to those seen in primary infection of the lung. In the eye, the equivalent of the primary complex in the lung is a severe keratoconjunctivitis with granulomatous inflammation of the preauricular lymph node. Ocular infection results from droplets entering the eye in an aerosol created when an infected patient coughs or by a laboratory accident. In the intestinal tract, the disease is usually caused by *M. bovis;* the primary focus is in the intestinal mucosa with granulomatous inflammation of the mesenteric lymph nodes draining that area of the bowel.

Reactivation (recrudescent) tuberculosis. Reactivation pulmonary tuberculosis is the result of rekindling of tuberculous inflammation in the apical zones of the lungs (Fig. 12-16). The reasons for this unique localization are still not fully understood. One suggestion is that the partial pressure of oxygen in the upper lobes favors the growth of *M. tuberculosis;* however, in some communities at high altitude, the incidence of apical tuberculosis is much higher than in those at sea level, suggesting that oxygen is not a factor.

Reactivation tuberculosis develops, rather surprisingly, in patients who have a considerable degree of cellular immunity, that is, who are tuberculin positive. The immune response, however, is unable to prevent the progression of the tuberculous lesions or can only do so after a period of many months or years.

The precise mechanisms that bring about reactivation of tuberculous infection are not known, but among known predisposing factors are the following:

1. Diabetes mellitus
2. Chronic alcoholism
3. Malignant disease, especially lymphoma (Chapter 13)
4. Corticosteroid therapy

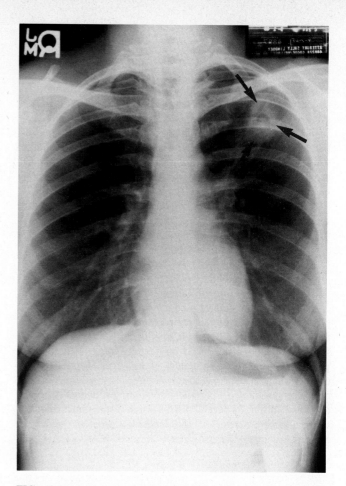

FIG. 12-16. Pulmonary tuberculosis. Radiograph of reactivation tuberculosis in the left upper zone. Central cavitation of the apical lesion can be seen. *(Courtesy of William Hayes, MD.)*

Reactivation of pulmonary tuberculosis in immunosuppressed patients is relatively uncommon. The characteristic features of reactivation tuberculosis are:

1. The lesions are fibrocaseous and form in the posterior aspects of the apices. Cavitation is a frequent sequel.
2. Progress of the lesions is fairly slow and takes place primarily via the lymphatics. Spread to distal hilar nodes, typical of primary tuberculosis is not a feature.

If healing takes place, it is by fibrosis and calcification over a long period. The complications of this form of tuberculosis are for the most part the same as those of primary infection: tuberculous bronchopneumonia, miliary tuberculosis, and tuberculous pleurisy. Blood spread of small numbers of organisms can cause localized tuberculous infection in such sites as bone, kidneys, the epididymis, and fallopian tubes. This type of dissemination is sometimes call *chronic metastatic tuberculosis.*

If there are large cavities and active proliferation of organisms, the resultant heavily infected sputum can carry mycobacteria upward to the bronchi and larynx, causing tuberculous bronchitis and laryngitis. If the bacilli are swallowed, tuberculous enteritis can develop.

Two other complications of reactivation tuberculosis are hemorrhage and amyloid disease. Hemorrhage results from erosion of blood vessels in tuberculous cavities. Elastic tissue

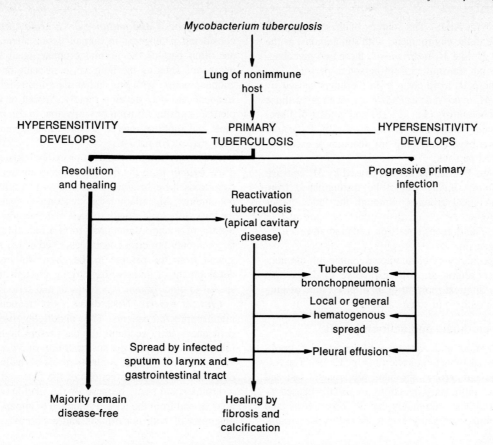

FIG. 12-17. Pathogenesis of pulmonary tuberculosis.

present in blood vessels is remarkably resistant to the destructive effects of caseation. Obliterative endarteritis also develops in the small arteries in the region of tuberculous foci. For these reasons, massive hemorrhage from a large vessel in a tuberculous cavity, which preceded the death of many characters in early novels, is very unusual. However, repeated minor hemorrhages that cause coughing up of blood-stained sputum (hemoptysis), are common.

As in several other, chronic longstanding inflammatory diseases, *amyloidosis* develops in some patients with prolonged advanced reactivation tuberculosis.

The pathogenesis of primary and reactivation tuberculosis is summarized in Fig. 12-17.

Clinical aspects. In 1980 in the United States, new cases of tuberculosis were detected at a rate of 12 per 100,000 of the population, about 1/150th of the incidence 75 years ago. The death rate in the United States in 1880 was around 400 per 100,000. In 1980 it had fallen to 1.5. These figures are the result of improved standards of living and the introduction, in the late 1940s, of specific chemotherapy.

The majority of primary tuberculous infections are symptomless; occasionally fever and malaise are present for a brief period. Reactivation tuberculosis is frequently symptomless in its early stages. With progression of the disease, the most common symptoms are fever and night sweats, weight loss, and malaise. Later cough, sometimes with hemoptysis, becomes more frequent.

The complications of both progressive primary and reactivation tuberculosis produce similar clinical manifestations.

Shortness of breath (dyspnea) is seen with tuberculous pneumonia and pleural effusion; chest pain may accompany early pleural involvement. The effects of spread of tuberculosis to kidneys, adrenal glands, bones, joints, and meninges are considered in later chapters.

The diagnosis of pulmonary tuberculosis is by chest radiograph, recognition and isolation of *M. tuberculosis* from sputum samples, and the use of the tuberculin reaction. Of these, isolating the organism is the most important in establishing a diagnosis. The treatment of tuberculosis is by chemotherapy. The main drug regimen at present is isoniazid and rifampin given for 9 months. Ethambutol or streptomycin can be substituted for rifampin. Currently in the United States, children and adults under 35 years of age who become tuberculin positive, but who have no overt disease, are treated with isoniazid alone for 6 to 12 months.

Other pulmonary mycobacterioses

In the last 40 years it has been increasingly recognized that mycobacteria other than *M. tuberculosis* can cause pulmonary disease. These organisms are now collectively referred to as the *nontuberculous mycobacteria* and by their specific names (Table 12-4).

Etiology and pathogenesis. The two most important species of nontuberculous mycobacteria, at least in the United States, are *M. kansasii* and *M. avium-intracellulare*. In some areas of the country (e.g., Dallas) *M. kansasii* may equal or exceed *M. tuberculosis* as the main cause of cavitary lung disease; *M. avium-intracellulare* is a frequent cause of pulmonary disease in patients with AIDS. The sources of these organisms are believed to be in the environment, with soil and dust as the likeliest sources. Unlike *M. tuberculosis,* these two mycobacterial species are not transmitted from person to person.

Pathology. The pathologic changes in the lungs caused by *M. kansasii* and *M. avium-intracellulare* are identical to those of reactivation tuberculosis (Fig. 12-18) and consist of fibrocaseous inflammatory change and cavity formation. Extension of these infections beyond the lung are uncommon except in immunosuppressed persons.

Clinical aspects. Pulmonary disease caused by *M. kansasii* and *M. avium-intracellulare* cannot be distinguished from tuberculosis on clinical grounds, although the latter causes much milder disease as a rule than either *M. kansasii* or *M. tuberculosis.* The diagnosis rests on isolation and identification of the organism.

Treatment is primarily by chemotherapy, although the nontuberculous mycobacteria are less responsive to drugs than *M. tuberculosis.* Surgical removal of an affected lobe of lung may improve the outlook in some cases.

Pulmonary nocardiosis and actinomycosis

Etiology. *Nocardia* and *Actinomyces* species are grampositive, filamentous branching bacteria (Fig. 12-19). The former are acid fast and aerobic; the latter are nonacid fast and anaerobic. Human pulmonary infections are usually caused by *N. asteroides* and less commonly by *N. brasiliensis* and *N. caviae.* Pulmonary actinomycosis is caused by *A. israelii.*

Pathogenesis and pathology. *Nocardia* species are usually considered pathogenic in human tissue; *Actinomyces* species are often part of the normal oropharyngeal flora. Nocardia organisms entering the lung cause an acute or subacute bronchopneumonia, with pus and abscess formation. Cavitation is frequent and may develop rapidly. Spread of infection to the pleurae, causing effusion or empyema, is common. Less common, but more serious is hematogenous spread to the brain, with abscess formation.

Pulmonary actinomycosis is probably initiated by aspiration of *A. israelii* from the oropharynx into an area of lung where conditions have become anaerobic as a result of collapse or pneumonia. An inflammatory response is usually induced in the lower lobes and slowly spreads to the pleurae. Dense tangled masses of actinomycetes may form a radiating pattern, which is commonly but erroneously described as *ray fungus.* Further spread from the pleurae to the chest wall may lead to the development of sinuses discharging through the skin. Blood spread to other organs is a frequent and serious complication.

Clinical aspects. Nocardiosis most frequently affects immunosuppressed patients. Thus underlying disease or immune deficiency partly accounts for the present high mortality rate (about 50%), despite the susceptibility of *Nocardia* species to the sulfonamide drugs. Actinomycosis of the lung has a worse outlook than similar infections of the face and neck or of the gastrointestinal tract, because of the likelihood of hematogenous spread from the lung. Prolonged treatment is needed. The diagnosis of both nocardiosis and actinomycosis depends on

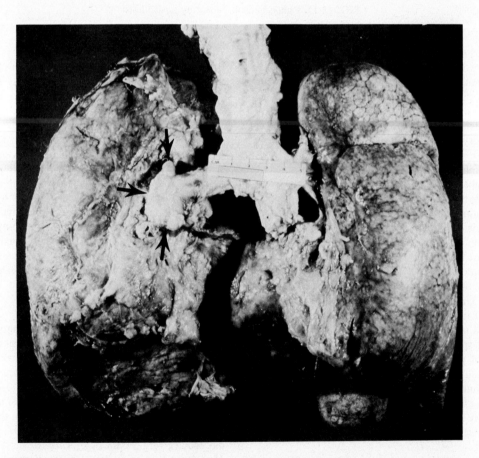

FIG. 12-18. Pulmonary infection by *Mycobacterium kansasii.* A large hilar caseating mass *(arrows)* is seen, and there is extensive thickening of the pleura of the right lung.

demonstration of the organisms in stained sputum smears and by culture under aerobic and anaerobic conditions, respectively. In actinomycosis, exudates containing yellow granules ("sulfur granules"), which consist of tangled masses of organisms, are a typical finding.

Pulmonary mycoses

Relatively few fungi are capable of causing systemic disease in humans. When they do, the term "deep mycoses" is often used to contrast them with the much more common superficial fungal infections of the skin and mucous membranes. Although deep mycotic infections may involve many organs, the lung is the route of infection in nearly all instances and is the organ most frequently affected. Most pulmonary mycotic infections cause pathologic changes that closely resemble pulmonary tuberculosis.

The important fungi causing pulmonary disease are:
1. *Histoplasma capsulatum*
2. *Coccidioides immitis*
3. *Blastomyces dermatitidis*
4. *Cryptococcus neoformans*
5. *Aspergillus fumigatus*

It is important to remember that most of these mycoses have a geographic distribution. They are particularly common in the United States and worldwide in patients who have AIDS but are otherwise rare in Europe.

Histoplasmosis. *H. capsulatum,* the fungus that causes histoplasmosis, exists as a yeast in infected human tissues and is usually observed within the cytoplasm of macrophages (Fig. 12-20). Infection is initiated in humans by the inhalation of dust contaminated with the yeast. Soil fertilized by bird and bat droppings that is disturbed in building site preparation or earth moving is a common source of infection in endemic areas. The organism is endemic in the United States, especially in the Mississippi and Ohio River valleys.

After alighting in the lungs the yeasts are phagocytosed by macrophages. After 1 to 2 weeks, hypersensitivity develops and a granuloma with central caseation appears at the site. When the number of organisms inhaled is low, the granuloma remains small and localized and heals by fibrosis and calcification. When large numbers of organisms are inhaled, an acute generalized reaction of variable severity follows. In the lung an acute interstitial pneumonitis is characteristic of the most acute type of reaction. Chronic pulmonary histoplasmosis is characterized by caseation, cavitation, and sometimes the formation of large air spaces. In the immunosuppressed, disseminated disease with granuloma formation can affect virtually any organ or tissue of the body.

Clinically, the disease has a widely variable presentation from insignificant infection to fulminating, fatal disease. Histoplasmosis is usually treated with amphotericin, although ketoconazole can be used for mild cases.

Coccidioidomycosis. Coccidioidomycosis (San Joaquin fever) is caused by *Coccidioides immitis,* a yeastlike fungus found in the western United States and parts of Central and South America.

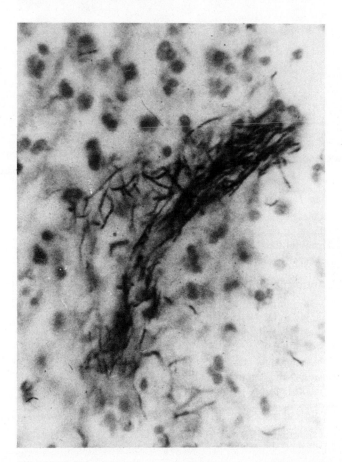

FIG. 12-19. Gram stain of pus containing *Nocardia asteroides*. Note the branching structure of the bacteria. *(From McCracken AW and Cawson RA: Clinical and oral microbiology, Washington DC, 1982, Hemisphere Publishing Corp.)*

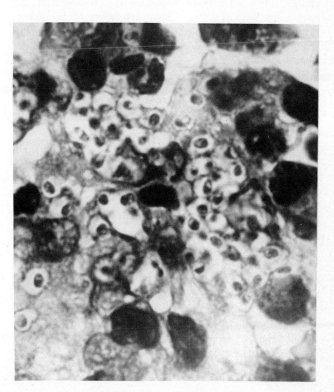

FIG. 12-20. Histoplasmosis. Tissue section showing macrophages and numerous intracellular capsulated yeast forms of *H. capsulatum. (From McCracken AW and Cawson RA: Clinical and oral microbiology, Washington DC, 1982, Hemisphere Publishing Corp.)*

Human infection follows inhalation of the highly infectious arthrospores. The pathologic changes in the lung resemble those of histoplasmosis with the addition of the characteristic spherules of *C. immitis,* which can be seen lying inside or outside of macrophages (Fig. 12-21). The disease follows one of three courses. First, in the majority of cases, the lesions heal with fibrosis and calcification. Second, the primary infection progresses, with the formation of cavitary lung lesions; sometimes the infection disseminates to other sites, including the meninges, a highly lethal complication. Third, after a period of quiescence, a chronic cavitary form of the disease may develop as old lesions reactivate and enlarge.

Clinically, the signs and symptoms range from those of transient minor illness to disseminated infection that may involve skin, bone, and central nervous system. The specific diagnosis is made by identification of *C. immitis* by microscopy and culture. Treatment is with amphotericin with miconazole as an alternative.

The main features of other mycoses involving the lung are summarized in Table 12-5.

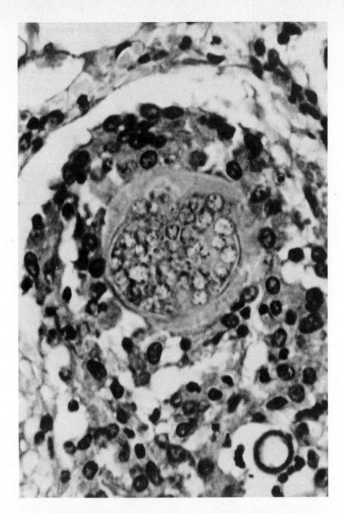

FIG. 12-21. Coccidioidomycosis. Lung section in which a characteristic thick-walled spherule containing many endospores is surrounded by an area of granulomatous inflammation. *(From McCracken AW and Cawson RA: Clinical and oral microbiology, Washington DC, 1982, Hemisphere Publishing Corp.)*

Respiratory failure

Respiratory failure is present when the mechanisms of respiration fail to maintain the partial pressures of oxygen and carbon dioxide within the normal range. A Po_2 less than 50 mm Hg or a Pco_2 greater than 50 mm Hg are indicative of respiratory failure. Lower Po_2 or higher Pco_2 levels can impair or injure the function of vital organs.

A detailed discussion of the altered physiology of respiratory failure is beyond the scope of this text. However, three mechanisms, acting either singly or sometimes in combination, are responsible for respiratory failure: (1) failure of pulmonary ventilation, (2) abnormalities of gaseous diffusion across the alveolar membranes, and (3) abnormal ventilation and perfusion.

The causes of respiratory failure are as follows:

Site of disease or injury	Cause
Central nervous system	Anesthesia, narcotic overdose
Chest wall	Trauma, flail chest
Pleura	Pneumothorax
Alveoli	Pneumonia, respiratory distress syndrome
Airways	Obstruction, asthma
Pulmonary vessels	Embolus
Heart	Congestive heart failure

Failure of pulmonary ventilation (hypoventilation)

Normal pulmonary ventilation, that is, the volume of gas taken into the lungs in 1 minute, is about 7000 ml in a healthy adult. Several diseases can compromise pulmonary ventilation, ranging from injury or intoxication affecting the respiratory centers or nerve supply to respiratory muscles to chest wall injuries and pleural diseases.

Abnormal diffusion

Any disease that affects the integrity of the alveolar membrane, the pulmonary capillary endothelium, or the interstitial tissue separating them will lead to impairment of the normal diffusion of oxygen and carbon dioxide. This can be seen, for example, in viral pneumonitis or pulmonary fibrosis. Recently the concept of *diffuse alveolar damage* (DAD) has been introduced to describe a sequence of pathologic events common to many of the diseases associated with abnormal diffusion. This concept is discussed later in the chapter.

Abnormal ventilation and perfusion

In addition to adequate pulmonary ventilation, the blood supply to the sites of gaseous exchange (i.e., perfusion of the alveolar capillary bed) is equally essential. The normal ratio of ventilation to perfusion is 1:1. Any pulmonary abnormality that alters this ratio sufficiently can lead to respiratory failure. Among the common conditions that alter the ventilation/perfusion ratio are pulmonary emboli, emphysema, and asthma.

Clinical aspects

Respiratory failure is characterized clinically by dyspnea, cyanosis, confused mental states, and disorders of cardiac rhythm. These are superimposed on the signs and symptoms of the underlying disease. There is hypoxemia and hypercapnia (increased Pco_2 in arterial blood). Treatment depends on the cause and is directed at maintaining adequate oxygenation of vital organs, using mechanical ventilation if necessary.

TABLE 12-5. Summary of the main features of pulmonary mycoses*

Causative fungus (disease)	Morphology in tissues	Pathology of typical pulmonary lesions	Progress of pulmonary lesions	Main sites of spread	Outcome
Histoplasma capsulatum (histoplasmosis)	2-3 μm yeast	Histiocytes, Langhans giant cells, caseation; fungus in histiocytes	Healing by fibrosis and calcification Chronic cavitary lung lesions	Adrenal glands; meninges; soft tissues of mouth, pharynx, and larynx	Most are asymptomatic or mild; high fatality rate in disseminated form
Coccidioides immitis (coccidioidomycosis)	20-100 μm spherule containing endospores	As for histoplasmosis with addition of polymorphic spherules in and outside histiocytes	Healing Progressive primary disease with cavitary lung lesions Delayed chronic lung infection	Meninges	Many asymptomatic; high fatality rate with meningeal involvement
Blastomyces dermatitidis (blastomycosis; N. American blastomycosis)	10 μm yeast	As for histoplasmosis with addition of polymorphic abscesses; fungus in and outside histiocytes	Progressive primary disease with lung abscesses and cavitation (uncommon)	Skin; bone (frequent)	?Asymptomatic; high fatality rate in disseminated disease
Cryptococcus neoformans (cryptococcosis)	3-8 μm yeastlike fungus	Mild granulomatous inflammatory changes; fungus inside or outside histiocytes	Rarely progressive	Meninges, especially in diabetics and immunosuppressed; occasionally skin and bone	Mortality rate about 40% in treated, 100% in untreated central nervous system disease
Aspergillus fumigatus (also *A. niger*) (aspergillosis)	Septate hyphae	Hypersensitivity pneumonitis; fungus ball; pneumonitis	Recurrent disease Slowly progressive Cavitation and blood vessel invasion	Brain, eye, kidney, heart valves	Varies according to type of disease; poor prognosis with pneumonia and disseminated forms
Paracoccidioides brasiliensis (S. American blastomycosis)	40 μm yeast	Granulomatous lesions of lung, skin, mouth, and lip in adults	Progressive often despite treatment	Skin, oral cavity	Poor prognosis in young patients; occasionally self-limiting

*All are common infections of patients with AIDS.

Diffuse alveolar damage

Diffuse alveolar damage (DAD) describes a predictable, although nonspecific, sequence of events that follows injury to the alveolar epithelium and endothelium from a wide variety of causes. Some of these are listed in the box at right. DAD is common to those severe, life-threatening, clinical states that are included in the *adult respiratory distress syndrome*.

Two stages of DAD have been recognized. In the acute, or exudative, stage there is interstitial pulmonary edema and hyaline membrane formation. This stage lasts approximately 1 week. Interstitial fibrosis develops in the organizing, or proliferative, phase, often with proliferation of type 2 pneumocytes. Both stages are reversible, however.

The basic causes of DAD are diverse and sometimes unknown. When DAD is the result of oxygen toxicity, the pulmonary injury has been attributed to the formation of superoxide anions and other toxic metabolies such as hydrogen peroxide.

The clinical features of DAD, regardless of cause, are severe hypoxemia and high mortality. The treatment is the same as that for acute respiratory failure.

Bronchiectasis
Definition and etiology

Bronchiectasis is characterized by permanent pathologic dilation of those bronchi which are normally greater than 2 mm in diameter. Apart from some rare congenital forms of the

---

EXAMPLES OF CAUSES OF DIFFUSE ALVEOLAR DAMAGE

Physical agents

Radiation
  X-radiation
  γ-Radiation
Heatstroke
Gases and fumes
  Oxygen
  Sulfur dioxide
  Smoke

Drugs and chemicals

Chemotherapeutic agents
  Ara-C
  Bleomycin
  Busulfan
  Methotrexate
Others
  Gold salts
  Heroin
  Nitrofurantoin
  Paraquat

Pathologic states

Altitude sickness
Drowning
Shock
  Oligemic
  Septic
  Cardiogenic
Uremia

Infectious disease

Bacterial
  M. pneumoniae
Viral
  Influenza
  Measles
  Parainfluenza
  Herpesviruses

disease, which are due to failure of alveolar tissue to develop, bronchiectasis is essentially a complication of a previous bronchial infection. Chronic infection and inflammation with acute inflammatory episodes invariably accompany the bronchial dilation.

Pathogenesis

Factors that predispose to bronchiectasis (Fig. 12-22) are:
1. Congenital defects in the lung

2. Bronchial obstruction with atelectasis (collapse of the lung)
3. Cystic fibrosis
4. Immunodeficiency disease
5. Necrotizing pulmonary infections

In congenital bronchiectasis, cystic dilations are present throughout the bronchial tree. Secretions collect in these dilations and become secondarily infected.

Unrelieved obstruction of the bronchi by such diverse causes

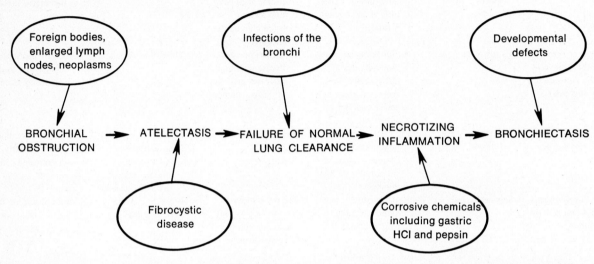

FIG. 12-22. Pathogenesis of bronchiectasis.

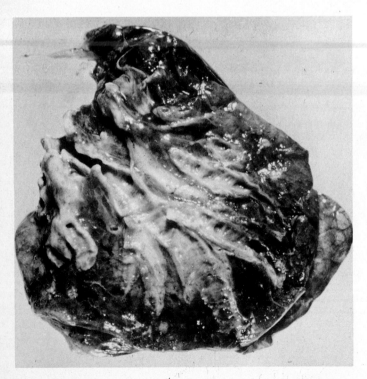

FIG. 12-23. Bronchiectasis. There is gross dilatation of the bronchi, which contain copious mucopurulent secretion. *(Courtesy Curator of the Gordon Museum, Guy's Hospital, London, England.)*

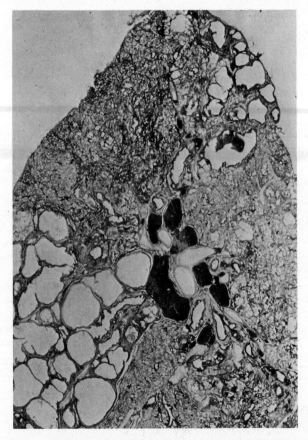

FIG. 12-24. Bronchiectasis. This whole lung section shows widely dilated airways, especially in the lower zones where the lung has a honeycomb appearance. *(Courtesy Curator of the Gordon Museum, Guy's Hospital, London, England.)*

as foreign bodies, enlarged lymph nodes, and neoplasms is followed by collapse of the lung segment supplied by that bronchus. Collapse (atelectasis) interferes with the normal pulmonary clearance mechanisms and predisposes to infection. In cystic fibrosis (Chapter 15) the bronchial secretions are thick and inspissated and impair pulmonary clearance, causing blockage of the bronchi with subsequent infection and resulting in bronchiectasis.

Bronchiectasis may complicate diseases in which there is necrotizing inflammation of the bronchi, such as influenza, measles, or, most important, whooping cough.

It seems likely, therefore, that the main predisposing factor to bronchiectasis is obstruction or impaired pulmonary clearance, which in turn is followed inevitably by stasis and the destructive effects of necrotizing inflammation.

Pathology

The essential elements of the bronchiectatic lung are abnormal dilation of the smaller caliber bronchi and acute and chronic inflammation (Fig. 12-23). The bronchi of the lower lobes are most frequently affected. The abnormal dilations can be saccular or cylindrical; the former usually affect the larger bronchi, the latter are seen in the smaller bronchi. These dilations give the lung a honeycomb appearance at autopsy (Fig. 12-24).

Histologically, there are abundant areas of acute and chronic inflammation in which collections of pus cells and sometimes red blood cells are prominent. Segments of bronchial epithelium that have undergone squamous metaplasia or have been destroyed are common. Destructive necrosis of the full thickness of the smaller bronchi may be seen. Healing is by fibrosis, but is usually ineffective and incomplete.

The complications of established bronchiectasis are frequent and common. They include:

1. Bronchopneumonia
2. Lung abscess
3. Disseminated infection with metastatic abscesses
4. Amyloid disease

Bronchopneumonia, discussed earlier in this chapter, occurs when bacterial infection from the bronchi spreads into lung parenchyma. The pneumonia is usually caused by mixed bacterial infection, especially by staphylococci, pneumococci, *H. influenzae*, and anaerobes. Lung abscess is usually a result of infection of a bronchiectatic area by one or more species of anaerobic bacteria derived from the upper respiratory tract or the oropharynx. Systemic spread of infection, especially to the brain, with formation of a cerebral abscess, is the most serious complication. In long-standing bronchiectasis, clubbing of the fingers is a common feature (Fig. 12-25) and ultimately amyloidosis may develop.

Clinical aspects

The accumulation of purulent secretions is responsible for the most characteristic symptom: a chronic cough producing purulent sputum that is most copious in the morning and often blood streaked. Persistence of active disease is associated with fever, weight loss, and anemia. Recurrent pneumonic episodes are common. Sudden worsening of the patient's condition suggests bronchopneumonia, or, if deterioration is associated with the appearance of putrid, offensive sputum, a lung abscess has probably developed. The diagnosis is usually established by bronchography, in which the abnormal bronchi are outlined by radiopaque dye (Fig. 12-26).

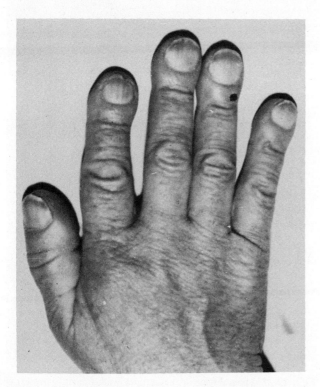

FIG. 12-25. Clubbing of the fingers is a striking physical finding in patients with long-standing bronchiectasis. (*Courtesy Curator of the Gordon Museum, Guy's Hospital, London, England.*)

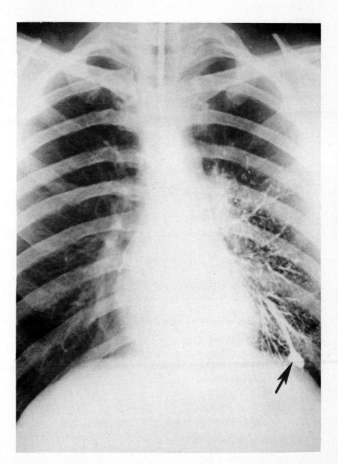

FIG. 12-26. Bronchiectasis. Radiopaque dye has filled a saccular bronchial dilation (*arrow*) in the left lower lobe.

Treatment is based on antibiotic therapy with adjuvant measures, particularly postural drainage, to improve the removal of bronchial secretions.

Aspiration pneumonia

Aspiration pneumonia results from the inhalation of certain foreign materials. Commonly inhaled substances that lead to aspiration pneumonia include gastric contents, food particles, infected tooth fragments, and contaminated water. Persons under anesthesia or those who are unconscious from injury, illness, or alcoholic intoxication are particularly liable to inhale these materials. Inhalation of contaminated water may complicate survival from drowning.

Aspiration pneumonia is pathologically a bronchopneumonia, often superimposed on chemical injury to the bronchial mucosa caused, for example, by gastric acid and pepsin. Blockage of a bronchus by aspirated material can lead to localized collapse of a lung segment, and the presence of anaerobic bacteria originating from the oropharynx can lead to lung abscess formation.

Lung abscess

A lung abscess is a localized area of destruction of the lung parenchyma containing pus.

Etiology and pathogenesis

The causes of lung abscess are numerous and are listed in the box below. Among the most common is the aspiration of infected materials, especially from the mouth and pharynx. Frequently this has two effects; first, the obstruction of a bronchus (for example, by a foreign body or tumor), and second, the introduction of oropharyngeal bacteria into the distal areas of the lung, which are normally sterile.

When aspirated material is derived from the oropharynx, it frequently contains abundant anaerobic bacteria. It is therefore not surprising that most lung abscesses are caused by anaerobic

organisms alone or mixed with a variety of aerobic bacteria. *Bacteroides melaninogenicus, Fusobacterium nucleatum (F. fusiforme)*, and anaerobic streptococci are the anaerobes usually responsible. Among the most frequent aerobic bacteria in lung abscesses are *S. aureus, K. pneumoniae,* and *Pseudomonas aeruginosa.*

Lung abscess is an important complication of impaired consciousness as a result of aspiration and an ineffective cough reflex. The patients most likely to be affected are those receiving anesthetics, especially for oral and upper respiratory tract surgery, and those who have taken overdoses of hypnotic drugs or alcohol. Aspiration is more likely when patients are recumbent. The aspirated materials readily reach the apex of the lower lobes and the posterior segment of the right upper lobe. These are common sites for lung abscesses. If gastric contents enter the lung by aspiration, there is chemical necrosis caused by hydrochloric acid and pepsin, which can initiate abscess formation. It should therefore be obvious that very similar mechanisms are responsible for aspiration pneumonia described previously and lung abscess.

Pathology

The pathologic changes include acute pyogenic inflammation, with central necrosis and liquefaction, resulting in a circumscribed cavity containing pus (Fig. 12-27). Unless the process is hyperacute, there is usually some attempt at localization of the abscess by a fibrous wall. In some infections, such as

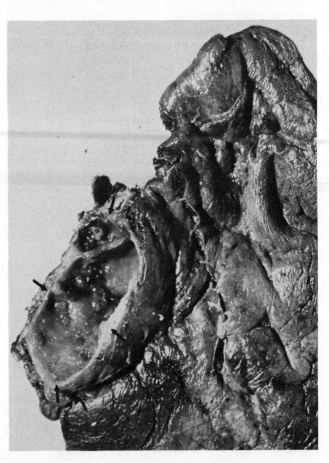

FIG. 12-27. Lung abscess. A large, thick-walled cavity *(arrows)* is shown in the periphery of the lung. The abscess contained foul-smelling pus caused by anaerobic infection.

CAUSES OF LUNG ABSCESS

In previously normal lung

1. Aspiration of infected materials
   a. Foreign bodies
   b. Infected oral and respiratory tract secretions
   c. Teeth
2. Aspiration of caustic materials
   a. Gastric pepsin and acid in vomitus

Associated with underlying pulmonary disease

1. Pulmonary infection
   a. Extension of bacterial or fungal pneumonia
   b. Complication of bronchiectasis
2. Pulmonary neoplasms
3. Pulmonary vasculitis
   a. Wegener's granulomatosis
   b. Polyarteritis nodosa

Associated with disease in other sites

1. Septic thrombophlebitis
2. Right-sided infective endocarditis

those caused by *K. pneumoniae*, multiloculated abscesses may form.

Clinical aspects

Many patients will initially have the acute symptoms of aspiration pneumonia such as fever, dry cough, and sometimes pleural pain. Despite antimicrobial treatment, an abscess may form and there is copious, foul-smelling sputum. At this stage, chest radiography may show the typical rounded shadow in which a horizontal fluid level can be seen. The symptoms of lung abscess may develop more insidiously, in which case the possibility of an underlying lung tumor should be considered. Much less frequently, lung abscesses are the result of infected thromboemboli from thrombophlebitis of the lower limbs or right-sided infective endocarditis, almost exclusively seen in persons addicted to intravenous drugs.

Other forms of pneumonitis

Inflammation of the lungs can be caused by a variety of agents other than the microorganisms considered earlier. These are listed in the box below.

Physical agents

In most instances the pathologic effects of physical agents are similar to those of DAD. Interstitial inflammation with hyaline membrane formation followed by fibrosis are common features.

In radiation pneumonitis, fibrosis may develop without preceding acute inflammatory changes (Chapter 3).

Hypersensitivity pneumonitis

Hypersensitivity reactions in the lungs to a wide range of microbial antigens, animal proteins, and chemical agents that can be present in inhaled dusts have been recognized, especially in persons engaged in certain occupations (Table 12-6). Examples of the causative agents, their sources and effects are listed in the same table. Hypersensitivity reactions to *Aspergillus* species are summarized in Table 12-5.

An example of hypersensitivity pneumonitis is *farmer's lung*, which is most often caused by hypersensitivity to the fungus *Micropolyspora faeni* or sometimes to *Thermoactinomyces vulgaris* or *T. sacchari*. The source of these organisms is rotting vegetable compost, and those affected are usually farmers, mushroom pickers, or sugar cane workers.

The pathologic changes in hypersensitivity pneumonitis consist of pulmonary nodules in which an assortment of inflammatory cells, including lymphocytes, plasma cells, histiocytes, neutrophils, and eosinophils are found. Multinucleate giant cells of the Langhans type may also be present. Inflammatory changes develop in the alveolar capillary walls and in the terminal bronchi.

Serum antibodies, usually of the IgG class, are demonstrable by the precipitin reaction, with the appropriate microbial antigens, in individuals who have farmer's lung. Immediate hypersensitivity reactions can also be shown in some individuals by skin testing.

Patients with this disease develop hypersensitivity symptoms within a few hours of exposure to the offending antigen. Fever, malaise, cough, and shortness of breath are typical, although the symptoms can vary in severity. A mild to moderate eosinophilia is common. The main therapeutic measure is the use of corticosteroids. Prevention is by industrial environmental protective measures or by avoiding exposure to the antigen.

Drug-induced pulmonary hypersensitivity

Several drugs can cause pulmonary hypersensitivity. Nitrofurantoin is the best documented of these drugs. Others include bleomycin, chlorpropamide, methotrexate, mephenesin, and penicillin.

The immune mechanisms by which pulmonary disease is produced by drugs are mediated by antibodies, cellular immunity, or both. Both acute and chronic reactions can follow the use of many of these drugs. In *acute reactions*, the disease is similar both pathologically and clinically to hypersensitivity pneumonitis due to microbial antigens. The *chronic reactions* are characterized by varying degrees of pulmonary fibrosis, as with the antineoplastic drugs bleomycin and methotrexate, or by persistent pulmonary infiltrates and pleural effusion, as associated with nitrofurantoin.

Eosinophilic pneumonitis

Pulmonary inflammatory infiltrates in which eosinophils are prominent are present in most forms of hypersensitivity pneumonitis. Eosinophils are particularly abundant in the lungs when they are infested with migrating parasitic larvae. The

---

NONINFECTIOUS CAUSES OF PULMONARY INFLAMMATION

Physical agents

Gases and vapors
Ionizing radiation
Thermal and blast injuries
Prolonged excessive oxygen
  therapy

Hypersensitivity reactions to:
Inhaled antigens
Drugs
Migrating worm larvae

Collagen-vascular diseases

Lupus erythematosus
Polyarteritis nodosa
Goodpasture's syndrome

Uremia

Disease of obscure or unknown cause

Sarcoidosis
Pulmonary alveolar proteinosis

TABLE 12-6. Causes and sources of hypersensitivity pneumonitis

Microbial, animal or chemical antigen	Source of antigen	Disease
Micropolyspora faeni; thermophilic actinomycetes	Moldy vegetation	Farmer's lung
	Moldy sugar cane	Bagassosis
	Mushroom compost	Mushroom worker's lung
Alternaria species	Moldy sawdust	Woodworker's lung
Pullularia species	Moldy sawdust	Sequoiosis
Penicillium casei	Moldy cheese	Cheesemaker's lung
Amebae (*Naegleria* and *Acanthamoeba*); *Aureobasidium* and *Thermactinomyces* species	Vaporizers, humidifiers, ventilation systems	Ventilation pneumonitis
Bird proteins	Avian droppings, dust	Bird fancier's lung
Phthalic anhydride	Plastic making	Plastic worker's lung

most common parasites affecting the lungs in this way are the nematodes (roundworms) *Ascaris lumbricoides* and hookworms. Large numbers of larvae migrate through the alveoli as they enter the air passages from the bloodstream en route to their final destination in the intestinal tract via the bronchi, trachea, and esophagus.

The characteristic pathologic feature is the appearance of large numbers of eosinophils in the alveoli and hence the sputum. The name *tropical pulmonary eosinophilia* (Weingarten's syndrome) has been applied to this form of pneumonitis.

Loeffler's syndrome

This condition is similar to tropical pulmonary eosinophilia and affects patients in whom no cause for pulmonary disease can be found. It is a benign self-limiting disease characterized by transient migratory eosinophilic pulmonary infiltrates. Patients have mild wheezing and cough together with eosinophilia in the peripheral blood.

Uremia

Uremic pneumonitis is a complication of renal failure. The cause is not known. The pathologic features are essentially those of DAD previously discussed. Chronic left ventricular failure may contribute to the pulmonary abnormalities, especially pulmonary edema.

Pulmonary diseases of obscure or unknown origin
Sarcoidosis

Sarcoidosis is a granulomatous inflammatory disease that affects many systems; the lungs, however, are the most frequently involved.

Etiology and pathogenesis. Numerous infectious agents, including *M. tuberculosis* and Epstein-Barr virus have been proposed, but no agent has yet been substantiated as the cause of the disease. Good evidence suggests an immunologic defect in sarcoidosis. Individuals with the disease have a depressed response to skin antigens, suggesting a T-cell deficit, and increased levels of serum immunoglobulins caused by B-cell overactivity. It is possible, therefore, that several agents, both infectious and noninfectious, interacting with a deranged immune response may cause sarcoidosis. Family studies have suggested that susceptibility to the disease may be inherited as a recessive characteristic.

Pathology. The characteristic feature of the disease is the sarcoid granuloma, which tends to be of uniform shape and size (Fig. 12-28) and consists of central histiocytes (epithelioid cells) with a surrounding collar of lymphocytes. Langhans' giant cells may be present, but caseation is absent.

Intracellular bodies within giant cells, including stellate (asteroid) bodies and calcified lamellar (Schaumann's*) bodies,

---

*J. Schaumann (1879-1953), Swedish dermatologist.

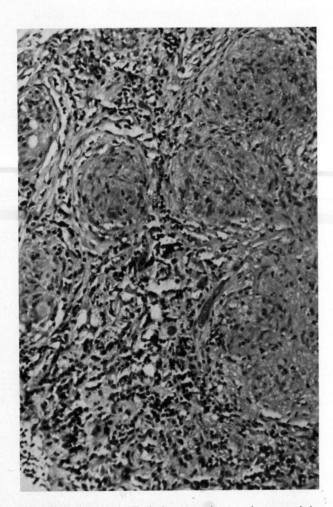

FIG. 12-28. Sarcoidosis. Typical noncaseating granulomas consisting of epithelioid cells and Langhans' giant cells.

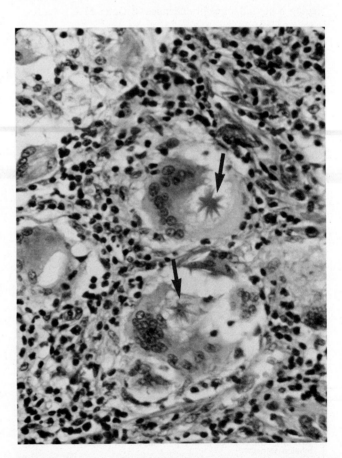

FIG. 12-29. Sarcoidosis. Photomicrograph showing multinucleate giant cells with prominent asteroid bodies *(arrows)* in the cytoplasm.

are described in sarcoidosis (Fig. 12-29). None, however, is diagnostic. Healing of sarcoid granulomas is by fibrosis.

The pathologic features are the same irrespective of the lesion site. In addition to the lungs and thoracic lymph nodes, tissues that may also be affected in order of decreasing frequency are skin, eyes, liver, and spleen. In a few instances, bones, joints, and peripheral nerves may be involved. Occasionally, swelling of the parotid or other salivary glands or the gingivae may be a feature of the disease (Chapter 14).

Abnormal T-cell and B-cell responses and disturbances of calcium metabolism may also be found. About one fourth of patients with sarcoidosis have raised levels of serum calcium (normal is 9 to 10.4 mg/dl), whereas others have hypercalciuria with normal serum calcium levels. These changes are probably caused by increased intestinal absorption of calcium. Abnormal calcium metabolism primarily affects the kidney, where deposition of calcium salts (nephrocalcinosis) may result in chronic renal failure.

Clinical aspects. Sarcoidosis is uncommon but affects blacks about 10 times more frequently than whites, both in the United States and Africa. However, the highest incidence of the disease is reported from Sweden. There are two clinical forms of sarcoidosis, *acute transient* and *chronic persistent*.

The most important initial acute effects of the disease are on the lungs. As a result, dyspnea and cough are the most common symptoms. When sarcoidosis progresses in a chronic fashion to extensive pulmonary fibrosis, cor pulmonale eventually develops. Erythema nodosum often accompanies sarcoidosis, but the most serious complications are renal failure and blindness. The former is the result of nephrocalcinosis; the latter is the result of granulomatous uveitis.

Sarcoidosis is difficult to distinguish from bacterial and fungal infections of the lungs and pulmonary malignancies. In this respect the Kveim skin test can be useful. The test consists of intradermal inoculation of a sterile suspension of human sarcoid tissue. In a positive case, biopsy of the resultant nodule, 4 to 6 weeks later, should show histologic findings typical of sarcoidosis. About 80% of patients have a positive Kveim test. However, some patients with regional enteritis (Crohn's disease) also react positively. The test is not available in the United States and lack of a standard reagent is a major drawback. Serum levels of angiotensin-converting enzyme (ACE) are elevated in patients with acute sarcoidosis; these levels decline when the disease is controlled by corticosteroid treatment. The serum lysozyme level is also elevated, and although this is not specific for sarcoidosis, it can also be used to monitor the effects of steroid treatment. The main aim of treatment is to prevent pulmonary fibrosis. Overall, the mortality rate is about 5%.

Alveolar proteinosis

Pulmonary alveolar proteinosis is a rare disease of unknown cause in which the alveoli fill with a lipoprotein material. No associated inflammatory or reactive process develops in the alveolar walls. Mild forms with recovery and severe forms with fatal respiratory failure or secondary infection by *Nocardia* species have been reported.

Asthma

Asthma (bronchial asthma) is a disease of the air passages characterized clinically by episodes of breathlessness, wheez-

ing, and cough as a result of reversible bronchiolar constriction, edema of the bronchial mucosa, and secretion of thick, viscid mucus.

Etiology and pathogenesis

Asthma may be caused by a variety of stimuli, but the underlying abnormality is hyperirritability of the bronchial tree in response to these stimuli. There are two broad groups of asthmatic patients: those who have allergic asthma and those who have idiosyncratic (intrinsic or idiopathic) asthma. Often the two cannot be differentiated, and multiple factors often initiate the asthmatic attack.

About one third of asthmatic patients are of the allergic type. In another third, an allergic component is frequently present. In persons with the idiosyncratic type, no personal or family history of allergy can be obtained.

Allergic asthma is often associated with a variety of other allergic manifestations, such as allergic rhinitis, urticaria, or eczema, in the patient or family members. Allergic asthma is often seasonal and develops in response to airborne antigens such as pollens and dust. Increased serum IgE is usual in these patients.

Chemical mediators of immediate hypersensitivity (Chapter 7) appear to be important in allergic asthma, but their interrelationships and the fundamental mechanisms that cause their release have not yet been clarified. One fundamental mechanism is that following sensitization to one or more allergens and the formation of specific IgE, mast cells in the respiratory tract become coated with IgE. When these cells are exposed again to allergens, the antigen and antibody (allergen and IgE) immediately interact and release mediators such as histamine, serotonin, and leukotrienes. These mediators cause bronchospasm and increased bronchial secretion and vascular permeability. Histamine and leukotrienes, meanwhile, may stimulate production of and be potentiated by, other mediators such as bradykinin and prostaglandins. Still other mediators are believed to be responsible for the attraction and participation of non–IgE sensitized cells in the reaction.

This theoretical explanation does not, however, apply to the idiosyncratic type of asthma, in which no IgE sensitization of pulmonary target cells takes place. One unifying theory that might explain both types of asthma suggests that the bronchoconstricting effects of many stimuli are opposed by the bronchodilating effects of β-adrenergic receptors in the bronchi. A defect in β-adrenergic activity would result in unopposed bronchoconstriction and the development of asthma. This defect would involve reduced cyclic AMP (cAMP) production, which might not only affect β-adrenergic receptors, but, by reducing cyclic nucleotides, would also stimulate the production of mediators. Among the most likely substances to cause reduced cellular levels of cAMP are the prostaglandins, which may play multiple roles in the pathogenesis of asthma.

In idiosyncratic asthma, the following factors may precipitate the attacks:
1. Infections
2. Airborne irritants or pollutants
3. Drugs
4. Physical exertion
5. Emotional stress

Infections, particularly acute upper respiratory tract infections, commonly initiate idiosyncratic asthma. Nonsteroid, antiinflammatory analgesics are known to precipitate or worsen asthmatic attacks in most patients. Some airborne pollutants such as sulfur dioxide, which is often present in smog, may be directly irritant.

Pathology

The bronchial and bronchiolar walls show the following features:

1. Widening of the submucous layer with a thickened basement membrane
2. Hypertrophy of smooth muscle fibers
3. Prominent active mucus-secreting glands

The bronchi contain mucous plugs in which eosinophils and granular crystals (Charcot-Leyden crystals) are present. The excessive, inspissated mucus is sometimes in the form of spiral strands (Curschmann's spirals). The alveoli are frequently over-distended, but in contrast with emphysema, no alveolar tissue is destroyed.

Clinical aspects

Asthma affects about 2% of the population of the United States and of most other countries. Most cases develop before the age of 40. Allergic asthma often starts in childhood, whereas idiosyncratic asthma often does not develop until adult life is reached. In this form of the disease several syndromes that indicate the precipitating causes are recognized:

1. Exercise-induced asthma, which occurs a few minutes after physical exertion is started
2. Cardiac asthma, which is bronchospasm resulting from fluid accumulation, as in congestive cardiac failure
3. Triad asthma, a form of idiosyncratic asthma associated with chronic rhinitis, polyp formation, and aspirin sensitivity

The asthmatic attack is characterized by wheezing, cough, and dyspnea. The breathing difficulty is in the expiratory phase of respiration because air can be expelled only with great effort against the ball-valve effect of narrowed airways and occluding plugs of mucus.

Asthmatic attacks last from minutes to many days. Prolonged attacks are called *status asthmaticus*, in which the most serious consequences of asthma are likely to develop. Death from cardiorespiratory failure is fortunately, rare, but severe hypoxia, pulmonary hypertension, atelectasis, and pneumothorax may accompany the prolonged asthmatic attack. Nevertheless, the overall death rate from asthma is significant.

Treatment consists of eliminating allergens, when possible, and drug therapy. Albuterol and aminophylline represent two classes of drugs that rapidly cause bronchodilation by elevating cAMP and suppressing mediators. Glucocorticoids are used when these drugs are ineffective. Cromolyn, a drug that prevents the degranulation of mast cells, has proved useful in the management of mild asthma.

Chronic bronchitis and emphysema

Chronic bronchitis, as defined by the American Thoracic Society, is a condition associated with excess tracheobronchial mucus production sufficient to cause cough with expectoration at least 2 consecutive years. Emphysema (a swelling caused by air) is defined by the same society as distention of the air spaces distal to the terminal bronchiole with destruction of the alveolar septae.

Chronic bronchitis and emphysema are by definition, two distinct entities, but they are very often found in the same patient. This is especially so in Great Britain where chronic bronchitis and emphysema are regarded as one disease, suggesting that the two conditions have a similar etiology in that part of the world. In other countries, including the United States, bronchitis without emphysema and vice versa are more common.

Etiology and pathogenesis

The factors associated with the development of chronic bronchitis and emphysema are:

1. Cigarette smoking
2. Atmospheric pollutants
3. Infection
4. Genetic factors

Smoking. Cigarette smoking has been frequently and convincingly shown, on statistical grounds, to be associated with chronic bronchitis and emphysema. Experimental studies have shown that inhaled cigarette smoke causes:

1. Inhibition of pulmonary mucociliary clearance
2. Inhibition of phagocytic activity by alveolar macrophages
3. Hyperplasia of bronchial mucous glands
4. Squamous metaplasia of the bronchi
5. Increased airway resistance as a result of increased bronchial smooth muscle tone

Fully developed emphysema has been produced in animals by exposing them to large amounts of tobacco smoke.

Pollutants. Pollutants are probably the single most important factor, especially those found in the environment of industrial areas or specific air contaminants associated with certain occupations such as workers in plastics manufacturing. These have similar effects to or may augment the effects of cigarette smoking.

Infection. The role of infections in the pathogenesis of chronic bronchitis is still unclear. The disease is rarely, if ever, the result of unresolved acute bronchitis. However, frequent isolation of bacteria such as *H. influenzae* and *S. pneumoniae* from respiratory secretions of those with chronic bronchitis has raised questions about the role of these organisms, which appear to be responsible for acute exacerbations.

Infection has also been postulated as a cause of emphysema by initiating inflammatory changes in the terminal bronchioles. These result in the destruction of related alveolar septae, possibly by damaging the blood vessels of the pulmonary acini.

Genetic factors. Genetic predisposition to emphysema is occasionally seen in persons who have an inherited deficiency of the enzyme α-1-antitrypsin. This enzyme is a protease inhibitor and its serum levels rise in the presence of many inflammatory reactions. The genes usually associated with α-1-antitrypsin abnormalities have been designated Z and S. Individuals who are homozygous for either of these genes (ZZ or SS) have extremely low levels of α-1-antitrypsin. Heterozygous individuals with an abnormal Z or S gene and a normal M gene usually have slightly or moderately reduced levels of the enzyme. The incidence of MS or MZ heterozygotes in the general population is about 10%, but is is not clear whether these individuals have a higher risk of developing emphysema.

The exact relationship between homozygous α-1-antitrypsin deficiency and the development of emphysema before the age of 40 is also not known. The enzyme is believed to protect the lung against proteolytic enzymes such as those released by inflammatory cells. Failure to inactivate these enzymes by antitrypsin results in destructive lung changes that lead in turn to emphysema.

In *cystic fibrosis* (Chapter 15), an inherited disorder of exocrine glands, inspissated secretions collect in the bronchial tree as a result of the effect of the disease on the bronchial glands. This predisposes to chronic bronchitis and later to bronchiectasis. Emphysema may also develop in cystic fibrosis, but this is usually of the compensatory variety or simple overdistention of a pulmonary segment caused by partial bronchial obstruction by thick mucus.

Pathology

On gross examination the lungs in emphysema are pale, distended, and bulging. The pallor is caused by widespread loss of blood vessels. The main histopathologic changes in chronic bronchitis are:

1. Hyperplasia of mucous glands and goblet cells with mucopurulent exudate in the bronchial lumen
2. Mucosal inflammation with infiltration by lymphocytes, macrophages, and polymorphonuclear leukocytes
3. Areas of squamous metaplasia in bronchial mucosa
4. Areas of fibrous healing leading to local distortion and narrowing of some bronchi

The classification of emphysema is controversial and is still unresolved. Emphysema without associated chronic bronchitis is sometimes called *primary emphysema*. In this form of the disease all parts of the pulmonary acini are affected: hence the term *panacinar emphysema* is frequently used. The dilated air spaces are small, usually less than 5 mm in diameter, and are found uniformly distributed throughout the lungs, although they tend to be more prominent in the lower lobes. There is little or no normal tissue between the dilated air spaces, which are sometimes called *emphysematous blebs* (bleb meaning blister).

Emphysema that accompanies chronic bronchitis is somewhat different in its form and distribution. The destructive process appears to be located in the terminal bronchioles that supply each acinus ("lobule"). The disease has been called *centrilobular* or more accurately *centriacinar emphysema* (Fig. 12-30). Not all acini are affected, but the dilated air spaces tend to be much larger than those in panacinar emphysema and are most prominent in the upper pulmonary segments. When air spaces reach a diameter greater than 1 cm, they are known as *bullae* (bubbles), and the disease is sometimes referred to as *bullous emphysema* (Fig. 12-31).

The distinction between one type of emphysema and another can only be made with confidence at autopsy. In the special technique of distention-fixation, the lungs are fixed by formaldehyde solution under pressure to retain their morphology. They may then be prepared by making full-length thin slices of the complete lung or lobe. The pattern of emphysema then becomes apparent (Fig. 12-30).

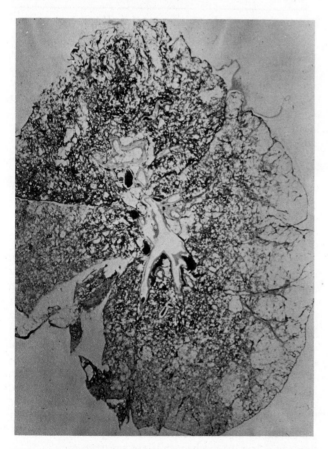

FIG. 12-30. Pulmonary emphysema. The whole lung section shows centrilobular emphysema. The destructive loss of alveolar tissue is especially evident at the periphery of the lung. Compare this with the appearance of normal lung in Fig. 12-4. *(Courtesy Curator of the Gordon Museum, Guy's Hospital, London, England.)*

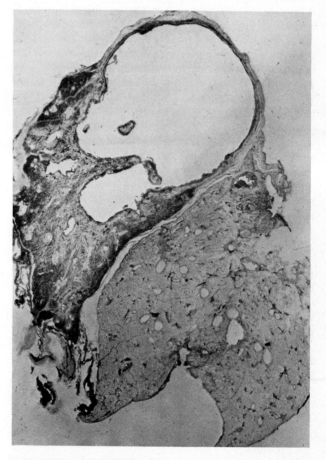

FIG. 12-31. Emphysema. A giant bulla replaces most of the upper lobe of the lung. *(Courtesy Curator of the Gordon Museum, Guy's Hospital, London, England.)*

Clinical aspects

The clinical aspects of chronic bronchitis and emphysema are considered separately later. Each, however, represents two ends of a wide spectrum of pulmonary disease in which the bronchitic or emphysematous component varies greatly from patient to patient. Common to both conditions is impaired oxygenation of the blood, retention of carbon dioxide, and constriction of the pulmonary vasculature. This effect, added to destructive vascular changes, leads to greatly increased vascular resistance in the pulmonary circulation. The vasoconstrictive effects of hypoxia are believed to be the main contributing factor to *pulmonary hypertension*. Pulmonary hypertension is most severe in chronic bronchitis and centrilobular emphysema and frequently leads to cor pulmonale and cardiac failure. Another effect of hypoxia is development of a compensatory erythrocytosis (polycythemia) with an increase in the packed cell volume (hematocrit) of the peripheral blood.

Chronic bronchitis is an extremely common disease. Its highest prevalence is in northwestern Europe and it has been reported in one sixth of the male population of Great Britain. When chronic bronchitis is the predominant disease, patients have a long history of persistent, productive cough. They are usually 50 or older and are almost invariably heavy smokers. As the bronchitis progresses and emphysematous changes develop, increasing breathlessness (dyspnea), cyanosis, and heart failure caused by cor pulmonale follow. Acute bronchial or bronchopneumonic infections are frequent serious complications superimposed on chronic bronchitis. Chronic bronchitis, with acute exacerbations, is a major component of cystic fibrosis in children (Chapter 15).

Pure primary emphysema is less common than chronic bronchitis, but is probably more prevalent in the United States than in Europe. The main symptom of emphysema is breathlessness on exertion. Cough is usually mild or minimal. The breathlessness is progressive and associated with diminished ability to expand the chest, an increased anteroposterior diameter (barrel chest), and the use of accessory muscles of respiration to aid ventilation. Cor pulmonale is unusual except as a late or terminal event. Pulmonary infections are likely to have disastrous results, causing acute respiratory failure and death.

The diagnosis of chronic bronchitis is made on the typical history of the illness; emphysema is diagnosed by the clinical and radiologic findings. The term *chronic obstructive pulmonary disease (COPD)* is sometimes applied to these conditions. Strictly defined, COPD is a condition in which there is chronic obstruction to the airflow in the lungs. Pulmonary function studies determine the presence and degree of obstruction. Hence COPD is a diagnosis based on altered pulmonary function. However, COPD is often used somewhat loosely as a synonym for the syndrome of chronic bronchitis and/or emphysema.

Management of chronic bronchitis and emphysema is difficult and complex because of the variable nature of the diseases and the fact that most of the pathologic changes are irreversible by the time the patient seeks medical aid. The principles of treatment involve:

1. Stopping the patient from smoking
2. Prompt antimicrobial treatment of acute pulmonary infections
3. Vaccine prophylaxis against influenza and pneumococcal infections
4. Bronchodilator drugs

Other forms of emphysema

The term *emphysema* is applied to a variety of other pulmonary conditions. In these contexts emphysema does not usually involve significant destruction of alveolar septae, but rather simple overdistention of the lungs. Emphysema of some degree is a common incidental finding at autopsy in older adults. It has been called *senile emphysema* and is of little significance. *Compensatory emphysema* is the overdistention of one part of a lung to compensate for loss of volume in an adjacent area. This type of emphysema is found near areas of collapse or scarring or when a portion of the lung has been surgically removed.

Mediastinal and surgical emphysema. These forms of emphysema are caused by air entering the mediastinum and tracking upward into the subcutaneous tissues of the neck, face, and axillae. Air may enter the mediastinum (1) by rupture or puncture of the trachea or esophagus by trauma or during a surgical procedure (surgical emphysema) or (2) by rupture of emphysematous bullae in the lung and spread of air to the mediastinum via vascular sheaths (spontaneous mediastinal emphysema). From the mediastinum, air tracks upward into the neck and can be felt beneath the skin where it produces a crackling sensation (crepitus) to the touch. The spontaneous variety is a benign, self-limiting condition. When subcutaneous or mediastinal emphysema is the result of tracheal or esophageal perforation, the main problem is the serious risk of mediastinal infection.

Pulmonary atelectasis and collapse

Although atelectasis is the term widely used to describe collapse of the lung, the exact meaning is failure of the lung to expand. This abnormality is strictly confined to the newborn, a condition known as *atelectasis neonatorum*, and is especially common in premature infants. The ability of the infant lung to expand and remain expanded is an important aspect of fetal maturity. The ability of the lungs to expand depends on the *surface activity* of the lungs, which can be assessed by determining the ratio of lecithin (L) to sphingomyelin (S) in amniotic fluid. An L/S ratio of 1 or less corresponds with a fetal age of 26 to 30 weeks. An infant delivered at this stage of maturity has serious respiratory problems because the lungs cannot expand normally. When the L/S ratio is 2 or more, the fetal age is approximately 35 to 36 weeks and normal lung surface activity can be expected.

The term atelectasis is also applied to an acquired condition in which normally aerated and expanded lungs collapse. The mechanisms causing collapse are compression of the lungs and obstruction of the airways with subsequent absorption of air below the obstruction. Compression of the lungs is caused mainly by fluid or air (or both) in the pleural cavity. Obstruction of the airway may be caused by obstruction of the bronchial lumen by a foreign body, secretions, or a neoplasm or compression of the bronchi by enlarged lymph nodes, a tumor, or an aneurysm. A serious postoperative complication associated with acute respiratory distress in which a whole lung or lobe suddenly collapses is called *acute massive collapse*. Some cases are caused by bronchial obstruction by respiratory tract secretions; in others the mechanism is not apparent.

On gross examination, the atelectatic lung is dark red, and the surface of the area of collapse is sunken below the level of the surrounding tissue. Microscopically, the picture is of closely packed collapsed alveoli. If the lung is not reinflated within a

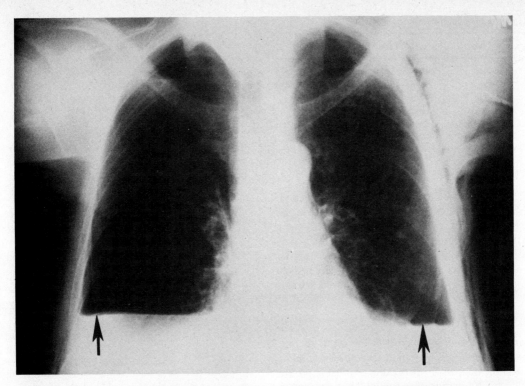

FIG. 12-32. Bilateral hydropneumothorax. Chest radiograph shows horizontal fluid levels in both pleural cavities. The patient had nephrotic syndrome.

few weeks, there is a high risk of fibrosis of the affected segment.

Pneumothorax

The presence of air in the pleural cavity is called pneumothorax. Normally the negative intrapleural pressure is between 2 and 8 cm of water. The introduction of air produces a positive pressure and collapse of the underlying lung.

Etiology and pathogenesis. The causes of pneumothorax are as follows:

1. Trauma to the chest wall, especially when ribs are fractured
2. Rupture of an abnormality of the pleural surface, producing a communication with the airways of the lung that may be caused by emphysema, lung abscess, tuberculous cavities, and sarcoidosis; pneumothorax resulting from these diseases is sometimes referred to as *secondary spontaneous pneumothorax*
3. Rarely, pulmonary neoplasms

The term *primary spontaneous pneumothorax* refers to the condition in which pneumothorax develops in a healthy subject with no known previous lung disease. However, many of these cases are the result of rupture of subpleural emphysematous blebs.

Rarely, the disease is the result of inherited defects of connective tissue, such as in Ehlers-Danlos or Marfan's syndrome. Spontaneous pneumothorax is occasionally associated with menstruation. It is speculated that in these rare cases there is underlying pulmonary endometriosis (Chapter 21).

A *tension pneumothorax* develops when a large amount of air enters the pleural cavity. The pressure exerted by the air closes the pleural tear in such a way that air under sufficient pressure (during coughing, for example) can enter the pleural cavity from the airways but cannot return. This valvelike mechanism can cause rapidly increasing intrapleural pressure, with serious or even fatal effects.

The effects of a pneumothorax are caused by the lateral pressure on the lungs and mediastinum and are most severe if a tension pneumothorax develops. Following are the effects:

1. Collapse of the lung on the affected side
2. Movement of the mediastinum away from the affected side
3. Interference with filling of the great veins and subsequent reduction of cardiac output

Clinical aspects. The onset of pneumothorax is sudden and dramatic. The individual experiences severe unilateral chest pain and acute breathlessness. The diagnosis is confirmed by clinical and radiologic evidence of a collapsed lung and shift of the mediastinum to the opposite side.

Most cases require decompression of the lung by insertion into the pleural cavity of a needle connected to a water-seal drain. When a tension pneumothorax is present, decompression may be lifesaving and must be performed immediately. About 50% of patients will have a single recurrence of the pneumothorax. Recurrent episodes are usually treated surgically.

Hydropneumothorax and pyopneumothorax are conditions in which fluid and pus, respectively, as well as air, are present in the pleural cavity (Fig. 12-32).

The pneumoconioses

The pneumoconioses comprise several pulmonary diseases caused by the inhalation of dusts. Not all dusts however, cause disease. As discussed in Chapter 8, the pulmonary defense

TABLE 12-7. Common pneumoconioses

Disease	Dust	Pulmonary pathology
Anthracosis	Coal dust	Bronchitis, pulmonary fibrosis
Asbestosis	Asbestos	Pulmonary fibrosis, lung and pleural malignant neoplasms
Berylliosis	Beryllium	Granulomatous inflammation
Byssinosis	Cotton and flax	Chronic airway obstruction
Silicosis	Silicon oxide	Pulmonary fibrosis

mechanisms rid the lungs of most inhaled particulate matter. However, if dust particles are in high enough concentration and of the right size, they may reach the alveoli. Particles ranging from 0.1 to 10 μm can cause pulmonary disease. Carbon particles, a constant component of air in industrial cities, appear to cause no adverse effects on the lungs except to color them black. The more important pneumoconioses are listed in Table 12-7.

Silicosis

Etiology and pathogenesis. Silicosis is the result of prolonged exposure of the lungs to high concentrations of silica particles (silicon dioxide, SiO_2). It is estimated that exposure to concentrations of 10^8 particles per cubic foot of air over 10 to 20 years is usually required for the development of most cases of overt silicosis. In some persons, however, the disease develops in 5 years or less. The pathologic effects of silica are believed to be the result of damage to macrophages. After phagocytosis of the inhaled particles, lysosomal damage in the macrophages causes release of lysosomal enzymes, which locally destroy lung tissue. These enzymes also cause death of the macrophages and the release of intracellular silica particles. The particles are phagocytosed by new macrophages and the process begins again, to be followed by fibrotic changes in the lung. The main stimulus to the development of collagen formation in this process was believed to be silicic acid, which forms on the surface of silica particles, but additional unknown substances appear to be necessary, since pure silica alone does not cause the changes described. Other possible causes of the pulmonary fibrosis include an immunologic reaction to the presence of silica.

Pathology. The pathologic features of silicosis (Fig. 12-33) are:

1. Accumulation of macrophages and multinucleate giant cells in the early stages of the disease
2. Development of progressively more fibrotic nodules throughout the lungs and under the pleurae; within these nodules, doubly refractive silica particles can be seen by polarized light microscopy

Clinical aspects. Silicosis is an occupational disease of miners and workers involved in sandblasting, polishing, and grinding processes. The main symptom is progressive breathlessness on exertion. Later, cor pulmonale may develop. Diagnosis is based on a long history of exposure to silica dust and the radiographic appearances in the lungs.

Asbestosis

A number of fibrous, hydrated silicates found in several mineral forms are referred to as asbestos. Of these silicates, chrysotile is a relatively fine flexible fiber, whereas crocidolite and amosite fibers are rigid, straight rods. These differences

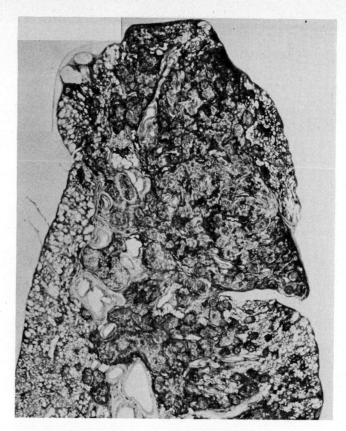

FIG. 12-33. Pulmonary silicosis. Whole lung section showing numerous fibrotic nodules with associated areas of emphysema. *(Courtesy Curator of the Gordon Museum, Guy's Hospital, London, England.)*

in physical properties may account for the more serious pathologic effects generally associated with crocidolite fibers, which, when inhaled, reach the periphery of the lungs.

Pathology. The changes caused by asbestos fibers are similar to those described in silicosis, but three other pathologic changes can be found in asbestosis:

1. Intense pleural thickening due to fibrosis.
2. The development of squamous cell carcinoma or adenocarcinoma of the lung in 10% to 15% of cases. When asbestosis is combined with heavy smoking, the risk of bronchogenic carcinoma is extremely high.
3. The development of malignant mesothelioma of the pleura. Mesothelioma develops in 2% to 10% of workers who have been exposed to asbestos (crocidolite or amosite) for long periods. The etiologic role (if any) of chrysotile in the genesis of this tumor is not known.

Most cases of malignant pleural mesothelioma are associated with exposure to asbestos, but a history of contact with asbestos is not always obtainable, or the period from contact to development of the tumor may take up to 50 years.

The lesions of pulmonary asbestosis are foci of loose fibrosis located around the bronchioles where the asbestos fibers alight. A characteristic microscopic feature is the asbestos (or ferruginous) body, an elongated, club-shaped structure measuring 40 to 50 μm in length and formed by the deposition of hemosiderin and glycoprotein around the asbestos fibers.

The widespread use of asbestos in insulating, textile, and acoustic materials and in automotive brakes is evident in the finding of asbestos fibers in nearly 40% of autopsies in the United States. Because of the association with malignant mesothelioma, the use of asbestos, especially crocidolite, in many industrial processes has been greatly curtailed.

Pulmonary fibrosis

Many diseases can lead to fibrous replacement of alveolar tissue, and ultimately to end-stage (honeycomb) lung and respiratory failure. DAD (Table 12-8) is an acute process that can lead to widespread pulmonary fibrosis. Other important causes of pulmonary fibrosis are:
1. Chronic interstitial pneumonias
2. Bronchiolitis obliterans organizing pneumonias

The former affects predominantly the pulmonary interstitium; the latter leads to plugging of the distal airways by connective tissue. Both groups of disorders, like DAD, may have an identifiable cause (such as infections, toxins, or collagen-vascular diseases) or may be idiopathic. They have an insidious onset and run a chronic course.

It is important to distinguish between the two forms of interstitial pneumonia. *Usual interstitial pneumonia* (formerly known as the Hamman-Rich syndrome*) affects the lungs in a widespread but patchy fashion. *Desquamative interstitial pneumonia* affects the lungs more uniformly. The former has a poorer prognosis than either desquamative interstitial pneumonia or bronchiolitis obliterans organizing pneumonia, mainly because it does not respond to corticosteroid treatment.

Neoplasms of the respiratory tract

There are many benign and malignant neoplasms of the respiratory tract. Carcinomas of the larynx and the lung are the most important groups of malignant tumors affecting humans. Malignant mesothelioma has already been mentioned because of its relationship with asbestosis, but it is rare. The bronchial carcinoid tumor is an uncommon pulmonary neoplasm that is of interest because of its association with the carcinoid syndrome (Chapter 13) and because it has a much better prognosis than most lung cancers.

Tumors of the larynx

Carcinoma of the larynx is by far the most important laryngeal neoplasm. It is 7 to 14 times more common in men than in women. Smoking, environmental pollution, and exposure to asbestos are among the likely contributing factors.

The vast majority of malignant tumors of the larynx are squamous (epidermoid) carcinomas. Carcinoma in situ, which is comparable in many ways to the same lesion of the uterine cervix, is recognized both with and without the presence of invasive carcinoma. On gross examination, invasive carcinomas are either papillary or form irregular, thickened areas in the larynx where the tumor has infiltrated. Tumors confined to the true vocal cords (intrinsic tumors) are likely to remain localized and do not readily metastasize to regional lymph nodes. Tumors extending beyond the vocal cords (extrinsic tumors) have a greater tendency to spread to lymph nodes. Distant metastases are uncommon.

Microscopically, typical nests of invasive keratinizing squamous cells are seen. Often the neighboring epithelium is hyperkeratotic or dysplastic or is the site of carcinoma in situ.

Other malignant tumors of the larynx are occasionally found. These tumors are more commonly associated with salivary glands, namely, mucoepidermoid and adenoid cystic carcinomas (Chapter 14).

Clinically, hoarseness is the common, early feature that leads to diagnosis. Small localized tumors may be cured by radiotherapy alone and carcinoma in situ by local excision. Intrinsic tumors are usually treated by laryngectomy a procedure that, although drastic, offers an 80% chance of a 5-year cure. Extrinsic tumors have a much poorer prognosis.

Tumors of the lung

Benign tumors of the lung are rare; the *pulmonary hamartoma* is perhaps the only noteworthy benign tumor. It consists of islands of mature cartilage in which smooth muscle, fat, and clefts lined with ciliated epithelium can be seen microscopically.

Bronchial adenoma is a grossly misleading term that has been used erroneously in the past to collectively describe a group of low-grade malignant tumors, namely, carcinoid tumors, adenoid cystic carcinomas, and mucoepidermoid carcinomas. It should no longer be used, since none of these neoplasms is benign.

Bronchogenic (bronchial) carcinoma is by far the most important of all pulmonary neoplasms. A classification of malignant pulmonary neoplasms based on that of the World Health Organization follows:

Squamous cell (epidermoid) carcinoma
Adenocarcinoma
Bronchioloalveolar carcinoma*
Adenosquamous carcinoma
Small cell (oat cell) carcinoma
Large cell carcinoma
Giant cell carcinoma
Mucous gland carcinoma
  Adenoid cystic carcinoma
  Mucoepidermoid carcinoma
Carcinoid tumor

Bronchogenic carcinoma

Bronchogenic carcinoma was a rare disease at the end of the 19th century, but it has now reached epidemic proportions, particularly in North America and western Europe. It is the most common malignant disease of men, accounting for one in every four male deaths from cancer. In 1984, in the United States, there were 118,000 deaths from lung cancer; roughly one third of these were women, for whom the mortality rate continues to rise toward that for men—a most depressingly undesirable trend toward sexual equality.

Etiology and pathogenesis. The known etiologic factors in bronchogenic carcinoma appear to be the following:
1. Cigarette smoking
2. Industrial atmospheric pollutants
3. Previous pulmonary fibrotic disease

Frequently these factors may be combined.

The role of heavy cigarette smoking is well documented. *Bronchogenic carcinoma is rare among nonsmokers.* The death rate in this disease in those who smoke 20 or more cigarettes a day is about seven times greater than in nonsmokers. Of a number of carcinogenic agents present in cigarette smoke, 3,4-

---

*L. Hamman (1887-1946), American physician; A.R. Rich (b. 1893), American pathologist.

*This tumor is also considered to be a form of adenocarcinoma.

benzpyrene is the most potent. The exact means by which these agents act is unclear, but it is believed that cell membrane–bound enzymes such as aryl hydrocarbon carboxylase convert the inhaled hydrocarbons (procarcinogens) to compounds (ultimate carcinogens) that cause the malignant changes in the bronchial epithelial cells. Although cigarettes are by far the most common etiologic agents, certain industrial pollutants are also associated with much higher risks of cancer. These include compounds of iron, nickel, and chromium and radon coming from rocks. The role of asbestos in pulmonary malignancy has already been mentioned in relation to both bronchial and pleural cancer.

The development of carcinomas in sites of chronic pulmonary fibrosis has been frequently described, especially in patients who have scleroderma (Chapter 16), but the reasons for this apparent relationship are unclear. These tumors are usually adenocarcinomas, and in some instances the abundant connective tissue stroma appears to be induced by the tumor, rather than play a causative role.

Pathology. The histologic varieties of carcinoma of the bronchus are listed on p. 265.

Malignant epithelial neoplasms of the lung appear to arise from cells that can differentiate along several lines normally present in the airways. Thus *squamous cell carcinomas* are found, as well as *adenocarcinomas* of different kinds, and neoplasms showing neuroendocrine differentiation, such as

carcinoid tumors. Mixed forms, such as adenosquamous carcinomas are not uncommon. Some carcinomas have no recognizable cell type by light microscopy and by convention are termed *undifferentiated carcinomas;* however, electron microscopy or immunohistochemistry may reveal limited squamous, glandular, or neuroendocrine differentiation.

Both small and large cell undifferentiated carcinomas are recognized; it is important to distinguish between them because small cell carcinomas, unlike other forms of lung carcinoma, tend to disseminate very early and widely.

Squamous cell carcinoma. Squamous cell (epidermoid) carcinoma comprises about 60% of all bronchogenic carcinomas; 80% of all epidermoid carcinomas are found in men. The anatomic location of these tumors is usually central, that is, near the hilum of the lung and at bifurcation points of the larger bronchi. These tumors frequently obstruct the bronchial lumen. As a result, the signs and symptoms of bronchial obstruction are demonstrable in nearly half of the patients with this tumor.

Epidermoid carcinoma begins with dysplastic changes in the bronchial mucosa, progressing to carcinoma in situ and finally to invasive carcinoma. The tumor grows into the bronchial lumen or may infiltrate beneath the bronchus and spread medially (Fig. 12-34). The tumor may ulcerate superficially or may compress or occlude the airway.

Local spread of the tumor may involve the mediastinal structures, including the superior vena cava, which may be severely compressed or obstructed. Apical tumors may spread directly into the chest wall (Fig. 12-35) or structures in the root of the neck *(Pancoast tumors)*. Many squamous cell tumors undergo central necrosis with formation of a cavity that often can be detected radiologically. Lymphatic spread to the hilar and prescalene lymph nodes is common; the latter are in a convenient

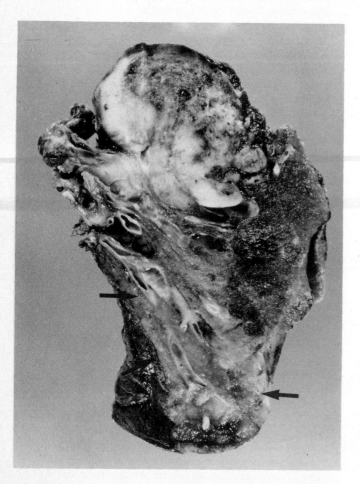

FIG. 12-34. Bronchogenic carcinoma. A tumor 4 cm in diameter is arising from and obstructing a large bronchus. The pale segment of lung *(arrows)* is an area of pneumonic consolidation.

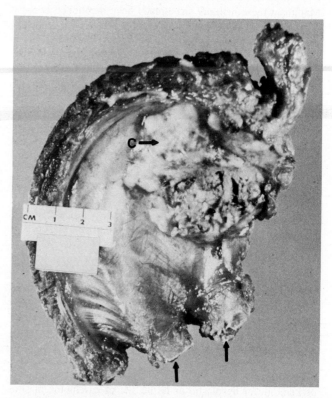

FIG. 12-35. Carcinoma of the bronchus. An apical carcinoma *(C)* is seen invading the pleura overlying the apex of the lung and the first two ribs (Pancoast syndrome).

site for performing a biopsy. Distant, bloodborne metastases are most frequently found in the adrenal glands, liver, bone, and brain. Histologically, the presence of keratin and the microscopic characteristics of carcinoma cells are the main diagnostic features.

Adenocarcinoma. 50% of all lung cancers in women are adenocarcinomas. A statistical relationship between adenocarcinoma and cigarette smoking has not been observed.

Adenocarcinomas are usually found in the periphery of the lung and they are the predominant tumor associated with pulmonary fibrosis ("scar carcinoma"). Histologically, the tumor has a glandular or papillary pattern and mucus is commonly present.

Bronchioloalveolar (alveolar cell, bronchiolar) carcinoma is an uncommon variety of adenocarcinoma that comprises 2% to 3% of all pulmonary neoplasms. The tumor appears to arise from cells in the distal airways and is therefore found in the periphery of the lungs (Fig. 12-36). Many of these tumors differentiate toward Clara cells, or type 2 pneumocytes, which are surfactant-producing cells. Bronchioloalveolar carcinoma can form discrete masses or may widely infiltrate the alveoli, producing a radiographic appearance that resembles pneumonia. The predominant histologic pattern is one of cuboidal or columnar epithelium that lines alveolar spaces (Fig. 12-37).

Bronchioloalveolar carcinoma has not been related to cigarette smoking. Clinically, it behaves like other adenocarcinomas, although the localized forms may have a slightly better prognosis.

Adenosquamous carcinoma. Adenosquamous carcinoma includes squamous carcinomas in which mucin production can be demonstrated or adenocarcinomas that have squamous elements; 8% to 10% of malignant lung tumors can be included in this group.

Small cell (oat cell) carcinoma. This distinctive tumor generally arises in the proximal airways and comprises about 10% of lung cancers. It consists of small compact cells, with a high nucleus/cytoplasm ratio (Fig. 12-38). The cells can be round, oval, or polygonal. The association of small cell tumors with various endocrine syndromes reflects the neuroendocrine differentiation found in many of these tumors. Almost all small cell tumors are found in males, of whom 85% to 90% are cigarette smokers. Small cell tumors are highly malignant and disseminate early and widely. Sometimes they are more localized at the time of diagnosis and may respond to chemotherapy.

Large cell undifferentiated carcinoma (including giant cell carcinoma). Large cell carcinomas (Fig. 12-39) are mainly peripheral in location and have been referred to previously. Their prognosis is generally related to their stage, size, and degree of spread when the diagnosis is made.

Adenoid cystic and mucoepidermoid carcinomas. These uncommon lung tumors arise from minor salivary glands in the respiratory tract. Both tumors have similar histologic appearances when they arise in the major salivary glands (Chapter 14) and have a poor prognosis.

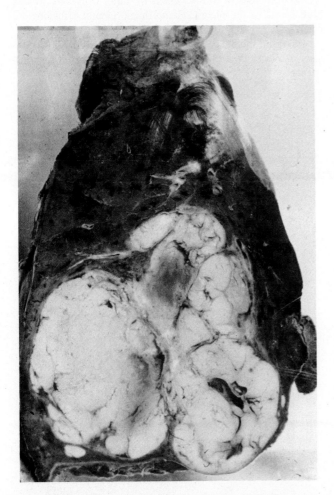

FIG. 12-36. Alveolar cell carcinoma of the lung. This large tumor has arisen in the periphery of the lung and has spread widely through the alveoli. *(Courtesy Curator of the Gordon Museum, Guy's Hospital, London, England.)*

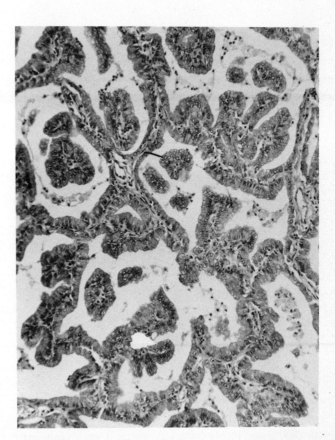

FIG. 12-37. Alveolar cell carcinoma of the lung. Tall, columnar, mucus-producing cells line the terminal air spaces.

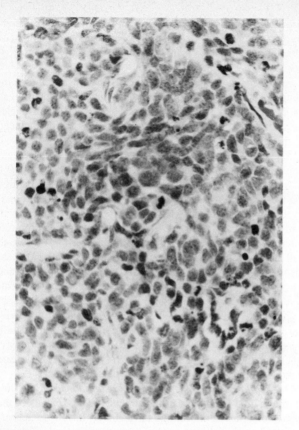

FIG. 12-38. Small cell carcinoma of the lung. The typical cells in this tumor are small, with a high nucleus/cytoplasm ratio, sometimes resembling lymphocytes.

Carcinoid tumors. Carcinoid tumors of the lung have in the past been referred to as *bronchial adenomas.* They are slowly invasive and destructive and may metastasize. Carcinoids form about 4% of all bronchial neoplasms. They are found beneath intact mucosa, mainly in the main bronchi, as solitary highly vascular tumors. Carcinoid tumors may metastasize to the liver and give rise to the *carcinoid syndrome.* This syndrome of skin flushing, diarrhea, cardiac valvular lesions, and bronchospasm is due to release from the tumor of highly active substances, including 5-hydroxytryptamine, histamine, bradykinin, adrenocorticotropic hormone, and a polypeptide (P substance). The carcinoid syndrome is further discussed in Chapter 13. Some small cell carcinomas may also exhibit neuroendocrine differentiation and cause the carcinoid syndrome.

The outlook after surgical resection is good; 70% to 80% of patients survive 10 years after resection.

Tumors of serous membranes. Both *localized* and *diffuse* forms of neoplasia may arise in serous membranes. The localized forms include fibroma (benign) and fibrosarcoma (malignant), which appear to arise from submesothelial connective tissue elements. Diffuse neoplasms of serous membranes are almost invariably *malignant mesotheliomas.* These may have an epithelial, sarcomatous, or biphasic (mixed) histologic pattern. *Malignant mesotheliomas* are uncommon tumors except in association with exposure to asbestos. The tumors form multiple nodules or diffuse sheets of tumor cells that involve both layers of the pleura. Hemorrhagic pleural effusions are often associated. The sarcomatous type is highly cellular, with pleomorphic spindle cells; the epithelial form (Fig. 12-40) consists of nests, cords, or acini of tumor cells set in a fibrous stroma.

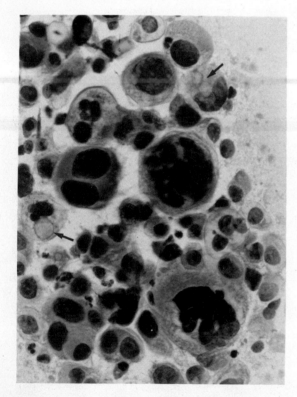

FIG. 12-39. Anaplastic large cell carcinoma of the lung (fine needle aspiration smear). There is striking pleomorphism and hyperchromasia. Vacuoles are present in some cells *(arrows)* suggesting that this may be a poorly differentiated adenocarcinoma.

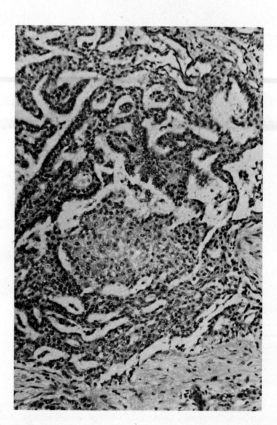

FIG. 12-40. Pleural mesothelioma forming slitlike spaces with papillary projections.

The prognosis in all malignant forms of mesothelioma is poor.

Clinical aspects

Carcinoma of the lung can appear clinically in many ways; however, lack of clinical signs and symptoms until the disease is well advanced is a major obstacle to early diagnosis. The clinical effects include weight loss, cough, pulmonary collapse distal to the tumor, and involvement of the pleura with chest pain and effusion. These may be accompanied by complications such as superior vena cava obstruction, endocrine effects of the tumor, and metastasis to other organs, especially the brain, liver, and bone. In some cases the clinical picture can be dom-inated by extrapulmonary syndromes related to the primary tumor or its metastases. These systemic syndromes are listed in Table 12-8. Asymptomatic tumors are not infrequently detected by radiographs of the chest or by sputum cytologic examination performed as a screening process. The diagnosis is established by histologic examination of tissue obtained by biopsy usually either by fine needle aspiration or at the time of bronchoscopy. It is customary to stage lung carcinomas on the basis of their size, the presence of lymph node metastases, and metastases to other organs. Depending on the stage of the disease, the treatment usually consists of surgical resection and/or radiotherapy. Chemotherapy may be combined with either of these two modalities, particularly in the treatment of small cell carcinomas. Despite improvements in surgery, radiotherapy, and chemotherapy, the prognosis in most cases of lung cancer is poor. The overall 5-year survival rate, even after apparent curative resection is only around 30%.

Metastatic tumors of the lung

The lung is a common site of tumor metastases. The primary tumors that commonly spread to the lungs are listed in Table 12-9.

TABLE 12-8. Systemic syndromes and abnormalities associated with bronchogenic carcinoma

Effects	Syndrome or abnormality
Hormonal	Cushing's syndrome
	Inappropriate secretion of antidiuretic hormone
	Gynecomastia
	Carcinoid syndrome
Metabolic	Hypercalcemia
Hematologic	Anemia
	Thrombocytopenic purpura
	Leukemoid reactions
Skin and connective tissue	Dermatomyositis
	Acanthosis nigricans
	Finger clubbing
Neurologic	Peripheral neuritis
Vascular	Nonbacterial thrombotic endocarditis

TABLE 12-9. Tumors that commonly metastasize to the lungs

Source	Type of tumor
Bone	Sarcoma
Breast	Adenocarcinoma
Colon	Adenocarcinoma
Kidney	Renal cell carcinoma
Prostate gland	Adenocarcinoma
Skin	Melanoma
Stomach	Adenocarcinoma
Uterus	Choriocarcinoma

Selected readings

Claypool WD, Rogers RM, and Matuschak GM: Update on the clinical diagnosis, management and pathogenesis of pulmonary alveolar proteinosis (phospholipidosis), Chest 85:550, 1984.

Craighead JE: Current pathogenetic concepts of diffuse malignant mesothelioma, Hum Pathol 18:544, 1987.

Edelstein PH and Meyer RD: Legionnaire's disease: a review, Chest 85:114, 1984.

Gail BG and Lenfant CJM: Cells of the lung: biology and clinical applications, Am Rev Respir Dis 133:943, 1986.

Hurt R and Bates M: Carcinoid tumors of the bronchus, Thorax 36:617, 1984.

Johanson WG and Harris GD: Aspiration pneumonia, aerobic infections, and lung abscess, Med Clin North Am 64:385, 1980.

Katzenstein A-LA and Askin FB: Diffuse alveolar damage. In Surgical pathology of nonneoplastic lung disease, Philadelphia, 1982, WB Saunders Co.

Reed CE: The pathogenesis of asthma, Med Clin North Am 58:53, 1974.

Schuyler M and Salvaggio JE: Hypersensitivity pneumonitis, Semin Respir Med 5:246, 1984.

Sheppard D: Adverse pulmonary effects of air pollution, Immunol Allerg Pract 6:25, 1984.

Silverberg E and Lubera J: Cancer statistics, 1987, CA 37:2, 1987.

Snider GL: Chronic obstructive pulmonary disease, Am Rev Respir Dis 133:942, 1986.

Sobin LH: The histologic classification of lung tumors, Hum Pathol 14:1020, 1983.

Yesner R: Small cell tumors of the lung, Am J Surg Pathol 7:775, 1983.

CHAPTER 13

Diseases of the blood and lymphatic system

Diseases of the blood are major afflictions. The anemias, particularly those resulting from lack of essential nutrients, are among the most common diseases. The leukemias, on the other hand, are quite rare, but partly because of their potentially lethal nature, command a great deal of attention from clinicians, researchers, and the public. Hemostatic derangements can greatly affect the outcome of all forms of surgical treatment. Transfusion of blood and its components, in addition to its importance in the treatment of injuries and blood diseases, has helped to change the face of cardiovascular surgery and the transplantation of major organs, such as the heart, liver, and kidney. However, the great benefits of blood and blood component therapy have been tempered by the recognition that it can transmit hepatitis and human immunodeficiency viruses.

Commonly used hematologic measurements

Many elements of the blood can be quantified either by counting or by biochemical or immunologic methods, many of which will be referred to throughout this chapter. The commonly used measurements are listed in Table 13-1. Significant deviations from the "normal," or reference, values for these measurements are characteristic of diseases of the hemolymphatic system itself or can be secondary to diseases of other organ systems.

DISORDERS OF RED BLOOD CELLS

ANEMIA

Anemia, which literally means "no blood," can be defined as a reduction in the mass of circulating red blood cells. Since this is a difficult quantity to measure, more practical definitions are required. These are based on the normal values given in Table 13-1. Anemia can be defined as a reduction below normal of the blood hemoglobin concentration, which may be reflected in reduction of the volume of packed red blood cells (hematocrit) and/or the red blood cell count. It is important, however, to consider patients' age and sex and even the altitude at which they live before basing a diagnosis of anemia on these values. Thus a hemoglobin concentration of 14.2 g/dL may be considered normal for an adult female, but can indicate severe anemia in a newborn infant.

Laboratory investigation

Investigation of anemia first requires a careful review of the patient's history and a physical examination, as discussed later. Determination of the degree and type of anemia depends on laboratory measurements. In addition to those listed in Table 13-1, that is, hemoglobin, red blood cell count, and hemato-

crit,* it is customary to calculate corpuscular constants from these values. Thus:

1. Mean corpuscular volume (MCV) =
$$\frac{\text{Hematocrit (\%)} \times 10}{\text{Red blood cell count (in millions}/\mu\text{L)}}$$
and gives a numerical assessment of mean red blood cell size in femtoliters (fL). (A femtoliter = 10^{-15} L.)

2. Mean corpuscular hemoglobin (MCH) =
$$\frac{\text{Hemoglobin (g/dL)}}{\text{Red blood cell count (in millions}/\mu\text{L)}}$$
and is the hemoglobin content of the average red blood cell in picograms (pg).

3. Mean corpuscular hemoglobin concentration (MCHC) =
$$\frac{\text{Hemoglobin (g/dL)} \times 100}{\text{Hematocrit (\%)}}$$
and is the average concentration of hemoglobin in a given volume of packed red blood cells in grams per deciliter (g/dL).

These constants can be determined automatically by electronic blood counting instruments, which are more precise and accurate than visual counting methods. Yet another value that is calculated by one electronic counter (current Coulter† instruments) is the *red cell distribution width* (RDW). The RDW is the coefficient of variation of the red blood cell volume distribution and has been used by some hematologists as an aid to the classification of anemias. In simple terms, however, the hemoglobin and MCV are the most useful guides to the cause of an anemia. Reference values for these hematologic constants are given in Table 13-1.

In addition to determining the hematologic constants, the most valuable procedure in the laboratory evaluation of all blood diseases is the examination of a stained peripheral smear by an experienced, knowledgeable observer. Further valuable information is obtained from a reticulocyte count and microscopic examination of the bone marrow. It is usual to obtain both a marrow biopsy specimen and an aspirated sample. The former preserves the anatomic relationships and the proportions of the various cellular elements; the latter is used to examine the cytologic details of the hemopoietic tissue. The importance of a complete history and thorough physical examination must not be forgotten.

Morphologic classification of red blood cells

Characteristics of red blood cells, based on their size and hemoglobin content, are commonly used to describe and classify anemias:

_____

*The percentage of packed red blood cells in a volume of blood after centrifugation.
†Coulter Electronics, Hialeah, Fla.

TABLE 13-1. Commonly used hematologic measurements and their reference values

Measurement	Reference values
Hemoglobin	
Adult males	16.0 ± 2 g/dL
Adult females	14.0 ± 2 g/dL
Newborn infants	19.5 ± 5 g/dL
Red blood cells	
Adult males	5.4 ± 0.8 million/μL
Adult females	4.8 ± 0.6 million/μL
Newborn infants	5.1 ± 1.0 million/μL
White blood cells	
Total white blood cells	4300-10,000/μL
Neutrophils	1500-6000/μL
Eosinophils	1-700/μL
Basophils	1-150/μL
Lymphocytes	1500-4000/μL
Monocytes	200-1000/μL
Platelets	140,000-400,000/μL
Hematocrit (packed cell volume)	
Adult males	47 ± 5 mL/dL
Adult females	42 ± 5 ml/dL
Red blood cell indices ("absolute values")	
Mean corpuscular volume (MCV)	90 ± fL/red blood cell
Mean corpuscular hemoglobin (MCH)	30 ± 3 pg
Mean corpuscular hemoglobin concentration (MCHC)	34 ± 2 g/dL

1. *Normocytic:* Red blood cells of normal size
2. *Microcytic:* Red blood cells smaller than normal
3. *Macrocytic:* Red blood cells larger than normal
4. *Normochromic:* Red blood cells with normal hemoglobin content
5. *Hypochromic:* Red blood cells with diminished hemoglobin content

The terms *poikilocytosis* and *anisocytosis* mean variations in the red cell shape and size, respectively. For example, a microcytic, hypochromic anemia usually indicates iron deficiency. Other terms describing red blood cell morphology are listed in Table 13-2.

General aspects of anemia

Anemia is not a disease of itself. It is the result of a wide variety of mechanisms that manifest themselves as a fall below normal of hemoglobin, hematocrit, and red blood cell count. Recognition of anemia demands that the underlying cause be ascertained to enable the disease to be managed effectively. The cause may be relatively simple to detect and readily correctable when anemia is found, for example, in a menstruating woman eating an iron-poor diet. On the other hand, it may have ominous implications when detected in a child or an adult male, since cancer is an important cause. There are many causes of anemia, and their recognition may necessitate extensive investigation of the patient; the treatment of anemia may therefore vary greatly from case to case.

General clinical aspects. Despite many causes and different specific signs and symptoms related to these causes, all anemias

TABLE 13-2. Morphologic abnormalities of erythrocytes

Abnormal erythrocyte	Description	Associated disorders
Acanthocyte	Irregular shape with one or two spiny projections	Some anemias and liver disorders
Echinocyte (burr cell)	Irregular shape with many spiny projections	Uremia; common artifact
Elliptocyte	Elongated with rounded ends	Hereditary elliptocytosis; some normal smears
Leptocyte (target cell)	Thin cell with outer rim and central zone of hemoglobin resembling target	Abnormalities of hemoglobin, e.g., thalassemia and postsplenectomy
Reticulocyte	Young red blood cell staining bluish due to RNA	Normal; increased after hemorrhage, hemolysis, and anemias receiving treatment
Schistocyte	Fragmented cell, often helmet shaped	Certain hemolytic diseases
Spherocyte	Spherical cell with reduced diameter and loss of central pallor	Hereditary spherocytosis
Stomatocyte	Central mouth-shaped cleft	Hereditary stomatocytosis; occasional artefact

of significant degree have clinical effects in common. Many reflect the following cardiovascular changes caused by the reduced oxygen-carrying capacity of anemic blood:

1. Tachycardia (a rapid heart rate), which combined with an increased stroke volume, causes palpitations as a manifestation of increased cardiac activity.
2. Dyspnea (shortness of breath) and rapid onset of fatigue on exertion are typical of severe anemia.
3. Cardiac systolic murmurs.
4. Faintness, dizziness, headache, and irritability.
5. Pallor of the skin, although commonly associated with anemia, is an unreliable guide to its presence. Palmar creases, nail beds, and oral mucosa are more reliable sites for the recognition of pallor, but there is no substitute for an accurate hemoglobin estimation to determine the degree of anemia.

Causes of anemia

The main causes of anemia are blood loss, increased cell destruction (hemolytic anemia), and decreased red blood cell production (hypoplastic or aplastic anemia). In some anemias, more than one of these causes can contribute to the pathogenesis.

Hemorrhage is the most common cause of anemia, although in acute massive bleeding, anemia is of secondary importance to the immediate effects, particularly shock, and is not immediately detectable.

Chronic blood loss may be considered physiologic in menstruating women and does not become significant unless dietary iron intake or absorption is insufficient to compensate for the loss. However, the most common sites of chronic blood loss include the uterus, mainly through menstrual loss, and the gastrointestinal tract, from peptic ulceration, hemorrhoids, and chronic aspirin ingestion. Infestation by bloodsucking hookworms is a major cause of blood loss in many parts of the world. The important manifestations of chronic blood loss are largely those of iron deficiency, which is considered below.

Iron deficiency anemia

The most common cause of anemia is lack of iron. In the United States more than half of all infants and pregnant women are affected, as are 13% of *all* adult women. The prevalence is even higher in other countries.

Etiology. Iron deficiency is a manifestation of some other disorder, but three mechanisms alone or in combination cause iron deficiency:

1. Increased demand for iron, as in growing children and pregnant women
2. Loss of iron through hemorrhage, either physiologic, as in menstruating women, or from some pathologic cause
3. Insufficient iron intake either because of low levels of dietary iron or the inability to absorb the iron available

Iron metabolism. Under normal conditions, the daily dietary intake of iron is about 15 mg, of which 4% to 7% is absorbed from the upper small intestine. After absorption, iron is conveyed in ferric form bound to a plasma globulin, *transferrin,* to the marrow for synthesis of red blood cell hemoglobin. Normal iron levels in the plasma range from 50 to 165 μg/dL. Iron is also transported for incorporation into myoglobin and iron-dependent enzyme systems. The amount of transferrin can be measured directly or as *total iron-binding capacity* (TIBC), which measures the sum of the serum iron bound to transferrin and the unsaturated transferrin. The normal TIBC is about 330 μg/dL; transferrin is normally 20% to 45% saturated with iron. Iron is stored in the macrophage-monocyte system of the liver, spleen, and marrow, and in hepatocytes iron is stored in the

form of hemosiderin and ferritin. Minute quantities (normally 10 to 200 ng/dL) of ferritin are also present in plasma. Healthy males have about 1 g of stored iron; in females the stores are normally less than half this amount. The body carefully hoards iron, and in health males lose only about 1 mg a day or less from normal loss of renal, mucosal, and cutaneous epithelium. Menstruating women have an unavoidable iron loss of 18 mg/month (an average of 0.6 mg/day). During pregnancy a mother will lose between approximately 500 and 1000 mg of iron to the fetus.

The following can therefore be concluded:

1. Iron deficiency in men is unusual and commonly reflects blood loss, especially from the gastrointestinal tract, or rarely in the United States or Britain, dietary deficiency of iron.
2. Because of physiologic iron loss and much lower levels of stored iron, menstruating women are much more likely to develop iron deficiency as a result of inadequate iron intake. The physiologic demands of pregnancy greatly enhance the likelihood of iron deficiency.

Pathogenesis. In iron-deficient states, the stored iron is used first, and when these reserves are exhausted, anemia develops. The levels of iron and ferritin in the serum fall and as less iron becomes available, the TIBC increases. In the peripheral blood, the red blood cells become smaller and their hemoglobin content is reduced.

On a stained blood smear, the red cells are microcytic and hypochromic, with only a small stained rim of hemoglobin at the periphery of the cell (Fig. 13-1). In severe cases, some red blood cells are elongated and pencil or cigar shaped. The MCV and MCH are reduced. The marrow responds by producing increased numbers of normoblasts. However, hemoglobinization of these cells is impaired, and stainable iron, normally

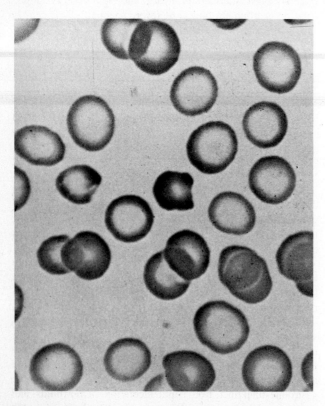

FIG. 13-1. Iron-deficiency anemia, blood film. The red blood cells are hypochromic, with only a small rim of dark-staining hemoglobin in each cell.

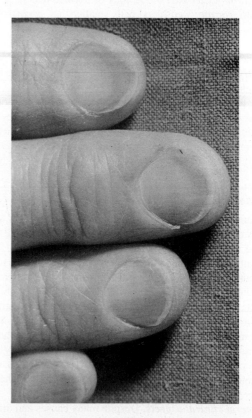

FIG. 13-2. Koilonychia (spoon-shaped nails) as a result of long-standing iron deficiency anemia.

present in the marrow, is greatly reduced or absent because of depleted iron stores.

Clinical effects. Symptoms of iron deficiency are often inconspicuous or absent. In addition to the symptoms common to all anemias, symptomatic patients have spoon-shaped nails (koilonychia) (Fig. 13-2), and a smooth, atrophic tongue may develop in severe cases (Fig. 13-3). Occasionally, in the Paterson-Kelly syndrome these are associated with dysphagia and esophageal webs (Chapter 14).

Once the diagnosis of iron deficiency has been established, management of the patient consists of determining the underlying causes, correcting or treating these causes, and giving iron. This will restore the blood picture to normal unless absorption is poor or the underlying disorder has not been eradicated. Early evidence that anemia is responding to iron is anincrease in the reticulocyte count. An increase in hemoglobin level should follow soon after.

Sideroblastic anemias

In sideroblastic anemia the marrow has normoblasts containing excessive amounts of iron arranged in ringlike fashion around their nuclei.

Sideroblastic anemias are believed to be due to a defect in the synthesis of the heme fraction of hemoglobin, although the exact cause is not known. Inherited and acquired forms are recognized. The *inherited* form is seen in children who develop the signs and symptoms of iron overloading and anemia. Enlargement of the liver and spleen and a microcytic, hypochromic anemia are the main findings. A similar clinical picture is seen in the *acquired* form of the disease, which may arise without any obvious cause (primary type) or as a result of chronic alcoholism or the use of certain drugs (secondary type). Sideroblastic anemia may also be associated with chronic inflammatory states, myeloproliferative disorders, and megaloblastic anemias, which are described later in this chapter. The

marrow in these cases contains at least 15% to 20% ring sideroblasts.

The main danger in sideroblastic anemia, especially in the inherited form, is from iron overload and its effects on the liver and heart (see the discussion on hemochromatosis in this chapter), especially if blood transfusions have been given to maintain an acceptable hemoglobin level.

It is usual to give pyridoxine (vitamin B_6) to patients with sideroblastic anemias. This vitamin is effective when inflammation or infection is the cause and can help correct the anemia when it is secondary to the use of antituberculous drugs or chronic alcoholism. In other forms of this anemia, pyridoxine may result in partial improvement.

Megaloblastic anemias

Anemias characterized by the presence of megaloblasts in the bone marrow and macrocytes in the peripheral blood are referred to as megaloblastic anemias. A *megaloblast*, as defined by Paul Erlich* in 1880, is an abnormal red blood cell precursor (Fig. 13-4). It is larger than its normoblastic counterpart, both in cell and nuclear size. Its chromatin is finely dispersed and

---

*P. Erlich (1854-1915), German microbiologist.

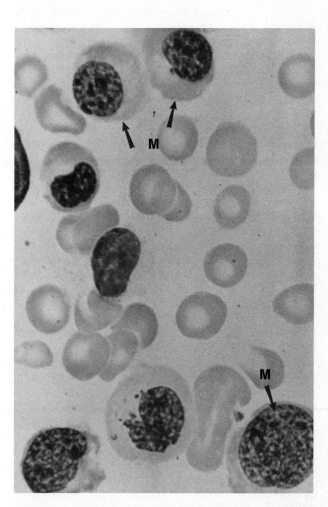

FIG. 13-4. Pernicious anemia, bone marrow. The abnormal red blood cell precursors (megaloblasts) *(M)* are much larger than normal; the nucleus/cytoplasm ratio is increased, and the chromatin of the nucleus is finely dispersed.

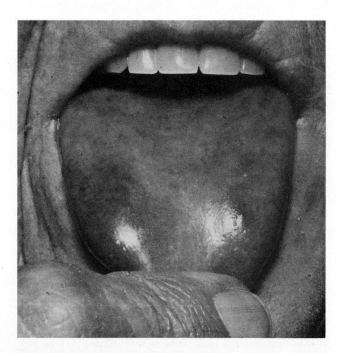

FIG. 13-3. The tongue in the Paterson-Kelly syndrome. The tongue is smooth and shiny, with loss of normal papillae.

MAIN CAUSES OF FOLATE DEFICIENCY

1. Dietary deficiency
2. Malabsorption syndromes (e.g., celiac disease)
3. Increased demands
   a. Pregnancy and childhood
   b. Hemolytic diseases (e.g., thalassemia)
4. Drugs
   a. Folate antagonists (e.g., methotrexate)
   b. Anticonvulsants
   c. Oral contraceptives
   d. Alcoholism
5. Liver disease (e.g., cirrhosis)

MAIN CAUSES OF COBALAMIN DEFICIENCY

1. Dietary deficiency (strict vegetarian diet)
2. Intrinsic factor deficiency
   a. Pernicious (addisonian) anemia
   b. Gastric resection
3. Intestinal defects
   a. Malabsorption syndromes (e.g., celiac disease)
   b. Terminal ileal resection
   c. Regional enteritis (Crohn's disease)
4. Parasitic
   a. Fish tapeworm infestation

---

there is dissociation between the slow maturation of the nucleus and the faster maturation of the cytoplasm.

Megaloblastic anemias are a consequence of disordered deoxyribonucleic acid (DNA) synthesis. However, other cells, particularly those with a rapid turnover, are also affected by this process; the cells of the gastrointestinal tract and white blood cells are examples.

There are many causes of megaloblastic anemia, but the defect is fundamentally a lack of folic acid or cobalamin (cyanocobalamin; vitamin B_{12}) or sometimes both.

Folate and cobalamin metabolism. Dietary folates (pterylglutamates) are found in considerable quantities in green vegetables, yeasts, and liver. Adults require a minimum of 50 μg/day. Folates are absorbed mainly in the jejunum and are transported bound to plasma protein to their sites of utilization. Only small amounts are stored in the liver, so that deficiencies can develop rapidly over a few weeks. Small amounts are excreted in the bile and the urine.

Cobalamin is present in meat, milk, and eggs. In the stomach cobalamin is released from its dietary source and combines initially with *R protein* present in the gastric secretion. The cobalamin is detached from this binder protein in the duodenum by pancreatic proteases, after which it is free to combine with *intrinsic factor* (IF). In this form it is conveyed to the terminal ileum, where in the presence of divalent cations, the cobalamin-IF complex attaches to the mucosal cell surface. Following dissociation, cobalamin is taken into the mucosal cell, from where it enters the bloodstream and is transported, bound to a plasma protein (transcobalamin II), to its sites of utilization. Up to 3 mg of cobalamin are normally stored in the adult liver. Small amounts of cobalamin are lost via the bile and the urine. The normal daily requirement to replace this loss is about 1 μg/day. Both folic acid and cobalamin are essential for normal DNA synthesis (Fig. 13-5).

Folic acid deficiency. Folic acid deficiency is a common cause of anemia and the most common cause of megaloblastic anemia. Conditions that lead to folate deficiency are listed in the box above. Leafy vegetables (folium literally means "a leaf") are an important source of folates but dietary deficiency is not a common cause of this form of megaloblastic anemia. The main causes are (1) pregnancy, (2) alcoholism, (3) folate-inhibiting drugs, and (4) intestinal malabsorption.

Pathogenesis. Since the body stores very little folic acid, the effects of deficiency can develop rapidly. As previously mentioned, cell nuclei throughout the body can be affected. In the peripheral blood, large oval macrocytes appear; that is, their MCV is increased. Enlarged neutrophil polymorphonu-

clear leukocytes (also known as macropolycytes) are seen. These cells characteristically have hypersegmented nuclei (Fig. 13-6), which reflects abnormal DNA synthesis. This morphologic finding can often be seen while the serum folate levels are still normal. Nuclear hypersegmentation is therefore an early indication of folate deficiency. The marrow is hypercellular. Most striking are the megaloblasts and giant metamyelocytes, precursors of the macrocytes and macropolycytes already described. Amounts of iron are usually increased, since iron is not being used. There may, however, be coexisting iron deficiency in some cases.

Clinical aspects. The symptoms are those of anemia in general. A painful, smooth red tongue, is a common oral manifestation, but aphthous stomatitis can be a troublesome complication (Fig. 13-7). The diagnosis rests on the morphology of the peripheral blood and marrow and estimation of the serum folate levels, which fall below the lower limit of normal of 7 ng/mL.

Folic acid deficiency is managed by treating the underlying cause and administering folic acid.

Cobalamin (vitamin B_{12}) deficiency. There are many causes of cobalamin deficiency, which leads to megaloblastic anemia (see the box above). When deficiency is the result of lack of IF due to autoimmune gastric atrophy, the term *pernicious anemia* is often used. This term derives from the severe degenerative disease of the spinal cord that can complicate this form of anemia. Pernicious anemia was first described in 1855 by Thomas Addison* of Guy's Hospital, London.

Pathogenesis. The main cause of cobalamin deficiency is gastric atrophy (Chapter 14), which results in a lack of IF secretion. Without IF, dietary cobalamin cannot be absorbed in the distal ileum. Autoantibodies to parietal cells and to IF are major abnormalities found in this disease.

Surgical removal of major portions of the stomach also leads to cobalamin deficiency, as does resection of the terminal ileum. Since dietary deficiency of cobalamin is rare and the normal liver has large stores, the onset of megaloblastic anemia following gastric or lower ileal resection may be delayed for 2 or more years.

The hematologic changes are very similar to those found in folic acid deficiency.

Clinical aspects. The combination of megaloblastic anemia and gastric atrophy is characteristic of pernicious anemia.

---

*Addisonian anemia must not be confused with Addison's disease (hypoadrenalism) described by the same physician (Chapter 18), but both diseases can be present in the same patient.

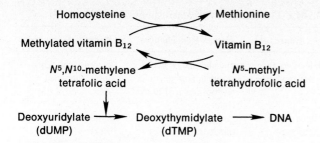

Homocysteine → Methionine
Methylated vitamin B_{12} ⇄ Vitamin B_{12}
N^5,N^{10}-methylene tetrafolic acid ⇄ N^5-methyl-tetrahydrofolic acid
Deoxyuridylate (dUMP) → Deoxythymidylate (dTMP) → DNA

FIG. 13-5. Role of folic acid and vitamin B_{12} in DNA synthesis. N^5, N^{10}-methylene tetrafolic acid is a cofactor required for conversion of dUMP to dTMP.

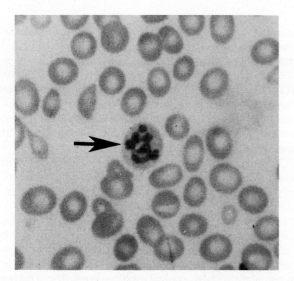

FIG. 13-6. Peripheral blood smear in megaloblastic anemia. The red blood cells are enlarged and oval. The polymorphonuclear leukocyte is also larger than normal, and there is excessive segmentation of the nucleus (macropolycyte) *(arrow)*. This hematologic picture can be seen in either folic acid or vitamin B_{12} deficiency.

Along with general symptoms of anemia, glossitis and complaints of a burning sensation in the tongue are common. Usually the tongue is smooth and shiny, but occasionally small shallow ulcers can be seen. In severe cases the skin can take on a lemon-yellow tint. One major difference from folate deficiency is that neurologic abnormalities commonly develop in untreated persons. These abnormalities are due to demyelination of the posterior and lateral columns of the spinal cord (subacute combined degeneration) and peripheral neuropathy. The effects of spinal cord degeneration may be made worse by giving folic acid.

The diagnosis of pernicious anemia is based on the findings of a megaloblastic anemia and levels of cobalamin below 100 pg/L together with evidence of autoimmune gastric atrophy. Distinction can be made between those causes of megaloblastic anemia of gastric origin and other causes by means of the *Schilling test.*

This test measures the urinary excretion of radioactive cobalamin (^{57}Co) after oral administration. Normally 7% or more of the oral dose of cobalamin is excreted in 24 hours. If urinary excretion is less than 7%, IF is given orally with another oral dose of radioactive cobalamin, and the urinary excretion of

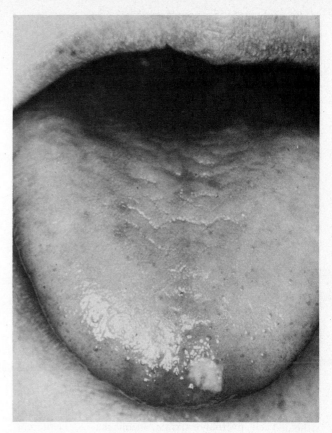

FIG. 13-7. Folic acid deficiency. This patient had megaloblastic anemia due to folic deficiency secondary to prolonged treatment with phenytoin. The main complaint in this case was recurrent oral and genital ulceration (Behçet's syndrome), which responded dramatically when folic acid was given.

^{57}Co is repeated. If the result of this second stage of the test is normal, the defect lies in the stomach; if it is abnormal, the cause is usually in the ileum.

Parenteral administration of cobalamin rapidly corrects the hematologic abnormalities. The first evidence of a good response is *reticulocytosis,* which is soon followed by a rise in hemoglobin level and restoration of normal morphology. The abnormalities in the nervous system may be irreversible. When the anemia is due to other causes, such as blind loop syndrome or fish tapeworm infestation, appropriate treatment of these causes is obviously required.

Hemolytic anemias

Hemolytic anemias result from a reduction in the life span of red blood cells from a normal of about 120 days. Thus the mechanism is one of accelerated red blood cell destruction. In hemolytic anemias, red blood cell destruction takes place in the macrophage-monocyte system and, to a lesser extent, within blood vessels. Worldwide the most common cause of hemolytic anemia is malaria.

Evidence for hemolysis

Many stigmata resulting from the increased destruction of red blood cells are described, but their absence does not necessarily exclude hemolysis. Indeed, because of the enormous

---

MAIN CAUSES OF HEMOLYTIC ANEMIA

A. Inherited disorders of red blood cells
   1. Abnormalities of the red blood cell membrane
      a. Hereditary spherocytosis
      b. Hereditary elliptocytosis
   2. Abnormalities of red blood cell enzymes
      a. Glucose-6-phosphate dehydrogenase deficiency
      b. Pyruvic kinase deficiency
   3. Abnormalities of hemoglobin synthesis
      a. Hemoglobinopathies, including sickle cell disease, HbC disease
      b. Thalassemias: α-, β-, other forms
      c. Combined hemoglobinopathies and thalassemia
      d. Unstable hemoglobins
B. Acquired disorders of red blood cells
   1. Antibody-induced hemolysis
      a. Alloantibodies (e.g., isoimmune disease)
      b. Drug-induced antibodies
      c. Autoimmune hemolytic anemia
   2. Infective causes (e.g., malaria, viral infections)
   3. Mechanical causes (e.g., cardiovascular prosthesis)
   4. Renal disease
   5. Paroxysmal nocturnal hemoglobinuria

TABLE 13-3. Summary of other causes of anemia

Cause	Hematologic changes	Probable mechanisms
Infections and inflammation	Normochromic or hypochromic; normocytic or microcytic (mild to moderate)	Defective iron utilization, shortened red blood cell survival
Chronic renal disease	Normochromic, normocytic (moderate to severe)	Shortened red blood cell survival; defective erythropoietin production
Chronic alcoholism	Macrocytic (moderate to severe)	Folate deficiency; hemolysis

reserve capacity of the marrow to increase its production of red blood cells fivefold or sixfold, anemia may not be present, even though excessive hemolysis is taking place.

Hemolysis may be indicated by the following:

1. Increased hemoglobin breakdown, leading to increased unconjugated serum bilirubin, urinary urobilinogen, and sometimes jaundice
2. Damaged red blood cells, which often become spherocytic or fragmented
3. Marrow response to increased breakdown of cells, which results in erythroid hyperplasia, sometimes sufficient to expand the surrounding bone
4. Appearance of increased numbers of young red blood cells (reticulocytes or normoblasts) in the peripheral blood

Hemolysis may also result in the presence of hemoglobin in the plasma. Here hemoglobin binds to haptoglobin (an α_2-globulin) until the binding sites are saturated. Saturation is followed by the appearance of hemoglobin in the urine. The presence of hemosiderin in the urine also indicates hemolytic disease. The final arbiter of abnormal hemolysis, however, is the demonstration of a shortened red blood cell life span by methods that determine the rate of decay of red blood cells coated with radiochromium.

There are many causes of hemolytic anemia, both hereditary and acquired. Most are listed in the box above. The more common and important causes will be considered in detail; the salient features of others are discussed briefly or summarized in Table 13-3.

Hereditary hemolytic anemias

Defects of red blood cell membrane. Of the eight or more abnormalities of the red blood cell membrane, *hereditary spherocytosis* is the most common, especially in northern European populations and their descendants.

The underlying defect appears to be in the skeleton of the eythrocyte membrane. Abnormalities of spectrin, a major component of the inner layer of the red blood cell membrane, have been described (Chapter 2). The red blood cells are small, spherical, and more fragile than normal. The survival time can be as short as 5 to 10 days. Destruction of the abnormally shaped cells takes place in the spleen, which enlarges as a result. The marrow responds by erythroid hyperplasia. In many patients the excessive hemolysis leads to formation of bile pigment gallstones.

Clinically, the effects of hereditary spherocytosis vary greatly. The patient may have no symptoms, but more often the symptoms of mild chronic anemia are present. Sometimes acute aplastic crises develop, with falling numbers of all blood cells and marrow hypoplasia. The main treatment is splenectomy, which essentially cures the effects of the disease without affecting the underlying red blood cell abnormality.

Hereditary elliptocytosis and *stomatocytosis* (Table 13-2) have similar effects to hereditary spherocytosis. The underlying causes appear to be abnormalities of proteins in the red blood cell membrane.

Glucose-6-phosphate dehydrogenase deficiency. Inherited deficiencies of many red blood cell enzymes involved in the glycolytic pathway, the pentose monophosphate shunt, and nucleotide synthesis have been described. Of these, the most common is glucose-6-phosphate dehydrogenase (G6PD) deficiency.

Oxidation of G6PD is the initial step in the red cell pentose monophosphate shunt, whose main function is to generate reduced nicotinamide adenine dinucleotidyl phosphate (NADPH) and pentoses:

$$\text{Glucose-6-phosphate} + \text{NADP} \xrightarrow{\text{G6PD}} \text{6-phosphogluconate} + \text{NADPH} + \text{H}^+$$

NADPH protects the red blood cell against injury by oxidants; for example, by antimalarial drugs such as primaquine. Scores of variants of G6PD have been described, but most of these function normally. For example, the so-called A+ variant, which is found in 20% of blacks, functions normally, whereas the A− variant (which affects about 15% of black American males) is a functionally abnormal gene.

G6PD deficiency is inherited as an X-linked characteristic. Generally, males are affected and females are asymptomatic carriers. In the presence of oxidant drugs, such as the antimalarials primaquine and quinine, the antimicrobials nitrofurantoin and sulfonamides, and the analgesics aspirin and phenacetin, hemolysis may develop. Hemolysis may also be precipitated by acute infections.

When hemolysis is due to the ingestion of the *Vicia fava* bean, the condition is called *favism*. Although G6PD deficiency is present in these cases, the disease is believed to be due to another, although unknown, genetic abnormality.

Clinically, patients with G6PD deficiency rapidly develop falling hemoglobin and hematocrit values during an acute infective illness or on exposure to an oxidant drug. There is no specific treatment and it is rarely necessary to give blood to correct the anemia. The main aim is to prevent the patient from again receiving oxidant drugs.

Disorders of hemoglobin

The function of hemoglobin is to transport oxygen from the lungs for release in the tissues. The hemoglobin molecule consists of the protein globin, which forms 97% of the molecule, and four iron-containing heme groups. Normal globin is composed of two identical α-chains, each containing 141 amino acids; the other pair of chains consists of 146 amino acids. Depending on the stage of life, several different (non-α-) chains are paired with the α-chains, although the configuration of the non-α-chains is very similar. The composition of "normal" hemoglobins is shown in Table 13-4.

Normal hemoglobins. In adults most hemoglobin is in the form of hemoglobin A (Hb A: $\alpha_2\beta_2$). About 2% of normal hemoglobin is in the form of Hb A_2 ($\alpha_2\delta_2$). In the fetus a different hemoglobin, Hb F (fetal Hb: $\alpha_2\gamma_2$), which normally disappears in early infancy, is found. Three minor components of Hb A (Hb A_{1a}, Hb A_{1b}, Hb A_{1c}), especially Hb A_{1c}, are important in the management of patients with diabetes mellitus. They are called *glycosylated hemoglobins* because they are attached to a carbohydrate moiety. Their significance is discussed in Chapter 18.

Two other hemoglobins, Hb Gower 1 ($\zeta_2\epsilon_2$) and Hb Portland ($\zeta_2\gamma_2$), are present in small quantities in very early embryonic life, in addition to Hb Gower 2 ($\alpha_2\zeta_2$) (Table 13-4).

Individual globin chains are under genetic control. The α-chain genes are on chromosome 16 and consist of four genes (two pairs of allelic genes) that normally produce two identical α-chains. The β- and δ-chains are each controlled by one pair of genes on chromosome 11. Each pair is responsible for the production of a slightly different γ-chain. In one γ-chain ($^G\gamma$) glycine is present at position 136; in the other ($^A\gamma$) it is replaced by alanine.

Hemoglobin variants. Scores of inherited variants of the molecular structure of hemoglobin have been described. These affect the globin fraction of the molecule and usually consist of the substitution of one amino acid in the polypeptide chains for another. In many cases, the resultant hemoglobin, despite its abnormal composition, is functionally as capable of transporting oxygen as Hb A. In some, however, the abnormal hemoglobin makes the red blood cells more fragile. The pathologic effects can be serious because of the excessive destruction of red blood cells.

In some instances the abnormal amino acid sequences interfere with the affinity of the hemoglobin molecule for oxygen, because they affect the binding of heme iron to the globin chain. Such abnormalities are associated with cyanosis due to the formation of methemoglobin and are called the *M hemoglobins*.

The rate and quantity of globin chain synthesis are genetically controlled, as is the switch of production of one chain to another during embryonic and fetal life. When the rate and quantity of globin production are abnormal, the disorders known as *thalassemias* result.

TABLE 13-4. The physiologic ("normal") hemoglobins

Stage of development	Hemoglobin	Globin chains
Embryo	Gower 1	$\zeta_2\epsilon_2$
	Gower 2	$\alpha_2\epsilon_2$
	Portland 1	$\zeta_2\gamma_2$
Fetus	Hb F	$\alpha_2\gamma_2$
Adult	Hb A	$\alpha_2\beta_2$
	Hb A_2	$\alpha_2\delta_2$

Another group of abnormal hemoglobins is due to an amino acid substitution affecting the region of heme attachment, leading to irreversible oxidation of the molecule and the formation of Heinz* bodies in the red blood cells. This is seen with *unstable hemoglobins* such as Hb Seattle. Thus the main abnormalities of globin synthesis are due to amino acid substitutions, leading to hemolysis from (1) tactoid or crystal formation, as in Hb S, (2) abnormal oxygen affinity and methemoglobin formation, as in Hb M, (3) the abnormal rate of production of normal globin chains, as in the thalassemias, and (4) unstable hemoglobin formation.

Sickle cell diseases

Hereditary disorders in which Hb S replaces Hb A are called sickle cell diseases. Hb S is a hemoglobin in which, at position 6 in the β-chain of the globin molecule, glutamic acid is substituted for valine. This seemingly minor change in the amino acid sequence of globin has profound effects on the properties of hemoglobin. Although Hb S transports oxygen efficiently, it is much less soluble than Hb A, especially when oxygen tension is lowered. Under these conditions, Hb S tends to form long, slender masses (tactoids). Tactoids appear to be the result of molecular polymerization and realignment into a multistranded helical fiber. This molecular rearrangement distorts red blood cells into sickle-shaped forms, which can be demonstrated in vitro and in vivo.

In vitro sickling is produced by treating blood containing Hb S with a reducing agent such as sodium metabisulfite (Fig. 13-8). In vivo sickling is responsible for the chemical and pathologic effects in the disease.

Hb S can also be detected, as can other hemoglobin variants, by electrophoretic mobility. Electrophoresis is a standard method for investigating abnormal hemoglobins, which, under the influence of an electric current and different supporting media and pH, migrate at different rates (Fig. 13-9).

There are two major sickling syndromes:

1. Homozygous: *Sickle cell anemia*
2. Heterozygous: *Sickle cell trait*

The sickling syndromes are found most commonly in black populations that originated in the tropical regions of Africa. Nearly 10% of black Americans carry the Hb S gene and about 0.2% are homozygotes; that is, have sickle cell anemia.

Sickle cell anemia. This disease is the result of inheritance of homozygous Hb S. In affected individuals Hb S forms about 80% to 100% of their total hemoglobin, and any conditions of

---

*R. Heinz (1865-1924), German pathologist. Heinz bodies are highly refractile particles of denatured hemoglobin.

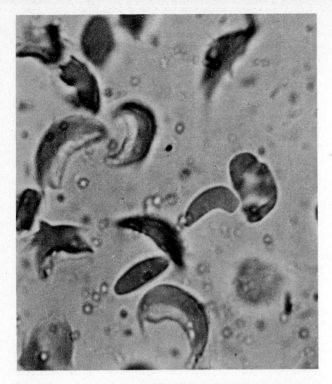

FIG. 13-8. The sickling phenomenon. Red blood cells from a patient with homozygous Hb S disease have been mixed with reducing agents, which cause the cells to become elongated and pointed or shaped like a holly leaf.

reduced intravascular oxygen tension can cause the sickling phenomenon in vivo.

Pathogenesis. The immediate results of sickling are hemolytic anemia and capillary obstruction due to microthrombi formation. Both these processes tend to worsen the hypoxia, with further sickling and red blood cell destruction. Damaged red blood cells are trapped in the spleen and contribute to its enlargement, which starts in infancy. Infarction of the spleen may become so complete that it is eventually replaced by an atrophic fibrous mass. This has been called *autosplenectomy* and is usually seen in children. The lack of a functioning spleen results in greatly increased susceptibility to certain infections such as those caused by *Streptococcus pneumoniae.* Vascular obstruction can affect almost any site in the body, including the lungs and the central nervous system with appropriately severe consequences.

Hematologic findings. In summary, these are:

1. Moderate to severe anemia, which is of the normocytic, normochromic type, unless another abnormality such as iron deficiency complicates the disease.
2. Wide variations in size and shape of red blood cells, some of which may appear sickle shaped in a stained blood smear.
3. Reticulocytosis.
4. Neutrophil polymorphonuclear leukocytosis, a common occurrence.
5. Erythroid hyperplasia in the marrow.
6. Positive sickling test.

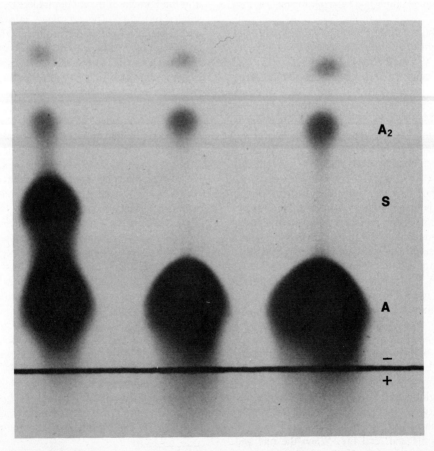

FIG. 13-9. Hemoglobin electrophoresis in sickle cell disease. The migration of Hb S is compared with that of hemoglobin A *(A).* A$_2$ is the normal minor hemoglobin A$_2$.

7. Characteristic hemoglobin electrophoretic pattern. The amount of Hb S can vary considerably as previously mentioned. When it is less than 100%, the balance is made up by fetal hemoglobin (Hb F).

Clinical aspects. The severity of symptoms is variable. In those individuals in whom the amount of fetal hemoglobin is high (20% to 30%) the disease may be very mild. This is seen, for example, in sickle cell disease affecting Mediterranean races. In the most severe forms, symptoms can begin in the first year of life; most commonly they are due to anemia. Slight jaundice reflecting the hemolytic process may be present.

During the course of the disease, starting as early as the first year of life, there are crises marked by fever and severe bone, joint, and abdominal pain due to infarctions. These may mimic a variety of other illnesses. Patients, especially children, with sickle cell anemia are susceptible to certain infections, including pneumococcal disease, salmonella osteomyelitis, and bacterial meningitis.

Expansion of the medullary cavity of bones, reflecting the increased erythroid hyperplasia of the marrow, can be seen on radiographs. The outlook for patients with sickle cell anemia is best when they have coexisting thalassemia or genes for high fetal hemoglobin. In severe forms of sickle cell anemia, death is common in the first year of life.

Pregnancy in a woman with sickle cell disease presents serious risks both to the fetus and to the woman. Fetal death, spontaneous abortion, and neonatal death are all common hazards; cardiac failure, cerebral thrombosis, and pulmonary embolus are the main maternal complications.

Patients with sickle cell anemia should not be given a general anesthetic unless there is no alternative, because of the risk of severe hemolysis and multiple infarctions. If general anesthesia is unavoidable, every effort must be made to avoid hypoxia. Even then there is a risk of hemolysis and infarction. Those with sickle cell trait (described in the following section) are also liable to develop hemolysis if they become hypoxic.

Sickle cell trait. The heterozygous carriers of the S gene are asymptomatic as a rule, except in unusual circumstances in which they are exposed to low oxygen tension, such as may happen during anesthesia. Hb S forms about 25% to 40% of their total hemoglobin; the remainder is mainly Hb A. The marriage of two heterozygotes (AS × AS) means that there is a 1 in 4 chance of a homozygous offspring.

Other abnormal hemoglobins. Among the several hundred abnormal hemoglobins described, some are associated with disease. These include (1) homozygous forms such as Hb C disease (CC), (2) forms in which the patient inherits a sickle cell gene from one parent and an abnormal hemoglobin gene (Hb C, for example) from the other, resulting in Hb SC disease, and (3) combinations of abnormal hemoglobins and thalassemia, for example, sickle cell thalassemia.

Hemoglobin C. Hb C ($\alpha_2\beta_2^{6\ Glu\rightarrow Lys}$) is seen in blacks and a homozygous form is associated with chronic hemolytic anemia and splenomegaly. Hb C$_{Harlem}$ has a similar β-chain abnormality to Hb C but has an additional amino acid substitution. This hemoglobin, when present with Hb S in a double heterozygote (Hb SC$_{Harlem}$), produces a clinical picture that is identical to that of homozygous Hb S disease. A similar effect is seen in persons who are doubly heterozygous for Hb O$_{Arab}$ ($\alpha_2\beta_2^{121\ Glu\rightarrow Lys}$) and Hb S.

Hemoglobin E. Hb E ($\alpha_2\beta_2^{26\ Glu\rightarrow Lys}$) is a hemoglobin variant that is benign in the homozygous form or when heterozygous with Hb A. However, heterozygous Hb E associated with some forms of thalassemia (Hb E/β^0-thal or Hb E/δ-β-thal) is accompanied by severe anemia.

M hemoglobins. This group of hemoglobins, of which Hb M$_{Saskatoon}$ is an example, have amino acid substitutions that affect the attachment of globin to heme and consequently the ability to keep iron in a reduced state. The subsequent methemoglobinemia makes the patient appear cyanotic. Recognition of this condition in infants is important to prevent unnecessary investigation of presumed congenital heart disease.

Thalassemia

Thalassemia (literally "sea in blood") is an inherited disorder of hemoglobin synthesis. The rate and quantity of globin chain production are under genetic control. Normally when Hb F synthesis stops shortly after birth, production of α-chains is balanced by β-chains to form Hb A and by a small amount of δ-chains to form Hb A$_2$ ($\alpha_2\beta_2$). The ratio of α- to δ-chain production is normally controlled at 40:1. The defect in thalassemia, that is, the presence of the thal gene, results in a variety of quantitative disorders of globin chain production that can affect any of the four normal globin chains (α, β, γ, and δ).

The genetic defects in thalassemia cause a complete or partial failure of production of the messenger ribonucleic acid (mRNA) involved in globin chain synthesis. Because any of the chains can be affected, α-, β-, γ- and δ-thalassemias are found, and thalassemia affecting both δ- and β-chains in one individual has also been described. γ- and δ-thalassemias are of little clinical importance.

α-Thalassemia. As previously discussed, α-chain production is regulated by four genes, two of which are inherited from each parent. One or more of these genes may be abnormal, and each set of abnormalities has different clinical implications, ranging from the asymptomatic carrier to fetal death (Table 13-5). In the more severe forms of α-thalassemia, since there is a major deficiency of α-chains, β- and γ-chains form tetramers with themselves ($\beta_2 + \beta_2$; $\gamma_2 + \gamma_2$), giving rise to Hb H (β_4) and hemoglobin Bart's (γ_4).

A clinically important form of α-thalassemia is Hb H disease, in which three of the four α-chain genes are abnormal. Hb H is an unstable molecule, and the disease is characterized by severe hemolytic anemia and the presence of inclusion bodies consisting of Hb H in about 0.2% of red blood cells.

β-Thalassemia. β-Thalassemia can be inherited as a homozygous or heterozygous disorder. Some cases have been described in most parts of the world, but it is particularly common in the Mediterranean littoral, especially among Italians and Greeks. Although only two genes for β-thalassemia exist, many different types of gene have been described; as a result, there are about 250 forms of β-thalassemia. Three important examples are considered here:

1. β^0-Thalassemia, in which β-chain synthesis is completely suppressed
2. β^+-Thalassemia, in which β-chain synthesis is greatly reduced; this type is characteristically seen in Mediterranean populations (here abbreviated β^+_{Med})
3. β^+-Thalassemia, in which there is a less severe reduction of β-chain synthesis; this type is found in black Americans (here abbreviated β^+_{Am})

TABLE 13-5. α-Thalassemia

Number of normal α -genes	Number of abnormal α -genes or gene deletions	Genotype	Disease	Hemoglobin
4	0	Normal	None	Hb A and A$_2$
3	1	α$^+$-Thal Heterozygote	None (carrier)	1%-2% Hb Bart's
2	2 (on same chain)	α^0-Thal Heterozygote	α-Thal minor	3%-10% Hb Bart's
2	2 (1 on each chain)	α^0-Thal Homozygote	α-Thal minor	3%-10% Hb Bart's
1	3 (2 on one chain, 1 on other)	α^0-Thal/α$^+$-Thal	Hb H disease	20%-30% Hb Bart's
0	4	α^0-Thal Homozygote	α-Thal major*	>80% Hb Bart's

*Associated with hydrops fetalis.

Each of these types can be homozygous or heterozygous. The homozygous forms, β^{0}β^0 and β$^+$$_{Med}$β$^+$$_{Med}$, have the most serious clinical effects and are referred to as *thalassemia major.* Heterozygous forms ββ^0, ββ$^+$$_{Med}$, and ββ$^+$$_{Am}$ have much milder clinical effects and are referred to as *thalassemia minor.* Homozygous β$^+$$_{Am}$β$^+$$_{Am}$ has moderately severe clinical effects and is called *thalassemia intermedia.*

Pathology. The pathologic changes in a person with thalassemia are caused by hemolysis, and the changes are most severe in thalassemia major. In a typical case, the following changes develop insidiously during the first or second year of life:

1. Splenomegaly
2. Mild jaundice
3. Skeletal changes due to erythroid hyperplasia in the marrow, particularly in the skull (Fig. 13-10) and in the malar bones, where expansion results in a mongoloid appearance
4. Pigment gallstones
5. Progressive anemia

Hematologic findings. Anemia occurs in thalassemia, and sometimes the hemoglobin level may fall to 3 g/dL. The red blood cells are microcytic and hypochromic and many have a target-like appearance. Normoblasts are plentiful in the peripheral blood. Reticulocytosis and polymorphonuclear leukocytosis are common.

The marrow, in response to increased demand, is intensely hyperplastic with a predominance of normoblasts that tend to be smaller than normal (micronormoblasts). Since hemoglobin synthesis is defective, iron is commonly present in increased amounts, especially if futile attempts have been made to correct the anemia by giving iron.

In thalassemia major, the amounts of fetal hemoglobin (Hb F) are greatly increased (up to 98%), with Hb A$_2$ levels as high as 10%. In thalassemia minor, Hb F forms up to 5% and Hb A$_2$ up to 8% of the total hemoglobin, the remainder being Hb A. In thalassemia intermedia, Hb F forms up to 40% and Hb A$_2$ up to 5% of total hemoglobin.

Clinical aspects. Depending on the severity, children with thalassemia may die in early childhood or survive into adult life. Death can be caused by intercurrent infection, the effects of severe anemia, or excessive iron or blood transfusion therapy, which deposits large amounts of iron in the heart and causes cardiac failure. The careful use of blood transfusions and the administration of folic acid are the only worthwhile treatments, but these are only palliative.

δ-β-*Thalassemia.* δ-β-Thalassemia results from the impaired synthesis of both δ- and β-chains. The disorder can be homozygous or heterozygous. Clinically, the homozygous form behaves like thalassemia intermedia, since normal γ-chain synthesis allows high levels of Hb F to be formed. The heterozygotes behave clinically like thalassemia minor.

Only the main examples of thalassemia involving β-chain abnormalities have been described here. These abnormalities are also associated with abnormal hemoglobins, such as Hb C/thal or Hb D/thal. The affected individuals are often asymptomatic and require no treatment.

Acquired hemolytic anemias

The acquired hemolytic anemias almost exclusively are due to extraerythrocytic causes, unlike the inherited abnormalities in which the defects are present in the red blood cell itself. There are many causes of acquired hemolytic anemia (p. 276); only a few will be discussed here.

Malaria. Malaria is one of the most common causes of anemia in the world. After many years of successful control, the disease is now epidemic in many countries from which it had almost disappeared 25 years ago. The malarial parasite causes hemolytic anemia by two processes. First, it enters the red blood cell and, on completion of the erythrocytic phase of its cycle, causes lysis of the cell.

In *falciparum malaria,* the number of parasitized cells can be so great that red blood cell destruction can lead to profound anemia within a few days. Second, probably as a result of stimulation by malarial antigens, macrophage activity greatly increases, especially in the spleen. One of the effects of this, which further enhances the anemia, is the destruction of nonparasitized red blood cells.

Antibody-mediated hemolytic anemia. Antibodies that cause in vivo hemolysis are of three main types:

1. Antibodies that cause hemolytic transfusion reactions to incompatible transfused blood and rhesus incompatibility

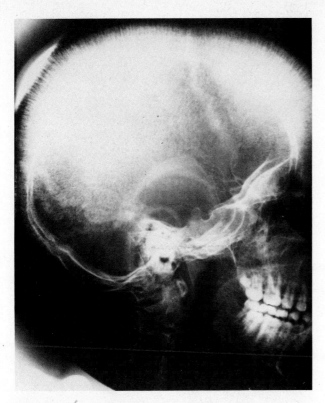

FIG. 13-10. Radiograph of the skull in β-thalassemia. The intense hemopoietic activity in the marrow of the skull causes the diploë to expand and perpendicular bony trabeculae to form. These give a characteristic hair-on-end appearance to the skull.

between mother and fetus. The latter condition is known as *isoimmune disease of the newborn* or *erythroblastosis fetalis.*

2. Autoantibodies that are formed during a variety of diseases, such as viral infections, malignant diseases, and collagen-vascular diseases.
3. Drug-induced antibodies.

Isoimmune disease of the newborn. This condition results from blood group incompatibility between mother and fetus. Fetal red blood cells can enter the maternal circulation during delivery, and, if mother and fetus have different blood groups, stimulate maternal antibodies. In subsequent pregnancies, maternal antibodies can cross the placenta and react with fetal red blood cell antigens, causing hemolysis and varying degrees of damage to the fetus.

The most common fetomaternal incompatibilities involve antigens and antibodies of the ABO blood group system. In the United States, ABO incompatibilities are usually of little clinical consequence, but this is apparently not the case in Central Africa, where ABO incompatibilities are an important cause of erythroblastosis fetalis. In western countries, Rh system incompatibilities tend to be more serious. Severe effects on the fetus are not usually seen until the second or, more commonly, the third pregnancy, when high concentrations of antibody have built up in the maternal circulation.

Pathology. The pathologic effects are due to hemolysis. In the most extreme cases, the fetus is stillborn and grossly edematous due to circulatory failure. This condition is known as *hydrops fetalis.* In infants who survive birth, hemolysis may

be of varying degrees of severity. Jaundice may be obvious at birth or may develop shortly after. The danger from high bilirubin levels, especially in excess of 20 mg/dL is that *kernicterus* may develop. This is yellow staining of the basal ganglia, cerebral cortex, and other parts of the nervous system by bilirubin. Kernicterus causes destruction of neural tissue in areas where high bilirubin levels are allowed to persist, leading to mental defects.

The peripheral blood and bone marrow respond to the hemolysis by producing many normoblasts (erythroblasts); hence the term *erythroblastosis.*

Vital to the diagnosis, treatment, and prevention of isoimmune disease are the direct and indirect antiglobulin or Coombs' tests.* The *direct test* detects maternal antibodies on the surface of the infant's red blood cells. It is performed on cord blood and is essential for the diagnosis of isoimmune disease. The *indirect test* detects maternal antibodies to the infant's red blood cells in maternal serum and is the method by which later isoimmune disease of the infant may be predicted during pregnancy.

Clinical aspects. Entry of incompatible fetal red blood cells into the maternal circulation takes place during delivery. The number of red blood cells is very small, and timely administration of specific anti-D immunoglobulin can eliminate the foreign cells and prevent Rh sensitization.

When isoimmune disease develops, the usual management is to exchange the infant's blood for transfused blood. The most important reason for exchange transfusion is the prevention of kernicterus.

Autoimmune hemolytic anemias

During the course of several diseases, the patient may develop antibodies against his or her own red blood cells. Such antibodies are produced in certain infections (e.g., mycoplasmal pneumonia), connective tissue diseases, and malignancies, particularly the lymphoproliferative type. Sometimes these antibodies act at body temperature *(warm antibodies)* or less commonly when the patient is exposed to cold. In the latter condition, the resulting hemolytic activity of *cold antibodies* may be severe enough to cause hemoglobin to appear in the urine. This condition is known as *paroxysmal cold hemoglobinuria.* Formerly associated with syphilis, it is now usually seen as a rare complication of viral infections.

The responsible antibody is directed against the P blood group antigen and is known as the *Donath-Landsteiner* antibody.†

The hemolytic anemias associated with lymphoproliferative disorders often present special problems of management. The antibodies responsible for hemolysis very frequently have blood group specificity, particularly for the Rh system. For this reason, when these patients require blood transfusion, it may be very difficult or even impossible to obtain compatible blood.

Drug-induced hemolytic anemia

Many drugs have been implicated as causes of hemolytic anemia. Commonly prescribed examples include quinidine, cephalosporins, penicillins (rarely), and particularly methyl-

---

*R.R.A. Coombs, contemporary English immunologist.
†J. Donath (1870-1950), German physician; K. Landsteiner (1868-1943), German physician.

dopa. Mechanisms that are known to cause drug-induced hemolytic anemias include:

1. The drug stimulates production of an antibody with which it forms an immune complex. This complex capriciously attaches to the red blood cell, which becomes the site for complement-mediated hemolysis.
2. Penicillin, for example, adsorbs to the surface of the red blood cell, where it combines with antibody. This renders the cell highly susceptible to phagocytosis and, to a much lesser extent, intravascular hemolysis.
3. Adsorption of the drug, such as cephalosporin, to the surface of the red blood cell alters the cell membrane so that it becomes fragile and more easily lysed.
4. By unknown means methyldopa stimulates an autoantibody, often with Rh specificity, which then attaches to the red blood cell antigen, causing hemolysis.

The direct antiglobulin test is positive in all of these mechanisms.

Paroxysmal nocturnal hemoglobinuria

Paroxysmal nocturnal hemoglobinuria (PNH) is an acquired disorder of red blood cells characterized by intravascular hemolysis that increases during sleep.

The cause of the abnormality is not known, but it renders the red blood cells more liable to complement-mediated hemolysis. However, populations of red blood cells with different susceptibilities to complement have been detected in individual patients.

Clinically, patients with PNH are usually between 20 and 30 years of age and have a period of pancytopenia before the onset of hemolysis. The hemolysis is chronic, intravascular, and increased during or immediately after sleep. The disease has periods of remission and relapse and is associated with an increased risk of thrombosis. The effects of chronic hemolysis include anemia and increased susceptibility to infection. A few cases terminate in myeloproliferative diseases, such as leukemia or myelofibrosis.

The diagnosis is usually based on a positive *acid-serum test,* in which the patient's red blood cells undergo 10% to 50% lysis when placed in acidified serum. The presence of hemosiderin in the urine is also a typical finding.

The treatment of PNH is unsatisfactory; corticosteroids have had some success, and transfusion with thawed red blood cells that have been stored frozen has been useful for correction of the anemia.

Aplastic (hypoplastic) anemia and agranulocytosis

Anemia due to failure of the marrow to produce new cells is called *aplastic anemia* (Fig. 13-11). Although this name suggests failure of red blood cell production, all elements of the marrow fail because the basic damage is to the pleuripotential marrow stem cells. The term *pancytopenia* means a diminution in numbers of all cellular elements of the marrow secondary to a variety of causes, including vitamin B$_{12}$ and folate deficiency and myelofibrosis.

When red blood cell production fails alone, a rare condition in both children and adults, the term *red blood cell aplasia* is applied.

Agranulocytosis describes the failure of granulocytic white blood cell production in the marrow. Since agranulocytosis may either be a component of aplastic anemia or a disease in its own right, it is convenient to consider these two conditions

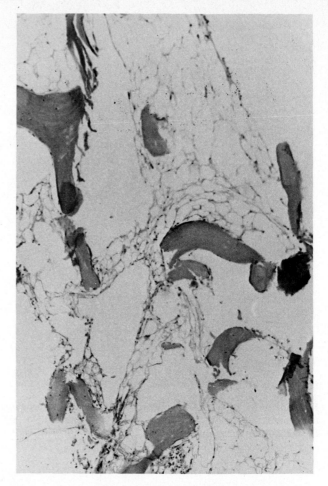

FIG. 13-11. Aplastic anemia. In this needle biopsy specimen of the bone marrow, there is complete absence of hemopoietic tissue. The marrow contains only a few strands of connective tissue and fat.

together, even though anemia is not a feature of pure agranulocytosis. Also, there are great similarities between the causes of the two diseases.

Aplastic anemia

Etiology. The causes of aplastic anemia include:

1. Idiopathic types (i.e., cause unknown)
2. Exposure to ionizing radiation
3. Myelotoxic agents, such as benzene and cytotoxic drugs
4. Numerous drugs
5. Other diseases, such as hepatitis, systemic lupus erythematosus, panhypopituitarism, and PNH

In many cases no acceptable cause can be found for the disease. A distinction can be drawn between the effects on the marrow of cytotoxic drugs, which are deliberately used to destroy neoplastic cells, and other drugs, which are not consistently myelotoxic. As examples of the latter group, chloramphenicol and phenylbutazone can be used without ill effects in most cases, but in a few instances, sudden, unpredictable, and irreversible failure of the marrow may develop. The effects of the cytotoxic drugs are dose related, whereas those due to chloramphenicol and other drugs are usually unrelated to the dose given.

Pathogenesis. The effects of aplastic anemia are due to anemia, neutropenia, and thrombocytopenia. Anemia gives rise to pallor, weakness, and dyspnea. Neutropenia causes fever, ulcerative pharyngitis, and liability to severe bacterial infections.

Thrombocytopenia causes hemorrhage, especially from the gingivae, nose, and skin. Purpura is often an early sign of aplastic anemia.

Clinical aspects. The diagnosis depends on careful assessment of the peripheral blood and bone marrow and the exclusion of other diseases that can produce similar findings, such as myeloproliferative disorders and pernicious anemia. Some patients recover when the drug is stopped. In others the disease is unresponsive to treatment and can be rapidly fatal. In treatment, infection control and blood transfusions are important. Marrow transplantation is used as a means of restoring hemopoietic function when more conservative measures have failed. This procedure has significantly improved survival but only in patients below the age of 30.

Agranulocytosis

Reduction of granulocytic white blood cells *(neutropenia)* is a fairly frequent effect of many drugs and is also associated with several diseases, such as pernicious anemia, malaria, and typhoid fever. Complete cessation of granulocyte production *(agranulocytosis)* is rare and is usually caused by an idiosyncratic reaction to drugs, including analgesics, antiinflammatory agents, some antibiotics (particularly cotrimoxazole), and phenothiazine tranquilizers.

The mechanisms that cause agranulocytosis are poorly understood but may include a direct toxic effect on white blood cell precursors or destruction of granulocytes by antibodies.

In agranulocytosis the white blood cell count falls below 2000 to 3000/μL, and neutrophils are absent from the peripheral blood or marrow smears. The patient develops an acute illness, with fever and oral, pharyngeal, and sometimes perianal ulceration, often during a course of drug treatment. There is a great risk of systemic bacterial infections. Recovery is usual but not invariable when the offending treatment is stopped. Treatment is directed largely at preventing infection while the marrow recovers.

Other causes of anemia

There are many other causes of anemia; some of these are summarized in Table 13-3.

POLYCYTHEMIA

An increase in the number of red blood cells per microliter above the normal upper limit for age and sex is called polycythemia. Strictly speaking, the name applies to all cells in the blood, but it has been reserved for increases in red blood cells only.

Relative polycythemia is due to reduction in the proportion of plasma to red blood cells, as might be seen in dehydration. *Absolute polycythemia* is a compensatory mechanism to a variety of conditions and disorders, particularly those which cause hypoxia, such as living at high altitudes or congenital heart disease. This form of polycythemia may also be due to diseases that stimulate the production of erythropoietin, such as cancer of the kidney or liver. *Erythropoietin* is formed in the kidney; it is a glycoprotein that acts on committed stem cells in the marrow to stimulate the formation of red blood cell precursors.

Polycythemia rubra vera

Polycythemia rubra vera (polycythemia vera) is a rare disease of unknown cause in which there is excessive formation of

TABLE 13-6. The myeloproliferative disorders

Major cell series involved	*Disease*
Myeloid	Chronic myeloid leukemia
Erythroid	Polycythemia rubra vera
Megakaryocyte	Thrombocythemia
Fibroblast	Myelofibrosis

red blood cells, blood platelets, and granulocytes.

Polycythemia vera is considered to be one form of a larger group of diseases characterized by uncontrolled proliferation of bone marrow elements, known as the *myeloproliferative disorders* (Table 13-6). These disorders have much in common; a relentless and eventually fatal outcome and an ability to change from one disease to another are characteristic. For example, it is common for patients with polycythemia vera to have coincident thrombocytosis (a very high platelet count). Some polycythemics develop myeloid leukemia as a terminal event; others develop sclerosis of the marrow with abnormal proliferation of fibroblasts and myeloblasts.

Pathogenesis. Polycythemia vera is currently believed to result from the proliferation of an abnormal clone of primitive stem cells. The effect is a gross overproduction of red blood cells, which is responsible for the pathologic changes that develop during the course of the disease. The principal changes follow:

1. Increase in blood volume, leading to congestion of all organs, especially the liver and spleen
2. Increase in blood viscosity associated with a tendency to thrombosis; as a result, infarcts are found in the kidney, spleen, and heart
3. Bleeding tendency due to several factors, including defective platelet function
4. Increased content of uric acid in the blood because of high turnover of nucleic acids from normoblasts and megakaryocytes in the hyperactive marrow; this may lead to gout in a minority of patients

Hematologic findings. In polycythemia rubra vera the blood is thick and viscous. The hemoglobin level ranges from 18 to 24 g/dL and the red blood cell count is 7 to 9 million/μL or higher. The hematocrit value may be as high as 70%, the white blood cell count is often moderately raised, and in many patients the platelet count may exceed 500,000/μL. Typically the alkaline phosphatase activity of the leukocytes is increased. The bone marrow is hyperplastic and replaces much of the marrow fat. All series of cells in the marrow are hyperplastic, especially normoblasts and megakaryocytes.

Clinical aspects. When fully developed, polycythemia vera causes the patient's complexion to be deep, dusky red. Cyanosis results from failure to oxygenate all of the excessive numbers of erythrocytes. The combination of this plethoric appearance with enlargement of the spleen and the hematologic findings described is characteristic.

Patients are usually over the age of 50; both sexes are affected, males more often than females. The tendencies to thrombosis and hemorrhage may affect the nervous system, the alimentary tract, or other sites and cause a wide range of symptoms. Headaches, visual defects, weakness, and gastrointestinal bleeding are common complaints. Thrombotic manifestations account for about one third of the deaths, hemorrhage for about 15%. Some patients die after developing myeloid leukemia, others from the effects of myelofibrosis.

Depending on the severity of the disease, it is treated by either the administration of radiophosphorus, by venesection, or by a combination of both methods. Some patients have been treated successfully with alkylating agents such as busulfan; the long-term effects, however, are not known. Since the introduction of radiophosphorus and the judicious use of venesection, the expectation of life in polycythemia vera has increased so that many patients survive more than 10 years from the time of diagnosis. However, more patients survive only long enough to succumb to the effects of myelofibrosis or leukemia.

DISORDERS OF WHITE BLOOD CELLS

The main function of white blood cells is defense, particularly against microorganisms and foreign substances. Another group of white blood cells, the platelets, protects against hemorrhage. The white blood cell functions are described in Chapters 5 and 7, and commonly accepted reference values for white blood cells are given in Table 13-1.

Increases or decreases in the number of circulating white blood cells accompany many diseases. The most common cause of *leukocytosis* (increased number of white blood cells above 10,000/μL of blood) is infection, especially, although not exclusively, that caused by pyogenic bacteria, to which the main response is an increase in segmented neutrophils. Parasite infestations, particularly the larval stages of various worms, frequently result in increased numbers of circulating eosinophils *(eosinophilia)*. Viral infections cause variable responses in white blood cells, depending on the nature of the virus and the stage of the illness. Segmented neutrophils frequently increase slightly but temporarily in many viral infections. Increasing numbers of lymphocytes *(lymphocytosis)* with atypical morphology *(atypical lymphocytosis)* are associated with certain

viruses, particularly Epstein-Barr virus and cytomegalovirus.

Sometimes tremendous increases in the number of circulating white blood cells to 50,000/μL or more are associated with certain infections, such as tuberculosis. This increase is called a *leukemoid reaction* and must be distinguished from the more sinister disease of leukemia.

Leukopenia is defined as a reduced number of leukocytes below normal for the patient's age, sex, and race. An adult with a white blood count less than 4000/μL is leukopenic. Neutrophils are most frequently affected; a severe reduction to less than 500/μL (agranulocytosis) has already been discussed. *Neutropenia* is the reduction of neutrophils to fewer than 1750/μL. Neutropenia is frequently an adverse reaction to drugs and may sometimes be a manifestation of leukemia. Selective neutropenia is an adverse effect of many drugs, including amidopyrine and antimicrobials, particularly the sulfonamides and cotrimoxazole. Eosinophils and lymphocytes are selectively decreased by adrenocorticosteroids. *Lymphopenia* (less than 1000 lymphocytes/μL) is a typical feature of human immunodeficiency virus infection.

Cyclic neutropenia is a rare condition in which the neutrophil count falls sometimes to zero every 2 to 5 weeks. The cause is not known, but the effect is to curtail or arrest the myeloid series of cells at the stem cell level. Most of those affected are asymptomatic, although a few may have serious consequences as a result of infection. The disease has to be distinguished from agranulocytosis, which in most cases, is a much more serious condition.

The main malignant diseases of white blood cells are the leukemias, Hodgkin's and non-Hodgkin's lymphoma, and the plasma cell dyscrasias, particularly multiple myeloma. The most obvious effects of leukemia are on blood cells and the manifestations of the disease are due to these effects. By contrast, the lymphomas and the plasma cell dyscrasias are more likely to manifest as tumoral masses.

TABLE 13-7. A classification of leukemias

Type	FAB* notation
Acute	
Myeloid	
Undifferentiated	M1
Myelocytic	M2
Promyelocytic	M3
Myelomonocytic	M4
Monocytic	M5
Erythroleukemic	M6
Megakaryocytic	M7
Lymphocytic	
Pre-B or null cell	L1
T-cell	L2†
B-cell	L3
Chronic	
Myeloid	
Lymphocytic	
Unclassified	
Hairy cell leukemia (leukemic reticuloendotheliosis)‡	

*French-American-British classification.
†Some cases of pre-B and null cell acute lymphocytic leukemia are included in L2.
‡Currently believed to be a B-cell lymphoproliferative disorder.

LEUKEMIA

Leukemia is a diffuse proliferation of neoplastic hemopoietic cells that infiltrate the bone marrow and other tissues of the body, particularly the blood. The majority of leukemias are either acute or chronic, lymphocytic or myeloid. The remainder are rare varieties (Table 13-7).

Originally the terms *acute* and *chronic* described the clinical course of the leukemias, but they now have a somewhat different meaning. *Acute leukemias* are those in which the cell type is poorly differentiated, and its lineage is very difficult to identify morphologically. By contrast, *chronic leukemias* are those in which the cell type is more mature and readily identified. Untreated acute leukemias run a fatal course in a few months; patients with chronic myeloid leukemia survive about 3 to 4 years without treatment, whereas those with chronic lymphocytic leukemia can survive for many years.

Classification

The classification of leukemias is still controversial. A simplified classification is shown in Table 13-7. A further subdivision of the acute leukemias, the FAB (French-American-British) classification shown in the same table, has been in use for several years. This system divides acute myeloid leukemia into seven types (M1 through M7) and acute lymphocytic leukemia into three types (L1, L2, L3).

Etiology

The cause of human leukemia remains a mystery. Viruses are known to cause leukemia in fowl, felines, and rodents, and this has led to much speculation on the possible viral etiology of leukemia in humans. Recently a class of retroviruses, the human T-lymphotropic viruses (HTLV), have been shown to be responsible for certain T-cell leukemias and lymphomas; the mechanisms remain to be elucidated.

Alkylating drugs such as chlorambucil and cyclophosphamide are now accepted as causing leukemia. Paradoxically, they may also be used to treat the disease. Industrial exposure to benzene is at least a potential cause of leukemia. Ionizing radiation can cause leukemia as has been shown in atomic bomb survivors or those subjected to therapeutic bone irradiation for nonmalignant disease. Some observations seem to support a role for genetic factors in the etiology of some leukemias; about 8% of cases have a familial incidence. Leukemia is also at least 15 times more common in patients with Down's syndrome (trisomy 21) than in normal individuals, and the vast majority of patients with chronic myeloid leukemia have an abnormal (Philadelphia) chromosome.

Acute leukemia

Although acute leukemia can be divided into several types (Table 13-7), it is more practical to consider the acute forms of the disease as one clinical entity. This is because in Europe and the United States, the majority of acute leukemias, especially in children, are of the lymphocytic (lymphoblastic) type, and the clinical manifestations are the same regardless of the cell type.

Pathogenesis and pathology

Acute leukemia proliferation of cells gives rise to the following:

1. Displacement by neoplastic cells of normal erythropoietic cells and competition for essential nutrients; anemia is therefore an invariable consequence
2. Depression of platelet production by similar mechanisms, causing purpura and hemorrhagic tendencies, which are often among the early manifestations of the disease
3. Impairment of cellular defense mechanisms due to displacement of normal white blood cells by neoplastic cells, leading to greatly increased susceptibility to infection
4. Leukemic cell invasion of the liver, spleen, and lymph nodes, which become enlarged as a result

Hematologic findings

Anemia, which is often severe, and thrombocytopenia, usually to less than 50,000 platelets/μL, are almost invariable findings. The white blood cell count frequently ranges from 25,000 to 40,000/μL, but much higher values may be found. On some occasions, (sometimes called an *aleukemic* or *sub-leukemic* phase) leukopenia is present and the peripheral blood smear may look unremarkable. However, a few primitive cells can often be found if the white cells are concentrated by centrifugation ("buffy coat" preparation). This aleukemic phase is due to a temporary failure of the release of cells from the marrow, in which the characteristic changes of leukemia can be found.

The presence of primitive (blast) cells in the peripheral blood is a typical finding, but determination of the cell series to which these immature cells belong may be very difficult (Fig. 13-

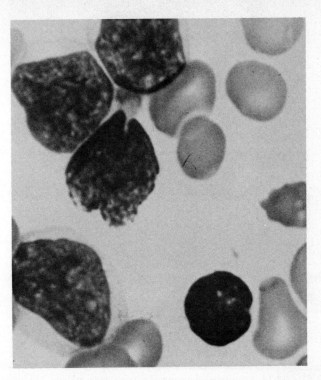

FIG. 13-12. Acute leukemia. Determining the cell of origin on morphologic grounds is difficult. This case was diagnosed as acute lymphocytic leukemia.

12). Marrow aspiration and biopsy are essential investigations. The marrow is usually crowded with blast cells, which form at least 30% or more of the marrow population. Red blood cell and platelet precursors are reduced.

The predominant cells in *acute myeloid leukemia* can be of several types (Table 13-7). Minimally differentiated myeloid cells or promyelocytes may predominate in some cases; in others, mixtures of immature monocytes and myelocytes may be present *(myelomonocytic leukemia)* (Fig. 13-13).

The demonstration of needlelike eosinophilic inclusions, called Auer rods* (or bodies), in the cytoplasm of leukemic cells distinguishes acute myeloid leukemia (Figs. 13-14 and 13-15). These rods appear to originate from lysosomes in myeloid cells. However, they may be absent, so that histochemical and other methods may be needed to differentiate myeloid cells from lymphoid or monocytic cells. For example, terminal deoxynucleotidyl transferase (tDT), which is involved in DNA synthesis, is present in lymphoblasts but rarely in myeloblasts. Again, in 70% of the cases of lymphoblastic leukemia in children, the common lymphocytic antigen (CALLA) can be demonstrated. Raised levels of muramidase (lysozyme) in plasma and urine are found in myeloid or myelomonocytic forms of acute leukemia.

In acute lymphoblastic leukemia (ALL) (Fig. 13-16), it can also be determined if the lymphoblasts have T or B cell immunophenotypic markers. Acute B-cell leukemias are very rare; T-cell types are more common, but the majority are neither T nor B cells and are called *null cells* (Table 13-7). However, recent data would indicate that these are pre-B cells in most cases.

---

*J. Auer (1875-1948), American physician.

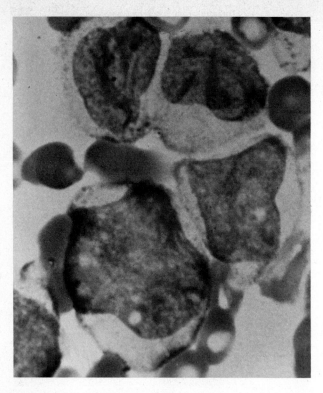

FIG. 13-13. Acute myelomonocytic leukemia, bone marrow. The cells resemble early monocytes but are regarded as being of myeloid origin.

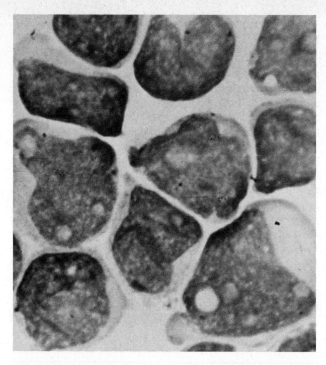

FIG. 13-14. Acute myeloid leukemia, bone marrow. The leukemic cells differ only slightly from those of acute lymphocytic leukemia. They are slightly larger and the nuclei stain less darkly. The presence of Auer rods (Fig. 13-15) is a diagnostic feature of myeloid leukemia.

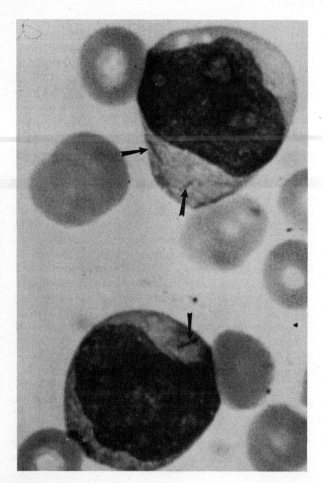

FIG. 13-15. Acute myeloid leukemia. Smear of the bone marrow shows two myeloblasts in which elongated crystalline bodies *(arrows)* can be seen. These are Auer rods, a morphologic feature of this form of leukemia.

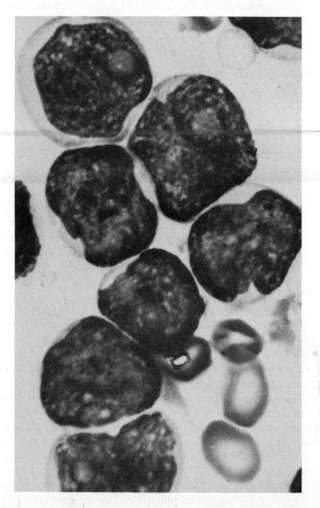

FIG. 13-16. Acute lymphocytic leukemia. The bone marrow is packed with lymphoblasts. Note the prominent nucleoli.

Clinical aspects

Acute leukemia is generally thought of as a disease of children, but there are just as many adult cases. The main difference is that in adults acute leukemia is usually of the myeloid rather than the lymphocytic type.

The common clinical manifestations are anemia, fever, and hemorrhage (Fig. 13-17). Oropharyngeal infections and enlarged lymph nodes are fairly frequent presenting symptoms. The onset of the disease is more sudden in children than in adults. Weakness and a sickly pallor, not entirely explicable by the degree of anemia alone, are common in children. Purpura, bleeding from the gums, and epistaxis are frequent (Fig. 13-18). Pharyngitis or a coldlike illness may be the initial manifestations, as may oral ulceration and oral or gingival infection. Gingival swelling is typically associated with acute myeloid and monocytic leukemia (Fig. 13-19). Enlargement of the liver, spleen, and lymph nodes is frequent.

The diagnosis is established from the hematologic findings, but because of its implications for treatment and prognosis, the diagnosis should never be made lightly or without due consideration of other diagnostic possibilities.

Treatment is still unsatisfactory, despite numerous therapeutic regimens. Nevertheless, increasing numbers of children with ALL have survived more than 5 years following intensive chemotherapy and radiotherapy, including treatment to attack leukemic deposits in the central nervous system. Survival for more than 3 years can be expected in more than half of these patients, especially after successful bone marrow transplantation, but claims for a cure of leukemia by current methods are still premature.

Chronic myeloid leukemia

Chronic myeloid leukemia (CML) involves the granulocytic series of white blood cells, and in over 90% of patients is associated with the presence of the Philadelphia (Ph₁) chromosome. This chromosome abnormality is due to the translocation of a portion of one of the long arms of chromosome 22 to chromosome 9. The abnormality is not confined to the granulocytes but is present in megakaryocytes and normoblasts. Its presence is known to precede the development of leukemia. The cause of this chromosome abnormality is not known.

Pathogenesis and pathology

The pathologic changes in CML are similar to those in other leukemias. Anemia due to displacement of erythroid elements of the marrow and competition for nutrients is typical. Invasion of the spleen by leukemic cells is massive, leading to spectacular splenomegaly. The spleen may reach 5 kg in weight (normal is 250 g). It is grayish-white because of generalized infiltration of the organ by leukemic cells. Liver infiltration may

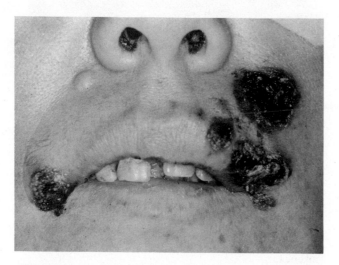

FIG. 13-17. Necrotic hemorrhagic perioral lesions in terminal acute leukemia.

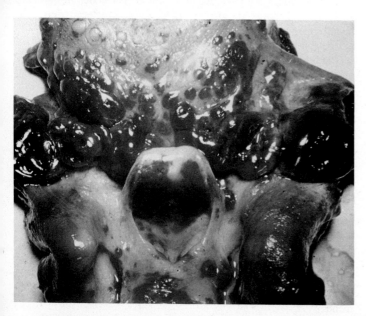

FIG. 13-18. Severe submucous hemorrhage into the pharynx and larynx in acute leukemia. The patient was severely thrombocytopenic.

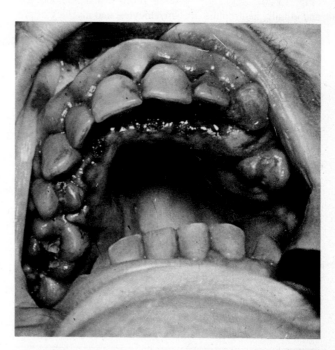

FIG. 13-19. Hypertrophy and bleeding of the gingivae in acute leukemia. There is ulceration along the lingual margin of the gingivae and purpura of the buccal mucosa. (*From Cawson RA: Essentials of dental surgery and pathology, ed 3, Edinburgh, Scotland, 1978, Churchill Livingstone.*)

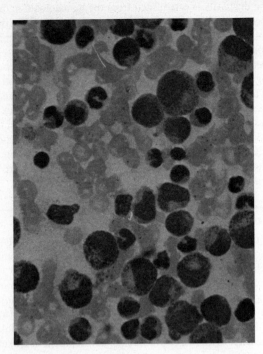

FIG. 13-20. Chronic myeloid leukemia, peripheral blood smear. The number of white blood cells is greatly increased. These are mainly mature granulocytes or late granulocyte precursors.

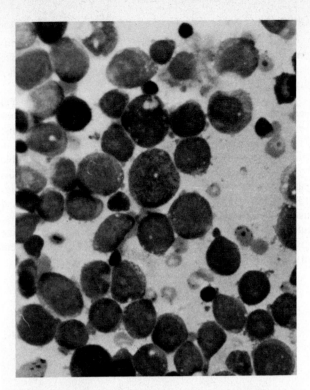

FIG. 13-21. Chronic myeloid leukemia, bone marrow. The marrow contains large numbers of myeloblasts and myelocytes.

also be found, but is less obvious. Leukemic cells may be scattered throughout the liver sinusoids and portal tracts.

Hematologic findings

Anemia is usual. The white blood cell count is very high (Fig. 13-20), frequently between 100,000 and 500,000/µL, and initially neutrophils, metamyelocytes, and myelocytes predominate. Myeloblasts are relatively few until terminal stages of the disease, when the number of platelets is usually decreased. The marrow (Fig. 13-21) is hyperplastic because of the great increase in myeloid series of cells, especially myelocytes. The Ph_1 chromosome can usually be demonstrated in special preparations of the marrow.

Clinical aspects

The onset of CML is insidious and becomes clinically apparent when the effects of anemia develop. Signs of hemorrhage due to thrombocytopenia may be found but are usually late manifestations.

Among a variety of other signs and symptoms that can be present, enlargement of the spleen is the most constant and often the sole physical finding.

CML is fatal, often within 3 years of onset. In about 70% of cases the terminal stage of the disease is similar to that seen in acute myeloid leukemia, with the appearance of large numbers of blast cells (a blast crisis) in the peripheral blood. Death is from the usual consequences of leukemia—infection, hemorrhage, and anemia.

Chronic lymphocytic leukemia

Chronic lymphocytic leukemia (CLL) shows considerable variation in its behavior compared with other forms of leukemia. Whereas other leukemias follow an inexorable downhill

course, many patients with CLL have a relatively benign disease, which may show little change over many years, so much so that an older patient may live out the normal expectation of life. Others, however, have a course similar to CML. CLL is a disease of middle and old age. There is a considerable body of opinion that CLL is totally different from all other forms of leukemia.

Pathogenesis and pathology

Enlargement of lymph nodes is the main pathologic change. Superficial nodes are most apparent, but deeper nodes in the abdomen and thorax are also enlarged. Pressure effects from nodal enlargement are rare. Splenic and hepatic enlargement is frequent but moderate.

The lymphoid tissue in the tonsils and salivary and lacrimal glands may be involved by the leukemic process. This is a cause of *Mikulicz' syndrome** (chronic enlargement of the lacrimal and salivary glands). The lymph nodes show similar pathologic changes as in well-differentiated lymphoma described later in this chapter.

Hematologic findings

Anemia is variable and often absent. When present, it may be due to causes other than diminished erythrocyte production. Of patients with CLL, 15% have a hemolytic anemia of the acquired immune type.

Most characteristic is the increase in lymphocytes (Fig. 13-22) in the peripheral blood to 50,000 or even to 250,000/µL in many cases. These lymphocytes are small and appear mature, so that the smear has a uniform appearance. The marrow shows an increase in lymphoid cells and a decrease in its other elements.

---

*J. von Mikulicz-Radecki (1850-1905), German surgeon.

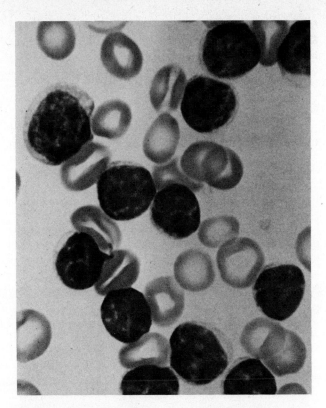

FIG. 13-22. Chronic lymphocytic leukemia, peripheral blood. Large numbers of mature lymphocytes are present; the lymphocyte count was 80,000/μL.

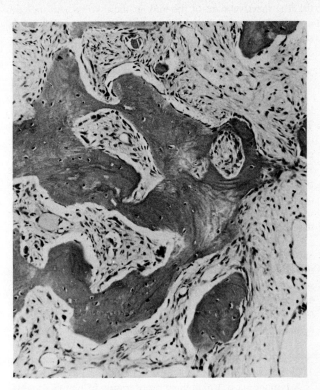

FIG. 13-23. Myelofibrosis. The marrow cavity in this bone marrow biopsy specimen contains no hemopoietic tissue. It has been totally repalced by vascular connective tissue.

In the majority of cases of CLL, the lymphocytes are of the B-cell type; the remainder are of T-cell origin.

Clinical aspects

The disease is insidious in onset, often asymptomatic in its early stages, and not uncommonly comes as an unexpected and unpleasant incidental finding during a routine medical examination.

Enlargement of lymph nodes is the most common complaint, but fever, spontaneous bleeding, or respiratory tract infections may bring the patient to the physician. Some patients appear to live in a state of truce with their disease for many years and form a "benign" group; others survive 3 to 5 years from onset. Although no curative treatment exists, palliative methods using radiotherapy and chemotherapy may keep the patient relatively symptom free until very late in the disease.

Myelofibrosis

Myelofibrosis (myelosclerosis, agnogenic myeloid metaplasia) describes a pathologic increase in the connective tissue of the bone marrow. It may be:
1. A primary neoplastic proliferation of the stromal mesenchymal cells of the marrow
2. Secondary to other bone marrow diseases
   a. Metastatic carcinoma
   b. Leukemia
   c. Polycythemia vera
   d. Hodgkin's disease

The close association of myelofibrosis with leukemia and polycythemia is responsible for its inclusion among the myeloproliferative disorders (Table 13-6).

Pathogenesis and pathology

There is still considerable debate whether myelofibrosis is a neoplastic process related to leukemia or a specific proliferative response of the marrow to injury.

The replacement of hemopoietic cells by fibrous tissue is compensated by hemopoiesis in other sites (Fig. 13-23). This extramedullary hemopoiesis is most prominent in the spleen, which may enlarge five to ten times its normal size, but without change in its normal microscopic architecture. The hemopoietic tissue may produce normal proportions of each cell series or a predominance or red or white blood cell precursors. Extramedullary hemopoiesis is also found in the liver and lymph nodes. This is believed to be due to primitive stem cell proliferation and a manifestation of the disease itself, rather than a purely compensatory development of normal marrow outside its usual site.

Anemia is usual and is due mostly to replacement of erythropoietic elements in the marrow and ineffective erythropoiesis.

Hematologic findings

The blood picture in myelofibrosis is typically *leukoerythroblastic anemia*, that is, an anemia accompanied by the presence of immature red and white blood cells in the peripheral blood. Many red blood cells are characteristically pear shaped or elliptical. Reticulocytes and normoblasts are common. The white blood cell count is raised in most cases and may be as high as 50,000/μL. Early granulocytes, including a few myeloblasts, may be seen.

The marrow biopsy shows a variable increase in fibrous tissue stroma and reticulin fibers and generally a decrease in hemopoietic tissue. Nevertheless, a few hyperplastic areas of marrow can be seen, and this may mislead the observer as to the true inactive state of the bulk of the marrow. An increase in the amount of trabecular bone *(osteosclerosis)* may be observed in marrow biopsy, especially in the later stages of the disease.

Clinical aspects

Myelofibrosis has an insidious onset, mostly in middle to late adult life, and usually runs a chronic course of 5 to 7 years. The main clinical findings are due to anemia and the effects of splenic enlargement. These may be superimposed on the effects of associated disease, particularly polycythemia vera. Bleeding from the nose and into the skin is frequent in the late stages, usually because of thrombocytopenia. The diagnosis is confirmed by marrow biopsy. Needle aspiration of the marrow usually results in a "dry tap," and this in itself may suggest the diagnosis.

Treatment of myelofibrosis is unsatisfactory, although the administration of androgens has been of benefit in some patients. Blood transfusion is necessary when anemia becomes severe. However, the benefits of blood seem to diminish with each transfusion. The disease may end with infection, cardiac failure, hemorrhage, or the development of acute myeloid leukemia.

THE LYMPHOMAS

A lymphoma is a malignant proliferation of lymphoid cells. Although this term as currently used implies malignancy, it is not infrequent to find the term *malignant lymphoma* in the literature, even though these diseases have no true benign counterparts.

The classification of the lymphomas has both fascinated and confused pathologists and clinicians for many years. It is still a subject that can stimulate heated debate. More recent classifications have tended toward simplicity rather than complexity, a sign, it is hoped, of increased understanding on the part of the classifiers. The two main divisions of lymphomas are Hodgkin's disease (Hodgkin's lymphoma) and lymphoma (non-Hodgkin's lymphoma).

Hodgkin's disease includes several variants that differ both in histologic appearance and clinical prognosis. The non-Hodgkin's lymphomas, by contrast, are a less distinct and highly variable group of malignant disorders of lymph nodes.

Little is known of the etiology, but there is increased susceptibility to lymphomas in the following conditions:
1. Primary immunodeficiency
2. Immunosuppressive treatment
3. AIDS
4. Connective tissue disorders, particularly rheumatoid arthritis

Hodgkin's disease (Hodgkin's lymphoma)

This malignant disease, which primarily affects lymph nodes, was first described by Thomas Hodgkin* of Guy's Hospital in England in 1832. The cause of Hodgkin's disease is unknown. Whether it is a lymphoma is open to argument, since the basic abnormality does not appear to be in the lymphocyte,

*Just prior to this, Hodgkin was curator of Guy's Hospital Pathology Museum. Many illustrations in this book are courtesy of his present successor in that office.

but is the presence of an abnormal cell (the Dorothy Reed, or Reed-Sternberg cell) among the cells of the lymph nodes. The latter show a variety of histologic pictures associated with this unusual cell. For the most part, however, Hodgkin's disease behaves as a malignant disease of lymphoid tissue.

Classification

The *histologic classification* most widely used is that of Lukes et al. (1966) (see the box below). In general, this clas-

---

HISTOLOGIC CLASSIFICATION OF HODGKIN'S DISEASE

1. Lymphocytic predominance
   a. Nodular
   b. Diffuse
2. Nodular sclerosis
3. Mixed cellularity
4. Lymphocyte depletion

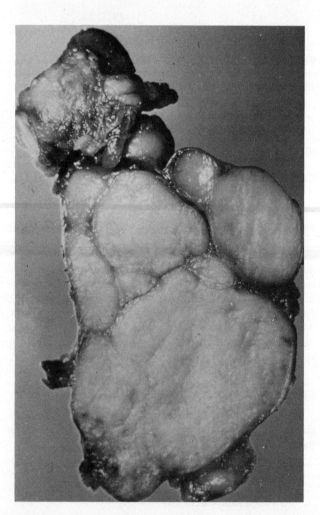

FIG. 13-24. A mass of lymph nodes in Hodgkin's disease. The nodes are greatly enlarged. Their cut surface has a uniform appearance, and each enlarged node remains well demarcated. *(Courtesy Curator of the Gordon Museum, Guy's Hospital, London, England.)*

sification emphasizes the role of the normal lymphocyte in defense of the host, since the greater proportion of these cells present, the more favorable the outlook for the patient.

Pathogenesis and pathology

The origin of the Reed-Sternberg (RS) cell that characterizes Hodgkin's disease has been a matter of speculation for many years. Recently it was proposed that RS cells arise from the interdigitating reticulum cells of lymph nodes. These cells have a variety of properties in common with the RS cell, including similar histochemical and immunologic markers. However, in the lymphocytic preponderance (nodular) type of Hodgkin's disease, good evidence suggests that the RS cell is of B-cell origin. The exact origin of this enigmatic cell, therefore, is still unresolved.

That there is severe derangement of the normal cellular defense mechanisms in Hodgkin's disease is undisputed, but the cause (or causes) is unknown. A viral agent has been postulated, mainly on epidemiologic grounds, but direct evidence is lacking.

The disease begins in lymph nodes (Fig. 13-24) and is often first seen in the neck. Typically, lymph node groups become involved by contiguous spread.

The enlarged nodes are firm, smooth, discrete, and rubbery. Later the spleen, marrow, and liver become infiltrated by the lymphomatous process (Fig. 13-25). In certain sites, such as the mediastinum, masses of enlarged lymph nodes press on the surrounding anatomic structures.

The essential diagnostic histologic feature of Hodgkin's disease is the RS cell, which is 15 to 40 μm in diameter, usually with a bilobed or multilobed nucleus. Although this cell is the sine qua non of Hodgkin's disease, it sometimes may be difficult to find while cells of identical morphology have been described in infectious mononucleosis and other diseases.

The patterns of cells found together with RS cells form the basis for the histologic classification of Lukes et al. A characteristic of all patterns is the complete or partial obliteration of the normal lymph node architecture. Another is that one histologic type may change to another less favorable variety during the course of the disease.

Four histologic patterns of the disease are recognized in this classification (see the box on p. 290). In the pattern of *lymphocytic predominance,* large numbers of lymphocytes arranged in sheets or nodules in the lymph nodes are characteristic, with a few RS cells that are often difficult to find. In *nodular sclerosis,* well-defined bands of collagen traverse the nodes; lymphocytes and histiocytes in varying proportions are present, but again morphologically typical RS cells are relatively scarce. In the *mixed cellularity* type, RS cells are more abundant and are found among a mixture of lymphocytes, histiocytes, neutrophils, eosinophils, and plasma cells (Fig. 13-26). The *lymphocyte depletion* type is self-explanatory. RS cells are common in a setting of strands of eosinophilic material in which all other cellular elements, especially lymphocytes are greatly reduced in number (Fig. 13-27).

It must be remembered that the cellular picture is highly variable, and it usually requires an expert and experienced pathologist, not merely to determine what form of the disease is present, but even to differentiate Hodgkin's disease from other lymphomas in some cases.

Clinical aspects

Patients with Hodgkin's disease may be of any age but are usually between ages 20 and 40. Males are affected two or three times more often than females. These patients commonly have enlarged lymph nodes, especially in the neck (Fig. 13-28). In the course of the disease, fever, weight loss, weakness, and anemia can develop, plus a variety of signs and symptoms referable to virtually every system may be present at the time of diagnosis.

Patients with Hodgkin's disease are prone to develop a wide range of *opportunistic infections,* including cryptococcosis, toxoplasmosis, and infections by the herpes group of viruses as a consequence of their disordered immune response.

The diagnosis can only be made by histologic examination, preferably of lymph nodes.

Systems of clinical staging of the disease have been developed and are based upon the number of lymph node groups involved, their site, involvement of other organs, and whether

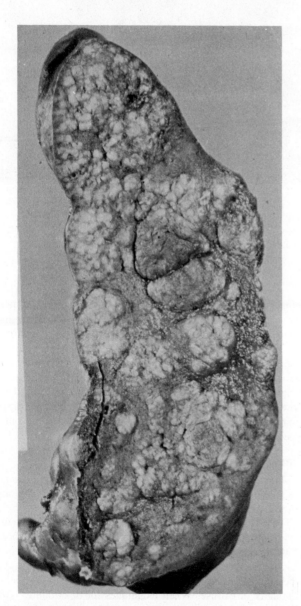

FIG. 13-25. Hodgkin's disease. The spleen is enlarged and studded with lymphomatous deposits. *(Courtesy Curator of the Gordon Museum, Guy's Hospital, London, England.)*

FIG. 13-26. A, Lymph node in Hodgkin's disease (mixed cellularity type). A typical RS cell is present and is the diagnostic feature of this disease. The remaining cells are a mixture of mature lymphocytes, histiocytes, and a few plasma cells. **B,** Lymph node in Hodgkin's disease showing an RS cell highly magnified. The bilobed nucleus with large, inclusion-like nucleoli are characteristic of this cell.

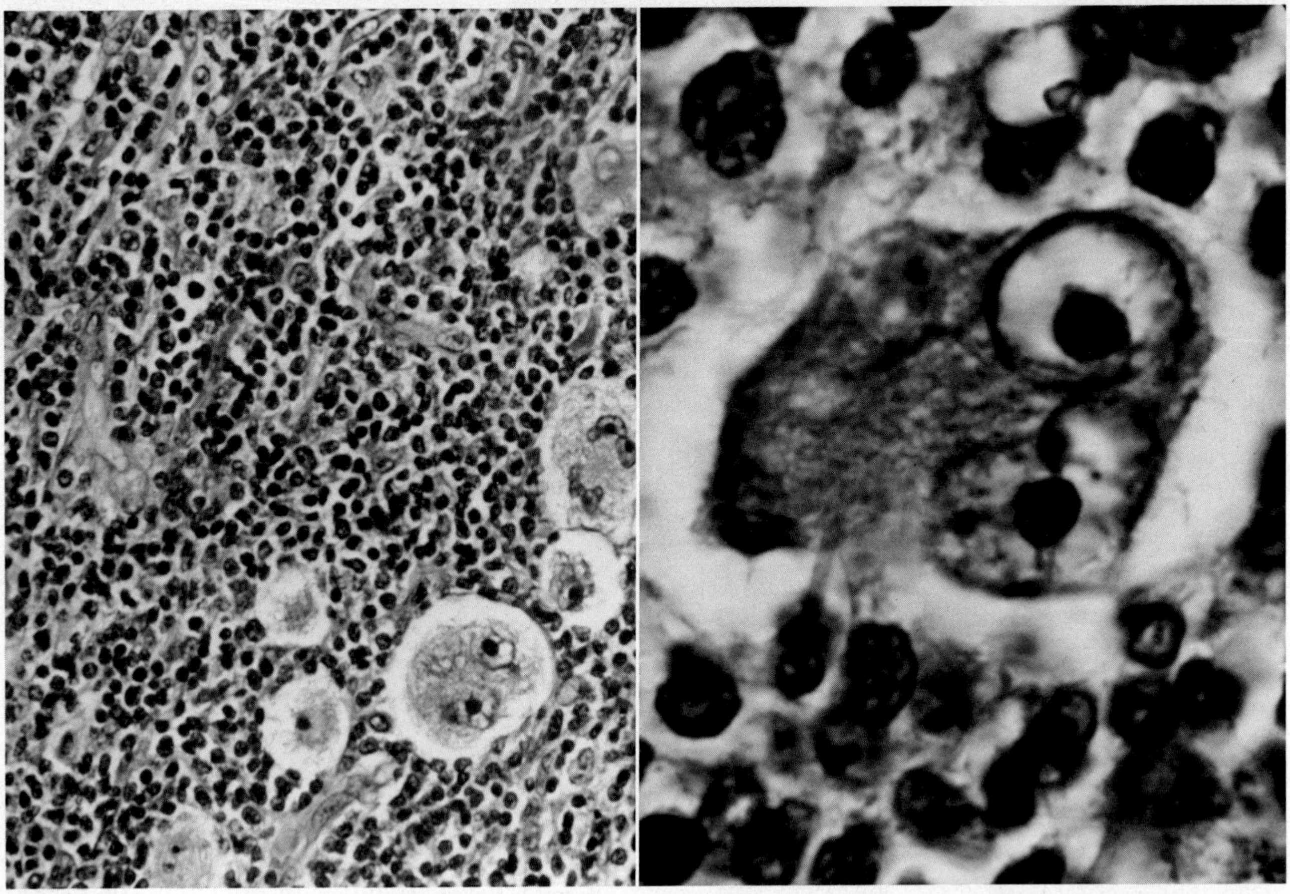

fever, weight loss, and night sweats are present. The purpose of staging is to allow selection of the optimal therapeutic regimen and to permit valid comparison of the results of different forms of treatment. The system almost exclusively used in the United States is the Ann Arbor Staging Classification (Carbone et al., 1971).

The outlook in Hodgkin's disease, once invariably fatal, has changed dramatically for the better in recent years. Radiotherapy and chemotherapy are the principal methods of treatment. The necessary investigative methods for staging are carried out before treatment. Five-year disease-free survivals are reported in 40% to 90% of patients treated by radiotherapy, depending on the stage. Even in the most serious and disseminated forms of the disease, combined chemotherapy with drugs such as alkylating agents, vincristine, and prednisone allows significant numbers of patients to survive 5 years or more without evidence of the disease.

Non-Hodgkin's lymphomas

Non-Hodgkin's lymphomas (NHLs) are malignant neoplasms that can arise wherever lymphoid tissue is present, but mainly in the lymph nodes. NHLs are heterogeneous; most carry immunophenotypic markers for B cells. A minority appear to originate from T cells or from macrophages or are of indeter-

minate origin. The cause or causes of NHLs are for the most part unknown. A viral etiology is frequently suggested, and indeed two of these diseases, adult T-cell leukemia-lymphoma and Burkitt's lymphoma, are possibly due to viruses.

Adult T-cell leukemia-lymphoma is etiologically linked to the oncogenic retrovirus HTLV 1. Strong epidemiologic evidence indicates that Burkitt's lymphoma may be caused by Epstein-Barr virus possibly in association with endemic falciparum malaria. There is still no convincing evidence that other types of NHL are caused by viruses.

Classification

Many classifications of NHLs have been proposed, indicating the uncertainty of our current understanding of this group of diseases.

The main purpose of classifying NHLs is to provide a sound basis for prognosis and compare the effects of different methods of treatment. One early, but still widely used classification (Rappaport, 1966), shown in Table 13-8, is based on the cell type and its degree of differentiation and whether the process is nodular or diffuse. When techniques for determining lymphocyte surface markers became available, Lukes and Collins (1974) used this together with lymph node imprints to classify NHLs according to whether they were of B-cell, T-cell, or undetermined origin and by histologic appearances. In Europe

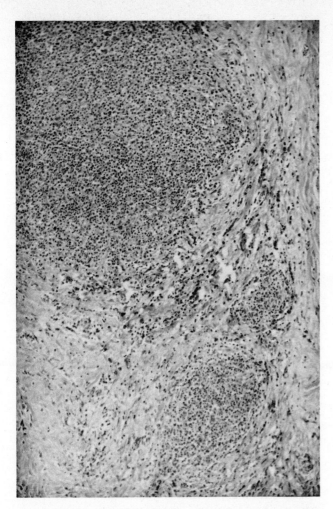

FIG. 13-27. Nodular sclerosing Hodgkin's disease. Well-defined, pale-staining bands of collagen separate collections of lymphocytes and histiocytes arranged in nodules of varying sizes.

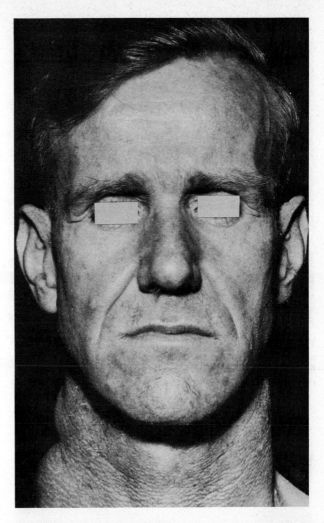

FIG. 13-28. Hodgkin's disease. Cervical lymph nodes are enlarged but have remained discrete from each other. (Compare with Fig. 13-30.) *(Courtesy Curator of the Gordon Museum, Guy's Hospital, London, England.)*

the Kiel classification (Gerard-Marchant et al., 1974) is favored. Its essential feature is the division of NHLs into low- and high-grade malignancies, with further categories in each division based on histologic features. More recently, a "working formulation" for NHL was proposed by the National Cancer Institute (1982) (Table 13-8). This designates NHLs as "malignant lymphomas," divides them into low-, intermediate- and high-grade malignancies, and subdivides each grade by cell morphology.

Pathology

In most cases the disease begins in the lymph nodes, especially those in the neck, groin, and axillae. In later stages other organs, especially the liver and spleen, are often infiltrated by malignant lymphocytic cells.

Lymphocytic lymphoma. Lymphocytic lymphomas comprise about 45% to 50% of all non-Hodgkin's lymphomas and are predominantly B-cell neoplasms. The *diffuse, well-differentiated type* has a pattern of sheets of small, mature-looking lymphoctes (Fig. 13-29). Many of these cases also have large numbers of lymphocytes in the blood or frank lymphocytic leukemia.

In the *poorly differentiated type*, which can have either a

diffuse or a nodular pattern, the lymphocytes are still small but their nuclei are cleaved rather than round. In the diffuse variety, about one third of cases have involvement of the oropharyngeal tissues.

Mixed small- and large-cell (lymphocytic and histiocytic) lymphoma. Again, both diffuse and nodular forms are recognized. The abnormal cells consist of a mixture of small cleaved lymphocytes and larger histiocyte-like cells, the latter forming between 20% and 50% of the cell population. The follicular form is of B-cell origin. The diffuse form can be composed of either B cells, T cells, or untypeable lymphocytes. Between 5% and 10% of all NHLs are of the mixed variety.

Large-cell (histiocytic) lymphoma. Histiocytic lymphomas make up about 30% of NHLs. Almost all have a diffuse pattern, consisting of large B or T cells, which morphologically resemble pleomorphic histiocytes. Thus the name histiocytic lymphoma is a misleading contradiction in terms. However, in some cases of NHL, the cells are of true histiocytic rather than lymphocytic origin. This is but one example of the difficulties encountered in classifying these lymphomas.

Lymphoblastic lymphoma. This type of NHL is uncommon in adults. It consists of diffusely arranged large primitive lymphoblasts.

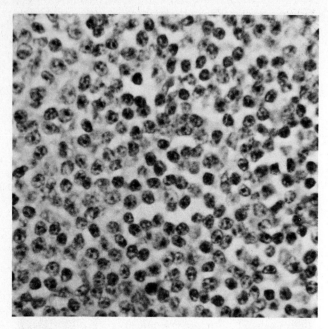

FIG. 13-29. A sea of small lymphocytes seen populating a lymph node in chronic lymphocytic leukemia. The histologic appearance of the lymph nodes in well-differentiated lymphocytic lymphoma is identical.

TABLE 13-8. Rappaport classification of non-Hodgkin's lymphoma compared with the National Cancer Institute's working formulation (abbreviated)*

Rappaport classification	Working formulation†
Well-differentiated lympho-cytic lymphoma	Low-grade malignant lymphoma: diffuse, small lymphocytic
Poorly differentiated lympho-cytic lymphoma	Low-grade malignant lymphoma: follicular, small (C) cell
Mixed lymphoma, nodular	Low-grade malignant lymphoma: follicular, small (C) and large cell
Histiocytic lymphoma, nodular	Intermediate-grade malignant lymphoma; nodular, large cell
Poorly differentiated lympho-cytic lymphoma, diffuse	Intermediate-grade malignant lymphoma: diffuse, small (C) cell
Mixed lymphoma, diffuse	Intermediate-grade malignant lymphoma: diffuse, small and large cell
Histiocytic lymphoma, diffuse	Intermediate-grade malignant lymphoma: diffuse, large (C and NC) cell
Histiocytic lymphoma, diffuse	High-grade malignant lymphoma: diffuse, large cell immunoblastic
Lymphoblastic lymphoma	High-grade malignant lymphoma: diffuse, lymphoblastic
Undifferentiated lymphoma Burkitt's and non-Burkitt's	High-grade malignant lymphoma: diffuse, small (C) cell

*Adapted from the Report of the Working Committee: National Cancer Institute sponsored study of classification of non-Hodgkin's lymphomas: Summary and description of a working formulation for clinical usage, Cancer 49:2112, 1982.
†C, Cleaved cell; NC, noncleaved cell.

Small-cell (undifferentiated) lymphoma. Two subtypes of undifferentiated lymphoma are recognized: Burkitt's and non-Burkitt's.

Burkitt's lymphoma is endemic in east central Africa. It is characteristically found in children, and unlike other lymphomas it typically arises in the mandible or maxilla, forming a large, destructive, expansile mass. An uncommon sporadic form of Burkitt's lymphoma is seen in the United States (American Burkitt's lymphoma). This form of the disease, by contrast with the African form, usually arises in the intestines and has no association with Epstein-Barr virus. Both variants have an identical histologic picture of large, rounded cells with a thin peripheral ring of cytoplasm, interspersed with large clear histiocytes, giving a "starry sky" appearance to histologic preparations. However, this pattern is not unique to Burkitt's lymphoma and may be seen in other histologic types.

The *non-Burkitt's* type consists of more pleomorphic cells with uncleaved nuclei and has a similar prognosis.

Clinical aspects

Most patients with NHLs, except those with African Burkitt's and lymphoblastic lymphomas, are in middle to late adult life and often have a history of lupus erythematosus, Sjögren's syndrome, rheumatoid arthritis, or congenital or acquired immune defects. It is now a well-recognized complication in patients who have had renal transplants or who have AIDS. Enlarged lymph nodes is a common early complaint (Fig. 13-30), but in persons with AIDS, lymphomas often develop in unusual sites, such as the brain, mouth, or salivary glands. Later in the disease, a wide variety of symptoms can develop, in addition to fever and weight loss.

Clinical staging similar to that used for Hodgkin's disease

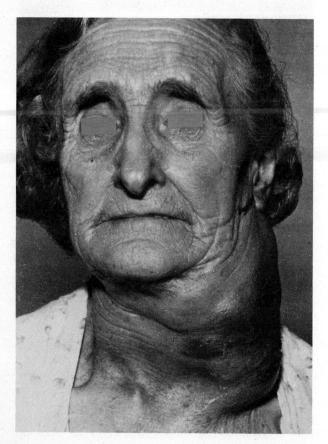

FIG. 13-30. Lymphoma in a 72-year-old woman. The malignant lymph nodes on the left side of the neck have formed a continuous mass in which individual nodes cannot easily be distinguished. *(Courtesy Curator of the Gordon Museum, Guy's Hospital, London, England.)*

has been developed, depending on the lymph node groups and/or organs and the presense of systemic symptoms. Generally, the outlook in NHLs is much less favorable than in Hodgkin's disease. With newer forms of chemotherapy, the outlook in well-differentiated, nodular, and large-cell lymphomas has improved considerably, but the long-term prognosis is still poor.

Other forms of lymphoma
Mycosis fungoides

Mycosis fungoides (Chapter 9) is a T-cell lymphoma that primarily involves the skin. It begins as a rash that can resemble a variety of other skin diseases. However, the disease can spread to involve lymph nodes, spleen, and liver, and the skin lesions may develop into tumor masses. At this stage the disease closely resembles histiocytic lymphoma. As with most forms of NHL, treatment is unsatisfactory and the disease is fatal, usually in 3 to 4 years.

Sézary's syndrome

This syndrome has many similarities to mycosis fungoides. It is characterized by chronic, itching, red skin lesions, which histologically show infiltration of the dermis by mononuclear cells and abnormal lymphocytes (Sézary cells) of T-cell origin. The syndrome therefore can be regarded as a form of lymphocytic T-cell lymphoma. Treatment with α-interferon is reported to give significant improvement in some cases.

Hairy cell leukemia (leukemic reticuloendotheliosis)

This disease should now be regarded as a lymphoproliferative disorder of the B-cell type. In one well-documented case, human T-lymphotropic virus 2 (HTLV-2) has been isolated. The significance of this finding is yet to be determined. The name reflects the presence in the peripheral blood of lymphocytes with thin cytoplasmic projections. Splenomegaly, pancytopenia and bone marrow infiltration are typical presenting features.

In the past, splenectomy was the treatment of choice, especially in the early stages of the disease. However, excellent responses to α-interferon have been reported, and this now appears to be the treatment of choice.

PLASMA CELL DYSCRASIAS

Multiple myeloma

Multiple myeloma is a malignant neoplasm of plasma cells and their precursors. The cause is unknown, and although viral particles have been demonstrated in myeloma tissue, they are more likely to be passengers than causative agents.

Pathogenesis and pathology

The basic abnormality in myeloma is a malignant clone of plasma cells developing in the marrow. These cells have two characteristic effects:
1. They invade and multiply in bone and other tissues.
2. They usually show aberrant production of immunoglobulins (paraproteins).

During the course of the disease, collections of neoplastic plasma cells proliferate in many parts of the skeleton. The vertebral column, ribs, and skull are most frequently involved. The areas affected contain soft reddish tissue and appear on radiographs as punched-out defects in bone. Alternatively,

more diffuse proliferation of plasma cells in the marrow can result in osteoporosis.

Microscopically, this tissue consists of large numbers of plasma cells in varying stages of maturity (Fig. 13-31). The cells may also be found as an infiltrate in liver, spleen, lymph nodes, and other organs.

In most, but not all cases of myeloma, specific immunoglobulins are produced. These abnormal proteins are the product of single clones of neoplastic cells. When detected by laboratory methods, the term *monoclonal gammopathy* is often applied (Table 13-9). The most common immunoglobulin produced is IgG, which is readily detected in plasma by electrophoresis (Fig. 13-32) and characterized by immunoelectrophoresis. An excessive production of light chains over heavy chains is frequently found; when this happens, the light chains appear in the urine as *Bence Jones protein*. These light chains can be readily categorized as either κ- or λ-chains by immunoelectrophoresis. Thus an IgA-λ myeloma is one in which the abnormal

TABLE 13-9. Plasma cell dyscrasia and immunoglobulin production

Disease	Immunoglobulins or polypeptides produced
Multiple myeloma	IgG, IgA (rarely IgE, IgD), Bence Jones protein
Macroglobulinemia (Waldenström's)	IgM
Heavy chain disease	γ-, α-, μ-Chains
Benign monoclonal gammopathy	IgA, IgG

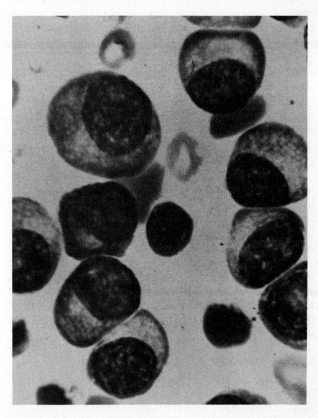

FIG. 13-31. Marrow in multiple myeloma. A high-power view of the bone marrow shows a collection of malignant plasma cells.

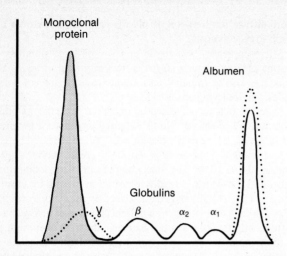

FIG. 13-32. Electrophoretogram of serum from a patient with monoclonal gammopathy. Note the very large monoclonal protein band *(shaded area)* in the γ-globulin region. The normal electrophoretic pattern is shown by dotted lines.

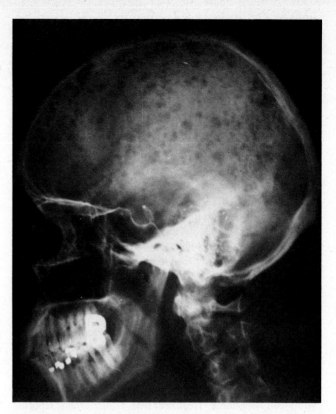

FIG. 13-33. Radiograph of the skull in multiple myeloma. The vault of the skull has numerous opacities due to the osteolytic effect of myelomatous deposits.

clone of plasma cells produces immunoglobulin of the IgA class with an excess of λ-chains.

The kidney is involved to varying degrees in myeloma. The term *myeloma kidney* applies to a pale kidney in which, microscopically, dilated ducts containing protein alternate with atrophic ducts or those in which giant cells are frequent. The means by which light chains cause renal injury is unknown. Renal impairment eventually affects about 75% of all patients with myeloma and is the immediate cause of death in 15% to 20% of cases.

The central nervous system is involved in one third of patients. Compression of the spinal cord or nerve roots because of masses of myeloma cells and diffuse involvement of the meninges, causing a myeloma meningitis, are the main serious effects.

Depending on the properties and amount of the abnormal protein present in the plasma, there may be an increase in the blood viscosity to such a degree that it causes serious effects. This is most likely to be associated with an IgM-producing myeloma, but it can also be seen with IgA and IgG paraproteins. The clinical effects are grouped under the name *hyperviscosity syndrome,* as discussed later.

In some patients the physical properties of the abnormal immunoglobulins can be altered by cold, which causes them to precipitate or gel. These proteins are called *cryoglobulins* and are usually IgM or IgG or complexes containing IgM or IgG. The clinical effects of these cold-precipitating proteins are due to interruption of blood flow and hypoxia.

Amyloidosis (Chapter 2) affects up to 10% of patients with myeloma, and the amyloid protein has amino acid sequences akin to those of the monoclonal light chains produced by the tumor. In myeloma the amyloid is characteristically deposited in the heart, kidney, and tendon sheaths and less frequently in the liver, lungs, and spleen.

Clinical aspects

Multiple myeloma is a disease predominantly of middle and late life and affects males twice as often as females. The earlier signs of the disease are due to anemia, infections, especially of the lung, and renal dysfunction. The effects of the hyperviscosity syndrome, including congestive heart failure, visual

and central nervous system disturbances, and hemorrhage into skin and alimentary tract, may be superimposed. The onset of painful bone lesions is a relatively late manifestation.

The diagnosis is made by radiographs (Fig. 13-33), biopsy of the lesions, and protein analysis of blood and urine.

Although many therapeutic regimens have been introduced, with some amelioration of the disease process, myeloma still remains a slowly progressive fatal disease.

Solitary myeloma (plasmacytoma)

There is doubt whether this rare lesion represents a single focus of multiple myeloma or whether it is another entity. Despite histologic similarities, the behavior of solitary myeloma is somewhat different from that of multiple myeloma.

Two types are described. One involves bone (intraosseous type), the other soft tissue (extramedullary type). Intraosseous myelomas are most often found in the femur, ribs, and vertebrae; extramedullary forms are seen in the upper respiratory tract and oral cavity. Any age group may be affected, males more often than females. The first symptoms are usually pain or swelling or both. Intraosseous lesions on radiographic examination have ill-defined margins because of bone destruction. In the mouth and nasopharynx, the extramedullary type forms red sessile or polypoid swellings.

Hyperimmunoglobulinemia or anemia characteristic of multiple myeloma are usually absent in solitary myeloma as is Bence Jones protein in the urine. The presence of any of these abnormalities should initiate a radiologic survey to detect other sites of myeloma. Myelomas are found more frequently if the initial lesion is located in bone rather than in soft tissue. Multiple myeloma is likely to develop in about half the cases of intraosseous disease, and in 10% to 15% of extramedullary forms, although many more can appear after several decades. The prognosis is favorable if the disorder is truly localized and is not associated with disseminated disease.

Waldenström's macroglobulinemia

This rare disease typically consists of enlargement of the lymph nodes, liver, and spleen associated with proliferation of plasmacytoid lymphocytes, which secrete excessive amounts of IgM. This monoclonal protein is present in the plasma, and the atypical lymphocytes appear in the peripheral blood.

Patients with Waldenström's macroglobulinemia have an increased tendency to infection and hemorrhage, and the effects of hyperviscosity syndrome and/or cryoglobulins can be superimposed on anemia and sometimes thrombocytopenia.

Generally, the outlook in this disease is much more favorable than in multiple myeloma. Plasmapheresis, that is, the removal of blood plasma and replacement of the patient's red blood cells, can greatly ameliorate the effects of hyperviscosity.

Heavy chain diseases

This is an uncommon group of disorders that resemble macroglobulinemia, except that monoclonal proteins resembling Fc fragments of heavy chains are secreted by the abnormal plasma cells. Abnormal proteins resembling the Fc fragments of IgG, IgM, IgA, and IgD (γ-, μ-, α- and δ-chains) have been described, of which γ–heavy chain disease (Franklin's disease) is perhaps the best known. Clinically, heavy chain diseases resemble macroglobulinemia, but generally have a poorer prognosis.

Monoclonal gammopathy of undetermined significance

Some elderly patients who are otherwise asymptomatic produce excessive amounts of immunoglobulin. It is important that this abnormality is not attributed to myeloma or other dysproteinosis simply because of elevated serum immunoglobulin levels and a monoclonal electrophoretic pattern. Generally those who have a monoclonal gammopathy that has no apparent clinical significance (benign monoclonal gammopathy) are over 70 years of age and have immunoglobulins of 2 g/dL or less. These patients need no treatment; however, since it is possible that some may be in the early stages of a more serious form of gammopathy, they should be examined periodically.

LANGERHANS' HISTIOCYTOSIS (HISTIOCYTOSIS X)

This name is applied to three fairly distinctive diseases of unknown cause that are characterized by proliferation of Langerhans' cells of the macrophage-monocyte system. These cells can be identified by immunophenotypic markers or by electron microscopic demonstration of Birbeck's granules (Fig. 13-34). Langerhans' histiocytosis comprises:

1. Letterer-Siwe disease
2. Multifocal eosinophilic granuloma (Hand-Schuller-Christian disease)
3. Solitary eosinophilic granuloma

Whether these three diseases are justifiably included under one title is very much open to question. Letterer-Siwe disease

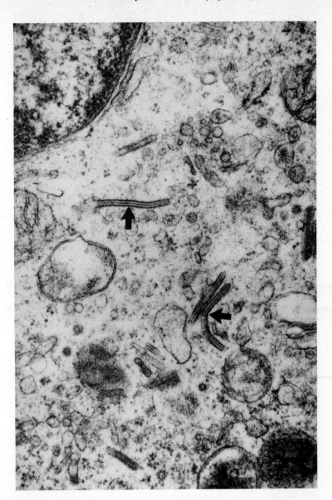

FIG. 13-34. Electron micrograph of Langerhans' cell showing several Birbeck's granules *(arrows)*, which are characteristic of these cells, in the cytoplasm. Typically these granules are rod shaped and resemble a zipper.

has many similarities to the lymphomas and involves proliferation of poorly differentiated histiocytes. The multifocal and solitary forms of eosinophilic granuloma appear to be variants of the same pathologic process in which a prolific response of mature histiocytes may be multifocal or unifocal, respectively. The principal pathologic and clinical features are given in Table 13-10.

SWELLING OF CERVICAL LYMPH NODES

Diseases of the lymphatic system are frequently characterized by lymphadenopathy (enlargement of lymph nodes). The lymph nodes of the neck are perhaps the most common clinically apparent site of lymphatic disease. Cervical lymphadenopathy is therefore a common and sometimes difficult problem of differential diagnosis.

The main causes of enlarged cervical lymph nodes follow:
1. Inflammatory swellings
   a. Infections of the oropharynx, particularly arising from tonsils, teeth, and periodontal tissues
   b. Infectious mononucleosis
   c. Herpes simplex
   d. Acquired immunodeficiency syndrome
   e. Nontuberculous and tuberculous mycobacterial disease (Fig. 13-35)

f. Syphilis, primary and secondary
g. Cat-scratch disease
2. Neoplastic swellings
  a. Lymphatic spread of cancer from mouth or naso-pharynx
  b. Lymphoma, Hodgkin's and non-Hodgkin's
  c. Lymphocytic leukemia

Infectious mononucleosis

Infectious mononucleosis is a generalized infection of lymphoid tissue. Pathologically, it is characterized by the following:

1. Hyperplasia of lymphoid tissue in lymph nodes and other sites
2. Abnormal lymphocytes in lymphoid tissue and peripheral blood

3. The development of heterophile antibodies and antibodies to the Epstein-Barr virus (EBV)

Etiology

It is now generally accepted that EBV, a member of the herpesvirus family, is the cause of infectious mononucleosis. The following are included in the supporting evidence:

1. Accidental infection of laboratory workers with EBV has caused typical infectious mononucleosis.
2. Experimental infection of squirrel monkeys with leukocytes infected with EBV produces typical antibodies in the serum of those animals and emphasizes the cell association of the virus.
3. In the early weeks of infectious mononucleosis specific EBV antibodies of the IgM class appear.
4. Various antibodies against EBV are present throughout and after the illness.

TABLE 13-10. Features of Langerhans' histiocytosis (histiocytosis X)

Disease	Age group	Pathology	Prognosis
Letterer-Siwe	<3 years	Proliferation of poorly differentiated histiocytes, involving spleen, liver, lymph nodes, skin: pancytopenia in blood and marrow	Rapidly fatal
Multifocal eosinophilic granuloma (Hand-Schuller-Christian; HSC)	<5 years	Proliferation of more mature histiocytes in bone, spleen, liver, lung, lymph nodes associated with eosinophils and lymphocytes; diabetes insipidus and exophthalmos in 25% due to pressure effects of skull lesions	Good with treatment
Solitary eosinophilic granuloma	Children, young adults	Solitary lesion with similar histologic appearance as HSC; usually found in skull, jaws, ribs, pelvis, femur, vertebrae	Excellent with treatment

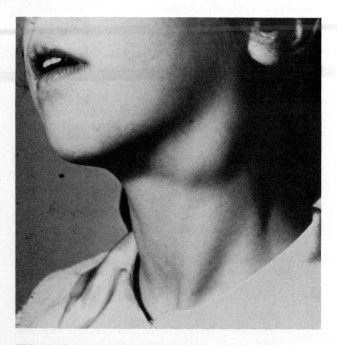

FIG. 13-35. Tuberculous lymphadenitis. The large painless swelling of the tonsillar lymph node is soft and fluctuant, with no evidence of acute inflammation ("cold abscess"). The tuberculin skin test was strongly positive. (*Courtesy Curator of the Gordon Museum, Guy's Hospital, London, England.*)

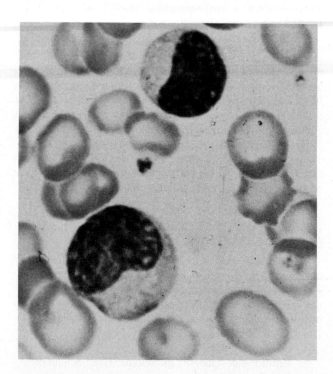

FIG. 13-36. Infectious mononucleosis. This peripheral blood smear shows two atypical lymphocytes, which are characteristic of the disease.

Pathology

Early in the disease both B- and T-lymphocytes are stimulated by viral infection and undergo hyperplasia; later, only T-lymphocytes are affected. The result is hyperplasia of lymphoid tissue in lymph nodes, tonsils and adenoids, and spleen. In histologic sections from these sites, collections of atypical lymphocytes are common, especially around small blood vessels, and can mimic lymphoma or Hodgkin's disease. Similar cells have been described in foci in the marrow and the liver.

Hematologic findings

The importance of the blood picture in infectious mononucleosis is to distinguish it from that of leukemia. The two have clinical and morphologic similarities that sometimes make it difficult to distinguish them from one another. The characteristic finding in infectious mononucleosis is absolute lymphocytosis (Fig. 13-36). At least 20% of the lymphocytes are of the atypical variety. These cells are large, with an oval or kidney-shaped nucleus and a characteristic deep blue cytoplasm. Usually the total white blood cell count is between 10,000 and 20,000/μL. The hemoglobin is usually normal,

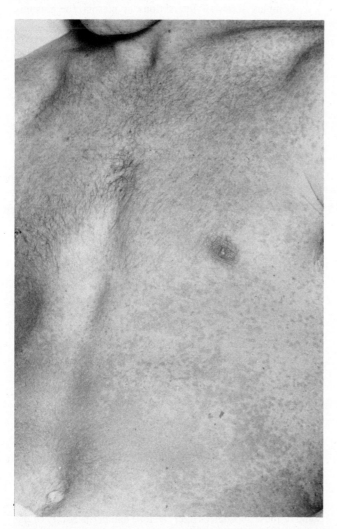

FIG. 13-37. Infectious mononucleosis. This patient has a prominent macular rash. Such rashes are not always present in infectious mononucleosis or may be faint and transient. *(Courtesy Curator of the Gordon Museum, Guy's Hospital, London, England.)*

but there may be a reduction in the platelet count. Rarely, thrombocytopenia may be severe, resulting in purpura.

Serology

The serologic changes are due to specific and nonspecific B-cell stimulation. A *heterophile antibody* is one that interacts with the cells of another species. In infectious mononucleosis the heterophile antibody agglutinates the red blood cells of sheep and other ungulates. Such an antibody is present in about half the patients in the first week of the illness, and this increases to about 80% by the fifth or sixth week. Antibodies to several EBV antigens can be demonstrated in virtually every patient, but have no relationship to the heterophile antibody.

Clinical aspects

A wide range of clinical effects can be attributed to infection by EBV. The vast majority of cases develop acute mononucleosis. A much smaller group has been recognized recently as having chronic forms of mononucleosis. Rarely, when individuals who have an X-linked defect in T- and killer lymphocyte function become infected with EBV, serious or fatal disease is the outcome. This inherited defect is called *X-linked lymphoproliferative syndrome*.

The typical features of acute infectious mononucleosis are fever, exudative tonsillitis, lymphadenopathy, rash (Fig. 13-37), and splenomegaly. Petechiae at the junction of the hard and soft palate are common. Liver function is almost invariably abnormal when tested biochemically, but jaundice is rare and always mild. The disease is often self-limiting within 3 to 6 weeks. Complications are rare and are usually in the nervous system. Guillain-Barré syndrome is perhaps the most serious complication (Chapter 18).

Physicians have reluctantly recognized chronic infectious mononucleosis, or perhaps more accurately, chronic EBV infection, because of the vague nature of the illness and the relative lack of definitive signs and symptoms. However, it is now accepted that after EBV infection, certain individuals, mainly adults in their twenties, develop a syndrome of low-grade fever, fatigue, and lethargy lasting up to a year or more. The main objective evidence for this syndrome is serologic; namely, an antibody titer to the early antigen of EBV of greater than 5 (1:5) and against viral capsid antigen of 160 or greater. There is no specific treatment for either the acute or chronic form of this disease. However, recognizing chronic EBV infection may be a valuable diagnostic achievement if it prevents unnecessary investigations or the presumption of psychiatric illness.

Cat-scratch disease

Cat-scratch disease is an illness of varying severity that usually follows a scratch by a cat. It may also follow puncture of skin by a plant thorn, but of course, the plant may have been infected by a passing cat! Recent evidence based on special staining and immunologic methods points to an unspecified bacterium in the primary lesions and lymph nodes as the causative organism.

In a typical case, the inflammatory reaction at the site of the skin injury is trivial, but after 1 to 2 weeks or occasionally after several months, the regional lymph nodes, usually in the neck, become painful, enlarged, red, and tense. The enlargement is sometimes gross. The lymph nodes soften and become fluctuant and suppurate in at least half the cases.

Histologically, the lymph nodes show a distinctive granulomatous reaction consisting of irregular or stellate abscess formation, containing in its center debris and fragments of leukocyte nuclei. Around the periphery histiocytes and fibroblasts proliferate, sometimes with giant cells. There is also a peripheral rim of lymphocytes and plasma cells. Although this histologic picture is distinctive, an identical histologic appearance is found in *lymphogranuloma venereum,* and *tularemia.* The diagnosis of cat-scratch disease is supported by a skin test (Rose-Hanger test). The antigen for this test consists of sterilized cat-scratch pus. Staining of affected lymph node tissue sections with the Warthin-Starry silver stain may show the suspected agent within the stellate abscesses or close to small blood vessels. The organisms appear as black-staining, pleomorphic rods. Culture of the organisms has not been consistently successful.

Cat-scratch disease is usually benign and self-limiting, with only mild systemic symptoms. Occasionally symptoms are more severe, with conjunctivitis (Parinaud's syndrome) or hyperpyrexia. In the vast majority of cases there is spontaneous remission, but death from meningitis has been reported.

SPLENOMEGALY

Enlargement of the spleen (splenomegaly) accompanies many pathologic processes. Rarely do these processes arise primarily in the spleen itself. Clinically, an enlarged spleen is an important physical sign that may indicate any of a wide range of diseases. The main cause of splenomegaly are listed in the box below.

CAUSES OF SPLENOMEGALY

I. Infective
   a. Parasitic
      1. Malaria
      2. Leishmaniasis
      3. Schistosomiasis
   b. Fungal
      1. Histoplasmosis
   c. Bacterial
      1. Brucellosis
      2. Infective endocarditis
   d. Viral
      1. Cytomegalovirus
      2. Infectious mononucleosis
   e. Infective
      1. Sarcoidosis
II. Circulatory
   a. Portal hypertension from any cause
III. Collagen-vascular disease
   a. Juvenile rheumatoid arthritis
   b. Systemic lupus erythematosis
IV. Hematologic disease
   a. Hemolytic anemias
   b. Leukemias: lymphomas
   c. Myeloproliferative disorders
V. Metabolic abnormalities
   a. Gaucher's disease
   b. Glycogen storage disease
   c. Niemann-Pick disease

DISORDERS OF HEMOSTASIS

Normal hemostatic mechanisms

If an ideal specification for human hemostatic mechanisms were to be written, it might be as follows:
1. Blood should remain liquid in the normal intact person.
2. When vessels are damaged, the response must be rapid enough to prevent major blood loss, be confined to the area of injury only, and permit final restoration of vessel wall integrity and blood flow.

Despite the complex reactions required of the hemostatic processes by this specification, the astonishing fact is that in the normal person they are indeed achieved unless the injury to blood vessels is very severe. In these circumstances, the specification must permit the assistance of a surgeon to control bleeding.

Processes contributing to the hemostatic process are:
1. Blood vessels contract proximal to the bleeding site, conserving blood and promoting stasis.
2. Platelets adhere to the blood vessel wall at the site of injury and to each other, forming an initial plug in the damaged vessel.
3. Fibrin is deposited at the injury site as a result of a complex series of interactions of plasma components, resulting in the conversion of fibrinogen to fibrin.
4. Retraction of the fibrin-platelet mass around the injury site is caused by contractile proteins produced by platelets.
5. Excessive amounts of fibrin are removed by a fibrinolytic mechanism, which comes into play almost simultaneously with coagulation.
6. The vascular integrity is restored by fibroblastic activity and endothelial proliferation.

To fully appreciate this sequence of events and its significance when abnormal, it is necessary to understand in more detail the role of platelets, fibrin formation, and fibrinolysis.

Platelets in hemostasis

Platelets are derived from the cytoplasm of mature megakaryocytes in the marrow; it is believed that their production is regulated by a hormone, *thrombopoietin.* The main function of platelets is in the hemostatic process. When endothelium is damaged, platelets rapidly adhere to it and to each other, thus forming a plug for damaged vessels. In the first stage of platelet adherence several stimuli cause platelets to become stickier by altering their surface properties. This effect may be initiated by exposure to collagen, thrombin, or antigen-antibody complexes. Prostaglandins can affect platelet activation either by stimulation of the process by thromboxane A_2 or inhibition by prostacyclin. Platelet activation is mediated by adenosine diphosphate (ADP) derived from tissue, red blood cells, or other platelets (Fig. 13-38).

At this point the reaction is still reversible, but under the influence of thrombin, an irreversible stage is reached when the platelets form a sticky mass in the damaged vessel. These irreversibly altered platelets not only seem to provide a nidus on their surface for coagulation to take place but also release factors affecting hemostasis in their immediate environment. Some of these substances alter the tone and permeability of the blood vessels, some promote the retraction of formed clots, and others have important effects on coagulation. These factors include platelet factors 3 and 4. Platelet factor 3 is not a biologic

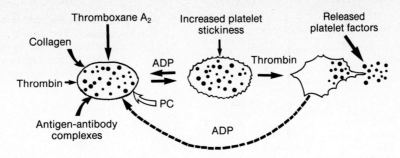

FIG. 13-38. Diagram of platelet aggregation by antigen-antibody complexes, thrombin, or thromboxane A_2. The process is inhibited by prostacyclin *(PC)*. *ADP*, Adenosine diphosphate.

compound; rather, it describes an alteration in the platelet surface properties that can then act as a catalytic site for the coagulation process. Platelet factor 4 is a protein, which binds to heparin and neutralizes its anticoagulant effect. ADP is also released by irreversibly altered platelets and can then activate more platelets.

Normal coagulation

Fibrinogen is present in circulating blood as a soluble protein. The result of the coagulation process is its conversion to insoluble polymerized fibrin. The development of our understanding of this remarkable process still goes on and much remains to be learned.

The current terminology of the various factors involved in coagulation is given in Table 13-11. In the 1960s a hypothesis of blood coagulation was proposed that likened the process to an electronic cascade, rather than a waterfall, in that it allowed for increasing velocity and amplification of reactions at different stages (McFarlane, 1964; Davie and Ratnoff, 1964). Although some of the assumptions made in this hypothesis have had to be revised, it had considerable practical value in the clinical investigation and treatment of hemostatic disorders. More recent investigations have shown that components of the kallikrein-kinin system (Chapter 6) also have a role in coagulation. The coagulation scheme given in Fig. 13-39 is a modification of the cascade mechanism and takes into account that certain procoagulant proteins are zymogens capable of being converted to active enzymes. For example, inactive factor XII is converted to an active enzyme, factor XIIa. Basic to this hypothesis and now generally accepted are the two pathways of coagulation, the intrinsic and the extrinsic.

The *extrinsic pathway* is activated by tissue factor released from damaged cells. It may also be activated by kallikrein and other proteolytic activators. This pathway can be mimicked in vitro by the addition of phospholipid-rich materials called *thromboplastins* and calcium salts to plasma. Thromboplastins are usually prepared from mammalian brain. This in vitro procedure is the basis for the prothrombin time test, which is used extensively in the investigation and management of hemostatic disorders.

The intrinsic pathway is activated by exposure of blood to certain abnormal surfaces. In vivo, collagen or fibrin can initiate the intrinsic pathway as can kallikrein in the presence of Fitzgerald factor (high molecular weight kininogen); in vitro a similar effect can be achieved by exposing plasma to kaolin or glass and adding calcium salts. The partial thromboplastin time, discussed later in this chapter, is based on such a procedure. Fitzgerald and Fletcher factors, which are involved in the initial stages of the intrinsic pathway, are components of the kallikrein-kinin system (Chapter 4) and form yet another link between fundamental mechanisms of defense—coagulation and inflammation. Both intrinsic and extrinsic pathways converge to a final common pathway that begins with the activation of factor X and ends with the formation of insoluble polymerized fibrin. Calcium ions and platelet factor 3 (PF3) are essential at several stages of the coagulation process.

Fibrinolysis

There are mechanisms that break down fibrinogen and fibrin. A scheme of fibrinolysis is shown in Fig. 6-8. This scheme, like that of coagulation, also involves inactive precursors that are converted to active enzymes. The conversion of plasminogen, an inactive plasma β-globulin to the powerful proteolytic enzyme plasmin, is the penultimate step and is followed by fibrinolysis. It is noteworthy that conversion of factor XII to XIIa is involved in the early stages of both coagulation and fibrinolysis.

Physiologically, the fibrinolytic system should be in balance with the production of fibrin. There should therefore be neither excessive deposition of fibrin nor excessive destruction of fibrin or fibrinogen. If there is a great imbalance between coagulation and fibrinolysis, the consequences may be very serious. This may happen as a result of several pathologic states. The consequent abnormalities of coagulation and fibrinolysis have been

TABLE 13-11. Coagulation factors and synonyms

Factor	Synonym
I	Fibrinogen
II	Prothrombin
IIa	Thrombin
III	Tissue thromboplastin
IV	Calcium ions
V	Ac-globulin
VII	Proconvertin, stable factor
VIII	Antihemophilic factor (globulin)
IX	Antihemophilic factor B; Christmas factor
X	Stuart-Prower factor
XI	Plasma prothrombin antecedent (PTA)
XII	Hageman factor
XIII	Fibrin-stabilizing factor
Fitzgerald	High molecular weight kininogen (HMWK)
Fletcher	Prekallikrein

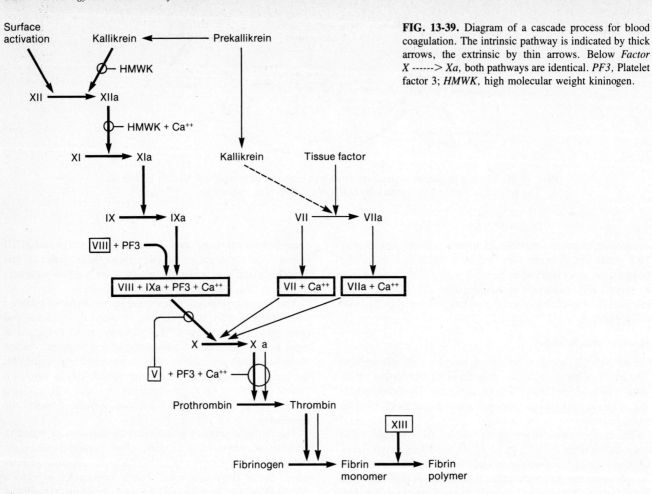

FIG. 13-39. Diagram of a cascade process for blood coagulation. The intrinsic pathway is indicated by thick arrows, the extrinsic by thin arrows. Below *Factor X ------> Xa*, both pathways are identical. *PF3*, Platelet factor 3; *HMWK*, high molecular weight kininogen.

TABLE 13-12. Basic laboratory tests for assessment of hemostasis*

Test	Function
Bleeding time	Platelet function and capillary vessel integrity
Prothrombin time (PT)	Extrinsic coagulation pathway
Activated partial thromboplastin time (APTT)	Intrinsic coagulation pathway
Fibrin split products	Fibrinolytic system activity
Platelet count	Platelet production and consumption
Platelet function tests	Mainly aggregation (by ADP, ristocetin, and other compounds)

*The whole blood clotting time test is uninformative and obsolete; however, visual observation of a clotting sample for the appearance, retraction, or speed of lysis of the clot can be clinically valuable.

TABLE 13-13. Interpretation of combined prothrombin and activated partial thromboplastin times

PT	APTT	Interpretation
Normal	Normal	Normal coagulation
Prolonged	Normal	Extrinsic abnormality above X->Xa
Normal	Prolonged	Intrinsic abnormality above X->Xa
Prolonged	Prolonged	Abnormality below X->Xa or multifactor abnormality

included under the commonly used but inadequate term, disseminated intravascular coagulation, described later.

Controlling mechanisms of coagulation

Equally important to the coagulation and fibrinolytic pathways are the mechanisms that control them and about which much less is known. Recently, however, *protein C*, a vitamin K–dependent glycoprotein, has been shown to have controlling properties on coagulation and fibrinolysis. Another recent discovery is *thrombomodulin*, a protein that appears to be responsible for binding thrombin to endothelial surfaces. Protein C is activated by thrombin alone or by a thrombin-thrombomodulin complex; activated protein C (protein Ca) has several effects, including inactivating factors Va and VIIIa and promotion of thrombolytic activity. Inactivation of factors Va and VIIIa is enhanced by a coenzyme to protein C, known as *protein S*.

Cases of protein C and protein S deficiency have already been described. These rare individuals have thrombotic and thromboembolic disease. Much remains to be learned of the role of these controller substances in coagulation and fibrinolysis.

Assessment of hemostatic function

Numerous tests have been devised to assess the function of the four contributing components of the hemostatic process, that is, blood vessels, platelets, coagulation, and fibrinolysis. Tests for the specific activity of controlling factors such as proteins C and S are not yet generally available.

Table 13-12 lists the more common tests and their functions. These investigations require considerable technical expertise to perform reliably, and test results must always be interpreted in light of the patient's history and physical findings.

Although a detailed discussion of these tests is not appropriate here, two tests already mentioned—the prothrombin time and the activated partial thromboplastin time—are of fundamental value in the investigation of patients and are worth further consideration.

The prothrombin time (PT) is the time taken for a clot to form when citrated plasma is mixed with a standardized tissue extract, such as animal brain and calcium ions. The normal PT is usually around 12 seconds and measures the activity of all the factors in the extrinsic pathway (*thin lines*, Fig. 13-38).

The partial thromboplastin time (PTT) is the time taken for a clot to form when citrated plasma (which has been mixed with kaolin and phospholipid to activate factor XII) is clotted with calcium ions. This test is also (and more accurately) known as the *cephalin-kaolin time*. The "normal" PTT is between 32 and 46 seconds and measures the function of the intrinsic pathway (*thick line*, Fig. 13-39). Prolongation of the PTT usually indicates a defect along that pathway. By combining the results of the PT and PTT an assessment can be made of the stage in the coagulation pathway at which an abnormality is present (Table 13-13).

HEMORRHAGIC DISORDERS

Disease characterized by hemorrhage can be due to defects in one or more of the factors that contribute to normal hemostasis, that is, the blood vessels, platelets, and coagulation. Vascular defects, however, are an uncommon cause of hemorrhagic disease.

Purpura is subcutaneous bleeding. An ecchymosis, or bruise, is a localized area of purpura caused by a blow. A *hematoma* by contrast, is a mass formed of effused blood.

Purpura and bruising are cardinal signs of many diseases that are characterized by platelet deficiency or defects or, more rarely, by vascular defects. It is important to distinguish between the purpuras and diseases in which the coagulation pathways are intact. In platelet or vascular abnormalities, bleeding after trauma may be excessive but eventually stops spontaneously. When coagulation mechanisms are abnormal (i.e., a coagulopathy is present), especially in hemophilia, bleeding may be delayed in onset, but then is prolonged and, if untreated, may eventually be fatal. Patients with coagulopathies have normal vessels and platelets; it is therefore possible to perform a venepuncture on a hemophiliac without causing serious hemorrhage. Von Willebrand's disease, described later, is an exception to these generalizations. This disease has both a platelet abnormality and a clotting factor deficiency (factor VIII). In most cases, the platelet defect predominates and purpura is the usual consequence.

Hemorrhagic diseases due to vascular defects

There are numerous causes of bleeding due to vascular defects but most of them are rare. Among the more important are:

1. Anaphylactoid purpura
2. Symptomatic purpura
3. Senile purpura

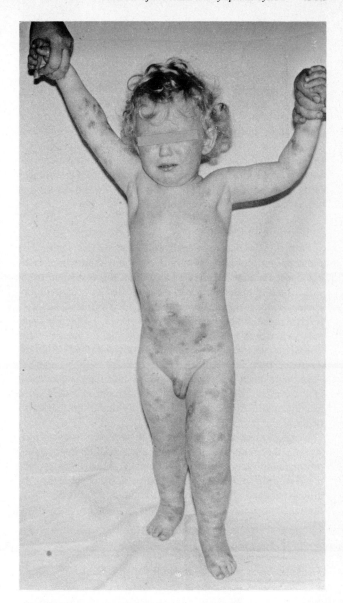

FIG. 13-40. Henoch-Schönlein purpura. The purpuric rash in this disease is typically on the lower abdomen and legs.

4. Hereditary telangiectasia

In these and other vascular defects bleeding is usually into the skin as *petechiae,* which are tiny pinpoint hemorrhages, or as bruising. Bleeding into joints, muscles, and the gastrointestinal tract is unusual.

Anaphylactoid purpura

Anaphylactoid purpura (Henoch-Schönlein purpura*), mainly found in children 12 years old or younger, is characterized by a generalized vasculitis that appears to be caused by a hypersensitivity reaction. Like rheumatic fever, it may be preceded by streptococcal pharyngitis. Other precipitating conditions include vaccinations, respiratory tract infections, and insect bites. Remarkably, the main effects of anaphylactoid purpura are on the lower part of the body (Fig. 13-40). Bleeding

*E. Henoch (1820-1910), German physician; J. Schönlein (1793-1864), German physician.

into the intestine wall causes abdominal colic. Joint pains are typically present, and about half the patients develop glomerulonephritis, with hematuria and proteinuria.

The pathogenesis of this disease is still not known, but evidence suggests that it may be due to IgA immune complexes. The pathologic changes in the skin lesions are nonspecific and consist of acute vasculitis, platelet thrombi, and perivascular hemorrhage. In the kidney, there is focal or diffuse glomerulonephritis with deposits of immunoglobulins, fibrin, and C3 fragment of complement in the mesangium. Most patients recover completely, although many have one or two recurrences of the disease before it finally resolves. A few, however, may progress to chronic glomerulonephritis.

Symptomatic purpura

Severe infections, particularly those with septicemia, can cause purpuric rashes. Purpura is especially common in meningococcemia and infective endocarditis, but is also an occasional finding in scarlet fever, measles, and infectious mononucleosis. It is also a feature of exotic infections such as Lassa fever, dengue, and other hemorrhagic fevers. Purpura is common in newborn infants who have congenital cytomegalovirus disease or rubella. In can also be a manifestation of AIDS, as discussed later.

In some instances, purpura due to infection is the result of toxic effects on the capillary endothelium; in others, such as congenital rubella, it is at least partly due to thrombocytopenia.

Drugs of many classes may produce purpura as a side effect. Among the more common drugs are antiinflammatory-antiprostaglandin agents and antihistamines. Most cases are the result of drug idiosyncrasies and purpura disappears when the drug is stopped. Purpuric drug reactions may also be due to thrombocytopenia, if they injure the bone marrow or act as haptens (Chapter 7).

Scurvy is one of the diseases in which purpura is common. Scurvy is due to severe deficiency of ascorbic acid (vitamin C), resulting in impairment of synthesis of collagen, dentine, osteoid, and intercellular substance. The pathogenesis is discussed in Chapter 5. Some patients will also have a normochromic, normocytic anemia due to the lack of vitamin C affecting hemopoiesis.

Senile purpura

This is the most common form of purpura and is found with increasing frequency in men and women from the sixth decade on. Pathologically, there is atrophy of skin collagen, mainly on the extensor aspects of the hands and forearms. The resultant loss of support for small vessels makes them readily damaged by minor trauma. The main significance of the abnormality is that is must be distinguished from more serious causes of purpura.

Hereditary telangiectasia (Osler-Weber-Rendu disease)*

This uncommon disease is inherited as an autosomal dominant trait and is characterized by widespread abnormalities, especially in small veins. These vessels are thin and deficient in extravascular collagen and form tangled masses lined by flat endothelial cells. These vessels lack normal contractility and thus one of the important hemostatic mechanisms. The vascular lesions are found in skin and mucous membranes throughout the body, including the nose and mouth (Fig. 13-41), bronchi, gastrointestinal tract, and vagina.

Clinically, the severity of the disease varies. In more serious cases, bleeding, especially from the nose, may result in anemia, severe bleeding, and even death.

---

*Sir W. Osler (1849-1919), Canadian physician; F.P. Weber (1850-1960), English physician; H. Rendu (1844-1902), French physician.

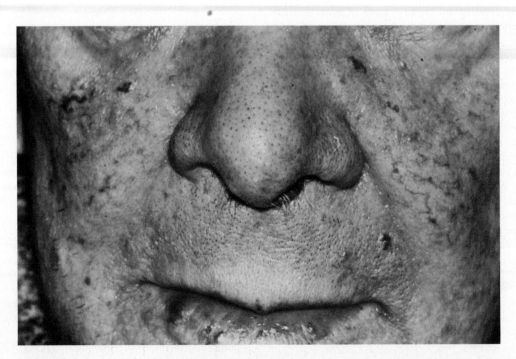

FIG. 13-41. Hereditary capillary telangiectasis. Characteristic angiomatoid lesions are present on the lips and face. *(Courtesy Curator of the Gordon Museum, Guy's Hospital, London, England.)*

Hemorrhagic diseases due to platelet defects
General considerations

Platelets may be defective in number or function. Reduction of blood platelets to less than 100,000/μL is called *thrombocytopenia*. However, it should be noted that even with electronic blood cell counters, there may be errors in platelet counting. Low platelet counts should always be correlated with examination of a stained blood smear. There is no fixed relationship between platelet count and tendency to hemorrhage, but spontaneous bleeding is uncommon unless the platelet count falls below 40,000/μL.

Platelets perform the following functions:

1. Form a hemostatic plug
2. Have a major function in coagulation
3. Are essential for clot retraction
4. Maintain endothelial integrity

Defects in these functions may cause hemorrhagic disease.

Most causes of thrombocytopenia can be assigned to either decreased production or increased destruction of platelets. A few are of complex or unknown cause. Common causes are:

1. Drugs, which are the most common
2. Autoimmune disease (idiopathic thrombocytopenic purpura)
3. Other blood diseases
   a. Aplastic anemia
   b. Megaloblastic anemia
   c. Leukemia
4. Infections
5. Disseminated intravascular coagulation

Drug-induced thrombocytopenia

At least 60 drugs can cause thrombocytopenia; 100 more have been associated with thrombocytopenia but necessary evidence is still lacking. Some drugs, such as quindine, for unknown reasons, stimulate the production of antibodies to platelets. Platelets that have been sensitized by these antibodies are

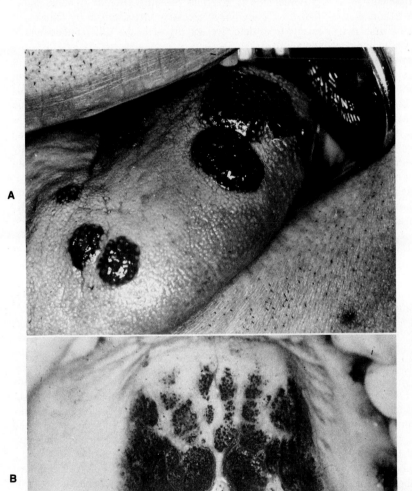

FIG. 13-42. Striking purpuric spots on the tongue **(A)** and palate **(B)** in a patient with idiopathic thrombocytopenic purpura. *(From Cawson RA: Essentials of dental surgery, ed 3, Edinburgh, Scotland, 1978, Churchill Livingstone.)*

then removed from the circulation by the macrophage-mono-cyte system, leading to thrombocytopenia. Other drugs act as haptens and when attached to a carrier molecule become antigenic and stimulate antibodies. These attach nonspecifically to platelets, which are then removed from the circulation by action of macrophages.

Clinically, the effects of drug-induced thrombocytopenia vary, from a mild chronic condition to a rapidly developing severe disease with oral mucous membrane hemorrhage, as can be seen with quinidine.

Idiopathic thrombocytopenic purpura

Pathogenesis. Although the basic cause is unknown, the pathogenesis of idiopathic thrombocytopenic purpura (ITP) in most cases depends on the presence of platelet IgG antibodies on the surface of the platelet. This results in the sequestration of platelets in large numbers in the spleen and liver. Thus splenectomy may only partially reduce the degree of platelet deficiency. However, since the spleen may be a source of the platelet antibody, its removal may be justified in patients in whom the disease persists beyond 3 months despite treatment.

In ITP the platelets are reduced and the bleeding time is prolonged. The bone marrow contains many normal-looking or large megakaryocytes, but special techniques may show that they are antibody coated. ITP is a common feature of AIDS.

Clinical aspects. Spontaneous bleeding, especially into the skin, is the most frequent manifestation (Fig. 13-42). In children, in whom the disorder is more acute, cerebral hemorrhage is the greatest threat, especially early in the illness. A chronic form of the disease in which bleeding persists beyond 6 months usually affects young adult women. Most patients with the acute form of the disease recover in time, regardless of treatment. These patients are usually managed with corticosteriods and platelet transfusions when necessary. The more chronic cases may respond to splenectomy. The use of aspirin and dental procedures should be avoided in these patients because of the risk of severe hemorrhage. Between 10% and 20% are unresponsive to treatment currently available.

Defects in platelet function

Platelet function can be defective in the following ways:
1. Adhesion may be diminished
2. Primary aggregation may be impaired
3. Release of ADP (Fig. 13-38) may be defective

Defects may be inherited or acquired; the former are uncommon. One example is the Bernard-Soulier syndrome in which platelet adhesiveness is defective because of abnormalities of the cell membrane glycoprotein 1b. The platelets may be greatly enlarged and reduced in number. Severe bleeding may result from these platelet abnormalities.

Abnormal platelet aggregation is characteristic of *thrombasthenia* (Glanzmann's disease). Here the defect lies in glycoproteins IIb and IIIa on the platelet cell membrane. This results in a prolonged bleeding time and greatly impaired aggregation of platelets, when they are exposed to ADP in vitro.

Thrombasthenia can give rise to severe bleeding into skin, mucous membranes and soft tissues in almost any site in the body. Surgery of any kind in these patients can lead to life-threatening bleeding. Even when clots form, the clot retraction mechanism fails.

Defective release of ADP by platelets is most commonly associated with drugs. Aspirin is by far the most important because of its universal use; others inlcude indomethacin and phenylbutazone. Aspirin blocks the synthesis of cyclic endo-peroxidase, thereby inhibiting the synthesis of thromboxane A2, a potent stimulator of platelet activation.

This effect is permanent for the life of each platelet affected by aspirin. The importance of avoiding aspirin in any condition in which there is a bleeding tendency should be self-evident. Aspirin prolongs the bleeding time in normal persons and alone can occasionally cause postoperative bleeding.

DEFECTS OF COAGULATION

Defects of coagulation are inherited or acquired. The important inherited disorders are hemophilia A and B and von Willebrand's syndrome. Among the acquired disorders are those caused by vitamin K deficiency, liver disease, anticoagulant therapy, and the complex syndrome of disseminated intravascular coagulopathy.

Hemophilia A

Hemophilia is a serious bleeding disorder of males transmitted as a sex-linked recessive characteristic by females; it results from defective activity of factor VIII (antihemophilic globulin).

Factor VIII is an unstable glycoprotein currently believed to be synthesized in the liver. Factor VIII is a vital procoagulant component of the intrinsic coagulation pathway. It usually circulates in plasma, forming a complex with another very large protein molecule, the von Willebrand factor (vWF), which is discussed later. Factor VIII is found in freshly drawn human plasma, but has no activity in serum, and its activity is rapidly lost unless plasma is kept frozen. Current terminology relating to factor VIII and its properties is as follows:
1. The procoagulant protein is designated factor VIII and circulates noncovalently bonded to vWF, forming a VIII/vWF complex.
2. When factor VIII participates in immune reactions, it is called *factor VIII antigen* (VIII:Ag).
3. When factor VIII coagulant activity or function is assessed, it is called *factor VIII coagulant* (VIII:C).
4. When factor VIII coagulant activity (VIII:C) is lost after normal plasma clots, factor VIII:Ag is still present.

Pathogenesis and pathology

The pathologic effects of hemophilia are directly due to recurrent hemorrhages, which can be either spontaneous or the result of trauma. In severely affected patients, bleeding into joints and muscles, especially of the lower limb, can cause destructive changes (Fig. 13-43). Initially intracapsular joint hemorrhages can result in pain and limitation of movement, followed by fibrous and eventually bony ankylosis of major joints. Intramuscular bleeding leads to fibrous contracture of muscles; this combined with joint changes leads to crippling deformities.

Clinical aspects

Hemophilia is believed to affect about 1 in 25,000 of the population. A newborn infant with hemophilia shows little evidence of the disease unless some operative procedure, such as circumcision is attempted. Severe bruising, often from minimal trauma, is common in young children. Typically, there is a delay between the injury and the onset of bleeding, since platelet function is normal (Fig. 13-44). Bleeding into critical areas, especially into the brain, may be rapidly fatal. Spontaneous bleeding into joints develops only when factor VIII:C level is less than 5%.

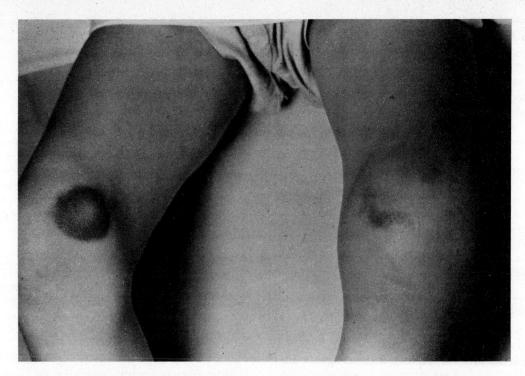

FIG. 13-43. Hemophilia. There is swelling of the right knee joint due to hemarthrosis and bruising on the right. Hemarthrosis is a frequent and serious complication of hemophilia. *(Courtesy Curator of the Gordon Museum, Guy's Hospital, London, England.)*

In the more severe forms of the disease the diagnosis is suggested by the history of spontaneous bruising or bleeding. A family history of hemophilia is lacking in about 40% of cases. The significant laboratory findings that establish the diagnosis are a prolonged APTT (with a normal PT) and greatly reduced levels of factor VIII:C.

Successful management of the hemophiliac patient may require the orchestrated skills of hematologists, surgeons, dentists, and other clinical disciplines expert in the management of the disease.

Specific treatment is to infuse factor VIII in the form of a lyophilized (freeze-dried) concentrate or as cryoprecipitate. One serious risk in treatment has been the transmission of human immunodeficiency virus (HIV) and the later development of AIDS. This risk has largely been removed by heat treatment of factor VIII concentrates, a procedure that inactivates HIV. It does not, however, affect hepatitis B or non-A, non-B hepatitis viruses, which can also be transmitted by these blood products.

About 7% of severe hemophiliacs develop antibodies to factor VIII. This creates great difficulties in treatment, since these antibodies inactivate to a variable degree, any factor VIII that has been given. Mild hemophiliacs may also be treated with 1-desamino-8-D-arginine vasopressin (DDAVP), a drug that appears to cause release of factor VIII, thus raising its levels in the circulation.

Surgical treatment, including dental surgery, should not be performed on hemophiliacs until they have received sufficient factor VIII to prevent hemorrhage. Factor VIII administration should be continued until healing is well advanced. The addition of epsilon-aminocaproic acid, an antifibrinolytic agent, reduces the amount of factor VIII that needs to be given for surgical treatment.

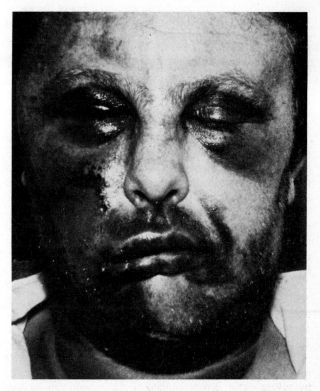

FIG. 13-44. Extensive deep soft tissue bleeding in patient with hemophilia following a local anesthetic injection. *(From Cawson RA: Essentials of dental surgery and pathology, ed 3, Edinburgh, Scotland, 1978, Churchill Livingstone.)*

Factor IX deficiency

Factor IX deficiency (Christmas disease,* hemophilia B), like hemophilia, is also a sex-linked recessive coagulation defect, but is about six times less common. One form of the disease (factor IX, Seattle 2) has been shown to be the result of a single adenine nucleotide deletion.

Factor IX deficiency is indistinguishable from hemophilia A, but it is essential that the nature of the defect be determined by factor IX assay in the laboratory, since the disease must be treated by replacement of factor IX and not by factor VIII, which is useless in these circumstances.

Factor IX is more stable than factor VIII, but is difficult and expensive to concentrate from donor blood. Plasma is a useful source of factor IX for the treatment of patients with hemophilia B. The risks of transmission of HIV and hepatitis viruses in the treatment of hemophilia B are similar to those in hemophilia A.

Other coagulation factor deficiencies

Inherited deficiencies or defects have been described for virtually all coagulant factors, including fibrinogen. Clinically, they are less severe than hemophilia A or B, but there is considerable variation from patient to patient. As with other bleeding disorders, the patient's history is the most important part of the investigation, followed by appropriate laboratory tests, which should include specific assays.

Von Willebrand's syndrome

Von Willebrand's syndrome describes a related group of inherited disorders that are due to abnormalities of the factor VIII molecule and in which purpura is the common clinical manifestation. Von Willebrand's syndrome differs from hemophilia in two main ways:

1. It is inherited as an autosomal dominant or occasionally autosomal recessive characteristic.
2. Both factor VIII:Ag and factor VIII:C are usually reduced in this syndrome, although either can occasionally be normal.

Based on the levels of factor VIII subunits, the mode of inheritance, and the results of platelet aggregation and other laboratory studies, eight subtypes of the syndrome have been recognized to date. In all varieties, there is abnormal endothelial and platelet function as well as factor VIII abnormalities.

Clinically, the syndrome is characterized by purpura, epistaxis, menorrhagia in women, and rapid onset of abnormal bleeding after surgery or trauma. Patients who inherit the disease as an autosomal recessive trait are the most severely affected.

All types of the syndrome have prolonged bleeding time and APTT with a normal PT. The platelet count is normal but platelet aggregation in the presence of ristocetin is usually abnormal. The von Willebrand factor, factors VIII:Ag, and VIII:C are reduced in several types.

The disease, however, is often mild and many cases do not require treatment. In more severe forms, bleeding is controlled by giving either cryoprecipitate or the vasopressin analog, DDVAP.

Remarkably, when patients are given cryoprecipitate or fresh plasma, their autologous production of factor VIII:C begins to

---

*Named after Martin Christmas, the first patient reported.

rise over the following 24 hours. It is thought that the transfused vWF stimulates the synthesis of factor VIII:C and protects its elimination.

Acquired defects of coagulation
Vitamin K deficiency

Vitamin K (from the German *koagulierung,* coagulation) is the precursor of prothrombin (factor II), and factors VII, IX, and X. Deficiency of vitamin K can cause severe hemorrhage. The deficiency may be the result of malabsorption, prolonged administration of oral antibiotics, and prolonged parenteral nutrition (hyperalimentation). The diagnostic feature of vitamin K deficiency is a prolonged PT corrected to normal by parenteral administration of vitamin K.

Liver disease

Severe liver disease is a frequent cause of impaired coagulation. It appears to be a combined effect of decreased hepatic synthesis of procoagulant proteins and an increased activity of proteolytic enzymes that the liver has failed to inactivate or remove.

Anticoagulant drugs

Drugs that interfere with coagulation are commonly used for the management of patients with thromboembolic disease. The two most important drugs are coumadin, which reduces the levels of factors II, VII, IX, and X, and heparin, which indirectly interferes with the coagulation cascade by its interaction with antithrombin, a plasma thrombin inhibitor. Through this interaction, heparin, even in low doses, inactivates other coagulation factors, particularly factor X.

Disseminated intravascular coagulopathy

This is a complex syndrome caused by a widespread triggering of coagulation and fibrinolysis within the circulation. Disseminated intravascular coagulation (DIC) can only be detected with certainty by use of a variety of laboratory procedures. However, experts disagree as to which laboratory tests best identify the condition, so a generally accepted definition on these grounds has not yet been formulated. It is now generally agreed that laboratory evidence of decreased fibrinogen and platelets, with an increase in the degradation products of fibrinogen and physical damage to circulating red blood cells, are typical findings.

Etiology. The triggering mechanism for DIC is the introduction into the circulation of various foreign substances, which may be the result of such diverse injuries as trauma, incompatible blood transfusion, or snakebite (see the box on p. 309).

DIC may also be associated with diseases in which tissue necrosis is severe, such as transplant rejection and hepatic necrosis. Severe infections, especially those caused by gram-negative bacteria, can trigger DIC as a result of release of bacterial endotoxin (Chapter 8). During childbirth or complicated abortions, amniotic fluid or even fragments of embryonic tissue may enter the circulation and initiate intravascular clotting. In incompatible blood transfusion, the transfused cells are lysed by antibody and complement, and the membranes of the lysed cells may trigger the coagulation system.

Pathogenesis and pathology. When intravascular coagulation begins on a large scale, excessive amounts of proteolytic enzymes, such as factor Xa and thrombin are generated. This causes widespread conversion of fibrinogen to fibrin in small blood vessels. Within a short time, circulating fibrinogen levels

---

COMMON CAUSES OF DISSEMINATED INTRAVASCULAR COAGULOPATHY

1. Incompatible blood transfusion
2. Severe trauma
3. Cardiopulmonary bypass
4. Obstetric complications
   a. Placenta previa
   b. Amniotic fluid embolus
   c. Intrauterine death
5. Bacteremia
   a. Gram-negative bacilli
   b. Meningococci
6. Disseminated carcinoma from the prostate, lung, or pancreas
7. Acute leukemia

---

fall as consumption outstrips production. Concurrently, there is intravascular aggregation of platelets, which are then removed from the circulation.

Although this is an oversimplified explanation, it can be seen that the results of DIC may be the following:

1. Fibrin is deposited in capillaries.
2. Plasma fibrinogen and other coagulation factors, including factors IX and XI, prekallikrein (Fletcher factor) and high molecular weight kininogen (Fig. 13-39) are reduced. This process is sometimes referred to as *consumption coagulopathy.*
3. The number of circulating platelets is reduced.

The above list is only part of the story. There is often simultaneous activation of the fibrinolytic process (Fig. 6-8) due to activator substances entering the bloodstream. Their effect is to convert plasminogen to plasmin. Plasmin may then lyse formed fibrin clots, as well as soluble fibrinogen. The hemorrhagic component of DIC results from:

1. Dissolution of clots, causing bleeding from wound sites.
2. A fall in the levels of circulating fibrinogen.
3. An increase in the amount of breakdown products of fibrin and fibrinogen. These *fibrin split products (fibrin degradation products)* are themselves anticoagulant and can increase the bleeding tendency.

When fibrin is deposited in small vessels, red blood cells are forced through the fibrin strands, causing physical damage to the red blood cells. The presence of these fragmented red cells (schistocytes) in the peripheral blood smear can often be demonstrated in DIC.

Intravascular clotting and fibrinolysis are commonly found together. Usually, one of the two processes predominates, but can be replaced by the other, so that a patient can have alternating episodes of clotting and bleeding. This variable behavior on the part of the coagulation and fibrinolytic systems, *when they are pathologically activated,* accounts for the difficulties in defining DIC and understanding its behavior in individual patients.

The pathologic consequences of DIC are superimposed on serious underlying diseases or trauma. Both acute and chronic forms of DIC are described. Generally, these terms apply to the speed of onset of the condition. For example, a chronic form of DIC may accompany acute myelocytic leukemia. However, chemotherapy, which is accompanied by release of products of cell destruction, may precipitate a severe acute form of DIC.

Shock is a frequent accompaniment of acute DIC and may present the most immediate danger to the patient. Excessive bleeding from sites of trauma, surgical wounds, or venepuncture is common. In severe cases, there may be signs of small vessel occlusion in the central nervous system.

Clinical aspects. The clinical picture is variable and confirmation of DIC rests on an expert performance and interpretation of laboratory tests of hemostatic function.

The management of DIC is first to recognize and vigorously treat the underlying cause and then to counteract shock. Heparin, platelet infusions, and transfusion of specific clotting factors have all been used to deal with the hemostatic defects. In view of the diverse nature of the causes and course of DIC, each case must be managed differently, and no single therapeutic regimen can be recommended.

Selected readings

Bateman CJ: Sideroblastic anemia, Arch Intern Med 140:1278, 1980.

Bennett JM et al: Proposed criteria for the classification of acute myeloid leukemia, Ann Intern Med 103:460, 1985.

Camitta BM, Storb R, and Thomas ED: Aplastic anemia: pathogenesis diagnosis, treatment, and prognosis, N Engl J Med 306:645, 712, 1981.

Carbone P et al: Report of the Committee on Hodgkin's staging classification, Cancer Res 31:1860, 1971.

Clouse LH and Comp PC: The regulation of hemostasis: the protein C system, N Engl J Med 314:1298, 1987.

Conley CL: Polycythemia vera, Hosp Pract 21:107, 1987.

Dacie JV: Autoimmune hemolytic anemia, Arch Intern Med 135:1293, 1975.

Davie EW and Ratnoff OD: Waterfall sequence for intrinsic blood clotting, Science 145:310, 1964.

de la Chapelle A: Chromosome anomalies in hematologic malignancies, Hosp Pract 21:121, 1986.

Fishleder AJ and Hoffman GC: A practical approach to the detection of hemoglobinopathies. I. The introduction and thalassemia syndromes, Lab Med 18:368, 1987.

Freireich EJ: Adult acute leukemia, Hosp Pract 21:91, 1986.

Gerard-Merchant R et al: Classification of non-Hodgkin's lymphoma, Lancet 2:406, 1974.

Gould J and Wu K: Coagulopathies in cancer, Tex Med 83:58, 1987.

Hart WN, Farber L, and Cadman E: Non-Hodgkin's lymphoma for the nononcologist, JAMA 253:1431, 1985.

Kaplan HS: Hodgkin's disease: biology, treatment, prognosis, Blood 57:813, 1981.

Karadia CP and Donaldson RM Jr: Disorders of cobalamin (vitamin B_{12}) absorption and transport, Annu Rev Med 36:93, 1985.

Knowles DM II: The human T-cell leukemias, Hum Pathol 17:14, 1986.

Kyle RA: Treatment of multiple myeloma, N Engl J Med 310:1382, 1984.

Lukes RJ and Collins RD: Immunologic characterisation of malignant lymphomas, Cancer 34:1488, 1974.

Lukes RJ et al: Hodgkin's disease: Report of Nomenclature Committee, Cancer Res 26:1311, 1966.

McFarlane RG: An enzyme cascade in the blood clotting mechanism and its function as a biochemical amplifier, Nature 202:498, 1964.

Nachman RL: Von Willebrand's disease: a clinical and molecular enigma, West J Med 136:319, 1982.

Purtilo DT: Epstein-Barr virus: the spectrum of its manifestations in human beings, South Med J 80:943, 1987.

Rappaport H: Tumors of the hemopoietic system. In Atlas of tumor pathology, fascicle 8, Washington DC, 1966, Armed Forces Institute of Pathology.

Report of the Working Committee: National Cancer Institute sponsored study of classification of non-Hodgkin's lymphomas: Summary and description of a working formulation for clinical usage, Cancer 49:2112, 1982.

Valentine WN, Tanaka KR, and Pagera DE: Hemolytic anemias and erythrocyte enzymopathies, Ann Intern Med 103:245, 1985.

CHAPTER 14

Diseases of the gastrointestinal tract

Diseases of the gastrointestinal tract are common, important, and varied in character. Historically speaking, gastrointestinal tract infections such as the dysenteries, cholera, and typhoid fever have caused huge epidemics throughout the world and remain a serious problem in developing countries. Even in the Western World few persons have managed to avoid infectious enteritis ("food poisoning") at some time in their lives. More serious problems are the widespread morbidity and not insignificant mortality caused by peptic ulcer. Cancer of the stomach and colon are among the more common forms of cancer that account for thousands of deaths each year in the United States alone.

Although the mouth forms the upper end of the gastrointestinal tract, diseases of the gastrointestinal tract rarely have obvious or significant manifestations in the mouth, apart from furring of the tongue, which is a nonspecific feature of many gastrointestinal tract disorders and various febrile illnesses.

Disease of the teeth (dental caries) and of the periodontal tissues are the most common human gastrointestinal tract diseases and are almost universal in developed countries. These diseases, although troublesome, rarely have serious effects on general health, but under certain circumstances bacteria from such sources can give rise to severe infections, particularly infective endocarditis (Chapter 11).

Anatomic and functional aspects

The anterior part of the mouth, which forms the entry to the gastrointestinal tract, has the same embryologic origin as the skin and shares many of the latter's diseases (Chapter 19). However, it serves for preparation of food by chewing and for initiation of swallowing. The mouth and teeth are also necessary for speech. The teeth can also, if necessary, also serve as weapons, and a human bite is particularly dangerous because of the great numbers of pathogens from periodontal pockets that can infect the wound.

The mouth is lined by stratified squamous epithelium that is only significantly keratinized on the dorsum of the tongue. It contains many minor salivary glands and the major salivary glands also empty into it. The saliva contains amylase, but this contributes little to digestion and its main function is lubricatory and defensive by helping to wash microbes towards the stomach. The saliva also contains IgA, but this too appears to have no significant protective function.

The muscles of the mouth are all voluntary apart from a little smooth muscle in the walls of blood vessels. This is in contrast to the rest of the gastrointestinal tract where there is only smooth muscle in the wall and the innervation (to maintain peristalsis) is autonomic.

The esophagus is also lined by stratified squamous epithelium and has a rich venous plexus in its walls which also contains mucous glands. It is continuous with the stomach at the lower esophageal sphincter.

The stomach has a lining of tubular glands which secrete mucus in the cardiac (junctional) mucosa but secrete acid pepsin in the body area. The gastric mucosa is protected from its digestive secretions by mucus secretion and bicarbonate ions; these form the mucosal barrier to which prostaglandin activity contributes. The gastric acid also has useful antibacterial activity.

Digestion is initiated in the stomach but few substances are digested. The stomach serves largely as a reservoir for and to propel onward food to the intestine. However, important functions of the stomach are the secretion of *intrinsic factor,* which is essential for the absorption of vitamin B_{12} in the small intestine. In addition, endocrine cells in the glandular layer of the gastric lining secrete vasoactive and other peptides as discussed later.

The small intestine is the main site of digestion of food to which end, intestinal glands, pancreatic secretions, and bile contribute. To present as large as possible an area for absorption, the jejunal mucosa is villous and the ileum is thrown into folds. The small intestine also has an autonomic innervation essential for peristalsis.

Endocrine cells secreting a variety of peptides are also present in the intestinal mucosa. In addition, there is lymphoid tissue in the intestinal wall much of which is aggregated in such sites as Peyer's patches and forms the gut (or mucosa) associated lymphoid tissue (GALT or MALT) as discussed later.

The small intestine ends at the ileocecal valve (strictly speaking, a sphincter). A few centimeters distal to the latter is the appendix, which is a diverticulum of the upper cecum with little function apart from its endocrine secretions.

The large intestine comprises the cecum, colon, and rectum. The lining is largely of mucous cells that line crypts. The function of the colon is mainly storage, fluid reabsorption, and excretion particularly of indigestible parts of the diet. Unlike the small intestine, which has a small indigenous bacterial flora, the large intestine has a vast bacterial population, which forms a significant part of the feces. In the newborn, the gut bacteria perform an essential function in synthesizing vitamin K (Chapter 13), which is absorbed with the help of bile in the small intestine. The bowel bacteria help to break down undigested food but otherwise seem to have little useful function in man and are a positive threat to life if the bowel perforates and peritonitis results.

Immunologic functions of the gut

The gastrointestinal tract needs to defend itself against very many kinds of assault ranging from microbes which have survived the gastric acid, to foods, and any toxic substances that they contain.

TABLE 14-1. Gut peptides

Peptide	*Origin*	*Action*
Gastrin	Gut	Stimulates gastric secretion
Cholecystokinin	Gut, brain	Stimulates gall bladder contraction; stimulates pancreatic enzyme secretion
Glucagon	Pancreas	Regulates carbohydrate metabolism
Enteroglucagon	Gut, brain	Trophic to gut; slows intestinal transit
Secretin	Gut	Stimulates pancreatic H_2CO_3 secretion
Gastric inhibitory polypeptide (GIP)	Small intestine	Stimulates insulin secretion; inhibits gastric acid secretion
Vasoactive intestinal polypeptide (VIP)	Central and peripheral nervous systems	Stimulates muscle relaxation, vasodilatation, secretion
Motilin	Small intestine	Stimulates gut motility
Pancreatic polypeptide	Pancreas	Inhibits pancreatic enzyme secretion and gall bladder contraction
Somatostatin	Gut, pancreas, thyroid, brain	Inhibits release of many peptides and hormones
Neurotensin	Gut, adrenal, brain	Vasodilatation; inhibits gastric secretion

The main immunologic defenses of the gut are secretory IgA and the gut-associated lymphoid tissue (GALT). Modified enterocytes (M cells) overlie lymphoid tissue (either in isolated follicles or aggregated in Peyer's patches) and transport antigens to macrophages, which process the material for presentation to the lymphocytes. IgA production is a typical response, and this immunoglobulin is transported across the lamina propria into the gut as dimers bound by a J chain and with a secretory component. A major function of IgA is to block the adherence of microbes to the gut wall.

In addition, there are intraepithelial effector (T) lymphocytes. The latter bear the CD4 (helper) or CD8 (cytotoxic) markers; in addition, there are natural killer (NK) lymphocytes. These, along with the cytotoxic T cells, probably contribute to defense against viral infections.

The intestinal lymphoid tissue is essentially a protective immunologic organ; therefore the gastrointestinal tract is a relatively rare target of immunologically mediated diseases. Food allergy is rare and the main autoimmune disease of the gastrointestinal tract is atrophic gastritis leading to pernicious anemia (Chapter 13); celiac disease appears to be an immunologic reaction, but the mechanisms are obscure.

Gut peptides. The gastrointestinal mucosa contains endocrine cells that secrete specific peptide hormones. These peptides control particular aspects of gastrointestinal function and may also have other effects. Neoplasms can also arise from these cells as described later.

The actions of the gut peptides are summarized in Table 14-1.

Disturbances of gut peptide levels are often of use in clarifying the pathogenesis or diagnosis of gastrointestinal diseases. Some of the more important examples are summarized in Table 14-2.

Investigation of gastrointestinal tract disease

The main techniques for investigation of gastrointestinal tract disease are as follows:

1. Physical examination helps to localize symptoms by finding points of tenderness, enlarged organs, or palpable masses.
2. Radiography is an essential part of the investigation of most complaints that arise from the digestive tract. Ra-

TABLE 14-2. Gut peptides in disease

Peptide	*Raised levels*	*Low levels*
Gastrin	Inhibitors of acid production*	—
	Gastrinomas	
Pancreatic polypeptide	Large bowel resection	Steatorrhea
Enteroglucagon	Steatorrhea	Large bowel resection, celiac disease
Motilin	Acute enteritis and diarrhea	—
Glucagon	Glucagonomas	—
Vasoactive intestinal peptide	Vipomas	—

*H2 antihistamines (cimetidine), vagotomy, antral resection, pernicious anemia (very high gastrin levels)

diographs may need to be taken with the patient in a variety of positions, and contrast media usually need to be used to reveal abnormalities such as ulcers and tumors.

3. Fiberoptic endoscopy allows the interior of the gastrointestinal tract to be clearly visualized. This makes it possible to quickly distinguish a cancer of the stomach from a peptic ulcer because a biopsy specimen can be taken at the same time. Endoscopy is now regarded as a routine investigation for most cases of gastrointestinal tract bleeding. Endoscopy has shown that nonspecific symptoms ("indigestion"), thought to have no organic cause, are in actuality due to peptic ulcer, carcinoma, or other lesions in an unexpectedly high proportion of patients.
4. Sigmoidoscopy is an important method of investigating cancer and other diseases of the colon. About 50% of colonic tumors can be visualized by this means. The colon can also be examined by fiberoptic endoscopy.
5. Biopsy is an essential supplement to endoscopy of any type, particularly in detecting the presence and type of malignant disease.
6. Secretion and absorption studies are of various types and include, for example, measurement of gastric acid secretion or the detection of malabsorption by the use of D-xylose.

7. Chemical studies are applied to feces for the detection of abnormal constituents such as occult blood or fat.
8. Microscopic investigation and bacterial culture are essential methods for investigation of infective diarrhea. The detection of intestinal parasites is based almost entirely on fecal examination.

Congenital anomalies of the gastrointestinal tract

Many congenital malformations of the gastrointestinal tract are possible but most are rare. The following are some important examples.

Esophageal stenosis

Congenital narrowing of the esophagus is uncommon. It causes dysphagia and early difficulty in feeding. Esophageal stenosis can also be acquired as a result for example of swallowing caustics or Barrett's esophagus and fibrosis.

Barrett's esophagus

Replacement of the normal squamous epithelial lining by columnar cells (the so-called Barrett's esophagus) is occasionally congenital and is discussed in more detail later.

Congenital hypertrophic pyloric stenosis

Congenital hypertrophic pyloric stenosis is a familial disorder which particularly affects males and may be found in approximately one in 500 live births.

Hypertrophied pyloric musculature forms an obstructive mass, which causes regurgitation of food, starting in the first week of life. A muscle splitting operation is curative.

Acquired pyloric stenosis is usually a complication of persistent peptic ulceration and usually causes regurgitation starting in middle age as discussed later.

Meckel's diverticulum

Meckel's diverticulum may reach a size of several centimeters or be no more than a mere cord, found proximal to the ileocecal valve. It is a remnant of the omphalomesenteric duct and its chief importance is that it can contain areas of gastric mucosa. The latter can ulcerate to cause pain and bleeding or perforate.

Other congenital diverticulae of the small intestine are relatively common but do not contain gastric mucosa or cause symptoms until late in life.

Congenital megacolon (Hirschsprung's disease)

Hirschsprung's disease is characterized by absence of ganglion cells due to failure of development of Meissner's and Auerbach's plexuses* along a variable length of the colon. The consequence is loss of peristalsis and paralytic obstruction particularly of the rectum and rectosigmoid colon.

Distention may be so rapid and severe as to cause thinning of the intestinal wall and extension of dilatation as far back as the small intestine. If less acute the bowel wall can undergo compensatory hypertrophy.

Clinically, the obstruction becomes apparent soon after birth as failure of passage of meconium, constipation and then vomiting and abdominal distension. Infection of the obstructed co-

---

*G. Meissner (1829-1905), German anatomist and physiologist; L. Auerbach (1828-1897), German neuropathologist.

lon, disturbance of fluid and electrolyte balance, and perforation are the chief threats to life.

Acquired (toxic) megacolon is chiefly a complication of fulminating ulcerative colitis or, less often, of Crohn's disease as discussed later. It can also result from severe infections such as typhoid fever or cholera causing extensive damage to the bowel wall.

Diseases of the mouth

Because the mouth is involved in gastrointestinal tract disease only to a limited extent, diseases of the oral cavity are presented only briefly in this chapter. Disease of the teeth and their supporting tissues account for most oral symptoms.

Dental caries

Dental caries is a bacterial infection and one of the most common of all diseases. Strains of *Streptococcus mutans* are widely believed to be the most important agents. The pathogenesis comprises:

1. Production of acid by bacteria, mainly from sugar, which must be available at frequent intervals to maintain a sufficiently low pH
2. Bacterial plaque, which consists mainly of adhesive polyglucans synthesized from sugars by bacteria enmeshed within it and prevents acid from diffusing away or being quickly buffered; plaque is cariogenic when deposited thickly in stagnation areas

The main factor known to affect the resistance of the teeth to bacteria is the fluoride ion. Where the drinking water contains at least 1 ppm of fluoride, caries activity is reduced by about 60%. Caries is not a disease of malnutrition. Where sugar is not eaten because of poverty, for instance, caries is uncommon although large amounts of carbohydrates are eaten. There is no evidence that so-called protective foods, such as dairy products or vitamin D, have any preventive effect. Caries can be most safely and effectively abolished by stopping the eating of refined sugar.

Pathology. The essential features of the pathology of dental caries are destruction of the calcified tissues of the teeth by acid, followed by invasion of the damaged tissue by bacteria.

Sequels of dental caries. After the dentin has been penetrated, bacteria can infect the pulp to cause pulpitis. Infection can spread from the pulp to the jaw and beyond with a wide variety of possible effects such as toothache.

Acute necrotizing ulcerative gingivitis

Acute necrotizing ulcerative gingivitis (ANUG) mainly affects young adults, many of whom are heavy smokers. It is an anaerobic infection, and direct smears from the depth of the lesion show *Borrelia vincentii* and fusobacteria in great numbers.

Clinically, ANUG is characterized by necrotizing ulceration, starting at the tips of the interdental papillae, spreading laterally along the gingival margins, and sometimes spreading deeply to destroy the interdental papillae and the crest of the alveolar bone.

Chronic gingivitis

Chronic gingivitis is a response to bacterial plaque at the gingival margins. It is widely believed that this inflammatory change initiates the destructive changes of the supporting tissues characteristic of chronic periodontitis. There is increasing interest in the activities of anaerobes and gram-negative bacteria such as *Bacteroides* species, clostridia, fusobacteria, and *Eikenella corrodens*. Many of these organisms produce enzymes, such as collagenase, capable of inflicting tissue damage and causing severe infections in other parts of the body.

Periodontitis

Periodontitis (pyorrhea), like dental caries, is almost universal. It is the chief cause of tooth loss in adults. Periodontitis is a chronic inflammatory disease that starts at the gingival margins (gingivitis) but goes on to destruction of the bone supporting the teeth and ultimately to loosening and loss of teeth.

Diseases of the oral mucous membrane

The oral mucous membrane is involved in mucocutaneous and other diseases (Chapter 19), but it is comparatively rarely affected by diseases of the gastrointestinal tract. The tongue is involved in many mucosal diseases, but there are some diseases peculiar to the tongue, of which the most important is glossitis resulting from anemia.

Oral leukoplakia and premalignant lesions

Leukoplakia is a purely clinical term used to describe a white, thickened area of the mucosa. The appearance of these plaques is a result of increased formation of keratin (hyperkeratosis). Causes include chronic abrasion, smoking, chronic candidosis, lichen planus, and rarely, now, syphilis. In many cases no cause can be found. The histologic changes vary from minor degrees of hyperplasia without significant disturbances of cell maturation to dysplasia or carcinoma in situ.

The importance of these lesions is that the risk of malignant change is increased, and a small minority of these lesions prove ultimately to be precancerous. The level of risk of malignant change is difficult to assess in individual cases.

In the past leukoplakia of the dorsum of the tongue was a well-recognized complication of tertiary syphilis and was relatively common. Estimates of the frequency of malignant changes in syphilitic leukoplakia have ranged from 30% to 100%, and it is probable that this has given rise to the impression that most oral leukoplakias are likely to be premalignant. However, surveys indicate that the risk of malignant change in leukoplakias is small unless there is histologic evidence of epithelial dysplasia.

Hairy leukoplakia. This recently described condition is seen in patients with human immunodeficiency virus (HIV) infection and may be followed by full-blown acquired immunodeficiency syndrome (AIDS) in 50% or more of those affected. Unlike oral thrush, hairy leukoplakia appears to be specific to HIV infection and may therefore be an important prognostic indicator.

Hairy leukoplakia was so called because fine filaments of keratin may protrude from the white plaque. This feature is, however, by no means always present and the lesion typically forms a soft white plaque with a corrugated surface and is most commonly distributed along the lateral margins or sometimes the ventral surface of the tongue.

Microscopically, hairy leukoplakia is characterized by a warty parakeratotic epithelial surface, acanthosis, and a scanty inflammatory infiltrate in the underlying connective tissue. Candidal infection may be associated in some cases, but the most striking feature is the presence of prominent subcorneal

koilocytes. The latter are large clear cells with shrunken darkly staining nuclei. Absolute confirmation of the diagnosis is reportedly made by detection of Epstein-Barr virus antigens in the epithelial cells where, it appears that the virus replicates.

Hairy leukoplakia may regress spontaneously or persist. It has been reported to respond to gancyclovir, an experimental antiviral drug effective against Epstein-Barr virus.

Erythroplasia. *Erythroplasia* is a clinical term for lesions of the oral mucosa that are red and often have a velvety excoriated appearance. These lesions are considerably less common than leukoplakias. They more frequently prove histologically to be dysplasia, carcinoma in situ, or invasive carcinoma. Lesions of this type (erythroplasia of Queyrat) also affect genital mucous membranes.

Cancer of the lip and mouth

Cancer of the mouth and lip account for approximately 2% of all cancers in the United States.

Etiology. Little is known about the cause of cancer of the mouth, but lip cancer is a hazard of prolonged exposure to sunlight. Outdoor workers, such as farmers and cattle hands, are particularly at risk. The risk is much increased in fair-skinned people, as natural pigmentation is protective. Therefore, cancer of the lip is more common in hot countries with a large population of fair-skinned people such as the southern United States and Australia. In the United States it has been calculated that the incidence of lip cancer doubles for every increment of 250 miles nearer the equator. Fishermen are also a high-risk group for lip cancer, but in this group some factor other than exposure to sunshine may be involved.

In the United States cancer of the mouth is ascribed to heavy cigarette smoking and excessive consumption of alcohol. However, it is remarkable that the great increase in cigarette smoking and alcohol consumption in Great Britain has not been associated with any comparable increase in mouth cancer but, rather, with a decline in its frequency.

However, the promotion and increasing use of so-called smokeless tobacco, held in the buccal pouch in the same manner as snuff dipping in the Southern United States, is causing concern. Use of tobacco in this way over a long period causes leukoplakia and is associated with an increased incidence of oral cancer. However, evidence has been presented to show that the incidence of oral cancer in the United States is increasing and that this increase started before widespread use of smokeless tobacco.

The incidence of oral cancer in India and Sri Lanka (Ceylon) is enormously high and in many parts of these countries is one of the most common kinds of cancer. Many believe that the disease is associated with the habit of so-called betel chewing. Betel usually consists of a mixture of areca nut, tobacco dust, and lime wrapped in a betel leaf.

Pathology. Oral cancers are well-differentiated squamous cell carcinomas in about 95% of cases. Spread is by local invasion and by the lymphatic system to the regional lymph nodes. The close proximity of so many vital structures of the head and neck means that these tumors need not spread far to cause dangerous complications and that sufficiently wide excision is difficult. The mortality rate from these tumors is high.

Clinical aspects. Lip cancer is overall more common than intraoral cancer; the tongue is the most frequently affected site in the mouth. The disease is age-related. Most patients are over 40, and the peak incidence is between ages 60 and 70. Lip cancer can, however, develop at a much earlier age in those frequently exposed to strong sunlight. A persistent crusting nodule on the lip, even as small as 5 mm across, is a carcinoma until proven otherwise by biopsy.

Early oral cancers are painless and inconspicuous so that the clinician needs to be unusually alert. In the later stages local invasion by the growth can cause gross tissue destruction. Severe pain, fixation of the tongue, and difficulty in speech and swallowing are characteristic. In neglected cases hemorrhage from an eroded vessel or sepsis and cachexia are well-recognized causes of death.

Treatment is by wide excision or radiotherapy, alone or in combination. The prognosis is poor except for lesions treated in the very early stages.

The 5-year survival rate for cancer of the lip is nearly 80%, but for cancer of the tongue only about a third of the patients survive for up to 5 years. The further back the lesion is, the worse the prognosis, almost certainly because of late diagnosis.

Diseases of the salivary glands
Salivary calculi (stones)

Stones occasionally form in salivary glands or ducts; at least 80% are in the submandibular gland. The stone is often fusiform and may obstruct a duct. This can lead to infection, pain, and swelling of the gland. Characteristically, pain is related to eating, when the smell or taste of food stimulates salivary secretion.

Salivary gland cysts (mucoceles)

The most common type of salivary gland cyst is seen on the lip and is usually the result of damage to the duct by a minor injury. Saliva leaks into the adjacent tissues until a pool of fluid collects and is surrounded by connective tissue. It is not (pedantically speaking) a cyst because it lacks an epithelial lining. Less often, a retention cyst is caused by obstruction of the duct of a minor gland and has an epithelial lining. Clinically these lesions typically form fluid-filled, thin-roofed swellings that are bluish in color. *Ranula* is the name given to a large cyst or mucocele of salivary gland origin in the floor of the mouth.

Mumps (acute epidemic parotitis)

Mumps virus, like measles virus, is one of the paramyxovirus group. It causes an acute febrile viral infection, usually in childhood, that affects the parotid glands (Fig. 14-1) and sometimes other organs. Once acquired, immunity to mumps is generally lifelong.

Microscopically, mumps is characterized by what appears to be widespread disintegration of acinar cells, a dense lymphocytic infiltrate and small hemorrhages. Despite the acinar damage, full functional recovery of the gland is the rule (as is the case when other glands are involved) so that necrosis must presumably be minimal.

The incubation period is about 3 weeks. Before the swelling appears there are usually 1 or 2 days of malaise and fever. Both parotid glands usually become swollen, either simultaneously or in succession.

Other major salivary glands may also be involved. The swelling usually subsides in about a week and there is no disability. In adults, other glands are more frequently affected. Orchitis and pancreatitis are recognized complications, and virtually any other gland can be affected, although permanent glandular dysfunction virtually never follows. However, mumps can cause

sensorineural deafness and rare complications are meningoencephalitis or myocarditis which can be fatal. Mumps virus is one of the few viruses causing meningitis that can be consistently isolated from the cerebrospinal fluid.

Acute ascending parotitis

Bacteria can infect the parotid glands by ascending their ducts, but they are normally prevented from doing so by the flow of saliva. Ascending sialadenitis is therefore a complication of dryness of the mouth (xerostomia), either as a complication of general dehydration or of salivary gland disease, particularly Sjögren's syndrome or irradiation damage. Debilitating disease and septicemia are also contributory causes in hospitalized patients. The main infecting agent is *Staphylococcus aureus* or sometimes *Streptococcus pneumoniae*.

Clinically, the parotid gland becomes red, swollen, and tender. There may be abscess formation. Treatment consists of adequate doses of systemic antibiotics and drainage as necessary.

Chronic sialadenitis

Chronic sialadenitis is usually a complication of obstruction of the ducts either by calculi or occasionally by a tumor. There is atrophy of salivary tissue associated with a chronic inflammatory cellular infiltrate. There is also dilatation of the obstructed ducts. There are usually no symptoms.

Irradiation damage

The salivary glands are particularly sensitive to irradiation, and radiotherapy for oral cancer usually damages the salivary glands, often irreparably. There is atrophy of the glandular acini and replacement fibrosis. A dry mouth is, therefore, a common and unpleasant side-effect and leads to rapid and severe dental caries and often periodontitis. It is particularly important to stop this rapid destruction of the teeth because extractions bring danger of severe and intractable osteomyelitis of the irradiation-damaged jaws (Chapter 17).

Sjögren's syndrome

Sjögren's syndrome* is an inflammatory disease of salivary and lacrimal glands. It is typically (but not always) associated with rheumatoid arthritis or one of the other collagen disorders. Sjögren's syndrome is believed to affect at least 10% of patients with rheumatoid arthritis. The latter, in turn, is estimated to affect approximately 2% of the population of the United States. Sjögren's syndrome is a common and important cause of dry mouth (xerostomia). The same disease causing a dry mouth and dry eyes in the absence of rheumatoid arthritis is known as *sicca (dry) syndrome*.

The pathology and immunologic features have been discussed in Chapter 7. Clinically, most patients are of middle age or over, and women are predominantly affected. Dryness of the mouth is troublesome (Figs. 14-2 and 14-3), and if there are standing teeth, dental caries and periodontitis are accelerated. Xerostomia also causes changes in the oral microflora, particularly overgrowth of staphylococci and *Candida albicans*. *C. albicans* causes inflammation and soreness of the oral mucous membrane and, usually, angular stomatitis.

The treatment of Sjögren's syndrome is symptomatic only. Irradiation or immunosuppressive treatment may provide temporary, symptomatic relief, but they are contraindicated be-

---

*Henrik Sjögren (b. 1899), Swedish ophthalmologist.

cause they may increase the risk of malignant change. It is imperative that the patient have an ophthalmologic examination to exclude keratoconjunctivitis sicca. This condition is initially asymptomatic, but it can ultimately damage or destroy the eyesight. A complication of Sjögren's syndrome is malignant lymphoma.

Other diseases of the salivary glands

Chronic infections such as tuberculosis or (in the past especially) syphilis can involve the salivary glands but are rare.

Salivary glands are one of the sites of predilection for *sarcoidosis* (Chapter 12) which can occasionally cause a parotid swelling. When there are clinical and radiographic signs of sarcoidosis, biopsy of minor (labial) salivary glands frequently shows typical granuloma formation, which enables the diagnosis to be confirmed readily and may obviate more major invasive methods of diagnosis.

*Mikulicz disease** is the term given to the rare condition of bilateral enlargement of the salivary and lacrimal glands of unknown cause but which has the microscopic features of lymphoepithelial lesion, discussed below. Some make a distinction between this disorder and a clinically similar facial swelling caused by identifiable diseases of these glands, such as sa-

---

*J. von Mikulicz-Radecki (1850-1905), German surgeon.

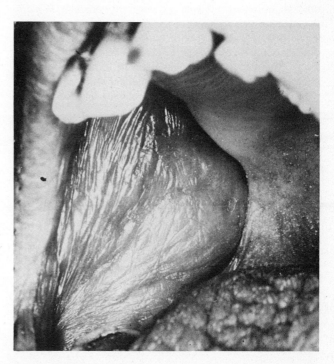

FIG. 14-2. Sjögren's syndrome. In this exceptionally severe case there is total absence of saliva. The oral mucosa is dry and parchment-like.

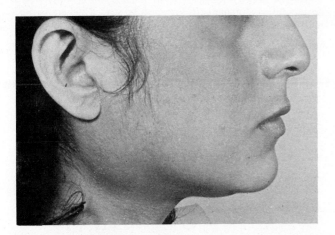

FIG. 14-1. Infective parotitis (mumps). The swollen parotid gland fills the normal depression behind the angle of the jaw.

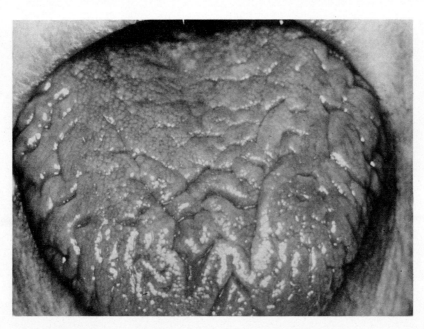

FIG. 14-3. Sjögren's syndrome. The change of the surface pattern of the tongue to this corrugated appearance is typical of long-standing disease.

croidosis, lymphomas, tuberculosis, or syphilis, which they term Mikulicz syndrome.

Graft-versus-host disease (Chapter 7) typically involves the salivary glands causing a Sjögren-like syndrome (as described earlier) with dryness of the mouth and eyes.

Parotitis can be a feature of AIDS particularly in children. A dry mouth (sicca) syndrome can result.

Salivary gland tumors

These small glands produce a remarkable variety of tumors, although overall the tumors are not very common. Modern classifications, such as that of the World Health Organization, recognize seven main types of tumors and several subsidiary varieties. Only the more important examples are discussed here. The pleomorphic adenoma (mixed salivary tumor) accounts for at least 70% of the tumors, while the main malignant salivary gland tumors are adenoid cystic carcinoma and adenocarcinomas.

Pleomorphic adenoma. Pleomorphic adenoma is a benign tumor and is so called because of the wide variety of histologic appearances it produces; although there are many common features, hardly any two pleomorphic adenomas look alike.

The tumor is partly encapsulated, but projections of tumor tissue beyond the confines of the capsule may lead to incomplete surgical removal and recurrence.

Histologically, common features (Fig. 14-4) include the following:
1. Multiple ductlike structures
2. Sheets of polygonal, darkly staining epithelial cells
3. Squamous metaplasia with keratin formation

4. Variable amounts of stroma that may have several forms, including a myxomatous or cartilaginous appearance

It is now generally believed that the mixed appearance of pleomorphic adenoma is the result of proliferation of epithelial and myoepithelial cells. The latter proliferate to produce the various types of stroma.

Recurrence of pleomorphic adenoma may be the result of attempts at enucleation of a tumor which lacks a complete capsule. Despite the surgical difficulties in the parotid region and the hazard to the facial nerve, partial or total parotidectomy is required as residual tumor can lead to recurrence. Tumor cells spilled into the incision can also seed to produce multiple tumor foci in the neck.

Warthin's tumor* (cystadenoma lymphomatosum, adenolymphoma). Warthin's tumor is the most common type of monomorphic adenoma. It affects the parotid glands, where it forms nearly 15% of tumors. CT and MRI scans indicate that multiple foci are more common than was previously suspected.

The histologic appearances are highly characteristic; tall, eosinophilic columnar cells line cystlike spaces and are backed by a dense lymphocytic stroma. Either component may predominate.

The name, *adenolymphoma,* although internationally accepted, is highly misleading as the tumor is not a lymphoma and is benign.

Other monomorphic adenomas. Monomorphic adenomas differ from pleomorphic adenomas in that there is a single epithelial cell type and no formation of connective tissue

*A.S. Warthin (1866-1933), American pathologist.

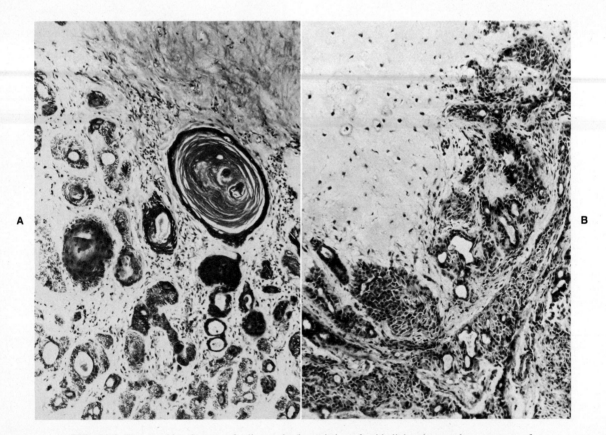

FIG. 14-4. Pleomorphic adenoma of salivary gland consisting of epithelial and stromal components of varying appearance. **A,** The epithelium forms nests and ducts and may undergo squamous metaplasia (**B**).

stromal structures. They form between 5% and 10% of salivary gland tumors.

Mucoepidermoid carcinoma. Mucoepidermoid carcinoma accounts for less than 2% of tumors of major salivary glands, but a far higher proportion of minor gland tumors. Microscopically, the two components are mucous cells, often surrounding small cysts, and sheets of epidermoid cells (Fig. 14-5). A minority of these tumors show frankly malignant microscopic features, but even the best differentiated and apparently benign tumors can occasionally be invasive.

Mucoepidermoid carcinoma is termed mucoepidermoid tumor in the World Health Organization classification since its behavior (like that of acinic cell carcinoma/tumor described below) is in general more benign than true carcinomas. Nevertheless, the behavior of both mucoepidermoid and acinic cell carcinomas is unpredictable from the microscopic appearances and degree of differentiation.

Acinic cell carcinoma. Acinic cell carcinoma is a rare type of salivary gland tumor that consists microscopically of sheets of basophilic, granular serous-type cells, sometimes with an acinar arrangement but without ducts. Multiple clear spaces are common and may be so numerous as to give a lacy appearance.

Microscopically, benign-appearing acinic cell carcinomas, like mucoepidermoid carcinomas, can occasionally be inva-

sive; but there are also frankly malignant variants with loss of differentiation, gross nuclear hyperchromatism, and pleomorphism.

Adenoid cystic carcinoma. Adenoid cystic carcinoma forms only about 2% of parotid tumors but relatively, considerably more frequent in other glands particularly the sublingual. Microscopically, the most characteristic pattern is of small dark cells forming rounded islands with a cribriform (Swiss cheese) pattern (Fig. 14-6). This tumor is invasive and also has a strong tendency to spread perineurally. Complete excision is therefore difficult so that wide excision followed by radiotherapy is usually the preferred treatment. However, the risk of recurrence, particularly in the long term, is high.

Other carcinomas. Adenocarcinoma and malignant change in a pleomorphic adenoma are the main examples. Squamous cell carcinomas are rare. Carcinoma in pleomorphic adenoma is one of the rare examples of malignant change in a previously benign tumor. It is recognizable microscopically by the presence of carcinoma within or adjacent to typical pleomorphic adenoma. Clinically, a long-standing tumor typically shows sudden acceleration of growth rate and the onset of pain or other symptoms.

Other (nonepithelial) salivary gland tumors. The most common nonepithelial tumorlike lesion of salivary glands is the (so-called) *benign lymphoepithelial lesion* (BLL). Microscop-

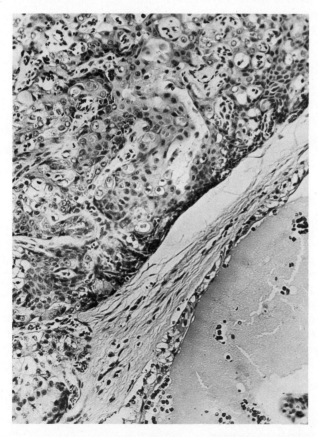

FIG. 14-5. Mucoepidermoid carcinoma of salivary gland shows the two essential components: epidermoid (squamous) epithelium (top and to the left) and mucous cells that have produced a microcyst of mucinous material (bottom right). *(From Cawson RA: Essentials of dental surgery and pathology, ed. 3, Edinburgh, Scotland, 1978, Churchill Livingstone.)*

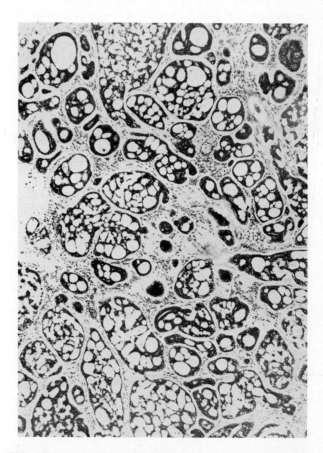

FIG. 14-6. Adenoid cystic carcinoma of salivary gland that was invading the periodontal ligament. This highly malignant tumor shows a characteristic pattern of tumor cells forming rounded islands perforated by small "holes" (cribriform or Swiss cheese pattern).

ically, there is replacement of acini by sheets of lymphocytes, among which islands of duct epithelium survive and proliferate to produce "epimyoepithelial" islands; these, however, lack myoepithelial cells.

Exactly the same picture is seen in the late stages of Sjögren's syndrome, and it is uncertain whether or not they are the same entity. Despite the title "benign," lymphoma can develop in a significant proportion of cases of BLL and this may happen in 20% or more such lesions.

Although uncommon, the most frequent nonepithelial salivary gland tumors are lymphomas. Other mesenchymal tumors, such as neurofibromas, may be seen but are rare.

Juvenile hemangioma. In childhood a salivary swelling, sometimes pulsatile in nature, can be caused by an hemangioma in which glandular tissue is largely replaced by a mass of capillaries. This may be so great as to form a vascular shunt which can rarely lead to high output heart failure. These tumors are probably hamartomatous and occasionally resolve spontaneously. Others, however, infiltrate local structures and recur after excision.

Clinical aspects. The incidence of salivary gland tumors is probably less than 3 per 100,000 of the population. Women tend to be affected slightly more frequently than men. The peak age of incidence for benign tumors appears to be about 40, but even children are occasionally affected. Malignant tumors tend to develop later, usually in the fifth or sixth decade. The parotid gland (Fig. 14-7) is affected in at least 70% of cases. Pleomorphic adenoma is the most frequently found salivary gland tumor overall, but about 12% of parotid tumors are malignant.

Salivary gland tumors usually cause firm, sometimes lobulated swellings. Benign and malignant tumors cannot be reliably distinguished clinically. Adenomas, however, grow very slowly and are painless. Pain and rapid growth are strongly suggestive of malignancy. In the case of the parotid, a facial

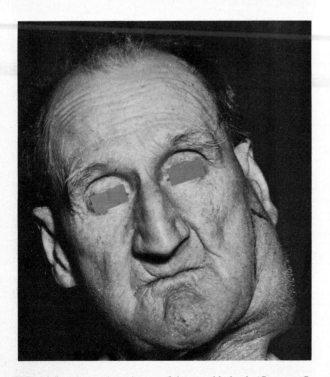

FIG. 14-7. Advanced carcinoma of the parotid gland. *(Courtesy Curator of the Gordon Museum, Guy's Hospital, London, England.)*

nerve palsy or ulceration of the overlying skin is also characteristic of malignant tumors.

Microscopic examination is essential for diagnosis. Treatment is preferably by wide excision, supplemented if necessary by radiotherapy for malignant tumors.

Tonsillitis and pharyngitis: sore throat

Streptococcal pharyngitis is caused by hemolytic, usually Group A, streptococci, which cause acute inflammation with redness and swelling of the tonsil and adjacent pharynx. There is often a superficial whitish exudate and suppuration can follow. The onset is sudden with fever, malaise, leukocytosis, and difficulty in swallowing as a result of pain.

If the causative streptococci produce erythrogenic toxin and the patient is nonimmune, a characteristic rash develops. The disease is then known as *scarlet fever.* The importance of streptococcal sore throat is that in susceptible subjects it can be followed by rheumatic fever, acute glomerulonephritis, or Henoch-Schönlein purpura. The infection responds well to penicillin.

Viral infections

Viral infections are considerably more common than streptococcal sore throat, but definitive virologic diagnoses are seldom practical. Adenoviruses are the main cause. Pharyngitis and tonsillitis are usually transient and without other ill-effects.

Herpangina. Herpangina is caused by coxsackieviruses belonging to Group A, which cause painful inflammation, vesiculation, and ulceration of the soft palate, the fauces, and pharynx. Fever and malaise are frequent.

Systemic viral infections. The common viral respiratory tract diseases (such as influenza and the common cold), measles, and rubella often start with pharyngitis, but this may only be a minor feature.

Infectious mononucleosis. This common infection caused by the Epstein-Barr virus (EBV) is characterized in about 50% of cases by severe sore throat as a result of involvement of the tonsillar lymphoid tissue and often by petechiae on the soft palate. There is widespread lymphadenopathy, but diagnosis depends on hematologic and serologic investigation (Chapter 13).

Diphtheria

Diphtheria is caused by toxinogenic strains of *Corynebacterium diphtheriae,* which predominantly remain localized to the pharynx and tonsils. Diphtheria was at one time common and should be of little more than historic interest now because it is preventable by immunization. However, there have been two epidemics in Texas, where large numbers of the population had not been immunized, and the disease is still common in other parts of the world. The pathologic changes of diphtheria are entirely a result of the local and general effects of the toxin, which interferes with synthesis of enzymes concerned with fatty acid metabolism. Locally, the toxin causes superficial necrotizing ulceration and formation of a grayish pseudomembrane. This consists of necrotic mucosal cells and fibrin and a central area containing *C. diphtheriae.*

Clinically, local symptoms are a moderately sore throat and swelling of the neck as a result of lymphadenitis. The main effects of diphtheria toxin are nerve paralyses, especially of cranial nerves, toxic myocarditis, and death. Death, especially in young children, can also be caused by spread of the membrane along the surface of the larynx, causing respiratory tract obstruction and asphyxia.

Vincent's angina

Vincent's angina is a rare type of pharyngeal ulceration that may mimic the local lesions of diphtheria. It is caused by the same fusospirochetal complex that causes acute necrotizing ulcerative gingivitis. Clinically, there is grayish ulceration of the pharynx, but typically there are no severe systemic effects.

Leukemia and agranulocytosis

One of the characteristic manifestations of leukemia or severe neutropenia is necrotizing ulceration of the pharynx or oral cavity. When the tonsils and pharynx are predominantly involved, the disease must be distinguished from infective pharyngitis as described earlier. Therefore, blood examination is an essential investigation.

Diseases of the esophagus

The main complaint caused by disease of the esophagus is difficulty in swallowing *(dysphagia)*, for which there are many causes. The most important disease of the esophagus is carcinoma, which has a very high mortality rate.

Achalasia (cardiospasm)

Achalasia is characterized by weak and uncoordinated peristaltic activity of the esophagus caused by impaired cholinergic innervation. The tone and motility of the esophagus are diminished. The esophagogastric sphincter remains permanently contracted, a condition called *cardiospasm*.

Pathology. The ganglion cells of Auerbach's plexus may be few or absent, while in other cases no defect can be found, and the underlying condition seems to be a functional parasympathetic disorder.

The body of the esophagus (Fig. 14-8) is generally flaccid and can become greatly distended (megaesophagus). Eventually, stasis of food proximal to the contracted esophagogastric sphincter causes chronic esophagitis. This can, in turn, cause nonspecific ulceration and fibrotic thickening. This is also thought to contribute, ultimately, to the development of carcinoma in some patients.

Clinical aspects. Symptoms can start at almost any age, but adults are particularly affected. The main symptom is gradually worsening dysphagia, but occasionally dysphagia seems to start suddenly. As the disease progresses, there is a tendency for the patient to regurgitate undigested food, particularly when lying down. This may cause aspiration pneumonia. Finally, obstruction may become complete.

The majority of cases can be relieved by forceful dilatation and a muscle-splitting operation at the esophagogastric junction.

Esophageal webs and strictures

An *esophageal web* is a membrane that can partially obstruct the esophagus, while a *stricture* is a narrowing often caused by scarring and contracture. The most common type of nonmalignant stricture is usually the result of chronic esophagitis in a hiatus hernia. A web in the postcricoid region of the esophagus is a feature of the syndrome of atrophic glossitis, dysphagia, and hypochromic anemia (sideropenic dysphagia)

described by Paterson and Kelly* but often incorrectly referred to as *Plummer-Vinson syndrome*. Women are almost exclusively affected. The proliferative changes at the upper end of the esophagus predispose to carcinoma at this site, but these patients also have a high risk of oral cancer. Cancer of the esophagus is otherwise a disease mainly of men and in men affects the middle or lower end of the esophagus.

Hiatus hernia

Hiatus hernia is, strictly speaking, a disease of the stomach rather than the esophagus. The stomach slides up through the esophageal hiatus of the diaphragm, but in the majority of cases, the esophagus appears to be short, and the esophagogastric junction lies above the diaphragm. In about 10% of cases there is a paraesophageal hernia where part of the stomach has herniated up through the diaphragm beside the esophagus.

Etiology and pathology. The cause of hiatus hernia is unknown. Obesity and advancing age are often thought to be contributory factors, but this is not certain. Hiatus hernia itself causes no physical abnormalities, but reflux esophagitis is common and may eventually cause an esophageal stricture.

---

*D.R. Paterson (1863-1939), English ENT surgeon; A. Brown-Kelly (1865-1944), English ENT surgeon.

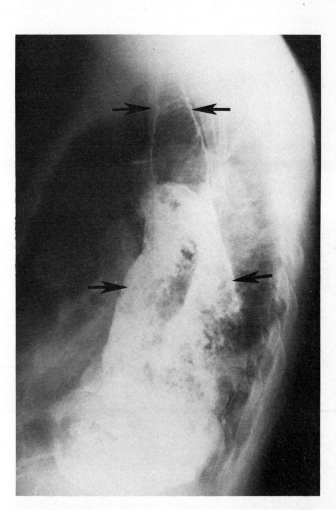

FIG. 14-8. Radiograph of achalasia. The gross dilatation *(arrows)* of the esophagus is outlined by barium.

Clinical aspects. Hiatus hernias appear to be extremely common and, depending on criteria of diagnosis, may affect from 10% to 40% of otherwise normal people. Whether a sliding hiatus hernia is of any clinical significance has long been a matter of controversy. About 50% of patients have no symptoms, and in most others, symptoms are variable. There is also little correlation between symptoms and objective radiographic findings. The typical symptoms of hiatus hernia are retrosternal pain (heartburn) and occasionally reflux of gastric juices into the mouth. Symptoms are characteristically most severe when the patient is bending forward. Paraesophageal hernia sometimes causes burning pain and reflux or bloating and belching after meals.

Esophageal varices

Dilated and elongated veins (Fig. 14-9) are a complication of portal hypertension, secondary to chronic obstructive liver disease (cirrhosis). They are an important cause of vomiting of blood (hematemesis), particularly in alcoholics with cirrhosis of the liver (Chapter 15).

Mallory-Weiss syndrome*

Esophageal lacerations causing severe hematemesis account for about 5% of cases of massive upper gastrointestinal tract

---

*G.K. Mallory (b. 1900), American pathologist; S. Weiss (1898-1942), American pathologist.

bleeding. The patients are often alcoholics, but lacerations can also result from increased intraesophagogastric pressure from any cause, particularly vomiting. The tears are of varying depth and lie near the esophagogastric junction. The diagnosis can only be made with certainty using fiberoptic endoscopy.

Barrett's esophagus

*Barrett's esophagus** is the term given to replacement of the normal squamous epithelium in the lower end of the esophagus by columnar epithelium (Fig. 14-10). Barrett's esophagus is found in 10% to 20% of patients screened for esophagitis and in up to 45% of patients with chronic strictures caused by scarred peptic ulcers of the esophagus.

Barrett's esophagus may occasionally be congenital and found in children; but, in the majority of patients, it appears to be secondary to gastroesophageal reflux. It is commonly found therefore at about the age of 60 and (like peptic ulcer) is more common in men.

Microscopically, the epithelium of Barrett's esophagus may be simple columnar structures, of gastric fundus or small intestine type.

Clinically, the chief symptoms may be those of an associated reflux esophagitis or result from esophageal peptic ulceration or stricture. However, the chief hazard is that of carcinomatous

---

*N.R. Barrett (1903-1979), English surgeon.

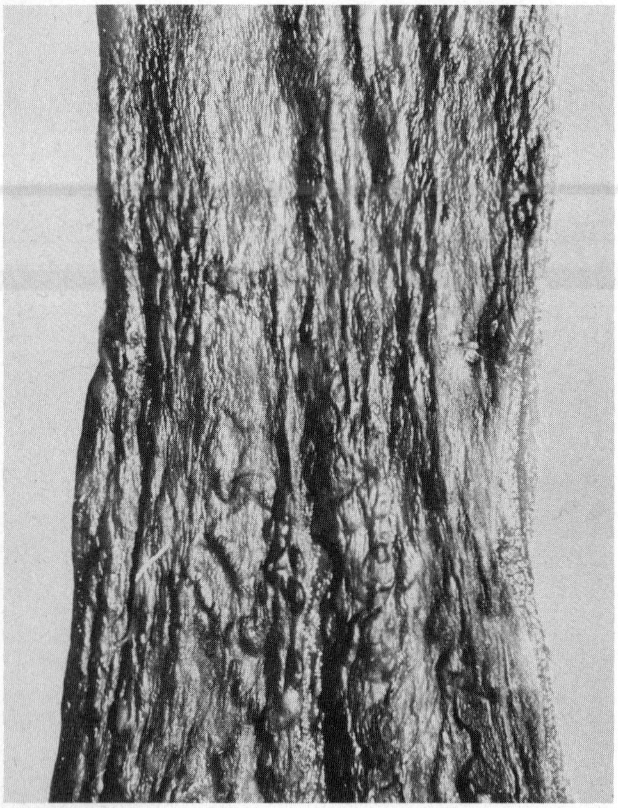

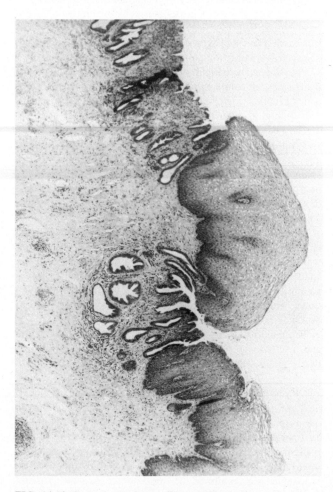

FIG. 14-9. Esophageal varices. The normal appearance of the esophageal wall is almost obliterated by the elongated, tortuous, and distended veins secondary to cirrhosis of the liver and portal obstruction. *(Courtesy Curator of the Gordon Museum, Guy's Hospital, London, England.)*

FIG. 14-10. Barrett's esophagus. The normal squamous epithelium is replaced in part by glandular epithelium formed of columnar cells.

change, which recent surveys have shown to be 30-fold to 40-fold greater than in the normal esophagus. Unlike the latter, carcinoma in Barrett's esophagus is an adenocarcinoma which is typically preceded by dysplastic change.

Repeated follow-up endoscopic examinations are required when Barrett's esophagus has been detected; biopsy examinations are needed when dysplasia or carcinomatous change is suspected. Symptoms of Barrett's esophagus can be relieved by use of cimetidine or other H2 receptor blockers, or antacids, but whether this causes regression of anything more than the inflammatory changes is uncertain.

Esophagitis

Inflammation of the esophagus has a variety of causes, but so-called reflux esophagitis due to hiatus hernia is by far the most common. The causes of esophagitis include the following:

1. Reflux esophagitis associated with hiatus hernia.
2. Ingestion of irritants. This may be a result of accidental or suicidal swallowing of corrosives such as phenolic antiseptics, strong acids, or alkalis. Chronic alcoholism may also be a cause.
3. Infection. Occasionally the esophagus may be involved in spread of infection from mediastinitis or pericarditis. Candidosis of the esophagus, often a result of spread from the oral cavity, is increasingly common in immunosuppressed or otherwise debilitated patients.
4. Peptic ulceration. This develops in ectopic gastric mucosa in the esophagus.
5. Prolonged gastric intubation.
6. Paterson-Kelly syndrome.
7. Uremia. This is characterized by dystrophic changes in the epithelium of the upper gastrointestinal tract. In addition, there is usually severe debility and often superimposed infection.

In many cases, apart from hiatus hernia and Paterson-Kelly syndrome, esophagitis is a terminal event. The characteristic symptoms are burning substernal pain and dysphagia.

Tumors of the esophagus

Benign neoplasms are uncommon and relatively unimportant. A leiomyoma, papilloma, or occasionally an adenoma may cause obstruction, but these are rare and operable. Carcinoma is, by far, the most common and important esophageal tumor.

Carcinoma of the esophagus. Carcinoma of the esophagus is a fatal disease. The importance of this disease emphasizes the need to investigate dysphagia, especially in older patients.

Etiology. A wide variety of factors appear to contribute to the development of carcinoma of the esophagus. The main factors are as follows:

1. *Environmental.* In some areas of the world, the incidence of esophageal cancer is enormously high, sometimes more than 200 times the incidence seen in the United States or Great Britain. These areas include the shores of the Caspian Sea, some parts of eastern and southern Africa, Curacao, and an extensive belt extending from the Middle East through central Asia to northern China.
2. *Alcohol.* The frequency of esophageal cancer among heavy drinkers is estimated as approximately 25 times higher than in nondrinkers. The form in which the alcohol is taken is important, and in Brittany where a crude form of apple brandy (calvados) is drunk, esophageal cancer

is much more prevalent than in other parts of France. It is possible, therefore, that other components of alcoholic drinks, rather than alcohol itself, cause the disease.

3. *Esophageal stasis and inflammation.* With longstanding esophageal stasis, such as in achalasia, the risk of carcinoma appears to be at least 10 times higher than in the general population. There is a similar risk to those who have ingested corrosive fluids, who suffer from reflux esophagitis, or who have ectopic gastric mucosa in the esophagus.
4. *Paterson-Kelly syndrome.* Carcinoma that follows Paterson-Kelly syndrome is unusual both in that it predominantly affects women and is sited at the upper end of the esophagus. Many patients with upper esophageal carcinoma may have some features of this syndrome. It is also estimated that about 16% of patients with Paterson-Kelly syndrome develop carcinoma of the esophagus or mouth.

Pathology. Most (90%) malignant esophageal tumors are typical squamous cell carcinomas (Fig. 14-11). The remainder, particularly at the lower end of the esophagus, are adenocarcinomas, presumably arising from acquired glandular tissue in the esophageal wall. The middle third of the esophagus is affected in about 50% of the cases, with the remainder approximately equally distributed in the upper and lower thirds. The initial lesion is small and plaquelike. The lesion may then encircle or extend deeply to the submucosa. It can progress in

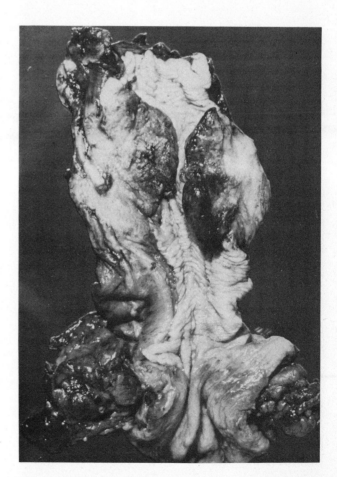

FIG. 14-11. Large ulcerating squamous cell carcinoma forming a thick constricting ring in the esophagus. *(Courtesy Curator of the Gordon Museum, Guy's Hospital, London, England.)*

one of the following ways: ulceration, formation of a polypoid mass, or infiltrative growth throughout the esophagus converting it into a thickened, rigid tube. Spread is mostly local, and metastases are late.

Clinical aspects. Carcinoma of the esophagus accounts for about 7% of all cancer deaths in males. It affects those over middle age, and men are affected approximately four times more frequently than women.

Carcinoma of the esophagus (Fig. 14-12) has an insidious onset, and the first symptom is usually dysphagia, which is often delayed until the tumor is well established. Weight loss is a common consequence. Other symptoms, such as hoarseness, cough, or hiccups, develop as a result of irritation of adjacent structures. Erosion of a blood vessel can cause severe hemorrhage.

Partly because of the insidious course and partly because of the close proximity to so many vital structures, treatment is rarely satisfactory. The prognosis is one of the worst for any form of cancer. The 5-year survival rate is usually about 7%, but better results are claimed in some series as a result of the use of modern techniques. Nevertheless, it is still one of the nastier ways to die.

Leiomyosarcoma. Leiomyosarcoma is a rare tumor, but it is the most common malignant nonepithelial tumor of the esophagus. Grossly, a leiomyosarcoma usually forms a submucosal mass, which protrudes into the lumen of the esophagus and may ulcerate.

Histologically, leiomyosarcomas usually show a pattern of interlacing strands of spindle-shaped cells with large darkly staining nuclei. Varying degrees of nuclear abnormality and numbers of mitoses may be present. The tumor invades deeply and metastasizes mainly to the lungs and liver. The overall prognosis is poor.

Leiomyomas and leiomyosarcomas can also affect the stomach and rectum, but they are exceedingly rare in the small intestine. Their gross and microscopic features and behavior are essentially the same as when the esophagus is affected.

Dysphagia

Dysphagia is one of the most important symptoms of diseases of the esophagus. The causes of dysphagia can be summarized as follows:

1. *Painful conditions of the oropharynx.* Acute tonsillitis, pharyngitis, and the immediate effects of tonsillectomy are the most common causes of inhibition of swallowing. Severe painful ulceration, such as herpangina, which particularly affects the back of the mouth or oropharynx, is an occasional cause. A rare cause is glossopharyngeal neuralgia, where initiation of swallowing provokes almost unbearably severe neuralgic pain.
2. *Obstruction.* The site is usually in the esophagus. There may be a stricture secondary to esophagitis or, more important, a carcinoma. In the case of Paterson-Kelly syndrome, an esophageal web forms an obstruction at the upper end of the esophagus.
3. *Mechanical interference with the muscles of deglutition.* Extensive infiltration of the tongue, particularly the posterior third, or of the esophageal wall by carcinoma interferes with the muscular activity of swallowing.
4. *Paralytic conditions.* Paralysis of the muscles of swallowing is a feature of acute poliomyelitis affecting the brain stem and can also be a feature of pseudobulbar palsy (Chapter 20).
5. *Neuromuscular incoordination.* Achalasia of the cardia is the main example.
6. *Neuroses.* Anxiety states may be associated with symptoms of difficulty in swallowing. Hallucinations of a foreign body embedded in the throat are more likely to be a feature of schizophrenia. Difficulty in swallowing may also be hysterical, and in this condition greater difficulty in swallowing fluids than solids is a characteristic complaint.

Diseases of the stomach
Gastritis

The term *gastritis,* like indigestion or liverishness, is used widely by the lay public and occasionally by physicians as a catchall for minor abdominal symptoms such as vague epigastric discomfort and mild nausea. In pathologic terms, gastritis can be classified as follows:

1. Acute gastritis
2. Chronic gastritis
   a. Simple atrophic
   b. Autoimmune

Acute gastritis. Acute gastritis is usually a response to the ingestion of irritants. The most common of these are alcohol and aspirin.

Pathogenesis and pathology. In mild acute gastritis there is little obvious structural change, although there is probably a

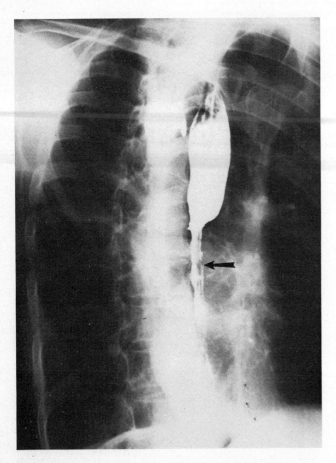

FIG. 14-12. Radiograph of carcinoma of the esophagus. There is an irregular constriction of the esophagus caused by carcinoma and dilatation above tumor.

more rapid turnover of mucosal cells. In more severe cases inflammation with mucosal edema and hyperemia develop. Severe gastritis, caused by aspirin or alcohol for example, is characterized by erosions of the gastric mucosa, causing hemorrhage of varying severity.

Aspirin is a potent gastric irritant. It can occasionally precipitate torrential gastric bleeding even in the absence of preexisting gastric ulceration. Antiinflammatory analgesics such as aspirin have a damaging effect on gastric epithelium by inhibiting prostaglandin synthesis. Inhibition of platelet aggregation by aspirin can also aggravate the bleeding. Too much alcohol, followed by aspirin to deal with hangover, can be dangerous because of the combined effects of the two irritants. Aspirin is probably better avoided in patients who have peptic ulcers or who are heavy drinkers.

Acute gastritis is usually transient and causes minimal symptoms, but there may be acute erosive hemorrhagic gastritis and bleeding, particularly after aspirin or alcohol ingestion.

Chronic gastritis. Atrophic gastritis is very common and may affect about 10% of the general population. In many cases it causes no symptoms. The incidence increases with age; excessive indulgence in alcohol and smoking probably also contribute. No symptoms can be reliably ascribed to the mucosal changes.

Etiology and pathogenesis. The cause of atrophy of the gastric mucosa is unknown, but there appear to be two types. The most common is so-called simple atrophic gastritis, characterized by patchy atrophic changes in the gastric mucosa with gradual and incomplete reduction of acid and pepsin secretion.

Autoimmune gastritis is characterized by widespread progressive and irreversible atrophy of both acid-secreting and pepsin-secreting cells, together with thinning of the stomach wall. In these patients and in asymptomatic relatives there is a significant incidence of antibodies to gastric parietal cells.

Autoimmune atrophic gastritis leads to failure of secretion of intrinsic factor and megaloblastic (pernicious) anemia (Chapter 13). One of the diagnostic features of pernicious anemia is therefore total failure of gastric secretion; no acid is secreted, even in response to histamine. Antibodies are also formed against intrinsic factor.

Pathology. The mucosa is thin; mucosal glands are few and mainly mucus secreting. Areas of mucosa may undergo metaplasia to an intestinal type while the submucosa is typically infiltrated by chronic inflammatory cells.

Peptic ulceration

Peptic ulceration, which includes both gastric and duodenal ulcers, is one of the most common causes of chronic ill health in the Western world today. It is also a common cause of acute surgical emergencies, particularly gastric bleeding or perforation, both of which have a significant mortality.

It is suggested that about 10% of the population may have peptic ulcers although symptoms may be mild ("indigestion") or even absent.

Etiology. Peptic ulceration develops only in sites exposed to acid-pepsin and therefore affects the stomach, duodenum (approximately equally), or occasionally the esophagus when ectopic gastric mucosa is present. It does not develop when there is complete achlorhydria, and usually ulcers heal when gastric secretion is blocked by drugs as discussed later.

The essential etiologic mechanism in peptic ulceration is not therefore the presence of acid-pepsin but failure of the mucosal barrier to protect against it. Contrary to popular belief the level of gastric acid production does not bear any direct relationship to ulcer formation in otherwise normal persons. Excessive gastric acid production is detectable in only 20% of cases of duodenal ulceration while patients with gastric ulcer have lower peak and basal amounts of acid than normal subjects though there is wide overlap. There is also no evidence for excessive production of proteolytic enzymes in this disease.

Acid-pepsin secretion is under the control of the hormone, gastrin, which is released in response to eating. Under conditions of excessive gastrin secretion as in the *Zollinger-Ellison syndrome,** caused by a gastrin-secreting tumor of the pancreas, gastric acid production is so high as to overcome the mucosal defenses and make peptic ulceration an invariable consequence. With this exception, there is no evidence of excessive gastrin secretion in patients with peptic ulceration.

Protection of the gastric mucosa against acid-pepsin attack depends on (1) an adequate mucosal blood supply, (2) a normal rate of mucosal cell replacement, (3) mucus production, and (4) bicarbonate formation. A major factor in maintaining mucosal protection is prostagladin E (PGE) and prostacyclin secretion in gastric fluid. Experimentally, administration of a PGE 1 analog also accelerates the healing of peptic ulcers, whereas nonsteroidal antiinflammatory drugs such as aspirin and its analogs, which (like cigarette smoking) act by inhibiting prostaglandin synthesis, can precipitate or aggravate peptic ulcer. Other antiulcer drugs such as sucralfate or colloidal bismuth, which enhance mucosal defenses, combat the effects of cigarette smoking better than drugs that inhibit gastric acid production and help to confirm the essential role of the gastric mucosal barrier in protecting against peptic ulceration.

Evidence is also accumulating that bacteria may cause antral mucosal damage and contribute to peptic ulcer disease. *Campylobacter pylori* appears to be associated with antral gastritis and can be found in the epithelium adjoining peptic ulcers. Circulating and local antibody titers to this bacterium also correlate well with gastritis or peptic ulcer; furthermore, a volunteer who swallowed a culture of *C. pylori* developed antral gastritis, although further progress of the latter was aborted by antibiotic treatment.

In addition there is a minor genetic contribution to susceptibility to peptic ulceration: gastric ulcers are more common in those with blood group A and duodenal ulcers more common in blood group O.

Pathology. Gastric ulcers can form virtually anywhere in the stomach, but the lesser curve is the single most common site and the majority of ulcers are close to the pylorus. Duodenal ulcers mostly form in the duodenal bulb or cap.

Peptic ulcers are usually round and sharply defined or punched out with vertical or overhanging walls and a smooth base (Fig. 14-13). The majority are 2 cm or less in diameter. Fibrosis secondary to inflammation causes scarring and puckering of the mucosa in a radiating pattern round the crater.

The microscopic appearances (Fig. 14-14) vary according to the ulcers' activity or chronicity. On the surface of an active ulcer there is a thin layer of necrotic debris with an underlying mixed infiltration of inflammatory cells with neutrophils predominating (Fig. 14-15). More deeply, there is granulation tissue infiltrated by histiocytes while the floor is formed of fibrous tissue. The degree of penetration is variable; the ulcer may extend through the whole thickness of the stomach wall,

---

*R.M. Zollinger (b. 1903), American surgeon; E.H. Ellison (1918-1970), American surgeon.

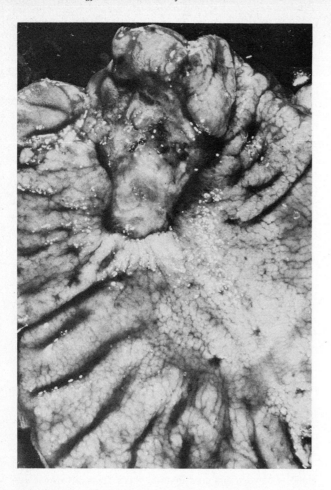

but endarteritis of the vessels in the base of the ulcer helps to prevent the majority of patients from bleeding too often or too severely.

With increasing chronicity there is greater fibrosis, scarring and distortion (Fig. 14-16).

Clinical aspects. Peptic and, particularly, duodenal ulcers are more common in men. The peak age incidence for duodenal ulcer is in the fourth and fifth decades but about 10 years later for gastric ulcer. Symptoms are highly variable but epigastric pain is typical. In the case of duodenal ulcer this may simulate hunger pain and be relieved by food; gastric ulcer pain is more variable, less likely to be relieved by food, and may be referred through to the back. However, gastric ulcers cannot be distinguished from duodenal ulcers by the symptoms alone and often there is only discomfort and "indigestion." In some cases the first indication of the presence of an ulcer is a severe hemorrhage or other complication.

Healing of peptic ulcer can be accelerated by the cessation of cigarette smoking, bed rest, antacids, and attention to the diet and many patients with mild symptoms manage in this way. Treatment of peptic ulceration, however, has been revolutionized by the drugs such as cimetidine, which block gastric histamine (H2) receptors and the secretion of acid-pepsin. Treatment may sometimes have to be continued for long periods as withdrawal of the drug may be followed by relapse, particularly of duodenal ulcers, but fortunately adverse effects of

FIG. 14-13. Large chronic peptic ulcer. The base of the ulcer has eroded through to the pancreas.

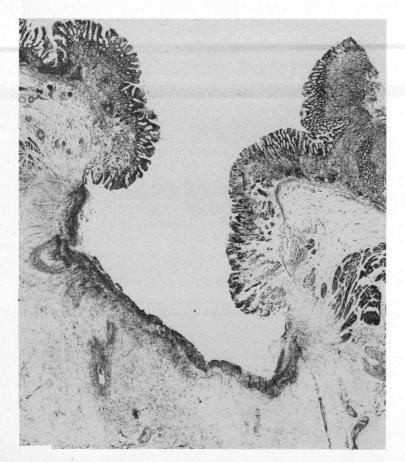

FIG. 14-14. Chronic peptic ulcer. The undermined edges of the ulcer and destruction of the glandular layer, the submucosa, and muscular layer can be seen. The ulcer has eroded half way through a large vessel, but obliterative endarteritis has prevented any bleeding.

these drugs are rare. There is also a variety of other drugs as suggested earlier which help to improve the mucosal defenses. As a result, surgery (partial gastrectomy) for peptic ulcer is now reserved for those few cases which fail to respond to vigorous medical treatment.

Complications. The main complications of peptic ulcer are (1) bleeding, (2) perforation, and (3) obstruction. Carcinoma is not a complication of peptic ulcer itself but occasionally develops long after ulcer surgery and is not a complication of duodenal ulcer.

Bleeding. Major gastric bleeding causing hematemesis may start without previous symptoms or warning of any sort. Precipitating factors can be overindulgence in alcohol (particularly spirits) or aspirin. Stools dark with blood (melena) are another consequence of bleeding from an ulcer, whether or not there has been hematemesis. Occult blood in the feces from minor bleeding is common, can cause iron deficiency anemia but can only be detected chemically. Massive bleeding from a peptic ulcer is a major emergency with a mortality of up to 10%.

Perforation. About 5% of peptic ulcers (almost exclusively in men) may perforate and, like bleeding, this may be without any warning. The result is release of intensely irritating acid-pepsin into the abdominal cavity and acute peritonitis. There is acute sometimes excruciating upper abdominal pain followed by reflex, boardlike rigidity of the abdominal muscles and sometimes nausea and vomiting. Immediate surgery is essential.

Obstruction. The chief cause is scarring, secondary to inflammation in the region of the pylorus. Pyloric stenosis results.

Hypertrophic pyloric stenosis

As mentioned earlier, hypertrophic pyloric stenosis is a developmental anomaly with an estimated frequency of 3/1000 live births. In adults, pyloric stenosis is usually associated with a gastric ulcer nearby; but in some cases there is no apparent cause, and it is possible that developmental stenosis may not become symptomatic until later in life.

Stenosis secondary to gastric ulceration is the result of extensive fibrosis associated with muscular hypertrophy; this can reduce the pylorus to a mere pinhole. Clinically, the result is persistent vomiting and gastric acid loss, which can lead to metabolic alkalosis. Malnutrition is also severe in affected infants but surgical correction is curative in either type.

Carcinoma of the stomach

Cancer of the stomach accounts for approximately 15,000 deaths a year in the United States but the mortality rate has declined sharply over the past 40 years. Cancer of the stomach is considerably more common in males and in some other countries.

Etiology. Like most forms of cancer, carcinoma of the stomach is a disease of advancing age. Etiological factors, especially

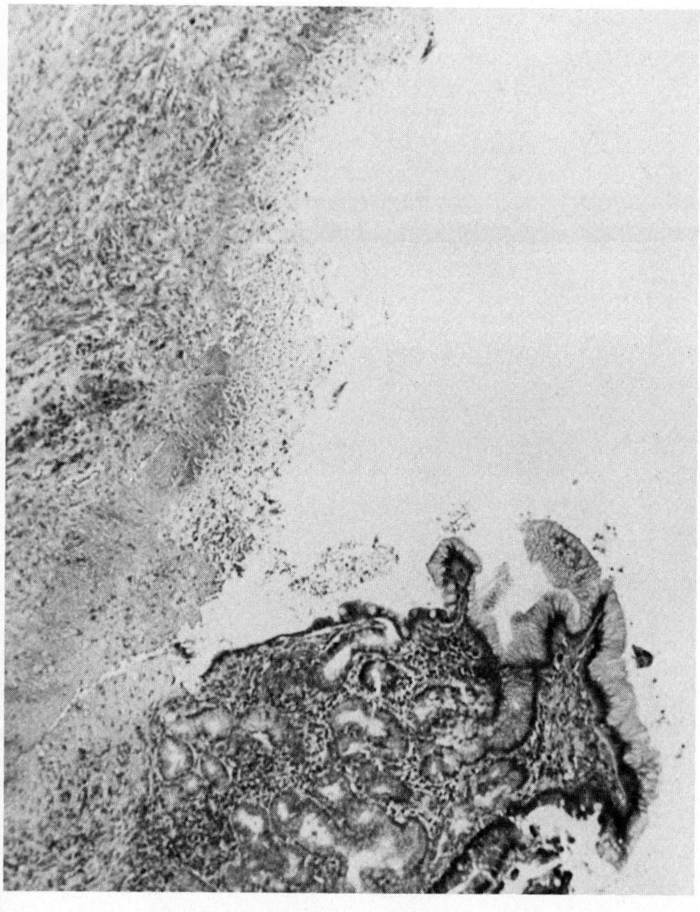

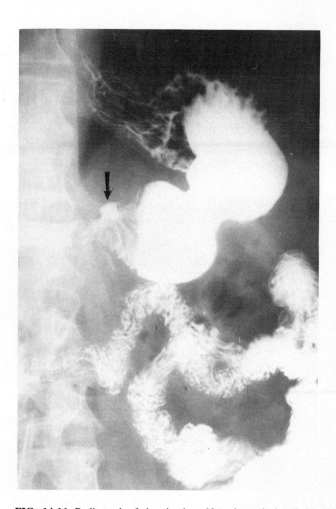

FIG. 14-15. Chronic peptic ulcer. There is localized destruction of the gastric mucosa. The floor of the ulcer contains necrotic cellular debris deep to which is granulation tissue.

FIG. 14-16. Radiograph of chronic ulcer. Note the typical radiating mucosal folds converging on the ulcer crater *(arrow)*.

some dietary components, particularly smoked foods and nitrates or nitrites, are suspected of contributing.

In some countries such as Chile and Colombia, the incidence of stomach cancer appears to correlate with the levels of nitrate intake. The problem of dietary nitrate intake is however complex. In Louisiana, Britain, Japan, and Canada patients with gastric cancer appear to have had a lower exposure to nitrate than populations at low risk from this disease. Also in many populations, a high nitrate intake may result from a high consumption of vegetables; in such cases a concomitant high intake of vitamin C, an inhibitor of N-nitrosation, may be protective. Further, as pointed out in Chapter 6, tobacco is a more important source of nitrates than foods in the Western World.

In South America by contrast, the drinking water can contain nitrate concentrations of several hundred mg per liter and dietary deficiencies may be contributory.

N-nitrosation is likely to be promoted by achlorhydria, by specific protein substrates or by deficiency of inhibitors of nitrosation. A few items of diet are also known to produce potent mutagens after treatment with nitrates. Such compounds have been isolated from some types of Japanese soy sauce, preserved fish and fava beans which are a staple item of diet in Colombia where, as in Japan, the incidence of cancer of the stomach is exceptionally high.

The high incidence of stomach cancer in Finland and Japan may be partly due to dietary habits or to a genetic effect. For example, Japanese living in the United States have an incidence of gastric carcinoma between that of Americans and that of Japanese living in Japan and this may indicate that both factors are contributory.

Few conditions of the stomach appear to be premalignant, but chronic atrophic gastritis, associated with pernicious anemia, increases susceptibility to stomach cancer. Though this accounts for only a tiny minority of cases 75% of patients with gastric cancer have hypochlorhydria and atrophic gastritis is frequently associated.

Nevertheless, achlorhydria alone does not appear to increase susceptibility to gastric cancer, so that anxiety about this risk in those taking acid-inhibiting drugs (such as cimetidine for peptic ulceration) appears to be unfounded.

Malignant change is rare in peptic ulcer and the latter is not regarded as premalignant. Paradoxically, however, there appears to be an increased risk of gastric carcinoma long after gastrectomy for a benign ulcer. Further there is epidemiologic evidence that heavy cigarette smoking, which increases susceptibility to peptic ulceration, is also associated with an increased risk of stomach cancer.

The etiology of stomach cancer therefore remains unclear but both environmental and genetic factors appear to play a part.

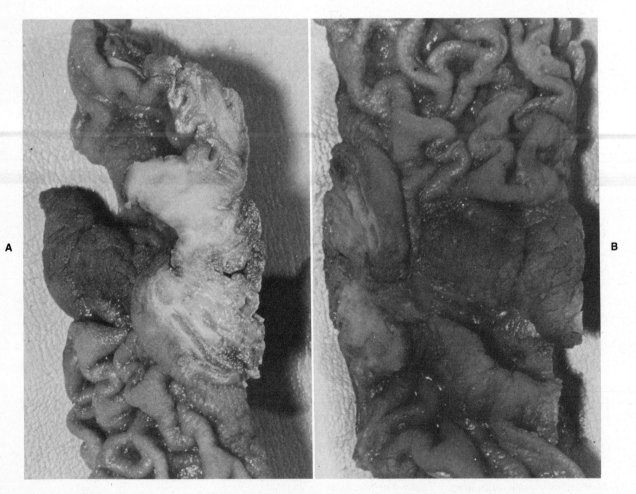

FIG. 14-17. Carcinoma of the stomach. These two views show both the proliferative changes and ulceration (**A**) and also invasion through the stomach wall to the subserosa (**B**). (*Courtesy Curator of the Gordon Museum, Guy's Hospital, London, England.*)

Pathology. Carcinoma of the stomach is an adenocarcinoma and usually takes one of three forms namely; (1) ulceration, (2) a polypoid mass, or uncommonly, (3) diffuse infiltration (*linitis plastica*).

The ulcerative type of tumor usually affects the greater curve of the stomach. Like malignant ulcers in other sites, it has raised, irregular margins and a rough, slough-covered floor. The polypoid type forms a rounded, cauliflower-like growth that grows outward into the lumen of the stomach more often than it infiltrates the wall.

The infiltrative type of growth spreads through the stomach wall in a uniform fashion, producing neither obvious ulceration nor localized swelling (Fig. 14-17). The stomach wall loses its normal mucosal folds and becomes a smooth, thickened, rigid sac, described as a leather-bottle stomach.

These morphologically different types of carcinoma are mainly adenocarcinomas and are usually well differentiated. However, they differ in their prognosis, as discussed later.

Clinical aspects. Gastric cancer is insidious, and the diagnosis is rarely made at an early stage because the stomach can accommodate a large mass without symptoms. Oddly enough, failure of early diagnosis rarely effects the prognosis, provided the tumor grows slowly. Symptoms may either be caused directly by the growth itself or alternatively by secondary deposits in various sites.

Gastric symptoms are often vague. They include loss of appetite and weight, or epigastric pain. A tumor near the cardia can cause dysphagia, while a growth near the pylorus can cause vomiting as a result of obstruction (Fig. 14-18). The tumor usually causes gradual leakage of blood, which leads to iron-deficiency anemia. Occasionally, the growth perforates the stomach wall, causing peritonitis as the first sign of the disease.

Secondary spread of the tumor is usually to the liver, and occasionally this may be the cause of the first symptoms. The most common effects are obvious hepatomegaly or ascites. Another manifestation is involvement of the lymph nodes; one characteristic site is at the base of the neck in the supraclavicular fossa. Occasionally, there is widespread peritoneal seeding of growth and gross accumulation of peritoneal fluid. Transperitoneal spread with secondary growth in the ovary (Krukenberg tumor*) or rectovesical pouch is well recognized. Diagnosis is usually suggested by radiography after a barium meal and is confirmed by endoscopy and biopsy.

Diseases of the intestinal tract

Many diseases of the intestinal tract such as the all too common infections, and Crohn's disease involve both small and large intestines. There are, nevertheless, certain differences in disease patterns between these two parts of the intestinal tract—particularly in that carcinomas are common in the large intestine but rare in the small intestine, whereas malabsorption syndromes are a common effect of very many diseases of the small intestine but not of the large intestine which has no digestive function.

Malabsorption syndromes

There are many causes of malabsorption syndromes, the characteristic feature of which is failure of absorption of one or, more usually, several constituents of the diet. The causes can be divided broadly into (1) primary disorders of the small intestine and (2) deficiency of digestive enzymes or bile salts. In many of the malabsorption syndromes, a multiplicity of mechanisms operate and in some cases the precise nature of some of these is uncertain. Important causes are summarized in the following list†:

1. Impaired digestive function
   a. Pancreatic diseases or resection
   b. Reduced bile salts
      (1) Parenchymal liver disease
      (2) Cholestasis
      (3) Bacterial destruction of bile salts
      (4) Drugs which bind or precipitate bile salts
   c. Postgastrectomy
2. Intestinal infections
   a. Tropical sprue
   b. Whipple's disease
   c. Blind loop syndrome
   d. Chronic giardiasis
   e. AIDS (various infections)
3. Reduced absorptive area
   a. Ileal resection
4. Defective mucosal absorption
   a. Lymphatic obstruction
   b. Congestive cardiac failure
   c. Celiac disease
   d. Crohn's disease
   e. Tropical sprue
   f. Disaccharidase deficiency
   g. Radiation damage
   h. Amyloidosis
   i. Systemic sclerosis
5. Unknown mechanisms
   a. AIDS enteropathy

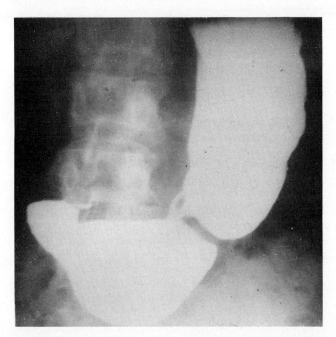

FIG. 14-18. Hourglass stomach. This appearance is occasionally produced by intense fibrous contracture secondary to peptic ulceration. The severe degree of obstruction thus caused will be evident. This type of deformity can also rarely be caused by a carcinoma. (*Courtesy Curator of the Gordon Museum, Guy's Hospital, London, England.*)

*E.F. Krukenberg (1871-1946), German pathologist.

†NOTE: In some of these disorders, a variety of mechanisms may be operating: in others, the precise mechanisms involved are uncertain.

In the Western world, malabsorption is most commonly the result of celiac disease (defective absorption), pancreatic disease (impaired digestion of fat and protein) (Chapter 15), or small bowel resection (reduced absorptive surface and sometimes bile acid deficiency). Worldwide, particularly in parts of Asia, tropical sprue is more important.

Malabsorption and wasting are a common complication of bowel disease in AIDS as discussed later.

Effects of malabsorption. Typical manifestations of malabsorption are as follow:

1. Diarrhea and steatorrhea (fatty diarrhea) caused by increased fecal fat and water—Serum cholesterol is decreased secondarily.
2. Weight loss, muscle wasting and fatigue caused by increased nitrogen and fat excretion and impaired glucose absorption
3. Stunting of growth in children caused by protein deficiency
4. Anemia resulting from impaired iron, vitamin B_{12} or folate absorption
5. Calcium loss leading to paresthesias and tetany, and osteomalacia or osteoporosis
6. Malabsorption of fats leading to failure of absorption of vitamin K and bleeding tendencies caused by reduced prothrombin formation
7. Failure of absorption of other fat-soluble vitamins, A, D and E
8. Edema resulting from protein loss and hypoalbuminemia
9. Stomatitis or glossitis resulting from deficiencies of B group vitamins

Gastric dysfunction. The most common example of gastric dysfunction is the dumping syndrome (excessively rapid transit of food through the intestine) as a consequence of gastrectomy.

An important effect of gastrectomy is the reduction or loss of intrinsic factor secretion. This can lead to failure of ileal absorption of vitamin B_{12} and, eventually, pernicious anemia (Chapter 13).

Pancreatic disease. Inadequate secretion of pancreatic enzymes causes defective absorption of protein and fats as for example in cystic fibrosis.

Hepatobiliary disease. Deficiency of bile salts reaching the intestine can seriously impair absorption of fats and fat-soluble vitamins. In addition bacteria or drugs can bind or inactivate bile salts. Pancreatic and hepatobiliary diseases are discussed in Chapter 15.

Intestinal disease. Important examples are Crohn's disease and its complications, and celiac disease. Intestinal resection and bypass operations substantially reduce the area for absorption and impair digestive function. Scleroderma, amyloid or lymphoma are examples of rare causes of malabsorption.

Infections. Under certain conditions, bacteria can proliferate in the bowel and impair absorption, as in tropical sprue and Whipple's disease as discussed later. In *blind loop syndrome* also, part of the bowel becomes cut off from the normal flow of gastrointestinal contents, either as a result of operative treatment or of adhesions. The effect is to form what is functionally a diverticulum, in which bacteria can proliferate. Malabsorption in such circumstances, can result from microbial deconjugation of bile salts, destruction of disaccharidase, damage to the brush borders, uptake of vitamin B_{12} by the bacteria and probably other mechanisms.

Clinical aspects. The manifestations of malabsorption are multifarious as indicated earlier and highly variable. Typical features however are fatty diarrhea (steatorrhea) (Fig. 14-19) with frequent passage of bulky, foul smelling stools, loss of weight or failure of growth, and the effects of vitamin deficiencies and other deficiencies. Anemia is common and may result from impaired vitamin B_{12}, folate or iron absorption. Deficiency of these substances or less often of other B group vitamins can cause sore tongue.

Despite these many possibilities, malabsorption may also be virtually asymptomatic and celiac disease, for example, may not be recognized until adult life is reached.

Celiac disease (gluten sensitive enteropathy, nontropical sprue)

Celiac disease appears to result from an immunologic reaction of an undefined kind to gluten. Gluten is the protein of wheat, and rye particularly, that binds the starch particles together and makes breadmaking possible. There is some evidence for a genetic component in the etiology and there is a significant association with HLA B8, Dw3 and Dw4.

The rapid deterioration of small bowel function on exposure to gluten and the response to a gluten-free diet are the main features suggesting an immunologic reaction. There is also extensive lymphocytic and plasma cell infiltration of the lamina propria of the jejunum in active disease and local synthesis of anti-α gliadin antibodies. Nevertheless, an immunologic basis to this disease is by no means certain as there is also evidence that gluten is toxic to the intestine in susceptible persons.

Pathology. The jejunal wall is heavily infiltrated with lymphocytes and plasma cells. There is rapid atrophy of the intestinal villi, which become short and blunt (partial villous atrophy) or may disappear. Absorption is impaired accordingly.

Clinical features. Although celiac disease starts in childhood, it is frequently not recognized until adolescence, early adult life, or sometimes until middle age. Severe disease causes permanent stunting of growth, but even this may not lead immediately to the diagnosis.

Failure of diagnosis of celiac disease is largely the result of the extreme variety of initial complaints. Only a minority have the typical symptoms of fatty diarrhea (or this may not be recognized as abnormal), loss of weight and other signs of malnutrition. The main complaints are more often the result of secondary effects, particularly anemia, edema, tetany or occasionally sore tongue.

Diagnosis of celiac disease can be confirmed by failure to absorb D-xylose, jejunal biopsy showing villous atrophy and, finally by response to a gluten-free diet. The latter is dramatic in effects but may be difficult to maintain. In children three jejunal biopsies (initial, after gluten withdrawal and after reexposure to gluten) are required because of the need to confirm the diagnosis with certainty, to avoid the hazard of stunting of growth and to distinguish celiac disease from causes of transient mucosal damage and malabsorption in this age group.

Complications. Dermatitis herpetiformis (Chapter 19), an itchy papulovesicular skin eruption, may be associated with celiac disease and also responds partially or completely to a gluten-free diet.

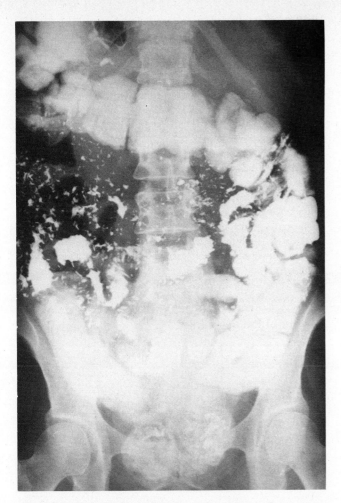

FIG. 14-19. Radiograph of barium study in malabsorption syndrome. The small bowel has lost its normal mucosal pattern, and the excess fat has caused the barium to form flocculent masses.

Gastrointestinal lymphoma is another possible complication, which is suggested by unexpected deterioration of gastrointestinal symptoms after good control or by fever, abdominal pain, and blood in the stools.

Tropical sprue (postinfective tropical malabsorption)

Tropical sprue (sprue is another name for fatty diarrhea) is most common in India, Southeast Asia, northern South America, and in travelers from those countries, but in only a few small areas of Africa. The disease is characterized by chronic malabsorption following an acute gastrointestinal infection.

Microbiology and pathology. There is colonization of the intestinal lumen by aerobic enterobacteriaceae but the picture varies with the country of origin. The microbial mechanisms causing malabsorption are varied as discussed earlier, but it seems likely that acute infection initiates the process by causing enterocyte damage. Enteroglucagon is then liberated and causes bowel stasis which, in turn, promotes bacterial colonization. Failure of absorption of folate which starts at an early stage hampers enterocyte repair and is perpetuated by continued malabsorption. This vicious circle persists until the bac- growth is eliminated and folate stores are made up.

Microscopically, intestinal abnormalities similar to those of celiac disease develop in some patients but in others no significant changes are apparent.

Tropical sprue usually responds to administration of folate (which hastens enterocyte recovery) and tetracycline, together with additional dietary supplementation as necessary.

Whipple's disease

Whipple's disease is an uncommon cause of malabsorption due to an infection of the gut but having widespread systemic effects. Whipple's disease typically affects white males usually in middle age.

In typical cases the wall of the small intestine becomes thickened and the villi are distended by macrophages to the extent that the gross appearance of the lining has been likened to a bearskin rug.

Microscopically, the intestinal mucosa is packed with foamy macrophages containing large granules which stain intensely with periodic Schiff reagent. Unidentified bacilli can be found in and among the macrophages, in neutrophils, in the intestinal epithelial cells and in macrophages in other tissues such as synovia or the central nervous system. Malabsorption in this disease seems mainly to be due to impairment of intestinal wall function and lymphatic obstruction.

Clinically, there are the signs and symptoms of malabsorption in typical cases or the picture may be dominated by the effects of the disease on other organs. Such effects include arthritis, central nervous system manifestations and skin hyperpigmentation.

Whipple's disease was formerly fatal and confirmation of the diagnosis is essential as the disease responds to treatment with trimethoprim-sulfamethoxazole and dietary supplementation as necessary.

Disaccharidase deficiency

The most common type of disaccharidase deficiency is lactase deficiency of which there is an uncommon hereditary type and an exceedingly common, late-onset type in adults. Lactase deficiency is frequently also associated with primary intestinal mucosal diseases and other causes of malabsorption, including infections such as giardiasis.

Congenital lactase deficiency causes acid diarrhea, as a result of production of lactic acid by bowel bacteria from undigested lactose, and failure to thrive until lactose is eliminated from the diet.

Adult lactase deficiency is characterized by symptoms varying from mild abdominal distention and a bloated sensation, to severe diarrhea.

There is no apparent abnormality of the intestinal mucosa in either the congenital or late-onset types of primary lactase deficiency.

Diagnosis is by detection of excess production of hydrogen (present on the breath) by gas chromatography and confirmed by withdrawal of and reexposure to lactose.

Crohn's disease

Crohn's disease typically affects the terminal ileum and can cause malabsorption. However, it can produce a clinical picture which may be difficult to differentiate from ulcerative colitis, as discussed later.

Appendicitis

Acute appendicitis is one of the most common causes of acute gastrointestinal tract pain. It causes appreciable mortality because it is so common and because, if not treated early, perforation and peritonitis are dangerous complications.

Etiology and pathology. The cause of acute appendicitis is not known. It is generally assumed that the precipitating event is obstruction of the lumen of the appendix by some material such as hardened feces. It is presumed that inflammatory changes, distention, and superimposed infection then follow. Cultures of acutely inflamed appendices usually, however, yield only normal bowel organisms, although this is not to say that they cannot be pathogenic in these circumstances.

Early acute appendicitis (Fig. 14-20) is characterized by progressive infiltration of the wall of the appendix with acute inflammatory cells together with congestion and edema. These early inflammatory changes can progress to acute suppuration and eventually necrosis (gangrene) of the appendix.

Complications. Complications are the result of gangrene and rupture of the appendix and include the following:
1. Generalized peritonitis
2. Abscess formation (locally or beneath the diaphragm)
3. Thrombosis of the portal venous drainage or pylephlebitis
4. Hepatic abscess as a consequence of transport of infection via the portal vein
5. Septicemia

Clinical aspects. Appendicitis is most common in adolescents and young adults, but persons of any age can be affected. Typically, acute appendicitis develops over the course of 24 to 48 hours with mild discomfort in the center of the abdomen together with loss of appetite, nausea, and vomiting. Later, as the overlying peritoneum becomes involved, pain becomes localized to the lower right quadrant of the abdomen and assumes a deep, aching character. There is tenderness on palpation and reflex guarding by the muscles of the abdominal wall. Increasingly severe pain and tenderness together with fever and leukocytosis are an indication of peritonitis even before the appendix ruptures.

These clinical features are by no means always so clear-cut as to make the diagnosis certain. In many cases the features are atypical, and there is frequently confusion between acute appendicitis and other abdominal inflammatory disorders. Delay can, however, be fatal; surgical intervention is, therefore, mandatory even before a firm diagnosis is made. Delay in surgical intervention, which allows gangrene to develop, results in a mortality rate of over 10%.

Tumors of the small intestine

Benign tumors. Adenomas are rare but when present can undergo malignant change. Leiomyomas and lipomas are benign connective tissue tumors which are occasionally found.

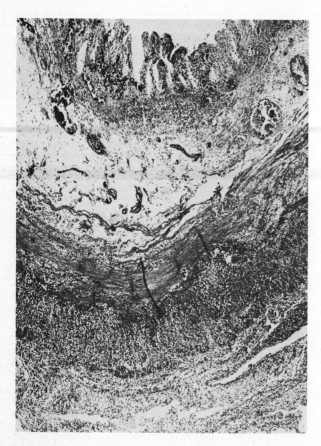

FIG. 14-20. Acute appendicitis. In this late stage the glandular epithelium *(top)* has been destroyed, but the outline of the crypts can still be seen. Inflammation has extended through the wall of the appendix to the serosa at the bottom of the picture.

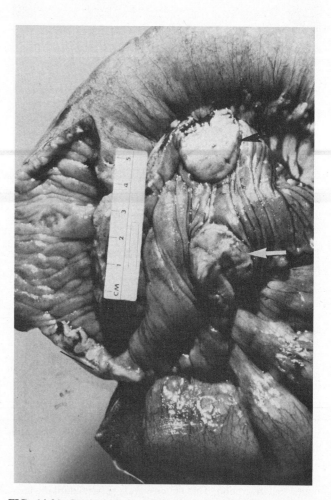

FIG. 14-21. Carcinoid tumor of the small intestine. Two small carcinoids *(arrows)* are seen in the mesenteric border of the ileum.

Carcinomas (adenocarcinomas) of the small intestine are rare. Typically such tumors encircle the intestinal wall and gradually obstruct it to cause nausea, vomiting, abdominal cramps, and loss of weight. Less often the tumor forms a fungating mass. Metastases have usually spread to the liver by the time the diagnosis has been made.

Endocrine tumors (carcinoids, argentaffinomas)

Carcinoids (the term is retained here for convenience) were so-called because of their lesser malignancy than the more common adenocarcinomas. Carcinoids are, however, morphologically distinct from carcinomas and are endocrine in nature. The endocrine cells are derived from stem cells (not from neuroendocrine cells as formerly thought) and take up silver stains; they are consequently also known as *argentaffinomas*. The parent cells have also been termed *APUD* (amine precursor uptake and decarboxylation) cells, which are widespread. In animals carcinoids have been induced by administration of drugs which inhibit gastric acid secretion. The latter, it is suggested, may stimulate gut endocrine cells by feedback stimulation of gastrin secretion.

Carcinoids are rare tumors that most commonly arise in the appendix. Carcinoid tumors secrete polypeptide hormones and amines, such as serotonin, which can have vasoactive and various other effects on many organ systems (carcinoid syndrome), particularly when widespread metastases develop.

Similar endocrine tumors can arise occasionally from the stomach, colon or rectum, or lungs or bronchi. However 77% of carcinoids arise from the appendix and most of the remainder from the small intestine. The pattern of hormones secreted by carcinoids and their ability to cause carcinoid syndrome depends on their embryologic origin. A characteristic feature of carcinoid tumors is that the clinical endocrine effects remain responsive to inhibitors as discussed later.

Pathology. Carcinoids usually form discrete firm submucosal plaques or nodules an inch or two across (Fig. 14-21). They are sometimes multifocal. The overlying mucosa usually remains intact, but the underlying muscle layer and serosa tend to be invaded and sometimes penetrated.

The tumor is typically a pale yellowish-brown color when cut across. Histologically, the pattern is variable, but there are often darkly staining epithelial cells of uniform size and arranged in strands or nests, sometimes with a poorly defined glandular pattern.

Granules of yellowish-brown pigment are present in the cytoplasm of the tumor cells and silver stains produce a fine black, granular pattern throughout the cells (Fig. 14-22).

The effects of carcinoid tumors are partly mediated by 5-hydroxytryptamine (serotonin) which gives rise to the diarrhea, bronchoconstriction and edema. Kallikrein, tachykinins such as substance P, and prostaglandins are also produced and probably mediate vasodilatation; they may also contribute to the diarrhea.

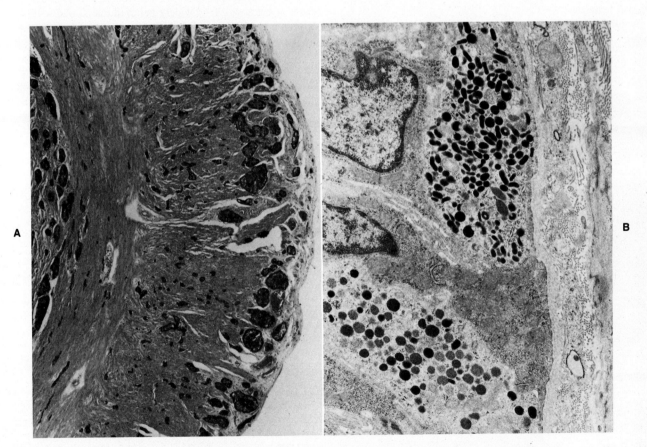

FIG. 14-22. A, Carcinoid tumor of the appendix. The specimen has been stained with silver salts, which the APUD cells have taken up and appear black as a result. **B,** Electronmicrograph of ileum showing two types of endocrine cells from which carcinoid tumors arise. These cells are characterized by their content of strikingly electron-dense granules.

Clinical aspects. Carcinoid tumors are more common in women (Fig. 14-23) and, when in the appendix, tend to arise before middle age. They occasionally invade deeply or cause partial or complete obstruction.

Since overt carcinoid syndrome usually results from a tumor that has already metastasized, curative surgery is not possible. Resection of the main tumor mass has a useful palliative effect, and many of the effects of carcinoid mediators can be controlled by somatostatin (Chapter 18) or its analogs, which inhibit the release of peptide hormones.

The relatively benign behavior of carcinoids is shown by the 5-year survival rate of 99% for those arising from the appendix irrespective of stage.

Tumors producing gut peptides (gastrinomas, glucagonomas, vipomas and others) mostly arise in the pancreas (Chapter 15).

Gastrointestinal lymphomas. Lymphomas of the gastrointestinal tract mostly arise in the stomach or small intestine. In the stomach, lymphomas represent about 5% of malignant neoplasms.

Lymphomas of the small intestine are of very varied types but are usually B cell tumors, having originated in gut-associated lymphoid tissue. They may be primary or secondary, single or multiple and be isolated lesions or associated with other diseases. A special type is the so-called Mediterranean lymphoma first described in Israel and associated with production of abnormal IgA which lacks alpha light chains. Persistent diarrhea, malabsorption, and abdominal pain are typical clinical features.

Small intestine lymphomas otherwise give rise to nodular masses or annular strictures and are most commonly immu-

noblastic or lymphoblastic (large noncleaved cell) types, but their categorization has caused considerable controversy.

Immunoproliferative small intestinal disease (IPSID). Immunoproliferative small intestine disease is also most common in the Middle East and lands bordering the Mediterranean. Male children and young adults are chiefly affected. Malabsorption, diarrhea, and loss of weight are typical symptoms. They are associated with an abnormal bowel flora and clinical improvement follows treatment with tetracycline.

Microscopically, the lamina propria of the small intestine is densely infiltrated with lymphocytes and plasma cells, whereas the villi and crypts become obliterated.

Despite the response to tetracycline, a high proportion of patients develop intestinal lymphomas.

Diseases of the large intestine
Crohn's disease (regional ileitis, regional enteritis)

Crohn's disease* is an uncommon cause of intestinal tract disease. It is characterized by a chronic relapsing course and the formation of granulomatous, sarcoidlike lesions in the intestinal wall. Although Crohn modestly proposed the name *regional ileitis,* this disease can also cause regional enteritis and affect many other sites, both in the gastrointestinal tract (including the mouth) and outside the gastrointestinal tract altogether.

Etiology. In spite of great interest in this disease and the amount of effort that has been put into its investigation, the cause is unknown. It is widely believed that Crohn's disease is immunologically mediated, and the main thrust of recent research has been in this direction. One factor suggestive of such a mechanism is the formation of sarcoidlike follicles in the intestinal wall in Crohn's disease. Similar follicles are typical both of sarcoidosis and tuberculosis where immunologic phenomena are associated.

Abnormalities of mucosal immunity are variable and inconsistent, however, and defects of cell-mediated immunity seem largely to be secondary to malnutrition. There is some response by Crohn's disease to immunosuppressive treatment although these drugs are by no means curative.

*B.B. Crohn (b. 1884), American physician.

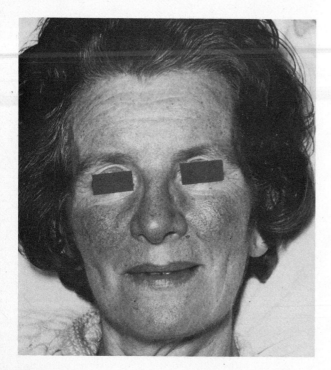

FIG. 14-23. Carcinoid flush. The symmetrical area of erythema extending across both cheeks and the nose is a result of the effects of the vasomotor amines produced by the tumor. (*Courtesy Curator of the Gordon Museum, Guy's Hospital, London, England.*)

TABLE 14-3. Distinguishing features of Crohn's disease and ulcerative colitis

Crohn's disease	*Ulcerative colitis*
Ileum especially, but any part of intestine	Colon
Segmental	Diffuse
Transmural	Superficial
Ulceration mild	Ulceration severe
Fibrosis severe	Fibrosis minimal
Chronic granulomatous (sarcoidlike) reaction	Nonspecific inflammation
Extraintestinal lesions common (e.g., mouth, skin) and of similar type	Extraintestinal lesions less common and of a different type (e.g., ankylosing spondylitis)
Surgery often followed by involvement of adjacent intestine	Surgery usually curative
Carcinoma not common	Carcinoma common late sequel

The main alternative theory is that Crohn's disease is infective, possibly as a result of some unidentified and elusive virus. Recent studies have suggested that adenoviruses or enterovirus-like agents may be implicated, but because these viruses are not infrequent, harmless passengers in humans, their significance is as yet unproven. Immunologic mechanisms may also, however, play a part even if the underlying cause is an infection.

Another controversial aspect of Crohn's disease is its relationship to sarcoidosis and ulcerative colitis. The granulomas of Crohn's disease are histologically somewhat similar to those of sarcoidosis, while clinically there may sometimes be some difficulty in distinguishing Crohn's disease from ulcerative colitis so that some workers believe that they are both manifestations of the same disease. However, current opinion, based on (1) the epidemiologic features, (2) the anatomic distribution of lesions, and (3) the response to surgical excision, is that Crohn's disease and ulcerative colitis are distinct entities. The etiology of sarcoidosis and ulcerative colitis are, unfortunately, also as obscure as that of Crohn's disease. Crohn's disease and ulcerative colitis are compared in Table 14-3.

Inexplicably the prevalence of Crohn's disease appears to be increasing in some parts of the world and declining in others.

Pathology. Crohn's disease involves the terminal ileum in the great majority (70%) of cases. In some cases the colon is involved, usually with the ileum as well.

The lesions are strikingly segmental and patchy. They involve the entire thickness of the wall at one point, but then skip a length of bowel, leaving an intervening normal segment. The characteristic change is progressive thickening of the bowel wall caused by fibrosis and narrowing of the lumen (Fig. 14-24). In addition, there are often proliferative changes in the mucosa, giving it a cobblestone appearance and causing varying degrees of ulceration.

Histologically there are granulomas and extensive lymphocytic infiltrates in the submucosa (Fig. 14-25). Any mucosal ulceration is associated with a more severe inflammatory reaction. The inflammatory changes advance to progressive fibrosis and thickening or obstruction of the bowel (Fig. 14-26). Microfistula formation is common.

Clinical aspects. Symptoms are variable, and often the diagnosis is not made until the disease is well established. The onset is often before the age of 20. Chronic intermittent diarrhea and episodes of colic are common early signs. Later there is loss of weight and sometimes melena. Malabsorption can cause

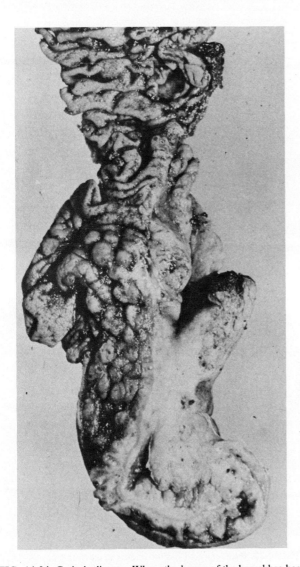

FIG. 14-24. Crohn's disease. Where the lumen of the bowel has been opened, the cobblestone appearance shows in strong contrast to the normal ridged appearance of the unaffected area above. Part of the bowel wall has been sectioned to demonstrate the gross thickening and narrowing of the lumen.

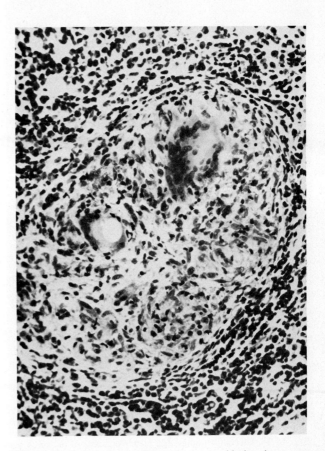

FIG. 14-25. Crohn's disease. Biopsy from an oral lesion shows a typical rounded granuloma. It consists of histiocytes and two multinucleate giant cells and is surrounded by a dense lymphocytic infiltrate. The patient developed Crohn's disease of the bowel a considerable time after this biopsy suggested the diagnosis.

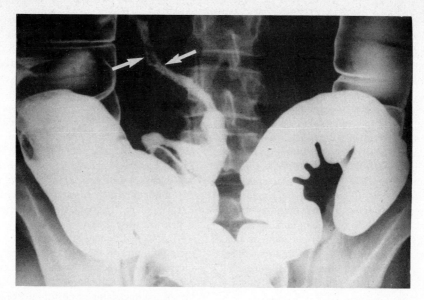

FIG. 14-26. Crohn's disease. This barium study shows the long narrow segment of ileum *(arrows)*, a typical feature caused by chronic inflammation and fibrosis.

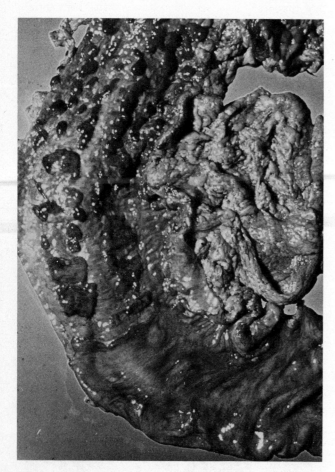

FIG. 14-27. Ulcerative colitis. The glandular lining of the colon has been destroyed, leaving an almost featureless atrophic epithelium with scattered hemorrhagic nodules caused by inflammatory hyperplasia. The appearances are those of ulcerative colitis during a period of remission. *(Courtesy Curator of the Gordon Museum, Guy's Hospital, London, England.)*

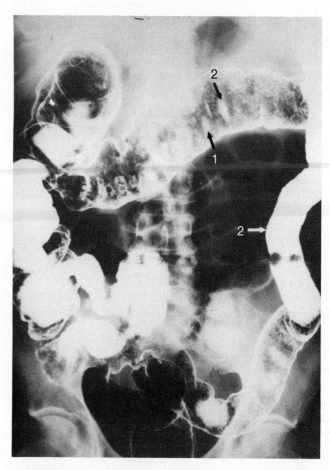

FIG. 14-28. Radiograph of barium enema in ulcerative colitis. There is complete loss of mucosal pattern *(1)* and pooling of barium in areas of deep ulceration *(2)*.

anemia and deficiency of vitamin B$_{12}$, folic acid, or iron in various combinations. Low-grade fever and malaise often accompany bowel symptoms. Serious complications are obstruction of the bowel or perforation. Crohn's disease can rarely cause characteristic oral lesions.

Complications include arthritis, iritis, hepatic dysfunction (caused by disturbance of enterohepatic circulation), perianal and other fistulas, and malabsorption.

With long-standing colorectal involvement (present in only 5% of patients with Crohn's disease) there is an increased risk of carcinoma in this area.

Crohn's disease pursues a chronic remittent course punctuated by relapses and periods of apparent recovery, but the progress tends to be slowly or rapidly downhill.

Treatment is not very satisfactory. Immunosuppressive drugs, particularly corticosteroids are frequently necessary and the antibacterial and antinflammatory drug, sulfasalazine is frequently helpful. Complications, such as anemia, must be managed as they develop. Surgery may be necessary, particularly if the disease causes intractable diarrhea or obstruction. The disease recurs after resection in about 50% of patients but may take 10 to 15 years before symptoms become troublesome again. Resection may not incidentally abolish extraintestinal symptoms such as arthritis.

Ulcerative colitis

Ulcerative colitis is now one of the most common causes of persistent, severe bowel disease. It has an estimated annual incidence in most populations of Anglo-Saxon origin of 5 to 10 per 100,000, while the prevalence of the disease in NW Europe is 70 to 90 per 100,000.

Etiology. The cause of ulcerative colitis is unknown, but it is believed by many to be immunologically mediated. Specific antibodies against various components of colonic mucous cells can be detected in most patients. Such antibodies are also found in unaffected relatives and do not appear to be pathogenic. Antibodies to lipopolysaccharide of intestinal epithelial cells also cross react with *Escherichia coli*, but their significance is unknown. Lymphocytes from patients with ulcerative colitis are however cytotoxic for colonic epithelial cells in vitro. However, despite the variety of immunologic abnormalities that have been reported none (as in Crohn's disease) have been consistently found and there are no immunologic tests of value in the diagnosis.

Whether there is an infective basis for ulcerative colitis remains an open question. There is some response to antibacterial drugs, but the evidence for an infective cause is not strong. Infection is not, however, incompatible with immunologic abnormalities as the main operative mechanisms.

A significant number of patients with ulcerative colitis have deep-seated personality disorders. Psychopathologic factors, however, explain little about the mechanism of the disease, and it must also be difficult to remain serene and emotionally stable when suffering from persistent, painful diarrhea.

Pathology. Ulcerative colitis predominantly affects the descending colon and often starts in the rectosigmoid. This is in contrast to Crohn's disease, which usually affects the ileum and ascending colon. Ulcerative colitis is confined to the colon, but it can cause secondary, so-called backwash ileitis. The characteristic feature is inflammation localized to the mucosa and submucosa, together with destruction of the epithelium (Fig. 14-27).

Early changes are infiltration by lymphocytes and neutrophils and necrosis of some mucosal cells. Microabscesses form by accumulation of polymorphonuclear leukocytes in the mucosal glands or crypts and extend to produce progressively larger areas of superficial ulceration. In severe cases the ulcers can erode through muscle or even perforate the bowel wall. In the worst cases almost the entire intestinal mucosa can be lost. Unlike Crohn's disease, fibrosis is not prominent, but pseudopolyps, which consist of nodules of hyperplastic granulation tissue surrounded by denuded mucosa, may form in large numbers (Fig. 14-28).

Complications. Complications include the following:
1. *Anemia.* This is mainly a result of blood loss and can be severe. Debility and loss of weight are almost inevitable.
2. *Cancer.* Proliferative changes in the bowel have a high premalignant potential. Probably about 30% of patients who have had the disease for 12 years or more develop colonic cancer.
3. *Toxic megacolon.* In unusually acute severe disease, necrosis of the colon can be so widespread that the lining virtually disintegrates, and bowel function fails. Diarrhea suddenly stops, and the colon rapidly dilates. This is known as toxic megacolon and is a life-threatening emergency.
4. *Bleeding.* Massive hemorrhage and perforation leading to peritonitis can develop, but they are less common.
5. *Extraintestinal changes.* These include arthritis resembling ankylosing spondylitis (Chapter 17), ocular lesions, skin disease, thrombophlebitis, or liver disease.

Clinical features. Ulcerative colitis most often starts in early adult life in an insidious fashion with painless diarrhea, which however becomes persistent and characterized by the passage of blood and mucus in the stools. In more severe cases there is bloody diarrhea, colic and lower abdominal pain, fever, loss of weight, whereas in a few patients, the onset is explosive with violent uncontrollable diarrhea causing severe fluid and electrolyte loss.

The course of the disease is highly variable, but usually chronic and relapsing. In some, it persists with relentless but more or less controllable diarrhea. Sulfasalazine, metronidazole or corticosteroid enemas will often mitigate such cases.

The outcome is equally variable and dependent on the severity of the disease. At the least it is distressing and can be disabling; at worst, death can result from bowel cancer or other complications. For this reason, excision of the affected length of bowel (colectomy) may be necessary for disease which is severe or persists for more than 10 years. Colectomy is often curative.

Diverticular disease

Small outpouchings of colonic mucosa and submucosa can herniate between the main muscle bundles and are called *diverticula*. These herniations often form in large numbers and become increasingly common with age. The term *diverticulosis* applies simply to the presence of many diverticula; *diverticulitis* means that inflammation has become superimposed. The two terms, however, are often loosely used as synonyms.

Etiology, pathogenesis, and pathology. It is probable that some individuals have congenital areas of weakness in the bowel wall, which makes them susceptible to diverticular disease. It is widely believed, however, that these abnormalities are predominantly dietary in origin and caused by the low residue diet that is now characteristic of modern industrialized society. Diverticulosis is almost unknown in those living on primitive diets with a high fiber content. Experimentally, rats can develop diverticulosis when fed a low residue diet. It is therefore postulated that a low residue diet delays the passage of food residues along the colon and also requires more powerful contraction of the sigmoid colon to move feces into the rectum. The high intracolonic pressures thus generated cause hypertrophy of the muscle and herniation of intervening colonic lining between the muscle bundles.

The diverticula appear as multiple, closely placed, rounded pouches from a few millimeters up to a centimeter in diameter along the margins of the tenia coli and principally affect the sigmoid colon (Fig. 14-29). These herniations have little or no muscle in their walls.

Diverticulitis was thought (like appendicitis) to be caused by impaction of fecal material in the orifice of a diverticulum and subsequent inflammatory changes. However, diverticulitis is caused by minute perforations of the thin walls of the diverticula leading to localized, pericolic inflammatory changes. Generalized peritonitis is a rare complication. To further complicate the picture, diverticular disease can be painful even in the absence of detectable inflammation.

Complications. Acute inflammation can supervene, and acute diverticulitis causes acute abdominal pain, fever, and tenderness. Abscess formation or, rarely, peritonitis can be consequences. Inflamed diverticula become surrounded by edematous fibrofatty tissue. Later, fibrosis may become more extensive, or a palpable fibrofatty mass can form.

Clinical aspects. Diverticular disease (Fig. 14-30) is common but rarely causes symptoms. It is often a fortuitous radiologic finding. When signs and symptoms develop, they often consist of colicky pain and either constipation or diarrhea, sometimes with blood in the stools. There is little correlation between the clinical manifestations and the radiologic or pathologic changes. A distinction between diverticulosis and diverticulitis is often academic.

When diverticular disease causes pain, a change in bowel habit, and an inflammatory mass, it is often a problem to distinguish it from carcinoma of the colon.

It is believed that diverticular disease can be controlled in most cases by means of a high fiber diet. Surgery is only necessary when complications develop.

Hernia

A hernia is the protrusion of a knuckle or loop of intestine, or less often, an abdominal viscus, through a weak point in the abdominal wall. The protrusion is covered by parietal peritoneum, which forms the lining of the hernia sac.

The most common type of hernia is of the small intestine through the inguinal canal. It is for all practical purposes a disease only of males. In the earliest stages, the hernia may

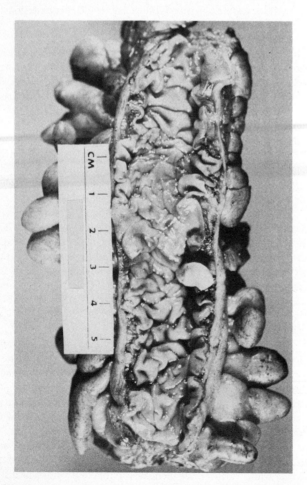

FIG. 14-29. Diverticular disease of the colon. There are many saclike diverticula protruding from the peritoneal surface of the colon. Some of the diverticula are mildly inflamed.

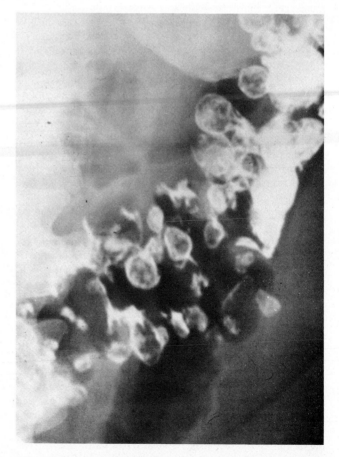

FIG. 14-30. Diverticular disease. The multiple spherical diverticula are clearly defined by the barium contrast medium in this radiograph. (*Courtesy Curator of the Gordon Museum, Guy's Hospital, London, England.*)

only appear when intraabdominal pressure is raised, particularly as a result of coughing or straining physically. The hernia can then usually be reduced, that is, returned to the abdominal cavity. Many hernias, particularly inguinal hernias, cause only minor symptoms and are tolerated for years. Nevertheless, they can give rise to serious complications. Adhesions can form so that the intestine is trapped in its sac and cannot be reduced. Occasionally, twisting of the neck of the hernia cuts off first the venous drainage and then the arterial blood supply. The hernia is then described as *strangulated* and if untreated becomes infarcted as a consequence. Infarction followed by gangrene causes intestinal tract obstruction, which rapidly progresses to peritonitis. This, therefore, constitutes an abdominal emergency requiring immediate surgical treatment.

Intestinal obstruction

Cessation of movement of the bowel contents can be a result of mechanical obstruction or paralysis of peristalsis. Causes of mechanical obstruction are tumors, strictures, or, less often, hernias or intussusception.

Paralytic obstruction is often termed *ileus*. It can result from peritonitis or, commonly, from excessive handling of the bowel during surgery in which case it is usually only temporary.

Effects of obstruction. If obstruction is mechanical, peristalsis is maintained and increased above the level of the obstruction, which the muscular contraction is unable to overcome. This causes severe colic.

The second consequence of obstruction is constipation, while accumulation of intestinal contents above the obstruction causes vomiting. In addition, bacterial fermentation of the static bowel contents produces large volumes of gas and abdominal distention (Fig. 14-31). Paralytic ileus, on the other hand, causes less severe symptoms, because there are no violent peristaltic contractions. Although there is no pain, there is constipation, gas formation, and vomiting.

The treatment of obstruction is to relieve any mechanical block or to treat peritonitis if this is the cause. Continuous suction is also set up to remove the static bowel contents and intravenous fluids are given to replace lost fluids and electrolytes. Suction and intravenous fluids alone usually relieve temporary ileus following abdominal surgery.

Volvulus

The mesentery, which supports most of the small intestinal parts and the colon, can become twisted; this is called a *volvulus*. Twisting of the mesentery obstructs first the venous drainage and then the arterial blood supply, causing infarction of the affected length of intestine. There is then acute severe abdominal pain, and immediate surgical intervention is needed. The damaged intestine usually has to be resected.

Intussusception

Intussusception is the term given to the telescoping of a segment of intestine into the intestine immediately beyond. The invaginated portion of intestine is dragged onward by peristaltic action and treated, in effect, like normal intestinal contents

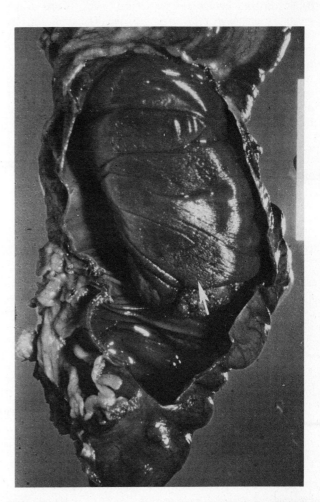

FIG. 14-32. Intussusception. The colon has been opened to show the segment of ileum *(arrow)* that has invaginated into the colon. The ileum is deeply congested because of strangulation of its blood supply. *(Courtesy Curator of the Gordon Museum, Guy's Hospital, London, England.)*

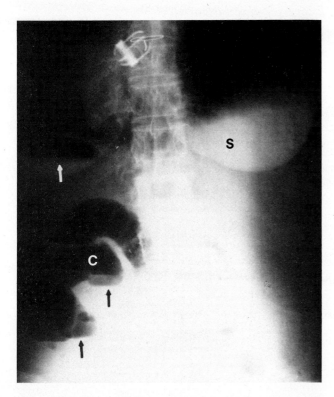

FIG. 14-31. Radiograph of acute intestinal obstruction. The stomach *(S)* and colon *(C)* are empty, and there are multiple horizontal fluid levels *(arrows)* typical of this condition.

(Fig. 14-32). In adults the process is usually initiated by the pull of peristalsis on a tumor of the bowel wall. In children, on the other hand, intussusception appears to happen spontaneously. The consequences of intussusception include intestinal obstruction and infarction of the affected bowel as a result of the blood vessels of the mesentery being also dragged into the distal segment and becoming obstructed.

Infections of the gastrointestinal tract

Gastrointestinal tract infections are among the most common illnesses affecting humans. There are many causes, and it is no exaggeration to say that gastrointestinal tract infections have had vast political and economic consequences. Dysentery has often caused more casualties to armies in the field than gunfire, and it was only in World War II that field sanitation was sufficiently well developed to control these epidemics. Epidemics of cholera have sometimes decimated populations. At the present time, traveller's diarrhea (turista, Montezuma's revenge, Delhi belly) is an important factor limiting tourism in many countries, especially in South and Central America and the Far East. It deprives these countries of hundreds of millions of dollars of much needed revenue.

The control of gastrointestinal tract infections, which until the nineteenth century were the cause of vast and lethal epidemics in both Europe and the United States, is one of the greatest triumphs of preventive medicine. The credit for this belongs mainly to sanitary engineers. The achievement is even more remarkable when it is appreciated that the successful abolition of water-borne diseases was achieved even before it was known that bacteria were the cause. Many more lives have been saved as a consequence of the apparently simple expedient of keeping feces out of drinking water than has been achieved by the use of antibiotics.

The causes of gastrointestinal tract infections are summarized in Table 14-4. Clinically, however, these diseases can be categorized as follows, although in several cases the pathogenic mechanisms overlap:

1. Infective diarrhea (including turista)
2. Cholera
3. Bacillary dysentery
4. Amebic dysentery and giardiasis
5. Viral gastroenteritis
6. Typhoid (enteric) fever

In recent years a wide variety of intestinal infections have become apparent in, and sometimes as the predominant feature of, AIDS as discussed later.

Infective diarrhea (including turista). The cause of travelers' or tourists' diarrhea has long remained a mystery. However, the most common single cause, accounting for about 30% of cases, is toxigenic strains of *Escherichia coli.* Causative agents vary from country to country, but in Africa and South America, for example, the infectious agents, so far identified include rotaviruses, Norwalk agent, Shigella, Salmonellae, *Giardia lamblia,* and *Entamoeba histolytica.* Yet other possible causes include different viruses, Campylobacter species, *Aeromonas hydrophila, Vibrio parahemolyticus, Plesiomonas shigelloides,* and Cryptosporidia (see Table 14-4).

Overall, the most effective prophylactic antibacterial agent is trimethoprim-sulfamethoxazole, the value of which has been established in extensive trials.

Coliform diarrhea, which is one of the most common forms, has effects that vary according to the strains involved. These changes depend on the production by some strains of an enterotoxin or, in the case of some Mexican strains of *E. coli,* by invasion of the intestinal mucosa. This, in turn, causes inflammation, ulceration, and bleeding.

An enterotoxin is an exotoxin that is released by the bacterium into and acts on the intestinal mucosa. One mechanism of action of the enterotoxins of many of these intestinal pathogens depends on their enhancement of the conversation of adenosine triphosphate (ATP) to cyclic AMP. This conversion is normally mediated by adenylcyclase, and this activity is greatly increased by enterotoxin (Chapter 8).

The result is active transport of water and salt through the bowel into the lumen of the intestinal tract. The rapid accumulation of fluid causes acute diarrhea. Several other mechanisms of production of diarrhea have been discovered more recently.

TABLE 14-4. Causes of infective diarrhea

	Agent	Pathogenesis	Remarks
Bacterial	*E. coli* (many strains)	Enterotoxin production	Mode of action as for *V. cholerae*
	Vibrio cholerae (including El Tor strain)	Enterotoxin that augments cAMP production	
	V. parahaemolyticus	As for *V. cholerae*	Marine organism; seafood infection
	S. aureus	Toxin production	Acts centrally usually < 4 hours after ingestion
	Clostridium perfringens	Toxin production	Acts locally after > 4 hours
	Salmonella species	Mucosal penetration	
	Shigella species	Mucosal ulceration and invasion	*S. shigae* most severe form of bacillary dysentery
	E. coli (some Mexican strains)	Mucosal invasion	Pathologic changes closely resemble bacillary dysentery
	Campylobacter jejuni	Mucosal invasion and ulceration	Acute exudative, bloody, enteritis
Viral	Gastroenteritis virus A	Cell invasion	Also known as Norwalk agent
	Gastroenteritis virus B	Cell invasion	Rotavirus or reo-like virus
Protozoal	*Entamoeba histolytica*	Mucosal ulceration	
	Giardia lamblia	Not known	
	Dientamoeba fragilis	Not known	
	Balantidium coli	Mucosal ulceration	Pig pathogen
	Cryptospiridium sp.	?Interference with absorption	Community epidemics. A severe complication of AIDS

The mechanism of staphylococcal food poisoning is different. Certain lysogenic strains of *S. aureus* produce enterotoxin, which can form in food during storage when the temperature and other factors are favorable. Ingestion of toxin-containing food, therefore, gives rise to diarrhea and vomiting of such rapid onset that it may start even before the meal has finished. This enterotoxin acts centrally on the chemoreceptor trigger zone in the brain. Clostridial diarrhea is usually caused by *Clostridium perfringens*, which also produces an enterotoxin. This is elaborated within the intestines, and diarrhea develops after a latent period, usually of more than 4 hours.

Diarrhea after eating shellfish is common and may be caused by *Vibrio parahaemolyticus*, which also produces enterotoxin.

Cholera. Cholera is caused by *Vibrio cholerae*. In the past it has caused vast epidemics, and the epidemic of 1867 to 1873 caused over a million deaths in Europe alone. Until relatively recently, cholera in India, the usual source of the disease, caused an annual mortality of over 300,000. Strangely in spite of its terrifying reputation, cholera is a preventable disease, and effective treatment has been known since the nineteenth century.

Epidemiology. The epidemics of cholera that take place today are mainly caused by the El Tor vibrio (named after a pilgrim quarantine station on the Red Sea), which has now spread virtually all over the world and has caused epidemics as far apart as Vietnam and southern Europe within the past decade. The success of the El Tor vibrio in continuing to spread across the world is a result of its greater ability to survive outside the body in food and water or within the intestine or gallbladder of symptom-free carriers. In 1978 an outbreak of cholera was reported in Louisiana and was apparently associated with seafood.

Pathology. The cholera vibrios do not invade the intestinal wall or cause any pathologic changes visible by light microscopy but secrete an enterotoxin, which by a mechanism similar to that of *E. coli* causes a violent outpouring of water and salts into the bowel lumen.

Clinical aspects. Cholera is characterized by profuse, uncontrollable watery diarrhea, abdominal cramps, and vomiting. The stools are pale and flecked with mucus (rice water stools).

The mortality from cholera results from severe dehydration and electrolyte imbalance. Intravenous replacement of fluids and electrolytes is rapidly effective, and cholera is then self-limiting. Fluid and salt replacement by mouth is often also effective.

The lethality of cholera is a result of the fact that it is most common in hot countries where the patients may already be dehydrated and are also often undernourished. Medical care is often also inadequate, and as a result the mortality rate can be as high as 30%. By contrast, healthy people with a normal level of gastric acid can often safely visit choleraic areas. Nevertheless, a raging cholera epidemic is not a feature likely to attract the average tourist to any tropical paradise.

A vaccine of killed organisms is available but is relatively inefficient.

Dysentery. Dysentery literally means a disorder of the bowels, but it has come to mean bloody diarrhea. Two forms of dysentery are caused by infectious agents:

1. Bacillary dysentery, which is caused by members of the genus *Shigella* or, rarely, invasive strains of *E. coli*
2. Amebic dysentery

Bacillary dysentery. The common form of dysentery is caused by various *Shigella* species (shigellosis). Worldwide *S. sonnei* is the most common cause, while a *S. dysenteriae* type 1 *(S. shigae)* causes the most severe disease.

PATHOGENESIS AND PATHOLOGY. Infection is acquired by eating contaminated food. In the early stages of the disease, the organisms produce enterotoxin similar to that produced by *E. coli* and *V. cholerae*. This may produce initial mild watery diarrhea, especially in infants. The organisms invade the mucosa of the lower ileum and colon, where they excite an acute pyogenic response. There is then local necrosis, ulceration of the mucosa, and pus formation. The effect of these inflammatory changes is that blood and mucus are passed in the stools; microscopic examination shows large numbers of leukocytes. Invasive strains of *E. coli* produce very similar pathologic changes.

CLINICAL ASPECTS. Bacillary dysentery is characterized by fever, abdominal pain, and bloody diarrhea. Its severity depends on the causative organism. Most cases are mild, but the disease is severe in debilitated individuals or when *S. dysenteriae* is the cause. This organism has caused severe epidemics in many Central American countries. The diagnosis is made by demonstrating red cells and leukocytes in the stools and culturing the causative organism. The disease responds well to one of several antibiotics.

Campylobacter infections. Animals are the reservoir of infection for most species of which *C. jejuni* is most important for humans. Campylobacter is as common as Salmonellae and more common than Shigellae as a cause of diarrhea.

C. jejuni, in particular, causes diarrhea, abdominal cramps and fever, and the symptoms may mimic acute appendicitis. The organism invades the epithelium of the small intestine and provokes inflammation which leads to the appearance of red and white cells in the excreta. Exotoxins and endotoxins are also produced but their actions are not known.

C. fetus subspecies *fetus* is uncommonly isolated from the stools but can cause septicemia in immunodeficient patients. As mentioned earlier *C. pyloris* has been implicated in gastritis and as a possible contributor to peptic ulceration.

Campylobacters are sensitive to many of the broad spectrum antibiotics.

Amebic dysentery. Amebic dysentery is caused by the protozoon *Entamoeba histolytica*, but about 10% of the population of the United States are estimated to harbor this organism without ill effect. In a minority, by contrast this protozoon can cause chronic or even fulminating diarrhea.

Pathogenic strains of *Entamoeba histolytica* can be distinguished from noninvasive strains by their isoenzyme patterns (zymodemes). Both invasive and noninvasive strains of *E. histolytica* are common in homosexual males.

E. histolytica is transmitted in the form of a cyst as a result of fecal contamination of water or food. Once in the bowel, the ameboid forms are released and invade the crypts of the glands of the colon. The amebae produce pore-forming proteins (Chapter 2), which enable them to penetrate the epithelium but not the muscle layer. Between the muscle and the epithelium, therefore, the amebae multiply and burrow widely to produce characteristic undermined ulceration. There is, however, relatively little inflammatory infiltration until secondary bacterial infection develops. In some patients chronic infection produces a localized inflammatory mass called an *ameboma*. Its main significance is its close resemblance to colonic cancer both clinically and radiologically.

Clinical aspects. The most frequent manifestation is diarrhea, together with abdominal cramps and occasionally melena.

Constitutional symptoms can be relatively slight or absent unless there is secondary bacterial infection. Amebae can penetrate the vessels and are carried by the portal blood to the liver where they produce abscesses. Patients with amebic abscesses have widely fluctuating fever, appear very ill, and may die if treatment is not given. Even with large abscesses, treatment with chloroquine or metronidazole is often remarkably successful.

Giardiasis. Giardiasis is a protozoan infection caused by *Giardia lamblia*. It is a relatively frequent cause of gastroenteritis in some areas, particularly in Russia and some parts of the United States, such as Colorado. In chronic cases, giardiasis causes malabsorption syndrome. The mechanisms of pathogenesis are complex and may include such factors as changes in intestinal motility, competition for nutrients, and interference with mucosal enzyme systems.

Viral gastroenteritis. In adults viral gastroenteritis is mainly caused by gastroenteritis virus A (Norwalk agent), which causes diarrhea and vomiting. Viral gastroenteritis due to gastroenteritis virus B (rotaviruses) is particularly common in children under 5 years old. It usually causes a brief illness characterized by diarrhea and vomiting. The disease frequently affects family members in rapid succession during winter months, and has been called "epidemic winter vomiting disease."

The pathologic mechanisms of these diseases are not known and the virus can only be recognized in the stools by electron microscopy or sophisticated immunologic procedures.

Enteric fever. Enteric fever is caused by *Salmonella typhi* and a few other *Salmonella* species. Typhoid is the most serious and important enteric fever. The disease is usually transmitted by fecal contamination of water or (less often) food. The sources of the organisms are symptomless carriers who transmit the infection, particularly if they become food handlers. The essential feature of enteric fevers is that bacteremia is an obligatory event (Fig. 14-33).

Pathology. The incubation period is from 10 to 14 days. During this time the organisms are localized and proliferate in the lymphoid tissue of the gastrointestinal tract, particularly Peyer's patches. After about a week, the mucosa overlying the hyperplastic lymphoid tissue becomes necrotic, causing elliptical ulcers.

At the end of the incubation period, the bacteria enter the bloodstream and spread widely throughout the reticuloendothelial system with consequences such as enlargement of the liver and spleen. The typical cellular response in enteric fever is by the macrophages, which undergo proliferation in the spleen and other lymphoid tissues.

Clinical aspects. The patient becomes severely ill with rising fever and severe malaise. During the first week a characteristic rash consisting of erythematous macules (rose spots) appears. Leukopenia and bradycardia are also characteristic. In the second week of illness, high fever continues, and abdominal pain and progressive exhaustion develop. During the third week, there is a high risk of intestinal tract and other complications. Mononuclear cells can be found in the stools, but diagnosis depends on culture of the infecting organism from blood, stools, or urine. Diagnosis can be confirmed by a rising titer of antibody during the second and third weeks. The main complications of typhoid are intestinal hemorrhage and perforation of the bowel wall.

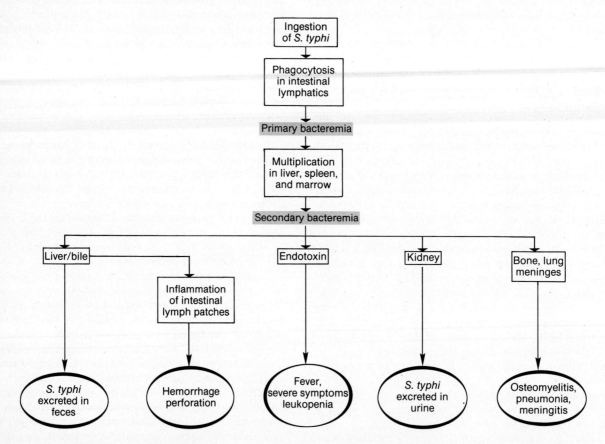

FIG. 14-33. Diagram of pathogenesis of enteric fevers. *(From McCracken AW and Cawson RA: Clinical and oral microbiology, Washington DC, 1982, Hemisphere Publishing Corp.)*

Cholecystitis is a frequent and important complication in that it may have the effect of establishing a persistent carrier state. Such symptomless carriers can remain as potential sources of further outbreaks in some cases for many years after.

The mortality rate from this disease is about 10% overall in untreated cases. Although this has been reduced by antibiotics, such as chloramphenicol and cotrimoxazole, these drugs are not completely reliable in that there are now chloramphenicol-resistant strains of *S. typhi*. These have infected some hundred thousand patients in Mexico in recent years and caused at least 14,000 deaths. The proliferation of these antibiotic-resistant organisms in countries such as Mexico, India, Thailand, and Vietnam is aided by uncontrolled and indiscriminate sale of antibiotics.

Antibiotic-associated colitis

Many antibiotics, including the penicillins, can occasionally cause colitis. The most severe of these is staphylococcal enterocolitis, usually caused by prolonged heavy doses of tetracyclines, particularly after bowel surgery. In this case the inhibition of most of the normal bowel flora allows pathogenic staphylococci to proliferate in vast numbers, causing destruction of the bowel wall, violent bloody diarrhea, and death. Now that the cause is recognized, this is rare.

Lincomycin, clindamycin, and other antimicrobial drugs can

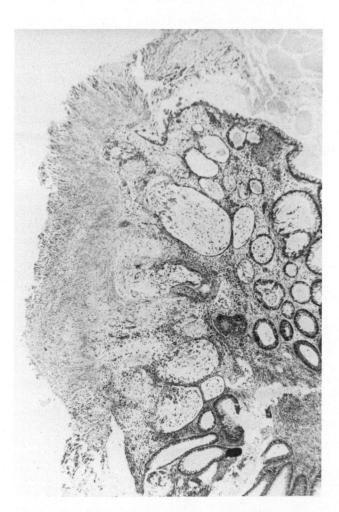

FIG. 14-34. Pseudomembranous colitis. Note the mushroom-shaped cap of fibrinoinflammatory exudate overlying dilated crypts of colonic mucosa.

cause mild diarrhea relatively frequently and occasionally fatal colitis, but this now seems preventable. Colitis following the use of these drugs appears to be the result of relative resistance of toxinogenic anaerobic bacteria, particularly *Clostridium difficile,* which proliferates when competitors are eliminated. Other antibiotics have a less broad spectrum of activity, especially against anaerobes, allow the survival of more competitors to *C. difficile,* which cannot so readily proliferate as a consequence.

The lesions are characterized by acute inflammation of the intestinal mucosa, destruction of the epithelium, and a characteristic mushrooming of inflammatory exudate from the damaged bowel into the lumen (Fig. 14-34).

Clinically, there is painful diarrhea with passage of mucus. In some cases, especially in elderly debilitated patients, there is passage of pseudomembranous material (necrotic mucosa) and blood. It occasionally results in death.

Antibiotic colitis can be prevented by giving vancomycin orally. The disease responds quickly to this treatment in most cases.

Clostridium difficile is also now recognized as a cause of nosocomial infectious diarrhea in chronic-care wards. In one study, approximately one third of patients' stools were positive for *C. difficile* or its toxin on admission.

Botulism

Clostridium botulinum produces the most potent exotoxin known. The organism is a natural inhabitant of the soil; hence, a source of the disease is home-canned vegetables that are contaminated by soil and inadequately sterilized. Botulism is also a hazard to Eskimos for whom a gourmet item is rotting seal meat.

In the United States, there are usually about 15 minor outbreaks of botulism annually, but these typically affect only a few people.

Like other forms of food poisoning, botulism is characterized initially by nausea and vomiting, but the exotoxin, absorbed through the bowel wall, causes widespread muscular paralysis terminating in respiratory failure. The consequences depend on the amount of preformed toxin ingested, but the mortality rate is approximately 65%. Botulism can also be contracted by infection of skin wounds (wound botulism), but this is even more uncommon.

Proliferation of the organism in the intestinal tract of young infants may lead to botulism, and it has been postulated as a cause of some cases of sudden infant death (SID, crib death) syndrome.

Gastrointestinal disease in AIDS

The gastrointestinal tract is involved in approximately 50% of AIDS patients and in a higher proportion of male homosexuals with this disease. Gastrointestinal involvement also appears to be particularly common in AIDS in Africa where the nickname "slim disease" has resulted from the wasting secondary to persistent diarrhea. A contributory factor in Africa is the greater prevalence of enteric infections and infestations to which AIDS patients are particularly vulnerable.

Gastrointestinal involvement in AIDS commonly leads to diarrhea, malabsorption, weight loss, and bleeding. These are usually the result of infections or (less often) tumors but there is also a so-called nonspecific enteropathy having these same effects, but for which no cause has yet been found.

Melena or more commonly occult blood loss is a frequent

sign in AIDS and can result from any of the infections causing colitis or proctitis; cytomegalovirus which can cause giant ulcers in any part of the gastrointestinal tract is also a major cause, as discussed below. Kaposi's sarcoma is another important source of intestinal bleeding.

Infections. Gastrointestinal infections in AIDS include both those to which most male homosexuals are susceptible and those resulting from immunodeficiency.

Common gastrointestinal infections presumably spread mainly by anogenital contact among non-AIDS homosexuals include:

1. Enteritis—Shigellosis, amebiasis, and giardiasis are the main examples.
2. Proctitis—Campylobacter, neisseria, chlamydia, and herpes simplex are the main causes.

In addition, hepatitis caused by hepatitis B and other viruses is common in this group and tends to be particularly severe. A high incidence of hepatocellular carcinoma secondary to hepatitis B has also been reported among male homosexuals.

AIDS patients are also susceptible to opportunistic gastrointestinal infections such as the following.

Cryptosporidiosis. This coccidian parasite has been known for many years to cause infections in animals but has only recently been identified as a cause of diarrhea and possibly cholecystitis or pancreatitis in humans.

The parasites are 2 to 5 μm diameter, spherical and intracellular in the intestinal epithelium, especially in the villi of the small bowel. Oocysts excreted in the feces are the probable infective agents and can be detected by their acid-fast staining. Persons in contact with farm and other animals are chiefly at risk, but the pathogenesis of cryptosporidial infection is unknown.

In otherwise normal persons, specific treament of the mild, self-limiting gastroenteritis and diarrhea is neither required nor available.

Cryptosporidiosis is a common, potentially lethal hazard for AIDS patients in areas where sanitation is poor; it causes persistent diarrhea, malabsorption, nausea, vomiting and abdominal pain. There is excessive intestinal secretion and thickening of the small bowel folds. There is no effective treatment.

Isospora belli, a sporozoon related to *Cryptosporidium* can also cause self-limiting diarrhea in normal hosts but chronic watery diarrhea, abdominal pain and loss of weight in AIDS patients. It is less common in the United States than in Haiti and some other countries, probably as a result of fecal contamination of water and food there. The response to trimethoprim-sulfamethoxazole is good but relapse is common.

Microsporidiosis. Microsporidia are rare intracellular parasites which were thought unlikely to cause human disease until the outbreak of AIDS. Infection probably results from ingestion of minute spores each of which contains a coiled polar filament or tubule, which can be seen by electron microscopy. Within the intestinal tract, the filament is extruded and may inject the infective body (the sporoplasm) into the host cell.

Microsporidiosis is yet another cause of persistent diarrhea in AIDS patients but has also been reported as a cause of myocarditis in such a patient. Microsporidia can also cause disseminated infections; they have been identified in many tissues, but their recognition has been hampered by their small size, similar to that of bacteria. Some genera, such as *Encephalitozoon* can only be recognized with certainty by electron microscopy.

Mycobacterium avium-intracellulare causes among other changes retroperitoneal and mesenteric lymphadenopathy but can also infect the small bowel to cause diarrhea, malabsorption and wasting. Microscopy shows numerous PAS positive macrophages and acid-fast bacilli but (as is common in AIDS) no granuloma formation.

Candida albicans causes oral thrush (a common premonitory sign of AIDS, indicative of developing immunodeficiency) and esophagitis. Esophagoscopy shows white plaques and often ulceration or proliferative changes producing nodularity of the mucosa. The response to antifungal drugs depends on the depth of the immunodeficiency.

Cytomegalovirus (CMV) among other effects, can infect any part of the gastrointestinal tract and ulceration has been described in the esophagus, terminal ileum and colon in AIDS patients. CMV inclusion bodies were present in these lesions. Diffuse colitis with raised yellow plaques containing CMV, have also been reported.

AIDS enteropathy. A subgroup of AIDS patients have diarrhea, wasting and often signs of malabsorption but lack any evidence of intestinal infection or neoplasia. Jejunal biopsy findings include partial villous atrophy, crypt hyperplasia and

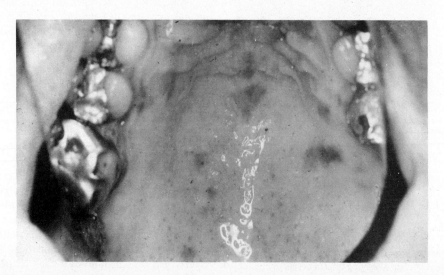

FIG. 14-35. Peutz-Jeghers syndrome. The patchy pigmentation of the oral mucosa resembling freckles is typical and usually associated with multiple polyposis of the small intestine.

lymphocytic infiltration of the lamina propria. However, such findings can also be made in AIDS patients without diarrhea and occasionally in asymptomatic male homosexuals. It is possible that the symptoms are secondary to IgA deficiency which is found in 50% of AIDS patients, and which may facilitate the entry of unidentified microorganisms. Alternatively, the widespread immunologic disturbances of AIDS may possibly give rise to a syndrome resembling celiac disease.

Tumors of the large intestine

Tumors of the large intestine, both benign and malignant are very common: colonic cancer, as discussed later is among the most important human malignancies.

Colorectal polyps. A *polyp* is a lesion that protrudes from a mucosal surface and colorectal polyps consist of proliferating glandular tissue. Colorectal polyps can be (1) nonneoplastic and (2) neoplastic.

Nonneoplastic polyps. Juvenile polyps are hamartomatous lesions found mainly in the rectosigmoid colon. They are typically solitary, and consist mainly of a disorderly collection of mucus-secreting glands. Inflammatory cells are often present in superficial eroded areas and in the lamina propria. Dysplastic changes which can progress to cancer may develop in the epithelium of these lesions.

*Peutz-Jeghers polyps.** The Peutz-Jeghers syndrome is characterized by multiple, harmartomatous polyps up to 3 cm in diameter. They are most numerous in the small intestine but are also found in the large intestine. Pigmentation of the mouth (Fig. 14-35) and perioral region is associated. This pigmentation, which resembles normal freckles is almost diagnostic of Peutz-Jeghers syndrome. The polyps are composed of a variety of mature intestinal epithelial cells, including absorptive, goblet, and neuroendocrine cells.

The chief complication of this disorder is intussusception. Malignant change is not a significant risk.

Hyperplastic polyps. Hyperplastic polyps are the result of a true hyperplasia of cells in the proliferative zone of the glandular crypts. In this area the cells become compressed and numerous mitotic figures may be present. However, the cells differentiate and mature normally. Hyperplastic polyps are small and do not appear to be premalignant.

Neoplastic polyps. Adenomatous polyps of the colon (Fig. 14-36) are true adenomas and can have various gross and microscopic appearances. Some are pedunculated, and some are sessile, and histologically, the pattern can be composed of tubules (Fig. 14-37), villi or mixtures of the two.

---

*J.L.A. Peutz, Dutch physician; H. Jeghers, American physician.

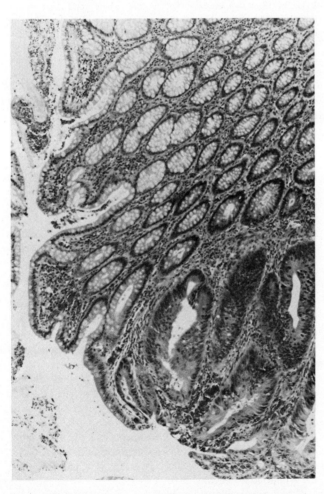

FIG. 14-36. Tubular adenoma of the colon. Colonic mucosa showing gradual transition from normal mucus-secreting epithelium above to crypts lined by neoplastic (tubular adenomatous) epithelium below.

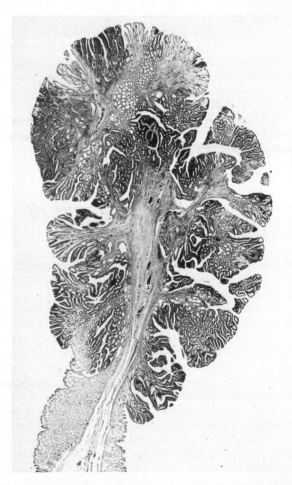

FIG. 14-37. Adenomatous polyp of colon. The neoplastic glandular tissue is supported by a vascular core, but although proliferation of the acini has produced a complex pattern of infolding, there is no invasion of the underlying tissue as is seen later in the carcinomatous polyp.

Adenomatous polyps of the colon can undergo malignant change.

Hereditary polyposis coli. Several rare syndromes are described in which multiple polyps of the colon are a prominent feature. Examples are Peutz-Jeghers syndrome (described on p. 343), familial polyposis coli and Gardner's syndrome.

Familial polyposis is characterized by vast numbers of polyps in both large and small intestine, particularly the former (Fig. 14-38). Sooner or later, in all cases, malignant change develops in one of the colonic polyps.

In *Gardner's syndrome,* * polyposis of the colon is associated with extracolonic neoplasms, particularly of the skin, soft tissues, mesentery, thyroid and duodenum. Dental abnormalities including mandibular exostoses, odontomas, and multiple unerupted teeth may also be associated.

Cancer of the colon and rectum

The colon is the most common site of cancer in men and women combined, and, as a cause of death, is second only to carcinoma of the bronchus in men and carcinoma of the breast in women. Colonic cancer accounts for about 20% of all cancer deaths; this amounted to 60,000 deaths in 1985.

Etiology and pathogenesis. Carcinomatous change in colonic polyps in the various hereditary syndromes, mentioned earlier, accounts for only a very small proportion of cancers of the colon. Probably most cancers develop in nonfamilial adenomatosis but even this may have a genetic component as discussed later.

Carcinoma of the colon is in general a disease of affluent, westernized countries and is common in the United States, Britain, and the rest of Europe. The incidence in Japan is intermediate between those countries and the more poverty-stricken peoples such as those of Africa, India, and some parts of South America.

Currently there is great concern about the role of diet in the etiology of colorectal cancer and epidemiologic studies have drawn attention to the association between the incidence of these tumors and dietary fat and fiber intake. One theory is that dietary fat enhances cholesterol and bile acid synthesis by the liver. The increased amounts of these sterols may then be converted by the bowel bacteria to potentially toxic metabolites. Fiber is thought to be protective by absorbing fats, by lowering sterol concentrations in the bowel and, by accelerating bowel transit, thus limiting the time that toxic substances can act on the lining. Animal experiments lend some support to such hypotheses but the role of diet in the etiology of colorectal cancer in humans is far from clear.

Bowel cancer genes. Bowel cancer may be genetically determined in familial adenomatous polyposis. In this disorder the gene has been localized on the long arm of chromosome 5; recently a somatic mutation on this chromosome has been found in cases of the common, nonfamilial type of colorectal cancer. This genetic abnormality may contribute to the etiology of bowel cancer by such mechanisms as failure to prevent tissue overgrowth and formation of bowel polyps, which, in turn, could become malignant as a result of environmental factors.

Pathology. The growth takes one of two main gross forms, either polypoid (cauliflower-like) (Fig. 14-39) or infiltrative (encircling the bowel) (Fig. 14-40).

The rectum and sigmoid colon (Fig. 14-41) are the main sites in about 75% of cases. The majority of the remainder form in the cecum and ascending and descending colon. The

*E.J. Gardner (b. 1909), American geneticist.

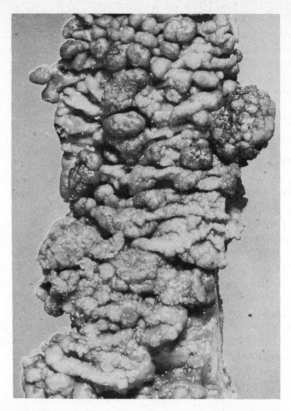

FIG. 14-38. Polyposis coli. The normal rugose appearance of the bowel wall has been obliterated by vast numbers of polyps. Several of these are large and irregular as a result of carcinomatous change. *(Courtesy Curator of the Gordon Museum, Guy's Hospital, London, England.)*

transverse colon and flexure are least often affected. Irrespective of its site in the bowel or its gross form, this tumor is usually a well-differentiated adenocarcinoma (Fig. 14-42) and produces mucin.

With cancer of the ascending colon, the growth is usually polypoid (Fig. 14-43) and quickly ulcerates, but obstruction develops relatively slowly. Growths in the left (descending) colon, by contrast, tend to be infiltrative, forming a stringlike constriction and causing early obstruction.

Clinical aspects. Constipation or change of bowel habit is usually the earliest sign and is a result of obstruction, particularly of the descending colon. The feces, which are held back, tend to liquefy by bacterial action, and this causes a short bout of diarrhea. Alternating diarrhea and constipation are, therefore, typical of cancer of the colon. Obvious blood in the stools is common with left colon cancer, but right-sided lesions tend to cause dark stools in which blood and mucus are mixed. Anemia as a result of blood loss or sometimes abdominal pain can also develop.

As the tumor spreads, it invades the bowel wall locally and extends to the regional lymph nodes. Thereafter, metastasis to the liver is very common, but a variety of other sites can be affected.

Surgery is the main form of treatment, and when the tumor is confined within the bowel, resection gives a 5-year survival rate of between 75% and 80%. This falls to about 25% once the lymph nodes become involved.

Carcinoembryonic antigen (CEA) is a characteristic antigen of embryonic tissues that has normally disappeared at birth. It is not found in normal adult tissue, but it is produced by about

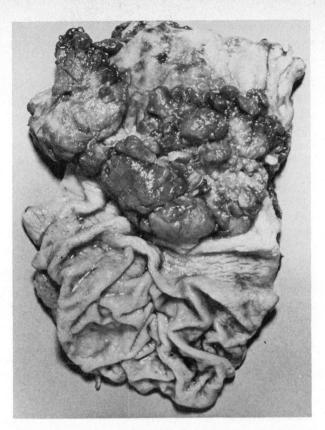

FIG. 14-39. Carcinoma of the colon. This carcinoma has produced an exophytic (cauliflower) proliferative mass. *(Courtesy Curator of the Gordon Museum, Guy's Hospital, London, England.)*

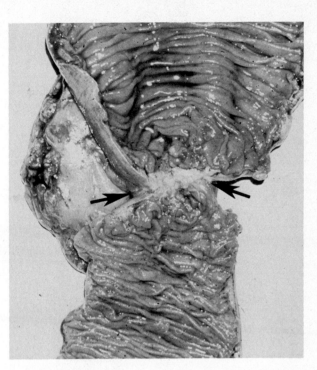

FIG. 14-40. Pursestring carcinoma of the colon. The tumor is small but has caused severe fibrous contracture and obstruction. *(Courtesy Curator of the Gordon Museum, Guy's Hospital, London, England.)*

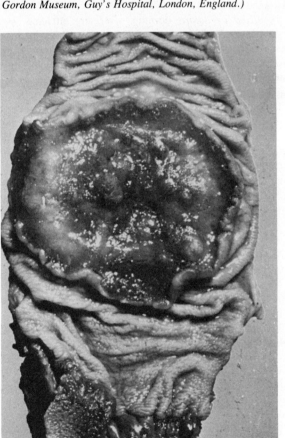

FIG. 14-41. Carcinoma of the rectum. The carcinoma has destroyed the typical architecture of the rectal mucosa and produced a typical malignant ulcer. *(Courtesy Curator of the Gordon Museum, Guy's Hospital, London, England.)*

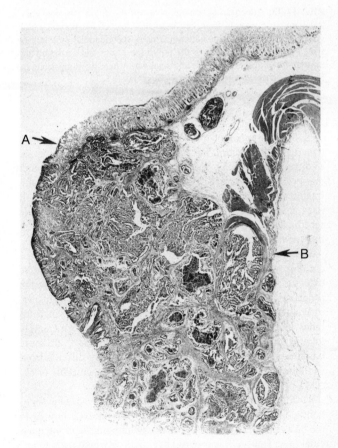

FIG. 14-42. Adenocarcinoma of the colon. Normal glandular epithelium abruptly changes to carcinoma, which has undermined the normal glands *(A)*, involved the full thickness of the intestinal wall, and destroyed the muscle layer to reach the subserous coat *(B)*.

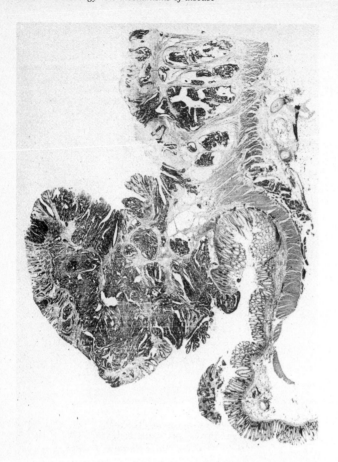

FIG. 14-43. Adenocarcinomatous polyp of the colon. Normal glandular mucosa extends from below to the base of the polyp, which consists of darkly staining carcinoma cells, the glandular structure of which is still evident. Above the polyp the tumor has destroyed the normal lining and invaded the intestinal wall where the tumor cells lie among clear areas formed by their secretions.

75% of carcinomas of the colon and also of the stomach and pancreas. Its detection has not been found to be a reliable aid to diagnosis, as it also appears in association with many other malignant and nonmalignant conditions. On the other hand, treatment of colon cancer causes a fall in the CEA level. It rises again as recurrence develops, and estimation of CEA in serum can, therefore, be a useful guide to the effectiveness of treatment.

Grading of colonic cancer. Colonic cancer is graded according to the degree of histological differentiation and the extent of spread; both are related (statistically speaking) to the prognosis. DNA cytometry may also be useful prognostically.

Well-differentiated adenocarcinomas show well defined tubules and nuclei of uniform size and shape. Intermediately tubules are recognizable but irregular and the nuclei are more variable in size, shape, and staining. In poorly differentiated carcinomas, glandular structures are barely recognizable or absent.

Different methods of surgical staging are in use. One time-honored method is that of Duke: Duke's A—growth limited to the bowel wall; Duke's B—growth extending through the muscular layer (muscularis propria) but not involving lymph nodes; Duke's C—involving lymph nodes. The prognosis deteriorates sharply with involvement of lymph nodes and further still with increasing numbers of lymph nodes involved.

Gastrointestinal neoplasms in AIDS

Kaposi's sarcoma (Chapter 11) involves the bowel in 50% of patients with AIDS in whom it produces raised bluish-purple nodules visible on endoscopy, as well as in the oral cavity. Kaposi's sarcoma of the bowel is frequently asymptomatic but has been reported to cause persistent diarrhea with sigmoidoscopic appearances resembling ulcerative colitis.

Lymphoma of the gastrointestinal tract can affect the mouth, salivary glands or esophagus (all otherwise rare sites for these tumors) in AIDS and may be found in 15% to 20% of such patients. More recently anorectal lymphomas have been described in patients with AIDS and since they are otherwise so rare, are a finding of possible diagnostic importance. In the esophagus lymphomas can cause dysphagia and appears on endoscopy as polyps, multicentric masses or ulcers. The diagnosis is confirmed by biopsy which typically shows either large cell or immunoblastic lymphoma.

Carcinomas either cloacogenic (anorectal) or oral have been described in AIDS patients but do not appear to be a common complication of the disease.

Diseases of the peritoneum and mesenteries
Peritonitis

Inflammation of the peritoneum can be localized or generalized.

Localized peritonitis develops over any inflamed viscus. Causes include acute appendicitis and peptic ulceration, Crohn's disease or diverticulitis. The inflamed peritoneum produces a fibrinous exudate which tends to isolate the inflammatory or infective process. In addition, the greater omentum tends to surround and adhere to the area. Later, organization of the exudate leads to formation of fibrous adhesions.

Generalized peritonitis is usually the result of perforation of the bowel or less often, of spread of infection from the pelvic organs, penetrating injuries or invasive medical procedures. Perforation of a peptic ulcer causes an intensely irritating and painful "chemical" peritonitis which later becomes infected.

Microbiology and pathology. Peritonitis resulting from perforation of the bowel is typically a mixed, predominantly anaerobic and coliform infection. Infection from the pelvic organs is by a variety of microbes and may be gonococcal or chlamydial or caused by hemolytic streptococci in the case of puerperal infection.

Specific infections of the peritoneum such as tuberculosis or actinomycosis are now exceedingly rare.

Microscopically, there is a typical acute inflammatory reaction with engorgement of peritoneal blood vessels and infiltration by leukocytes. The serous surface becomes covered by fibrinous exudate following desquamation of the mesothelial cells and granulation tissue starts to form. At the same time fluid exudate accumulates in the peritoneal cavity and infection spreads via the lymphatics until the whole peritoneal cavity is involved.

Clinically, extensive, acute peritonitis causes a severe illness, with fever, and often shock and paralytic ileus. The mortality is high unless surgical intervention is prompt and effective.

Complications. The usual consequence of peritonitis is paralytic ileus, probably caused by injury to Auerbach's plexus, and complete bowel obstruction. The gut becomes distended with gas and toxic products are absorbed through the bowel wall rendered anoxic by venous stasis.

Septicemia is another possible complication but death from peritonitis is now more often the result of paralytic ileus.

Abscess formation either subphrenic or pelvic can follow in those that survive the acute phase of peritonitis. These abscesses may be difficult to detect but give rise to signs of infection, namely, fever, malaise, and leukocytosis which should prompt a search for their source.

Peritoneal adhesions can be a late complication as a result of fibrous healing of the fibrinous exudate and in severe cases can form straplike bands of connective tissue, which may tie down a viscus or obstruct the intestine.

Only minor adhesions should result from the healing of surgical incisions but in the past, particularly, talc or starch powder used on surgical gloves acted as an irritant and even "clean" abdominal surgery could result in extensive adhesions. In many cases of peritonitis, however, the serous surface recovers its normal structure.

Sclerosing peritonitis. Sclerosing peritonitis is a recently described condition caused by beta-blocking drugs, particularly practolol but, rarely others.

Histologically, there is progressive deposition of fibrous tissue predominantly in the peritoneum of the small bowel, immediately deep to the mesothelium. Eventually the peritoneal cavity can become obliterated by thick vascular fibrous tissue. The retroperitoneal region is not involved.

Retroperitoneal fibrosis

Retroperitoneal fibrosis is usually of unknown cause and particularly affects men of middle age or greater. Fibrosis typically begins round the lower abdominal aorta and spreads upwards, laterally and less often downwards towards the pelvis. Ultimately an ill-defined mass either diffuse or nodular forms and causes symptoms particularly when it reaches and obstructs the ureters.

Histologically, at the advancing edge of the lesion, there is typically a mixed predominantly mononuclear inflammatory infiltrate. Behind this there is active fibroblastic proliferation and centrally in the most mature areas, dense, poorly cellular collagenous fibrous tissue. In addition, sclerosing phlebitis is reported to be a characteristic finding and venous obstruction may develop.

Although an association with connective tissue diseases has been reported, retroperitoneal fibrosis is not a characteristic feature of systemic sclerosis. The only agent known to cause retroperitoneal fibrosis (as well as endocardial and pleural fibrosis) is the anti-migrainous drug methysergide—a substance chemically related to the hallucinogen LSD.

Tumors of the peritoneum

A variety of tumors can arise in the peritoneum but are uncommon. *Mesotheliomas* of the peritoneum are also uncommon. They may be localized or diffuse and show great variety of histologic appearances. Papillary, fibrous, adenomatoid, cystic, epithelial, sarcomatoid, and mixed types have been described. Diffuse types may be associated with exposure to asbestos.

Selected readings

Baker RW and Peppercorn MA: Gastrointestinal ailments of homosexual men, Medicine 61:390, 1982.

Bresalier RS and Kim YS: Diet and colon cancer, N Engl J Med 313:1413, 1985.

Cook GC: Aetiology and pathogenesis of postinfective tropical malabsorption (tropical sprue), Lancet i:721, 1984.

Cooper BT and Read AE: Coeliac disease and lymphoma, Quarterly J Med 63 (new series):269, .

Fletcher RH: Carcinoembryonic antigen, Ann Intern Med 104:66, 1986.

Forman D: Gastric cancer, diet, and nitrate exposure, Br Med J 294:528, 1987.

Greenspan D and Greenspan JS et al: Relation of hairy leukoplakia to infection with the human immunodeficiency virus and the risk of developing aids, J Infect Dis 155:475, 1987.

Greenspan JS and Greenspan D et al: Replication of Epstein-Barr virus within the epithelial cells of "hairy" leukoplakia, an AIDS-associated lesion, N Engl J Med 313:1564, 1985.

Glynn J: Tropical sprue—its aetiology and pathogenesis, J Royal Soc Med 79:599, 1986.

Greutzfeldt W and Stockmann F: Carcinoids and carcinoid syndrome, Am J Med 82:(suppl 5B)4, 1987.

Heading RC: Barrett's oesophagus, Br Med J 294:461, 1987.

Heaton KW: Aetiology of acute appendicitis, Br Med J 294:1632, 1987.

Hornick RB: Peptic ulcer disease: a bacterial infection? N Engl J Med 316:1598, 1987.

Moore JRL and LaMont JT: Colorectal cancer: risk factors and screening strategies, Arch Intern Med 144:1819, 1984.

Oates JA: The carcinoid syndrome, N Engl J Med 315:702, 1986.

Polak JM and Bloom SR: Regulatory peptides: key factors in the control of bodily functions, Br Med J 286:1461, 1983.

Quimby GF, Bonnice CA, and Burstein SH et al: Active smoking depresses prostaglandin synthesis in human gastric mucosa, Ann Intern Med 104:616, 1986.

Sachs G, Tache Y, and Debas HT et al: Control of gastric secretion, Am J Med 83:307, 1987.

Santangelo WC and Krejs GJ: Southwestern Internal Medicine Conference: Gastrointestinal manifestations of the acquired immunodeficiency syndrome, Am J Med Sc 292:328, 1986.

Schattenkerk ME, Obertop H, and Mud HJ: Survival after resection for carcinoma of the oesophagus, Br J Surg 74:165, 1987.

Shklar G: Oral leukoplakia, N Engl J Med 315:1544, 1986.

Smart HL and Mayberry JF: Epidemiologic studies of mortality in patients with ulcerative colitis, Arch Intern Med 146:651, 1986.

Spechler SJ: Barrett's esophagus, N Engl J Med 315:362, 1986.

Targan SR (moderator): Immunologic mechanisms in intestinal diseases, Ann Intern Med 106:853, 1987.

CHAPTER 15

Diseases of the liver, biliary tract, and pancreas

THE LIVER
Anatomy and histology

The normal adult liver weighs about 1500 g and occupies much of the upper right quadrant of the abdomen. About three fourths of its mass lies in the right lobe; one fourth lies in the left lobe.

There is still controversy over the fine details of the basic microscopic structure (Fig. 15-1) of the functional unit of the liver. For many years the *lobule* has been regarded as the functional unit which consists of cords or plates of liver cells radiating from a central vein to the portal tracts, several of which are situated on the periphery of a lobule. The central vein is connected to a portal venule and hepatic arteriole by a sinusoid lined with phagocytic Kupffer cells. Also lying between the liver cells are the bile canaliculi which convey bile to the bile duct system. Blood flow is from the portal tracts towards the central vein and there is mixing of portal venous blood with hepatic arterial blood in the liver sinusoids. Bile flows in a direction opposite to that of the blood flow.

In the last 20 years, the concept of the liver *acinus* as the functional unit of the liver has gained wide acceptance. The complex hepatic acinus is a three dimensional structure, composed of 3 or more simple acini, in which the portal tract is considered to be the central axis from which the blood flows from the portal vein and hepatic arteriole via the sinusoids to the hepatic venules. The simple acinus is divided into three zones: zone 1, in which the liver cells are close to the portal tracts, zone 2, an intermediate area and zone 3 which comprises the liver cells in the regions around the hepatic veins (Fig. 15-2).

The zones of the acinus correspond to the following:
1. Zones of decreasing oxygenation, with oxygen concentration being highest in zone 1 and lowest in zone 3
2. Distribution of enzymes within liver cells
3. Distribution of liver cell injury caused by ischemia or toxins

Thus it is presently believed that viewing the liver as being composed of acini rather than lobules corresponds much more closely to the microscopic changes seen in liver diseases.

Liver functions

The liver has multiple functions, most of which are vital for normal body metabolism. It is the main site for protein synthesis, amino acid metabolism, and urea production. It is also the main site of essential stages of lipid metabolism, including formation of free fatty acids, cholesterol, phospholipids, and triglycerides. It is an important site of glycogen formation and storage and has a major role in detoxification of metabolic products as well as many drugs. In addition to glycogen, other essential substances such as vitamins K and B12 (cobalamin) are stored there. It follows that damage to liver cells can have profound effects on the essential metabolic processes of the body.

Bilirubin metabolism

Liver cells also have an essential function in the formation of bile and the metabolism of bilirubin (Fig. 15-3). The bilirubin, which is largely formed in the spleen by breakdown of red cell hemoglobin is conveyed to the liver bound to albumin. In this form bilirubin is unconjugated. Bilirubin enters the liver

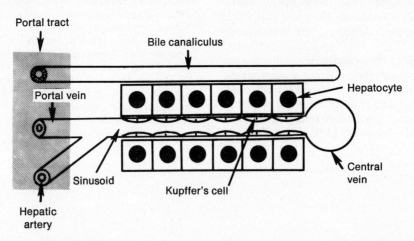

FIG. 15-1. Diagram of relationships between the hepatocytes, biliary system, and hepatic blood vessels.

cell where it combines with glucuronic acid to form *conjugated* bilirubin, which enters the biliary tract.

In the normal person, the total amount of bilirubin present in the blood consists of both conjugated and unconjugated forms and is present in the blood in concentrations up to 1 mg/dL of serum. Of this, 0.25 mg or less/dL of serum is present as conjugated bilirubin. Raised levels of unconjugated bilirubin are generally the result of increased breakdown of red cells (hemolytic anemias) while raised conjugated bilirubin levels follow obstruction to the outflow of bile. Raised levels of both forms of bilirubin in the blood are seen when inflammatory diseases of liver cells are present. Here, damage to the liver cell can first, interfere with conjugation, and second, cause the liver cells to swell resulting in obstruction to bile flow in the canaliculi.

Hepatic enzymes

Numerous enzymes are present in liver cells. They are responsible for catalyzing its complex metabolic processes. Damage to liver cells releases these enzymes into the bloodstream where they can be measured and the levels compared with those found in healthy individuals. Among several enzymes which can be measured in serum to assess the nature and degree of hepatic injury are the following:

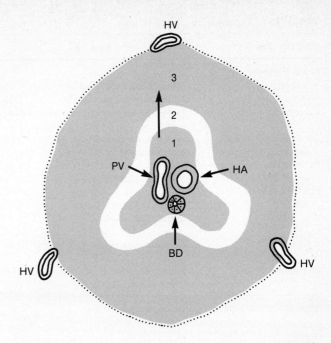

FIG. 15-2. Diagram of a simple liver acinus, showing the relationship of the portal tract containing portal vein *(PV)*, hepatic artery *(HA)* and bile duct *(BD)* to the hepatic veins *(HV)*, and the three acinar zones. The direction of blood flow is from *zone 1* to *zone 3*.

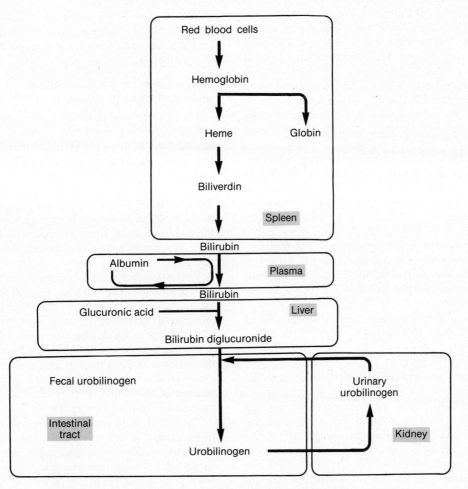

FIG. 15-3. Diagram of formation of bilirubin and the enterohepatic circulation.

TABLE 15-1. The main liver function tests

Test	Function assessed	Reference values	Examples of abnormalities
Serum bilirubin			
Indirect	Mainly breakdown of RBC's	1 mg or less per dL serum	Increased in hemolytic anemia
Direct	Mainly ability to excrete bile	0.25 mg or less per dL serum	Increased in obstructive jaundice
Urinary bile	Reflects ability of liver to excrete bile	Normally negative	Positive in obstructive jaundice
Serum alkaline phosphatase	Liver enzyme synthesis and biliary excretion	50 to 136 u/L	Increased in metastatic cancer to liver and in obstructive jaundice
Serum alanine aminotransferase* (ALT)	Liver cell amino acid metabolism and permeability	5 to 35 u/L	Increased in viral hepatitis
Serum proteins			
Albumin	Synthesis of protein in liver	5.5 to 8 g/dL	—
	Synthesis of albumin	3.5 to 5 g/dL	Decreased in hepatic cirrhosis and necrosis
Globulin	Synthesis of globulin	2 to 3.5 g/dL	Increased in hepatic cirrhosis and chronic hepatitis
Prothrombin time	Activity of factors II, V, VII, and X synthesized in the liver	12 seconds with 12 second control	Prolonged in many liver diseases and in patients taking coumadin

*Formerly serum glutamic pyruvic transaminase (SGPT).

1. *Aminotransferases (transaminases)*—Of many enzymes used to evaluate liver cell damage by chemical methods, measuring the serum levels of aspartate aminotransferase (AST) or alanine aminotransferase (ALT) have proved most useful. ALT is a particularly sensitive measure of liver cell damage. The normally low levels of AST and ALT are significantly raised when hepatocytes are injured, as in viral hepatitis, and resolution of the injury is accompanied by a return of the serum enzyme to normal values.
2. *Lactic dehydrogenase (LDH)* is an enzyme present in many tissues. However, one of its 5 isoenzymes, LDH5, is present in high concentration in liver cells and skeletal muscle. In the absence of skeletal muscle damage, raised levels of LDH5 indicate liver injury.
3. *Alkaline phosphatase* is also present in many tissues especially in bone, intestine and placenta, as well as liver cells. However, in the absence of bone disease and pregnancy, raised levels of alkaline phosphatase are usually caused by impairment of the liver's excretory function.
4. *Other liver enzymes*—Gamma glutamyl transpeptidase (GGT) is a very sensitive indicator of minor degrees of liver cell damage. 5′ nucleotidase has a similar significance to alkaline phosphatase but is less specific for hepatic dysfunction.

Other methods of testing the wide range of liver functions are summarized in Table 15-1.

Investigation of liver disease

Among the many procedures that have been devised, the following are important:

Radiologic methods. A wide range of radiologic methods are now available for investigation of the liver and biliary system. These include computerized tomography (CT scanning), sonography, the use of radioactive tracers and radiocontrast methods.

Liver biopsy. Small portions of liver tissue can be removed either by a percutaneous needle biopsy or at operation, by removal of a larger piece of liver. Subsequent histologic ex-

mination, sometimes combined with microbiologic methods when infectious agents are suspected, can give important clues to the nature of a hepatic illness.

Biochemical methods. Among numerous methods devised, the levels of serum bilirubin, serum proteins, both total and individual, and serum enzyme levels already discussed, are most commonly employed. Liver dysfunction may also be reflected in abnormalities of blood coagulation tests (see Table 15-1).

General clinical manifestations of liver disease

The liver has great reserves. It may suffer moderate damage without producing symptoms to indicate that there has been any damage. Perhaps the most common clinical evidence of liver disease is the appearance of jaundice (icterus).

Jaundice is a yellow discoloration of the skin and ocular sclerae, which develops when the serum bilirubin level exceeds 2 to 2.5 mg/dL. Jaundice is frequently accompanied by itching. In the newborn infant persistent high levels of unconjugated bilirubin such as are found in isoimmune disease of the newborn are toxic to brain tissue and produce *kernicterus* (Chapter 13).

The end result of some liver diseases, particularly of cirrhosis is liver failure, which is usually a lethal process, and has numerous clinical manifestations. These include a deep red appearance of the hands (liver palms), numerous small branching blood vessels in the skin (spider nevi), and gynecomastia.

The last is enlargement of the male breasts and is caused by the presence of estrogens that have persisted due to failure of the inactivating mechanisms in the liver. In addition, abnormalities in the central nervous system, kidneys, blood, and gastrointestinal tract may develop.

The effects on the central nervous system range from tremor of the hands ("liver flap") to a comatose state (hepatic coma). The cause of hepatic encephalopathy is not known although the shunting of large quantities of portal blood into the systemic circulation appears to play a major role. This is reflected in raised levels of ammonia in the blood. This, however, is an indicator of the condition rather than a cause.

Liver failure may be associated with renal failure in the *hepatorenal syndrome*. The cause of the renal failure appears to be, at least in part, the result of failure of a liver-dependent mechanism that exerts control over renal cortical blood flow. Other contributory factors may include the presence of high circulating levels of aldosterone and the severe ascites which is present in these patients. The precise cause is, however, unknown. Despite the absence of any obvious structural damage to the kidney, recovery from this syndrome is rare.

Many changes in the blood result from liver failure. Diminished plasma protein synthesis may lead to hypoprothrombinemia and a tendency to hemorrhage. Anemia is common although the underlying causes may be complex. Both hemolytic and sideroblastic anemias (Chapter 13) can be found.

Peptic ulceration may develop in liver failure possibly as a result of the effects of increased gastrin secretion.

Jaundice

Jaundice has already been described as being caused by hyperbilirubinemia. The causes of jaundice are many and it is necessary to review the metabolism of bilirubin in order to understand them.

Bilirubin is presented to the liver cell in unconjugated form bound to albumin. Released from albumin it then enters the liver cell where its intracellular transport is facilitated by protein binding enzymes (ligandins). Within the endoplasmic reticulum, bilirubin, which is poorly water soluble, is combined with glucuronic acid under the influence of glucuronyl transferase, forming a water-soluble diglucuronide. Most bilirubin is excreted as a diglucuronide. Small amounts of monoglucuronide and traces of an unconjugated water soluble isomer of bilirubin may also enter the bile canaliculi. Bilirubin is finally conveyed to the duodenum by the biliary apparatus (Fig. 15-4).

Jaundice may be caused by abnormalities at any stage of formation and excretion of bilirubin from the breakdown of red blood cells to the entrance of bile into the intestinal tract. The causes of jaundice are as follows:

1. Excessive production of bilirubin
   a. Hemolytic anemias
2. Interference with uptake of bilirubin by hepatocytes
   a. Sepsis
   b. Drugs
3. Impaired conjugation with glucuronic acid
   a. "Physiologic" jaundice of newborn
   b. Hereditary deficiencies of glucuronyl transferase activity: Gilbert's syndrome; Crigler-Najjar syndrome
   c. Drug interference with transferase activity: chloramphenicol
   d. Liver cell disease: viral hepatitis; hepatic cirrhosis
4. Impaired secretion of bilirubin
   a. Familial disorders: Dubin-Johnson syndrome; Rotor syndrome
   b. Liver cell disease
   c. Drug interference: male and female hormones
5. Mechanical obstruction to biliary outflow
   a. Biliary stones, tumors, parasites
   b. Pancreatic carcinoma; enlarged lymph nodes
   c. Bile duct stricture

Excessive hemolysis. Excessive hemolysis results in jaundice. Numerous mechanisms are known (Chapter 13) and include the effects of antibodies, especially in blood transfusion reactions, defects in the red cell envelope, and heritable abnormalities of the hemoglobin molecule and erythrocytic en-

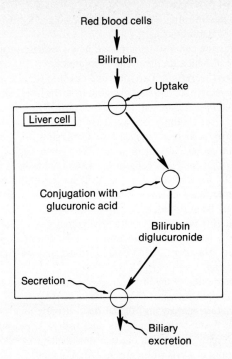

FIG. 15-4. Uptake, conjugation, secretion, and excretion of bilirubin.

zymes. Increased breakdown of red blood cell precursors, typical of *ineffective erythropoiesis,* can also cause excessive production of bilirubin.

Defective uptake of bilirubin. Uptake of unconjugated bilirubin by liver cells with subsequent jaundice is sometimes seen in patients with severe sepsis, though the mechanism is unknown. One antihelminthic drug, flavispadic acid, can cause jaundice by competing for liver cell ligandins. The antibiotic novobiocin appears to act in a similar manner.

Impaired conjugation with glucuronic acid. The most common example is "physiologic" jaundice of the newborn. Virtually every infant experiences a brief period of hyperbilirubinemia due to a low level of activity of glucuronyl tranferase in the first few days of life. The resultant jaundice is usually slight and resolves spontaneously in a few days. The process may be enhanced in premature infants in whom high levels of unconjugated bilirubin may accumulate. When the bilirubin level reaches 20 mg/dL or higher there is a high risk that kernicterus with subsequent nervous system injury may develop. Exposing the infant to ultraviolet light, which causes soluble isomers of bilirubin to form, usually controls the hyperbilirubinemia until the infant's own transferase reaches normal levels.

Inherited abnormalities of bilirubin conjugation are fairly rare. *Gilbert's syndrome* is a benign condition in which there is a moderate increase in blood levels of unconjugated bilirubin with no apparent ill effects other than mild jaundice. The serum bilirubin rarely exceeds 5 mg/dL. Some patients may show evidence of concurrent mild hemolysis, others do not.

More severe effects of abnormal conjugation are seen in the *Crigler-Najjar syndrome*. There are two variants. First, an absence of glucuronyl transferase causes severe, and eventually fatal hyperbilirubinemia. Liver transplantation is the only possible treatment. Second, a partial deficiency of the enzyme results in moderately increased levels of bilirubin (usually less than 20 mg/dL). This is a relatively benign form of the disease, in which the bilirubin levels can often be controlled by administration of barbiturates.

Conjugation can also be impaired in any disease (e.g., viral hepatitis) in which the liver cell is injured.

Impaired secretion. Two inherited conditions are characterized by defective secretion of bilirubin from the liver cell. These are the *Dubin-Johnson* and *Rotor* syndromes. The exact causes of these excretion abnormalities are not known. Both are characterized by moderately raised levels of conjugated bilirubin, but symptoms are absent or minor. The main distinguishing feature is that the liver cells in the Dubin-Johnson syndrome are heavily pigmented with an intracellular lipofuscin-like pigment, while those in Rotor syndrome are not. This difference has not yet been explained.

Obstructive jaundice. Obstructive jaundice is caused when the outflow of bile to the duodenum via the common bile duct is blocked. Blockage of the common duct may be caused by the following:

1. Obstruction of the lumen by gallstones, bile duct tumors, or certain parasites (e.g., *Ascaris lumbricoides*)
2. Stricture (narrowing) of the duct, usually as a result of scar tissue formation in the duct wall
3. External pressure on the bile duct system by pancreatic tumors or cysts or enlarging lymph nodes

Metabolic effects of hyperbilirubinemia. When jaundice is due to accumulation of *unconjugated bilirubin* due to hemolysis and the liver cells are undamaged, there is increased conjugation activity in response to the increased load. The excess conjugated bilirubin is excreted into the intestine where it is converted by bacterial action into urobilinogen, thus raising the levels of fecal urobilinogen. Excess urobilinogen absorbed from the intestinal tract is detectable in increased quantities in the urine.

In obstructive jaundice as a result, for instance, of a stone lodged in the common bile duct, entry of bile into the duodenum partly or completely stops. As a result, the blood levels of *conjugated bilirubin* are increased. The absence of bile entering the duodenum leads to the formation of pale, clay colored stools. The excess of bile (conjugated bilirubin) in the blood spills over into the urine which becomes dark greenish-brown. By contrast with states of excessive hemolysis, there is no conversion of bilirubin to urobilinogen in the intestine and the urinary urobilinogen is decreased.

When the liver parenchyma is involved in a diffuse inflammatory process, such as viral hepatitis, the effects of both obstructive and intrahepatic jaundice are seen. First, obstruction of the bile canaliculi is caused by swelling of the liver cells. Second, conjugation and/or secretion of bile from the liver cell is impaired, as a result of cell injury. Thus, depending on the stage of the disease, jaundice may be the result of raised blood levels of either conjugated or unconjugated bilirubin or both.

Diseases of the liver
Hepatitis

Hepatitis is a term that is usually used to describe a diffuse inflammatory process that affects the whole liver. Localized inflammatory lesions such as seen in pyogenic infections of the liver, for example, are best described as liver abscesses and not as hepatitis. The main causes of hepatitis are (1) viral infections and (2) toxic substances and drugs. Most of these agents cause acute inflammation though some can cause more

chronic inflammatory disease. Cirrhosis of the liver, for example, which is discussed later in this chapter, can be a sequel to acute hepatitis, due either to viral infection or toxic substances. Etiologic agents of hepatitis are as follows:

Infective
1. Enteroviruses
   a. Coxsackieviruses
   b. Hepatitis A virus
2. Flavivirus
   a. Yellow fever
3. Herpesviruses
   a. Cytomegalovirus
   b. Epstein-Barr virus
   c. Herpes simplex virus
4. Unclassified or unidentified
   a. Hepatitis B virus
   b. Delta hepatitis virus
   c. Non-A, non-B agents

Drugs and toxic substances
1. Acetaminophen
2. Alcohol
3. Carbon tetrachloride
4. Chlorpromazine
5. Chlorothiazide
6. Halothane
7. Isoniazid
8. Methyldopa
9. Phenytoin

Viral hepatitis

Many different viruses can infect the liver resulting in hepatitis (see previous list). It is customary, however, to reserve the term *viral hepatitis* for a group of very similar diseases caused by the following infectious agents: hepatitis A virus (HAV), hepatitis B virus (HBV), non-A, non-B (NANB) agents, and delta agent. These agents, either alone, or in the case of delta agent in concert with HBV, can cause pathologic changes in the liver and clinical illnesses which are often extremely difficult to distinguish from each other. However, recent advances in clinical laboratory methods have made it possible to identify HAV and HBV infections. Tests which can identify infections by NANB and delta agents are not yet generally available.

Etiologic agents

Hepatitis A virus (HAV). Hepatitis A virus is a small (27 nm) non-enveloped RNA virus. Its size and structure are very similar to those of other small RNA viruses whose habitat is the human intestinal tract, i.e., the enteroviruses. The virus has been grown with difficulty in cell culture. Routine laboratory methods of virus identification have not been developed, but methods of demonstrating IgM antibodies to HAV are generally available.

Hepatitis B virus (HBV). HBV, by contrast, is a larger (42 nm) enveloped DNA virus. HBV has not yet been cultivated but its etiologic role in hepatitis, like that of HAV, is now certain.

During the replication of HBV in the liver, surface antigen (HBsAg) is expressed on the outer surface of the viral envelope. However, large amounts of this antigen, far in excess of that required for synthesis of complete virus particles, are produced in the liver. This antigen forms filamentous and spherical aggregates in blood and body fluids, where it can readily be detected serologically. The presence of HBsAg in the blood is evidence that the patient has active hepatitis B or is a carrier of the virus.

Other antigens that can be detected serologically are as follows:

1. Hepatitis B core antigen (HBcAg) largely consists of double stranded desoxyribonucleoprotein.
2. Hepatitis e antigen (HBeAg) is a soluble internal antigen associated with replicating HBV particles. Its exact chemical nature is still undetermined. It is found in association with HBsAg and can be regarded as a measure of *infectivity*. Thus persons who are HBsAg and HBeAg positive are considered to be more highly infective than those who are merely HBsAg positive.
3. DNA polymerase is closely associated with HBcAg.

Specific antibodies to HBs and HBe antigens can be found in patient's serum, depending on the clinical stage of the infection. These are discussed later in this section.

Non-A, non-B hepatitis viruses (NANB). Now that hepatitis A and B can be specifically identified, it has become apparent that many patients who have typical viral hepatitis have no evidence of infection by either of these two agents. These patients are currently considered to have non-A, non-B hepatitis and epidemiologic studies indicate that these NANB agents can cause two forms of infection:

1. A disease with some of the characteristics of hepatitis B including transmission by the parenteral route—Two viruses have been postulated as causing this form of hepatitis which appears to account for most cases of posttransfusion hepatitis in the United States and Europe.
2. Epidemic NANB hepatitis which appears to be spread in a manner similar to hepatitis A, namely by the orofecal route—Outbreaks have been reported from Africa and Asia. So far the epidemiology suggests that epidemic NANB hepatitis is caused by a single virus.

There are currently no laboratory tests for the detection of NANB agents. Diagnosis is based first on exclusion of HAV and HBV infection, and second on the epidemiologic data.

Hepatitis D virus (Delta agent). Hepatitis D virus (HDV) is a defective RNA virus, which requires hepatitis B virus (HBV) for its transmission, expression and replication. The viral particle is about 35 nm in diameter with a nucleocapsid (HDAg) and an envelope on which HBsAg among other proteins can be found. Infection by HDV appears to take place in one of three ways:

1. Simultaneous acute infection by HDV and HBV
2. Superinfection of HBV carriers by HDV
3. Chronic HDV infection superimposed upon chronic hepatitis B

Although the full clinical range of effects of HDV infections is still incomplete, the clinical effects are very similar to those described for hepatitis B, but in significant numbers of patients the disease tends to be more severe.

Pathology of viral hepatitis. The pathologic effects of the various hepatitis viruses on the liver are very similar. Infection by HAV, HBV and NANB viruses can cause structural alterations in the liver that range from minor derangements to massive death of liver cells. The most severe changes are likely to be seen in HBV infection especially when there is simultaneous or sequential infection with delta agent.

Coinciding with the onset of symptoms, there is enlargement of the liver. Histologically, the cells throughout the liver are affected to varying degrees. Those in the region of the hepatic venules (zone 3) (Fig. 15-2) tend to be the most severely affected. Swelling of the liver cells (ballooning degeneration) is a prominent histologic feature. Depending on the severity of the disease, a variable number of liver cells die. This process of individual liver cell death is the unique process called *apoptosis* discussed in Chapter 2. *Apoptosis* is characterized by shrinkage of the hepatocyte, progressive eosinophilia and expulsion of the nucleus. The residual structure is known as a Councilman body.* These changes distort the architecture of the liver so that the histologic appearance may show little resemblance to normal. The reticulin "skeleton" of the liver, however, is not disrupted. Collections of lymphocytes, macrophages and occasional polymorphs are found in the portal tracts and in surrounding areas of dead or dying liver cells. Scattered foci of regenerating liver cells may be found and the Kupffer cells become hyperplastic.

In cases of hepatitis B, using special stains such as orcein, viral antigens can be located within the liver cell. HBcAg is found in the nucleus and HBsAg within the cytoplasm of infected hepatocytes.

In most cases of viral hepatitis, as the symptoms subside, the hepatic abnormalities begin to improve. Death of liver cells diminishes and the inflammatory infiltrates decrease. The surviving cells undergo hyperplastic changes and multinucleate liver cells are commonly present.

In some cases, the process is more severe, with areas of liver cell necrosis extending from around one hepatic venule to another, often referred to as "bridging necrosis" (strictly, apoptosis). This is accompanied by varying degrees of disruption of the reticulin framework of the liver. Even with these severe changes, restoration of hepatic architecture can take place in some cases. However, in others, resolution is accompanied by fibrosis and permanent disruption of the structure of the liver. These more severe pathologic changes are more likely to be due to HBV or NANB viruses than HAV, and particularly, delta agent.

Occasionally there is widespread destruction of liver cells with collapse of the liver architecture. This process is called *acute massive necrosis* (Fig. 15-5), and if it is severe enough, death from acute hepatic failure follows in a few days to a few weeks. If the patient survives necrotic areas are replaced by coarse bands of fibrous tissue resulting in *postnecrotic scarring*. In this condition, the liver is divided by bands of collagen into large, pale, irregularly shaped lobules.

Massive necrosis of the liver can also result from certain drugs and chemical agents, including carbon tetrachloride and the general anesthetic agent halothane, particularly as a consequence of repeated administration of this anesthetic at short intervals.

Sequelae of viral hepatitis. Despite the similarities in the pathologic processes seen in the liver, there are important differences between hepatitis A and other forms of viral hepatitis in the outcome of the disease. In hepatitis A, recovery within a few weeks is the rule and fulminating hepatitis with fatal hepatic necrosis is seldom seen. Hepatic necrosis is usually a complication of HBV infection, particularly when there is coincident infection with delta agent; or less frequently, it is the result of transfusion-related NANB hepatitis.

The outcome of hepatitis B is shown in Fig. 15-6. In about

---

*William T. Councilman (1854-1933), American pathologist.

10% of cases viral synthesis continues beyond 6 months and, as a consequence, HBsAg persists in blood and body fluids. This group of patients falls into three categories:

1. Asymptomatic carriers of HBV
2. Chronic persistent hepatitis
3. Chronic active hepatitis

The outcome of NANB hepatitis is similar but a much higher proportion of patients appear to develop chronic hepatitis and its sequelae.

Asymptomatic carriers. Following clinical recovery from acute hepatitis, some individuals continue to be positive for HBsAg, and are therefore capable of transmitting HBV in the appropriate circumstances. Others may be carriers but have no clinical history of viral hepatitis, because the initial infection was asymptomatic. The carrier state is most likely to develop in premature infants, in immunosuppressed individuals and in

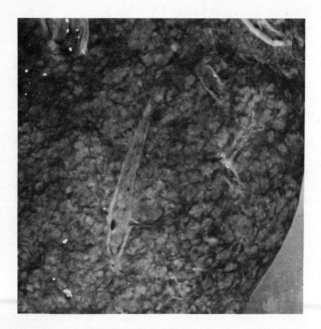

FIG. 15-5. Acute massive necrosis of the liver. The cut surface of the liver shows complete necrosis of the parenchyma. The cause in this case was thought to be halothane anesthesia.

Down's syndrome. For unknown reasons, carriers fail to form antibody against HBsAg. For equally unknown reasons, some eventually develop anti-HBsAg thus ending the carrier state: others do not and may remain carriers for life. Those carriers who are positive for both HBsAg and HBeAg are considered to be highly infectious.

Chronic persistent hepatitis. In this form of chronic hepatitis symptoms are usually minimal, but serologic abnormalities are present and include the following:

1. Seropositivity for (a) HBsAg and/or (b) antibody to HBcAg
2. Moderately elevated serum levels of aminotransferases

About 3% to 4% of all patients with hepatitis B will develop chronic persistent hepatitis. About half of all patients with NANB hepatitis will also develop persistent hepatitis; in these cases raised hepatic enzyme levels are the only current means of recognizing the disease other than liver biopsy.

The histologic picture in persistent hepatitis is that seen in mild hepatitis B. The significant histologic finding is that the cells at the periphery of the lobule (the limiting plate) remain intact. There is a mild chronic inflammatory infiltrate in the portal tracts but there are no fibrotic changes.

It is thought that while some cases of persistent hepatitis eventually resolve spontaneously others may progress to more severe forms of liver disease. The factors responsible for this form of hepatitis are not known but as with the carrier state, it seems likely that it is due to impairment of the immune response.

Chronic active hepatitis. Chronic active hepatitis is a serious sequel of viral hepatitis, often due to HBV but NANB agents appear to be emerging as the main cause of this disease. There is also evidence that methyldopa and possibly other drugs may cause a similar liver disease. The term *chronic aggressive hepatitis* is also used for this disease and serves to emphasize its seriousness.

Abnormal cell-mediated and humoral responses appear to have an important role in chronic active hepatitis. This is supported by the following:

1. The disease is frequently accompanied by immunologically-mediated conditions such as autoimmune thyroiditis and Sjögren's syndrome.
2. Tests for lupus erythematosus and other "collagen-vascular" diseases are frequently positive.

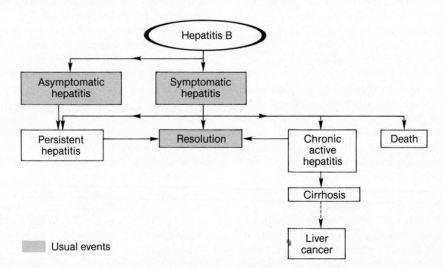

FIG. 15-6. Diagram of pathogenesis and outcome of HBV infection. *(From McCracken AW and Cawson RA: Clinical and oral microbiology, Washington DC, 1982, Hemisphere Publishing Corp.)*

3. Most patients fail to produce antibodies to HBsAg.
4. Considerable success in the management of these patients has been achieved with immunosuppressive treatment.

Histologically (Fig. 15-7), the disease differs from persistent hepatitis mainly in the disruption of the limiting plate with destruction of liver cells at sites where parenchyma and connective tissue meet ("piecemeal necrosis") and the development of fibrosis suggestive of early cirrhosis. When HBV infection is the cause viral particles may be demonstrable in the cell nuclei.

The outcome of chronic active hepatitis appears to be any one of the following:

1. Progression to liver failure
2. Slowly progressive disease leading to cirrhosis
3. Possible resolution and recovery in some cases

Clinical aspects of viral hepatitis. Clinically, as well as pathologically, there is considerable overlapping of hepatitis A, B, and non A-non B. These three infections are rarely distinguishable without laboratory and epidemiologic information. Generally speaking, hepatitis A is the mildest and its complications are rare; hepatitis B is the most serious with a higher risk of complications and death; NANB hepatitis more closely resembles hepatitis B, but the true fatality rate is still uncertain.

The onset of symptoms is often abrupt in hepatitis A, more insidious in the other forms of the disease. Other properties of hepatitis A are compared with hepatitis B and NANB in Table 15-2.

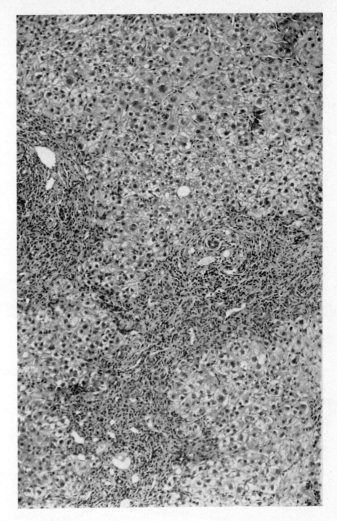

FIG. 15-7. Liver biopsy in chronic active hepatitis. The portal areas are greatly expanded due to fibrosis and lymphocytic infiltration, and are becoming confluent.

TABLE 15-2. Comparison of properties of hepatitis A, B and non-A, non-B virus

		HAV	*HBV*	*NANB*
Virus	Nucleic acid	RNA	DNA	?
	Envelope	None	Present	?
	Virus or antigens in			
	Blood	Days	Months to years	*Possibly months to years
	Stool	Weeks	Present	†Probably
	Saliva	—	Present	?
Clinical aspects	Incubation period	15-50 days	40-180 days	35-70 days
	Age of patient	Children, young adults	Any age	Any age
	Route of infection	Orofecal, but may be parenteral	Parenteral but orofecal fairly common	*Parenteral and †Orofecal fairly common
	Complications	Very rare	Common	Fairly common
	Mortality rate	>0.1%	Up to 10%	?
	Laboratory tests	No	Yes: for antigens and antibodies	No
	Carrier state	No	Yes	Yes
Prevention	Gamma globulin	Prevents jaundice	High titer HB immune globulin	None
	Vaccine	No	Inactivated vaccine	
Disinfection	Heat at 56°C for 30 min	Virus resistant	Virus resistant	?
	Heat at 121°C for 15 min	Infectivity lost	Infectivity lost	Infectivity lost
	Sodium hypochlorite for 30 min	Infectivity lost	Infectivity lost	? Infectivity lost

*Parenterally transmitted type
†Epidemic type

In typical cases, headache and myalgia precede jaundice, fever, and anorexia. The liver is slightly enlarged and tender, and the serum aminotransferase (transaminase) levels are greatly increased. When jaundice appears, nausea, anorexia and vomiting continue and there is further increase in the size and tenderness of the liver. The stools are pale and the urine is dark. In the early stages of hepatitis B, up to 20% of patients will develop an immunologically-mediated illness, characterized by polyarthralgia and urticaria. This syndrome is occasionally seen in hepatitis A. Polyarteritis nodosa or glomerulonephritis may also develop in hepatitis B. These abnormalities are thought to be immune complex mediated.

In most cases, with bed rest, most symptoms subside after the jaundice has cleared. Appetite and a feeling of well-being gradually return. Complete recovery in most cases is expected in 4 to 6 weeks unless complications already described develop. Weakness and fatiguability may persist longer in hepatitis B.

Normal response

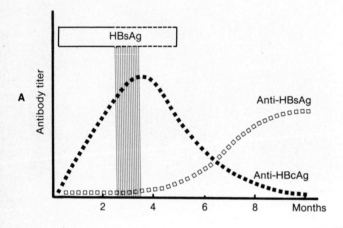

Carrier state

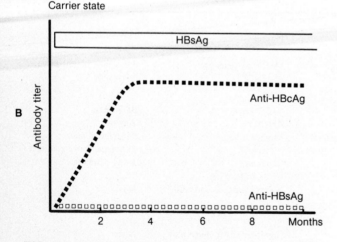

FIG. 15-8. Serologic responses in hepatitis B. **A,** "Normal" response shows the disappearance of HBsAg as anti-HBsAg appears; the shaded area is a "window" of time during which, occasionally, neither HBsAg nor anti-HbsAg are detectable. During this period, detection of anti-HBcAg is the only laboratory evidence of infection. **B,** The carrier state in which no anti-HBsAg is formed and HBsAg persists. *(Modified from McCracken AW and Cawson RA: Clinical and oral microbiology, Washington DC, 1982, Hemisphere Publishing Corp.)*

No specific treatment is available. Even the benefits of complete bed rest in the early stages, which has been recommended for many years, are unproven.

The specific diagnosis of hepatitis A is made by serologic demonstration of anti-HAV IgM; that of hepatitis B can be made most convincingly by the presence of anti-HBcAg IgM in the serum; alternatively, a positive HBsAg test also indicates active HBV infection. The serologic responses in hepatitis B are illustrated in Fig. 15-8. NANB hepatitis is diagnosed by exclusion and history.

Active immunization using purified inactivated HBsAg is an effective and safe method of protecting against HBV. Since delta agent is entirely dependent on pre-existing or concurrent infection with HBV, successful vaccination against HBV also confers immunity to delta agent. Adverse reactions to the vaccine are minor and it is recommended for all health care workers.

Nonimmune individuals who are exposed parenterally to HBV infection should receive high titer hepatitis B immune globulin (HBIG) which confers a high degree of passive immunity. These individuals should also receive active vaccination. In situations where exposure to hepatitis B is slight or questionable, prophylaxis with serum immune globulin is currently recommended. This prophylactic method is also effective for passive immunization against hepatitis A.

Transfused blood and blood products, particularly fibrinogen and factors VIII and IX are the main sources of HBV and NANB hepatitis. Although testing of blood donors for evidence of HBV has greatly reduced the risk of hepatitis B, the lack of specific tests for NANB agents is still a serious deficiency. In an attempt to detect donors who might harbor NANB agents, many blood transfusion centers now test donor blood for abnormal levels of aminotransferases and reject those with elevated levels.

There is an epidemiologic relationship between HBV and liver cancer as discussed later in this chapter.

Reye's syndrome

Reye's syndrome of fatty liver and encephalopathy is an unusual complication of influenza B and occasionally other viral diseases, including influenza A, chickenpox and measles. Children below the age of fifteen are affected.

Etiology. Although viruses, especially influenza B, appear to be the main cause, the use of aspirin to treat the symptoms of viral infections increases the risk of developing the syndrome. However, it should be noted that Reye's syndrome can develop in children who have not taken aspirin.

Pathology. There is extensive small-droplet fat accumulation in the liver. Ultrastructural examination reveals injury to the mitochondria which become swollen and pleomorphic and to the rough endoplasmic reticulum of the liver cells. In some cases there is necrosis of liver cells in zone 3. Fatty change similar to that seen in the liver is present in renal tubular cells. In the central nervous system, the main findings are cerebral edema and neuronal degeneration (Chapter 20).

Clinical aspects. The onset of Reye's syndrome is around the third day of the viral illness and is marked by vomiting, convulsions and coma. The liver is enlarged but there is no jaundice. There is no specific treatment and about half the patients die of liver failure. Treatment consists of correcting hypoglycemia resulting from failure of glucose 6-phosphatase function with glucose and controlling cerebral edema with mannitol infusions. It is now recommended that aspirin should not be given to children with febrile viral illnesses.

Cirrhosis

Cirrhosis refers to widespread diffuse scarring of the liver. It is accompanied by some degree of regeneration of liver cells (regeneration nodules), which are, however, structurally and functionally deranged. The World Health Organization defines cirrhosis as a diffuse process characterized by fibrosis and conversion of normal liver architecture into structurally abnormal nodules. The causes of cirrhosis are listed as follows:

1. Congenital
   a. α-1-Antitrypsin deficiency
   b. Galactosemia
   c. Glycogen storage disease
   d. Hemochromatosis
   e. Hepatolenticular degeneration (Wilson's disease)
2. Acquired
   a. Alcohol
   b. Chronic biliary obstruction
   c. Chronic hepatitis
   d. Following massive hepatic necrosis
   e. Hyperalimentation (total parenteral nutrition)
   f. Sarcoidosis
   g. Schistosomiasis
   h. Venoocclusive disease

However, it should be noted that at least 80% of cases comprise only three types. These are the following:

1. Alcoholic cirrhosis
2. Postnecrotic (posthepatitic) cirrhosis
3. Biliary cirrhosis

Alcoholic cirrhosis

Prolonged and excessive intake of alcohol can lead to cirrhosis of the liver. The vast majority of patients with clinical and pathologic evidence of cirrhosis have a long history of alcohol abuse. However, although the mechanisms by which acute exposure to alcohol can damage the liver causing fatty change are known, the processes that lead to liver cell destruction and fibrosis typical of cirrhosis are not. Decreased intake of proteins and vitamins, frequently seen in alcoholics, may contribute to the development of cirrhosis; nevertheless, in the absence of alcohol, malnutrition does not cause cirrhosis.

Fatty change has been described earlier (Chapter 2). In brief, the effects of ethanol on hepatic lipid metabolism appear to be as follows:

1. Increased synthesis of fatty acids and triglycerides
2. Reduced oxidative breakdown of fatty acids
3. Direct toxic effect of ethanol on hepatic mitochondria which further inhibits fatty acid oxidation

These effects are generally reversible when ethanol is stopped. However, with continued intake of large amounts of alcohol over many years, a point is reached when liver cells are irreversibly damaged and diffuse fibrosis begins.

As the disease progresses, strands of fine fibrous tissue appear, linking the portal tracts, hence *portal cirrhosis*. Liver cells contain collections of amorphous pink-staining material termed *Mallory bodies* formerly called "hyalin" bodies (Chapter 2) (Fig. 15-9). Foci containing acute inflammatory cells are often present at this stage, during which the liver may be slightly enlarged. With further progression there is loss of fat,

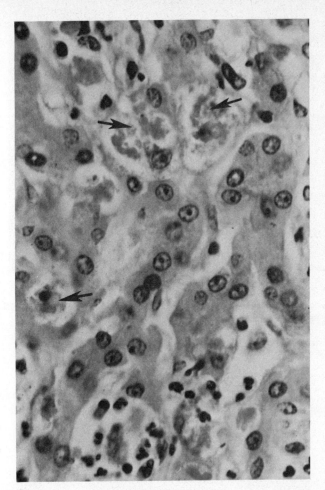

FIG. 15-9. Liver in alcoholic cirrhosis. The cytoplasm of many liver cells contains Mallory bodies *(arrows)*. Small foci of inflammatory cells are present.

shrinkage of the liver, and increasing fibrous tissue resulting in loss of the normal liver lobules and their associated portal tracts. They are replaced by collections of healthy looking but functionally compromised liver cells called *regeneration nodules*. There is also proliferation of small non-functioning bile ducts. Finally, the liver is shrunken and is composed of small nodules separated by fibrous bands. The liver surface has a rough, irregular appearance reminiscent of coarse grained leather. The term *micronodular* cirrhosis is sometimes used to describe this appearance. However, it is only a descriptive term and a micronodular pattern can be seen in cirrhosis due to other causes such as hemachromatosis.

With destruction of the portal tracts, there is increased pressure within the portal system *(portal hypertension)*. As portal venous pressure increases, several abnormalities may follow:

1. Progressive enlargement of the spleen
2. Varicosities at the sites of portosystemic venous anastomoses (e.g., at the lower end of the esophagus or rectum)
3. Ascites

Postnecrotic (posthepatitic) cirrhosis

Postnecrotic cirrhosis (Figs. 15-10 and 15-11) has already been described as a sequel to massive necrosis of the liver and viral hepatitis.

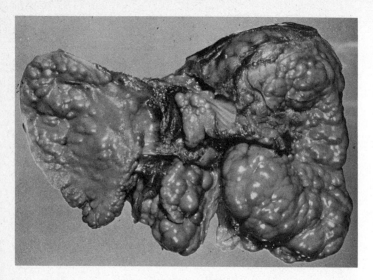

FIG. 15-10. Postnecrotic scarring of the liver. The liver weighed 1100 g. It was shrunken with a coarse, irregular surface as a result of bands of fibrous tissue interspersed with regeneration nodules. The liver is viewed from behind and below. *(Courtesy Curator of the Gordon Museum, Guy's Hospital, London, England.)*

Biliary cirrhosis

Biliary cirrhosis is usually a sequel to ascending inflammatory disease of the biliary tract following chronic obstruction of the biliary outflow. This is due, for example, to congenital biliary atresia or sometimes to biliary calculi. However, some cases of biliary cirrhosis arise with no evidence of any biliary obstruction. These patients are usually women aged 40 to 50 years and the term *primary biliary cirrhosis* is given to this form of the disease. Its cause is unknown, although some form of immune mechanism is possible, as various autoantibodies are associated.

The liver in biliary cirrhosis is usually normal in size, but increasing content of bile as a result of biliary obstruction may result in a green liver. Fibrosis begins around the small bile ducts, which often contain static bile (biliary thrombi), and which undergo proliferation. Fine strands of fibrous tissue containing lymphocytes and plasma cells, connect the portal tracts. Involvement of the portal venous system is slight so that portal hypertension and its sequelae may only appear at very late stages of the disease.

Clinical aspects of cirrhosis

Alcoholic cirrhosis is a common and serious disease. It has a variable clinical course and is frequently asymptomatic even in well-advanced stages. The effects of cirrhosis are a result of either portal hypertension and its effects or impairment of liver function or both.

Pathologic dilatation of veins is common, particularly in the esophagus and rectum, causing esophageal varices and hemorrhoids. Rupture of esophageal varices results in serious or catastrophic hemorrhage. Blood loss from hemorrhoids frequently contributes to anemia. Fluid in the peritoneal cavity (ascites) is a frequent though late manifestation of portal hypertension. It causes abdominal swelling and may be serious enough to embarrass respiration. Jaundice may or may not be present. Because of the severe derangement of liver function, patients with cirrhosis may react badly to some drugs. Drugs which are metabolized by the liver include the barbiturates, hypnotics, and intravenous anesthetics. Impaired liver function can greatly delay the excretion of these agents, thus dangerously prolonging and deepening anesthesia.

Patients with cirrhosis are subject to abnormal bleeding because of impaired synthesis of essential clotting factors. Death in alcoholic cirrhosis is the result of rupture of varices, liver failure, and/or intercurrent infection. There is an increased risk of hepatocellular carcinoma in patients with cirrhosis. The evidence of an association is most convincing when cirrhosis is the result of chronic hepatitis B virus infection.

Other forms of cirrhosis

There are several conditions where the deposition of abnormal substances or excessive quantities of physiologic substances lead to fibrosis and functional derangement of the liver (see list on p. 357). Two examples will be discussed: hemochromatosis and hepatolenticular degeneration.

Hemochromatosis. Hemochromatosis is a disorder of iron storage in which the liver, pancreas, skin and other organs are involved by excessive deposition of hemosiderin. The cause is excessive intestinal absorption of iron throughout life, although the nature of the metabolic abnormality is not known. However, it may have a genetic basis since about three-quarters of patients belong to HLA type A3.

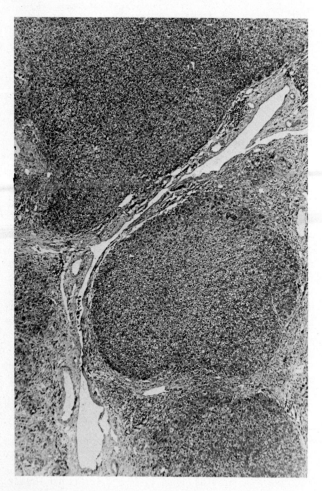

FIG. 15-11. Hepatic cirrhosis showing portions of several large regeneration nodules separated by fibrous tissue septa.

The presence of excessive iron in all cell types in the liver stimulates the formation of fibrous tissue. A similar process results in interstitial fibrosis in the pancreas. The pancreatic injury is associated with the development of diabetes mellitus, while iron deposition in the skin results in a brownish pigmentation. The term *bronze diabetes* has been used to describe the syndrome. The disease is a slow chronic process, and the effects of long term treatment by repeated phlebotomy appear to slow the process sufficiently to extend the survival time of most patients to 8 years or more. A very similar disease is seen in thalassemia if iron and blood transfusion therapy are used excessively.

Hepatolenticular degeneration. Hepatolenticular degeneration (Wilson's disease*) is the result of an inherited defect of copper metabolism.

Normally, copper in the body is maintained at a very low level by its excretion into the bile. In this disease, there is (1) deficiency of *ceruloplasmin*—a plasma protein responsible for copper transport—and (2) a possible defect in hepatic lysosomes which results in failure of copper excretion in bile. As a consequence, copper levels in blood are very low. In the liver cells the copper concentration increases, disrupting those hepatic enzyme systems which require only trace amounts of copper. As a result, excessive amounts of copper cations are present in the liver and begin to accumulate in other organs, most significantly in many parts of the central nervous system. The hepatic changes caused by excessive copper are first, fatty change, followed by death of liver cells and hepatic fibrosis. Copper deposition in the nervous system causes widespread death of neurons.

The diagnosis is confirmed by finding low levels of serum ceruloplasmin (usually less than 20 mg/dL), and the disease is treated by removing copper using the chelating agent D-penicillamine.

Tumors of the liver

The most common tumors of the liver are metastatic (Fig. 15-12), particularly from primary cancers of the breast and gastrointestinal tract. Nearly one half of all patients dying of cancer have hepatic metastases at autopsy. Benign primary tumors of the liver are uncommon and are of two types: (1) adenoma and (2) hemangioma. *Adenomas* are collections of cells closely resembling normal hepatocytes. An increased incidence of adenomas and hemangiomas has been reported in women taking oral contraceptive drugs. *Hemangiomas* usually consist of fairly large endothelial lined blood spaces. The main danger of these tumors is hemorrhage during liver biopsy if they are large and their identity is not suspected or from spontaneous intraperitoneal hemorrhage.

Liver cancer

Primary malignant tumors of the liver arise from (1) bile ducts (cholangiocarcinoma), (2) liver cells (hepatoma or hepatocellular carcinoma), or (3) blood vessels (angiosarcoma). These tumors are uncommon in the Western world, but they are common in Africa. Hepatoma is about four times as common as cholangiocarcinoma. Angiosarcoma is very rare and is associated with industrial exposure to vinyl chloride or with the radiopaque substance thorotrast. Predisposing factors for hepatoma include the following:

*Kinnear Wilson (1874-1936), English neurologist.

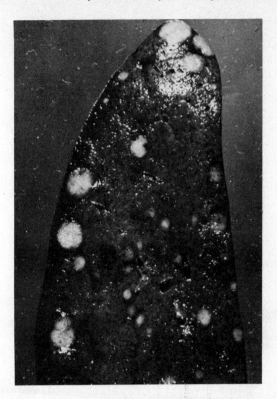

FIG. 15-12. Multiple hepatic metastases from carcinoma of the breast. *(Courtesy Curator of the Gordon Museum, Guy's Hospital, London, England.)*

1. Chronic liver disease especially when associated with persistent hepatitis B virus infection (Fig. 15-13)
2. Exposure to carcinogenic substances such as
   (a) Aflatoxins of *Aspergillus flavus*
   (b) Benzene, toluene, and their derivatives

An increased incidence of liver cancer has also been reported in patients who have received long term androgen therapy.

Although it is customary to divide liver carcinomas into hepatocellular carcinomas and cholangiocarcinomas, this is somewhat artificial since elements of both may be found in the same tumor.

Hepatocellular carcinomas are composed of atypical cells that resemble those of normal liver and are arranged in cords with intervening sinusoids and sometimes biliary epithelium.

Many patients who have hepatocellular carcinoma have raised serum levels of α-1-fetoprotein, an embryonic globulin which reappears in their serum. The presence of this substance has been used as an aid in diagnosis.

Cholangiocarcinomas differ from hepatomas in several ways. They are not associated with cirrhosis but are usually found in patients with chronic liver fluke infestation, cases of which are confined to Asiatic countries where the consumption of raw freshwater fish is common. Cholangiocarcinomas are composed of cells which form irregular tubular structures resembling bile ducts.

Few patients survive primary liver cancer beyond five years because there is no effective therapy. Partial resection of the liver and liver transplantation have been attempted so far with limited success.

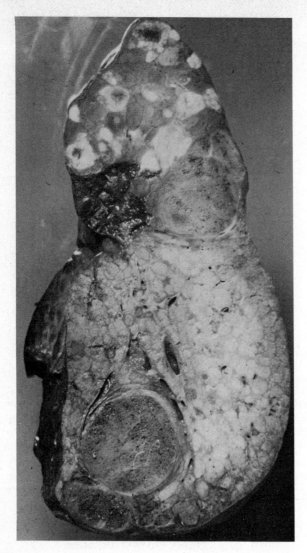

FIG. 15-13. Primary carcinoma of the liver arising in a case of hepatic cirrhosis. *(Courtesy Curator of the Gordon Museum, Guy's Hospital, London, England.)*

Vascular disease of the liver

Among the vascular diseases which affect the liver are (1) portal hypertension (already discussed)—of which cirrhosis is the main cause, (2) chronic venous congestion resulting from cardiac failure as described in Chapter 11, (3) venoocclusive disease resulting from the ingestion of senechial alkaloids, and rarely, (4) thrombosis of hepatic veins as seen in the Budd-Chiari syndrome.

Venoocclusive disease of the liver is the result of ingestion of alkaloids of the plant genus *Senechio* and related genera. These plants are used to make "bush teas," which are part of folk medicine in Jamaica and other Caribbean islands. They cause death of liver cells and replacement by fibrous tissue around the hepatic venules, eventually leading to a form of cirrhosis.

Budd-Chiari syndrome* is the result of endophlebitis of the hepatic vein, resulting in thrombosis and venous occlusion. No

---

**George Budd (1808-1882), English physician; Hans Chiari (1851-1916), German pathologist.

obvious precipitating cause may be found, but in some cases the syndrome is associated with polycythemia rubra vera (Chapter 13) or with metastatic cancer. The effects of the occlusion when severe and clinically apparent are to cause acute abdominal pain, severe shock, and ascites. The liver in this syndrome is enlarged, with variable areas of severe congestion, hemorrhage and necrosis. The fully developed syndrome usually has a fatal outcome. Liver transplantation has had some success in treating this disease.

Liver transplantation

Over the last 25 years, techniques for the transplantation of the liver have been developed with continually improving survival. Currently the longest living survivor received the transplant 20 years ago. The best results are presently in children with, for example, congenital anomalies of the bile duct system or inherited metabolic diseases that lead to cirrhosis. Liver transplants are also performed in cases of cirrhosis, and in some cases of subacute hepatic necrosis. Advanced alcoholic liver disease, hepatitis B surface antigenemia and the presence of delta agent are among contraindications to transplantation.

Although the liver is relatively resistant to immune rejection, acute rejection is common, but chronic rejection is a less frequent adverse response. The use of the immunosuppressant cyclosporine appears to have improved the results of liver transplantation but it has important side effects including hepatic and renal toxicity.

The pathologic changes that accompany early acute rejection include endophlebitis of the hepatic and portal venules, infiltration of the portal tracts by lymphocytes and eosinophils, with liver cell necrosis in some cases. In established acute rejection, larger areas of hepatic necrosis may be seen. In chronic rejection the portal tracts are infiltrated with lymphocytes and eosinophils, and cholestasis with biliary thrombi is often present.

Scarcity of suitable donors, the high order of technical facilities, surgical skill, and sophisticated support services required for liver transplantation, together with its very high cost (at least $50,000 to $60,000 a case) make it a controversial procedure even after 25 years.

Summary of hepatic diseases

1. The most common sign of hepatic injury is jaundice, which, however, may also result from extrahepatic causes such as excessive hemolysis or obstruction of the biliary tract.
2. Liver injury with or without jaundice is often reflected in abnormalities of liver function as determined by a wide range of biochemical tests such as elevated serum aminotransferases.
3. The common intrahepatic causes of jaundice are as follows:
   a. Viral hepatitis and its sequelae
   b. Abnormalities of bilirubin metabolism
   c. Toxic effects of drugs such as halothane
   d. Late stages of hepatic cirrhosis
4. The principal known causes of viral hepatitis are hepatitis viruses A, B, and NANB. Although these infections have many common features, hepatitis B tends to be the most severe with the greatest risk of complications especially when there is coincident delta agent infection. NANB hepatitis is now the most common cause of posttransfusion hepatitis in the United States and Europe.

5. The common causes of hepatic cirrhosis are as follows:
   a. Prolonged, excessive ethanol intake
   b. Previous unresolved acute and chronic hepatitis
   c. Biliary obstruction with ascending infection
6. The main consequences of hepatic cirrhosis are as follows:
   a. Portal hypertension with splenomegaly, esophageal varices, hemorrhoids, and ascites as later complications
   b. Liver failure with coma
   c. Possible predisposition to liver cancer
7. Aspects of liver disease of clinical importance include the following:
   a. Viral hepatitis B can be transmitted during many surgical, medical and dental procedures. The disease is preventable by vaccination, screening of blood donors, and rigorous application of established standards for personal techniques and environmental disinfection.
   b. Halothane can occasionally cause severe liver damage. The risk is increased if administration is repeated at short intervals.
   c. Patients with chronic liver disease or who are recovering from viral hepatitis or obstructive jaundice may have severe hemorrhagic tendencies.
   d. Patients with impaired liver function metabolize many drugs slowly. Therefore certain drugs, especially intravenous anesthetics, can be dangerous.
8. Portal hypertension, of which hepatic cirrhosis is the main cause, and chronic hepatic venous congestion of cardiac failure are the main circulatory disturbances of the liver. The consequences of portal hypertension are serious and include venous varicosities, especially of the esophagus, and ascites.
9. Transplantation of the liver in some cases of irreversible hepatic disease is now a fairly frequent procedure. Careful selection of cases is essential but survival rates continue to improve. Rejection is less of a problem with liver transplantation than with other organs.
10. The causes of liver enlargement are listed as follows:
    a. Inflammatory and infective
       (1) Viral hepatitis
       (2) Cirrhosis
       (3) Bacterial infections (e.g., brucellosis)
       (4) Parasitic infections
           (a) Amebic liver abscess
           (b) Hydatid disease
           (c) Leishmaniasis
    b. Abnormal depositions
       (1) Fatty liver (e.g., Reye's syndrome)
       (2) Storage diseases
           (a) Galactosemia
           (b) Glycogen
           (c) Neiman-Pick disease
           (d) Wilson's disease
    c. Biliary obstruction from any cause
    d. Vascular causes
       (1) Congestive cardiac failure
       (2) Hepatic vein occlusion (Budd-Chiari syndrome)
       (3) Venoocclusive disease
    e. Neoplastic
       (1) Primary and metastatic tumors
       (2) Leukemic and lymphomatous infiltration

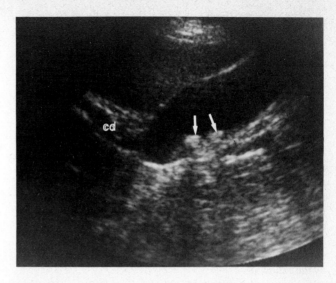

FIG. 15-14. Gallbladder sonogram. Two gallstones *(arrows)* are shown lying in the body of the gallbladder. (*cd*, cystic duct.)

THE BILIARY TRACT

Diseases of the biliary tract

The common and important diseases of the biliary tract are caused by the presence of stones, inflammation, or a combination of both. Primary malignant tumors of the gallbladder, duct system and the ampulla of Vater* are rare. Congenital anomalies affecting the anatomic arrangement of the biliary tract are probably fairly common. Many do not affect the normal function of the gallbladder and ducts but are exceedingly important to the surgeon performing biliary surgery. *Atresia of the bile ducts* (partial or total obliteration) is important since it is now potentially treatable by liver transplantation.

Investigation of the biliary tract

Radiology is the main method of investigation. Biliary stones containing calcium may show on plain films of the upper abdomen, but radiocontrast methods and sonography provide more information. The main radiographic procedures are the cholecystogram which outlines the gallbladder and its contents following orally administered contrast medium, and the cholangiogram in which intravenous contrast medium outlines the hepatic duct system. Gallbladder ultrasound is a rapid accurate method which can detect most gallstones with little or no risk or discomfort to the patient (Fig. 15-14).

Cholelithiasis and cholecystitis

Both cholecystitis and cholelithiasis (Fig. 15-15) are common afflictions, but their causes are still uncertain. Whether inflammation of the gallbladder (cholecystitis) precedes biliary stone formation (cholelithiasis) or vice versa presents a similar dilemma to deciding the precedence of the hen over the egg. Separate consideration is therefore artificial but it serves to simplify their description.

Cholelithiasis (gallstones, biliary calculi). Gallstones are common. About 20 million people in the United States harbor gallstones, the highest incidence being in the American Indian population. However, many people who harbor these mineral

---

*Abraham Vater (1684-1751), German anatomist.

occupants of the gallbladder are unaware of their presence. Gallstones are almost three times more common in women than in men. They are especially common in obese, multiparous women over the age of 40 and in young women taking estrogen contraceptive pills over a long period.

The varieties of gallstones are listed in Table 15-3, but most stones are of the mixed variety. The mechanisms by which stones form are discussed in Chapter 2. However, it is worth briefly reviewing the factors which promote the formation of (1) cholesterol and mixed stones and (2) pure pigment stones (Figs. 15-16 and 15-17).

Pathogenesis. The factors favoring the formation of cholesterol stones are those which disturb the normal quantitative relationships between cholesterol, bile acids and lecithin, which are responsible for maintaining cholesterol in soluble form. Disturbance of these relationships can result in the formation of lithogenic (stone-producing) bile, and this may be caused by the following:

1. Increased secretion of cholesterol in bile
2. Decrease in bile salt and phospholipid secretion by the liver
3. An abnormal enterohepatic circulation
4. Decrease in activity of cholesterol 7 alpha hydroxylase in the liver

Increased secretion of cholesterol is associated with obesity, use of certain drugs (e.g., clofibrate used to lower blood levels of lipoproteins), and diabetes mellitus. Reduction of bile salts can be the result of metabolic abnormalities impairing the for-

mation of bile salts from cholesterol. When ileal disease is present, reabsorption of bile salts and phospholipids from the small bowel may be seriously impaired. Bile acid synthesis requires cholesterol 7 alpha hydroxylase; this enzyme is frequently reduced in patients with mixed or cholesterol stones.

Although the mechanisms which result in the formation of bile that is supersaturated with cholesterol are known, the processes which lead to actual stone formation have not been completely elucidated. However, it appears from experimental

TABLE 15-3. Constituents and size of gallstones

Type of stone	*Contents*	*Size*
Pure stones* (20% to 25%)	Cholesterol	Up to 6 cm
	Bile pigment (calcium bilirubinate)	Up to 1 cm
	Calcium carbonate	Up to 2 cm
Mixed stones (75% to 80%)	Cholesterol, bilirubinate, calcium salts	Up to 2 cm

* Includes those stones which have a major component of a single substance with a small core or shell of different composition.

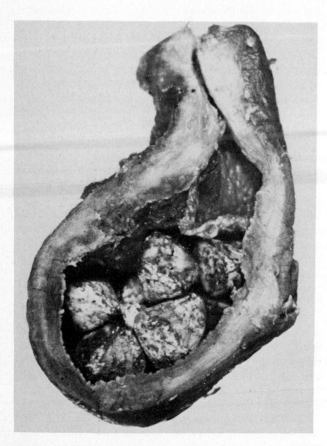

FIG. 15-15. Chronic cholecystitis and cholelithiasis. The gallbladder wall is very thick as a result of chronic inflammation and fibrosis and contains several mixed stones. (*Courtesy Curator of the Gordon Museum, Guy's Hospital, London, England.*)

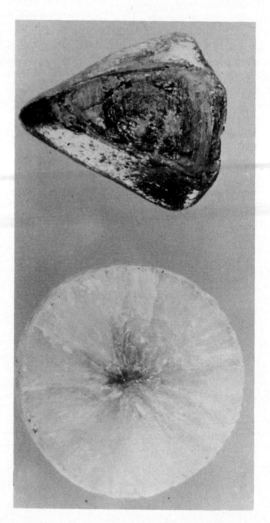

FIG. 15-16. Gallstones. A multifaceted mixed stone is shown above and the crystalline structure of a pure cholesterol stone below.

evidence, that the sequential stages of gallstone formation are (1) nucleation, (2) crystallization of cholesterol monohydrate, and (3) continued growth of these crystals to form stones. It has been recently proposed that gallbladder mucus may serve as a nidus for the initial formation of a nucleus of cholesterol crystals (nucleation) after which further crystallization leading to macroscopic stone formation can proceed.

Pigment stones consist of calcium bilirubinate and are probably due to increased amounts of insoluble conjugated bilirubin entering the bile. Pigment stones are most common in oriental countries. In western countries the predisposing factors include chronic hemolytic diseases, chronic biliary infection, and alcoholic cirrhosis.

Clinical aspects. Gallstones are very often asymptomatic; however, they may enter the duct system causing pain and obstruction or they may be associated with infection, especially of the gallbladder. Passage of a stone through the cystic duct into the common bile duct is usually accompanied by severe upper right quadrant pain (biliary colic). Persistence of obstruction of the common duct leads to obstructive jaundice and eventually to ascending biliary infection (ascending cholangitis). When this happens, there is also fever and painful liver enlargement. Surgical relief of the obstruction combined with antimicrobial treatment of the bacterial infection is indicated.

Longstanding obstruction of the cystic duct occasionally results in the distension of the gallbladder by mucus with formation of a *mucocele.*

Treatment of cholelithiasis is usually by surgical removal. Other methods include attempting to dissolve gallstones by bile acids (chenodiol) or by methyl tertiary butyl ether (MBTE); or by extracorporeal shockwave therapy (lithotripter). Surgery remains the treatment of choice. Chenodiol therapy is slow, has limited application and is still experimental.

Cholecystitis. More than 90% of patients who have acute or chronic inflammation of the gallbladder also have gallstones, which often obstruct the cystic duct. Inflammation of the gallbladder without stones is the exception. It is, nevertheless, a feature of typhoid fever.

The pathologic changes are those of acute pyogenic inflammation of the wall of the gallbladder (Fig. 15-18). If untreated, inflammation may progress to abscess formation and rupture of the gallbladder; or the gallbladder may become distended with pus (empyema).

Clinically, acute cholecystitis is suggested when a patient develops severe, upper, right-sided abdominal pain, fever, and vomiting, with or without slight jaundice. Typically, the pain is referred to the right shoulder or scapula. Acute tenderness can be elicited over the tip of the ninth costal cartilage.

If cholecystectomy is not performed in the acute stage of the disease, nearly half of the patients will develop complications such as (1) rupture of the gallbladder, with resulting peritonitis, or (2) fistula formation caused by adherence of the gallbladder to another structure such as the duodenum, colon, or stomach. In most cases, therefore, surgery is the treatment of choice.

Repeated attacks of mild or severe cholecystitis result in chronic inflammation of the gallbladder. Pathologically, the

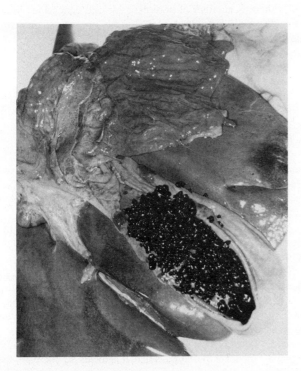

FIG. 15-17. The gallbladder has been opened to show a mass of small pigment stones. *(Courtesy Curator of the Gordon Museum, Guy's Hospital, London, England.)*

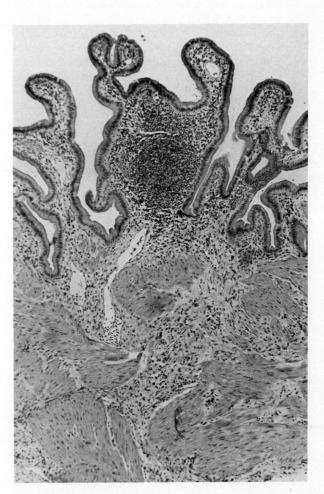

FIG. 15-18. Chronic nonspecific cholecystitis is characterized by chronic inflammatory cell infiltrates as seen here in the mucosa and an increase in fibrous tissue in the gallbladder wall.

gallbladder wall in chronic cholecystitis becomes fibrous and thickened with resultant contraction of the size of the organ. Gallstones are often present.

The symptoms are variable with upper abdominal pain the most frequent. Intolerance of fatty foods is a common complaint. Many of the complications of cholelithiasis and acute cholecystitis may supervene. The diagnosis of chronic cholecystitis is often less clear-cut than in the acute form of the disease, and has to be distinguished from other abdominal inflammatory conditions such as peptic ulceration. The diagnosis rests mainly on the radiologic findings and the treatment is usually surgical removal of the gallbladder.

Cholesterolosis of the gallbladder. Cholesterolosis is characterized by accumulation of cholesterol within macrophages in the submucosa of the gallbladder. The yellow flecks of cholesterol against the red mucosal background impart the appearance of a ripe strawberry—hence the term *strawberry gallbladder.* This condition until very recently has been dismissed as a harmless curiosity, but this conclusion may be wrong. Cholesterolosis has now been associated with symptoms typical of gallbladder disease but without radiologic or sonographic evidence of gallbladder abnormalities.

Summary of gallbladder disease

1. Cholelithiasis and cholecystitis are frequently coincident diseases of the biliary tract.
2. The events in cholesterol stone formation are (a) inherited or metabolic defects leading to supersaturation of the bile with cholesterol and (b) nucleation and growth of cholesterol crystals eventually forming macroscopic stones.
3. Both cholecystitis and cholelithiasis are characterized by upper right abdominal pain. Obstructive jaundice caused by stones in the biliary tract is a potentially severe complication.

THE PANCREAS
Anatomy

The pancreas lies with its head in the C of the duodenum and extends pennant-like across the back of the abdominal cavity where its tail contacts the spleen. The lower third of the common bile duct passes through the head of the pancreas en route to the duodenum. This is an important relationship when pancreatic cancer develops.

Pancreatic functions

The exocrine functions are as follows:
1. Synthesis of proteins, mainly precursors of enzymes such as trypsin, amylase and lipase
2. Secretion of water and electrolytes, especially bicarbonate

Endocrine secretions, which are discussed in Chapter 18, are secretion of (1) insulin by beta cells of islet tissue, (2) glucagon by alpha cells, (3) somatostatin by delta cells, and (4) pancreatic polypeptide by PP cells. Each of the preceding cell types can occasionally give rise to tumors.

Investigation of the pancreas

Investigation of pancreatic disease has been greatly facilitated by modern techniques. Among the more useful are the following:

1. Measurement of pancreatic enzymes, particularly amylase and lipase in the serum
2. Radiologic methods include sonography, computerized tomography (CT), and angiography
3. Fecal examination for evidence of impaired proteolytic and lipolytic activity

Diseases of the pancreas
Acute pancreatitis

Despite numerous hypotheses, the cause of acute pancreatitis is unknown. Its frequent association with biliary tract disease and acute excessive intake of alcohol is well known. Other etiologic factors include the following:
1. Viral infections
2. Hyperlipidemias
3. Abdominal injury
4. Drugs such as the thiazides
5. Hypercalcemia associated with hyperparathyroidism
6. Hypothermia

Pathogenesis and pathology. One etiologic factor may be mechanical or functional obstruction of the ampulla of Vater leading to retrograde flow of bile into the pancreatic duct system with subsequent enzymic injury to pancreatic tissue. Whatever may be the initiating stimulus, the effect is proteolytic destruction of the pancreas by the action of its own enzymes—an example of suicide of an organ. As a result of this self-destructive process (Fig. 15-19) pancreatic enzymes are released into the peritoneum. Because of lipase activity on peritoneal fat, *enzymic fat necrosis* develops. Fatty acids released by lipase combine with calcium to form soaps, which excite foci of intense inflammation in the peritoneum.

The process may involve all or part of the pancreas, which becomes swollen, necrotic and often hemorrhagic. Histologically, there is necrosis of both exocrine and endocrine tissue. In cases associated with biliary disease or acute alcoholism, the inflammatory necrosis tends to develop around the pancreatic ducts. This is often accompanied by thrombosis of pancreatic vessels leading to ischemic necrosis superimposed on the autolytic effects of pancreatic enzymes.

In other cases necrosis is confined to the peripheral zones of the pancreatic lobules. Here, the initiating event appears to be interruption of the blood supply to the pancreas with resulting ischemic necrosis.

Clinical aspects. The sudden severe chemical damage to the pancreas and peritoneum is often reflected in the dramatic and life-threatening clinical picture. Typical consequences are severe, relentless abdominal pain, accompanied by fever, tachycardia, shock, and intestinal ileus.

Abnormally high levels of amylase can be detected in the blood and urine 8 to 12 hours after onset. Similar although slower increases in serum lipase levels can be detected.

The outlook in acute pancreatitis depends on the extent of the necrotic process and the quality of clinical management. The chief danger in the early phase of the illness is prolonged refractory hypotension (shock); the main danger in the later phase is secondary suppurative bacterial infection.

Success depends on early diagnosis, so that surgery can be avoided whenever possible, since it appears to increase the complications. Treatment is, therefore conservative and consists of relief of pain, control of hypotension, and possibly reduction of pancreatic secretions with atropine.

About 25% of patients die. Some develop pancreatic *pseudocysts* as a result of pancreatic secretion becoming sealed off in a sac formed by adherent layers of peritoneum. Others have repeated mild attacks of pancreatitis or develop a slower insidious inflammatory process that results in chronic pancreatitis.

Chronic pancreatitis

Most cases of chronic pancreatitis are alcoholics and the disease often accompanies alcoholic cirrhosis. The main pathologic process is generalized fibrosis of the pancreas affecting

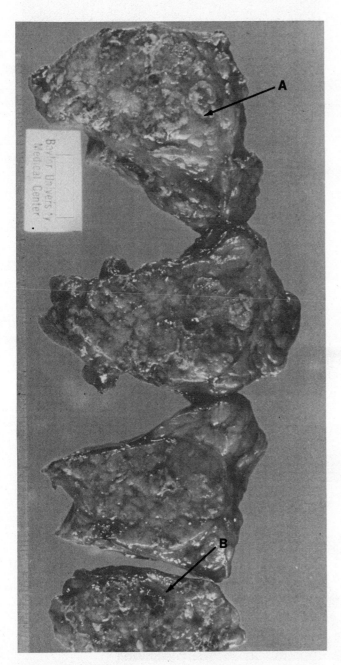

FIG. 15-19. Acute pancreatitis. The pancreas has been sectioned to show areas of necrosis *(A)* and hemorrhage *(B)*.

mainly the exocrine tissue. Reduction in pancreatic secretions leads to excessive fat in the stools (pancreatic steatorrhea).

Cystic fibrosis (fibrocystic disease of the pancreas; mucoviscidosis)

Cystic fibrosis is a serious disease in which the function of exocrine glands in many parts of the body is deranged. The pancreas is always severely affected, but many organs may be involved to varying degrees. These include the following:

1. The lungs, which are usually seriously damaged
2. The mucous glands of the gastrointestinal tract
3. The salivary glands, especially the mainly mucus producing submaxillary glands
4. The biliary tract
5. The sweat glands of the skin

Etiology and pathogenesis. Cystic fibrosis is inherited as an autosomal recessive abnormality. It is found in 1:1500 caucasian births in the United States; it is ten times less common in the black population. The precise nature of the basic defect is not known, but current hypothesis suggests that an inability of chloride ions to cross the cytoplasmic membrane of exocrine cells results in failure to resorb sodium ions. This at least would explain the increase in sodium concentration of sweat present in cystic fibrosis.

In the pancreas, the ducts become blocked with inspissated secretions. The acinar tissue atrophies and is replaced by fibrofatty tissue; cystic dilatation of the ducts develops (hence the term *cystic fibrosis*). The effects of this destruction of the exocrine pancreatic tissue are (1) steatorrhea and (2) malabsorption, especially of fat-soluble vitamins.

In the lungs, the viscid secretions impair normal lung clearance mechanisms, obstruct the bronchi, and predispose to recurrent infections. Chronic bronchitis and bronchiectasis with episodes of acute inflammatory lung disease are typical. Chronic sinusitis, for similar reasons, is found in association with the pulmonary disease.

In the gastrointestinal tract the viscid secretions of the mucous glands, when combined with the severe pancreatic insufficiency, may obstruct the intestinal tract with inspissated materials. When this takes place in very young children, it is called *meconium ileus.*

Biliary involvement is uncommon, but the obstructive effects of the inspissated bile may cause biliary cirrhosis in a few cases.

Abnormally functioning sweat glands are present in nearly all cases of cystic fibrosis. The concentrations of sodium and chloride in sweat are greatly increased. This, combined with malabsorption of minerals, may cause serious sodium depletion in these patients especially in warm weather.

In patients surviving into adult life, a few cases of amyloidosis have been reported.

Pathology. The pancreatic changes in cystic fibrosis (Fig. 15-20) are as follows:

1. Numerous dilated pancreatic ducts containing plugs of mucus
2. Absence of pancreatic acini
3. Squamous metaplasia of the duct epithelium if malabsorption of vitamin A is severe
4. Fibrofatty stroma in which the islet cells are still intact

Clinical aspects. Cystic fibrosis is a serious incurable disease of children. The main clinical effects are malnutrition as a result

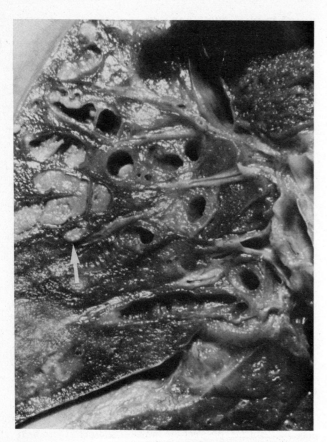

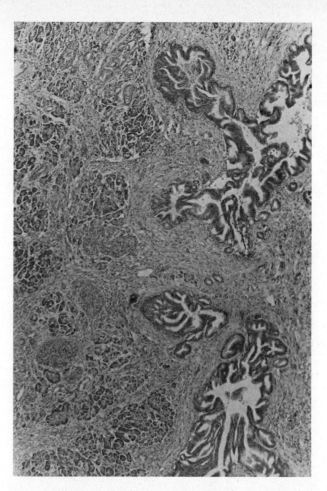

FIG. 15-20. The lung in mucoviscidosis. Thick, inspissated secretions can be seen filling the widely dilated bronchi *(arrow)*.

FIG. 15-21. Adenocarcinoma of the pancreas. Neoplastic ductal tissue, showing a complex papillary pattern, is seen on the right.

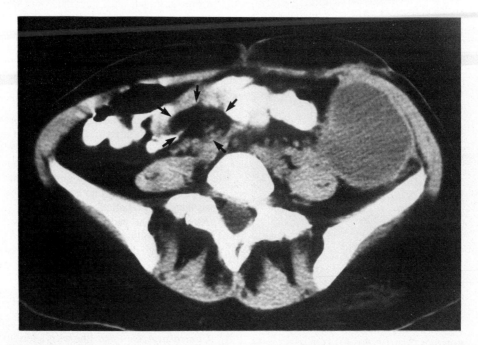

FIG. 15-22. Computerized tomogram. Transverse section through the abdomen shows a large carcinoma of the pancreas *(arrows)*.

of the severe pancreatic insufficiency and acute-on-chronic pulmonary infections. The diagnosis is based on these findings together with the elevation of sweat chloride and sodium and biopsy of affected tissue e.g. intestinal biopsy. Patients with cystic fibrosis require long-term management with dietary supplements of vitamins and salt and treatment of acute and chronic bronchial infections. Oral administration of pancreatic enzymes can help improve intestinal symptoms due to steatorrhea.

Pancreatic tumors

Benign tumors of the pancreas are rare and most, such as lipomas and fibromas, are not unique to the pancreas. Cystadenomas which are generally large tumors are typical but uncommon and benign.

Tumors of the endocrine portion of the pancreas are discussed in Chapter 18.

The important malignant tumor of the pancreas is the *adenocarcinoma*. This lethal tumor is most common in the seventh decade of life. In two thirds of cases, the tumor arises in the head of the pancreas where its expansile or invasive effects frequently obstruct the outflow of bile relatively early in the disease, causing jaundice. Tumors of the body and tail are usually quite large and widespread by the time they are detected.

Microscopically, adenocarcinomas of the pancreas usually have a typical, well-differentiated glandular pattern with abundant fibrous stroma (Fig. 15-21). There is often direct spread to adjacent organs; metastases are common in lymph nodes, lungs, and bone.

Clinical aspects. The main clinical features of carcinoma of the head of the pancreas are deep-seated abdominal and back pain preceding or concurrent with progressive obstructive jaundice. Some patients, for unknown reasons, develop paraneoplastic syndromes such as thrombophlebitis, peripheral neuritis, and Eaton-Lambert syndrome (Chapter 17). The latter is a condition characterized by muscle weakness, which curiously, improves following exercise. The diagnosis of pancreatic carcinoma has been greatly assisted by CT scanning (Fig. 15-22) and percutaneous fine needle biopsy. The outlook for the patient, however, is bleak. Few patients survive for more than two years after laparotomy and the five year cure rate is practically zero. Operative removal of the pancreas has a high mortality rate (10% to 15%).

Summary

1. Acute pancreatitis is an abdominal emergency arising from acute necrosis of the organ and release of its enzymes into the peritoneal cavity. The disease is accompanied by elevations of serum and urinary amylase, and serum lipase levels.

2. Cystic fibrosis is an inherited defect of exocrine glands affecting the pancreatic and pulmonary secretions as well as those of the sweat glands and intestines. It is mainly a disease of children characterized by steatorrhea and pulmonary infection. Increased sweat chloride is a diagnostic feature.

3. Adenocarcinoma of the pancreas is a lethal malignancy in which the tumor frequently occludes the common bile duct leading to obstructive jaundice.

Selected readings

Anthony PP, Ishak KG, Poulsen HE et al: The morphology of cirrhosis, J Clin Pathol 31:395, 1978.

Bassendine MF: Hepatitis B virus and liver cell carcinoma. In Anthony PP and MacSween RNM, editors: Recent advances in histopathology, Edinburgh, 1984, Churchill Livingstone.

Bonino F and Smedile A: Delta agent (type D) hepatitis, Sem Liver Dis 6:28, 1986.

Bradley DW and Maynard JE: Etiology and natural history of posttransfusion and enterically transmitted non-A, non-B hepatitis, Sem Liver Dis 6:56, 1986.

Geokas MC: Acute pancreatitis, Ann Intern Med 103:86, 1985.

Gerber MA and Thung SN: Histology of the liver, Am J Surg Pathol 11:709, 1987.

Hollinger FB: Serologic evaluation of viral hepatitis, Hosp Pract 22:101, 1987.

Jacyna MR and Bouchier IAD: Cholesterosis: cause of "functional" disorders, Br Med J 295:619, 1987.

Kerr JFR, Searle J, and Halliday WJ et al: The nature of piecemeal necrosis of the liver in chronic active hepatitis, Lancet 2:827, 1979.

Kew MC: Hepatic tumors, Sem Liver Dis 4:89, 1984.

Patel KH and Thomas E: Carcinoma of the pancreas, Hosp Pract 22:131, 1987.

Redeker AG: Delta agent and hepatitis B, Ann Int Med 98:542, 1983.

Ruebner BH: Collagen formation and cirrhosis, Sem Liver Dis 6:212, 1986.

Schaffner F: Primary biliary cirrhosis, Curr Concepts Gastroenterol 8:14, 1983.

Searle J, Harmon BV, and Bishop CT et al: The significance of cell death by apoptosis in hepatobiliary disease, J Gastroenterol Hepatol 2:77, 1987.

Sherlock S: Patterns of hepatocyte injury in man, Lancet 1:782, 1982.

Sherlock S: Hepatic transplantation, South Med J 80:357, 1987.

Sherlock S, and Thomas HC: Delta virus hepatitis, J Hepatol 3:419, 1987.

Smith BF, LaMont TJ, and Small DM: The sequence of events in stone formation (editorial), Lab Invest 56:125, 1987.

Tavill AS and Bacon BR: Hemachromatosis, Hepatology 6:142, 1984.

Vyas GN and Blue HE: Hepatitis B virus infection, West J Med 140:754, 1984.

Weisberg HF: Pathogenesis of gallstones, Ann Clin Lab Sci 14:243, 1984.

Wollcoff AW: Bilirubin metabolism and hyperbilirubinemia, Sem Liver Dis 3:1, 1983.

Zuckerman AJ: The enigma of fulminant viral hepatitis, Hepatology 4:568, 1984.

CHAPTER 16

Diseases of the kidney and lower urinary tract

Renal diseases pose many problems for their victims and for medical science. Renal diseases can cause the kidneys to fail, ultimately leading to the death of the patient. In recent years, however, the artificial kidney has provided the means to support life by hemodialysis in the presence of renal failure. Renal transplantation has permitted the survival and return to productive life of many patients who would otherwise have died from renal disease.

Many problems in the pathogenesis and pathology of renal disease have been resolved by the application of electron microscopy and immunostaining techniques to the examination of renal biopsy material. Electron microscopy of normal and abnormal renal tissue has permitted satisfactory classification of many previously problematic renal lesions, especially those that affect the glomerulus. Immunofluorescence and immunoperoxidase staining methods have been used to demonstrate the presence and type of immune substances, such as immunoglobulins and complement, which are important in the pathogenesis of many glomerular diseases. These methods, in conjunction with light microscopy, are now generally regarded as essential for the diagnosis and management of renal diseases.

Approaches to classifying renal diseases

Most problems in classifying renal diseases relate to conditions which affect the structure and function of the nephron, and its associated vasculature and interstitium. By comparison, classifying, for example, renal neoplasms and calculi is relatively simple.

It is also unusual for the morphologic abnormalities to be limited to renal glomeruli, tubules, arteries, or interstitium, and disease affecting one of these structures is very likely to involve one or more of the others secondarily. However, renal diseases can be grouped according to the structure which is primarily or predominantly affected. Thus they can be classified as follows:
1. Glomerular
2. Tubular
3. Vascular
4. Interstitial

GLOMERULAR DISEASE
Descriptive terminology

Glomerulonephritis and *glomerulopathy* are terms commonly used to describe renal disorders primarily affecting glomeruli. These diseases fall into one of two categories:
1. The kidney is the sole or predominant organ affected.
2. Renal involvement is part of a multisystem disorder such as diabetes mellitus.

Basic considerations

In approaching the pathology of glomerular diseases for the first time, it is important to note that it is difficult to make clear cut distinctions of etiology, pathogenesis, pathology, and clinical presentation among the many conditions which affect the glomeruli. There is therefore no unanimous agreement on how best to classify glomerular disease. Nevertheless, the following are important to an understanding of renal diseases:
1. The kidney may be exposed to numerous noxious agents but it can only respond to injury in a limited number of ways. Thus, a single, distinctive, pathologic pattern can be produced by many different diseases. For example, the histologic and ultrastructural pattern of *membranous nephropathy*, described later, may be seen in the kidney in association with many diverse conditions: systemic

TABLE 16-1. WHO classification of lupus nephritis

Number	Description
Class I	Normal
Class II	Mesangial proliferation
Class III	Focal proliferation
Class IV	Diffuse proliferation
Class V	Membranous

TABLE 16-2. Glomerular diseases and their most common clinical presentations

Disease	Clinical presentation
Hematuria	IgA nephropathy Hereditary glomerulonephritis Thin basement membrane syndrome Anaphylactoid purpura
Acute nephritic syndrome	Postinfectious glomerulonephritis Focal glomerulonephritis Early crescentic glomerulonephritis
Proteinuria/nephrotic syndrome	Nil disease Mesangial proliferative glomerulonephritis Focal glomerulosclerosis Membranous nephropathy Membranoproliferative glomerulonephritis Preeclampsia/eclampsia Systemic diseases (diabetes, amyloidosis)
Acute renal failure	Crescentic glomerulonephritis Thrombotic microangiopathy
Chronic renal failure	"Chronic glomerulonephritis" (end-stage)

lupus erythematosus (SLE), syphilis, gold therapy, hepatitis B, or neoplasms are examples.

2. A single *disease* can produce several different morphologic patterns of renal injury. An excellent example is SLE, in which any one of six possible histologic patterns may be seen in the kidney (Table 16-1).

3. Similarly, the same clinical *syndrome* can result from a variety of renal lesions (Table 16-2). Thus the nephrotic syndrome (considered later) can be the result, for example, of any of the following conditions described later in this chapter:
   a. Membranous nephropathy
   b. Membranoproliferative glomerulonephritis
   c. Focal glomerulosclerosis
   d. Nil disease

Classification

No single classification of glomerular disease is completely satisfactory, though many have been proposed. Classification may be based on one of the following:
1. The morphology of structural changes in glomeruli
2. Pathogenetic mechanisms causing glomerular disease
3. Etiology of glomerular disease
4. Clinical presentation
A brief discussion of each classification follows.

Morphologic classification. Glomerular diseases can be classified according to the type of structural change seen in the glomeruli. Chief among these are the following:
1. *Proliferative changes*—Proliferative forms of glomerulonephritis are characterized by an *increase in the number of cells* in the glomerulus. The proliferative changes may involve (Fig. 16-1) the following:
   a. Extracapillary (epithelial) cells
   b. Intracapillary (endothelial and mesangial) cells
   c. Combinations of these two groups of cells
2. *Exudative changes*—There is exudation of inflammatory cells, usually polymorphonuclear leukocytes, into the glomerular tuft.

3. *Sclerosis—Sclerosis* is a term which describes a significant increase in the mesangial matrix, which is usually accompanied by obliteration of the lumina of glomerular capillaries.

Important morphologic distinctions can be made according to the *distribution* of the microscopic changes in the glomeruli, as follows:
1. With respect to the entire kidney
   a. *Generalized*—The changes affect most or all glomeruli.
   b. *Focal*—Usually fewer than half of the glomeruli are affected.
2. With respect to individual glomeruli
   a. *Diffuse*—The disease affects most, or all of the glomerulus.
   b. *Segmental*—Only part (usually less than one half) of the glomerulus is affected.

A simplified morphologic classification of glomerulopathies follows:
1. Proliferative
   a. Acute extracapillary proliferative glomerulonephritis (crescentic glomerulonephritis)
   b. Acute intracapillary proliferative and exudative glomerulonephritis (postinfectious glomerulonephritis)
   c. Chronic proliferative and sclerosing glomerulonephritis ("chronic glomerulonephritis")
   d. Focal and segmental proliferative/necrotizing glomerulonephritis
   e. Membranoproliferative glomerulonephritis
   f. Mesangioproliferative glomerulonephritis
2. Nonproliferative
   a. Amyloidosis
   b. Diabetic glomerulosclerosis
   c. Focal and segmental glomerulosclerosis
   d. Hereditary glomerulonephropathy (Alport's syndrome)
   e. Membranous nephropathy
   f. Nil disease (minimal change glomerulopathy)

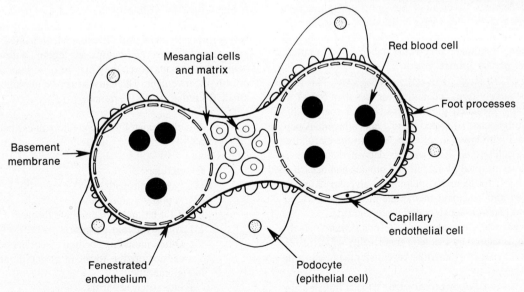

FIG. 16-1. Diagram of two glomerular capillary loops illustrating the relations of the three main cellular components of the glomerulus.

Pathogenetic classification. Another means of categorizing glomerular disease is based on the underlying pathogenetic mechanisms, which have largely been elucidated by correlating the findings of light microscopy with those of electron microscopy and immunostaining.

By this means glomerular disease can be divided into two categories: (1) immunologically mediated and (2) nonimmunologically mediated. Most, however, are immunologically mediated and are usually either of the *immune complex* type or *glomerular antibasement membrane antibody* type.

Immunologically mediated renal disease

IMMUNE COMPLEX-MEDIATED INJURY. This very common process is characterized by the presence of macromolecular antigen-antibody complexes in the glomeruli. These immune complexes may either (a) form in situ within the glomeruli or (b) be deposited there from the circulation. In the latter situation, the kidney is the victim of a disease process originating elsewhere in the body.

The antigens involved may be either *endogenous* (DNA, for example) or *exogenous* (environmental), such as microbial toxins, and the antigen-antibody complexes which they form, do not necessarily have any special affinity for renal structures. Their presence in the kidney is apparently the result of a normally highly negatively charged, glomerular capillary surface, attributable to proteoglycans, which have affinity for positively charged antigens.

Electron microscopy of the glomerulus can be used to determine the position of *immune deposits,* which, like the pattern of immunofluorescence, has an important bearing on pathologic diagnosis and clinical prognosis.

Subendothelial deposits of immune complexes are seen as large, electron-dense aggregates situated between the basement membrane and the endothelial cells. Because of their position, they usually cause rapid occlusion of the glomerular capillaries, resulting in severe impairment of renal function.

Subepithelial immune deposits are seen as smaller electron-dense aggregates caught between the podocytes and the basement membrane. They generally cause less severe or more slowly developing impairment of renal function.

Mesangial deposits lie clear of the peripheral glomerular capillary loops and therefore have little effect on glomerular function. Mesangial and subendothelial deposits result mainly from circulating immune complexes; subepithelial immune complexes are mainly formed in situ.

INJURY DUE TO ANTIBODIES TO BASEMENT MEMBRANE. This form of injury is relatively rare, accounting for less than 5% of all immunologically mediated glomerulopathies. Autoantibodies (usually of the IgG class) directed against noncollagenous peptides associated with type IV collagen, arise in the circulation by unknown mechanisms. They are then deposited along basement membranes of renal glomeruli and tubules and occasionally in other sites, for example, pulmonary alveolar basement membranes. In anti-basement membrane-mediated injury accumulations of electron-dense material are not seen.

Alport's syndrome, an example of the *nonimmunologically* mediated type, is caused by a genetic abnormality which results in defective synthesis of glomerular basement membrane components.

EFFECTS OF IMMUNE INJURY ON GLOMERULI. Once initiated, injury of the immune complex or anti-basement membrane antibody type is the result of both humoral and cellular activity. Thus immune activation of the *complement system* can lead to the following:

1. Immune lysis of glomerular cells
2. Production of activated complement components, leading to increased vascular permeability and/or chemotactic attraction of neutrophils and/or monocytes

Neutrophils and monocytes appear to contribute to glomerular injury by producing oxygen radicals and by releasing factors capable of enzymatically degrading the basement membranes. Alteration of the endothelial surface and exposure of matrix collagen can lead to initiation of intravascular coagulation and localized platelet aggregation. The net result of these events is to alter the structural and functional integrity of the glomerular capillaries. This leads to reduced glomerular filtration, increased permeability to plasma proteins, and movement of leukocytes and red cells outside the vascular compartment.

Etiologic classification. Despite our current knowledge of the pathogenesis of the glomerular diseases, their exact *etiology,* in most instances, is unknown. Attempts at etiologic classification are therefore, at present, unhelpful. Currently, clinical management is guided chiefly by knowledge of the morphology, rather than the cause of the glomerular disease.

Clinical classification. Glomerular (and other) renal diseases can be grouped according to their usual clinical manifestations (Table 16-2) and in this chapter are considered under the following headings:

1. Hematuria
2. The acute nephritic syndrome
3. Proteinuria and the nephrotic syndrome
4. Acute renal failure
5. Chronic renal failure

Conditions included under these headings also involve pathologic changes in structures other than the glomeruli. Thus, in some, renal tubules, vessels, or interstitial tissue may be primarily affected.

Glomerular diseases presenting as hematuria

Hematuria is defined as the presence of blood in the urine. It may either be visible to the naked eye or detectable only microscopically and may be painless or accompanied by pain. Not surprisingly, hematuria is often accompanied by some degree of proteinuria. The causes are legion, with close to 100 being listed in some texts; they may be of serious consequence, or only inconvenient. The causes may be classified as (a) prerenal, (b) renal, or (c) postrenal:

1. Prerenal
   a. Chiefly hematologic (coagulopathies, hemoglobinopathies)
2. Renal
   a. Glomerular
      (1) IgA nephropathy
      (2) Alport's syndrome
      (3) Thin basement membrane disease
      (4) Anaphylactoid purpura
      (5) Other, including "benign essential hematuria," focal necrotizing forms of glomerulonephritis
   b. Nonglomerular
      (1) Interstitial nephritis
      (2) Neoplasms
      (3) Polycystic kidneys
      (4) Trauma
      (5) Vascular pathology (e.g., infarcts)

3. Postrenal
   a. Calculi
   b. Foreign bodies (e.g., catheters)
   c. Neoplasms
   d. Trauma, including exercise-related hematuria
   e. Urinary tract infections

In those cases in which the hematuria, perhaps on the basis of red cell urinary casts, is traced to the kidneys, fully 50% of cases demonstrate no characteristic findings on renal biopsy ("benign essential hematuria"). The other 50% show a variety of glomerular lesions, the most characteristic of which are discussed below.

IgA nephropathy

The idiopathic type of IgA mesangial nephropathy (Berger's disease) is now recognized as being the *most frequent primary glomerular disease* in many countries throughout the world. It is an important cause of chronic renal failure and is estimated to account for around ten percent of patients on maintenance hemodialysis.

IgA nephropathy is found at all ages, but is most common in the second and third decades of life. It affects males more frequently than females. The common clinical presentation is either *asymptomatic microscopic hematuria and proteinuria, or macroscopic hematuria;* approximately one half of those with this disease have no symptoms. Episodes of gross hematuria are often closely associated with attacks of respiratory tract infection, or, less frequently, other *mucosal infections* (gastrointestinal or urinary tracts). The interval between the precipitating event and the appearance of gross hematuria is characteristically very short (24 to 48 hours).

The essential feature of IgA nephropathy is the *mesangial deposition of IgA,* diffuse in all glomeruli. In the great majority of cases C3 deposits, and in about half IgG deposits, are found distributed in a pattern similar to IgA, but always with a lesser intensity of fluorescence. Mesangial electron-dense deposits are present (Fig. 16-2). On light microscopy, the most frequent abnormality is mesangial widening, with a variable amount of increased mesangial cellularity which varies from minimal to focal and segmental to generalized and diffuse. With progression of the disease, there is increasing collapse of capillary loops and glomerular sclerosis, and ultimately a picture of "end-stage" kidney ("chronic glomerulonephritis") results. *Progression to chronic renal failure* is relentless, although the rapidity of this progression varies greatly. Some patients die from renal failure soon after diagnosis, whereas others have normal renal function more than 30 years after the first episode of gross hematuria; the most frequent clinical course is an indolent, slowly progressing chronic disease.

Pathogenesis. Since IgA is the principal immunoglobulin defense system in mucosal secretions, and since acute exacerbation of IgA nephropathy is frequently associated with mucosal infections, it is postulated that the IgA deposited in the glomerular mesangium is an antibody to antigens entering at mucosal sites. This is further supported by the fact that the mesangial IgA is of the *polymeric type,* normally present in mucosal secretions but usually only found in small amounts in the circulation. Indeed, high serum levels of polymeric IgA are found, particularly in the early stages and during exacerbations of the disease. Polymeric IgA is cleared with difficulty by the mesangial cells, leading to its prolonged retention at this site. This predisposition to produce high levels of circulating polymeric IgA, appears to be inherited because members of

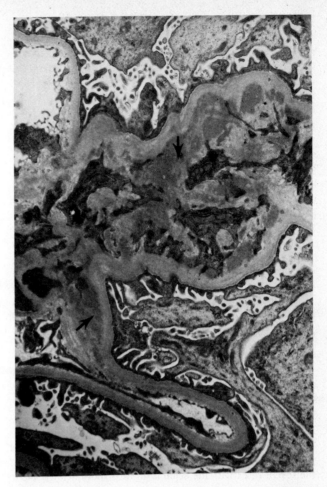

FIG. 16-2. Mesangial electron-dense deposits *(arrows).* From a case of IgA nephropathy.

patients' families, although asymptomatic, often demonstrate the abnormal IgA production.

The mere presence of mesangial IgA does not lead to progressive glomerular injury; IgA deposits have been found at necropsy in the mesangium of patients without microscopic evidence of glomerulonephritis. Experimental studies suggest that activation of the complement cascade, with the formation of *immune complexes* containing C3, is necessary to cause the proliferative lesions and subsequent glomerular sclerosis. This could also explain why relatives of patients with IgA nephropathy may have increased production of IgA without disease.

There is no proven treatment for IgA nephropathy. It recurs very frequently after transplantation, within one to four years. Interestingly, transplantation of donor kidneys with mesangial IgA deposits into patients with previous non-IgA-related disease results in disappearance of the deposits.

Alport's syndrome (hereditary glomerulonephritis)

Alport's syndrome is an autosomal dominantly inherited disease which begins in childhood with attacks of hematuria. The disease is found in both males and females but is considerably more severe in the former, often ending in renal failure by the time the patient reaches the late teens or early 20's. In females, the course is much milder and most live to old age. In addition to renal manifestations, the other characteristic feature of this syndrome is deafness.

Early in the disease, there may be no significant renal abnormalities on light microscopy. Electron microscopy, however, reveals a characteristic lesion in the glomeruli which consists of thickening and splitting of lamina densa of basement membranes (see Chapter 2). In some though not all patients, but particularly in children, stretches of basement membrane are thinned out rather than thickened. Thickening may possibly develop with progression of the disease, or these cases may be subgroups of the syndrome that do not show the typical basement membrane lesion.

Thin basement membrane syndrome

The *thin basement membrane syndrome* is also a familial disease characterized by recurrent attacks of hematuria. The glomeruli show no significant changes on light microscopy, but on electron microscopy considerable thinning of the basement membrane may be observed, with the lamina densa measuring one half to one third of normal thickness. Most cases appear to be nonprogressive, but some develop renal failure. The molecular defects responsible for the abnormal basement membrane formation may be related in some way to those producing Alport's syndrome.

Anaphylactoid purpura (Henoch-Schonlein purpura)

Anaphylactoid purpura is an acute illness characterized by petechial hemorrhages in the skin, hematuria, and sometimes also melena. The disease is most common in children but is also found in adults. Though renal involvement is common in anaphylactoid purpura, it is usually mild and only 5% to 10% of patients have significant renal disease. Those with milder forms of renal involvement present with hematuria, whereas the severe cases with the acute nephritic syndrome progress to renal failure.

Histologically, a spectrum of changes is seen, with some cases resembling IgA nephropathy, others resembling postinfectious glomerulonephritis, and the more severe forms exhibiting focal-segmental necrotizing lesions, leading to crescent formation. IgA-containing deposits are frequently found.

Glomerular diseases presenting as the acute nephritic syndrome

The acute nephritic syndrome is characterized by hematuria, diminished urinary output, retention of nitrogenous metabolic products (azotemia), and hypertension. It should not be confused with the nephrotic syndrome (Table 16-3).

Postinfectious glomerulonephritis

Synonyms for postinfectious glomerulonephritis, which is becoming distinctly uncommon in developed countries, include acute glomerulonephritis and acute intracapillary proliferative and exudative glomerulonephritis.

Postinfectious glomerulonephritis is usually, but not exclusively, a sequel to infection by certain types of streptococci. Other microorganisms, including staphylococci, pneumococci, and hepatitis B, measles and mumps viruses, can cause identical lesions in the kidney. When streptococci are the cause, the organisms belong to certain antigenic groups. Specifically, these streptococci belong to the Lancefield group A β-hemolytic streptococci and possess surface protein M antigens types 1, 4, 12, 49, and 57. Type 12 is known to produce a specific nephrotoxin that is independent of other products of streptococci.

Light microscopy shows that all glomeruli are involved in an inflammatory process characterized by swelling and increased cellularity of the glomerular tufts, due in part to the exudation of polymorphonuclear leukocytes. On electron microscopy (Fig. 16-3) there is also an increase in both mesangial and endothelial cells. Sometimes the third cellular element of the glomeruli, the epithelial cells, also proliferate and form crescent-shaped thickenings around the glomerulus. Beehive-shaped subepithelial deposits ("humps") containing IgG and complement are present early in the disease. Immunofluorescence shows a granular ("lumpy-bumpy") deposition of IgG and C3 along the glomerular basement membrane.

TABLE 16-3. Components and outcome of nephritic and nephrotic syndromes

Clinical findings	Syndrome	Possible outcome
Hematuria Oliguria Azotemia Hypertension	Nephritic syndrome	Recovery, persistent hypertension, or renal failure
Generalized edema Severe proteinuria Hypoalbuminemia Hyperlipidemia	Nephrotic syndrome	Recovery with steroid therapy or renal failure

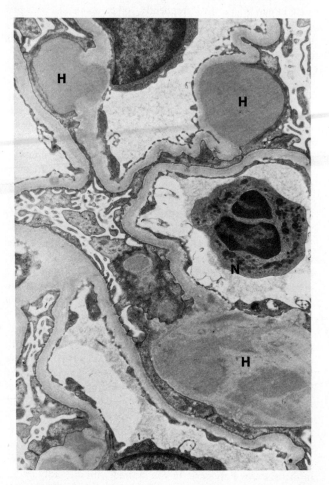

FIG. 16-3. Acute glomerulonephritis. Intramesangial and subepithelial humplike deposits are a characteristic feature *(H)*. One capillary contains a neutrophil *(N)*.

Many cases of postinfectious glomerulonephritis follow streptococcal infections of the pharynx or the skin (pyoderma) after a period of 1 to 4 weeks. Both adults and children are affected. The main clinical findings are hematuria, oliguria, edema of the face (periorbital), and, in about half the cases, hypertension (i.e., the nephritic syndrome). Red blood cells, red cell casts, and protein are present in the urine. β-hemolytic streptococci may still be isolated from the throat in some patients. In others, serologic evidence of antecedent streptococcal infection may be obtained from tests for various antibodies to streptococcal products. The most commonly used procedure is the antistreptolysin (ASO) titer, which is elevated in about half the patients. Higher percentages of positive results are reported for antibodies to streptococcal deoxyribonuclease and nicotinamide adenine dinucleotidase. Serum C3 is decreased in the acute phase.

Most patients with acute proliferative glomerulonephritis recover completely, but the urinary and morphologic abnormalities may persist for many months. A few patients, who sustain greater degrees of glomerular damage, progress to crescentic glomerulonephritis and rapidly developing renal failure. A disputed, but probably small, number progress to end-stage renal disease ("chronic glomerulonephritis") and chronic renal failure. Treatment is aimed at control of edema and hypertension until recovery takes place.

Focal necrotizing glomerulonephritis and early crescentic glomerulonephritis

The term *focal glomerulonephritis* implies that only some glomeruli (usually fewer than half) show glomerular tuft changes on light microscopy. These changes are usually also segmental in distribution—i.e., affect only a part (usually less than one half) of the glomerulus. It is important to note, however, that on electronmicroscopy and immunostaining there are usually diffuse and generalized glomerular abnormalities (i.e., the terms *focal* and *segmental* apply strictly to *light* microscopic appearances).

Two classes of focal glomerulonephritis, with very different prognostic implications, are distinguished:

1. The lesions consist of focal and segmental exaggeration of a mesangial cell proliferation that is present throughout glomeruli
2. Focal and segmental *necrotizing* lesions, usually accompanied by thrombosis of the associated tuft capillaries

The former class of lesion, which is exemplified by some cases of IgA nephropathy, usually presents with hematuria and is of a relatively benign nature (progressing gradually to glomerular scarring), whereas the necrotizing variety more typically presents with the acute nephritic syndrome and, because of leakage of plasma constituents into Bowman's space,* *frequently progresses to crescentic glomerulonephritis*, with rapidly developing renal failure.

Examples of diseases which may give rise to the necrotizing type of focal glomerulonephritis, and ultimately crescentic glomerulonephritis, are as follows:

1. Goodpasture's syndrome
2. Polyarteritis nodosa
3. Wegener's granulomatosis
4. Anaphylactoid purpura
5. Infective endocarditis

---

*Sir William Bowman (1816-1892), English physician.

The early stages of crescentic glomerulonephritides that are *not* preceded by focal necrotizing glomerulonephritis may also present with the acute nephritic syndrome prior to developing renal failure. These include the following:

1. Idiopathic crescentic glomerulonephritis,
2. Poststreptococcal crescentic glomerulonephritis, and
3. Crescentic subtypes of membranoproliferative glomerulonephritis.

The pathology of crescentic glomerulonephritis is discussed under "Acute Renal Failure."

Glomerular diseases presenting as proteinuria or the nephrotic syndrome

The nephrotic syndrome (see Table 16-3) consists of excessive quantities of protein in the urine, with consequent fall in serum albumin and generalized edema, and high levels of cholesterol in the blood. Many examples present with asymptomatic proteinuria before progressing to the full-blown nephrotic syndrome.

Increased loss of protein in the urine is often accompanied by thickening of glomerular capillary walls. This apparent paradox can be explained in the following way. It appears that the normal glomerular barrier to the filtration of circulating plasma proteins consists of two interdependent, but discrete, permeability functions. One of these is based on the negative (anionic) electrostatic charge that is a property of basement membrane constituents such as heparan sulfate proteoglycans, forming the *charge-selective permeability barrier;* the other is based on the size and shape of the protein molecule and the physical dimensions and density of the theoretical cylindrical "pores" in the capillary wall, and constitutes the *size-selective permeability barrier.*

In diseased membranes, polyanionic membrane constituent macromolecules lose their negative charges, resulting in loss of electrorepulsion of similarly charged molecules, particularly albumin, which thus gain passage through the basement membrane. Structural disorganization of the capillary wall in disease produces enlarged "pores," through which larger protein molecules, such as neutrally charged IgG, are allowed to pass.

Minimal change disease (Nil disease)

As the name suggests, the distinctive feature of this entity is the lack of obvious alterations in the glomeruli on light microscopy. The diagnosis is dependent on electron microscopy, which demonstrates diffuse effacement of the podocyte foot processes, but no evidence of immune deposits.

Despite the apparent normal appearance of the glomeruli microscopically, the kidneys themselves are grossly far from normal. The term *large, pale kidney* describes an appearance that is due partly to generalized renal edema and partly to the presence of lipids in tubular epithelial cells and interstitial macrophages (Fig. 16-4). These changes, which are also seen in the nephrotic syndrome due to other causes, follow the tubular reabsorption of lipids that have escaped into the glomerular filtrate through the abnormal capillary walls. The term *lipid nephrosis* has been employed in the past as a synonym for minimal change disease.

This condition presents chiefly in children and accounts for about 80% of cases of nephrotic syndrome in this age group. Although most often idiopathic, the lesion has also been observed in adults with lymphoma or renal cell carcinoma. Frequently, a viral upper respiratory tract infection immediately

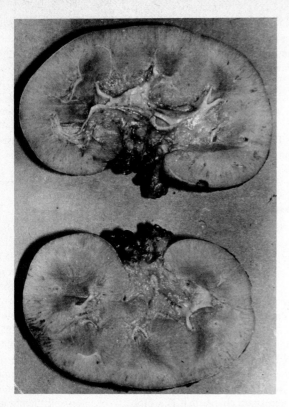

FIG. 16-4. The kidneys in lipoid nephrosis (minimal change disease). The kidneys are enlarged, pale, and edematous. The pallor is due to the excessive accumulation of lipids in the renal tubular cells. The patient had the nephrotic syndrome of edema, albuminuria, and hypercholesterolemia.

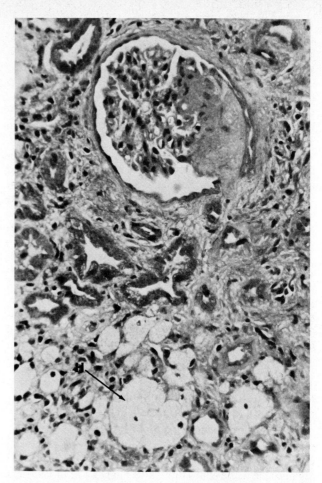

FIG. 16-5. Focal segmental sclerosis. Approximately one half of the glomerulus shown here appears sclerosed. Several lipid-rich foam cells are seen in the bottom part of the picture *(H)*.

precedes the onset of proteinuria. Various studies have suggested a role for immune mechanisms in the pathogenesis of this disease, including the possibility of diminished cell-mediated immunity, but the actual mechanism of injury remains unknown.

The disease generally runs a benign course, frequently with spontaneous remissions. The clinical and urinary changes respond well to corticosteroid therapy.

Mesangial proliferative (mesangioproliferative) glomerulonephritis

The mesangial proliferative pattern of injury is found on biopsy in approximately 10% of instances of idiopathic nephrotic syndrome in adults and 15% of children.

This lesion is characterized by a diffuse increase in mesangial cellularity *in the presence of essentially normal-appearing peripheral glomerular capillary walls.* It may be the result of diverse pathologic processes, may exhibit a range of immunostaining patterns, and present clinically in various ways. Other diseases previously discussed may show the same pattern. The most common of these is IgA nephropathy.

In those cases where the mesangial proliferative pattern is associated with proteinuria or the nephrotic syndrome, immunostaining is usually either negative, or shows IgM in the mesangium. Cases in which the mesangial cell proliferation is mild and which present with proteinuria have much in common with minimal change disease, and are probably a morphologic variant of this condition. In patients with more prominent mesangial proliferation and the full-blown nephrotic syndrome,

there is a tendency for persistence of proteinuria and gradual progression to renal failure. Biopsy of patients in this unfavorable category will usually show features of focal and segmental glomerulosclerosis, a description of which follows.

Focal and segmental glomerulosclerosis (focal sclerosis)

Focal sclerosis, as with most of the glomerular lesions discussed in this chapter, may be idiopathic or may be associated with defined etiologic factors. Thus the focal sclerosis pattern may be seen in association with "street" heroin abuse, vesicoureteral reflux, and acquired immunodeficiency syndrome, and is commonly seen in the late stages of a variety of other primary glomerular diseases that exhibit an unfavorable clinical course (progression to "chronic glomerulonephritis"). Many investigators believe that the idiopathic variety of focal sclerosis is a stage in the evolution of a subgroup of patients with minimal change disease or idiopathic mesangial proliferative glomerulonephritis.

In focal sclerosis (Fig. 16-5), there is a spotty, progressive obliteration of the glomerular capillary bed. Because the blood supply to the tubules passes through the glomeruli, sclerosis of glomeruli is associated with tubular atrophy, and accompanied by interstitial fibrosis and lymphoid infiltrates. In the idiopathic form, granular and nodular deposits of IgM and C3 are commonly found in the segmental sclerosing lesion, sug-

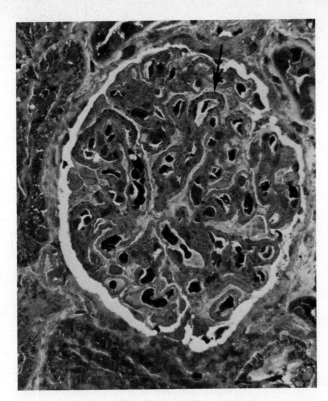

FIG. 16-6. Membranous nephropathy. There is severe diffuse thickening of glomerular capillary basement membranes *(arrow)*.

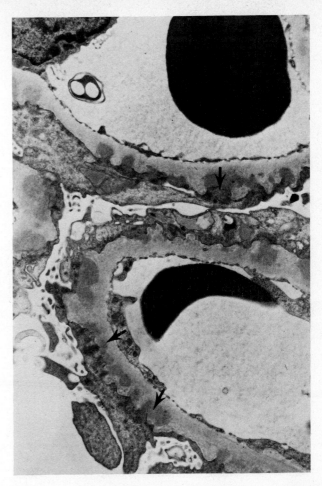

FIG. 16-7. Membranous nephropathy. Rows of small, subepithelial deposits *(arrows)* lie along the outer aspect of the basement membrane, separated by spike-like projections of the latter.

gesting an immune mechanism. By electron microscopy, collapse of capillary walls, accompanied by mesangial matrix increase, is seen. Unlike minimal change disease, there is little response to corticosteroid therapy, and slow progression to renal failure is the rule in most cases. Focal sclerosis is notorious for its tendency to recur in renal transplant recipients, occasionally within a few hours of transplantation.

Membranous nephropathy (membranous glomerulonephritis)

Membranous nephropathy accounts for 30 to 40 percent of cases of idiopathic nephrotic syndrome in adults, but is quite rare in children. It may also be associated with specific diseases or etiologic agents, such as systemic lupus erythematosus (see below), certain chronic infections (e.g., hepatitis B), solid tumors (e.g., melanoma and cancer of the colon and lung), or after exposure to heavy metals (gold, mercury) or drugs (penicillamine, captopril).

The membranous nephropathy pattern is characterized by predominant or exclusive involvement of the glomerular capillary wall, with little change, at least in early stages, in the mesangium. The glomerular capillary walls are thickened due to generalized and diffuse deposition of immune complexes on the epithelial side of the basement membrane and formation of "spikes" (projections of basement membrane) between the deposits (Figs. 16-6 and 16-7). These deposits are seen to contain IgG, sometimes IgM and complement. In a minority of cases a specific antigen may also be demonstrated.

In the majority of patients, membranous nephropathy runs a prolonged course, with progressive sclerosis of glomeruli and renal failure. Spontaneous complete remissions take place in some patients (mostly children), and partial remissions may be

induced by steroid therapy. The disease is often complicated by renal vein thrombosis.

Membranoproliferative (mesangiocapillary) glomerulonephritis (MPGN)

This disease usually presents in adolescence or early adult life. It typically presents with the nephrotic syndrome, although nephritic presentations, or combined nephritic-nephrotic features, are sometimes seen. The prognosis is uniformly poor, with universal progression to chronic renal failure over a period of 5 to 10 years. Light microscopy shows that (unlike mesangioproliferative glomerulonephritis) there are major abnormalities *both in the capillary walls and in the mesangial regions* of all glomeruli. There is a tendency for the serum C3 levels to be low in this condition and a fraction called C3 nephritic factor may also be identified in the serum.

In the most common type of MPGN (type I) there are large subendothelial and mesangial deposits (Fig. 16-8) of C3 which seem to stimulate mesangial cell proliferation and subsequent growth of mesangial cell cytoplasm around capillary walls between the endothelial cells and the basement membrane—*circumferential mesangial interposition.* The mesangial cell extensions secrete matrix, producing the appearance of a doubled basement membrane. The capillary lumens become progressively occluded and finally this leads to glomerular sclerosis

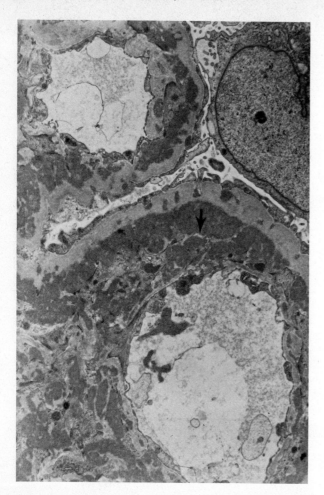

FIG. 16-8. Membranoproliferative glomerulonephritis showing large subendothelial *(arrow)* and mesangial deposits.

and nephron loss. (A similar mechanism of capillary lumen obliteration may be seen in other glomerular diseases with subendothelial deposits, such as some forms of systemic lupus erythematosus, paraproteinemias, and conditions resulting from intravascular coagulation; these are described elsewhere in this chapter.)

There is a less common type of MPGN called *linear-dense deposit disease (type II MPGN)* in which C3 is deposited *within* glomerular and tubular basement membranes, producing a striking and highly distinctive appearance on electron microscopy. Despite these differences in the morphology, the clinical features and prognosis are very similar to those of type I disease.

Preeclampsia/eclampsia

Preeclampsia/eclampsia is a condition of uncertain pathogenesis, peculiar to pregnancy, and falling into the broad clinical category termed toxemia of pregnancy, characterized by combinations of hypertension, proteinuria, and edema. Eclampsia is an accelerated form of preeclampsia, and seizures are a feature. Although moderate proteinuria is a cardinal feature of preeclampsia, the full-blown nephrotic syndrome develops only occasionally. Preeclampsia is uncommon before 20 weeks of gestation, and is usually found in the first pregnancy. The condition resolves dramatically following delivery.

Characteristic morphologic changes are seen in the glomeruli in preeclampsia/eclampsia. The features reflect a chronic, low-grade *intravascular coagulation,* and consist of prominent glomerular capillary endothelial cell swelling and vacuolation, with extreme narrowing of capillary lumina. These cells contain lipid droplets or myelinoid bodies, which may result from degradation of blood platelets. The subendothelial space is expanded by usually pale, amorphous deposits that stain for fibrin/fibrinogen. In more advanced cases, mesangial cell interposition may be seen. The severity of the glomerular lesions roughly corresponds to the degree of proteinuria.

Systemic diseases commonly affecting glomeruli

Diabetic nephropathy. Diabetes mellitus affects the structure and function of the kidney in many ways. The term *diabetic nephropathy* encompasses all of the lesions found in the kidney in this disease. It includes (1) hyaline arteriolonephrosclerosis, (2) chronic interstitial nephritis, (3) papillary necrosis, and (4) the glomerular lesions described below. Diabetic nephropathy develops in over 60% of patients with insulin-dependent (type I) diabetes mellitus and less frequently in type II diabetics.

Glomerular lesions, termed *diabetic glomerulosclerosis,* are particularly common and account for the majority of abnormal clinical findings referable to the kidney. They are morphologically identifiable 3 to 5 years after the onset of clinical diabetes. Proteinuria is the principal clinical manifestation of diabetic glomerular disease, only develops 13 to 20 years after onset of the disease but signals the onset of a steady downhill course to endstage diabetic renal disease. A full-blown nephrotic syndrome may precede the onset of renal failure. Careful control of blood sugar levels and systemic arterial blood pressure in the early stages of the disease (i.e., prior to the onset of proteinuria) may retard the onset or progression of glomerular lesions. Nonetheless, end-stage diabetic renal disease is today one of the most common indications for renal transplantation.

Morphologically, two forms of diabetic glomerulosclerosis, diffuse and nodular, are seen. In the more common, diffuse form, there is a mild diffuse increase in mesangial matrix accompanied by an increased width of the glomerular basement membrane. In the nodular type *(Kimmelstiel-Wilson lesion),* the mesangial matrix increase takes on a nodular form (see Fig. 18-29). At the periphery of the nodules, which are relatively acellular, open glomerular capillary loops are found. The pathogenesis of diabetic glomerulosclerosis is discussed briefly in Chapter 2.

Amyloidosis. Any form of amyloidosis (discussed in Chapter 2) may affect the glomeruli. Proteinuria, often pronounced, is the most common manifestation of renal involvement. Renal amyloidosis is a progressive disease for which there is no established treatment, and progression to endstage renal disease is the rule.

RENAL FAILURE AND ITS CAUSES

Renal failure (insufficiency) is a temporary or permanent state in which the kidneys' ability to excrete urine is lost or diminished. A number of other terms are frequently used synonymously with renal failure. *Oliguria* and *anuria* mean, respectively, that little, or no urine is being excreted by the kidney and therefore imply renal failure. The term *anephric* is sometimes used to describe total cessation of renal function. *Uremia* means literally that urinary products are present in the bloodstream. However, the term implies a complex clinical syndrome often marking the final stages of renal failure. Uremia, however, may arise from causes other than primary renal disease, but damage to the kidneys is an integral part of the pathogenesis. The causes of uremia and the causes of renal failure are therefore practically the same.

The term azotemia means that elevated levels of nitrogenous metabolites are present in the bloodstream, and it is used strictly to describe a biochemical abnormality. When azotemia becomes symptomatic, uremia is present.

Renal failure is a life-threatening state. It may be *acute* or *chronic*.

Acute renal failure

Whereas the nephritic and nephrotic syndromes mostly result from underlying glomerular pathology, in *acute renal failure* renal structural elements other than the glomeruli—particularly the tubules—are involved, and extrarenal factors come into play. Prerenal, renal, and postrenal causes of acute renal failure are recognized:

1. Prerenal
   a. Bilateral renal artery occlusion
   b. Cardiovascular failure
   c. Circulating pigments and nephrotoxins
   d. Hepatorenal syndrome
   e. Hypercalcemia
   f. Hypovolemia
2. Renal
   a. Acute interstitial nephritis
   b. Crescentic glomerulonephritis
   c. Intravascular coagulation states
3. Postrenal
   a. Extrarenal obstruction (e.g., cervical cancer, prostatism)
   b. Intrarenal obstruction (e.g., uric acid, Ig light chain casts)
   c. Trauma (bladder rupture)

It should be emphasized that frequently no, or minimal, morphologic alterations are observed on histologic examination of the kidneys, and in such instances the abnormalities are limited to a functional level. The best-defined renal lesions in acute renal failure are next discussed in turn.

Acute tubular necrosis

The most common general cause of acute renal failure is *renal ischemia*. Clinical conditions associated with renal ischemia include shock due to severe hemorrhage and profound volume depletion, and operative procedures associated with interruption of renal circulation. Since normally about 1200 ml of blood/minute, or one fourth of the cardiac output, circulates through the kidneys to maintain normal function, it is not surprising that diminution of renal blood flow can have serious effects. These effects are most severe on the structures most sensitive to hypoxia, namely the convoluted tubules. *Nephrotoxic agents* are a frequent cause of acute renal failure. Aminoglycoside antibiotics and radiographic contrast agents are the leading nephrotoxic causes, the latter in patients with underlying renal disease. Release of large amounts of myoglobin or hemoglobin into the circulation, such as follow severe muscle injury or hemolysis respectively, is also an important cause of acute renal failure. Although myoglobin and hemoglobin are not directly nephrotoxic, it is thought that other muscle or red cell breakdown products may result in cell injury, and that the formation of myoglobin or hemoglobin casts may impair renal function through tubular blockage.

On histology, two main types of lesions are seen. Following *direct nephrotoxic injury,* there is uniform, diffuse necrosis of proximal tubular epithelial cells, with sparing of the basement membrane. In contrast following major *renal ischemia,* mild patchy necrosis is found throughout the nephron, most marked in tubular segments at the corticomedullary junction (hence the old synonym, 'lower nephron nephrosis'). Disruption of tubular basement membranes is also observed. Despite these histologic differences, the clinical courses of nephrotoxic and ischemic acute tubular necrosis are similar.

Despite a great deal of experimental work, the *intrarenal factors* that bring about the ischemia or hypoxia remain controversial. Intratubular casts, whether consisting of sloughed necrotic tubular cell debris, myoglobin, or hemoglobin, are a cardinal histologic feature of acute tubular necrosis. One theory suggests that casts and cellular debris obstruct the tubular lumina in acute renal failure and cause increases in intratubular pressure sufficient to decrease net filtration pressure. Another theory suggests that 'back-leak' of glomerular filtrate across damaged tubular epithelium is responsible for the azotemia. Third, proponents of a vascular basis suggest that marked decreases in renal perfusion pressure, severe afferent arteriolar constriction, or efferent arteriolar dilatation reduce glomerular flow and hydrostatic pressure sufficiently to diminish glomerular filtration. It is probable that all of these factors interact in producing acute renal failure.

Clinical manifestations. In addition to manifestations of the underlying cause of the tubular necrosis, the main clinical finding is a period of oliguria or anuria. Initially the patient passes a very small volume of urine, which may be as little as 40 to 50 ml/day. The anuric period varies from a few days to 2 months, provided that the patient can be kept alive by dialysis. Recovery is heralded by a diuretic phase in which there is a rapid return of urine flow. As one would expect, the longer oliguria persists, the more likely are complications. These are numerous and reflect the profound disturbances of electrolyte, fluid, and acid-base balance that follow oliguria. With increasing azotemia the patient becomes drowsy and weak. Most serious of all are the effects of excessive potassium, which usually accompanies acute renal failure caused by severe trauma or infection. Sudden death due to cardiac arrest is an ever-present danger when serum potassium levels exceed 9 mEq/L. Bacterial infections are frequent in acute renal failure, and neurologic disturbances that may progress to coma are grave complications.

The *management* of acute tubular necrosis must be in the hands of expert physicians and nurses. The aim is to maintain the patient in satisfactory general condition until tubular regeneration is complete and renal function is restored. Rigid control of fluid, electrolyte, and acid-base balance and careful nursing, especially to prevent infection, are important principles. When there is delay in restoration of renal function, especially if there is potassium intoxication, either peritoneal dialysis or hemodialysis (the artificial kidney) is necessary. These methods have improved the outlook in acute tubular necrosis, but overall mortality is still about 50% and reflects the severity of the underlying causes.

Bilateral renal cortical necrosis

Bilateral renal cortical necrosis is a much less common cause of acute renal failure than acute tubular necrosis and is obviously associated with a worse prognosis. It often leads to death or necessitates hemodialysis or renal transplantation.

Some cases with patchy involvement of the renal cortex have been known to recover.

The etiology of cortical necrosis is similar to that of tubular necrosis, but there is a marked association with obstetric complications, such as premature separation of the placenta during delivery or septic shock. The mechanisms that cause cortical necrosis are not entirely clear but are thought to involve renal ischemia, with prolonged and severe vascular spasm, with intravascular coagulation following terminal relaxation of vascular spasm.

The effect of the ischemic changes is that the entire renal cortex, or large portions of it, become necrotic (Fig. 16-9). The kidneys at autopsy are enlarged, and the superficial yellow necrotic cortex contrasts sharply with the darker congested medulla. Microscopically there is massive necrosis of virtually all nephrons, with both glomeruli and tubules involved. Large numbers of leukocytes collect in the renal medulla.

Acute uric acid nephropathy

Three kinds of lesions may be produced in the kidneys of persons with increased concentration of uric acid in the urine (hyperuricosuria). The first, *acute uric acid nephropathy,* is characterized by the precipitation of uric acid crystals in the presence of a low pH environment in the renal tubules. It is this type that may be accompanied by acute renal failure. This can be prevented by maintaining high urine volumes and a high urinary pH in persons with a tendency to hyperuricosuria; also, cancer patients may be treated with allopurinol, which blocks the formation of uric acid from nucleic acids, prior to chemotherapy, in which massive amounts of nucleic acids are released.

The second type of pathology, *uric acid nephrolithiasis,* results from similar mechanisms and is discussed in connection with urinary calculi further on in this chapter. In the third type of lesion, *chronic urate nephropathy,* interstitial urate precipitates, which form at a physiologic pH equivalent to that found in the blood or tissue fluid, are found in the renal interstitium of individuals who, usually due to tubular abnormalities, are underexcretors of uric acid. The urates are seen as interstitial crystalline deposits, termed tophi, in association with a chronic interstitial nephritis. Although this histologic picture may be associated with chronic renal failure, it is generally agreed that the urate deposition alone does not impair renal function and that renal failure, when it exists, is due to complicating factors such as hypertension, diabetes, or chronic lead toxicity (which results in defective tubular secretion of uric acid).

Causes of hyperuricemia and hyperuricosuria are discussed in connection with gout in Chapter 17.

Renal lesions in plasma cell dyscrasias

Plasma cell dyscrasias (Chapter 13), also referred to as monoclonal gammopathies or dysproteinemias, comprise several disorders characterized by the proliferation of a single clone of cells that produce excessive amounts of complete monoclonal immunoglobulin (Ig) proteins with or without free light chain proteins, or of light chain proteins alone. Multiple myeloma, which usually develops in individuals 50 years of age or older, is the most important member of this group of conditions and is associated with renal disease in a majority of cases. Renal dysfunction may be the first clinical manifestation of myeloma and is characterized by proteinuria with or without acute or chronic renal failure and/or by specific tubular functional defects such as Fanconi's syndrome. After infection,

renal failure is the second most common cause of death in these patients.

In plasma cell dyscrasias, aside from *neoplastic infiltration* of the kidneys, there are two major classes of nephropathy— those resulting from light chains and those resulting from cryoglobulins:

Immunoglobulin light chain nephropathies. Several types are recognized.

Bence-Jones cast nephropathy. The Bence-Jones cast nephropathy is the most common and characteristic form of "myeloma kidney." The main morphologic feature is the presence of numerous, large, intratubular casts, consisting of nephrotoxic Ig light chains, often surrounded by multinucleated giant cells. The tubular epithelial cells themselves tend to be atrophied or necrotic. This form of renal involvement is the type usually found in association with an acute renal failure presentation.

Light chain nodular glomerulosclerosis. In this entity, acellular mesangial nodules consisting of light chain deposits and

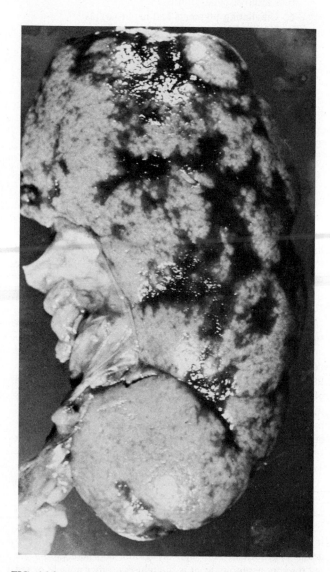

FIG. 16-9. Acute cortical necrosis causing renal failure. The surface of the kidney has alternating pale and dark areas due to necrosis of the renal cortex and hemorrhage into the necrotic areas. *(Courtesy Curator of the Gordon Museum, Guy's Hospital, London, England.)*

increased mesangial matrix, are found. This lesion mimics the Kimmelstiel-Wilson lesion of diabetic nephropathy.

Immunoglobulin light chain amyloidosis (AL). See Chapter 2.

Cryoglobulinemic glomerulonephropathy. Subendothelial cryoglobulin deposits, which are seen to consist of collections of tubular material on electron microscopy, result in a membranoproliferative-type picture. Circulating cryoglobulins are found not only in lymphoproliferative disorders, but also in autoimmune diseases and infections.

Acute interstitial nephritis

Infiltration of the interstitium by inflammatory cells, with edema or fibrosis, is a common accompaniment of several forms of glomerulonephritis. The term *interstitial nephritis* is, however, used only where these changes are found in the absence of primary glomerular damage. Because the interstitial inflammation is usually accompanied by varying degrees of tubular damage, some prefer the term tubulointerstitial nephritis. Interstitial nephritis is classified into *acute and chronic* forms, with some overlap between the two.

The major examples of *acute interstitial nephritis* are as follows:

1. Adverse reactions to drugs
2. Acute renal transplant rejection (cellular type)
3. Acute bacterial infections (acute pyelonephritis)

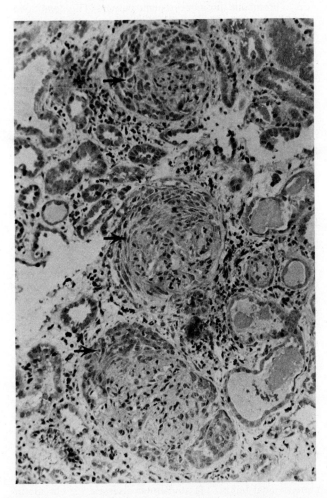

FIG. 16-10. Crescentic glomerulonephritis. The glomeruli shown here *(arrows)* have collapsed tufts surrounded by large, cellular crescents.

In acute interstitial nephritis, the interstitium is edematous. In acute bacterial infections, which are not usually associated with acute renal failure, the predominant inflammatory cells are neutrophils. (This cause of acute interstitial nephritis is discussed later under "Urinary Tract Infections.") The other major examples of acute interstitial nephritis, although they present as clinically acute disease (acute renal functional impairment), are characterized by interstitial infiltrates of lymphocytes, plasma cells, and histiocytes. Tubules may show varying degrees of atrophy or loss and actual necroses may be seen in some.

Adverse drug reactions causing acute interstitial nephritis may take the form of acute renal failure or worsening of an already present renal failure. Some are hypersensitivity reactions and accompanied by fever, skin rashes, eosinophilia, and hematuria. Drugs thought to act by this mechanism are those of the penicillin group (chiefly methicillin), rifampicin, diphenylhydantoin (dilantin), and phenindione (an anticoagulant). Other drug reactions appear to be dose dependent and include antibiotics such as amphotericin, colistin, polymyxin B, the cephalosporins, and gentamicin. Recovery may take place when the drug is withdrawn, but in some instances there may be permanent damage to the kidneys. *Renal transplant rejection* is discussed under "Chronic Renal Failure."

Crescentic glomerulonephritis

Crescentic glomerulonephritis is an uncommon, often lethal, form of glomerular injury which may be idiopathic or be associated with the conditions previously listed in the discussion on "Lesions Producing the Acute Nephritic Syndrome." When crescentic glomerulonephritis is associated with antiglomerular basement membrane antibody deposition, there is frequently accompanying injury to pulmonary alveolar basement membranes, resulting in life-threatening hemoptysis; this association constitutes the *Goodpasture syndrome.** (Pulmonary hemorrhage is, however, more frequently associated with forms of glomerulonephritis other than antiglomerular basement membrane disease, including anaphylactoid purpura, systemic lupus erythematosus, and Wegener's granulomatosis.) Crescentic glomerulonephritis is generally associated with rapid decline in renal function, and the clinical term *rapidly progressive glomerulonephritis* has been used synonymously with crescentic glomerulonephritis in the past.

The histologic hallmark of crescentic glomerulonephritis is the widespread formation of glomerular crescents (Fig. 16-10). This is due to massive proliferation of, initially, monocytes, and then epithelial cells, arranged in crescent-shaped masses within Bowman's space, with concomitant collapse and shrinkage of the glomerular tuft. The crescent formation is the consequence of severe injury to the glomerular tuft, allowing leakage of large proteins, such as fibrinogen, and the passage of cells, into Bowman's space. The cells of the crescent initially fulfill a phagocytic function, and subsequently assume the character of fibroblasts, secreting collagen. Cellular crescents become transformed into acellular fibrous crescents, which surround small, sclerosed tuft remnants.

Findings on immunostaining and electronmicroscopy vary with the underlying disease process. There may be (1) immune complexes (granular immunostaining and electron-dense deposits), (2) antiglomerular basement membrane antibodies (linear immunostaining), or (3) no detectable immune reactants.

---

*Ernest W. Goodpasture (1886-1960), American pathologist.

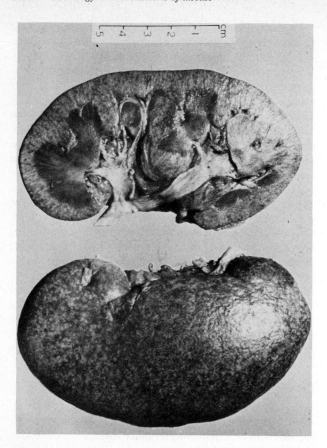

FIG. 16-11. Crescentic glomerulonephritis. The kidneys are normal in size, but the cortex and surface show many small, punctate hemorrhagic foci. *(Courtesy Curator of the Gordon Museum, Guy's Hospital, London, England.)*

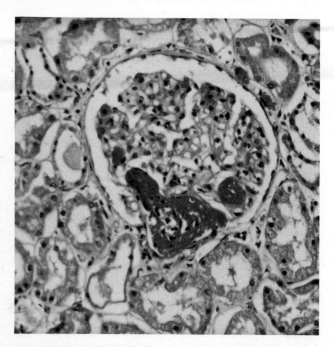

FIG. 16-12. Glomerulus showing segmental intracapillary thrombi. From a case of thrombotic microangiopathy in a renal transplant patient, possibly related to cyclosporine administration.

Fibrin deposition in relation to tufts and crescents is, however, a frequent finding in all types.

Many examples of crescentic glomerulonephritis are associated with vasculitis of small renal vessels. Gross examination in cases of crescentic glomerulonephritis shows enlarged kidneys with pale, smooth surfaces with multiple tiny hemorrhagic foci—the so-called "flea-bitten" kidneys (Fig. 16-11).

The more glomeruli that are affected, the worse the outlook for the patient. Patients with crescents in more than 50% to 75% of glomeruli rarely recover their renal function. These patients require hemodialysis and renal transplantation for survival.

Intravascular coagulation states involving the kidney

Factors such as the high vascularity and high perfusion pressure of the kidney make the kidney particularly susceptible to damage by intravascular coagulation (Chapter 13). Significant renal lesions (Fig. 16-12) may develop either as part of a systemic disorder of intravascular coagulation, or as a complication of a variety of renal diseases.

Systemic disorders causing intravascular coagulation and involving the small blood vessels in various parts of the body are collectively termed *thrombotic microangiopathy*. These include the following uncommon conditions:

1. Postpartum renal failure
2. Hemolytic-uremic syndrome
3. Thrombotic thrombocytopenic purpura (This condition is discussed in Chapter 13.)

Examples of *intravascular coagulation states confined to the kidney* are as follows:

1. Renal transplant rejection, humoral type
2. Malignant nephrosclerosis (the lesion of malignant hypertension)
3. Progressive systemic sclerosis (scleroderma)
4. The crescentic glomerulonephritides

The prognosis for recovery of renal function in florid, acute cases of intravascular coagulation is poor. Aggressive treatment, perhaps with anticoagulants, in less advanced cases may have some measure of success.

Chronic renal failure

As the name implies, chronic renal failure is a gradual process that takes place over many years. During this time there is an ongoing loss of functional nephrons from a variety of causes, previously listed. Hypertrophy of other nephrons is not sufficient to compensate for those which have been destroyed, so there is a gradually increasing impairment of renal function.

The initial pathologic changes that cause chronic renal failure are variable and depend on the underlying disease. Whatever the cause, there is irreversible destruction of nephrons. In the terminal stages of chronic failure, even after careful pathologic examination of the kidney at autopsy, it may be impossible to decide what was the original disease of the kidney. The term *end-stage kidney* is frequently (and conveniently) used as a catch-all to conceal our ignorance of the pathogenesis.

Causes of chronic renal failure

Three main classes of renal lesions are seen in patients with chronic renal failure: (1) glomerular diseases, (2) chronic interstitial nephritis, and (3) polycystic kidney disease.

Glomerular diseases. Many of the glomerular diseases described in this chapter slowly progress into a chronic form, in which most, or all, glomeruli eventually become sclerosed and nonfunctioning. In summary, the most important are as follows:

1. IgA nephropathy
2. Focal sclerosis
3. Membranoproliferative glomerulonephritis
4. Membranous nephropathy
5. Amyloidosis
6. Diabetic glomerulosclerosis

Some patients may have a well-documented history of renal disease. More commonly, the disease is insidious and is recognized only after an asymptomatic period of perhaps many years, when the effects of chronic failure begin to be felt. Some patients, on the other hand, experience an episode of symptoms of the nephrotic or nephritic syndrome during the course of the disease. Examination of renal biopsy specimens from patients presenting with chronic renal failure due to glomerular disease may reveal no traces of the underlying disease, and the term *chronic glomerulonephritis* is used in such instances for want of a more specific name.

The kidneys in chronic glomerulonephritis are usually symmetrically shrunken to half their normal size, and show a granular subcapsular surface, sometimes with cortical cysts being visible. The capsule strips with difficulty.

Microscopically, all components of the kidney, not only the glomeruli, are severely involved. The glomeruli typically are mostly sclerosed or fibrosed and appear hyalinized (Fig. 16-13), but some may show changes suggesting one of the underlying glomerular diseases listed. The glomerular population is decreased in number due to resorption of sclerosed glomeruli. The ultrastructure and immunofluorescence of residual glomeruli is highly variable, even from one nephron to another. Tubular atrophy is common, accounting in large part for the shrunken size of the kidneys, and there is interstitial fibrosis and lymphocytic infiltration. Dilatation of residual tubules, which often contain hyaline proteinaceous casts, may impart a thyroid-like appearance to portions of the kidney. Hypertensive arteriolosclerotic changes are common.

Chronic interstitial nephritis. In both acute and chronic forms of interstitial nephritis, the predominant interstitial cells may be lymphocytes, plasma cells, and histiocytes; however, in most cases of the acute form, there is edema of the interstitial tissue, whereas in chronic interstitial nephritis there is fibrosis of the interstitium.

Chronic interstitial nephritis has many causes, including the following:

1. Chronic pyelonephritis
2. Obstruction to outflow of urine (hydronephrosis)
3. Chronic rejection in renal transplants
4. Parenchymal changes consequent on papillary necrosis (e.g., in *analgesic nephropathy*)—This rare condition follows ingestion of large doses of antipyretic analgesics over long periods. The chronic interstitial nephritic changes in the cortex follow papillary necrosis which is probably the result of injury to small vessels in the renal papilla. Analgesic nephropathy may predispose to transitional cell carcinoma of the renal pelvis.

Polycystic kidney disease. This is discussed under "Developmental and Cystic Diseases of the Kidney."

Clinical manifestations of chronic renal failure

The effects of chronic renal failure are profound and widespread. Chiefly affected are the following:

1. Water and electrolyte balance
2. Acid-base balance
3. Calcium and phosphate metabolism
4. Hemopoiesis
5. Blood pressure

Water and electrolyte balance. Impairment of control of water excretion frequently results in an increased volume of urine with a fairly constant specific gravity (i.e., there is loss of concentrating properties of the kidney). In some forms of chronic renal failure there is excessive sodium loss (salt-losing nephritis) due to damage to the portion of the tubules responsible for sodium resorption; this is additional to the excess water loss already described. Eventually, however, in end-stage kidney disease there is inability to excrete either water or sodium.

Acid-base balance. Acid base mechanisms are damaged in chronic renal disease. Among these is an impairment of the tubular excretion of ammonium ions. There is consequent impairment of acid excretion, and acidosis develops.

Calcium and phosphorus metabolism. Calcium and phosphorus metabolism is impaired, resulting in generalized de-

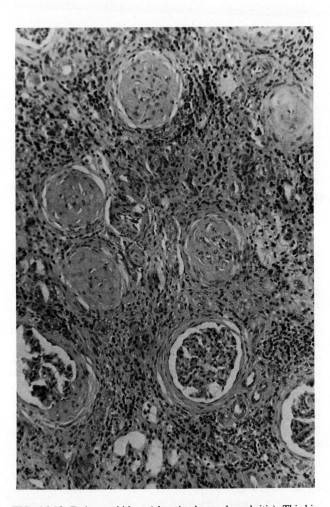

FIG. 16-13. End-stage kidney (chronic glomerulonephritis). This histologic appearance, common to a host of renal disorders, is characterized by extensive glomerular sclerosis, tubular atrophy, interstitial inflammation, and fibrosis.

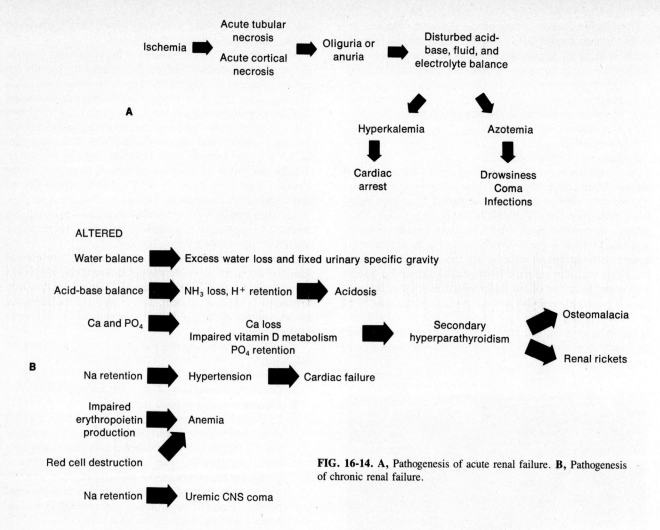

FIG. 16-14. A, Pathogenesis of acute renal failure. **B,** Pathogenesis of chronic renal failure.

mineralization of bone, or renal osteodystrophy. The contributing mechanisms are described in Chapter 16.

Hemopoiesis. Anemia is invariable in chronic renal failure. Two mechanisms are involved. In some cases the widespread damage to renal vascular endothelium results in mechanical damage to circulating red cells. This type of hemolytic anemia is sometimes called *microangiopathic anemia* and is characterized by the appearance of fragmented red blood cells in peripheral blood smears. The second mechanism is more common and is a hypoproliferative anemia secondary to deficient production of erythropoietin or its precursor by the kidney.

Blood pressure. Hypertension is almost invariably present in chronic renal failure. Sodium retention, which is a feature of advanced renal failure, is a major factor in promoting hypertension. The pathologic changes in blood vessels due to hypertension are a feature of the histology of the end-stage kidney (Chapter 10).

Clinical aspects

The onset of chronic renal failure is slow and silent. Initially the patient complains of nonspecific symptoms such as fatigue, weakness, anorexia, and nausea. Pallor and breathlessness due to the anemia are common. Later, as failure progresses, these symptoms worsen, and abnormalities of virtually all systems of the body may develop. This is the complex clinical state of uremia. Briefly, some of the common manifestations of the uremic state that affect the blood and cardiovascular and nervous systems, respectively, are as follows:

1. Anemia and a bleeding tendency
2. Hypertension, cardiac failure, pericarditis
3. Peripheral neuritis, lethargy, and coma

The effects of acute and chronic renal failure are summarized in Fig. 16-14.

Aspects of the management of chronic renal failure

The management of chronic renal failure is supportive and palliative. Before dialysis or renal transplantation became feasible, the disease was fatal. The current aim of management of chronic renal failure is to replace the diseased kidneys with a *transplant* in selected patients. The function of *dialysis* is to maintain patients until a suitable kidney donor (cadaver or living relative) is available, the quality of life with successful transplants being superior to that on dialysis. Not all patients with chronic renal failure are suitable for transplantation, and the outlook for many is still grim.

The major problems besetting patients with renal transplants are the following:

1. *Complications* resulting from chronic immunosuppression—These include increased incidence of infections and malignancies, and renal parenchymal injury as a result of toxicity due to cyclosporine.

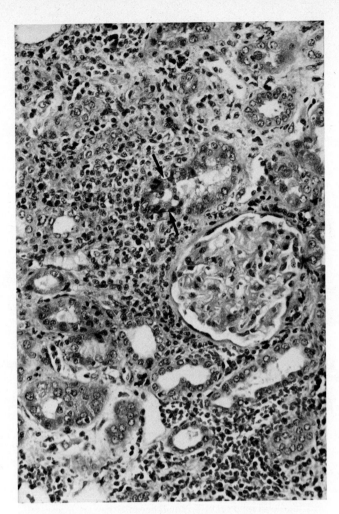

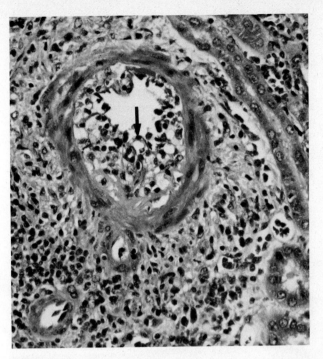

FIG. 16-16. Acute humoral (vascular) rejection. The large vessel is an interlobular arteriole showing an intimal lymphoid cellular infiltrate ("endothelialitis") *(arrow).* A slight interstitial infiltrate of lymphoid cells (cellular rejection) is also evident.

FIG. 16-15. Acute cellular (tubulointerstial) rejection. Dense lymphoid cellular infiltrates occupy the interstitium. Focally, there is infiltration of tubules ("tubulitis") *(arrows).*

2. *Recurrence* of the original disease in the graft—The lesions most likely to recur are membranoproliferative glomerulonephritis, focal glomerulosclerosis, antiglomerular basement membrane antibody nephritis, and oxalosis. For some reason, recurrence of lupus nephritis in transplanted kidneys is distinctly unusual.

3. *Rejection*—Three forms of renal transplant rejection are recognized, although there is some overlap between them.

Hyperacute rejection. Hyperacute rejection takes place within minutes to hours after graft vascularization and is mediated by circulating antibodies already present in the recipient. Grossly, the kidney is enlarged, flabby and cyanotic; these changes may be seen before the transplant operation has been completed. Light microscopy shows infiltration of glomeruli by neutrophils and changes of florid, acute intravascular coagulation.

Acute rejection. Acute rejection may take place at any time in an allograft but is most often found during the first two months following surgery. Macroscopically the kidney is usually enlarged and hemorrhagic. Histologically there is an acute interstitial nephritis characterized by a variable degree of interstitial lymphoplasmacytic cellular infiltration, with infiltra-

tion of tubules and resulting tubular destruction (Fig. 16-15). An acute endarteritis (Fig. 16-16), often with some degree of intravascular coagulation (humoral, or vascular, rejection), frequently accompanies the cellular, tubulointerstitial rejection component. Severe vascular changes may lead to renal infarction and loss of the graft.

Chronic rejection. Chronic rejection may begin as early as two months after transplantation or be delayed for up to 2 years. Once initiated, it is irreversible. Morphologically, it is characterized by widespread obliterative intimal thickening affecting small and large arteries, and by interstitial fibrosis, loss of tubules, and sometimes membranoproliferative-like glomerular changes that reflect a chronic, low-grade intravascular coagulation. Both humoral and cellular mechanisms play a role in causing the tubular destruction.

Patients who lose their graft due to rejection or other problems may be placed back on dialysis and may receive new grafts if they are suitable candidates.

Summary of glomerular diseases

The renal glomeruli may be injured by a variety of mechanisms, mainly immunologic, and attributable to causes such as infections or autoimmune disorders. In many cases, however, the cause is not known. There are several different kinds of glomerular lesions, and these may present clinically in a variety of ways, such as the nephritic or nephrotic syndromes. Severe injury to large numbers of glomeruli generally results in renal failure. Table 16-2 lists the most common glomerular diseases together with their usual modes of clinical presentation.

In investigating the pathologic changes by renal biopsy,

immunostaining is required to determine the presence and type of immunoglobulins and other reactants; electron microscopy is necessary to detect the sites of immune complexes and changes in renal ultrastructure that characterize different classes of glomerular diseases.

These investigations are essential for diagnosis and prognosis and the selection of appropriate methods of treatment, particularly when steroid therapy or renal transplantation are contemplated.

THE KIDNEY IN HYPERTENSION

Hypertension is fully discussed in Chapter 10. The kidney is affected by hypertensive vascular changes to a degree that varies with severity of the hypertension. Two forms of hypertensive nephrosclerosis are recognized. Borrowing from the language of tumor pathology, they are called *benign* and *malignant*, which indicate the relative severity and rate of progress.

In the benign form, the pathologic changes in the kidney are an exaggeration of those that develop with aging in normal, normotensive persons ("benign nephrosclerosis"). There is slight narrowing of small arteries and arterioles, with hyaline thickening of their walls, causing variable ischemia of nephrons. The results are glomerular tuft collapse, focal global sclerosis, and areas of tubular atrophy associated with fibrous scarring and lymphoid infiltrates (i.e., small foci of chronic interstitial nephritis). Grossly, these changes coupled with compensatory hypertrophy of groups of tubules result in kidneys with granular, scarred subcortical surfaces, and arteries with thickened walls stand out prominently (Fig. 16-17). Apart from mild proteinuria, the functional effects are minimal. The changes in the malignant form of hypertension ("malignant nephrosclerosis") are of greater consequence and severity. They are described in the section of this chapter dealing with "Acute Renal Failure."

DEVELOPMENTAL AND CYSTIC DISEASES OF THE KIDNEY

Renal dysgenesis refers to abnormal development of the kidney in regard to size, shape, or structure. This group of conditions overlaps with the cystic diseases of the kidney.

Renal dysgenesis

Renal dysplasia is defined as abnormal metanephric differentiation. Although it is diagnosed histologically, on the basis of primitive ducts and metaplastic cartilage, its diagnosis may be suggested on gross examination. There is incomplete development of both cortex and medulla, which may be diffuse, segmental, or focal. Cysts may or may not be present. *Aplasia* is an extreme form of dysplasia in which a small remnant of nonfunctioning dysplastic tissue is identified capping either a normal or an abnormal ureter. Dysplasia is discussed further under Cystic Diseases.

Agenesis refers to absence of the kidney.

Hypoplasia (oligonephronia) refers to a small kidney or segment of kidney with less than a normal number of nephrons. If dysplastic elements are present, then the term *hypodysplasia* is preferred. Kidneys or segments of kidneys associated with vesicoureteral reflux may be small because they are hypoplastic or hypodysplastic, or they have been affected by pyelonephritis or a combination of these conditions. When any of these conditions exist in association with vesicoureteral reflux the noncommittal term *reflux nephropathy* is used. Any class of reflux nephropathy may be associated with scarring of the renal parenchyma, proteinuria and, eventually, hypertension and renal insufficiency. Reflux nephropathy is considered further in connection with "Urinary Tract Infections."

Cystic diseases of the kidney

Cystic diseases of the kidney are a diverse and interesting group of disorders that are important because many lead to renal failure, some are associated with other important lesions, and several put the patient at increased risk for the development of renal malignancy.

Renal cysts are abnormal, saclike dilatations that may develop in various parts of the nephron (e.g., collecting tubules) and which are lined with epithelial cells. They may be visible macroscopically or only with the microscope. There may or may not be communication to glomeruli, collecting ducts, or calyces. Cystic diseases of the kidney are classified into genetic and nongenetic types. The major entities are named in the following list. Only the relatively more common or especially interesting varieties are discussed later:

1. Genetic
   a. Polycystic kidneys
   b. Juvenile nephronophthisis-medullary cystic disease complex
   c. Congenital nephrosis

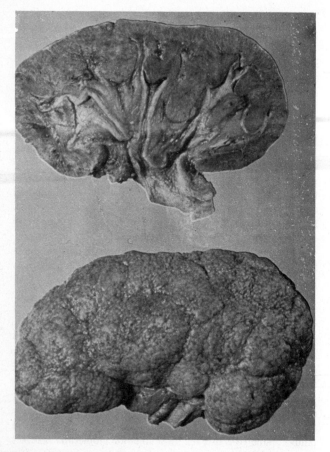

FIG. 16-17. Kidneys from a hypertensive patient, showing the typical features of benign nephrosclerosis. The kidneys show slight reduction of the cortical width, and the surfaces appear rough and finely scarred.

d. Cysts associated with multiple malformation syndromes
   (1) Mendelian (single gene) disorders
       (a) Autosomal dominant
           Tuberous sclerosis
           von Hippel-Lindau's disease
       (b) Autosomal recessive
           Meckel's syndrome
           Jeune's asphyxiating thoracic dystrophy
           Zellweger's cerebrohepatorenal syndrome
           Goldston's syndrome
           Lissencephaly, etc.
       (c) X-linked dominant: orofaciodigital syndrome, type I
   (2) Chromosome disorders
       Trisomy 21 (Down's syndrome)
       Trisomy 13 (Trisomy D, Patau's syndrome)
       Trisomy 18 (Trisomy E, Edwards' syndrome)
       Trisomy C
2. Nongenetic
   a. Multicystic dysplasia
   b. Multilocular cyst (multilocular cystic nephroma)
   c. Simple cysts
   d. Medullary sponge kidneys
   e. Acquired renal cystic disease in chronic hemodialysis patients
   f. Calyceal diverticulum (pyelogenic cyst)

Genetic cystic diseases

Polycystic diseases. Two forms of polycystic disease, traditionally called the *infantile* and *adult* types, have been identified. Both terms are misnomers, since the infantile form can manifest in adolescence and the adult form in infancy. The so-called infantile form is transmitted as an autosomal recessive trait and the adult form as an autosomal dominant trait.

Autosomal recessive polycystic kidney disease. The kidneys are large and show marked ectasia of the collecting ducts, which appear in a radial arrangement from the calyx to the capsule. The earlier the presentation the worse the prognosis. In those severely affected, there may be associated pulmonary hypoplasia and Potter facies (low-set ears, wide-set eyes, beaked nose), and in these patients renal failure develops rapidly postnatally. Congenital hepatic fibrosis is often associated with this form of cystic disease.

Autosomal dominant polycystic disease. This is the most common form of renal cystic disease, with a frequency of 1 per 1,000. It is characterized by bilateral involvement and progressive enlargement of renal cysts, which eventually occupy virtually the entire kidney (Fig. 16-18). Up to 50% of patients have cysts of the liver; cysts are found less frequently in other organs (pancreas, spleen, lungs, ovaries, and testes). *Aneurysms of the circle of Willis* (Chapter 10) develop in 10% to 40% of patients. The genetic mutation for dominant polycystic disease has been localized to the short arm of chromosome 16; the cysts have been demonstrated microscopically in the kidneys of fetuses electively aborted following prenatal diagnosis of the disorder. Despite this early development of the cysts, most cases present clinically (e.g., with renal failure or hypertension) during adult life. Prior to the era of dialysis and transplantation the mean age at death was about 50 years. Patients may die of a ruptured berry aneurysm before the onset of renal failure.

Juvenile nephronophthisis-renal medullary cystic disease complex. This complex is the leading cause of idiopathic renal failure among adolescents. The two forms of the disease are identical anatomically, differing only in their mode of genetic transmission. The major manifestations of the complex are small kidneys and progressive renal failure. Most examples demonstrate medullary cysts and virtually all show interstitial nephritis.

Congenital nephrosis. The importance of congenital nephrosis, an autosomal recessive disease, is its distinction from the minimal change nephrotic syndrome presenting in children. The latter condition responds to corticosteroid therapy, whereas congenital nephrosis progresses relentlessly to renal failure.

Nongenetic cystic diseases

Multicystic dysplasia. Multicystic dysplasia is the most common form of cystic disease in infants, and is also the most common cause of an abdominal mass in neonates. The kidneys range from being extremely large, crossing the midline, to extremely small or microscopic. Multicystic kidneys, as they are also known, are associated with a nonpatent drainage system in which there is either pelviinfundibular atresia, or an atretic or absent ureter. Contralateral hydronephrosis is present occasionally, which usually is owing to obstruction at the ureteropelvic junction. Bilateral disease is incompatible with life and can be associated with oligohydramnios, pulmonary hypoplasia and Potter facies. The unilateral form may be compatible with long survival, as hypertension or the development of neoplasia is rare.

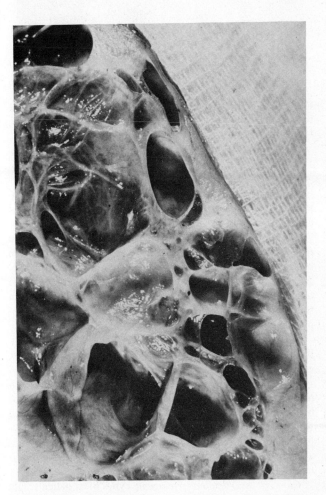

FIG. 16-18. Close-up view of the cut surface of a polycystic kidney of the so-called adult type. Note the total absence of normal renal tissue.

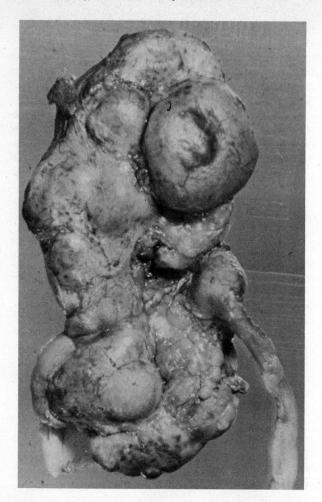

FIG. 16-19. End-stage kidney with several simple cysts visible on the surface. *(Courtesy Curator of the Gordon Museum, Guy's Hospital, London, England.)*

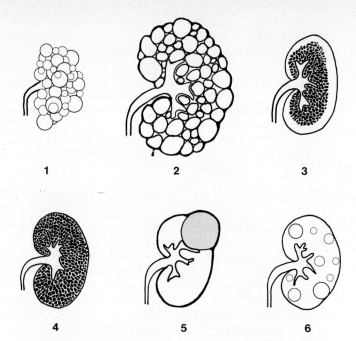

FIG. 16-20. Diagram representing several kinds of renal cysts. *1*, Multicystic dysplasia. The ureter is included for orientation, but is, in fact, generally absent. *2*, Polycystic disease, autosomal dominant type. *3*, Medullary sponge kidney. *4*, Polycystic disease, autosomal recessive type. *5*, Simple cyst. *6*, Acquired cystic disease (chronic hemodialysis).

Multilocular cyst (multilocular cystic nephroma). A multilocular cyst is part of the Wilms tumor spectrum (discussed under "Tumors of the Urinary Tract").

Simple cysts. Simple cysts (Fig. 16-19), the most common type found in the kidney, can be discovered anytime from infancy through adulthood but the incidence increases with age. At autopsy in adults older than 50 years more than 50% are found to have simple renal cysts. They average 3 to 4 cm in size. Their major importance lies in their ability to mimic neoplasms radiologically.

Medullary sponge kidney. Medullary sponge kidney is similar to the juvenile nephronophthisis-medullary cystic disease complex, but is not inherited.

Acquired renal cystic disease in chronic hemodialysis patients. The kidney with acquired cystic disease is characterized by cysts that are clearly visible on the subcapsular surface, and which are diffuse and can replace the entire parenchyma. Hyperplasia of the renal tubular epithelium is commonly associated, and there is a significantly increased risk for the development of renal adenocarcinoma.

Calyceal diverticulum (pyelogenic cyst). Most patients with calyceal diverticulum are asymptomatic, and the cyst is an incidental finding. Occasionally there may be complications such as calculi or infection, which resolve after excision of the diverticulum.

Some of the more common or characteristic kinds of renal cysts are shown diagramatically in Fig. 16-20.

URINARY TRACT OBSTRUCTION
Pathogenesis

The outflow of urine from the renal tract can be obstructed in many ways (Table 16-4). With so many causes, it is clear that the degree and duration of obstruction will vary, depending on the cause. During pregnancy, for example, there is temporary external pressure on the ureter until delivery. A slowly enlarging prostate, on the other hand, progressively increases the degree of obstruction. The effects of persistent chronic obstruction are borne by the ureters and by the kidney. When the blockage is below the insertion of the ureters into the bladder, the effects are bilateral. The dilatation of the ureters and the renal calyces results in *hydroureter* and *hydronephrosis,* respectively. Obstruction in the urethra or prostate initially causes bladder distension that, if unrelieved, leads to hydroureter and hydronephrosis (see Fig. 16-21).

The effects of the increased back pressure fall on the renal vessels, especially in the medulla, where tubular function is impaired.

Grossly, in the fully developed form of hydronephrosis the kidney substance is reduced to a thin rim of cortical tissue with loss of the renal papillae. The calyces and renal pelvis are markedly dilated. *Microscopically,* the picture is that of a chronic interstitial nephritis, with widespread loss of tubules, although some fairly normal glomeruli may persist late into the

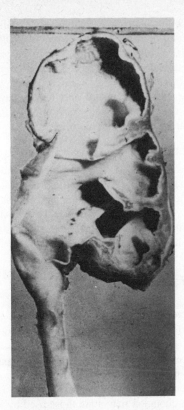

FIG. 16-21. Hydronephrosis caused by chronic enlargement of the prostate. The renal calyces are widely dilated, leaving only a rim of normal renal tissue. The ureter is also widely dilated. *(Courtesy Curator of the Gordon Museum, Guy's Hospital, London, England.)*

TABLE 16-4. Causes of urinary tract obstruction

Site	Disease or abnormality
Kidney	Polycystic kidney, calculus
Ureter	Calculus, vascular obstruction, blood clot, congenital valves, pregnant uterus, surgical misadventure
Bladder	Calculus, blood clot, primary or metastatic tumor, neurogenic causes
Prostate	Inflammation, benign hypertrophy, malignant tumor
Urethra	Phimosis, foreign body, urethritis

disease. These changes are seen when obstruction is fairly gradual. Sudden complete obstruction, as may occasionally happen when the ureter is inadvertently tied at surgery, results in cessation of renal function and atrophy within 2 or 3 weeks, with little in the way of hydronephrotic change. In the early stages of acute complete obstruction the glomerular filtrate is eventually reabsorbed by the lymphatic and vascular systems. This mechanism, however, soon fails, and the severe pressure effects on the renal vasculature result in cessation of glomerular function.

Clinical aspects

When the hydronephrosis is unilateral, it is frequently asymptomatic unless infection is also present. The symptoms of acute pyelonephritis, described later, then develop. Bilateral obstruction, if complete, requires immediate relief. It is best

to prevent hydronephrosis if possible by early surgical removal of any obstruction; if there is severe unilateral damage, removal of the affected kidney is necessary, provided that the other kidney functions adequately.

Urinary calculi

Stones (calculi) may be found in the renal calyces and pelvis, in the ureters, and in the bladder. Renal stones vary in size from tiny pieces of gravel to large solid masses that fill the calyces and pelvis of the kidney, forming the so-called staghorn calculi. The presence of stones in the kidney is called *nephrolithiasis*. This term should be distinguished from *nephrocalcinosis*, in which calcium salts are deposited throughout the substance of the kidney as a result of metabolic disturbances, but not in the large collecting passageways.

The incidence of urinary calculi in the United States is conservatively estimated to be 16 cases/10,000 population/year, or more than 350,000 cases/year, and there is evidence that the incidence is on the rise.

Composition of urinary calculi

In recent years considerable progress has been made in understanding the physicochemical and physiological basis for stone formation, and this has led to the formulation of new methods of treatment. The chemical composition of stones differs according to the causal mechanisms involved, and therefore it has become extremely important to know the *chemical composition* of calculi in order to select appropriate therapy; for recurrent stone formers, in particular, tailored therapeutic regimens can prevent recurrence and arrest the growth of calculi in many cases.

The most accurate methods for analyzing the composition of calculi are by optical crystallography and infrared spectroscopy. It is important that both the *nidus*, if present, as well as the *peripheral layers and shell*, be analyzed; the composition of the nidus provides information regarding initiating factors, and that of the other layers points to the nature of the growth factors. The frequency of the different kinds of stones is approximately as follows:

Composition of stone	Percent
Calcium oxalate	33
Calcium oxalate and calcium phosphate	34
Struvite (magnesium ammonium phosphate hexahydrate)	15
Uric acid	8
Calcium phosphate	6
Cystine	3
Miscellaneous	1

Etiology of calculi according to chemical type

Calcium stones. Calcium stones account for slightly less than three-quarters of all urinary calculi. They may be associated with a variety of metabolic disorders, often of an idiopathic nature. Three main classes of metabolic disturbance are recognized:

Hypercalciuria. This may be (1) idiopathic (the most common metabolic cause of stone formation), ascribed to either increased intestinal calcium absorption or impaired renal tubular reabsorption due to obscure mechanisms; (2) the result of hyperparathyroidism, causing excessive bone resorption; (3) the result of a variety of miscellaneous causes, including sarcoidosis.

Hyperoxaluria. Two conditions, in particular, are characterized by hyperoxaluria. The first, *primary hyperoxaluria,* usually appears in childhood, with recurrent formation of calcium oxalate stones and early renal failure. There is extensive intratubular oxalate crystal deposition, and widespread deposition of oxalate crystals throughout the body *(oxalosis).* More commonly, hyperoxaluria is found in patients with inflammatory bowel disease or after jejunoileal bypass surgery, and is due to increased absorption of dietary oxalate, which appears to be related to fat malabsorption.

Hyperuricosuria. The frequency of stones of this type is high among patients with gout, and the stones usually consist of calcium oxalate, perhaps with a nidus of crystalline uric acid.

Magnesium ammonium phosphate. *Magnesium ammonium phosphate ("triple phosphate" or "struvite")* stones are a result of infection. The underlying cause of such stone formation appears to be an infection of the urinary tract with urea-splitting organisms. Bacterial urease hydrolyzes urea, releasing ammonia and thereby increasing the urinary pH so that the urine becomes supersaturated with magnesium ammonium phosphate. The accompanying rise in urine osmolality probably contributes to the precipitation of crystallization-inhibiting glycosaminoglycans that are normally found dissolved in urine. Struvite (magnesium ammonium phosphate hexahydrate) forms the so-called "staghorn" calculi that develop in alkaline infected urine.

Uric acid stones. *Uric acid stones* develop with or without hyperuricemia (raised blood uric acid). In fact, the majority of those with a tendency to form uric acid stones do not have hyperuricemia but may have a persistently acid urine, usually with a high uric acid content (hyperuricosuria). Only one quarter of patients with uric acid stones are found to have gout.

Cystine stones. *Cystine stones* indicate *cystinuria,* a relatively harmless and rare hereditary disorder that prevents the renal tubular reabsorption of the amino acid cystine. Cystinuria should be distinguished from *cystinosis,* a potentially more serious disorder in which cystine deposits are found throughout the body, but in which urinary calculi rarely form. Cystinosis accompanies the serious childhood form of the *De Toni-Debre-Fanconi syndrome,* which consists essentially of rickets or osteomalacia (which is resistant to conventional doses of vitamin D), glycosuria, aminoaciduria, hyperphosphaturia, and very often acidosis and hypokalemia.

Results and complications of urinary calculi

The pathologic effects of stones are the results of obstruction and of predisposition to infection; Stasis in the urinary tract caused by stones inevitably leads to infection. Renal stones, provided they remain in situ, cause no symptoms until the effects of obstruction or infection supervene. Smaller stones, formed in the kidney and entering the ureter, lead to the symptoms of *renal colic.* This is among the most painful of human disorders. Often it is associated with difficulty in urination (dysuria). Approximately 80% of patients with urinary calculi spontaneously pass the stones.

Management of urinary calculi

Once the nature of the calculi being formed is determined, a rational approach to management can be formulated. Close attention to diet and the use of drugs aimed at changing the urinary pH or blocking the formation of crystallizing metabolites may retard or arrest the formation of calculi. In the 20% of individuals in whom the stones cannot be passed spontaneously, the use of a lithotripter, a recently developed device that shatters calculi with shock waves while the patient is immersed in water under general anesthetic, may be fruitful. Where renal damage due to obstruction and infection is advanced, nephrectomy may be required.

Bladder stones

Stones arising primarily in the bladder are much less common than renal calculi. They are closely associated with neurogenic bladder, a condition in which there is loss of voluntary neural control of bladder function, usually following trauma to the spinal cord. This leads to urinary retention and stasis, which appear to be major factors contributing to stone formation.

URINARY TRACT INFECTIONS
Definitions

Urinary tract infection includes a variety of conditions in which bacteria invade different parts of the normally sterile urinary tract. Nevertheless, a great deal of confusion and controversy still exists regarding the nomenclature, pathology, and pathogenesis of this common malady. This is partly because there is no generally agreed definition of terms. The following definitions in quotation marks are those used by Kunin.* *Urinary tract infection* includes "a wide variety of clinical entities whose common denominator is invasion of any of the tissues of the urinary tract from the renal cortex to the urethral meatus." *Pyelonephritis* is "an inflammatory process of the kidney and renal pelvis, and the term is often used to mean *bacterial pyelonephritis* "due to organisms other than *M. tuberculosis.*" Tuberculosis of the renal tract is discussed later in this chapter.

The term *acute bacterial pyelonephritis* is used in two contexts:

1. To describe a well-defined clinical syndrome, consisting of "fever, pain and tenderness in the flank, and bacteria and leukocytes in the urine. There may or may not be accompanying cystitis."
2. To define specific pathologic changes in the kidney that accompany the clinical picture just described

Chronic bacterial pyelonephritis is due to the presence of either "long-standing infection associated with active bacterial growth or the residuum of lesions produced in the past but not now active." This definition includes two variants:

1. Chronic active bacterial pyelonephritis in which there are symptoms associated with bacteria and inflammatory cells
2. Chronic inactive (healed) bacterial pyelonephritis in which the patients are symptom free and the urine contains no bacteria or inflammatory cells

It should be added, however, that the existence of these two entities is seriously disputed and that they are at best unusual pathologic states.

Significant bacteriuria is a term introduced on the basis of studies by Kass,† in which it was shown that there was a high degree of correlation between the presence of 10^5 or more

---

*Kunin CM: Detection, prevention and management of urinary tract infections, ed 2, Philadelphia, 1974, Lea & Febiger, p. 13.
†Kass EH: Bacteriuria and diagnosis of infection of the urinary tract, Arch Intern Med 100:709, 1957.

bacteria/ml of a midstream sample of urine obtained after adequate genital cleansing, and the presence of active infection in the urinary tract. The term is used to distinguish between bacteria in voided samples of urine due to actual infection of the urinary tract and bacteria introduced during sampling by contamination from vaginal, fecal, or urethral flora. Thus in a clean voided sample of urine a bacterial count of 10^5/ml has been called a "significant bacteriuria." When, on the other hand, urine is obtained aseptically, as by bladder puncture, the presence of any number of bacteria may be regarded as significant (i.e., indicates infection of the urinary tract). There are other exceptions too, as discussed later.

It is not uncommon, incidentally, to find more than 10^5 organisms/ml of urine in clean voided specimens from women who have no symptoms referrable to the urinary tract. This finding is called *asymptomatic bacteriuria*.

Etiology of urinary tract infections

The bacteria that cause urinary tract infection are almost exclusively aerobic organisms that inhabit the lower intestinal tract. By far the most common enteric bacterium infecting the urinary tract is *Escherichia coli*, although *Klebsiella* and *Proteus* species are also common. Two other organisms, *Pseudomonas aeruginosa* and *Streptococcus faecalis*, are quite common and very troublesome because of their resistance to many antibacterial drugs.

Infection is either hematogenous or ascends from the urethral meatus. The latter is by far the most important route. Blood-borne infections of the kidney are a complication of bacteremic illnesses.

Predisposing factors to ascending infections include any obstructive lesion leading to urinary stasis, but in many cases of urinary tract infection no obstruction can be found. Many of the latter can be traced to *vesicoureteral reflux*, consisting of a forceful reflux of urine up the ureters during the act of micturition. This is found as a not infrequent developmental anomaly in infants; if a bladder infection develops in a child with reflux, the infected urine will be propelled upwards to the kidney. In most cases the reflux disappears spontaneously as the infant grows up, but in a certain number, particularly those with severe reflux, the condition persists. Urinary tract infections are much more common in females. Factors such as the relative shortness of the female urethra and trauma to the urethra during intercourse have been postulated as accounting for this higher prevalence. Ureteric obstruction during pregnancy is another common predisposing factor.

Pathology of urinary tract infections

The pathologic entities that result from unmistakable microbial infection of tissues of the urinary tract are acute cystitis, acute pyelonephritis, and the dysuria-pyuria (urethral) syndrome. *Acute cystitis* (bladder inflammation) is frequently found without involvement of the kidney, but some degree of cystitis is usual when *acute pyelonephritis* is present. Of interest are findings that bacteria coming from the kidney are coated with immunoglobulins, whereas those from the bladder usually are not. This provides a means of differentiating pyelonephritis and cystitis and is an important distinction in view of the seriousness of the former and the relative mildness of the latter. However, in practical terms, this method lacks both sensitivity and specificity. The *dysuria-pyuria syndrome* is essentially due to inflammation of the urethra in women by one of several microbial agents.

Acute cystitis

Pathologic changes in the bladder wall are minimal in early cases and consist only of mucosal hyperemia in which modest numbers of acute inflammatory cells can be seen microscopically.

In uncomplicated cases these changes are completely reversible with proper treatment. In the presence of persistent infection, and especially with bladder outlet obstruction, more severe inflammation with hemorrhage and ulceration may develop. In long-standing cases chronic inflammation with fibrosis and rigidity of the bladder wall develop, and the term *chronic cystitis* may be appropriately applied.

A specific form of cystitis—acute viral hemorrhagic cystitis—has been described and linked to adenovirus type 16. This infection is seen in children, is characterized by hematuria, and is a benign self-limiting disease requiring no specific treatment.

Dysuria-pyuria syndrome (urethral syndrome)

Although many women who have dysuria with frequency and urgency will be found to have more than 10^5 bacteria/ml urine (and therefore, by definition, "significant bacteriuria"), up to 40% of women can have similar symptoms but urinary bacterial counts less than 10^5/ml. However, pyuria (i.e., >7 leukocytes/ml unspun urine) can be demonstrated in most of these cases, and the symptoms usually respond to antimicrobial therapy.

Women with this syndrome can be divided into three groups:
1. Bladder infection by enteric bacteria particularly *Escherichia coli* or by *Staphylococcus saprophyticus* at concentrations lower than those that are usually seen with bacterial cystitis
2. "Sterile" pyuria, caused mainly by *Chlamydia trachomatis* or sometimes *Neisseria gonorrhoeae*
3. Sterile pyuria of undetermined, possibly noninfectious origin—*Ureaplasma urealyticum* may account for some cases; chemical or traumatic irritation for others. In some instances, an accompanying bacterial or viral vaginitis may account for the urinary symptoms.

The diagnosis is made on the history, physical and pelvic examination, and quantitative urine culture, with special culture for chlamydia and gonococcus where required. The treatment depends on the cause; tetracycline is the antimicrobial agent used most for this syndrome.

Acute pyelonephritis

The acute inflammatory changes may be seen in one or both kidneys. The presence of multiple abscesses, scattered throughout the organ and readily seen beneath the capsule, is typical (Fig. 16-22).

Microscopically, the picture is that of an acute interstitial nephritis, with large numbers of neutrophils in an edematous interstitium. Abscesses consisting of small dense collections of polymorphonuclear leukocytes, and which can sometimes contain obvious microcolonies of bacteria, are typical of acute pyelonephritis (Fig. 16-23). Tubules are damaged and eventually destroyed by the inflammatory process, but the glomeruli withstand the infection well and may show no changes.

Involvement of the kidney in acute pyelonephritis is patchy, with frequent involvement of the upper and lower poles and sparing of the midsection of the kidney; the reason for this appears to be an anatomical peculiarity of the papillae at the poles of the kidney that permits the reflux of infected urine from the pelvicalyceal system into the renal tubules. Healing

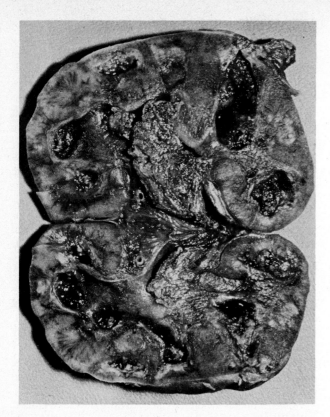

FIG. 16-22. Acute pyelonephritis. There are several large abscess cavities and numerous smaller abscesses throughout the kidney. *(Courtesy Curator of the Gordon Museum, Guy's Hospital, London, England.)*

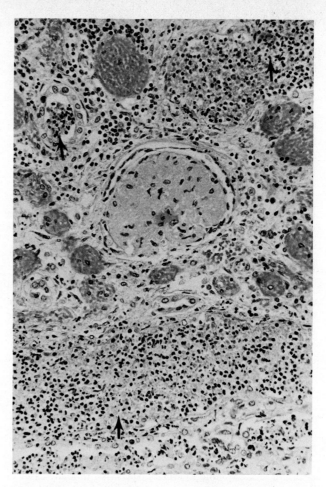

FIG. 16-23. Acute pyelonephritis. The tubules are filled with pus *(arrows)* and show extensive loss of epithelium.

produces scarring of the parenchyma, with chronic interstitial nephritis ("chronic pyelonephritis").

Clinical aspects. A typical attack of acute bacterial pyelonephritis causes fever, flank pain, pain and difficulty with urination, and bacteria and inflammatory cells in the urine. Diagnosis is confirmed by culture of the urine, and treatment is by adequate fluid intake and administration of an appropriate antimicrobial drug. In acute cystitis there is suprapubic discomfort, as well as frequent, painful, and difficult urination, and sometimes frank hematuria. Although it is a much less serious condition, acute cystitis is managed in a way similar to that of acute pyelonephritis. In both infections it is important that patient progress is followed carefully to ensure eradication of the infection.

Acute pyelonephritis and cystitis are two fairly well-defined entities, but not all patients with urinary tract infections may be so readily recognized and treated. Among the more troublesome aspects of urinary tract infection are the following:

1. Relapse of infection
2. Reinfection
3. Asymptomatic bacteriuria

Relapse of infection happens when infection by the same organism recurs following treatment. This implies that treatment has failed to eradicate the original bacterium.

Reinfection takes place when a different strain of bacterium causes another attack of urinary tract infection. In about 80% of patients another strain of *E. coli* is the usual reinfecting agent. Reinfection implies that the original factors leading to

bacterial infection are still operating but that the treatment of the first attack was successful.

Asymptomatic bacteriuria can usually be detected only by quantitative bacterial culture performed as a routine or survey procedure on a population. The significance of asymptomatic bacteriuria is still unclear. It is found almost exclusively in women, and the incidence seems to increase in lower socioeconomic groups and with parity. Studies in girls and women suggest the following:

1. Asymptomatic bacteriuria is usually benign and transient.
2. In a few cases it may progress to symptomatic infection of the urinary tract.
3. In pregnant women eradication of asymptomatic bacteriuria has been shown to prevent the development of overt pyelonephritis and can lower the prevalence of perinatal mortality.

Chronic pyelonephritis

Chronic pyelonephritis is the end result of a bacterial infection of the kidney. It may develop in association with interference to urinary outflow, or without demonstrable obstruction. In the obstructive variety, the kidney is damaged by a combination of obstruction and infection. The kidneys show generalized calyceal dilatation. In the nonobstructive type, which practically always follows vesicoureteric reflux, there is usually dilatation of only one or two calyces, usually at one or both poles, in association with an overlying, flat scar; the apparent reasons for this peculiar distribution have been mentioned previously. Whether or not reflux of sterile urine can produce the picture of chronic pyelonephritis is controversial.

Microscopically, chronic pyelonephritis is characterized by a chronic interstitial nephritis, with lymphoid infiltrates, fibrosis, dramatic loss of tubules, and, characteristically, "thyroid-like" areas where residual tubules are dilated and contain casts resembling thyroid colloid. The inflammatory changes involve the pelvis and calyces, as well as the scarred portions of the parenchyma. Although usually impossible to distinguish from "chronic glomerulonephritis" by needle biopsy, chronic pyelonephritis may be recognized at autopsy (it is an important cause of chronic renal failure) by the calyceal dilatation, flattening of associated papillae, and thinning and scarring of overlying areas of parenchyma, as well as the often asymmetrical appearance of the kidneys when left and right are compared.

Renal tract tuberculosis

M. tuberculosis spreads through the blood to the kidney from a focus usually in the lung. Such spread may take place during early primary infection, but the majority of cases appear to be the result of metastatic spread from apical lesions in reactivation tuberculosis.

The initial infection is in the renal cortex, where typical tuberculous granulomas develop. Involvement of the glomeruli results in bacilli being shed in the urine, which may carry infection to the ureters, the prostate, and the bladder. In males, further spread from the prostate may infect seminal vesicles and an epididymis. If undetected, tuberculous renal infection may eventually replace the kidney by a mass of caseation necrosis (tuberculous pyonephrosis).

Renal tuberculosis is frequently symptomless. Evidence of the infection may be detected in the urine, where sterile pyuria (pus in the urine with negative conventional bacteria cultures) is a common finding. Hematuria or proteinuria may sometimes be due to tuberculosis. The diagnosis is by culture of urine on specific media for *M. tuberculosis*. The treatment is antituberculous chemotherapy.

Summary of urinary tract obstruction and infection

The urinary tract can be obstructed by a variety of causes at any point from the renal pelvis to the distal urethra. Obstruction below the bladder leads to hypertrophy and dilatation of the bladder, dilatation of the ureters and renal pelvis, and hydronephrosis.

The presence of stones within the urinary tract may cause obstruction or acute renal colic (sometimes with hematuria), especially as they traverse the ureters.

Urinary tract infection is a common sequel to urinary obstruction. It may also develop in the absence of obstruction, especially in women, as a result of retrograde infection by enteric bacteria, and in children, as a result of vesicoureteric reflux. Urinary tract infection may affect the kidney or the bladder or both and is characterized by pain, fever, dysuria, the presence of more than 10^5 bacteria/ml of urine and often many pus cells. Asymptomatic infections are common in women and children.

The essential management is the early relief of obstruction and the use of antimicrobial drugs to eliminate infection.

TUMORS OF THE URINARY TRACT

The important primary urinary tract tumors are listed as follows:

1. *Renal parenchyma*
   a. Angiomyolipoma
   b. Tubular epithelial cell neoplasms
   c. Wilms' tumor (nephroblastoma) and related childhood neoplasms
2. *Urothelium* (renal pelvis, ureter, bladder, urethra)
   a. Transitional epithelial cell neoplasms
   b. Squamous cell carcinoma
   c. Adenocarcinoma

Renal parenchymal neoplasms

Angiomyolipoma of the kidney. Renal angiomyolipomas are uncommon benign lesions that are considered hamartomas rather than neoplasms. They are composed of mature adipose tissue, thick-walled blood vessels and smooth muscle in varying proportions. They are usually small and asymptomatic but are sometimes large and may give rise to hematuria, flank pain, or other symptoms. They usually present in the 3rd to 5th decades of life. About 50% of patients have *tuberous sclerosis* (Chapter 20), and about 80% of patients with tuberous sclerosis have angiomyolipomas. In the absence of tuberous sclerosis lesions are usually single and unilateral, whereas in patients with tuberous sclerosis they are frequently multiple and bilateral.

The advent of computerized tomography has made the preoperative diagnosis of these lesions possible, where previously, it was impossible to distinguish these neoplasms either clinically or radiologically from renal cell carcinomas. With more accurate diagnosis, observation or conservative surgery is now possible, and nephrectomy commonly performed in the past can be avoided.

Renal tubular epithelial neoplasms. The renal tubular epithelium gives rise to a spectrum of neoplasms that may be small or large, show minimal or marked atypia, and are composed of epithelial cells with variable cytoplasmic features. Small tumors (less than 3 cm) usually, but not always, fail to metastasize and have been termed, inaccurately, *adenomas*. Tumors (large or small) that are composed exclusively of oncocytic (mitochondrion-packed) cells showing minimal nuclear atypia very rarely metastasize and are called *oncocytomas*; they have a distinctive gross appearance, with a homogeneously brown cut surface surrounding a central, stellate, fibrous scar. All of the remaining tubular epithelial cell neoplasms are called *renal cell carcinomas*. Preliminary evidence indicates that, in some cases, renal oncocytomas can be distinguished from renal cell carcinomas preoperatively by magnetic resonance imaging.

Renal cell carcinoma. Renal cell carcinoma is by far the most common of all renal tumors and arises from the renal tubular epithelium. The old and fictitious theory that the tumor was derived from "rests" of suprarenal cells gave rise to the term *hypernephroma*. This should have disappeared from the literature but still lingers on. Other synonyms for this neoplasm include renal adenocarcinoma and Grawitz's tumor.

Renal carcinomas most commonly are found in the cortex. They may attain a size of several centimeters or more before

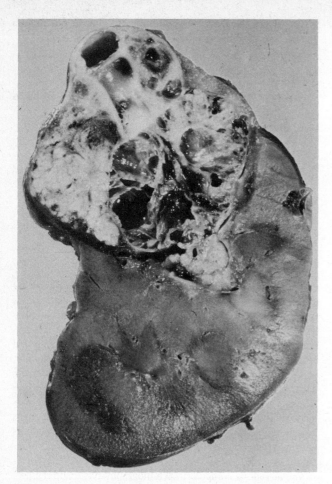

FIG. 16-24. Carcinoma of the kidney. A large renal cell carcinoma occupies the upper pole of the kidney. The tumor is characteristically pale but more cystic than is usual. *(Courtesy Curator of the Gordon Museum, Guy's Hospital, London, England.)*

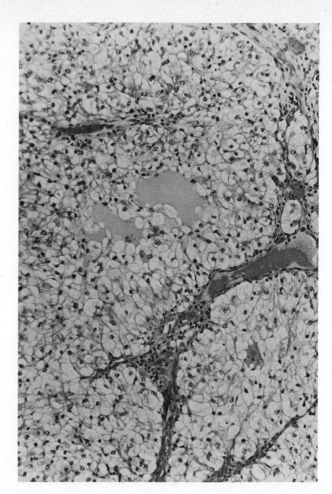

FIG. 16-25. Renal cell carcinoma. The tumor cells show the typical clear-cell appearance, which is due to their high cytoplasmic lipid and glycogen content.

their presence is suspected. The cut surface of the tumor is typically yellow, but this may be considerably altered by hemorrhage and necrosis. Most tumors are solid, but cystic degeneration, as well as true cystic components, are sometimes seen (Fig. 16-24). The tumor tends to invade blood vessels and commonly grows along the renal vein.

Microscopically, the cells are typically large, with abundant clear or pale cytoplasm (Fig. 16-25) rich in glycogen and, especially, fat, which imparts to the tumor its yellow naked-eye appearance. Less commonly, tumor cells have a granular, eosinophilic cytoplasm or may be spindly, or sarcoma-like. The latter variant is associated with more aggressive tumor behavior.

Renal cell carcinoma is a tumor of middle and late life. The invasive properties of the tumor give rise to its most common presenting symptom—hematuria. The hematuria is usually painless and variable in intensity. Some patients may complain of dull pain in the flank. Among other manifestations that may be encountered are the following: (1) about 20% of patients have fever, the origin of which is unknown; (2) a few patients develop polycythemia resulting from the elaboration of erythropoietin (Chapter 13); (3) a small percentage of cases may have hypertension, which is ascribed to the presence of perivascular renin-secreting cells in such neoplasms. (Similar cells, supposedly causing hypertension, have also been reported in

other kinds of renal tumors, and may themselves rarely give rise to hypertension-causing neoplasms.) Renal cell carcinomas metastasize, especially to lung, liver, bone, and the other kidney, but the development of metastases, like so many properties of this tumor, is unpredictable.

The treatment of renal cell carcinoma has traditionally been nephrectomy, although there is now a trend towards more conservative surgery in selected cases. As already mentioned, the behavior of this tumor can be unpredictable and it may be difficult to make a clear prognostication about its behavior after surgery. Large tumors invading blood vessels and removed with difficulty may not recur for many years, whereas small tumors readily removed at surgery may recur and kill the patient within a year or so. The role of DNA cytometry in predicting tumor behavior remains to be determined.

Nephroblastoma (Wilms tumor). This tumor is a complex embryonal neoplasm almost exclusively limited to children under 8 years and, although uncommon, accounts for one fifth of all childhood cancers.

Wilms tumors are large, frequently filling much of the abdominal cavity so that the most common presenting sign is an abdominal mass.

The typical Wilms tumor includes areas of renal blastema (embryonic renal tissue) with varying degrees of tubular and glomeruloid differentiation, often arranged in micronodules surrounded by a loose fibrous stroma. The tumor is commonly associated with nephroblastomatosis, a condition defined as persistence of metanephric blastema in a kidney beyond 36 weeks of gestation. The differentiation of these tumors forms a spectrum that corresponds to various stages of renal morphologic development, and more mature elements (e.g., simulating renal cell carcinoma) may sometimes be observed in Wilms tumors.

Although frequently massive, Wilms tumors are highly sensitive to radiotherapy and chemotherapy, and, when these are combined with surgery, about 75% of patients can expect to be cured. Prognosis mostly depends on two major factors: the histologic grade, and the stage of the neoplasm. Those with unfavorable histology (enlarged, hyperchromatic nuclei and abnormal mitotic figures) have a much less favorable prognosis and may develop metastases to abdominal lymph nodes, lungs, liver, and other sites.

Wilms tumor has a peak incidence between 2 and 4 years and is rarely seen in the newborn. It must be differentiated from a similar tumor, the *congenital mesoblastic nephroma*, which typically presents during the first 3 months of life and is usually cured by nephrectomy alone.

Urothelial neoplasms

Most neoplasms arising from urothelium differentiate along urothelial lines (i.e. are *transitional cell neoplasms*). A small percentage of squamous and gland-forming neoplasms are also seen, which is consistent with the capacity of urothelium, especially in chronic inflammatory states, to undergo squamous or glandular metaplasia.

The transitional epithelial cell neoplasms that arise in the renal pelvis are essentially the same lesions as are found in the ureters, urinary bladder, and urethra. In fact, they are not infrequently found arising in more than one of these sites in the same patient. This is because transitional cell neoplasms are not isolated lesions but part of a *field change* affecting the entire urinary tract to a greater or lesser degree, which also explains the high recurrence rate of transitional cell neoplasms following removal. Most of the description that follows pertains to the urinary bladder, where most of these neoplasms arise.

The cause of most bladder tumors is unknown. However, a very high incidence of bladder cancer has been found in aniline dye workers exposed to substances such as benzidine and xenylamine. An association has also been reported from Egypt between chronic bladder infestation by the blood fluke *Schistosoma haematobium* and bladder cancer, but these are often squamous cell carcinomas. Bladder cancer accounts for 2% of all malignancies in adults. It is 3 to 4 times more common in men than in women, with a peak incidence in the sixth decade.

Histologic and biologic spectrum of transitional cell neoplasia. Most transitional epithelial neoplasms begin as zones of epithelial hyperplasia. The hyperplastic epithelium may show only minimal nuclear atypia; alternatively, nuclear enlargement, pleomorphism, coarseness of chromatin, and frequent mitoses may be present. The former are termed *low-grade* lesions, the latter *high-grade* lesions. Both kinds may be either *flat* or *papillary*.

Low-grade flat lesions are sometimes termed *dysplastic*, and high-grade flat lesions *carcinoma in situ*. Only the latter tend to become invasive transitional cell carcinomas and to give rise to metastases. Low-grade papillary lesions, among which are lesions termed *papillomas*, behave in an essentially indolent fashion. The term *papillary transitional cell carcinoma* is re-

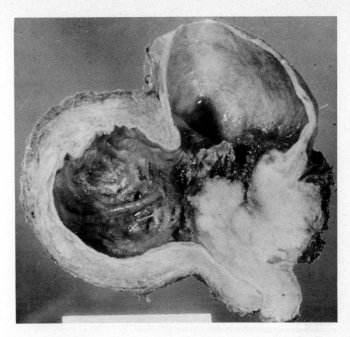

FIG. 16-26. Cancer of the bladder. The bladder has been sectioned to show a large tumor of the floor of the organ. There is hypertrophy of the bladder as a result of obstruction of urinary outflow by the tumor. *(Courtesy Curator of the Gordon Museum, Guy's Hospital, London, England.)*

served for high-grade papillary lesions, as only high-grade papillary lesions tend to become invasive and metastasize. In summary, the most important morphologic feature that determines whether a proliferative transitional epithelial lesion has an invasive potential is its *cytologic grade*, rather than its architecture. The outcome for the patient with infiltrating lesions depends on the *stage* of the disease (extent of spread), including the depth of infiltration into the bladder wall, the presence or absence of nodal involvement and whether there is concomitant unilateral or bilateral neoplasia in the upper urinary tract.

Urine cytology and *mucosal biopsy* obtained at cystoscopy are generally employed to determine whether a lesion is high-grade or low-grade, and whether the lesion is in situ or infiltrating. Although the majority of transitional epithelial lesions fall into these fairly well-defined categories, examples of intermediate grade lesions are sometimes encountered. In practice, most of these appear to exhibit a biologic behavior that more closely approximates that of the low-grade than the high-grade lesions. However, because of the observer subjectivity involved in grading these lesions by routine microscopy, the clinical application of objective techniques for assessing nuclear grade, in particular *DNA flow cytometry*, is being developed.

Invasive transitional cell carcinomas arising in flat lesions are sessile broad-based tumors that enlarge by invasion of the bladder wall (Fig. 16-26). Papillary lesions project into the lumen as they grow. The most frequent symptom is painless hematuria, often associated with difficulty in urination.

Low-grade papillary lesions can be removed locally using cystoscopy. A common regimen of treatment for invasive lesions is preoperative irradiation followed by total removal of the bladder and implantation of the ureters into a segment of the ileum. Intravesical BCG is being employed with some success in the management of superficially invasive bladder lesions at some centers.

Summary of renal tract tumors

Angiomyolipoma is an uncommon benign renal tumor sometimes associated with tuberous sclerosis and apt to be confused with renal cell carcinoma preoperatively.

Renal cell carcinoma is a common tumor of later life with a tendency to invade the renal veins, but with an otherwise unpredictable long-term behavior. It commonly causes painless hematuria and is usually treated by nephrectomy.

Wilms tumor is found mainly in children. It typically resembles the embryonal kidney histologically, but may also differentiate in a variety of other directions. The response of this tumor to surgery, radiotherapy, and chemotherapy is generally favorable.

Tumors of the renal pelvis and bladder are typically *transitional cell carcinomas*. Histologically, high-grade lesions tend to invade and metastasize readily and carry a generally unfavorable prognosis. Painless hematuria is the common symptom, and the treatment is primarily surgical.

Selected readings

Bannayan GA: Tumors of the kidney. In Forland M, editor: Nephrology, New York, 1983, Medical Examination Publishing Co., Inc.

Beckwith JB: Wilms' tumor and other renal tumors of childhood. In Finegold M, editor: Pathology of neoplasia in children and adolescents, Philadelphia, 1986, WB Saunders Co.

Ben-bassat M et al: The clinicopathologic features of cryoglobulinemic nephropathy, Am J Clin Pathol 79:147, 1983.

Blute MI, Malek RS, and Segura JW: Angiomyolipoma: clinical metamorphosis and concepts for management, J Urol 139:20, 1988.

Bowie WR: Urethritis and infections of the lower urinary tract, Urol Clin N Am 7:17, 1980.

Cohen AH and Border WA: Mesangial proliferative glomerulonephritis, Sem Nephrol 2:228, 1982.

Cohen AH and Nast CC: HIV-associated nephropathy: a unique combined glomerular, tubular, and interstitial lesion, Mod Pathol 1:87, 1988.

Consensus conference (National Institutes of Health, Bethesda, MD): Analgesic-associated kidney disease, JAMA 251:3123, 1984.

Cooper K and Bennett WM: Nephrotoxicity of common drugs used in clinical practice, Arch Intern Med 147:1213, 1987.

D'amico G: The commonest glomerulonephritis in the world: IgA nephropathy, Quart J Med 245:709, 1987.

Glassberg KI et al: Renal dysgenesis and cystic disease of the kidney: a report of the committee on terminology, nomenclature and classification, section on urology, American Academy of Pediatrics, J Urol 138:1085, 1987.

Heptinstall RH: Pathology of the kidney, ed 3, Boston, 1983, Little, Brown & Co.

Jordan AM, Weingarten J, and Murphy WM: Transitional cell neoplasms of the urinary bladder: Can biologic potential be predicted from histologic grading? Cancer 60:2766, 1987.

Kaysen GA et al: Mechanisms and consequences of proteinuria, Lab Invest 54:479, 1986.

Keown PA and Stiller CR: Kidney transplantion, Surg Clin N Am 66:517, 1986.

Kincaid-Smith P and Whitworth JA: The kidney: a clinico-pathological study, ed 2, Oxford, England, 1987, Blackwell Scientific Publications.

Lindop GBM and Lever AF: Anatomy of the renin-angiotensin system in the normal and pathological kidney, Histopathology 10:335, 1986.

Maierhofer WJ: Renal disease from excess uric acid, Postgrad Med 82:123, 1987.

McCluskey RT: Immunopathogenetic mechanisms in renal disease, Am J Kid Dis 10:172, 1987.

O'Brien WM, Rotolo JE, and Pahira JJ: New approaches in the treatment of renal calculi, Am Fam Phys 36:181, 1987.

Schwartz GL and Strong CG: Renal parenchymal involvement in essential hypertension, Med Clin N Am 71:843, 1987.

Sturgill BC, Tucker FL, and Bolton WK: Immunoglobulin light chain nephropathies, Pathol Ann 22(2):133, 1987.

Sutton RAL, editor: Urolithiasis, Min Electrol Metab 13:213, 1987.

CHAPTER 17

Diseases of the musculoskeletal system and related soft tissues

The musculoskeletal system comprises the bones, joints, and muscles. The joints, or periarticular tissues, are among the most common sources of symptoms (rheumatic complaints of various sorts), and the bones are also affected by a wide variety of diseases. Osteoporosis, for example, affects virtually everyone, particularly women, as age advances but only becomes apparent late in life as a predisposing cause of fractures of the neck of the femur or collapse of vertebrae.

The muscles, by contrast, are an infrequent site of disease. The most important are the muscular dystrophies, but even these are uncommon.

Calcium metabolism and its control

The skeleton forms the main bulk of calcium in the body and acts as a reservoir of calcium. The concentration of calcium in the plasma and other fluids depends on the following:

1. The amount of calcium absorbed from the intestine
2. The amount of calcium excreted in the urine
3. The equilibrium between mobilization of calcium from and its deposition in bone

The factors influencing these processes include the vitamin D content of the diet and the activities of parathyroid hormone and calcitonin (thyrocalcitonin) (Fig. 17-1). The calcium content of the diet seems less important, and, if absorption and metabolism are normal, the body is apparently able to adapt to a very low intake.

Vitamin D

The natural fat-soluble vitamin is cholecalciferol (vitamin D_3). Calciferol (vitamin D_2) is a semisynthetic product that can be used therapeutically. Ultraviolet light (in sunlight) also converts an inactive precursor (7-dehydrocholesterol) into vitamin D_3 in the skin.

Vitamin D_3 absorbed from the intestinal tract or skin is converted into active metabolites in the liver and kidney. These metabolites of vitamin D affect intestinal absorption of calcium, renal handling of calcium and phosphate, calcification of skeletal tissue, and contractility of voluntary muscle. A major effect of the active vitamin is to enhance absorption from dietary sources by potentiating intestinal transport of the calcium ion.

Calcium, together with phosphorus, is excreted by glomerular filtration. Vitamin D increases reabsorption of calcium from the renal tubule (returning it to the circulation) but decreases reabsorption of phosphate.

If there is a relative or absolute lack of vitamin D, calcification of the organic matrix of the bone is impaired, causing rickets in children or osteomalacia in adults.

As described earlier, chronic renal disease can also cause excessive mineral loss and renal rickets (Chapter 16), which is relatively resistant to correction by vitamin D.

Other effects of vitamin D deficiency are muscular weakness and hypocalcemia. This may be severe enough to cause tetany or convulsions.

Parathormone

The parathyroid gland secretes the peptide hormone parathormone (PTH). PTH is released in response to a fall in the blood calcium level, whereas a raised blood calcium level inhibits release of PTH.

PTH acts both on bone, intestinal absorption, and excretory mechanisms. PTH mobilizes calcium from bone and thus raises plasma calcium levels at the expense of bone calcium. Overactivity of the parathyroid glands due to hyperplasia or a PTH-producing tumor causes excessive calcium resorption from bone mainly by enhanced osteoclastic activity.

PTH potentiates the action of vitamin D in mediating absorption of calcium by the intestine. PTH also reduces the renal clearance of calcium by returning more of the calcium filtered out at the glomerulus to the plasma. The relative importance of these three functions of PTH has not yet been finally resolved.

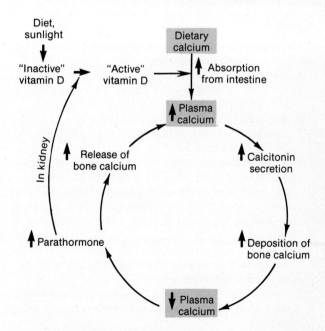

FIG. 17-1. Simplified diagram of interaction of calcium, calcitonin, vitamin D, and parathormone.

Calcitonin

This hormone is produced by the parafollicular cells of the thyroid gland and in many ways acts as an antagonist to PTH. The main action of calcitonin is inhibition of bone resorption with the result that both calcium and phosphorus levels in the plasma are lowered.

Calcitonin also opposes PTH in the kidney by increasing renal clearance of calcium and phosphorus. The physiologic role of calcitonin in calcium metabolism is nevertheless obscure in many ways. Its principal effect is to lower both plasma calcium and phosphate, and calcitonin production in turn is regulated by the serum calcium level. Hypercalcemia stimulates the release of calcitonin; hypocalcemia depresses it. On the other hand, changes in calcium and phosphate metabolism do not seem to follow calcitonin deficiency in totally thyroidectomized patients or of excess calcitonin secretion in patients with a calcitonin-secreting tumor (medullary carcinoma of the thyroid). Despite these facts, calcitonin combats bone loss in osteoporosis and Paget's disease. It is also effective in lowering the blood calcium level in hypercalcemic states.

Growth and other hormones

Growth hormone determines the length of the long bones during development, and overproduction of growth hormone during development produces a giant. Even in an adult, hypersecretion of growth hormone causes increase in the size of some bones, notably the mandible and bones of the hands and feet (acromegaly; Chapter 18).

Corticosteroids (glucocorticoids) cause loss of skeletal bone, presumably as a result of depression of synthesis of protein matrix. Osteoporosis is therefore a complication both of Cushing's syndrome and of prolonged heavy doses of corticosteroids.

Estrogens also have an effect on bone metabolism. As women age, estrogen secretion falls, and osteoporosis increases. The role of estrogen deficiency in osteoporosis is, however, controversial. Thyroid hormone appears also to affect serum calcium, and in severe thyrotoxicosis there is hypercalcemia, presumably due to increased bone resorption.

Summary

The main factors controlling blood calcium levels and bone metabolism include the following:

1. Dietary intake of vitamin D, together with vitamin D synthesis in the skin under the influence of sunlight, is a major factor.
2. The main function of vitamin D is to promote intestinal transport of calcium and phosphate to maintain their normal extracellular fluid levels.
3. Parathormone secretion is regulated by blood calcium levels; when these fall, PTH is secreted and accelerates the removal of calcium from bones to raise the blood calcium level. PTH acts synergistically with vitamin D to increase absorption and decrease renal excretion of calcium.
4. Calcitonin opposes the action of parathormone and lowers the blood calcium level mainly by increasing deposition of calcium in the bones.
5. Several other hormones, including estrogens and thyroxine, affect bone formation and metabolism to varying degrees.

Skeletal development, structure, and metabolism

Bone is a dynamic tissue that is being constantly remodeled throughout life. It is a reservoir of calcium, magnesium, phosphorus, sodium, and other ions necessary for many homeostatic functions.

The formation of bone depends on the deposition of calcium phosphate, both as hydroxyapatite and as amorphous calcium phosphate in a protein matrix (osteoid).

Osteoblasts secrete osteoid, which then becomes mineralized during bone development. The resorption of bone is carried out by multinucleated osteoclasts and mononuclear cells. During the growth period, bone develops by the remodeling and replacement of cartilage to form the long bones or, in the flat membrane bones, by mineralization of fibrous tissue.

Increase in the length of long bones depends on proliferation of cells of the epiphyseal cartilage. Increase in width and thickness is the result of deposition of bone by the periosteum. The rate of deposition of mineral in osteoid depends on the concentration of calcium and phosphorus ions in the plasma and extracellular fluid.

The matrix is collagenous and its formation therefore depends on normal collagen production (Chapter 2). Collagen appears to catalyze the deposition of calcium and phosphorus.

If the concentrations of calcium and phosphorus ions in the extracellular fluid fall below a critical level, mineralization of the bone matrix is reduced or stops.

When bone is resorbed, calcium and phosphorus ions are removed and released into the extracellular fluid. The mechanisms are not clear, but a fall in pH or the presence of chelating agents may be factors. Osteoclasts are rich in acid phosphatase, but the function of this enzyme in mineralization is not known. Osteoblasts, on the other hand, contain alkaline phosphatase, and the level of this enzyme in the serum rises when osteoblastic activity increases.

The rate of bone resorption is affected by several hormones, particularly parathyroid hormone and calcitonin. Bone resorption is also accelerated by the action of prostaglandins of the E series and osteoclast-activation by interleukin 1 (IL-1).

Fluoride, when incorporated into bone, replaces hydroxyl ions to form crystalline fluorapatite and decreases the proportion of amorphous calcium phosphate.

TABLE 17-1. Osteogenesis imperfecta subtypes

Type and heritance	Fractures	Teeth (DI)	Other features
I AD	Mild, early onset	+	Hypermobility, blue sclerae, thin aortic valves
II AR	Severe, multiple fractures	−	Lethal, usually stillborn, skull hardly ossified
III AR*	Progressive Crippling	−	Blue sclerae, reduced stature
IV AD	Severe	+	Stature reduced
V Various	Mild	***	Highly hypermobile joints

DI, Dentinogenesis imperfecta
*, Some are sporadic
***, Sometimes present

DISEASES OF THE MUSCULOSKELETAL SYSTEM

Genetic skeletal diseases

Osteogenesis imperfecta (brittle bone syndrome)

Osteogenesis imperfecta is characterized by brittle bones and is usually inherited as an autosomal dominant trait. The underlying defect is in type I collagen formation. At least five subtypes of this disorder are recognized (Table 17-1).

The general characteristics are that the bones are capable of growing to their normal length but are abnormally thin and weak (Fig. 17-2). Multiple fractures follow minimal or unnoticed trauma, and the most severe form (type II—autosomal recessive) is lethal as a result of multiple fractures in utero and almost complete failure of ossification of the skull.

About 80% of cases are type I. They suffer multiple fractures in childhood and usually therefore become grossly deformed (Fig. 17-3). The thin sclerae appear blue, and there is hearing loss resulting from overgrowth of soft spongy bone around the oval window or from fractures of the auditory ossicles. The joints tend also to be hypermobile and the aortic valves are thin. The teeth are frequently abnormally translucent with weak attachment of the enamel to the dentine (dentinogenesis imperfecta).

Microscopically, the bone is not merely reduced in amount but often woven in character (Fig. 17-4). The long bones typically have slender shafts but normal epiphyses, giving them a trumpetlike shape. Fracture healing is not delayed but usually leads to distortion of the bones.

Osteopetrosis

Osteopetrosis is a genetically heterogeneous group of disorders characterized by defective osteoclast function. As a consequence, there are failure of normal bone modeling, formation of abnormally dense bone with loss of differentiation between cortical and cancellous types, and complete or almost complete obliteration of medullary spaces. Anemia and widespread extramedullary hemopoiesis and other effects such as cranial

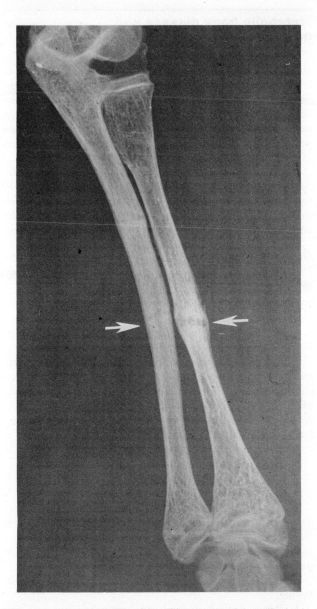

FIG. 17-2. Osteogenesis imperfecta. The bones are abnormally slender and have a delicate structure. There have been fractures through the middle of both the radius and the ulna, which have healed *(arrows)*.

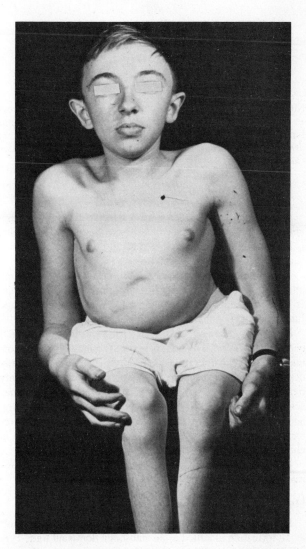

FIG. 17-3. Osteogenesis imperfecta. In this autosomal dominant disease, this boy has gross deformities as a result of multiple fractures.

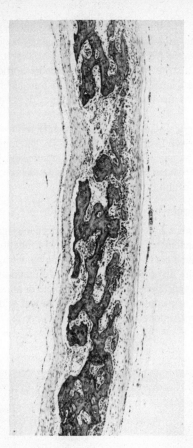

FIG. 17-4. Osteogenesis imperfecta. This section of the skull from an affected infant shows the thin, poorly formed bone and failure of formation of inner and outer tables. *(From Cawson, RA: Essentials of dental surgery and pathology, ed 3, Edinburgh, Scotland, 1978, Churchill Livingstone.)*

nerve compression can therefore result. The bones, although abnormally dense, are weak and fracture readily; osteomyelitis is a recognized complication as a result of the impaired blood supply.

Microscopically, in the less severe cases there may be an attempt to form normal lamellar bone but the medullary cavity is replaced with bone containing minute marrow spaces and little or no hemopoietic tissue.

Blindness, deafness, and facial palsy result from cranial nerve compression. The dominant type is compatible with normal survival with only occasional effects such as those already described, or even absence of symptoms, and discovered only by chance on routine radiography. Intermediate forms are characterized by ricketslike skeletal disease, renal tubular acidosis, and deficiency of carbonic anhydrase II. In the most severe, recessive type, hemopoiesis is so much impaired that death in childhood from anemia, hemorrhage or infections is usual.

Early onset osteopetrosis can be treated successfully by bone marrow transplantation.

Marfan's syndrome

Marfan's syndrome* is a relatively common defect of collagen formation inherited as an autosomal dominant trait. Typical features are a tall slender body habitus with arachnodactyly,

---
*J.A. Marfan (1858-1942), French pediatrician.

dislocations of the lens, and cardiovascular defects. It has been suggested that Abraham Lincoln had Marfan's syndrome because of his build and facial appearance, but this is contradicted by his broad strong hands.

The underlying defects include unstable cross-linkage and increased solubility of the collagen molecule or other defects in type I collagen, but they do not explain the abnormal skeletal morphology.

Clinically, there is considerable variation in expression of Marfan's syndrome. In addition to the typical body habitus, about 50% of patients have mild to severe ectopia lentis and up to 90% of patients have mitral valve prolapse and regurgitation. Aortic dilatation and regurgitation are less common but more serious, and the main cause of shortened expectation of life is aortic dissection (Chapter 10). Aortic and mitral valve dysfunction may be associated with hypermobile joints in some of these patients.

Metabolic bone disease and osteodystrophies

Bones can be affected by metabolic diseases, particularly, vitamin D deficiency. The underlying causes of such diseases are outside the skeleton and usually correctable. *Osteodystrophies* is a term sometimes given to bone diseases, which are neither inflammatory nor neoplastic but are caused by some intrinsic defect of bone formation or of skeletal maintenance activity. Some of these disorders are genetic while others are of unknown etiology.

In the study of metabolic bone disease, morphometric methods are valuable. Quantitation of bone mineral and its turnover can be carried out by means of quantitative image analysis microscopy, dual photon absorptiometry, and bone scintigraphy which allow progress of the disorder to be accurately evaluated.

Osteoporosis

Osteoporosis is characterized by loss of all elements of bone. It is an almost invariable consequence of aging, particularly in women. Although in itself asymptomatic, it is an important contributory cause of some 1,500,000 fractures in the elderly in the United States alone and is therefore of considerable public concern.

Etiology and pathogenesis. Two types of osteoporosis may be recognized. Type I mainly affects postmenopausal women and is characterized by accelerated loss particularly of trabecular bone. Type II mainly develops after the age of 70, affects women twice as frequently as males, and is characterized by both cortical and trabecular bone loss.

Factors determining osteoporosis include the following:
1. Aging (the most important factor)
2. Loss of estrogenic activity after the menopause
3. Initial (peak) bone mass

The initial bone mass is, in turn, affected by calcium intake earlier in life, fluoride content of the drinking water, physical activity, and race—whites, in general, have less bone mass than blacks. Calcium absorption also decreases with aging and parathyroid function may change.

Factors which can contribute to osteoporosis are the following:
1. Drugs, particularly long-term corticosteroids
2. Diseases causing increased bone loss
   a. Hyperthyroidism
   b. Cushing's syndrome

c. Lactase deficiency (low intake of milk products)

d. Hemiplegia

e. Early oophorectomy and subtotal gastrectomy

Biochemically, calcium absorption and metabolism of vitamin D [25-OH-D to 1,25(OH)$_2$] are decreased in both types of osteoporosis, whereas parathyroid function is decreased in type I but increased in type II.

After the age of about 40, bone loss usually begins, and there is slow loss particularly of trabecular bone which is metabolically more active. After menopause, women experience an accelerated loss of cortical bone for some years. Calcium absorption also decreases with aging. In addition, there may be increased serum levels of parathormone, but the role of calcitonin is uncertain.

However, the precise pathogenesis of the process and, in particular perhaps, the role of estrogens is unclear. Despite the far greater prevalence of osteoporosis in women and the acceleration of bone loss after oophorectomy, serum levels of sex steroids in postmenopausal women are not lower in those with osteoporosis compared with normal subjects.

Microscopically, bone remodeling appears to be a cyclic process. At the start of the cycle, osteoclasts appear and for about 2 weeks remove areas of trabecular or cortical bone. Osteoclasts are followed by osteoblasts that, depending on age, replace more or less of the resorbed bone with resulting increase or decrease in final bone mass. In slow (senile) osteoporosis replacement bone is deficient, whereas in accelerated, postmenopausal bone loss there is excessive osteoclastic activity. In either case the reduction in osteoblastic activity is probably the result of the decreased synthesis of several growth factors that appear to be regulators of bone remodeling activity. There is no significant qualitative abnormality of the bone, and no significant reduction in the ratio of the mineral to organic phases of the bone. This quantitative change is therefore most obvious microscopically, as decrease in the number and thinning of the trabeculae.

The progressive loss of bone in relation to its overall volume results in it becoming less dense radiographically. Recently, however, as mentioned earlier, more precise densitometry and quantitation of bone turnover is now possible by such methods as single or dual photon absorptiometry and quantitative computed tomography using single energy scanning.

Prevention. The process of osteoporosis can be slowed to some degree. Drugs currently approved for this purpose by the Food and Drug Administration are calcium, estrogens, and calcitonin, which decrease bone resorption and may induce a small increase in bone mass. However, estrogens carry with them the possible risks of cardiovascular disease and endometrial carcinoma. Fluoride and calcium supplementation increase bone mass but the toxic effects of the fluoride make such regimens unacceptable.

Rickets and osteomalacia

Rickets is a childhood disease characterized by defective mineralization particularly of epiphyseal cartilage in the developing bones. Osteomalacia has a similar pathogenesis but affects adults, in whom there is failure of bone replacement in the normal process of bone turnover.

Etiology and pathogenesis. Causes of or factors contributing to these diseases include the following:

1. Nutritional deficiency of vitamin D

2. Failure of vitamin D synthesis in the skin, due to lack of sunlight and marginal intake

3. Vitamin D loss in malabsorption syndromes

4. Renal disease with impaired vitamin D activation and decreased absorption of calcium

5. Inactivation of dietary vitamin D by phenytoin

6. Excessive calcium demands particularly as a result of pregnancy and lactation

The mechanism of production of osteomalacia by anticonvulsants is the induction of hepatic microsomal enzymes, which reduce 25-hydroxy vitamin D availability for renal hydroxylation.

In addition a group of rare polymorphous tumors of bone and soft tissues can cause osteomalacia or rickets.

Vitamin D is abundant in fish liver oil and to a lesser extent in animal livers, but only in small amounts in other natural components of the diet. Synthesis of vitamin D in the skin under the influence of sunlight is important. Rickets and osteomalacia can therefore result from a dietary deficiency in poorly nourished communities, but the disease is also seen in dark-skinned persons deprived of sunlight. Examples are certain strict Muslim communities who keep their infants indoors for long periods and immigrant populations living in areas, such as the northern parts of Britain, where there is relatively little sunlight. There is also evidence that, in this latter group, a contributory factor may be the eating of whole-meal flour, which contains substances such as phytates and fiber that bind to calcium and impair its absorption. Osteomalacia is most likely to develop in adult women as a result of the demands for calcium placed on them by pregnancy and lactation. If calcium absorption is marginal, this increased loss is sufficient to cause the disease.

Malabsorption states impair the absorption of all fats, including those containing vitamin D. Osteomalacia can therefore result from *steatorrhea* (fatty diarrhea) of any cause (Chapter 14).

Chronic renal insufficiency can cause osteomalacia, not merely because of excess calcium loss but also because the kidneys are probably no longer able to synthesize the active metabolite of vitamin D.

Pathology. The basic abnormality in both rickets and osteomalacia is defective mineralization of osteoid. An increased amount of osteoid matrix also forms, and as a result the bones may be thickened although inadequately mineralized.

The changes in rickets are complex because of its effects on endochondral ossification. These changes follow:

1. Failure of provisional calcification as a result of failure of mineralization of cartilage

2. Overgrowth of cartilage because of failure of cartilage cells to calcify, mature, and be removed (Fig. 17-5)

3. Deposition of osteoid matrix on persistent cartilage with the result that the architecture of the osteochondral junction becomes grossly disordered

4. Ingrowth of fibroblasts and capillaries into the osteochondral junction, increasing its disorganization

In radiographs the epiphyseal plates of the long bones are seen as thick, wide, uneven, and irregular (Fig. 17-6).

Clinical aspects. In rickets the bones become weak and readily deformed. The abnormally soft vault of the skull can be indented with a finger but springs back when the finger is removed (craniotabes). The chest is characteristically deformed. The costochondral junctions are swollen, producing the "rachitic rosary," whereas the lower ribs are indented at the site of the attachment of the diaphragm. In the absence of treatment, progressive deformities of the pelvis and extremities

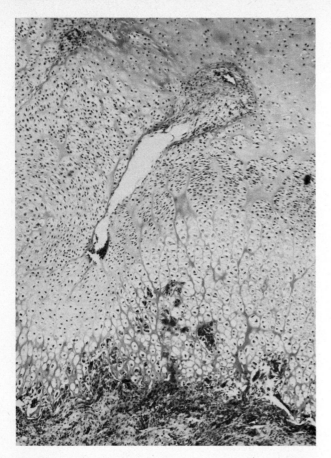

FIG. 17-5. Rickets. There is grossly irregular overgrowth of the epiphyseal cartilage and failure to form the uniform, parallel columns of cells that normally immediately precede provisional calcification, which is also absent. Calcification is replaced by proliferating connective tissue, which is invading the cartilage from its deep aspect. *(From Cawson RA: Essentials of dental surgery and pathology, ed 4, Edinburgh, Scotland, 1984, Churchill Livingstone.)*

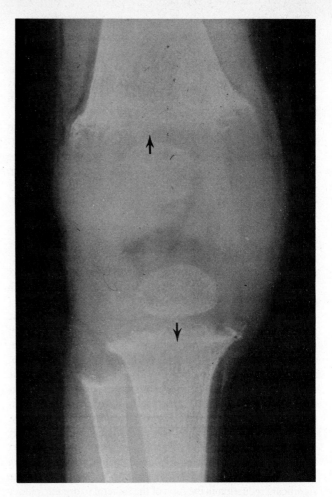

FIG. 17-6. Rickets. Note that the epiphyseal ends of the bones, particularly the tibia and fibula, are grossly irregular *(arrows)* due to failure of calcification but continued production of connective tissue. *(From Cawson RA: Essentials of dental surgery and pathology, ed 4, Edinburgh, Scotland, 1984, Churchill Livingstone.)*

develop (see Fig. 6-3). The bones also fracture easily but often incompletely (greenstick fractures).

In addition to having skeletal changes, infants and young children are often listless and irritable, and the muscles are weak and hypotonic. Eventually the child may become unable to walk without support.

Occasionally rickets can be so severe that the resulting hypocalcemia causes tetany, laryngeal spasm, or convulsions due to increased neuromuscular excitability.

In osteomalacia the osseous changes are essentially similar to those of rickets but predominantly affect membranous bone. Inadequate mineralization and an excess of unmineralized osteoid matrix produce weak bone with a coarse pattern. Deformity of weight-bearing bones is therefore the most obvious consequence.

The management of rickets and osteomalacia is to ensure an adequate intake of vitamin D and calcium. Complications, such as deformity of the bones, must also be treated.

Renal osteodystrophy

Renal osteodystrophy differs etiologically from dialysis osteodystrophy (see following discussion). However, both fre-

quently coexist, since patients in end-stage renal failure are likely to be maintained by dialysis.

Pathogenesis. Increased secretion of parathyroid hormone is detectable early in renal failure. The probable cause is progressive failure of phosphate excretion by the renal tubule. The resulting hyperphosphatemia leads to a reciprocal hypocalcemia and stimulation of parathyroid secretion, which for a time, can restore normal calcium homeostasis at the cost of bone resorption.

As insufficiency advances the kidney loses its ability to respond to parathyroid hormone. Severe hyperphosphatemia, hypocalcemia, and hyperparathyroidism result. The effect on the skeleton is accelerated bone turnover with an excess of resorption over replacement. In addition, there is incomplete calcification of osteoid, and osteomalacia results.

Histologically, there are increased numbers of osteoclasts and osteoblasts, deep Howship's lacunae, and an excess of osteoid. In addition, there is deposition of fibrous tissue in the marrow spaces (osteitis fibrosa) but only in close juxtaposition to the bone surfaces and hemopoiesis is not impaired.

Osteomalacia frequently also develops as a result of failure of the kidney to synthesize 1,25-hydroxy vitamin D, and this may be the prominent and more disabling feature.

Factors contributing to renal osteodystrophy include: (1) an increasingly negative calcium balance as a result of metabolic acidosis and (2) decreased intake of calcium in the form of dairy products.

Treatment of renal osteodystrophy is by control of serum phosphate by dietary restriction or administration of calcium carbonate, which will help to raise serum calcium levels and lessen bone loss.

Dialysis (aluminum-associated) bone disease

Although effective dialysis should restore normal calcium homeostasis, aluminum-associated bone disease may become superimposed on renal osteomalacia as a result of one of the following:
1. High aluminum content in the dialysis water
2. Increased intake of aluminum in antacids

Experimentally, aluminum injections will induce osteomalacia in normal animals, and removal of excess aluminum from dialysis fluids prevents the onset of this disease in humans.

Histologically, bone biopsies show that aluminum is deposited in the zone between the mineralized bone and osteoid. This suggests that the aluminum may interfere with the mineralization of osteoid. Aluminum is also deposited in bone in association with osteitis fibrosa but seems to have no effect on mineralization.

Clinically, the aggravation of renal osteodystrophy by aluminum causes bone pain and fragility. Aluminum dementia may be associated.

Transplant osteonecrosis

Another hazard for patients who have had renal or other transplants is aseptic necrosis of bone. This may affect 15% or more of transplant patients and becomes evident as bone pain after about 2 years. Weight-bearing bones are particularly affected. The most likely cause is the administration of corticosteroids, which can cause the following:
1. Aseptic necrosis of bone by unknown mechanisms
2. Osteoporosis by impairing protein metabolism

Patients on long-term corticosteroids for purposes other than organ transplantation also suffer bone loss by these mechanisms. Occasionally aseptic necrosis of bone has no apparent cause.

Dialysis arthropathy. In those who fail to receive a renal transplant, long-term survival on dialysis is frequently complicated by deposition in bones and synovia of recently characterized form of amyloid which is composed of β-2 microglobulin.

Clinically, there is carpal tunnel syndrome, pain, and stiffness—particularly of the shoulders, hips, hands, wrists and knees—which may be disabling. There is no treatment, but the disease can be prevented by use of a more porous dialysis membrane that allows excess β-2 microglobulin to escape.

Hyperparathyroidism

Overproduction of parathyroid hormone as a result of hyperplasia or a tumor of the gland can result in bone resorption, hypercalcemia, and tumorlike foci of giant cells which give the radiologic picture termed osteitis fibrosa cystica. These are shown in Figs. 18-22 and 18-23, and the condition is discussed further in that chapter.

Paget's disease (osteitis deformans)

This disease was described in 1867 by Sir James Paget* and is one of five diseases to which his name is attached. Paget's disease of bone is common and is characterized by localized or widespread distortion of the bony architecture as a result of an increased turnover of bone by both osteoclasts and osteoblasts. The effect of these changes is to produce thickening as well as weakening of the bones, which can distort under stress.

Etiology. Paget's disease affects mainly those of Anglo-Saxon descent and can be detected in some degree in 5% to 10%, although with considerable variation in prevalence from one area to another. There is also some evidence of a familial tendency.

There is no convincing evidence that the disease is (as Paget believed) inflammatory, and hypotheses that it might be hormonal or caused by a defect of collagen synthesis seem unacceptable because of the patchy distribution of the lesions with intervening areas of normal bone.

The possibility that Paget's disease might be infective is, however, suggested by reports of the ultrastructural and immunologic detection of intranuclear inclusions and of measles-related antigens in the osteoclasts.

If it can be established that Paget's disease has an infective component in its etiology, this might also explain the family clustering or variations in geographic distribution. However, the cause of Paget's disease currently remains controversial.

Pathology. The characteristic features are increased resorption and new bone formation, but, in the early stages at least, resorption predominates. Later, as the activity of the disease declines, there is progressively less resorption and eventually the formation of hard, dense, poorly vascularized bone (Fig. 17-7). This haphazard pattern of change also disturbs the gross architecture with the result that the differentiation between cortical and cancellous bone disappears.

The microscopic appearances are those of irregular destruction and reformation of bone, which destroys the normal haversian system (Fig. 17-8). Increased numbers of multinucleated osteoclasts and osteoblasts surround the margins of the bone trabeculae, and an irregular pattern of basophilic reversal lines is produced where bone resorption has stopped and new bone formation has started. This has been somewhat ineptly described as a *mosaic pattern*. The marrow spaces are filled with loose cellular fibroblastic connective tissue. The giant cells contain many more nuclei than typical osteoclasts and contain viral inclusions. The latter are not necessarily however the cause of the disease. Possible endogenous mediators of bone cell activity in Paget's disease have been investigated but without any conclusive result.

In addition to the bony changes, there is replacement of fatty and hemopoietic marrow with loose fibrous tissue and increased vascularity.

The disease may affect a single bone (monostotic) or be polyostotic. In the polyostotic type the axial skeleton is predominantly involved. The pelvis and sacrum are often the first site, but the process may involve the skull (Fig. 17-9), spine, and extremities. The monostotic type most often affects the tibia.

The affected bones are characteristically uniformly enlarged, thickened, relatively radiolucent, and can become bent under stress. In the early stages, particularly when the skull is in-

---

*Sir James Paget (1858-1942), English surgeon and pathologist.

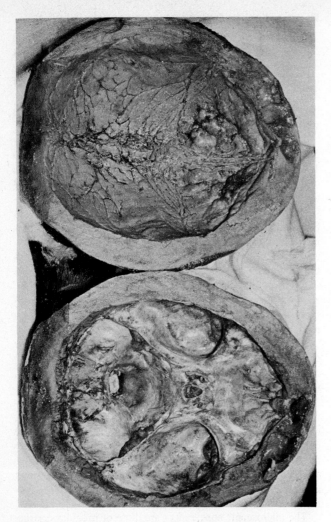

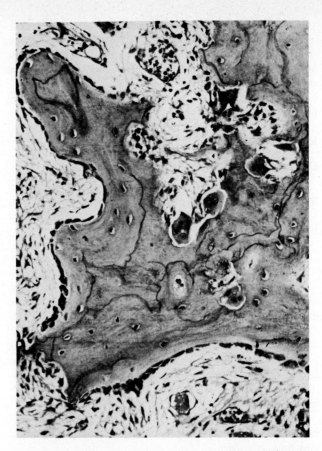

FIG. 17-8. Paget's disease. The bone is irregular due to repeated phases of resorption and reapposition, as shown by the dark irregular mosaic of reversal lines. The marrow has been replaced by fibrous connective tissue, and many osteoblasts and osteoclasts surround the bone edges.

FIG. 17-7. Paget's disease. The skull has become enlarged as a result of continued apposition of bone. At the same time the cortical plates have become obliterated, and the bone of the skull has become grossly thickened and featureless. *(Courtesy Curator of the Gordon Museum, Guy's Museum, London, England.)*

volved, large areas of radiolucency may be seen. In some cases there is intense pain, unresponsive to analgesics, in affected bones. The upper jaw is infrequently affected (Fig. 17-10) and the mandible hardly ever. Typical changes are gross, symmetric, rounded thickening of the alveolar ridge.

The increased osteoblastic and osteoclastic activity is reflected by the urine hydroxyproline and serum alkaline phosphatase levels, which can be higher than those in any other disease when lesions are widespread. Serum calcium and phosphate levels are typically normal.

Clinical aspects. Mild cases have no symptoms, and radiographic signs of the disease can be detected in about 1% of the population of the United States. Recent surveys have reported higher figures in Britain. Men are affected more frequently than women, and symptoms typically become apparent in the elderly.

A complication of Paget's disease, in addition to deformities or pathologic fractures, is compression of cranial nerves so that deafness or visual disturbances may result. Another complication is the greatly increased blood flow within the abnormal bone, which acts in effect as an arteriovenous fistula and can

ultimately cause heart failure. The most serious complication is the development of osteogenic sarcoma. This is unusual in that osteogenic sarcoma is otherwise a disease of younger people, but in Paget's disease it affects the elderly. The incidence of sarcomatous change varies in different studies. It is about 1% in cases with symptomatic Paget's disease but probably develops in no more than 0.1% of all cases of Paget's disease.

The lesions in the different parts of the body do not necessarily progress at the same rate or synchronously with one another. The extent of the disease is determined radiographically; the activity of the process is indicated by serum alkaline phosphatase and urine hydroxyproline levels, which can also be used as indices of the effectiveness of treatment.

In patients with symptoms sufficiently severe enough to require treatment a wide variety of drugs has been tried, including fluorides, glucagon, and mithramycin (a drug cytotoxic to osteoclasts), which are at least partially effective. Currently, however, the most promising agents are calcitonin and diphosphonates.

Fibrous dysplasia of bone

Fibrous dysplasia and related fibroosseous lesions form a controversial area of bone pathology. Fibrous dysplasia is probably most usefully defined as a developmental disorder characterized by early onset, active growth during childhood, and cessation of activity in adult life, when the remainder of the

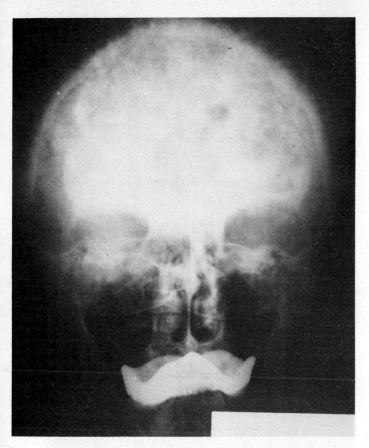

FIG. 17-9. Radiograph of the skull in Paget's disease. The vault is thickened, and there are areas of bone formation or destruction scattered irregularly throughout the skull, giving a moth-eaten appearance.

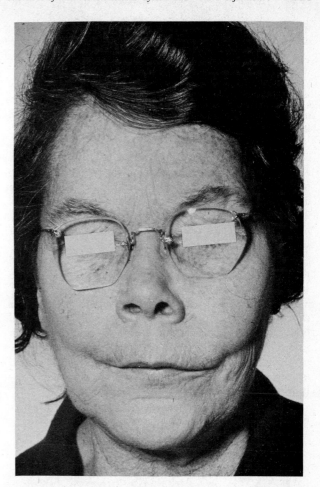

FIG. 17-10. Paget's disease of the maxilla. The maxillae are almost symmetrically enlarged. In the process the nostrils have been pulled outward, and the alar folds have become obliterated.

skeleton matures. In the initial stages one or more areas of bone are replaced by cellular connective tissue. The connective tissue is progressively replaced by woven bone until a mainly osseous, inactive lesion is left.

By no means all diseases thought to be fibrous dysplasia fit into such a well-defined pattern, however, and histologically similar lesions sometimes behave more like true neoplasms.

Monostotic fibrous dysplasia most often affects the facial bones, particularly the maxilla, and is discussed later. Less frequently, fibrous dysplasia is polyostotic.

Albright's syndrome* is the name given to polyostotic fibrous dysplasia characterized by multiple bone lesions, patchy pigmentation of the skin, and endocrine disturbances, particularly precocious puberty. Girls are mainly affected by this rare syndrome.

Acute osteomyelitis

Acute suppurative osteomyelitis is the most important infection of bone. Although at one time common, disabling, or lethal, it is now uncommon and has much less severe effects.

Acute osteomyelitis of a long bone is typically an infection of childhood and is the result of transient bacteremia from some primary focus of infection elsewhere. Osteomyelitis caused by direct infection as a result of an open fracture is now rare.

Acute osteomyelitis of the jaw is typically a complication of local (dental) infection and is discussed later.

---

*Fuller Albright (1900-1969), American physician.

Etiology and pathogenesis. The principal bacterium causing suppurative osteomyelitis is *Staphylococcus aureus.* Other agents are streptococci, pneumococci, gonococci, *Haemophilus influenzae,* coliform bacilli, and, less often, anaerobes. Salmonella osteomyelitis is a recognized complication of sickle cell disease.

The first main factor in the pathogenesis of typical acute osteomyelitis is bacteremia from a primary focus of infection. This may be, for example, a staphylococcal skin infection. Second, there has to be a vulnerable site, such as a hematoma, where the bacteria can settle and proliferate. This is provided by bleeding from the fragile vessels of the epiphyseal plate, where the rate of blood flow is slow and the vessel wall is readily torn by minor injuries. This is the usual site where acute osteomyelitis begins.

Pathology. Osteomyelitis is a typical acute inflammatory reaction involving the soft tissues within the marrow cavity and bone, but the process is modified by the hard tissue. The main features are:

1. Spread of infection and necrosis of bone
2. Bone resorption
3. New bone formation and repair

The acute inflammatory reaction is characterized by hyperemia and the outpouring of fluid exudate and inflammatory cells, especially polymorphonuclear leukocytes. The bone cannot stretch to accommodate the exudate, which as a consequence is forced further along the marrow spaces, spreading the infection. Vessels in the bony canals are also compressed and may thrombose. This obstruction to the blood supply and the effects of bacterial toxins cause an area of bone to die.

Bacteria proliferate freely, protected by this necrotic tissue. Dead bone can be recognized under the microscope by the absence of osteocytes from the lacunae and is associated with large numbers of polymorphonuclear leukocytes (Fig. 17-11).

At the junction between dead and living bone, osteoclasts resorb the bone and eventually separate it. Resorption of bone also forms sinuses through which pus can escape into the subperiosteal region. The periosteum, as a consequence, becomes distended with purulent exudate and stripped from the bone, thereby further reducing the blood supply. Later the periosteum may be perforated by pus, which can form a sinus through the soft tissues to discharge on the skin surface.

The dead bone is known as a *sequestrum* and corresponds to the dead tissue formed in severe infections of soft tissues, such as an abscess.

At the margins of the area of infection and inflammation, new bone starts to form as part of the healing reaction. New bone also forms under the periosteum, where it has been distended by pus (Fig. 17-12). In this way a complete casing of new bone, known as an *involucrum*, can form eventually around the original bone, but this is rare now that effective treatment is available.

Where bone has died, been separated, and removed, the gap fills with granulation tissue as in any other wound. Coarse,

fibrous bone forms in this connective tissue and is then gradually remodeled almost to the form of the original bone.

This classic picture of osteomyelitis of a long bone with extensive involucrum formation is only seen now in museum specimens.

Complications include extension into the adjacent joint causing suppurative arthritis, but this too is exceedingly rare. Rarely the infection becomes walled off by granulation tissue, forming a chronic localized abscess known as Brodie's abscess. This in turn becomes enclosed by bone as a result of reactive osteoblastic activity. Garré's sclerosing osteomyelitis is the name given to thickening of the periosteum and dense, subperiosteal new bone formation.

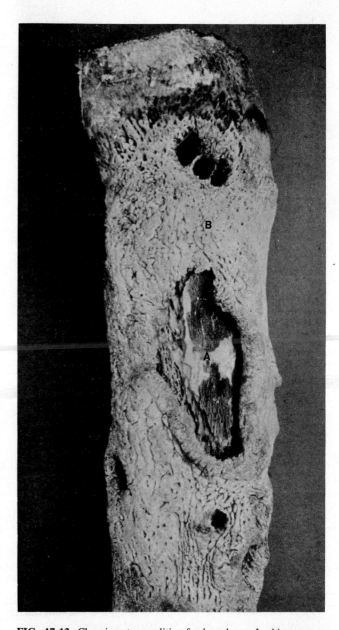

FIG. 17-12. Chronic osteomyelitis of a long bone. In this museum specimen of a case from the past, the original bone has become encased in an involucrum as a result of continued bone formation by the periosteum, which has become distended by pus. The involucrum is perforated by cloacae, which are the sinuses through which pus is discharged. In the center *(A)*, dead bone (sequestrum) can be seen within the involucrum *(B)*. *(Courtesy Curator of the Gordon Museum, Guy's Hospital, London, England.)*

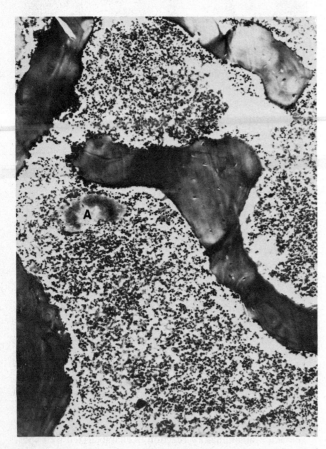

FIG. 17-11. Acute osteomyelitis. The bone trabeculae are necrotic, and their surface is rough and irregular due to earlier osteoclastic action. The marrow has been destroyed, and the bone trabeculae are surrounded by pus cells in which a colony of bacteria *(A)* can be seen.

Clinical aspects. Acute osteomyelitis causes a severe systemic febrile illness with severe bone pain, tenderness, redness, and swelling. Blood cultures are usually positive during the most acute phase. Bone sclerosis (seen as ill-defined areas of increased radiopacity) and bone destruction (seen as areas of increased radiolucency) are not seen in radiographs until after 10 days.

In the past, osteomyelitis was so persistent an infection that secondary amyloid formation was a recognized complication. Now the disease can be effectively managed by large doses of penicillin or other antibiotics and surgical drainage.

Osteomyelitis of the jaws. Although the jaws are part of the skull, osteomyelitis of the mandible, is usually a much less serious infection than when long bones are affected.

Patients are almost invariably adults, and the infection is dental in origin. Anaerobes or gram-negative enteric bacteria are the main organisms responsible, unless infection has resulted from an open fracture or gunshot wound.

Ischemia of the jaws following radiotherapy for cancer in this area makes the jaws susceptible to severe and intractable infection, which may result in necrosis of the overlying skin or mucosa and exposure of an extensive area of the mandible to the exterior. Even under such circumstances, however, there may be little systemic disturbance (Chapter 5).

Osteomyelitis of the maxilla in a newborn is a rare but recognized entity. It is thought to be secondary to local injury by the fingers of a physician or midwife during delivery.

Neoplasms and tumorlike lesions of bone

The most common tumors of bone are *metastatic* and have spread from sites such as the bronchus, breast, prostate, kidney, or thyroid and hence are carcinomas.

Primary bone tumors. Most primary tumors of bone are sarcomas and exhibit osseous and/or cartilaginous differentiation. Others are fibrous or formed from other normal soft tissue elements of bone such as blood vessels or nerves; they will not be discussed further here. The hemopoietic (lymphoreticular) tissues of the bone marrow (somewhat paradoxically) are not major sources of bone tumors, and the only important example is multiple myeloma (Chapter 13). Multiple myeloma is a multifocal, osteolytic tumor of plasma cells. Ewing's sarcoma is a rare undifferentiated mesenchymal sarcoma of bone, the cells of which resemble lymphoreticular cells. Despite the resemblance, this tumor is no longer believed to be of hemopoietic origin, as discussed later.

The infrequency of primary bone tumors can be judged by the fact that even in a center such as the Mayo Clinic fewer than 4,000 specimens had been seen in a period of 57 years.

A simplified classification of bone tumors follows:
1. Bone-forming tumors
   a. Benign
      (1) Osteoma
      (2) Osteoid osteoma and osteoblastoma
   b. Malignant
      (1) Osteosarcoma
2. Cartilage-forming tumors
   a. Benign
      (1) Osteochondroma
      (2) Enchondroma
      (3) Chondromyxoid fibroma
      (4) Chondroblastoma

   b. Malignant
      (1) Chondrosarcoma
3. Giant cell tumors
4. Lymphoreticular tumors
   a. Myeloma
   b. Lymphoma
   c. Eosinophilic granuloma
5. Vascular, neural, and other tumors
   a. Benign
      (1) Hemangioma
      (2) Neurofibroma and neurilemmoma
   b. Malignant
      (1) Angiosarcoma
      (2) Neurofibrosarcoma
      (3) Malignant fibrous histiocytoma
      (4) Undifferentiated and other sarcomas
      (5) Ewing's tumor

It should be noted first, that tumors of osseous tissues, notably osteosarcomas can form both bone and cartilage. Second, it is not always possible to make a firm distinction between benign and malignant bone tumors from their microscopical appearances alone. Apparently benign chondromas, in particular, sometimes prove to be chondrosarcomas. Giant cell tumors and fibrous histiocytomas show variable degrees of aggressiveness and propensity for recurrence.

It should be emphasized therefore that many of these tumors are morphologically similar, and microscopic diagnosis can be difficult. Therefore the diagnosis should always be based on the following:
1. Clinical history
2. Radiographic appearances
3. Histopathology
4. Biochemical investigations

Osteoma

Osteomas are usually regarded as hamartomas, although some may be true tumors. Osteomas form slowly growing, predominantly cancellous or lamellated masses on the surface of bones particularly of the craniofacial skeleton. Removal may be required for cosmetic reasons.

Osteochondroma (cartilage capped exostosis)

Osteochondromas differ from osteomas only in that they have an actively growing cap resembling epiphyseal cartilage, overlying a cancellous bony mass, and particularly affect the long bones.

These exostoses typically develop during childhood and growth of the cartilaginous cap usually ceases with skeletal maturation. Radiographically, they form a mushroomlike or cauliflowerlike opaque mass. Histologically, identical lesions are seen in the condition of multiple hereditary exostoses in which malignant change may occasionally develop.

Osteoid osteoma

Osteoid osteoma is a common tumor particularly of long bones and, although benign, is characteristically painful.

Microscopically, the center of the tumor consists of a nidus of highly vascular osteogenic connective tissue and consists of either fibroblastic connective tissue or a network of osteoid trabeculae, or is heavily calcified. The peripheral bone is usually sclerotic.

Clinical features. Over 95% of patients with this tumor are aged between 5 and 24; males are 2 to 3 times as frequently affected as women. The tibia and femur are the most common sites but may form in almost any bone, although rarely in the skull and jaws.

Pain is the main symptom and is sometimes severe. The typical radiographic appearance is a well-defined, rounded area of radiolucency with peripheral sclerosis, usually just deep to the cortical surface. The appearance may mimic sclerosing osteomyelitis.

The behavior of this tumor is unpredictable. Occasionally symptoms regress spontaneously; in other cases the lesion remains static or, rarely, increases in size. However, curettage is likely to lead to recurrence and a block of bone containing the tumor should be excised.

Osteoblastoma

This tumor is somewhat similar to the osteoid osteoma and is sometimes termed giant osteoid osteoma. It differs mainly in that it more frequently affects the vertebrae or bones of the fingers and tends to form larger masses than osteoid osteomas, and in its microscopic appearances.

Microscopically, osteoblastoma consists of highly cellular, vascular connective tissue and osteoid. Irregular trabeculae of bone and osteoid form in profusion, and the cellularity is such as sometimes to mimic, in some degree, an osteosarcoma except for the lack of nuclear pleomorphism or anaplasia.

Osteosarcoma (osteogenic sarcoma)

Osteosarcoma is the most common *primary* malignant tumor of bone.

Nothing is known of the etiology except that a few cases either develop in Paget's disease late in life or are a sequel of irradiation of bone. Bone sarcomas were a recognized complication of the ingestion of radioactive material used at one time in the painting of luminous watch dials.

Pathology. Osteosarcoma (Fig. 17-13) consists of malignant osteoblasts and a neoplastic stroma with osteoid, bone, or cartilage formed by the tumor cells. The malignant osteoblasts are also pleomorphic and hyperchromatic and may show bizarre mitoses. In some parts of the neoplasm, osteoid or bone may predominate. Other parts may consist mainly of neoplastic connective tissue or cartilage. Foci of multinucleated giant cells may also be seen.

In view of the wide varieties of appearance, the criterion for making the diagnosis of osteosarcoma is the formation of osteoid or immature bone. The prognosis, however, may be somewhat better in the predominantly fibroblastic or chondroblastic types of tumor.

Clinical aspects. The incidence of osteogenic sarcoma is not known precisely, but in Sweden it was found to affect less than five per million of the population. The peak age incidence is between 10 and 20 years, except in cases secondary to Paget's disease or irradiation. The disease is more common in males than females.

The metaphyses of long bones are predominantly affected, particularly the leg just above or below the knee joint. Osteosarcoma is rare in the jaws as compared with other bones.

The presenting symptoms are pain and swelling. The symptoms are usually of short duration, sometimes only for a few

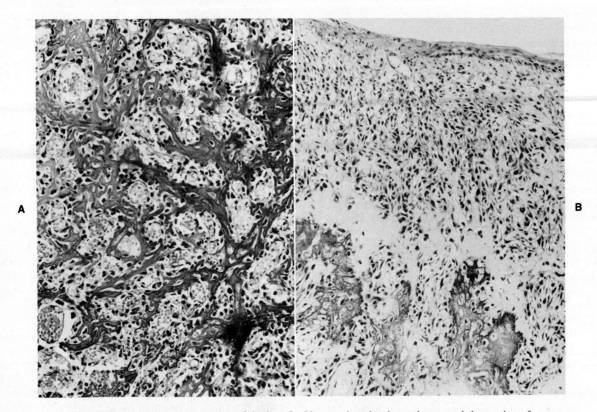

FIG. 17-13. A, Osteogenic sarcoma of the jaw. In this area there has been almost total destruction of the normal bone and replacement by a network of calcifying osteoid. Malignant osteoblasts are present in large numbers and are conspicuous by their widely variable size, form, and depth of staining. **B,** Osteogenic sarcoma. The dark, angular malignant osteoblasts extend up close under the oral epithelium. More deeply, tumor osteoid has formed.

weeks, but at most a matter of a few months. By then the tumor has usually already penetrated the cortex and is invading the surrounding soft tissues to form a large swelling. (Fig. 17-14).

The radiographic features are irregular and patchy bone destruction and new bone formation. As the tumor raises the periosteum from the cortex, long radiating spicules of new bone may form to produce an appearance known as sun-ray spiculation (Fig. 17-15).

Spread is predominantly by the bloodstream, almost exclusively to the lungs. Multiple rounded secondary deposits of varying degrees of radiopacity are characteristically formed and are known as cannonball metastases. Metastasis to the lung is present in more than 90% of fatal cases.

Diagnosis by biopsy is absolutely essential, since surgical treatment is drastic and must be carried out as soon as the diagnosis is confirmed.

The main line of treatment is traditionally surgical with the margins of the excision well away from the apparent area of the tumor. This may mean disarticulating the leg at the hip. More recently, cytotoxic chemotherapy has been used alone or in combination with excision. Five-year survival rates of up to 40% are now possible in some countries. Nevertheless, other factors such as earlier diagnosis have probably affected the prognosis in recent years.

Osteosarcoma subtypes. In addition to the variety of microscopic appearances, osteosarcomas are also subdivided according to site:

1. Medullary (the most common type)
2. Parosteal (juxtacortical)
3. Periosteal
4. Cortical

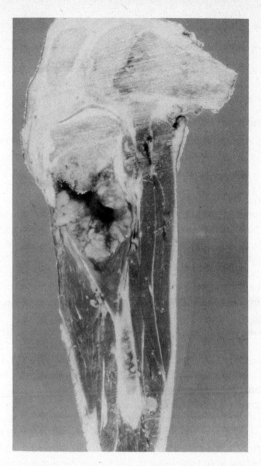

FIG. 17-14. Osteogenic sarcoma of the tibia. The tumor involves the metaphysis of the bone and extends into surrounding soft tissues.

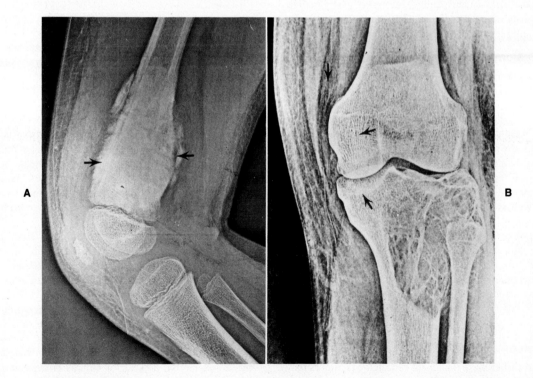

FIG. 17-15. Osteogenic sarcoma. These two xeroradiographs show the different appearances that may be seen. **A,** The tumor at the lower end of a child's humerus shows exstensive neoplastic new bone formation. **B,** Bone destruction is the predominant feature, but trabeculae of neoplastic new bone extend out into the soft tissues.

The last three subtypes tend to be better differentiated and have a somewhat better prognosis than the more common, medullary type.

Extraskeletal (soft tissue) osteosarcomas are another rare entity. They are morphologically identical to the osseous form, affect adults, and are highly malignant.

Chondroma

Chondroma is a benign tumor with, however, a tendency to recur after excision. It can be periosteal, or more frequently, within the bone (enchondroma). Multiple enchondromatosis (Ollier's disease) is an inborn anomaly of osseous development resulting in abnormal endochrondral ossification.

Chondromas are typically lobulated with a cut surface, which has the translucent bluish-white or yellowish appearance of cartilage. Microscopically, the cartilaginous structure is well defined and only slightly less regular than normal cartilage. However, it is important to examine as wide an area as possible to avoid missing a focus of sarcomatous change.

Clinically, adults are predominantly affected. Periosteal chondromas cause a swelling often with discomfort or pain. Enchondromas tend to be asymptomatic unless they are exceptionally large, and then they can cause pain or a pathologic fracture.

Chondromas form fairly well-defined radiolucent masses often containing calcifications.

Chondromas should be excised with as wide a margin of normal bone as possible, since they tend to recur. They can also undergo malignant change, although it is frequently difficult to distinguish a well-differentiated chondrosarcoma from a chondroma. In this situation, the size of the tumor is critical; cartilaginous tumors exceeding 6 cm are in all likelihood, malignant. Furthermore, tumors arising in the axial skeleton or long bones close to the torso, are usually malignant. Those in distal locations, such as hands and feet are usually benign. The risk of malignant transformation is substantially greater in patients with multiple enchondromatosis.

Chondroblastoma

This uncommon tumor, can be mistaken for a sarcoma. It particularly affects the epiphyseal regions of long bones of males between the ages of 10 and 20. The tumor usually forms a rounded or lobulated mass, which can be conspicuously destructive as well as expansive. Radiographically, the tumor appears as cloudy, relatively radiolucent mass containing flecks or cottonwool-like areas of radiopacity so that, in combination with the clinical features, malignancy is readily suspected.

Microscopically, chondroblastoma is typically a highly cellular tumor with great variation in the appearance of different fields.

The cells are predominantly rounded with conspicuous nucleoli but usually some spindle-shaped cells and often, giant cells are also seen. Separating the cells are areas of chondroid tissue with variable amounts of calcification.

The benign nature of this tumor is shown by its response to excision, but this should be complete if recurrence is to be avoided.

Chondrosarcoma

As implied earlier these malignant cartilaginous tumors may be primary or originate in chondromas.

Pathology. Chondrosarcomas within long bones cause expansion and destruction. The margins appear well defined but

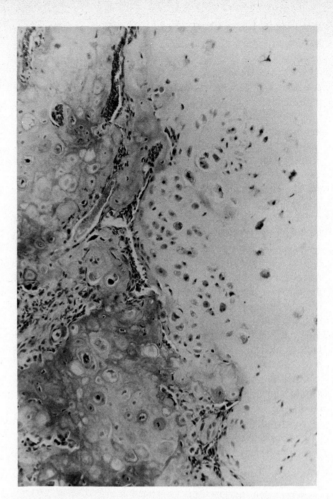

FIG. 17-16. Chondrosarcoma showing the disorderly and pleomorphic malignant chondrocytes.

often there is destruction of the cortex and spread into the soft tissues. The cut surface of the tumor usually appears lobulated and cartilaginous with flecks of calcification.

Microscopically, chondrosarcomas may be so well differentiated as to appear benign or so poorly differentiated as to be difficult to recognize as cartilaginous. A characteristic appearance is of poorly formed cartilage with variable staining and many nuclei (Fig. 17-16). The malignant chondrocytes are irregular in size and shape, whereas binucleate or even multinucleate chondrocytes are the hallmark of malignancy, especially if there is also mitotic activity. In the absence of such indicators, invasion of surrounding tissues confirms the malignancy of the tumor.

Microscopic diagnosis can be difficult, since chondrosarcomas must be distinguished from chondroblastic osteosarcomas which are more malignant. Foci of osteoid or bone formation must therefore be looked for by examining as great an area of tumor tissue as possible.

Clinically, chondrosarcomas are twice as common in men as in women; they are rare before the age of 20 years. The average age at the onset of symptoms is 45 years. Pain and swelling are typical effects but the less malignant, slowly growing tumors can be present for months or even years, and particularly when originating in the pelvis can reach an enormous size. Metastasis by the bloodstream is possible but a late feature.

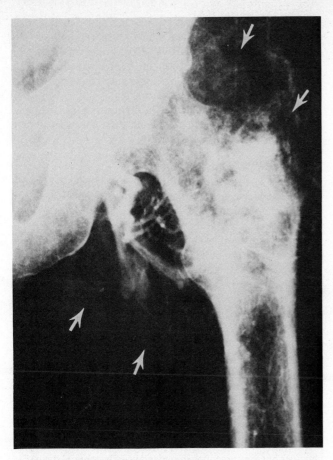

FIG. 17-17. Radiograph of chondrosarcoma of the head of a femur. The area in and around the hip joint is filled with a large tumor mass *(arrows)*. There is partial destruction of the femoral head and areas of new bone formation.

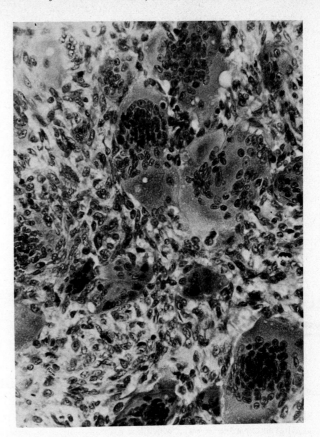

FIG. 17-18. Giant cell tumor of the tibia. The large multinucleate giant cells and the matrix of plump spindle-shaped cells can be seen.

The radiographic appearance (Fig. 17-17) is characteristic, namely a radiolucent, lobulated mass containing calcifications and projecting from, but also destroying, the bone of origin.

Treatment is by wide excision and this may necessitate removal of a limb. Chondrosarcomas also readily seed in the soft tissues after biopsy or inadequate excision so that local recurrence is relatively common and allowance must be made for reoperation.

The 10-year survival rates vary from 35% to about 70%.

Mesenchymal chondrosarcoma. Mensenchymal chondrosarcoma is an uncommon variant consisting essentially of poorly differentiated, malignant chondroblasts. Therefore it is not readily recognizable as a chondrosarcoma except for the fact that occasional small islands of poorly formed chondroid tissue can be found. These tumors have a worse prognosis than conventional chondrosarcomas.

Giant cell tumors of bone

Giant cell tumors of bone are uncommon, aggressive, or occasionally frankly malignant tumors that typically affect young adults. Despite their destructive nature these tumors show an expansile pattern of growth; however, reactive new bone formation by surrounding osseous tissue probably contributes to this progress.

Pathology. Microscopically the conspicuous feature is the many giant cells (Fig. 17-18); these resemble osteoclasts but tend to be larger and to contain many more nuclei, which may be crowded within the cytoplasm. Between the giant cells is a vascular stroma of plump spindle cells. These are the essential tumor cells, and they sometimes form the main mass of the tumor; giant cells may then be relatively scanty.

Malignancy is shown by pleomorphism and anaplasia of the stromal cells of any degree up to frank sarcomatous change. Nevertheless, even histologically benign giant cell tumors may prove difficult to control by any form of treatment and prognosis deteriorates with each recurrence.

Clinical aspects. Giant cell tumors are rare in the young and their highest incidence is in the third decade; unusually for bone tumors they are more common in women.

Most giant cell tumors arise from the epiphyseal or metaphyseal region of a long bone and most frequently either immediately above or below the knee. The characteristic radiographic appearance (Fig. 17-19) is a soap-bubblelike radiolucent mass expanding the end of the bone, but not extending beyond the epiphyseal plate. A little reactive, periosteal new bone formation may be associated.

Behavior is variable and somewhat unpredictable; however, those with sarcomatous features behave accordingly. Probably only about 50% of these tumors follow a completely benign course.

To avoid mutilation or deformity, treatment by curettage may be attempted but is followed by recurrence in at least 50% of cases; lower recurrence rates are reported with cryosurgery. With infiltrative tumors resection is preferable as radiotherapy is of little value, and if there is gross destruction, amputation may be unavoidable.

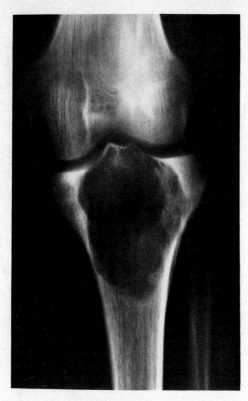

FIG. 17-19. Radiograph of a typical giant cell tumor of the tibia showing an expansile lesion in which fine trabeculation can be seen.

Giant cell tumors occasionally metastasize; spread is then by the bloodstream to the lungs. Although such an event is more probable in the case of poorly differentiated tumors it has also been reported in well-differentiated lesions.

Other giant cell lesions of bone

Giant cell tumors of bone must be distinguished from the following:
1. Giant cell-rich osteosarcomas
2. Giant cell lesions of hyperparathyroidism
3. Chondroblastoma
4. Central giant cell granulomas of the jaw
5. Giant cell lesions of Paget's disease
6. Cherubism
7. Aneurysmal bone cysts
8. Giant cell variant of fibrous histiocytoma

In the case of osteosarcomas, foci of giant cells may give a misleading impression but are only one feature of a far more pleomorphic picture than that of typical giant cell tumors.

Giant cell tumors of hyperparathyroidism tend to be multiple and associated with characteristic biochemical changes, particularly hypercalcemia (see Chapter 18). Giant cell granulomas of the jaws (which are not true neoplasms but probably reactive in nature) also tend to be difficult or impossible to distinguish by their microscopic features from true giant cell tumors but it is questionable whether any of the latter have been found in this site. Cherubism (formerly termed familial fibrous dysplasia) is an unusual giant cell lesion, histologically similar to the giant cell granuloma but appearing in childhood and symmetrically distributed; it is most common in the region of the angles of the jaws. It is an autosomal dominant trait but there are many sporadic cases. The lesions of cherubism tend to resolve spontaneously after adolescence.

The rare giant cell lesions of bone in Paget's disease also appear to be nonneoplastic and in many respects similar to the giant cell granulomas of the jaws. However, they are typically multifocal and are associated with the osseous and biochemical changes of Paget's disease. Unlike true giant cell tumors, these lesions appear to respond well to irradiation.

Giant cells may be numerous in fibrous dysplasia of bone or aneurysmal bone cysts but, overall, form only a small part of such lesions as discussed later.

Ewing's sarcoma

Ewing's sarcoma* is one of the most malignant neoplasms of bone but, fortunately, is rare. Its nature has long been controversial: it was thought by Ewing to arise from capillary endothelial cells. However, the tumor has been reported to be vimentin positive suggesting a connective tissue origin and that it arises from a primitive mesenchymal cell with no tendency to differentiation. It has also been reported that the tumor stains for neural markers; indeed in some cases the tumor has microscopic features somewhat similar to those of some neuroblastomas. This has led some to conclude that there can be neural differentiation in these aggressive neoplasms.

Pathology. Ewing's tumor usually arises in the medullary cavity of a long bone and spreads initially within this space before destroying the cortex and extending into the surrounding soft tissues. There is sometimes some reactive bone formation but no production of osteoid tissue by the tumor.

Microscopically, Ewing's sarcoma consists of nests of closely packed cells with large round nuclei but scanty cytoplasm with indistinct outlines. They superficially resemble lymphocytes but they are much larger and usually contain glycogen. These cells form broad bands and surround blood vessels often in an ill-defined rosettelike pattern. Unlike large cell lymphomas, Ewing's sarcoma lacks a framework of reticulin fibers between individual tumor cells.

Clinical features. Ewing's tumor is a disease of the young, most frequently between the ages of 10 and 30 years. The long bones of the arms or legs are the most common sites. Typical symptoms are pain and swelling which may eventually become severe enough to limit movement, but pathologic fracture is uncommon.

The radiographic features are nonspecific. They consist of a radiolucent area with bone destruction and patchy reactive bone formation. As with other bone tumors histologic examination is essential for diagnosis.

Anemia—and sometimes, leukocytosis—may be associated. Metastasis may be an early event. Metastasis is frequently atypical in that it is often to other bones, as well as to the liver, lungs, or even lymph nodes.

The choice of treatment depends on the age of the patient, the location of the tumor, and the stage of the disease. It usually consists of irradiation and/or cytotoxic chemotherapy. The 5 year survival rate is no more than 30% but varies with the anatomic site; the rare Ewing's sarcomas of the craniofacial skeleton for example have an unexpectedly good prognosis.

Fibrous histiocytoma of bone

Fibrous histiocytomas are described later among the soft tissue tumors, which share similar microscopic features and behavior. Fibrohistiocytic tumors form a rare group of neoplasms that can affect bone or soft tissues. They can be benign,

---

*James Ewing (1866-1943), American pathologist.

malignant, or intermediate in their behavior. Xanthogranulomas (xanthomas) are included in the benign category.

Malignant fibrous histiocytomas of bone affect an older age group than osteosarcomas. They are highly invasive and destructive tumors. Long bones are mainly affected and these tumors may occasionally complicate irradiation or Paget's disease of bone.

Microscopically, fibrous histiocytomas can present a variety of features but the essential characteristic is the presence of histiocyte-like cells among the tumor fibroblasts. The latter cells form tangled or knotted (storiform) patterns. In addition, there may be xanthomatous or myxoid areas or rarely a predominance of giant cells.

Clinically, fibrous histiocytomas have no distinctive features, but the malignant variants can cause local pain and can metastasize usually to the lungs.

Lymphoma of bone

Lymphomas form about 5% of primary bone tumors. They are mostly diffuse, large cell lymphomas (Chapter 13).

Clinical aspects. Males are affected at least twice as frequently as women. The long bones are usually affected and a large painful swelling often forms. Nevertheless, patients often appear surprisingly well until there is spread of tumor with extension into soft tissues or dissemination to other bones or lymphoid tissue.

The radiographic features of bone destruction with patchy reactive bone formation are nonspecific.

Overall, radiotherapy may be the most effective form of treatment, and 5-year survival rates of up to 50% have been reported.

Multiple myeloma

Multiple myeloma is an important although uncommon tumor affecting bone and is described in Chapter 13.

Secondary tumors of bone

As mentioned earlier metastatic tumors, which are virtually all carcinomas from various sites, are more common than primary tumors of bone. Since bones (apart from the jaws) normally contain no epithelial elements, epithelial tumors in most bones are, almost by definition, metastatic.

The bronchus and prostate are the most frequent sites of the primary tumors in males, whereas the breast is the most common site in females.

Bone metastases may be found in over 25% of patients dying from cancer but in 75% of those dying from cancer from the breast. The structure of metastases reproduces that of the primary tumor, but the effects on the bone varies. Metastases from the breast are usually osteolytic, producing areas of radiolucency with ragged margins. Metastases from the prostate can induce new bone formation and a sclerotic mass.

Bone metastases are sometimes the first sign of a neoplasm; back pain resembling rheumatism is a typical symptom or less frequently there may be a pathologic fracture.

Tumors and tumorlike lesions of the jaws

In terms of tumors, the jaws differ from the remainder of the skeleton in two important respects. First, primary bone tumors and even metastatic tumors are particularly uncommon in the jaws. Second, the jaws are the site of tumors which do not form in any other bones, namely odontogenic tumors which arise from remnants of tooth-forming tissues which in turn have originated embryologically from downgrowth of epithelium

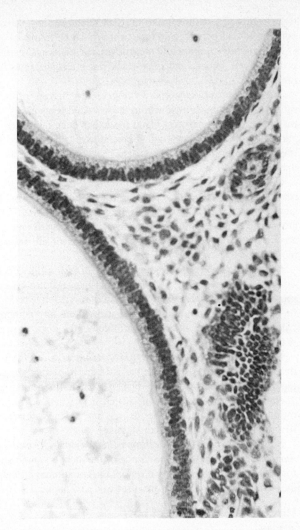

FIG. 17-20. Ameloblastoma. This shows the tall columnar ameloblast-like cells with epithelium resembling stellate-reticulum below the nuclear pole. At the opposite end of the ameloblast-like cells are cystic spaces formed by breakdown of the connective tissue matrix.

into the developing jaws. As mentioned earlier therefore there is the paradoxical situation that a primary tumor which is not osseous but of epithelial origin can form within the bone of the jaws. This odontogenic epithelium also gives rise to the many kinds of cysts of the jaws.

The jaws, more than any other bones are the site of lesions which are tumorlike in that they form chronic swellings and radiolucent areas, and include the following.

Primary odontogenic tumors. The most common and important of the primary odontogenic tumors is the ameloblastoma (Fig. 17-20) (formerly termed adamantinoma). It is a slowly invasive and locally destructive tumor but does not metastasize. Truly malignant ameloblastomas (or for that matter other, malignant odontogenic tumors) are so rare as to be little more than pathological curiosities.

Odontogenic mesenchymal tumors are considerably less common than the ameloblastomas while the ameloblastic fibroma (a rare entity) appears to be a true mixed tumor of epithelium and mesenchyme.

Odontomas. Odontomas are hamartomas of dental tissues of which a great variety exists. The complex composite odontome is most likely to resemble a tumor in that it can form a large confused cauliflowerlike mass of dental tissues. Mixed odontomas and odontogenic tumors may also be found.

Primary bone tumors and metastases. As mentioned earlier, primary bone tumors and metastases can affect the jaws but rarely do so.

Intraosseous salivary gland tumors. Very rarely, primary salivary gland tumors arise within the jaws and particularly the mandible. Ectopic salivary gland tissue has been described in various parts of the jaws and it seems likely that this is the origin of these intraosseous tumors. Their chief importance is that they should not be confused with metastatic tumors.

Cysts of the jaws. The vast majority of jaw cysts arise from remnants of odontogenic epithelium and probably form the single most common type of chronic swelling of bone. They are mostly true, epithelium-lined cysts and most frequently arise secondarily to inflammation at the apex of an infected tooth (radicular cyst).

Giant cell lesions of the jaws. Giant cell lesions have been discussed earlier and the only point that may need to be emphasized is that most are giant cell granulomas (reactive lesions) or, rarely, hyperparathyroidism and if there are any authenticated cases of true giant cell tumor affecting the jaws, they are pathological curiosities.

Fibrous dysplasia and other fibroosseous lesions. Fibrous dysplasia is discussed later but the jaws are important sites of the monostotic type of fibrous dysplasia. In addition there are uncommon fibroosseous lesions which may resemble fibrous dysplasia to a greater or lesser degree but which may behave like tumors and are difficult to classify.

Solitary eosinophilic granuloma (histiocytosis X) and solitary plasmacytoma. The jaw is one of the most common sites for solitary lesions of solitary eosinophilic granulomas although they are overall rare. They are discussed in Chapter 13.

Miscellaneous lesions of bone

Solitary (simple, unicameral) bone cyst. In spite of its name, this uncommon cavitating lesion of bone, unlike a true cyst, lacks an epithelial lining and is not always solitary.

Etiology. The cause is unknown. In the past these lesions have been ascribed to trauma or cystic change in a hematoma (hence the older names—hemorrhagic or traumatic bone cyst), but there is no acceptable evidence to support these theories.

Pathology. The cyst has a bony wall and a scanty fibrous lining, sometimes containing a few giant cells and often altered blood products adhering to the wall. The cysts contain fluid that ranges from clear and straw colored to frankly bloody.

Clinical aspects. Children and young adults are predominantly affected. The first symptom is either pain or swelling, and there is sometimes stiffness of the adjacent joint. The most common sites are the ends of the long bones, particularly the humerus or femur. These cysts cause pathologic fractures in up to 60% of cases.

Radiologically a solitary bone cyst forms a well-defined, rounded radiolucent area often with pseudoloculation due to trabeculation of the walls. Curettage and insertion of bone chips are probably the most widely used forms of treatment, but recurrence is common. Paradoxically, however, 15% of cysts that have caused fracture heal spontaneously.

Aneurysmal bone cysts. Aneurysmal bone cysts are uncommon. They are not true cysts but show replacement of bone by connective tissue containing large blood-filled spaces. The etiology is speculative, and these lesions are thought to be vascular malformations (which seems probable) or reactive change in a preexisting bone tumor.

Pathology. The lesion consists of a spongy or honeycomb mass of soft tissue containing blood-filled spaces replacing bone.

Histologically the blood-filled spaces are of varying size and usually separated by a cellular fibrous tissue septum. The latter often contains osteoid, giant cells, and altered blood products. This tissue is often highly cellular, and these proliferative changes may be mistaken for a sarcoma. The tissue must be carefully examined because these cysts can coexist with a variety of benign or malignant bone neoplasms.

Clinical aspects. The lesion is most common in the second and third decades, but the age range is wide. The growth rate is highly variable. Spread to an adjacent bone is an unusual but characteristic feature. Swelling, pain, and tenderness are typical symptoms. In one large series the leg was affected in nearly 30%, the spine in a little under 30%, and other bones considerably less frequently. The skull, including the jaw, was affected in 3%.

Radiographs show a rounded radiolucent area with a thin expanded cortex.

Treatment is by excision, but recurrence rates of up to 20% have been recorded, especially in younger patients. The rate of recurrence is apparently greatly reduced by using radiotherapy in addition to surgery. However, the development of sarcoma in irradiated aneurysmal bone cysts has also been described.

Diseases of joints
Congenital diseases affecting the joints

A variety of congenital abnormalities of joints, often genetically determined, are recognized. One of the most common is congenital dislocation of the hip and a similar disorder affects German Shepherd dogs as a result of excessive inbreeding.

In addition, the genetic disorders of collagen formation (Chapters 2 and 3) often cause the joints to be hypermobile. This may allow unusual agility in youth but frequently, the weak connective tissue support of the joints can lead to chronic arthritis in later life. Genetic disorders causing floppy joints include osteogenesis imperfecta, Marfan's syndrome (Chapter 3), and, particularly, Ehlers-Danlos syndrome.

Ehlers-Danlos syndrome

Ehlers-Danlos syndrome* is a genetically determined defect of collagen formation. Ten subtypes have now been identified and the majority are inherited as autosomal dominant traits. As yet the biochemical basis of the connective tissue of many of these subtypes has not yet been identified but prominent features are listed in Table 17-2. There is considerable variation in the predominant manifestations of the various subtypes as this table shows but typical characteristics include hypermobile joints, hyperextensible and often fragile skin with a susceptibility to easy bruising and in some cases more severe hemorrhagic tendencies due to weakness of blood vessel walls (see also Chapter 19).

---

*Edvard Ehlers (1863-1937), Danish dermatologist; Henri-Alexandre Danlos (1844-1912), French dermatologist.

TABLE 17-2. Ehlers-Danlos disease subtypes

Subtype and heritance	Joint mobility	Skin bruising	Other features
I (gravis) AD	+ +	+ +	Joint damage +, mitral valve prolapse
II (mitis) AD	+ (1)	+	Mitral valve prolapse
III (benign) hyper-mobile) AD	±	+	Dislocations, early arthritis, mitral valve prolapse
IV (ecchymotic) AR	(2)	+ + +	Severe purpura, CVAs (3)
V (sex-linked) XL	±	+	Joint damage
VI (ocular)	+ +	+	Weak cornea and sclera, early loss of sight and deafness, multiple dislocations, short stature
VII (AMC) AR	+ +	±	
VIII (periodontic) AD	±	±	Early loss of teeth, blue sclerae
IX (occipital horn syndrome) AR	±	±	Skeletal and urinary tract dysplasia
X (fibronectin deficiency) AR	±	±	Bleeding tendency

1, Hands and feet only; *2,* digits only; *3,* bleeding from major arteries; *CVAs,* cerebrovascular accidents; *AD,* autosomal dominant; *AR,* autosomal recessive; *SLR,* sex-linked recessive; *AMC,* arthrocalasis multiplex congenita.

Suppurative arthritis

Suppurative arthritis is uncommon. Most cases are probably the result of hematogenous spread of infection to the joints. Predisposing causes include the following:

1. Septicemia from any cause
2. Chronic debilitating disease, severe diabetes, chronic alcoholism, liver failure
3. Neoplastic disease with impaired immune responses
4. Immunosuppressive treatment
5. Severe long-standing rheumatoid arthritis
6. Intraarticular corticosteroid injections
7. Intravenous injections by drug addicts

Infection of the joints in rheumatoid arthritis may be due to the reduced antibacterial activity of the synovial fluid or in some cases to the use of corticosteroids.

Etiology and pathogenesis. *Staphylococcus aureus* is by far the most common cause and accounts for about 25% of cases in children. *Streptococcus pneumoniae* may account for 10% of cases in adults and 25% in children. Overall, however, as discussed later, gonococcal arthritis is probably more common in adults. Patients with depressed immune responses and drug addicts seem particularly at risk from infection by gram-negative bacilli, such as *Pseudomonas aeruginosa,* but fungal infection is an increasing problem.

Clinical aspects. Patients are febrile within the first few days of infection. Large joints, particularly the knee, are mainly affected. The joint is painful, tender, swollen, and limited in movement, but the disease can be polyarticular.

Diagnosis is confirmed by aspiration and culture of joint fluid, which usually contains large numbers of polymorphs. The basis of treatment is to give doses of antibiotics parenterally.

Despite the many potent antibiotics available, suppurative arthritis continues to cause chronic disability and death. Factors affecting prognosis are the duration of infection before treatment is started, the virulence of the infecting organism, and the condition of the patient at the time of the infection. Death rates are highest among patients with malignant disease, liver failure, or rheumatoid arthritis.

Gonococcal arthritis

Gonococcal infection appears now to be the most common cause of suppurative arthritis in young to middle-aged women. It is believed to account for 50% of cases among adults. Other forms of bacterial arthritis by contrast usually affect children, the debilitated, or elderly, and there is a slight male preponderance.

Gonococcal infection is typically polyarticular, affecting large and small joints, mainly of the limbs. Unlike other infections, tenosynovitis is common with gonococcal arthritis.

Gonococcal arthritis is often accompanied by a characteristic rash consisting of pustules with a necrotic umbilicated center.

The diagnosis of gonococcal infection can be made with certainty only by culture of synovial fluid or blood. Nevertheless, positive cultures are only obtained in a minority of cases.

Gonococcal arthritis, unlike other forms of suppurative arthritis, responds rapidly to penicillin with relief of pain within 2 to 4 days.

Tuberculous arthritis

Tuberculous arthritis is now a rare disease. The infection produces characteristic formation of tuberculous granulomas and destruction of joint tissues. The disease is chronic and usually monoarticular, often in weight-bearing joints. The tuberculin skin test is positive, and the diagnosis can be confirmed by aspiration and culture of joint fluid. The disease is treated with antituberculous drugs. The response is good if the disease has not caused severe joint destruction.

Lyme disease

Lyme disease is an infective arthritis caused by the spirochete *Borrelia burgdorferi.* The disease was named after the town of Lyme on the banks of the Connecticut river where it was first reported. It seems to be spreading widely in the United States and has been reported in Europe and Australia.

Etiology. *Borrelia burgdorferi* is transmitted to man mainly by the tick, *Ixodes damnosum,* but has also been isolated from mosquitoes and other insects as well as from a variety of animal hosts, particularly deer.

Clinically, Lyme disease is seasonal and develops in stages. The usual first symptoms are from a characteristic rash (erythema chronicum migrans) which spreads outwards in an annular pattern from the tick bite and is frequently associated with multiple secondary lesions. A small minority of patients first complain of neurological symptoms (Chapter 20) or muscular pain.

The most common persistent feature of Lyme disease is arthritis, which can develop within weeks or even years after acquisition of the infection. There is intermittent swelling of large joints, particularly the knees; this may be followed by chronic synovitis and in a minority, erosion of cartilage and bone.

Histologically, the synovial membrane is thickened and infiltrated by lymphocytes and plasma cells; neutrophils may be numerous in the synovial fluid. Spirochetes have been identified both in the inflamed synovium and in the synovial fluid.

Inflammation appears to be triggered by release of interleukin

I stimulated by lipopolysaccharide from the bacterium's cell wall. An early specific IgM response with peak titers 3 to 6 weeks after infection, and a slower IgG response develop. In more severe cases a more prolonged rise in specific IgM and cryoglobulins have been described. Those who are tissue type HLA DR2 appear to be more susceptible to cardiac and neurologic involvement.

Early treatment with penicillin will arrest the progress of Lyme disease but it has been reported that late complications are fewer or absent if tetracycline has been given.

Complications. Fewer than 10% of patients develop cardiac disease but rarely, death has resulted from pancarditis.

Other bacterial and reactive arthropathies

As mentioned in Chapter 11, arthritis is a prominent feature of the acute phase of rheumatic fever but not as a result of infection of the joints and there is no permanent joint damage. Arthritis may be the main early manifestation of infective endocarditis and be prominent in acute or chronic meningococcal infection. In all of the latter, synovitis is probably immune complex mediated.

Acute synovitis can be an occasional feature of infections with *Mycoplasma pneumoniae*. The clinical picture can mimic Reiter's disease but should be readily distinguishable by the serologic changes (Chapter 12).

Viral arthritis

Joint pain is a common feature of many viral infections such as influenza, hepatitis B or adult rubella. More recently, human parvoviruses (HPV) (Chapter 8) have been identified as a cause of arthralgia particularly in young women. The pathogenesis is unknown but, though there is speculation that it is immune complex mediated, some biopsy specimens have shown no inflammation and it is possible that there is direct viral invasion of the joints.

Serologic diagnosis of HPV arthralgia is useful to exclude more dangerous or destructive joint disease. HPV arthralgia is usually mild and self-limiting, but the possibility that these viruses can cause progressive joint damage cannot be excluded. However, it does not appear that they are a cause of rheumatoid arthritis.

Rheumatoid arthritis

Rheumatoid arthritis is a multisystem disease that can affect virtually any organ, but its most common and, usually, most troublesome manifestation is arthritis. A variety of serologic changes is associated (Chapter 7).

Rheumatoid arthritis is a common disease causing misery or disablement on an enormous scale; it typically affects people at their most productive period of life and frequently causes prolonged pain and limitation of mobility.

Etiology. Rheumatoid arthritis is one of the connective tissue (collagen vascular) diseases and appears to be immunologically mediated, probably as an immune complex reaction in the affected tissues as discussed in Chapter 7.

Pathology. The characteristic feature is synovitis. The synovial membrane is congested, thickened and often velvety in appearance. Granulation tissue (called *pannus* in this situation) spreads onto and replaces the articular cartilage, destroying its normal glistening white surface.

Microscopically the synovial membrane is highly vascular and shows chronic inflammatory changes with an infiltrate of lymphocytes and plasma cells (Fig. 17-21).

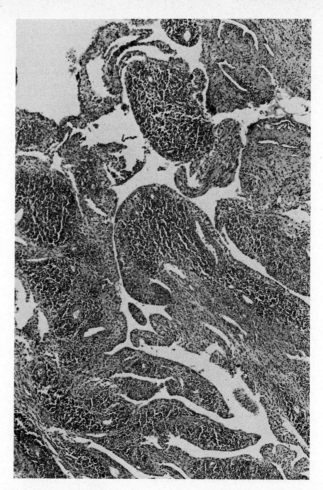

FIG. 17-21. Rheumatoid arthritis. The synovial villi are swollen by chronic inflammatory cell infiltrate. A similar appearance can be seen in villonodular synovitis.

Initially the synovial cells proliferate from a single-celled layer to several layers of columnar cells, and the synovium acquires a villous configuration.

The granulation tissues spreading over the articular cartilage erode its surface and eventually invade the immediately subjacent bone; the erosions can also form cystic cavities at the bone ends. The bone destruction and loss of cartilage finally cause the joint surfaces to disintegrate, but bony ankylosis is not ordinarily a complication.

At the other extreme the disease can be mild and of short duration. The changes are then no more than inflammatory thickening of the synovial membrane without damage to articular cartilage or bone.

In addition to the synovial membrane of joints, the similar lining of the tendon sheaths, at the wrist, fingers, or ankle, for instance, are often inflamed (tenosynovitis).

Rheumatoid nodules are common in severely affected patients and form under the skin, usually near the elbows (Fig. 17-22). These nodules consist of a core of necrotic fibrous tissue surrounded by a chronic inflammatory reaction. Similar inflammatory nodules can develop in many organs, producing a variety of systemic manifestations (Fig. 17-23).

Systemic complications of rheumatoid arthritis include arthritis, pleurisy, and pericarditis, heart failure, pneumonitis, hepatitis, and a variety of hematologic disorders. Sjögren's

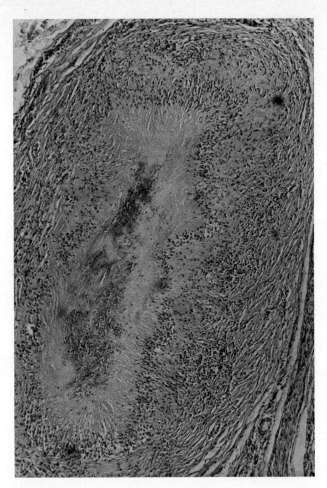

FIG. 17-22. Rheumatoid nodule (subcutaneous tissue). The central portion consists chiefly of degraded collagen-rich connective tissue ringed by histiocytes and fibroblasts in palisade arrangement.

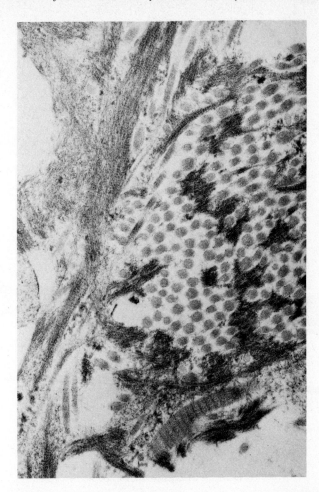

FIG. 17-23. Electron micrograph of a rheumatoid nodule showing the effects of collagenolytic activity on the collagen fibers. They have partially lost their compact structure, and many look as if they have been teased apart. *(Courtesy Curator of the Gordon Museum, Guy's Hospital, London, England.)*

syndrome is the most important ocular and oral complication and can endanger sight.

Clinical aspects. Rheumatoid arthritis has a worldwide distribution; in the United States it is estimated to affect about 3% of the population. Women are more often affected than men in a ratio of 3:1.

Rheumatoid arthritis varies from a mild and apparently self-limiting disorder to severe crippling disease with widespread destruction of joints and involvement of other tissues.

The disease most frequently starts between the ages of 30 and 40, but almost any age can be affected. The onset is usually insidious, often with a feeling of stiffness in the hands or feet, worse in the morning. Later there is aching pain, swelling, redness, and tenderness of the joints, particularly of the fingers. Movement becomes limited, and wasting of the adjacent muscles causes the joint swellings to become spindle shaped. In some cases the onset is acute, with joint pain, fever, and malaise.

Rheumatoid arthritis typically begins in the small joints of hands (Fig. 17-24) and feet; later involvement of the wrists, elbows, ankles, and knees is common. The disease tends to affect the body symmetrically. In severe cases progressive destruction causes instability and deformity of the joints.

Depending on the severity of the disease, common extra-articular features include subcutaneous nodules (Fig. 17-25),

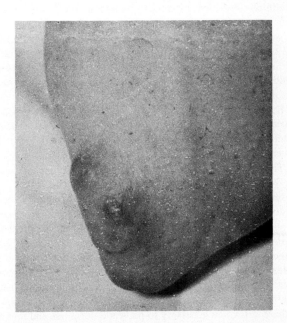

FIG. 17-24. A rheumatoid nodule on the elbow. *(Courtesy Curator of the Gordon Museum, Guy's Hospital, London, England.)*

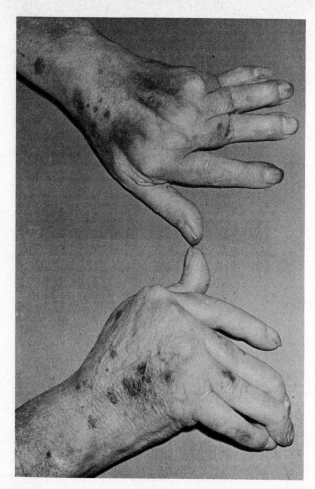

FIG. 17-25. Rheumatoid arthritis. In this advanced case there is typical ulnar deviation of the fingers. The dark patches on the skin are purpura resulting from corticosteroid treatment. A clinically similar picture of arthritis can be produced by psoriasis.

tendinitis, fever, loss of weight, enlargement of lymph nodes, and anemia.

Anemia is common and usually normochromic or mildly hypochromic. The cause may be the anemia of chronic inflammation; but there may also be chronic iron loss secondary to insidious gastrointestinal bleeding caused by aspirin or other antiinflammatory agents.

Radiographic features include widening of the joint space due to inflammation and exudate, erosions of the joint surfaces, osteoporosis of the bone adjacent to the joint cavity, and, in severe cases, cystic destruction of the bone ends.

The most important serologic changes, as described in Chapter 7, are rheumatoid factor and antinuclear factor.

Overall, the most useful drug in the management of rheumatoid arthritis is aspirin. Other antiinflammatory agents now available may cause less gastric irritation and also may have a more prolonged action. Gold salts and corticosteroids are also effective but, because of their severe side effects, are only used when simple antiinflammatory agents are ineffective. More recently penicillamine, a drug that affects collagen metabolism, has been used for selected cases. In addition to drugs, physiotherapy is often necessary to prevent deformities and muscle wasting and also to keep the patient mobile. The surgical correction of deformities may greatly alleviate crippling in advanced inactive disease.

Lupus erythematosus

Joint pain is the most common symptom in systemic lupus erythematosus (Chapter 7). Typically there is mild, flitting joint pain (arthralgia) often mistaken for early rheumatoid arthritis or rheumatic fever.

In many patients this progresses to polyarthritis, which especially affects the hands, wrists, knees, and ankles and resembles rheumatoid arthritis in many respects. Severe damage to joints and deformity are, however, rare in lupus erythematosus. In terms of prevalence, also, the latter is a minor cause of joint disease compared with rheumatoid arthritis.

Seronegative arthropathies

Seronegative arthropathies is a term frequently applied to a group of diseases characterized by arthritis, which is clinically and often histologically similar to rheumatoid arthritis. However, such diseases lack the serologic and other immunologic features of the latter, and there is little or no evidence for an immunopathogenesis. Also unlike rheumatoid arthritis, these diseases often have an association with HLA B27 and frequently affect males predominantly.

The seronegative arthropathies include:
1. Ankylosing spondylitis
2. Reiter's disease
3. Psoriatic arthropathy
4. Arthritis associated with inflammatory bowel disease
5. Behcet's syndrome
6. Some types of chronic juvenile arthritis

It has to be pointed out that, confusingly, the term *seronegative rheumatoid arthritis* is sometimes also used for proven rheumatoid arthritis but which lacks the usual (IgM) type of rheumatoid factor.

Ankylosing spondylitis

Ankylosing spondylitis is a relatively common chronic, progressive, inflammatory disease which particularly affects the spine and sacroiliac joints and has a strong tendency to cause bony fusion (ankylosis).

Etiology. There is a strong genetic factor and almost 90% of patients are HLA B27. Moreover, asymptomatic persons who are also HLA B27 have a high risk of developing ankylosing spondylitis. This unusually strong HLA association is often taken to imply that the disease is immunologically mediated despite the fact that no significant serologic abnormalities or autoimmune mechanisms have been demonstrated. Also unlike typical autoimmune diseases, ankylosing spondylitis shows a strong male predominance, and some 85% of patients are men. However, the pathologic changes in the synovia are similar to those of rheumatoid arthritis.

The etiology of ankylosing spondylitis is therefore unknown.

Pathology. The synovial changes in this disease are similar to those of rheumatoid arthritis, but there is in addition, inflammation at the sites of insertion of ligaments and tendons into bone. A serious complication is therefore ligamentous ossification and formation of bony bridges (syndesmophytes) between adjacent vertebral bodies and bony ankylosis of affected joints. A raised erythrocyte sedimentation rate (ESR) and mild anemia accompany the inflammatory changes. Other effects are iritis or iridocyclitis in about 25% of patients and carditis in about 10%.

Clinical aspects. The typical patient is a man of about 30 who develops insidiously increasing lower back pain and stiffness that is most severe in the morning but initially relieved by exercise. In some patients the first symptoms are from limb joints such as the hips or knees and these joints may be the most severely affected.

The most important effects are pain in and progressive limitation of movement of the back or hips. A minority progress to complete bony ankylosis of the spine, starting in the lumbosacral region but sometimes extending into the cervical spine. This is occasionally so severe as to force the chin down onto the chest and this together with involvement of the costovertebral joints can severely impede respiratory movement.

Fixation of the hip joints is another serious complication. Peripheral arthritis may be clinically indistinguishable from rheumatoid arthritis.

The radiographic findings include sacroiliitis, followed by ossification until the sacroiliac joints are completely obliterated. There is osteoporosis of the vertebral bodies, but obliteration of the anterior concavity so that they appear square. This together with calcification of the annulus fibrosus, gives rise to the bamboo spine appearance.

Complications include ocular, cardiovascular, respiratory or gastrointestinal disease, and there is a significant mortality as a result. Probably, however, the majority of patients with ankylosing spondylitis manage to continue a relatively normal life helped by antiinflammatory analgesics and exercises to maintain mobility.

Reiter's disease

Reiter's syndrome* comprises the triad of arthritis, urethritis and ophthalmitis, but the manifestations can be much more varied and the term Reiter's disease is now therefore preferred.

Reiter's disease appears to a postinfective, reactive syndrome which particularly follows enteric infections (as was the first case, described in a Prussian officer in World War I) by shigella, yersinia, salmonella, and campylobacter species. Alternatively, it can be postvenereal and be associated with chlamydial or mycoplasmal infections. About 80% of patients are HLA B27 and males are predominantly affected.

Microscopically, the synovia show nonspecific inflammation with a fibrin-rich exudate and a mixed inflammatory cell infiltrate. Hemosiderin from the breakdown of red cells may be deposited in the synovium but the histologic picture may be indistinguishable from that of rheumatoid arthritis.

Clinically, Reiter's disease attacks males between the ages of 18 and 40, with urethritis as the first sign, followed by

---

*Hans Reiter (1881-1969), German physician.

conjunctivitis and joint pains. Attacks average about 3 months duration and relapse is common; between 10% and 20% of patients develop permanent disability. The arthritis has features similar to ankylosing spondylitis; sacroiliitis is common and joints of the lower limb are mainly affected.

In addition to conjunctivitis, painful keratitis or iridocyclitis can develop. Mucocutaneous lesions in the mouth, or on the penis, palms or soles are common. The skin lesions are straw-colored, keratin-filled vesicles. Gross hyperkeratosis, particularly of the soles of the feet, may occasionally develop.

Treatment is mainly symptomatic but corticosteroids need to be given if uveitis develops.

Psoriatic arthropathy

This disease may closely resemble rheumatoid arthritis but for its association with psoriasis (Chapter 19) and lack of autoantibodies. It is usually also less severe. Some cases more closely resemble ankylosing spondylitis and about 45% of patients are HLA B27 positive. A somewhat characteristic feature of many cases but rare in other types of arthritis, is sausagelike inflammatory swelling of the fingers.

Behçet's syndrome

The typical manifestations of Behçet's syndrome are oral and genital ulcers and iritis. However, the syndrome is a multisystem disease which can affect a wide variety of organs.

Arthritis—particularly of the knees and ankles—may be present in up to 50% of patients. But the disease presents such wide variations in incidence and in the predominant clinical manifestations in different countries, that it is impossible to generalize. Indeed there are no absolute criteria for the diagnosis of Behçet's syndrome which is discussed more fully in Chapter 19.

Juvenile chronic arthritis

Juvenile chronic arthritis (often misleadingly termed juvenile rheumatoid arthritis) comprises a group of diseases of which four main types, and often, several subtypes, are usually recognized. Classification of these diseases has been further complicated by the variety of HLA associations that have been found (see Table 17-3).

Juvenile chronic arthritis is estimated to affect about one in 2,000 children. The main types involve either many joints (polyarticular) or few joints (pauciarticular) and may resemble rheumatoid arthritis (with similar serologic abnormalities), an-

---

TABLE 17-3. Juvenile arthritis

Disease*	Typical clinical features	Joints affected	HLA and immunologic findings	Outcome
Systemic (polyarticular)	Fever, rash; heart, liver, lymph nodes may be involved	Any, often destructive	—	1% to 2% mortality, can be severely crippling
Pauciarticular				
Subtype I	Iritis +	Large joints	DR 5, DR 8	Blindness in 10%
Subtype II	Iritis rarely	Mainly spinal	B 27 +	? progress to ankylosing spondylitis
Polyarticular				
Subtype I	Resembles adult RA	Symmetric	RF + DR4	Sometimes crippling
Subtype II	Malaise, low fever, anemia	Symmetric	RF neg	Milder disease

RF, Rheumatoid factor; *RA*, rheumatoid arthritis; *ANA*, antinuclear antibodies.
*All types except pauciarticular type II, more common in females.

kylosing spondylitis (with similar complications), or other types of adult arthritis. *Still's disease** is a term sometimes used for a severe form of juvenile arthritis (and occasionally, but even more confusingly, for all types of juvenile arthritis); it has a febrile onset, multisystem involvement, and a small but significant mortality.

Primary gout

Primary gout is an inborn disorder of metabolism of polygenic inheritance and characterized by (1) increased levels of uric acid in the blood (hyperuricemia), (2) deposition of urates in tissues, and (3) recurrent arthritis. Secondary gout is an acquired disorder resulting from increased production or reduced excretion of uric acid.

Etiology and pathogenesis. Uric acid, the end product of purine metabolism, is relatively insoluble, and uric acid levels in plasma and urine are close to saturation.

The main factors determining blood uric acid levels are (1) the rate of breakdown of endogenous purines, (2) the quantity of purines in the diet, and (3) the rate of renal clearance of uric acid.

Specific defects in uric acid metabolism leading to overproduction include enzyme deficiencies and impaired uric acid binding to plasma protein. Congenital absence of one of these enzymes, hypoxanthine-guanine phosphoribosyl transferase (HG-PRT) causes gross hyperuricemia and the rare Lesch-Nyhan syndrome (Chapter 20).

*Sir Frederick Still (1864-1941), English pediatrician.

In most cases of gout the specific biochemical defect is unknown. The effect, however, is overproduction of uric acid with or without reduced excretion. The upper levels of serum uric acid may be double or treble the normal.

Pathology. In acute gouty arthritis, crystals of urates are deposited in the synovial membrane. This stimulates acute inflammation and exudation of polymorphonuclear leukocytes into the joint. Phagocytosis of the crystals is followed by death of leukocytes, disruption of their lysosomes, release of unaltered crystals, and perpetuation of the inflammatory process (Fig. 17-26).

Chronic gout is characterized by the deposition of large masses of urate crystals (tophi) with surrounding inflammation. These deposits interfere with joint function and destroy the joint tissues, cartilage, and bone. The final result is a severe deforming polyarthritis (Fig. 17-27).

Extraarticular tophi are typically first seen in the helix of the ear as hard, pale, subcutaneous nodules. The overlying skin may become necrotic and allow semisolid masses of urate to be extruded (Figs. 17-28 and 17-29).

Renal disease is the most common complication, with the characteristic histologic finding of urate crystals and a giant cell reaction. Early tubular damage associated with an interstitial reaction causes a distinctive type of glomerulosclerosis. Renal failure is the eventual cause of death in 20% to 25% of gouty subjects. Most gouty patients, however, die of cardiac or cerebral vascular disease, and the incidence of coronary heart disease is about twice as high in patients with gout as in those with normal serum urate levels.

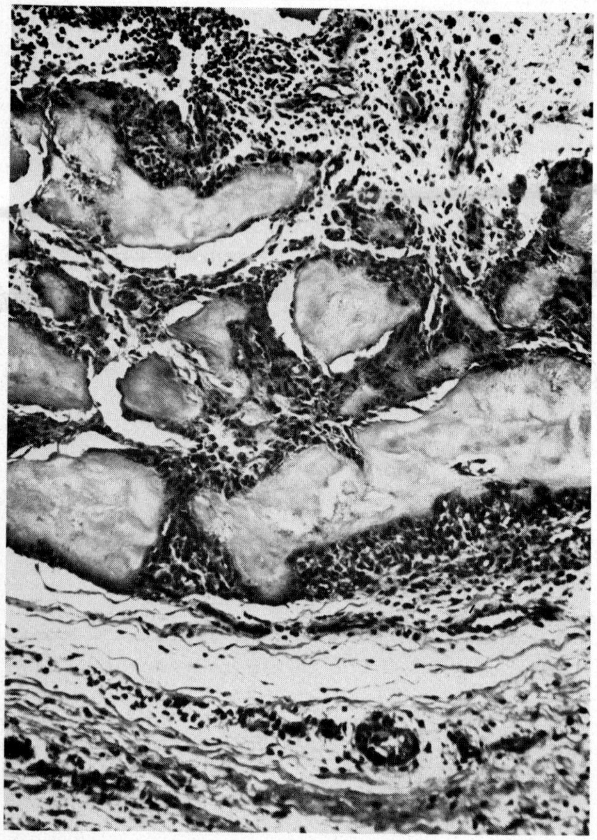

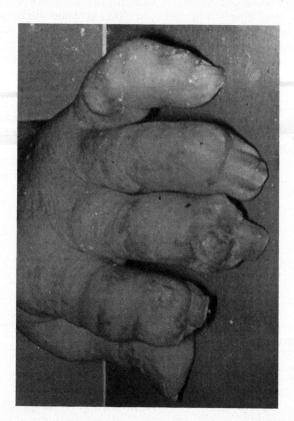

FIG. 17-26. Urate deposits in gout. The urate appears in irregular masses of pale, almost amorphous material surrounded by an intense inflammatory infiltrate.

FIG. 17-27. Gout. In this severe case there is gross swelling of the fingers. Over the terminal phalanges of several fingers are more localized swellings due to gouty tophi. *(Courtesy Curator of the Gordon Museum, Guy's Hospital, London, England.)*

Secondary gout

Hyperuricemia causing secondary gout is considerably more common than primary gout and can result from the following:

1. Increased purine turnover. The main cause is gross overproduction of nuclei, as in the myeloproliferative diseases.
2. Excessive cell breakdown. Radiotherapy especially can cause rapid breakdown of vast numbers of cells and their nuclei, precipitating or exacerbating an attack of gout.
3. Decreased urate excretion. Urate retention can result from renal disease or particularly from the administration of one of the thiazide diuretics, which now are probably the most frequent cause of gout.

Clinical aspects. Acute gout (Figs. 17-27 to 17-29) typically causes sudden and intense joint pain, usually in men around the ages of 30 to 35. A single joint, particularly the big toe, or occasionally a few joints are affected. The pain and inflammation may be severe enough to simulate bacterial cellulitis. There is often tachycardia, fever, leukocytosis, and raised serum uric acid levels. The acute attack usually settles in 1 or 2 weeks, but attacks can follow at intervals of weeks, months, or even longer.

In an acute attack, antiinflammatory analgesics are the first line of treatment. In the long term, uric acid levels can be lowered by increasing excretion with uricosuric drugs such as probenecid or with allopurinol which inhibits xanthine oxidase and decreases uric acid production.

Pseudogout (crystal arthropathy)

Pseudogout is the term given to pyrophosphate arthropathy, which differs from gout not merely in the type of crystal deposited, but also lacks the male predominance and usually develops in the middle-aged or elderly. A positive family history is not uncommon.

There may be episodic acute attacks or progressive degenerative joint disease. In acute cases, large joints (particularly the knee) are more often affected.

The diagnosis can be confirmed by detecting calcium pyrophosphate crystals in a synovial fluid specimen, using po-larized light microscopy. These crystals form rods, tablets or parallelapipeds.

Calcium apatite arthropathy is discussed in Chapter 2.

Osteoarthritis (osteoarthrosis)

The term *osteoarthritis* has long been considered inappropriate since it was thought to be an essentially degenerative disease. Therefore the term osteoarthrosis, was introduced. However, current research suggests that inflammation plays an important if not central role in the etiology. The etiology nevertheless appears—to say the least—complex.

Etiology. Osteoarthritis has traditionally been regarded as largely resulting from the effects of wear and tear on heavily stressed joints. It is, for example, one of the diseases of old age, and there has been a strong clinical impression that the disease was particularly common in the overstressed joints of the obese and those in physically stressful occupations. Nevertheless, reexamination of the incidence of osteoarthritis has not confirmed that the disease is more common in such groups. It also does not appear that osteoarthritis is more prone to develop in joints which lack adequate support as a result, for example, of paralytic poliomyelitis. Moreover the most commonly involved joints in osteoarthritis in the elderly (Heberden's nodes or more gross degenerative changes) are in the hands, even in nonmanual workers. Severe osteoarthritis in such sites can be completely painless.

Factors that predispose to osteoarthritis are derangements of the normal functional anatomy of the joint as a result, for example, of operations such as meniscectomy on the knee or of long standing rheumatoid arthritis. There also appears to be a strong familial predisposition to the disease.

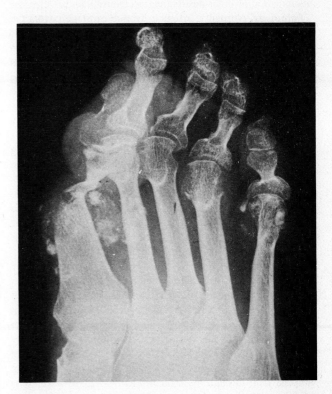

FIG. 17-29. Gout. There are gross arthritic changes in the metatar-sophalangeal joints. The first of these has been completely destroyed, and there is periarticular calcification around the others. *(Courtesy Curator of the Gordon Museum, Guy's Hospital, London, England.)*

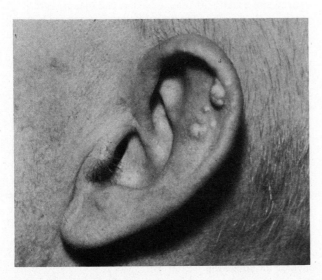

FIG. 17-28. Gouty tophi containing urate crystals in the subcutaneous tissue of the ear, a typical site. *(Courtesy Curator of the Gordon Museum, Guy's Hospital, London, England.)*

Contributory factors to the pathogenesis of osteoarthritis may therefore include the following:

1. Genetic factors
2. Systemic factors affecting cartilage metabolism
3. Aging
4. Abnormal types of stress on or internal derangements of the joint
5. Inflammation

Two views on the etiology of osteoarthritis currently predominate. First a variety of abnormal physical stresses on the joints cause cell injury and degradative changes in previously normal cartilage (and lead, ultimately, to its breakdown). In the alternative view, aging, genetic factors, metabolic disorders, inflammation, and possibly immunologic abnormalities may lead to abnormalities in joint cartilage (which as a result is unable to withstand abnormal stresses). Degenerative changes follow as a consequence.

More recent research has prompted the hypothesis that (in simplified terms) physical forces lead to disordered chondrocyte regulation and a net increase in protease activity. These degradative enzymes may then cause breakdown of the cartilage matrix and release of metabolic products which provoke inflammatory changes and phagocytosis of synovial cells (see also Chapter 2). Such inflammatory changes would contribute materially to joint damage.

Whatever the etiologic mechanisms are, it is important to distinguish the underlying causes from factors which accelerate its progress, once present, or which aggravate the process and so cause inflammation and pain.

The effects of nonsteroidal antiinflammatory drugs on cartilage metabolism in osteoarthritis are the subject of considerable current research and seem likely to clarify the role of inflammation or other destructive mechanisms in this disease.

Pathology. Normally, articular hyaline cartilage covers the bearing surface of the bone and is firmly attached to it by fibrous tissue (Fig. 17-30). The cartilage consists of chondrocytes in a firm translucent ground substance of mucopolysaccharides and collagen fibers. Cartilage has no intrinsic blood supply, and its nutrition is derived from the synovial fluid, not the underlying bone. Partly because of this lack of blood supply, cartilage is unable to regenerate, and damage is repaired mainly by proliferation of fibrocytes.

The earliest detectable lesion of osteoarthrosis is softening of the matrix of the articular cartilage due to loss of chondroitin sulfate from the superficial layers. This in turn leads to separation of superficial fibrils, often starting in the areas of the most severe stress. Fine flakes of cartilage split off into the joint space and undergo phagocytosis by synovial cells. This can cause a low-grade synovitis. For a time the deeper chondrocytes react by producing more chondroitin sulfate.

As degeneration of the articular cartilage progresses, bone changes develop. There is proliferation of bone, which becomes thickened as if compensating for the extra stress imposed on it following the loss of cartilage. New bone also forms at the joint margins, forming osteophytes. These changes appear to affect the response to stresses on the bone, and there is a tendency for the formation of microfractures of the trabeculae. Cystic spaces also form within the bone ends and can communicate with the joint through these microfractures. Joint movements produce pressure changes transmitted to these cystic spaces through the microfractures and cause the spaces to enlarge.

The first gross change to be seen is loss of the normal glis-

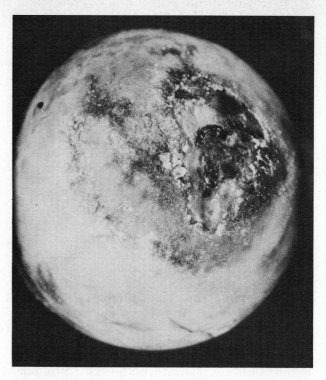

FIG. 17-30. Osteoarthritis of the femoral head. The smooth surface of articular cartilage has been destroyed and eroded, leaving a rough irregular surface of bone.

tening surface of the articular cartilage followed by patchy development of a soft and roughened surface. This advances until ulceration starts to expose the bone. The exposed bone is smooth at first but is unable to sustain the frictional stress of joint movement for long and as a consequence becomes increasingly roughened. Cysts also become exposed and collapse, while osteophytes continue to develop at the periphery until the joint structure is grossly deformed.

Clinical aspects. The clinical findings depend very much on associated factors such as obesity and preexisting joint damage. Patients are usually 50 years or older, and one or more joints are typically affected. The main symptom is pain with slowly progressive loss of movement and deformity. There is great variation in the rate of progress of the disease from one patient to another, and symptoms often show little relation to the severity of the radiographic or even the pathologic changes in the joint, except when major weight-bearing joints (particularly the hip or knee) are involved.

*Heberden's nodes** (Fig. 17-31) are common and produce highly characteristic pea-sized or larger protuberances. They are osteophytes in the margins of the joints at the base of the distal phalanx. They develop slowly with varying degrees of pain and are commonly associated with generalized osteoarthrosis. In addition to the distal interphalangeal joints, other joints of the hands and feet, the acromioclavicular, the knee, and the apophyseal joints of the spine are commonly affected, but the wrists usually escape.

The characteristic radiologic changes seen in osteoarthrosis include the following:

---

*William Heberden (1710-1801), English physician.

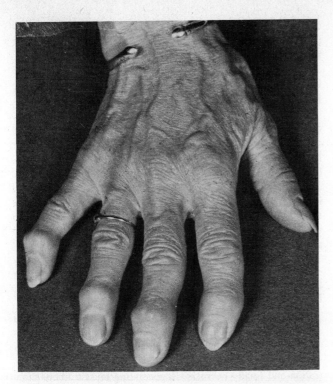

FIG. 17-31. Osteoarthritis. Heberden's nodes at the base of the terminal interphalangeal joints are readily seen. *(Courtesy Curator of the Gordon Museum, Guy's Hospital, London, England.)*

1. Narrowing of the joint space
2. Marginal osteophyte formation
3. Subchondral sclerosis
4. Bone cysts, which appear as rounded areas of translucency (varying in size from 1 to 2 mm up to a few centimeters) just under the joint surface
5. Deformity

Once the diagnosis has been confirmed, the main principles of treatment are rest and protection of the joints, reduction of obesity (if possible), and analgesics as necessary. Physiotherapy is necessary to prevent atrophy of muscles acting on the affected joints, to train patients to improve their gait and posture, and to use walking aids. Surgical replacement of the hip is often carried out.

Subgroups of osteoarthritis are recognizable, namely (1) generalized, (2) predominantly hip and spine, and (3) severe inflammatory and rapidly destructive disease. The patterns of joint involvement also apparently show some geographical variation and hip disease seems to be common in Western Europe, while knee involvement seems to be more common in Africa and China.

Prolapsed intervertebral disk

Back pain is a common cause of disability. The best known example, although it probably accounts for a relatively small proportion of cases, is mechanical derangement due to prolapse of an intervertebral disk, often called a "slipped disk."

Pathogenesis and pathology. An intervertebral disk consists essentially of a central core of stiff jelly (nucleus pulposus) surrounded by a fibrous elastic wall (annulus fibrosus).

Parts of the intervertebral disk often gradually degenerate and become weakened. Stress on a disk can rupture the elastic wall, allowing slow escape of some of the nucleus pulposus. The extruded material forms a swelling, which first stretches the posterior longitudinal ligament causing severe back pain. Stretching of one of the nerves emerging from the spinal canal causes pain, which usually radiates down the leg. The lowest lumbar disk or the next above is usually affected.

Clinical aspects. In a typical case, a few hours or days after jarring the back or unusual exertion, there is sudden agonizing pain in the lower back when stooping. The pain gradually lessons but after a few days radiates to the buttock and down to the foot.

In time, the extruded nuclear material loses water and gradually shrinks until no more than a fibrous scar is left. Natural healing can be helped by resting the back by confinement to bed or by supporting the spine with a plaster cast or surgical jacket.

Surgical treatment to excise the protruding tissue is justified when there is massive prolapse of the disk or the elastic wall of the disk is displaced as well. This usually produces dramatic relief of pain.

Acute lower back pain more often develops without radiologic evidence of extrusion of the nucleus pulposus or sciatic pain, but the cause is unknown. Although agonizingly severe at first, this tends to resolve spontaneously in 2 or 3 weeks.

Villonodular synovitis

Villonodular synovitis is an obscure condition in which there is villous proliferation of the synovium and deposition of hemosiderin. Giant cells are typically also present. The mass may involve the whole of the synovium of a joint cavity or a tendon sheath. A tumorlike mass may thus form, but usually does not extend beyond the confines of its structure of origin.

Rarely, however, large masses of this nature may erode bone and its tendency to recur after excision are features contributing to the belief that it was a benign tumor but the current consensus is that it is reactive in nature (see Fig. 17-21).

Giant cell tumor of tendon sheaths

Giant cell tumor of tendon sheaths is a common tumor that affects young and middle aged adults. It is usually seen as a small, raised, firm nodule on the finger; less common sites include the feet, ankle, and knee.

The pathogenesis is controversial; while most consider it to be a neoplasm some believe it is a reactive process and prefer the term *nodular tenosynovitis*.

Microscopically, it consists of round cells, phagocytic histiocytes and giant cells. Excision is usually curative; if incomplete there may be local recurrence.

Ganglion cysts

The so-called ganglion cyst is a common cystic swelling arising from a tendon sheath (often of the wrist) or a joint capsule.

The probable etiology is "myxoid degeneration" (see Chapter 2) of the tendon sheath connective tissue followed by cystic change and peripheral fibrosis.

Clinically, ganglia form tensely cystic nodules usually less than 2 cm in diameter. The traditional treatment is to burst them with a blow with the family Bible, but excision is less likely to be followed by recurrence.

Tumors of joints

Tumors can arise from any of the structures such as fibrous tissue or cartilage which contribute to the structure of joints, but rarely do so.

Synovial sarcoma is a rare tumor and, paradoxically, arises more commonly in the soft tissues adjacent to joints, such as tendons or tendon sheaths, rather than in joint cavities. It can also form in soft tissues unrelated to joints. The extremities, particularly the lower extremity, are most commonly involved: about 8% are in the head and neck region and occasionally the abdominal wall is the primary site.

Clinically, a typical manifestation of synovial sarcoma, is an insidiously growing, deep soft tissue mass which may eventually become painful and, if related to a joint, limit movement.

Microscopically, synovial sarcoma is unusual in that it is characteristically biphasic, consisting of both spindle cell and epithelial elements. The spindle cells are fibroblast-like while the epithelial cells, which stain positively with epithelial cell markers, are typically tall and columnar (Fig. 17-32).

The spindle cells usually form the bulk of the tumor and are usually uniform in appearance with plump nuclei and indistinct cytoplasm. They may form well orientated streams of cells resembling a well differentiated fibrosarcoma.

The epithelial cells can form a variety of arrangements such as whorls or solid cords, or line clefts or cystlike spaces when they may resemble normal synovium; alternatively they may

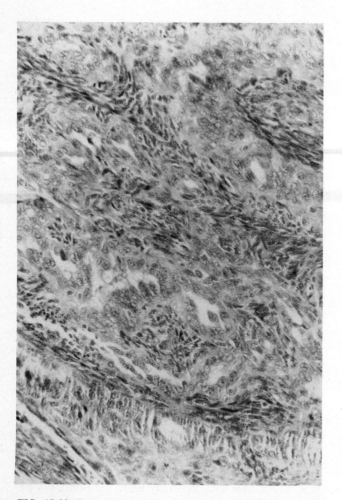

FIG. 17-32. Biphasic synovial sarcoma showing columnar epithelial cells surrounded by sarcomatous spindle-shaped cells.

confer a glandlike appearance to the area. Occasionally epithelial elements are so small in amount and difficult to find that the tumor is termed monophasic.

Varying degrees of calcification or even ossification develops in about 40% of these tumors and is an important radiologic feature.

The prognosis of synovial sarcoma is related to the degree of differentiation rather than to the relative amounts of the two cellular components, but despite its slow growth, the tumor has a poor prognosis and the reported 5 year survival rate varies between 25% and 50%. Wide excision is therefore necessary and radiotherapy may be beneficial, but since recurrences after limited resection may be delayed for a decade or more it is difficult to assess cure rates. Metastases are most frequently to the lungs, but sometimes to lymph nodes or occasionally to the bone marrow.

Diseases of muscle
Muscle changes in response to injury or disease

Degeneration and regeneration of muscle fibers as a result of injury, such as local infection or a tumor, is a common finding. Typical microscopic features of muscle degeneration include hyaline change with loss of cross-striations, vacuolization and finally necrosis. Regenerating muscle fibers show such changes as basophilia, indistinct striations, and variations of fiber size. The nuclei are increased in number, enlarged and often have prominent nuclei ("sarcolemmal giant cells"). Muscle degeneration and regeneration may often be seen side by side, but if the injury (such as irradiation damage) is sufficiently severe, there is no regeneration but merely replacement of muscle by fibrous tissue.

Giant cell arteritis: polymyalgia rheumatica

Polymyalgia rheumatica is one of the most common manifestations of giant cell arteritis (Chapter 10). The symptoms resemble arthritis but the pathologic changes are primarily in the blood vessels. Although there is ischemic muscle pain, significant muscle damage is not a feature.

Polymyalgia rheumatica is usually therefore included among the rheumatic diseases for symptomatic reasons only.

Clinically, women, usually after middle age, are predominantly affected. The chief symptoms are weakness and pain of the shoulder or pelvic girdles or both. Lethargy, fever, malaise, and loss of appetite and weight are usually associated and the ESR is greatly raised.

Cranial arteritis may also be associated and cause severe headache, and in 20% of patients, ischemic pain in the masticatory muscles, comparable to intermittent claudication.

The response to corticosteroids is good. These must also be given because of the risk of blindness if there is concommitant cranial arteritis.

Myasthenia gravis

Myasthenia gravis is a disorder of neuromuscular conduction which results in weakness of skeletal muscles and in the absence of treatment has a significant mortality. It is associated with disorders of the thymus in the great majority of cases and immunopathogenic mechanisms in this disease have been worked out in considerable detail.

Etiology and immunopathogenesis. The ultimate cause of myasthenia gravis is unknown but the evidence that the disease is autoimmune in nature is as follows:

1. Circulating autoantibodies to acetylcholine receptor proteins of neuromuscular end plates are present.
2. The titer of antibodies correlates well with the severity of the disease.
3. Acetylcholine receptor antibodies and complement are detectable at affected motor end plates.
4. Experimentally, myasthenia gravis can be induced in animals by injection of the following:
   a. Serum from patients with the disease
   b. Monoclonal antibodies to acetylcholine receptors
   c. Homologous acetylcholine receptor protein with resulting antibody formation
5. The thymus also contains acetylcholine receptor proteins and in the great majority of cases of myasthenia gravis, there is hyperplasia or a tumor of the thymus.
6. Thymectomy is usually curative.

Mysthenia gravis also has the characteristic general features of autoimmune diseases (Chapter 7). It is significantly more common in women and tends to be associated with other autoimmune diseases such as pemphigus vulgaris (Chapter 19) or, less often thyroiditis or pernicious anemia.

Pathology. Hyperplasia of the thymus is present in 70% and a thymoma is present in a further 10% of patients. In addition to the immunologic abnormalities, the motor end plates, can be seen by electron microscopy, to be abnormal. In particular there is loss of receptor sites and widening of the presynaptic cleft. By contrast the muscles appear normal both grossly and microscopically, and no more than small interstitial accumulations of inflammatory cells can be occasionally found.

Clinical aspects. Females are affected twice as frequently as men, and the peak age of onset is in the early 20's. The onset is late in those with thymic tumors (Chapter 18) and there is the rare syndrome of thymoma, myasthenia gravis, and pure red cell aplasia. Thymomas also tend to cause defective cell-mediated immunity so that manifestations of the latter and, in particular, candidosis can be associated with late onset myasthenia gravis.

The characteristic feature is increasing muscle weakness, aggravated by exercise particularly, and also other factors such as emotion, surgery, infections, or drugs such as the aminoglycoside antibiotics.

The muscle groups affected, in order of frequency, are (1) extraocular, (2) bulbar, (3) neck, (4) limb girdle, (5) distal limb, and (6) trunk. The course is highly variable but usually fluctuates, affecting one group of muscles more severely than the others and is frequently interrupted by spontaneous remissions which sometimes persist for years. The disease is rarely acutely or chronically progressive. Death from respiratory paralysis, which gave a 30% mortality before effective treatment became available, should not now be a significant risk. In patients with thymoma however, the tumor is the usual cause of death.

The diagnosis can be readily confirmed in most cases by showing the response to an anticholinesterase such as edrophonium. Acetylcholine receptor antibodies are found in about 90% of patients and can also be used to confirm the diagnosis.

Treatment (discovered by an English resident, Mary Walker, in an otherwise obscure London Hospital in 1936) is administration of anticholinesterase. However, thymectomy is probably the treatment of choice in young adults as it may confer permanent remission. Alternatively, immunosuppressive treatment or plasma exchange are usually effective, but like thymectomy, are not without difficulties or complications.

Other disorders of neuromuscular transmission. In the Eaton-Lambert syndrome there is defective release of acetylcholine at neuromuscular junctions associated usually with small cell carcinoma of the lung or occasionally with autoimmune diseases.

In botulism (Chapter 8), the toxin of *Clostridium botulinum* prevents the release of acetylcholine at the neuromuscular junction and widespread muscular, including respiratory paralysis results.

Myopathies

Myopathies (unlike myasthenia gravis) are diseases of muscle. They are also termed muscular dystrophies and include a great variety of disorders either genetic (primary) or secondary to systemic disease. The genetic myopathies include both diseases of muscles themselves and enzyme deficiencies (such as myophosphorylase deficiency) affecting muscles.

Their characteristic effect is weakening and atrophy (or pseudohypertrophy) of skeletal muscle. In the myotonic myopathies there is initially inability of muscles to relax fully before weakness and muscle atrophy develop. In the most severe (Duchenne) type, cardiomyopathy and early death are common.

The individual myopathies are uncommon or rare, but collectively are now the most common crippling diseases of childhood.

Muscular dystrophies

Pseudohypertrophic muscular dystrophy (Duchenne type*). This disease (Fig. 17-33) is inherited as a sex-linked recessive trait. Affected boys fail to walk normally, become disabled by the age of about 10, and usually die of respiratory failure before adulthood or later of cardiomyopathy.

At necropsy the muscles appear to be marbled with or largely replaced by fat. Microscopically, normal or necrotic and regenerating muscle fibers may be found, surrounded by fat.

Other myopathies are less severe and often compatible with a normal lifespan. They do not differ significantly in the pathological findings but rather in the groups of muscles predominantly affected.

Limb girdle muscular dystrophy. Males and females are affected in this simple recessive disease. The onset is typically in early adult life with progressive muscular weakness and pseudohypertrophy. The progress is variable; severe weakness may take 20 years to develop, but the expectation of life may be reduced.

Facioscapulohumeral muscular dystrophy. This autosomal dominant disease usually has its onset between 10 and 20 years. All the facial muscles, but particularly the orbicularis oris, are involved. However shoulder girdle weakness is sometimes the first sign. Most patients have a normal expectation of life and the prevalence of the disease is therefore relatively high.

The glycogen storage diseases. These genetic disorders, discussed in Chapter 3, cause muscle weakness as a result of defective glycogen metabolism. In the most common of these, myophosphorylase deficiency (McArdle's disease), there are typically, muscle cramps induced by exercise, and weakness associated with failure of lactic acid production, which can be used in diagnosis. Rhabdomyolysis can lead to myoglobinuria and renal failure. The other glycogen storage diseases produce distinctive clinical pictures also.

---

*G.B.A. Duchenne (1807-1875), French neurologist credited with being the first to use the biopsy in diagnosis.

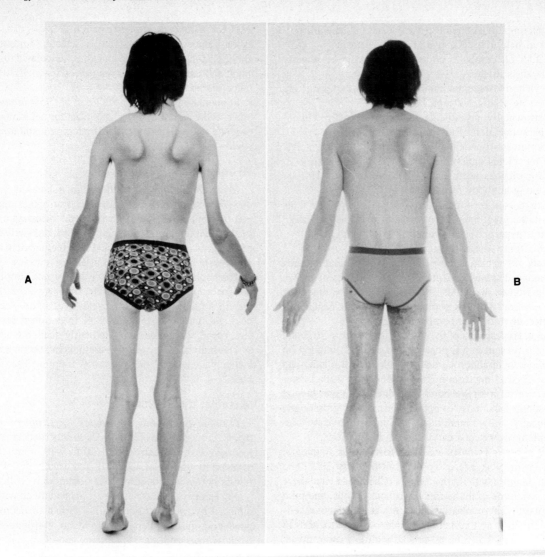

FIG. 17-33. Muscular dystrophy, pseudohypertrophic (Duchenne type). **A,** Obvious features are winging of the scapulae as a result of weakness of the muscles of the shoulder girdle and the pseudohypertrophy, particularly of the calves. **B,** Same patient in a photograph taken several years later. *(Courtesy Curator of the Gordon Museum, Guy's Hospital, London, England.)*

Congenital myopathies. These are rare conditions which can resemble the genetic myopathies clinically but which show characteristic abnormalities of muscle by light and electron microscopy. They are the main causes of "floppy baby syndrome" but do not necessarily shorten the expectation of life. Important examples of the congenital myopathies whose names indicate the main microscopic abnormalities in the muscle fibers are (1) rod body (nemaline), (2) centronuclear, and (3) mitochondrial myopathies.

Myotonic myopathies. As mentioned earlier the salient feature is slow relaxation of muscle after contraction. The most severe type is *myotonic muscular dystrophy (dystrophia myotonica),* an autosomal dominant disease, which causes widespread muscular weakness with more severe involvement of the muscles of the distal limbs, neck and face. Cataracts, endocrine disorders, cardiac disease, and other systemic disorders are often associated. Other myotonic disorders usually only involve the muscles and may not be significantly disabling.

Acquired myopathies. The most common of these is polymyositis as discussed below. Myopathy can also be secondary to a variety of endocrine disorders (particularly hyperthyroidism or hypothyroidism), bone diseases, and drugs (including alcohol) but is rarely a prominent feature clinically. Cardiac disease and other systemic disorders are often associated. Other myotonic disorders usually only involve the muscles and may not be significantly disabling.

Malignant hyperpyrexia. Malignant hyperpyrexia is a genetic disorder in which exposure to anesthetic agents and the muscle relaxant suxamethonium, particularly if prolonged, causes persistent muscle spasm and a progressive rise in body temperature which is not infrequently fatal. It is thought to be caused by sustained release of calcium ions and consequently prolongation of the myosin/actin reaction.

Polymyositis and dermatomyositis

Immunologic aspects of these inflammatory diseases of the muscles and skin have been discussed in Chapter 7.

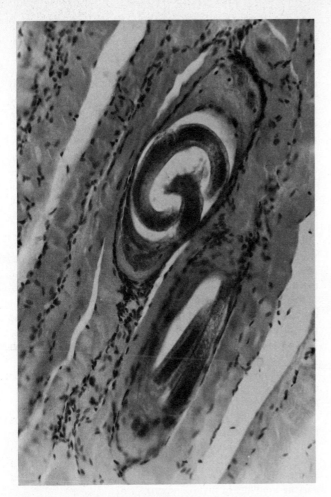

FIG. 17-34. Trichinosis. Larvae of *Trichinella spiralis* are shown encysting in striated muscle.

Pathology. The main features in approximate order of frequency are as follows:

1. Degeneration of muscle fibers associated with variable degrees of regeneration
2. Phagocytosis of necrotic muscle fibers
3. Interstitial infiltration of muscle by chronic inflammatory cells
4. Interstitial fibrosis and later, sometimes, calcinosis

Clinically, almost any age can be affected. Most patients are women between the ages of 50 and 60. The onset is typically insidious, usually with weakness of the girdle and proximal limb muscles, especially of the legs. Difficulty in speaking or swallowing can also develop.

In severe cases, weakness makes the patient bedridden and ultimately there can be atrophy, contracture and calcinosis of the muscles.

The most effective drugs are corticosteroids.

Trichinosis

Trichinosis is an infestation, particularly of muscles, caused by the larvae of the roundworm *Trichinella spiralis*. It is contracted by eating infected, inadequately cooked meat particularly pork or rarely, bear meat.

Trichinosis was at one time common in the United States but fewer than 50 cases were reported in 1985. Of these, the source was either grizzly bear or walrus meat in nearly 50% of the cases.

Pathogenesis and pathology. The larvae are encysted in the meat and are released by gastric digestion, after which they migrate to the intestines. The female worm liberates great numbers of larvae, which penetrate the intestinal wall to enter the bloodstream. Larvae are then deposited in skeletal muscle (Fig. 17-34).

The larvae penetrate muscle fibers causing myositis and infiltration mainly by lymphocytes and eosinophils. The larvae become coated with immune globulin and degenerating muscle. Later a fibrous reaction surrounds the larvae, which eventually become encysted but nevertheless remain viable for many years. After 1 or 2 years the cysts become calcified, and multiple foci can be seen in radiographs. Larvae do not encyst in the heart muscle but can cause severe interstitial myocarditis. The larvae seldom form cysts in the brain, but a granulomatous meningoencephalitis may develop.

Clinical aspects. In most cases the disease is mild or subclinical, indicating low levels of infiltration. At the other extreme there can be nausea, diarrhea, abdominal pain, and sometimes fever, as the larvae invade the intestine in large numbers. Hematogenous spread and invasion of muscles are often associated with fever, widespread muscle pain, tenderness, which may be prolonged, and edema.

Central nervous system involvement can cause a wide variety of changes, including meningoencephalitis and cranial or peripheral nerve palsies. Cardiac failure can result from severe myocardial infection, but the mortality overall is probably less than 2%. A high eosinophilia is characteristic.

The diagnosis can be confirmed by a muscle biopsy, which shows the coiled, encysted parasites within the muscle.

Thiabendazole sometimes produces clinical improvement, but there is no fully reliable treatment. Prevention is particularly important and consists of ensuring that pork and other meats are properly cooked.

Tumors of muscle

The main tumor of muscle is the rhabdomyosarcoma as rhabdomyomas are exceedingly rare. The so called abdominal desmoid tumor is relatively common but is a form of fibromatosis.

Rhabdomyoma. These tumors account for no more than 2% of all muscle tumors; they are most commonly found in the nasopharynx, tongue or other parts of the mouth where they produce symptomless swellings.

Microscopically, rhabdomyomas consists of large, rounded or polygonal cells with small nuclei and sometimes extensively vacuolated. In such cases the tumor appears largely fatty. Close examination and use of special stains however, clearly demonstrates regular striations in many of the cells.

Excision is curative.

Cardiac rhabdomyomas have essentially similar appearances but are regarded as hamartomas rather than true tumors. They are typically associated with tuberous sclerosis.

Rhabdomyosarcoma. This is one of the most common types of malignant soft tissue tumors in infants, children and adolescents. The most common sites are in the head and neck, particularly in the region of the orbit and in the oronasopharyngeal tissues. The paratesticular region is another important site but almost any area can be affected.

Clinically, rhabdomyosarcomas form rapidly growing, initially painless, soft tissue masses which soon invade and destroy any underlying bone. Symptoms and disability are determined largely by the site of origin of the tumor.

Microscopically, three main types of rhabdomyosarcoma, namely embryonal, alveolar, and pleomorphic, are recognized.

Embryonal rhabdomyosarcoma is the most common type and is predominantly found in children. Characteristic findings are cellular and myxoid areas, whilst the cells range in differentiation from nondescript small round cells to vacuolated rhabdomyoblasts as the result of their glycogen content. Rhabdomyoblasts are frequently strap, racquet or tadpole-shaped and cross striations may be shown by using a stain such as Masson's trichrome.

A variant of the embryonal rhabdomyosarcoma is the botryoid type which has a polypoid ("bunch of grapes") appearance and is mostly found in hollow organs or body cavities (Fig. 17-35). The superficial polypoid areas appear myxoid but elongated striated rhabdomyoblasts can be found.

Alveolar rhabdomyosarcoma has as its main microscopic feature, slitlike or more extensive spaces from the walls of which hang rounded or comma-shaped cells which are frequently also present in varying numbers in the spaces. The amount of intervening fibrous tissue is highly variable; elsewhere the tumor cells may be closely packed and multinucleate giant cells may be found.

Pleomorphic rhabdomyosarcoma is the most difficult to recognize microscopically. The cells are highly variable in size and shape and lack any orientation; the nuclei are mostly large with prominent nucleoli. Intracellular glycogen may be found with appropriate stains but cells with cross striations demonstrable with conventional stains may be difficult to find. Increasing numbers of these lesions have been found to be malignant fibrous histiocytomas on reassessment.

In diagnosis, cross striated cells may be difficult to find but electron microscopy can show the characteristic Z banding as well as thick (myosin) and thin (actin) fibrils. However, the latter two components may be detectable with monoclonal antibodies to myogenic proteins such as myoglobin or intermediate filament desmin.

Combination therapy appears to have brought a significant improvement in the prognosis. The current treatment of choice is therefore wide excision, radiotherapy and chemotherapy but the prognosis is still poor for group III (gross residual tumor after resection) and group IV (metastases already present at diagnosis) cases.

Untreated or incompletely treated rhabdomyosarcomas widely infiltrate and destroy adjacent tissues including bone. Metastases are mainly to the lungs, lymph nodes and bone marrow but a wide variety of organs can be involved.

Proliferative myositis. This is a rare tumorlike lesion that can justifiably be described as pseudosarcomatous and, in the past particularly, has been mistaken for a rhabdomyosarcoma. It is a counterpart of proliferative fasciitis but arises within muscle.

Clinically, proliferative myositis usually forms a painless mass that can grow significantly in size in a few days. Middle-aged adults are predominantly affected.

Microscopically, the mass is poorly defined and infiltrates the surrounding tissues. It consists of highly pleomorphic cells including giant, basophilic ganglion-like cells with large nuclei and prominent nucleoli. Occasional mitoses may be seen. In addition, there may be immature fibroblastlike spindle cells and varying amounts of myxoid matrix.

Excision is curative and there is less tendency to recurrence than in the case of the fibromatoses.

FIBROUS TUMORS AND TUMORLIKE LESIONS OF SOFT TISSUES

Fibrous tumors of soft tissues form a diverse group of proliferative disorders that differ widely in their behavior. Some are neoplastic whilst others are probably inflammatory, though their clinical and histologic features mimic true neoplasms.

Fibrous tumors of soft tissues can be simply classified as follows:

1. Benign fibroblastic proliferations, including fasciitis
2. Fibromatoses (superficial and deep)
3. Fibrosarcoma

This classification correlates well with clinical behavior in that (1) benign fibrous proliferations and superficial fibromatoses are usually small, localized and do not recur after excision; (2) deep fibromatoses (desmoid tumors) can reach a large size if untreated, are diffusely infiltrative and frequently recur; (3) fibrosarcoma is frankly malignant and has high rates of recurrence and metastasis.

Nodular fasciitis

Benign fibroblastic proliferations encompass a group of reactive and nonneoplastic inflammatory conditions which account for a high proportion of fibrous soft tissue lesions. They usually grow rapidly and form small nodules, thus the name nodular fasciitis.

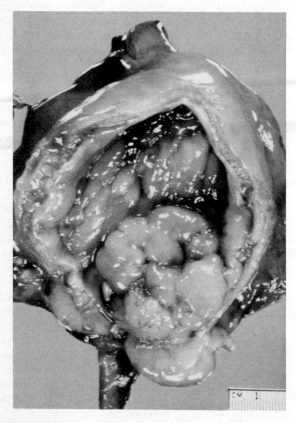

FIG. 17-35. Sarcoma botryoides, a variant of rhabdomyosarcoma of the urinary bladder in an 8-year-old boy. Note the polypoid appearance of the tumor.

Nodular fasciitis is typically a solitary lesion, less than 3 cm in size. It is most common between the ages of 20 and 35, but any age can be affected. The lesion is superficial, can involve any part of the body but has a predeliction for the forearms and chest wall.

Histologically, there is proliferation of fibroblasts which are arranged in short bundles. These are separated by loose "myxoid" stroma, rich in mucopolysaccharides and in which there are usually chronic inflammatory cells and microhemorrhages (Fig. 17-36). A fine reticulin meshwork may be gradually replaced by increasing amounts of collagen fibers as the lesion matures. The condition is self-limiting and local excision is curative.

Fibromatoses

The fibromatoses are divided into two major groups, namely, superficial and deep. Individual examples are named after their anatomic sites (palmar, plantar etc.).

Superficial fibromatoses are confined to the superficial fascial planes, are slow growing and small (1-2 cm in diameter). By contrast, deep fibromatoses *(desmoid tumors)* involve the musculoaponeurotic fascia, grow rapidly and can attain a large size. Malignant change in fibromatoses of any type is rare.

Superficial fibromatoses

Superficial fibromatoses mostly affect men; their incidence increases with age and is higher in diabetics. The role of trauma in the pathogenesis is controversial and their etiology is uncertain.

Superficial fibromatoses commonly form nodules which are frequently bilateral; several may develop at different times. They are often asymptomatic, but may cause dull aching or tingling sensations.

Histologically, these nodules are cellular and composed of parallel fascicles of uniform, spindle-shaped fibroblasts, separated by a collagenous stroma.

Local excision is curative.

Deep fibromatoses

These fibrous tumors are slow growing and deep seated in the connective tissue of muscles and their fascia. The most common sites are the muscles of the shoulder, chest wall, back and thighs of adolescents and young adults.

Abdominal fibromatosis (abdominal desmoid) involves the abdominal wall of women of childbearing age, particularly during or after pregnancy (Fig. 17-37).

Other forms of deep fibromatosis are intraabdominal and involve the mesentery or retroperitoneum (Fig. 17-38). Intra-

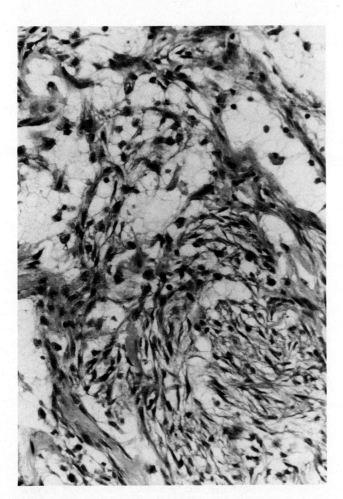

FIG. 17-36. Nodular fasciitis. Note the loose bundles of fibroblasts in a mucoid stroma containing chronic inflammatory cells.

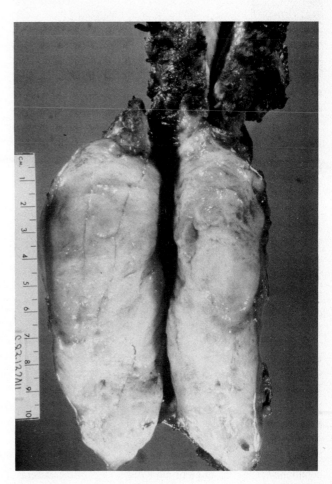

FIG. 17-37. Abdominal fibromatosis (desmoid tumor) resected from the anterior abdominal wall of a young woman. The lesion has a coarse trabeculated surface resembling dense scar tissue.

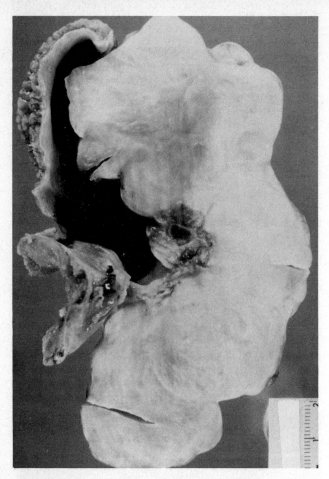

FIG. 17-38. Intraabdominal fibromatosis involving the mesentery and a segment of small intestine.

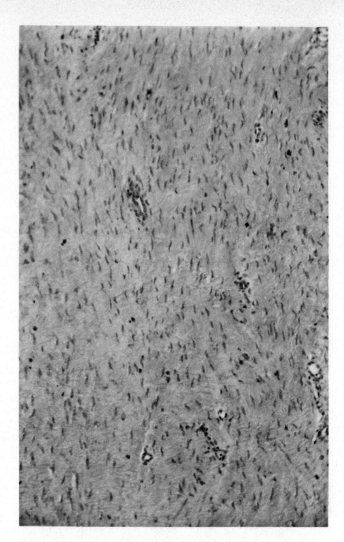

FIG. 17-39. Fibromatosis showing uniform slender fibroblasts in a dense collagenous stroma.

abdominal and other desmoids are present in an estimated 50% of cases of Gardner's syndrome (Chapter 14).

At the time of diagnosis, the majority of deep fibromatoses are between 5 and 20 cm in diameter. They are poorly circumscribed and may encroach on adjacent structures such as nerves or blood vessels.

Microscopically, these tumors consist of interlacing bundles of uniform, slender fibroblasts, separated by heavily collagenous stroma (Fig. 17-39). Some areas may be more cellular than others and infiltration of adjacent tissues, particularly muscle is often conspicuous; sarcolemmal giant cells may then give a false appearance of malignancy.

Treatment is by wide surgical excision, and because of their infiltrative nature, recurrence is common if excision is inadequate. These tumors do not metastasize however and, rarely, spontaneous regression has been reported.

Fibrosarcoma

A fibrosarcoma usually forms a slow-growing, deep-seated soft tissue mass, 3 to 8 cm in size (Fig. 17-40). The most common sites are the thigh or more distal parts of the extremities. It is most common between the ages of 35 to 55 years but almost any age can be affected. The tumor is firm and the cut surface appears well circumscribed.

Histologically, fibrosarcomas consist of parallel or intersecting fasicles and bundles of spindle fibroblasts, often form-

ing a herringbone pattern. The fibroblast nuclei are enlarged, oval or slender and hyperchomatic with scanty cytoplasm surrounding them (Fig. 17-41). Mitoses are usually evident. The amount of stroma and collagen formation is variable.

Treatment is by wide surgical excision and if this is less than complete the recurrence rate is 60%. Dissemination of fibrosarcomas is by the bloodstream, principally to the lungs. In children, the outcome is more favorable with substantially lower rates of recurrence and metastasis.

Fibrohistiocytic neoplasms

Fibrous histiocytomas have been relatively recently recognized as an entity, however their histogenesis remains controversial. This neoplasm shows the morphologic features of both fibroblasts and histiocytes, but the bulk of evidence indicates that the latter cells are poorly differentiated fibroblasts rather than true histiocytes.

Fibrous histiocytomas can be divided into 3 major groups: (1) benign, (2) intermediate or low grade malignant, and (3) malignant fibrous histiocytoma. Many tumors formerly categorized as pleomorphic fibrosarcomas and other sarcomas are now regarded as malignant fibrous histiocytomas.

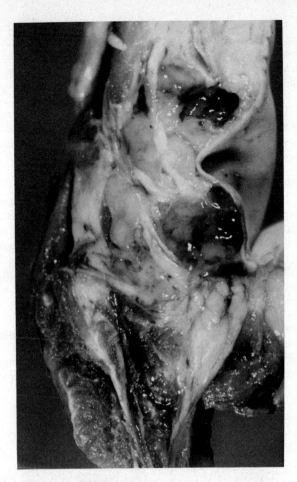

FIG. 17-40. Recurrent fibrosarcoma of the arm showing the typical infiltrative growth pattern and extension into the surrounding soft tissues, skeletal muscle, and skin.

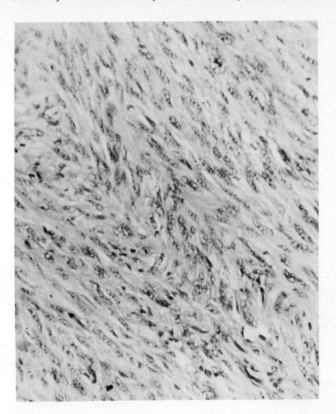

FIG. 17-41. Fibrosarcoma showing fascicles of poorly differentiated fibroblasts. The cellular pattern is irregular and mitotic figures are present.

Benign fibrous histiocytoma

Several alternative names have been given to this tumor; dermatofibroma or sclerosing hemangioma are the most widely used.

Benign fibrous histiocytoma usually affects the dermis and superficial subcutaneous tissues, and only rarely, deeper tissues. It is most common in the third and fourth decades, and appears as a solitary raised, sometimes pedunculated, red-brown nodule, a few millimeters to a few centimeters in diameter. Multiple nodules may form in a third of the cases.

Microscopically, the tumor is composed of tightly intermingled fibroblasts and histiocytes, typically, forming cartwheel or storiform (tangled) patterns (Fig. 17-42). Multinucleate giant cells, foam cells and hemosiderin-laden macrophages are common features and inflammatory cells are frequently associated.

Surgical excision is usually effective.

Dermatofibrosarcoma protuberans

Dermatofibroma protuberans (DFSP) resembles benign fibrous histiocytoma both clinically and histologically but is characteristically larger and represents the intermediate grade of this group of tumors. DFSP typically affects the trunk of young males between the ages of 20 to 40 years and forms a solitary, nodular subcutaneous mass of an average size of 5 cm. Other sites are the extremities and the head and neck region. Occasionally, multiple small nodules form and this is more frequent with recurrent tumors.

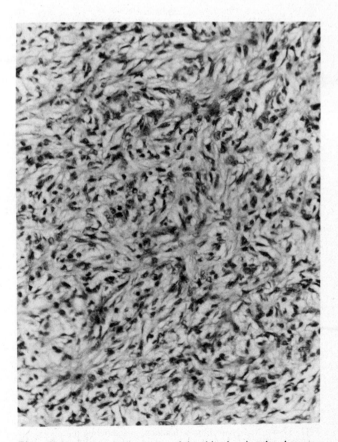

FIG. 17-42. Fibrous histiocytoma of the skin showing the characteristic storiform pattern consisting mainly of spindle-shaped fibroblasts.

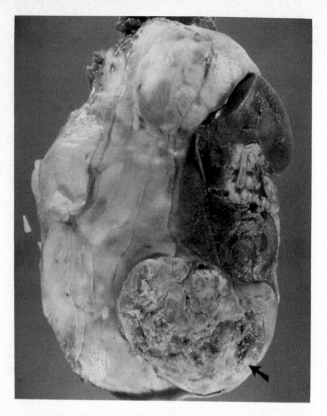

FIG. 17-43. Malignant fibrous histiocytoma of the retroperitoneum. The tumor surrounds the kidney and in its lower pole there is an area of necrosis *(arrow)* a frequent finding in these tumors.

Histologically, DFSP is diffusely infiltrative, extends into the epidermis and involves the adjacent dermis and subcutaneous tissue. It usually consists of compact, plump fibroblasts in a characteristic, uniform storiform pattern. Unlike the benign variant of this tumor, giant cells, foam cells and inflammatory cells are not common features.

DFSP is locally aggressive and has a high recurrence rate so that wide excision is necessary. A very few of these tumors (less than 1%) metastasize, usually to the lungs or regional lymph nodes.

Malignant fibrous histiocytoma

Malignant fibrous histiocytoma (MFH) is probably second only to liposarcoma as the most common type of sarcoma of late adult life. It usually arises in the deep soft tissues of the extremities or retroperitoneum, but occasionally involves bone or other tissues. The majority of MFHs are in men between 50 and 70 years but almost any age can be affected. The tumor grows slowly and is usually at least 5 cm in diameter at the time of diagnosis. Retroperitoneal tumors may grow up to 30 cm (Fig. 17-43).

Microscopically, MFH is pleomorphic and there are several histologic patterns. The most typical is an infiltrative pattern consisting of fascicles of spindle cells in a storiform arrangement, surrounding slitlike vessels and commonly intermingled

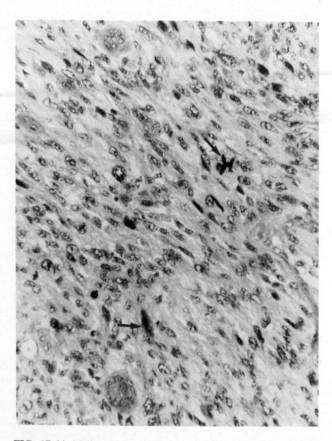

FIG. 17-44. Malignant fibrous histiocytoma showing the poorly differentiated sarcomatous cells, which vary in form from spindle shaped to large multinucleated giant cells. Note the hyperchromasia, pleomorphism, and the bizarre mitotic figures *(arrow)*.

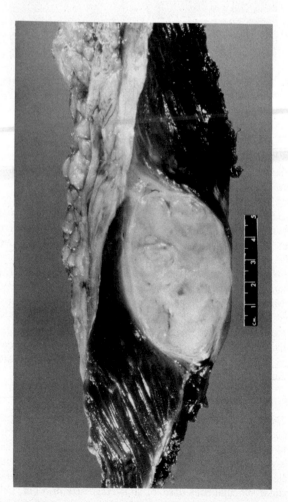

FIG. 17-45. Liposarcoma of the thigh in a 60-year-old man. Despite their malignant nature, these tumors, as shown here, tend to be well circumscribed. Note the fine lobular pattern.

with round or polygonal mononuclear cells. Some cells are multinucleate, giant, bizarre or foamy. Nuclear pleomorphism, anaplasia and high mitotic activity are frequent features (Fig. 17-44). The stroma varies from a compact collagenous matrix to loose myxoid tissue. In some types, many neutrophils, lymphocytes and xanthoma cells are present.

Malignant fibrous histiocytoma is a sarcoma of high malignant potential with recurrence rates of 40% to 70% and rates of metastasis of 40% to 50%. The prognosis depends on the depth, size and histologic type of the tumor. Spread, as with other sarcomas, is hematogenous and usually to the lungs.

Treatment is by wide resection supplemented by chemotherapy and/or radiotherapy.

Lipomatous tumors

Neoplasms of adipose tissue can be benign or malignant. The benign group includes several subgroups of which the most common is the *lipoma,* which is the most common mesenchymal tumor in humans. It is however rare in early life but of increasing incidence with age. The majority are found in the fifth and sixth decades, and more frequently in women and in the obese. Most of these tumors are solitary (rarely multiple), well circumscribed and superficial. The main sites are the back, shoulders and neck: deep, intramuscular or retroperitoneal tumors are rare.

Lipomas typically consist of mature adipose tissue surrounded by a thin capsule of fibrous tissue.

Lipomas are benign and respond to local excision. Recurrence is rare and malignant change is virtually unknown.

Lipoblastoma is the counterpart to lipoma in infancy and early childhood. It consists of irregular lobules of immature fat cells.

Liposarcoma is the most common sarcoma in later adult life with a peak incidence between 40 and 70 years of age; there is a slight male predominance. The tumor is typically deep seated and 5 to 20 cm across at the time of diagnosis. The most common sites in descending order of frequency are the thighs (Fig. 17-45), retroperitoneum and trunk. Retroperitoneal tumors can cause abdominal distension and compress the viscera or ureters. The tumor appears deceptively well circumscribed macroscopically as small, infiltrating tumor nodules can be seen microscopically.

Histologically, four main types, relating to the developmental stage of the lipoblast, have been characterized (Fig. 17-46). These are: (1) well differentiated, (2) myxoid, (3) round cell, and (4) pleomorphic. Myxoid liposarcoma is the most common and consists of lipoblasts with a signet-ring appearance (due to microscopic fat globules) in a delicate myxoid stroma with a prominent network of capillaries (Fig. 17-47). The most poorly differentiated (pleomorphic) liposarcomas are highly cellular. The cells vary widely in size and shape; they include deeply eosinophilic giant cells and so little fat as to make it difficult to recognize their lipoblastic origin.

The prognosis of liposarcoma depends on the histologic type, anatomic site and stage. Excision the first line of treatment,

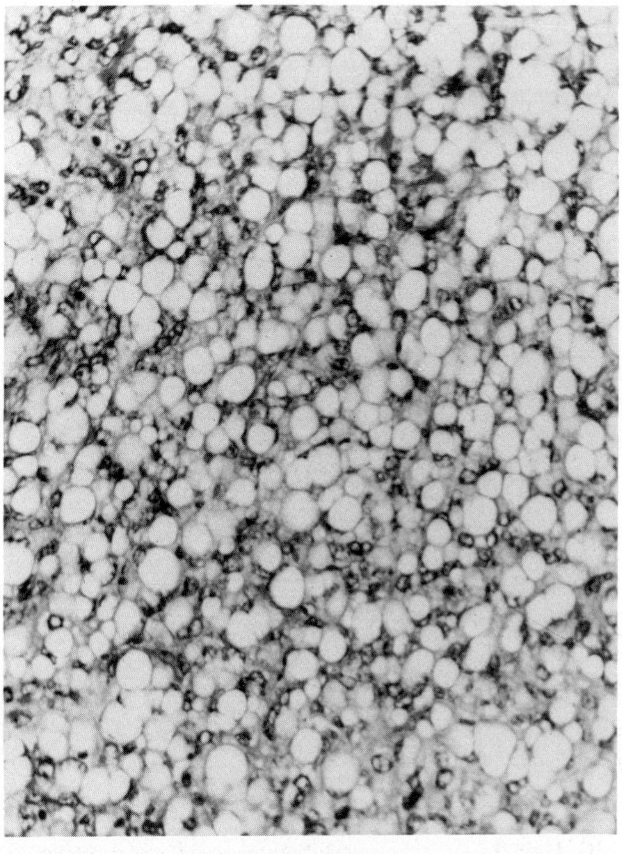

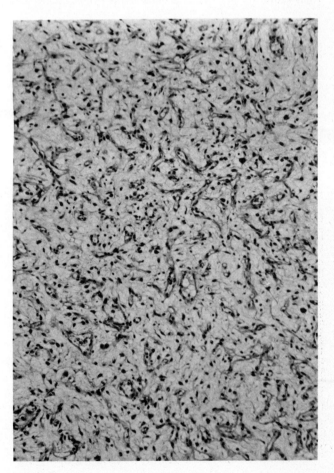

FIG. 17-46. Well-differentiated liposarcoma; a histologic pattern of this tumor in which the cells resemble lipoblasts.

FIG. 17-47. Myxoid liposarcoma; another histologic type that is characterized by a rich, fine vascular network and myxoid stroma.

but is difficult to achieve completely, especially from the ret-roperitoneal region; 50% to 70% of these tumors (all types) therefore recur. Adjunctive radiotherapy is however helpful particularly for myxoid liposarcomas. Poorly differentiated tumors metastasize to the lungs and other viscera.

Alveolar soft part sarcoma

Alveolar soft part sarcoma is a rare but distinct type of soft tissue sarcoma, the nature of which is unknown and controversial. It affects young people and its highest incidence is between the ages of 15 and 35; females are more frequently affected. The most common sites for this tumor are the head and neck region in children and the lower extremities in adults. It usually forms a painless, slow-growing poorly circumscribed mass.

Histologically, the tumor cells are typically arranged in nests of varying size, forming a well defined alveolar pattern and separated by fine fibrovascular network (Fig. 17-48). In some cases however the alveolar pattern is absent and the tumor cells form unbroken sheets. The individual cells are loosely cohesive, large, round or polygonal and have an eosinophilic, granular cytoplasm rich in glycogen. A characteristic feature is the presence of intracytoplasmic needle shaped crystals which stain strongly with periodic acid Schiff (PAS) and are apparently unique to this tumor. Ultrastructurally, these crystals are rhomboid with a regular lattice pattern.

Alveolar soft part sarcoma has a poor prognosis with a 5 year survival rate of only 60%. Metastases to the lung or brain may be the first manifestation of the tumor but metastases may also develop many years, even up to 30 years, after treatment. The latter is primarily surgical but supplemented by radiation and chemotherapy.

Epithelioid sarcoma

Epithelioid sarcoma is a rare distinctive soft tissue sarcoma that may be seen at all ages, but characteristically in young adults (15 to 35 years of age). It is primarily a tumor of the extremities particularly the distal parts of the upper extremity i.e. fingers, hands, and forearms. It presents as a subcutaneous or deeply seated nodule or group of nodules. Their size is extremely variable ranging from a few millimeters to several centimeters. Deeply seated tumor nodules are commonly attached to tendons or fascia.

Histologically, the tumor nodules show central necrosis and some may appear coalescent. The tumor cells vary in shape from large oval polygonal cells with abundant eosinophilic cytoplasm to elongated spindle shaped cells (Fig. 17-49). The sheets of polygonal tumor cells are responsible for the tumor's resemblence to an epithelial neoplasm—thus the designation "epithelioid sarcoma" and indeed, these cells stain positively with antisera to keratin as well as to vimentin. From a biologic point of view, this neoplasm is an extremely interesting example of a mesenchymal neoplasm exhibiting "epithelial" differentiation. This is the reverse of the process seen in examples of spindle cell or "sarcoma-like" differentiation in carcinomas.

Epithelioid sarcoma has a high recurrence (75%) and metastatic rates (50%). Metastasis is most commonly to regional lymph nodes and lungs.

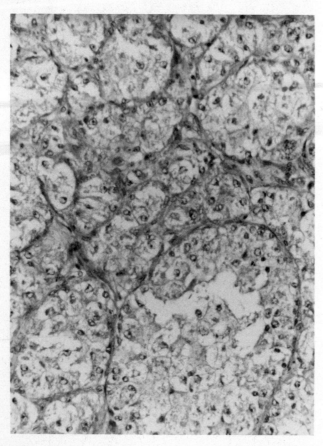

FIG. 17-48. Alveolar soft part sarcoma consisting of nests of varying size consisting of large granular tumor cells. Note the alveolar-like pattern.

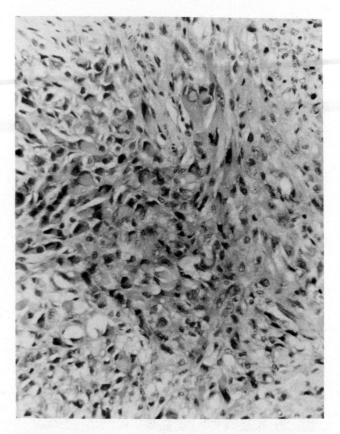

FIG. 17-49. Epithelioid sarcoma. Note the central oval and polygonal cells which resemble epithelial cells. At the periphery the tumor cells are elongated and spindle shaped. The tumor cells stain positively with antibodies to keratin.

Selected readings

Audran M and Kumar R: The physiology and pathophysiology of vitamin D, Mayo Clin Proc 60:851, 1985.

Cavazzana AO, Miser JS, and Jefferson J et al: Experimental evidence for a neural origin of Ewing's sarcoma of bone, Am J Path 127:507, 1987.

Chambers TJ: The pathobiology of the osteoclast, J Clin Pathol 38:241, 1985.

Consensus development conference: Prophylaxis and treatment of osteoporosis, Br Med J 295:914, 1987.

Drachman DB: Present and future treatment of myasthenia gravis, N Engl J Med 316:743, 1987.

Enzinger FM and Weiss SW: Soft tissue tumors, The CV Mosby Co. St. Louis, 1983.

Ducatman BS, Scheithauer BW, and Dahlin DC: Malignant bone tumors associated with neurofibromatosis, Mayo Clin Proc 58:578, 1983.

Huvos AG: Osteogenic sarcoma of bones and soft tissues in older persons: a clinicopathologic analysis of 117 patients older than 60 years, Cancer 57:1442, 1986.

Huvos AG, Woodard HQ, and Heilweil M: Postradiation malignant fibrous histiocytoma of bone: a clinicopathologic study of 20 patients, Am J Surg Path 10(1):9, 1986.

Maletz N, McMorrow LE, and Greco MA et al: Ewing's sarcoma: pathology, tissue culture, and cytogenetics, Cancer 58:252, 1986.

Minkin C and Shapiro IM: Osteoclasts, mononuclear phagocytes, and physiological bone resorption, Calcif Tissue Int 39:357, 1986.

Nakashima Y, Morishita S, and Kotoura Y et al: Malignant fibrous histiocytoma of bone: a review of 13 cases and an ultrastructural study, Cancer 55:2804, 1985.

Nakashima Y, Unni KK, and Shives TC et al: Mesenchymal chondrosarcoma of bone and soft tissue: a review of 111 cases, Cancer 57:2444, 1986.

Nathan CF: Secretory products of macrophages, J Clin Invest 79:319, 1987.

Navas-Palacios JJ, Aparicio-Duque R, and Valdes MD: On the histiogenesis of Ewing's sarcoma, Cancer 53:1882, 1984.

Osteosarcoma, Lancet ii:131, 1985.

Osteoporosis, Lancet ii:833, 1987.

Paget's disease of bone, Calcif Tissue Int 38:309, 1986.

Taylor WF, Ivins JC, and Pritchard DJ et al: Trends and variability in survival among patients with osteosarcoma: a 7-year update, Mayo Clin Proc 60:91, 1985.

Upchurch KS, Simon LS, and Schiller AL et al: Giant cell reparative granuloma of Paget's disease of bone: a unique clinical entity, Ann Intern Med 98:35, 1983.

Wald ER: Risk factors for osteomyelitis, Am J Med 78 (Suppl 6B) 206, 1985.

CHAPTER 18

Diseases of the endocrine system

The endocrine glands produce hormones that are essential regulators of functions ranging from body growth to autonomic activity. These hormones act in low concentrations on specific receptors in the target organs.

Hormonal function

Hormones have a regulatory function and probably primarily affect cellular enzyme systems. Most peptide hormones act on a receptor on the cell surface and activate adenyl cyclase ("second messenger"). This mediates the conversion of ATP to cyclic AMP (cAMP) in the cell cytoplasm. cAMP in turn, acts on an intracellular receptor to stimulate phosphorylation of cell proteins (Fig. 18-1). Other second messenger systems, such as cyclic GMP appear to act in a similar way.

Pathogenesis of endocrine diseases

Most endocrine diseases result from *overproduction* or *underproduction* of hormones, caused by disorders of the glands themselves or of their control mechanisms. In addition, the target organs may fail to respond to normally produced hormones by a variety of mechanisms such as deficiency or defects of hormone receptors, or post-receptor abnormalities, such as defective enzymic activity. Generally, however, overactivity of endocrine glands results from hyperplasia or tumor formation.

By far the most common endocrine diseases are diabetes mellitus and thyroid disorders; the remainder are uncommon.

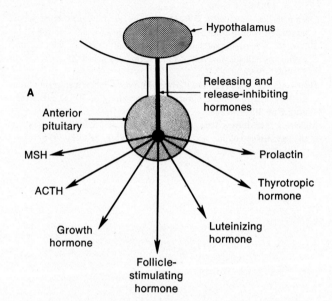

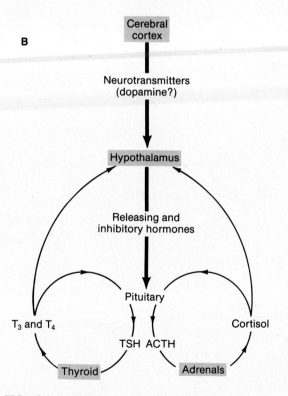

FIG. 18-2. **A,** Simplified scheme of interaction of the hypothalamus and the anterior pituitary. **B,** Endocrine biofeedback systems. For simplicity the interactions between the pituitary, thyroid, and adrenals only have been shown.

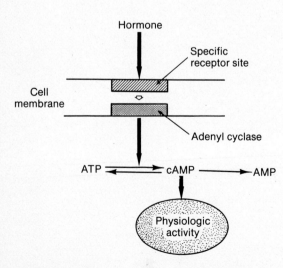

FIG. 18-1. Effect of hormones on adenylate cyclase.

Autoimmunity in endocrine deficiency diseases

Many of the endocrine deficiency diseases appear to be immunologically mediated, as aplasia of these glands is rare. There is good evidence for autoimmune processes being involved in thyroiditis, Addison's disease, and some cases of hypoparathyroidism and diabetes mellitus. Thyroiditis was in fact the disease which formed the basis for Witebsky's formulation of criteria for autoimmune disease.

Evidence for autoimmunity in endocrine deficiency diseases includes in many cases, the presence of organ-specific antibodies binding to components of secretory cells or others directed against the hormone, or both. Serum containing such autoantibodies, when injected into an animal may induce a similar disease, as shown by Witebsky in the case of thyroiditis. In addition, many of these endocrine deficiency disorders have the typical general characteristics of autoimmune diseases, namely they (1) are more common in women, (2) often have a familial tendency, and (3) tend to be associated with other autoimmune diseases; for example, there is a strong association between thyroiditis and pernicious anemia. Moreover, in the polyendocrinopathy syndrome discussed later, multiple autoimmune endocrine deficiencies, particularly Addison's disease and hypoparathyroidism develop in the same patient.

THE PITUITARY

Pituitary lesions can have a wide variety of effects because this gland produces many hormones that regulate the function of other endocrine glands (Fig. 18-2). Pituitary tumors, even when benign, can sometimes have severe effects. A growth at that site, for example, may compress the optic tracts and cause loss of visual fields.

Pituitary hormones and their control

Although, in the past three cell types have been identified in the anterior pituitary, it is now possible to recognize at least six main types by means of electron microscopy and immunohistochemical staining methods. The histologic staining properties of these cells when stained by the standard hematoxylin and eosin method, are outlined below. Many of these cells can, however, be identified with greater certainty with monoclonal antibodies to the hormones that they secrete:

1. Acidophils
   a. Growth hormone cells (somatotrophs)
   b. Prolactin cells (lactotrophs)
2. Basophils
   a. MSH-ACTH cells (melanocorticotrophs)
   b. TSH cells (thyrotrophs)
   c. FS-LH cells (gonadotrophs)
3. Chromophobes
   a. Poorly granulated cells of all varieties

There is preferential concentration of these specialized cells in different parts of the anterior pituitary. For example, the somatotrophs are located mainly in the lateral wings while corticotrophs are present in the central wedge.

Although chromophobes have little affinity for standard histologic stains, they do in fact synthesize hormones; however, the concentration of these hormones is not high enough to react histochemically. It is possible, too, that some pituitary cells are capable of producing more than one peptide, but it is technically very difficult to demonstrate this property.

Biochemical studies of the pituitary peptide hormones have shown that several are derived from a single precursor peptide. For example, in the anterior pituitary, proopiomelanocortin (POMC) is cleaved, yielding ACTH, β-lipotropin and β-endorphin (see Fig. 18-3). In the intermediate lobe, ACTH and β-lipotropin are almost entirely processed to α-melanocyte stimulating hormone (MSH) and β endorphin.

The posterior pituitary stores *vasopressin* (antidiuretic hormone) and *oxytocin,* which increases the force of uterine contraction. Vasopressin and oxytocin differ only by one amino acid in the side chain. Both hormones are secreted in the supraoptic and paraventricular nuclei, are attached to carrier substances, and travel down the axons of the hypothalamohypophyseal tract to the posterior lobe where they are stored.

Somatostatin. Somatostatin, a peptide, was first isolated from the hypothalamus as a product of specific neurons but has since been found in the anterior and posterior lobes of the pituitary, the gamma cells of the islets of Langerhans, gastric mucosal endocrine cells and many others.

Somatostatin inhibits the release of pituitary growth hormone and many other peptides but has no inhibitory effect on, for example, luteinizing or follicular stimulating hormones. There are specific receptors for somatostatin in many sites. Although its intracellular mode of action is not known, it could interfere with any of the several processes that mediate the physiologic action of hormones as summarized in Fig. 18-2, *A.* Nevertheless, although its physiologic function is still uncertain, it has been used therapeutically to control the effects of hormone-producing tumors such as carcinoids (Chapter 14), which have metastasized.

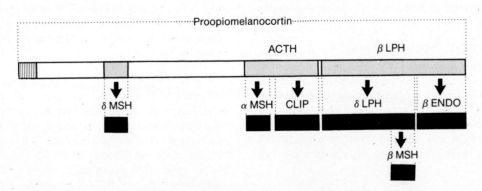

FIG. 18-3. Diagram showing the derivation of pituitary peptide hormones from a single precursor molecule. *ACTH,* adrenocorticotrophic hormone; *LPH,* lipotropic hormone; *MSH,* melanin-stimulating hormone; *CLIP,* corticotropin-like intermediate lobe peptide; *ENDO,* endorphin.

Hypopituitarism

Total failure of pituitary function (panhypopituitarism) is known as *Simmond's disease.** Hypopituitarism in the adult can be the result of any of the following:

1. Postpartum pituitary necrosis (Sheehan's syndrome)
2. A nonfunctioning pituitary tumor
3. Pituitary failure in late acromegaly
4. Hypophysectomy

Sheehan's syndrome†

Pathogenesis and pathology. Sheehan's syndrome appears to result from extensive thrombosis of the pituitary vessels together with hypotension secondary to blood loss during delivery. The blood supply to the anterior pituitary is dependent on the hypophyseal portal system, since the direct arterial blood supply alone is inadequate. Thus the pituitary is vulnerable to circulatory damage. Small infarcts are found in up to 3% of autopsy specimens, but at least 60% of the pituitary must be destroyed before clinical effects appear.

The pituitary also enlarges during pregnancy as a result of hyperplasia of prolactin-producing cells; it is then even more vulnerable to any decrease in blood supply.

In Sheehan's syndrome, almost the entire anterior pituitary can undergo necrosis, but the clinical effects depend on the degree of destruction. In the early stages the lesions appear either ischemic or hemorrhagic. The necrotic tissue gradually undergoes phagocytosis and is replaced by a fibrous scar.

Clinical aspects. The characteristic first signs of this disease are failure of both lactation and menstruation. The onset may be insidious and symptoms are variable. The main effects tend ultimately to be hypofunction of the thyroid, adrenals, and gonads. The diagnosis depends on the history and laboratory evidence of decreased plasma thyroid stimulating hormone (TSH), adrenocorticotropic hormone (ACTH), and gonadotropin levels. Treatment is mainly to maintain thyroid and adrenal function with thyroxine and corticosteroids respectively.

Nonfunctioning pituitary tumors

The most common are nonfunctioning adenomas and craniopharyngiomas (Chapter 20). These can cause pressure atrophy of the gland.

Hypophysectomy

Surgical removal of the pituitary was, in the past, performed mainly for hormone-responsive carcinomas of the breast when all else had failed. As effective antiestrogenic agents have become available, this operation is now rarely performed for this purpose.

Other syndromes of hypopituitarism

Prepubertal hypopituitarism. This syndrome is usually the result of a craniopharyngioma of early onset or a suprasellar cyst. The effect is dwarfism without distortion of normal body proportions and delay in or failure of sexual development.

Froelich's syndrome.‡ Froelich's syndrome is characterized by obesity of the trunk and failure of sexual development and may be associated with a tumor of the hypothalamic-pituitary area.

---

*M. Simmonds (1855-1957), German physician.
†H.L. Sheehan (b. 1900), English pathologist.
‡A. Froelich (1871-1953), Austrian/American physician.

Hormonal regulation of growth

Determination of body stature is multifactorial; genetic, nutritional, hormonal and other factors are involved. With respect to hormonal factors, pituitary growth hormone and sex steroids are the most important. Growth hormone, however, has no demonstrable effect on cartilage in vitro and appears, in vivo, to act indirectly by stimulating a mediator (somatomedin) at another site. Several somatomedins have now been isolated and purified. The most important of these appears to be *insulin-like growth factor (IGF) I*, also termed somatomedin C (SM-C), which promotes growth at the epiphyses and the normal pubertal growth spurt appears to depend on the combined actions of growth hormone, IGF I and sex steroids.

Plasma levels of somatomedin C may be used to assess growth hormone secretion and normal reference levels in relation to age and sex, have been established.

Short stature is regarded as a social stigma and can have undesirable psychologic effects; it can be primary (idiopathic) or result from such causes as damage to the pituitary during irradiation of an intracranial tumor.

Children who have growth hormone deficiency, have been successfully treated with human growth hormone, but some have developed Creutzfeldt-Jakob disease (a lethal brain disease caused by a "slow" virus) or have developed antibodies to the hormone. More recently, a biosynthetic growth hormone has been produced and this overcomes the hazard of transmitting infection.

There is often also a desire to treat children of short stature but without detectable abnormality; this would require long-term use of growth hormone, but a variety of hazards may ensue. Antibodies (both to the biosynthetic and the endogenous hormone) may form or diabetes, hypertension or even acromegaly might finally ensue. These hazards seem to be of a low order but have yet to be fully assessed.

Growth hormone releasing hormone (GHRH) is a peptide produced in the hypothalamus. GHRH is a possible alternative to growth hormone for the treatment of short stature.

Hyperpituitarism

Hyperpituitarism is most often caused by a hormone-secreting pituitary adenoma. The pathogenesis of pituitary adenomas remains unknown but there is growing evidence that 80% to 90% of these tumors arise de novo in the pituitary. The remaining 10% to 20% of cases are possibly the result of an underlying disorder of hypothalamic regulation.

Pituitary adenomas usually secrete only one hormone; overproduction of either GH or ACTH is the most important. Tumors producing MSH or TSH are very rare. The important effects of hyperpituitarism are acromegaly, Cushing's disease, or hyperprolactinemia.

Pituitary adenomas

These tumors arise from and consist of adenohypophyseal cells. Based on staining characteristics of the cell cytoplasm, they were divided previously into chromophobic, acidophilic, and basophilic types. This classification however, fails to identify the endocrine function of the adenoma cells. Advanced morphologic techniques including electron microscopy and immunochemistry, have led to a functional classification of pituitary adenomas, including the following*:

---

*They can be further classified by the degree of granulation of the cells.

1. Growth hormone cell adenoma (Fig. 18-4)
2. Prolactin cell adenoma
3. Mixed growth hormone-prolactin cell adenoma
4. Acidophilic stem cell adenoma
5. Corticotroph cell adenoma
6. Thyrotroph cell adenoma
7. Gonadotroph cell adenoma
8. Undifferentiated cell adenoma

Adenomas consisting of acidophilic stem cells or cells sparse in secretory granules are frequently nonfunctional.

Histologically, it is often difficult to distinguish between benign and malignant tumors, but the overwhelming majority are benign. An expanding benign tumor can extend beyond the sella turcica and give the appearance of invading adjacent tissues, such as dura, bone, vessels, and cranial nerves. These *invasive* adenomas, however, are regarded as benign. Evidence of local invasion may be seen in approximately 35% of all types of pituitary adenomas. By contrast, a minority of tumors can prove to be carcinomas, which histologically are cellular, pleomorphic tumors with increased mitosis and which can metastasize. Nevertheless, conclusions regarding the biologic behavior of these tumors cannot be drawn solely from their histologic appearances.

Gigantism and acromegaly

Both gigantism and acromegaly (literally, large extremities) are due to hypersecretion of growth hormone. They differ only in that gigantism develops before puberty. Excessive growth of the whole body is therefore characteristic of gigantism, whereas in acromegaly there is abnormal growth only in certain parts of the body. The rate of growth, particularly of cartilage, also depends on somatomedins but the relationship between somatomedin levels and growth hormone secretion is as yet unclear.

Gigantism. Gigantism is due to hypersecretion of growth hormone before closure of the epiphyses. Growth continues and the patient may become seven feet tall or more. (The "Bronx Giant," for instance, was nearly 8 feet tall and could not stand upright in his apartment. The soft tissues and viscera also increase proportionately in size.

In the later stages of the disease hypopituitarism, which causes weakness and abnormal fatigability, or some of the complications of acromegaly can develop. Treatment is essentially the same as that for acromegaly.

Acromegaly. Acromegaly is considerably more common than gigantism and, as a result of the conspicuous clinical features, particularly the facial changes is also the most readily recognizable endocrine disease.

Acromegaly is the result of a growth hormone-producing adenoma developing after the epiphyses have closed. The mandible, hands, feet, and some soft tissues, however, continue to grow. In rare instances, acromegaly may result from ectopic production of growth hormone-like peptide, usually by carcinoids or islet cell tumors.

Clinically, acromegaly (Fig. 18-5) is often instantly recognizable by a combination of the following:

1. Overgrowth of the mandible causing gross prognathism and separation of the teeth
2. Enlargement of the tongue
3. Coarse and thickened facial features
4. Enlarged, broad, spadelike fingers and enlarged feet
5. Enlarged viscera

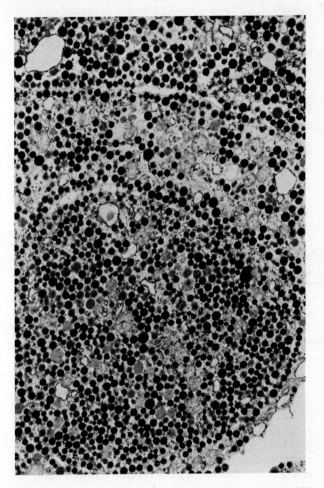

FIG. 18-4. Growth hormone (GH) cell adenoma. Numerous GH-containing secretory granules are demonstrated in this electron micrograph.

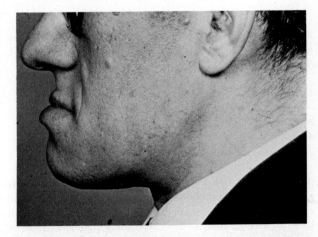

FIG. 18-5. Acromegaly. The lower jaw is grossly enlarged and prognathic and shows increased obliquity of the angle. The nose is also enlarged as a result of the soft tissue overgrowth of the face.

Complications of acromegaly include diabetes mellitus (since growth hormone has a diabetogenic action), headache, and visual defects as a result of the tumor expanding beyond the sella and pressing on the optic chiasma. This typically causes loss of the outer halves of the visual fields (bilateral hemianopia).*

Some pituitary tumors "burn out" with the result that hypopituitarism may follow acromegaly.

Diagnosis can be confirmed by radiologic or MRI evidence of a pituitary tumor and by assay of plasma growth hormone (after an oral glucose load) and somatomedin C levels.

Small adenomas can be removed surgically. Most are more than 1 cm in diameter and may need to be treated by irradiation or ablation of the pituitary. Replacement of adrenal, thyroid, and gonadal hormones is then needed.

Relapses after successful treatment are uncommon. In most surgically treated cases the disease is controlled rather than cured, as shown by the persistence of high somatomedin C levels in 30% to 50% of cases. Somatomedin analogs have now been shown to be effective in controlling growth hormone and there is preliminary evidence that they may cause the tumor to shrink.

Control of the pituitary tumor should result in some improvement in the soft tissue abnormality, but the bony changes do not regress. Orthognatic surgery is usually required and can produce a striking improvement in the patient's appearance and morale.

Prolactin-producing adenoma

Hyperprolactinemia is the most common hypothalamic-pituitary disorder. An important cause of the syndrome of non-puerperal galactorrhea (inappropriate secretion of milk), amenorrhea and infertility is a pituitary adenoma secondary to excessive prolactin releasing factor from the hypothalamus. This is now believed to be the most common type of pituitary adenoma.

Many drugs are associated with hyperprolactinemia; most produce this effect by their antidopaminergic action. Estrogens are known to stimulate lactotropic cells with consequent hyperprolactinemia. However, there is no conclusive evidence that women taking oral contraceptives have an increased incidence of prolactinomas.

Clinically, amenorrhea or infertility may be the main problem, and there may be no complaint of galactorrhea. If the breast is squeezed, however, milk usually appears at the nipple if there is hyperprolactinemia.

In men the disease is characterized by abnormal growth of the breasts (without the production of milk) and impotence.

Investigation is by radioimmunoassay (RIA) of prolactin and by high resolution computerized tomography (CT) scan and/or magnetic resonance imaging (MRI) of the pituitary fossa to demonstrate small tumors.

Bromocriptine, a dopamine agonist directly stimulates dopamine receptors on neuronal and pituitary cell membranes. It effectively controls prolactin hypersecretion and there is little risk of complications. Surgery may, however, be required when there is chiasmal compression endangering sight and before or during pregnancy when these adenomas may enlarge rapidly.

---

*Incidentally, an ingenious doctor has suggested that David's success against Goliath was due to the latter having been a pituitary giant with defective vision resulting from pressure of the tumor on his optic chiasma.

Posterior pituitary disease

Disease of the posterior pituitary is rare. The main disorder is diabetes insipidus.

Diabetes insipidus

The single most common cause of this disorder is a tumor or other infiltrative process. Next is surgical intervention, particularly hypophysectomy. Severe head injury may be a cause, but in some cases no cause can be found.

Clinically diabetes insipidus is characterized by polyuria, excessive thirst and polydipsia. Drinking makes up for the fluid loss, but if fluid intake is restricted, dehydration rapidly develops and can be fatal. The disease can be treated by hormone replacement. Vasopressin can be taken in the form of a nasal spray.

Inappropriate secretion of antidiuretic hormone (ADH)

Inappropriate secretion of ADH is characterized by continued release of ADH without regard to plasma osmolality. The effect of ADH is to prevent excretion of excess water, so that ingestion of fluid increases the extracellular fluid volume and a state of water intoxication results. One effect of this dilution of body fluids is a fall of serum sodium concentration (hyponatremia).

Inappropriate ADH secretion can result from a variety of diseases involving complex mechanisms. Examples include the following:

1. *Central nervous system disease*—Many diseases of the CNS can apparently stimulate the neurohypophysis to cause ADH secretion.
2. *Pulmonary disease*—Pulmonary tissue can synthesize ADH, particularly in the presence of severe infections, such as tuberculosis or pneumonia.
3. *Malignant tumors*—By far the most common cause is small cell carcinoma of the lung, which can synthesize ADH.
4. *Drugs*—Chlorpropamide (a hypoglycemic agent) may sensitize the kidney to ADH, while cytotoxic agents, may stimulate inappropriate ADH secretion.

Clinical aspects. Inappropriate ADH secretion causes water retention but rarely edema. There is usually increased weight, lethargy, and weakness, which can ultimately progress to convulsions and coma.

The cause of the disorder must be sought and rectified if possible. Restriction of water intake alone may be successful in early cases but in severe cases causing hyponatremia (low-sodium levels) more rapid correction is necessary. This may be achieved with the diuretic furosemide and electrolyte replacement. Alternative treatments which may be successful according to circumstances are demeclocycline, urea or lithium carbonate.

THE ADRENAL GLANDS

The adrenal cortical hormones and their mode of action are discussed here briefly.

Glucocorticoids, such as cortisol, increase gluconeogenesis, enhance glycogen mobilization, increase lipolysis, but depress protein synthesis. The overall effect is to raise the blood glucose level. Corticosteroids also have a wide variety of actions. Clinically, the effects of corticosteroid deficiency on the blood glucose are usually of trifling importance in comparison with the circulatory effects. Glucocorticoids also have antiinflammatory and immunosuppressive effects that appear to be unrelated to their basic physiologic actions but for which purpose they are widely used in therapeutics.

Mineralocorticoids, such as aldosterone, mainly affect electrolyte and water balance. In particular, they cause retention of sodium and water. Cortisol also has these effects but is less potent. Aldosterone is reported to be the most important hormone in keeping adrenalectomized animals alive and enabling them to resist stress. Adrenal sex hormones mainly affect the secondary sex characteristics.

The *adrenal medulla* produces mainly epinephrine (adrenaline) but also some norepinephrine (noradrenaline). Epinephrine forms about 80% of the stored catecholamines in the adrenal medulla. Norepinephrine is the mediator at sympathetic nerve endings and causes generalized vasoconstriction and increased blood pressure.

Epinephrine has a wide range of actions producing the "fight, fright, or flight" reaction, including increased force and rate of the heart, dilatation of vessels supplying voluntary muscle (but constriction of subcutaneous and splanchnic vessels), dilatation of the bronchioles, and mobilization of liver glycogen. The adrenal medulla is not, however, essential to life.

Although cortical and medullary secretions can interact in various ways, particularly in their effects on the blood pressure, they function as separate entities (see Chapter 10).

Hypofunction of the adrenal cortex

Hypofunction of the adrenal cortex can be due either to primary disease of the adrenals or more commonly to long-term corticosteroid treatment. Plasma corticosteroid levels exert feedback control of pituitary ACTH release. Long term corticosteroid treatment can therefore lead to atrophy of the cortex from which recovery is slow. Occasionally, hypoadrenalism is secondary to hypopituitarism and loss of ACTH secretion, as in Sheehan's syndrome.

Acute adrenocortical failure is the main feature of *Waterhouse-Friderichsen syndrome** as a result of hemorrhage into the gland and is usually the consequence of meningococcal or other overwhelming bacteremic infection.

Primary adrenocortical deficiency (Addison's disease†)

This disease, described originally in 1855 by Thomas Addison is due to atrophy or destruction of the adrenal cortices. In the past, the most common cause was tuberculosis, but this is now rare and idiopathic (autoimmune atrophy) predominates. The main infective cause of Addison's disease is now histoplasmosis, especially in immunodeficient patients, and, as a consequence, is seen as a complication of AIDS.

Pathogenesis and pathology. In tuberculous disease there is confluent caseous necrosis of the adrenal gland; there is granuloma formation and fibrosis is minimal, possibly due to the influence of corticosteroids. The disease may therefore progress locally and spread into adjacent soft tissues.

In idiopathic adrenal atrophy there is progressive lymphocytic and monocytic infiltration of the cortices and loss of their normal three layered structure. The cortices as a result, become shrunken and fibrotic, but the medullas remain intact.

Antibodies to adrenal microsomes are detectable in approximately 50% of patients and autoantibody binding to the secretory cells can be demonstrated by immunofluorescence microscopy. Prospective studies have shown that approximately 50% of persons who were clinically normal but had adrenal autoantibodies, developed Addison's disease within periods of one to 31 months.

Circulating autoantibodies can be found in 50% to 75% of patients. There is also an association with other types of autoimmune disease, particularly in the *polyendocrinopathy syndromes* (discussed later). These appear to be genetically determined.

The consequences of cortical insufficiency are due to a combination of effects. Predominant is sodium and fluid loss, which causes hypotension. Hyperkalemia, due to relative potassium retention, causes muscle weakness. Pigmentation is caused by raised melanocyte-stimulating hormone (MSH)* levels due to lack of cortical feedback control to the pituitary. Hypoglycemia probably contributes to the muscle weakness.

Clinical aspects. Addison's disease is rare. Women are affected by the idiopathic form at least twice as frequently as men. The main effects (in order of frequency) are (1) weakness, (2) pigmentation of skin and mucous membranes, (3) loss of weight, (4) anorexia, nausea, and vomiting, and (5) hypotension. Other features, such as abdominal pain, a craving for salt, constipation, or diarrhea, are much less frequent.

Muscle weakness (asthenia) is the most common and one of the most important symptoms. Eventually even the voice may become almost inaudible. Increased suntan-like pigmentation is usually also present and is most severe in normally pigmented areas such as the nipples. Within the mouth the pigment often resembles racial pigmentation, which has a predilection for the gingivae but can also affect the buccal mucosa.

Laboratory findings are low levels of serum sodium and chloride, and urinary 17-ketosteroids and 17-hydroxyketosteroids but levels of serum potassium and nonprotein nitrogen are raised. Plasma cortisol is at a low level or undetectable (and does not rise in response to administration of ACTH) while plasma ACTH levels are high. Eosinophilia and lymphocytosis are typically also present.

The diagnosis depends on these clinical and laboratory findings and exclusion of other causes of hypoadrenocorticism listed as follows:
1. Autoimmune adrenalitis
2. Infections
   a. Tuberculosis
   b. Histoplasmosis
   c. Meninogococcal septicemia (acute adrenal failure)
3. Bilateral adrenalectomy
4. Tumor metastases
5. Amyloidosis
6. Hemochromatosis
7. Granulomatous disease (rarely sarcoidosis)
8. Vascular damage (acute hemorrhage into the adrenals or adrenal vein thrombosis)
9. Congenital adrenal hypoplasia

---

*Rupert Waterhouse (1872-1958), English physician; Carl Friderichsen (b.1886), Danish pediatrician.
†Thomas Addison (1793-1860), English physician; contemporary and colleague of both Bright and Hodgkin.

*A breakdown product of ACTH (Fig. 18-3).

Nevertheless autoimmune adrenalitis is the main cause of adrenocortical hypofunction, but as mentioned earlier, infection should be considered in immunocompromised patients such as those with AIDS.

Specific hormone replacement is essential in adrenal insufficiency. Cortisone analogs are the mainstay of treatment. It is usually also necessary to give an aldosterone analog.

Acute adrenocortical insufficiency: adrenal crisis

Acute adrenal insufficiency is a life-threatening condition that may complicate chronic adrenocorticism as a result of excessive demands imposed on the system by infection or trauma. More commonly, it can result from similar stresses or sudden withdrawal of treatment in a patient receiving (for whatever cause) long-term corticosteroid treatment. Alternatively the syndrome can be caused by acute bilateral destruction of the adrenals by such causes as severe acute sepsis particularly, acute meningococcemia, or hemorrhage into the gland from other causes such as anticoagulant therapy. Clinically, in an addisonian crisis there is an acute exacerbation of symptoms with nausea, vomiting, and often diarrhea. Headache, lethargy, and confusion typically progress to coma as a result of acute hypotension. There may be fever and the features of the triggering disorder, such as dehydration. In the case of meningococcemia, purpura and other signs of this infection will appear.

Laboratory findings are low serum glucose and sodium, but high potassium and urea levels. Blood and urinary cortisol levels are very low—unlike primary adrenal disease, where plasma ACTH is greatly raised.

High doses of corticosteroids intravenously together with fluid replacement should be given and the cause sought and treated, particularly if it is an infection.

Secondary adrenocortical hypofunction

Hypopituitarism is a rare cause and is typically associated with other features of hypopituitarism, as discussed earlier. Otherwise, the essential features are similar to those of Addison's disease except that hyperpigmentation is absent because of failure of pituitary MSH secretion.

Diagnosis depends on tests for pituitary function and particularly on finding low plasma ACTH levels. On the other hand, ACTH stimulation will induce production of cortisol by the adrenals, but the effect may be delayed.

Corticosteroid-induced hypoadrenalism

Suppression of adrenal function as a result of long-term administration of corticosteroids is now, by far, the most important cause of adrenal hypofunction and is a common and serious problem.

Corticosteroids in themselves are not toxic and, for acute emergencies such as anaphylaxis or acute adrenal hypofunction, are given in enormous doses with beneficial effect. Given over the long term, by contrast, even minute doses of corticosteroids depress adrenocortical function. This state persists, and after cessation of such treatment, full adrenal function may not return to normal for 2 years.

The typical corticosteroid side effects, particularly susceptibility to infection, "moon face," and osteoporosis are sometimes evident; but affected patients otherwise appear well. Nevertheless, adrenal function is greatly impaired and stress has a severe effect. Since the adrenals are then unable to produce the sudden great increase in cortisol output that is needed, the blood pressure falls; within a few minutes the patient becomes unconscious resulting from severe hypotension and can quickly die.

The picture differs from adrenal crisis in Addison's disease in that there are none of the associated features, such as vomiting and abdominal pain, but the outcome is the same.

Even minor operations, are dangerous for these patients and have been fatal. Adequate preparation is therefore essential, and any patient at risk must have adequate replacement therapy with corticosteroids before operative treatment. If acute hypotension develops, immediate treatment with massive doses of intravenous corticosteroids, hospitalization, and administration of intravenous fluids are necessary.

Nelson's syndrome

Nelson's syndrome* follows bilateral adrenalectomy for Cushing's syndrome. It is characterized by an enlarging pituitary tumor and increasing pigmentation. Nelson's syndrome is due to continued growth of a pituitary adenoma (undetected when the diagnosis of Cushing's syndrome was made) and to lack of feedback control after removal of the adrenals.

Hyperfunction of the adrenal cortex

The main effects are Cushing's syndrome or disease (due to excessive cortisol production), adrenal virilism, and hyperaldosteronism (Conn's syndrome). They are all uncommon, particularly the latter.

Cushing's disease and Cushing's syndrome

In 1932 Harvey Cushing† described a disease characterized by hyperplasia of the adrenal cortex associated with pituitary "basophilism," in most cases caused by a small basophil adenoma of the pituitary.

Later it was found that the majority of patients with the clinical picture of Cushing's disease had bilateral adrenal hyperplasia but no detectable pituitary lesion. Controversy about the cause of this disease was eventually resolved by reserving the names *Cushing's disease* for primary pituitary disease and *Cushing's syndrome* for primary adrenocortical disease. Nevertheless, these terms are often used loosely or Cushing's syndrome is applied to both types of disease.

Cushing has, however, been vindicated in that, in the great majority of cases the syndrome is due to a minute tumor of the pituitary, invisible on conventional radiographs and detectable only by polytomography.

Thus there truly is a Cushing's disease *and*, less frequently, a Cushing's syndrome. Both are described together, since the majority of cases are due to bilateral adrenal hyperplasia secondary to ACTH production by the pituitary.

In addition to adrenal hyperplasia or tumor, Cushing's syndrome can be caused by abnormal (ectopic) ACTH production by neuroendocrine tumors such as carcinoids (Chapter 14), but more often by small cell carcinoma of the lung. Many of the features of Cushing's disease can also result from prolonged administration of high doses of corticosteroids as discussed later.

Pathology. Hyperplasia of the zona fasciculata of the adrenal cortex, usually secondary to a pituitary microadenoma, accounts for about 70% of cases. The cells of the zona fasciculata become enlarged and have pale, foamy or finely granular cy-

---

*D.H. Nelson (b.1925), American endocrinologist.
†H.W. Cushing (1869-1939), American neurosurgeon.

toplasm and a relatively small nucleus. Hyperplasia of the zona fasciculata may be so extreme as to compress the zona reticularis and glomerulosa and even penetrate to the medulla.

Hyperplasia resulting from excessive ACTH production is characterized by enlargement of the gland greater than that of simple hyperplasia, and the enlarged cells show depletion of lipids.

The changes caused by hypersecretion of corticosteroids are the result of sodium and fluid retention and increased protein catabolism leading to weakening of the subcutaneous connective tissue and osteoporosis. Focal depositions of fat are highly characteristic. Although there is increased gluconeogenesis and a tendency to hyperglycemia, diabetes mellitus is uncommon. There is also a tendency to virilization in women because of an overproduction of adrenal sex hormones.

Clinical aspects. The effects of overproduction of corticosteroids in order of frequency are (1) typical body habitus and increased body weight, (2) fatigability and weakness, (3) hypertension, (4) hirsutism, (5) amenorrhea and other signs of virilism, (6) cutaneous striae, (7) personality changes, (8) ecchymoses, and (9) edema.

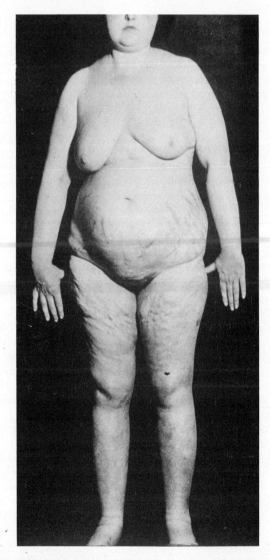

FIG. 18-6. Cushing's disease. This shows the typical body habitus, particularly the obesity of the trunk and abdominal striae. *(Courtesy Curator of the Gordon Museum, Guy's Hospital, London, England.)*

Women are affected more often than men in the ratio of 3:1. The onset is typically in the third or fourth decade.

The characteristic changes of body habitus are the development of a moonlike face, often with puffiness around the eyes, a ruddy complexion, a "buffalo" hump, and obesity of the trunk (Fig. 18-6). Osteoporosis resulting from decreased matrix production can occasionally be severe enough to cause collapse of vertebrae.

Diagnosis depends on showing increased cortisol production and then on determining whether this is secondary to a pituitary tumor secreting excessive ACTH. Administration of low doses of dexamethasone for 2 days, does not, unlike in normal persons, depress urinary 17-hydroxycorticosteroid excretion. Administration of high doses (2 mg 6 hourly) of dexamethasone causes urinary 17-hydroxycorticosteroid levels to fall to 50% of baseline levels in the case of Cushing's disease, where there is relative resistance to the normal negative feedback inhibition of ACTH by cortisol production. In Cushing's syndrome caused by adrenal tumors or ectopic ACTH production, there is no such inhibition by endogenous or administered corticosteroids. A variety of other tests is available to determine the precise cause of hypercortisolism.

Treatment of Cushing's disease by removal of the pituitary adenoma via the transsphenoidal approach is usually successful. In such cases the remainder of the pituitary remains intact and functional so that the patient is not dependent on corticosteroids and there is no risk of Nelson's syndrome (described earlier) developing. If adenomectomy fails, the treatment is the same as for Cushing's syndrome, namely bilateral adrenalectomy. Pharmacologic treatment using mitotane to destroy adrenal tissue or inhibitors of steroid synthesis such as metapyrone, is not always successful and adverse effects can be severe. A more promising, though as yet experimental approach is the use of a glucocorticoid receptor blocker. Such a drug seems likely also to be useful for unresectable adrenal carcinomas and preoperatively to lessen the risks of surgery in patients with Cushing's syndrome.

Tumors of the adrenal cortex
Adrenocortical adenoma

Adenomas usually form a single nodule but may less often be bilateral. Microscopically, the tumor consists of large, fairly uniform cells with abundant foamy, lipid-laden cytoplasm typically arranged in an organoid pattern and surrounded by fine fibrous septa.

The border between the tumor and the normal, well-demarcated zones of the remainder of the cortex is well defined. A fibrous capsule or a rim of compressed connective tissue surrounds the periphery. Most adenomas are functional and the resulting clinical syndrome depends on the hormone or its precursors produced by the tumor cells. The most common syndromes in decreasing order of frequency are (1) hyperaldosteronism, (2) Cushing's syndrome, (3) virilization, and (4) feminization.

Adrenal carcinoma

Adrenal carcinoma is characterized histologically, by cellular pleomorphism, increased numbers of mitoses, nuclear atypia, and multinucleated cells. Recognition of malignancy, however, depends on finding evidence of invasion and is confirmed, unfortunately too late, by the appearance of metastases. Adrenal carcinomas are frequently large when found. Carcinoma

accounts for 10% of cases of Cushing's syndrome in adults, and 45% of cases in children. The effects of hormone secreting tumors, in addition to local effects or metastases are Cushing's syndrome or adrenogenital syndrome; virilization is a common effect in children.

Adrenogenital syndromes

Adrenogenital syndromes in infancy or childhood are most frequently due to congenital adrenal hyperplasia or less often to a tumor secreting excessive amounts of androgens.

Congenital adrenal hyperplasia. Congenital adrenal hyperplasia comprises a group of inborn errors of metabolism, each characterized by a deficiency of one of the enzymes involved in the synthesis of cortisol. The most common type is 21-, 11-β-hydroxylase deficiency. In either case the resulting deficiency of cortisol production leads to increased ACTH with consequent overproduction of adrenal androgens.

The clinical effects in females are virilization, which can range from clitoral enlargement to formation of ambiguous external genitalia and female pseudohermaphroditism. In males there is premature virilization with overenlargement of the genitalia and accelerated growth—the so-called "Infant Hercules." In addition there is hypercortisolism. In 11-β-hydroxylase deficiency, hypertension due to excessive production of the cortisol precursor, desoxycorticosterone, which has strong mineralocorticoid properties, but glucocorticoid deficiency is associated.

The essential principles of management are to give a glucocorticoid in sufficient doses to suppress ACTH secretion and reverse the metabolic disorder, but a mineralocorticoid may have to be given in the salt-losing type. Early plastic surgery may be required for females with ambiguous genitalia.

Adrenogenital syndrome in adult females. This syndrome and other virilizing diseases in women can be caused by the following:

1. Hyperplasia or tumors of the adrenal cortex
2. Ovarian tumors or other disorders with overproduction of androgens, for example, polycystic ovarian disease
3. Drugs, particularly testosterone and anabolic steroids

Clinically, the effects include diminished or absent menstruation, deepening of the voice, hirsutism but with thinning of head hair, loss of feminine body contour and enlargement of the clitoris. Diabetes mellitus and obesity are often associated and when tumors are the cause they are frequently malignant.

Urinary 17-ketosteroids are raised in adrenal but not in extraadrenal diseases causing this syndrome. In the latter case, a variety of tests is required to determine the cause.

Management depends on the underlying cause. Early removal of malignant tumors may be curative as metastasis is often delayed.

Hyperaldosteronism

Overproduction of aldosterone is the result of overactivity of the zona glomerulosa as a result of hyperplasia or, more commonly, an adenoma. An aldosterone-producing carcinoma is rare. Under normal conditions aldosterone secretion is regulated mainly by the renin-angiotension system (Chapter 10) and only to a slight extent by ACTH.

Hyperaldosteronemia is due in the majority of cases to an adrenocortical adenoma (Conn's syndrome*) or less often nodular hyperplasia of the adrenal cortex. Aldosterone-producing

---

*J.W. Conn (b.1907), American physician.

adenomas consist of a mixture of cells which include lipid-filled clear cells and dense cells. Microscopically, some of these cells resemble those from the zona glomerulosa or zona fasciculata.

Laboratory findings include low serum potassium, hypernatremia, and alkalosis. Plasma and urinary aldosterone levels are high, whereas renin levels are low and do not rise in response to sodium depletion as they would in normal persons.

In addition there are typically also signs of renal damage resulting from the hypertension.

Clinical aspects. Conn's syndrome is characterized by (1) hypertension, (2) muscular weakness and other neurologic manifestations of hypokalemia, and (3) polyuria and thirst secondary to poor renal concentration. Hypertension is only moderately severe and related to an increased circulating volume. Edema is characteristically absent. Headaches are common and retinopathy often develops, but papilledema is rare.

Hyperaldosteronism is a rare cause of hypertension and overall accounts for only 1% to 2% of cases.

Treatment of a unilateral aldosterone-producing adenoma is usually by surgical removal, whereas bilateral adrenal hyperplasia is best treated with spironolactone, an aldosterone antagonist.

Hypoaldosteronism

Hypoaldosteronism is a rare disorder resulting from causes such as destruction of the zona glomerulosa, enzyme defects, or blockade of aldosterone production by drugs. There is sodium loss and hyperkalemia, which can cause cardiac arrhythmias.

THE ADRENAL MEDULLA

Hypofunction of the adrenal medulla has no apparent effect, and the only important disorder is a catecholamine-producing tumor known as *pheochromocytoma*.

Pheochromocytoma

Pheochromocytoma is an uncommon tumor. It is thought to be present in 0.5% of patients with hypertension and may be found in 0.1% of unselected autopsy specimens. The tumor derives its name from its affinity for chromium salts, which stain secretory granules brown due to the presence of catecholamines. Chromaffin tissue is widely distributed in the body at birth but mostly atrophies at puberty. Nevertheless, remnants can give rise to extraadrenal pheochromocytomas (paragangliomas: Chapter 20), for example, in parasympathetic ganglia.

Although pheochromocytomas are rare and sporadic, 10% to 15% are familial, either in isolation or in a variety of familial syndromes as follow:

1. Pheochromocytoma in multiple endocrine adenoma syndromes types II and III (p. 459)
2. Pheochromocytoma associated with neurofibromatosis (Chapter 19)
3. Pheochromocytoma associated with islet cell tumors of the pancreas
4. Pheochromocytoma in von Hippel-Lindau syndrome (hemangioblastomas of the retina and other parts of the nervous system) (see p. 463)

Pathology. Most pheochromocytomas are solitary. However, in about 10% of cases (particularly those of the familial type), there are multiple tumors. They may reach several thousand

grams in weight (Fig. 18-7), but the size of the tumor seems to bear little relation to the severity of the symptoms.

Histologically, pheochromocytomas show great variation in cell and nuclear size. The pattern may resemble that of the adrenal medulla or be less well defined. Both acidophil and basophil cells as well as cytoplasmic pigment granules of varying sizes are present. The epinephrine and norepinephrine granules can be distinguished by electron microscopy. Catecholamines can also be demonstrated in fresh tissue or in fixed tissues using monoclonal antibodies to specific proteins such as chromogranin and neuron-specific enolase.

Most pheochromocytomas are benign but malignant variants account for about 6% of these tumors and are sometimes also functional. The cellular pleomorphism of medullary adenomas makes microscopic recognition of carcinomas difficult and confirmation may depend on finding metastases.

Raised urinary levels of catecholamines and vanillylmandelic acid (VMA) are present in most cases. Plasma epinephrine and norepinephrine levels can also be measured during or just after an attack. Measurement of plasma catecholamines collected via a venous catheter can be used to localize the site of an extramedullary pheochromocytoma.

Clinical aspects. Pheochromocytomas most frequently cause symptoms in young adults but can develop at almost any age.

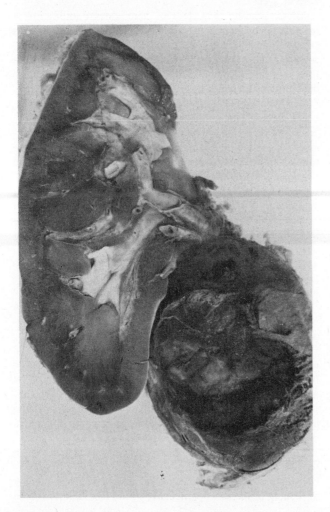

FIG. 18-7. Pleochromocytoma. The gross overgrowth of the adrenal medulla as a result of this tumor has distorted and displaced the entire gland toward the lower pole of the kidney. *(Courtesy Curator of the Gordon Museum, Guy's Hospital, London, England.)*

Typical features include (1) attacks of headache, (2) hypertension which is persistent in about 70% of patients, (3) postural tachycardia and hypotension, and (4) effects secondary to hypertension, such as proteinuria or occasionally, papilledema.

Hypertensive crises are often spontaneous but may be precipitated by physical exertion or emotional stress. These paroxysmal attacks are caused by sudden release, mainly of norepinephine, and the blood pressure often exceeds 250/150. Fatal complications are ventricular fibrillation, cerebral hemorrhage, or pulmonary edema. Shock or renal failure, resulting from the sudden fall in blood pressure, can follow an attack.

In a minority, the tumor is predominantly epinephrine-producing. This can cause paroxysms of hypotension (presumably because of the adrenergic effect on the large arterial bed of the muscles) and often glycosuria.

The treatment of choice is removal of the tumor, but adrenergic blockade with phenoxybenzamine and then a β-blocker to control hypertension and arrhythmias is essential pretreatment to reduce the operative hazards. Any other surgery should be postponed until the disease has been controlled. In the case of inoperable or malignant tumors, metyrosine (which blocks catecholamine synthesis) or prolonged phenoxybenzamine treatment can be given. After removal of a pheochromocytoma urinary catecholamine levels should be checked to ensure that no other such tumors are present.

THE THYROID

The thyroid gland controls a variety of metabolic processes by its hormones thyroxine (T4) and triiodothyronine (T3). In the blood T3 and T4 are transported bound to plasma proteins.

Control of thyroid function by the anterior pituitary is mediated by thyroid-stimulating hormone (TSH), which is regulated in turn by hypothalamic thyrotropin-releasing factor. Hypopituitarism, as in Sheehan's syndrome, can lead to hypothyroidism, but TSH-secreting tumors are extremely rare.

Thyroid hormone is an important determinant of development and of the metabolic rate, including oxidative reactions. Other effects of hypersecretion include increased sympathetic activity.

Hyperthyroidism and hypothyroidism are the main diseases of the thyroid. The gland may be enlarged (goiter) in either of these conditions. *Goiter* is a clinical term denoting any visible or palpable enlargement of the thyroid and does not indicate the functional activity of the gland or the nature of the pathologic process.

Recently, the technique of fine needle aspiration has been introduced as a diagnostic method in cases of thyroid enlargement. A very thin needle is inserted into the gland, cells are aspirated and cytologic preparations of the aspirate are examined. This simple procedure has proved increasingly useful in diagnosis and management of thyroid disease.

Simple (nontoxic) goiter

Simple goiter is the result of hyperplasia of thyroid follicles to compensate for impaired hormonal synthesis. In the process, the thyroid follicles can eventually lose their normal regularity of size and pattern (Fig. 18-8).

TSH secretion is not usually increased, as was at one time believed, and it is possible that defective hormone production may make the gland more sensitive to normal TSH levels.

The best known of the nontoxic goiters is the so-called *en-*

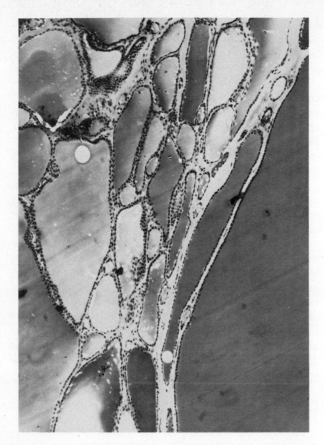

FIG. 18-8. Goiter. The thyroid acini are irregular in size and shape, and some are distended by gross accumulation of colloid.

demic (colloid) goiter caused by iodine deficiency or less often, by goitrogens that may be present in the soil.

In simple goiter, thyroid function is normal until the gland can no longer compensate for impaired hormone synthesis. The incidence of cretinism, described later, is however, higher among children of women with goiter.

A hyperactive focus in a simple goiter (*toxic nodular goiter* or "hot node") can develop and cause hyperthyroidism. Follicular cells differ in their ability to replicate, and it has been suggested that toxic nodular goiter is the outcome of preferential replication of follicular cells which have an intrinsic growth advantage. It is also not uncommon for these nodules to be multifocal.

Clinical aspects. There may be no symptoms, but goiter is disfiguring and if very large, can compress the esophagus or the trachea. Hemorrhage into a nodule can cause sudden swelling, pain, and acute pressure on adjacent structures (Fig. 18-9).

Any exogenous cause, such as iodine deficiency, should be remedied. Often no cause is found and the main line of treatment is to give levothyroxin to suppress thyroid function. The goiter then usually regresses. Nodular goiters, those which fail to respond or are causing compressive effects, may need to be treated by subtotal excision of the thyroid.

Hypothyroidism

Inadequate production of thyroid hormone (hypothyroidism) can result from a variety of causes. The main examples follow:

1. Thyroidal (primary)
   a. Developmental
   b. Hashimoto's thyroiditis
   c. Iodine deficiency
   d. Irradiation or thyroidectomy
   e. Antithyroid drugs
   f. Idiopathic
2. Suprathyroidal (secondary)
   a. Hypopituitarism

Hashimoto's disease (chronic lymphocytic thyroiditis)

As mentioned earlier, Hashimoto's thyroiditis* can be regarded as one of the most typical organ-specific autoimmune diseases.

Pathogenesis and pathology. A variety of immunologic abnormalities are found and include complement-fixing antibodies to thyroid microsomes and to thyroglobulin in most patients. Antithyroglobulin binding to colloid in the follicles and anti-microsomal antibodies to cytoplasmic components of thyroid parenchymal cells can be demonstrated by immunofluorescence. In addition, there is experimental evidence of cell-mediated damage to secretory tissue. There is also a strong genetic predisposition to the disease in individuals with HLA B8 or DR5 antigens.

Microscopically (Fig. 18-10), there is dense infiltration of the thyroid by lymphocytes and plasma cells. Hürthle cells (large eosinophilic cells with many mitochondria) are increased as a result of change in the follicular epithelial cells. These cells have high metabolic activity; nevertheless, hormonal production is inefficient.

The lymphocytic infiltrate goes on to form germinal follicles, while the epithelial follicles show a mixed picture of degeneration, regeneration or compensatory hyperplasia. As the disease progresses there is increasing fibrosis which, with the cellular infiltrate may cause the gland to become lobulated and asymmetrically enlarged (Fig. 18-11).

Hashimoto's disease has a significant association with other autoimmune diseases particularly pernicious anemia (Chapter 13) and 30% of patients have gastric parietal cell autoantibodies. There is also an association, but less often, with the connective tissue diseases. However, in the latter the associations are rather paradoxical in that antithyroid antibodies are commonly found particularly in Sjögren's syndrome but hypothyroidism rarely develops.

In the early stages of Hashimoto's disease, thyroid function is normal or occasionally, increased, but in most cases, hypothyroidism develops over an extended period of time.

Hypothyroidism is characterized by a low basal metabolic rate, raised plasma cholesterol levels, and depressed plasma T4 (thyroxin) levels. In primary thyroid disease the plasma TSH levels are increased, but in hypothyroidism secondary to hypopituitarism, TSH levels are abnormally low. Circulating auto antibodies are found in over 90% of patients with Hashimoto's disease.

Clinical aspects. Hypothyroidism is the general name given to the changes resulting from depressed thyroid activity. *Myxedema* is a severe form of the disease characterized by a doughy thickening of the skin, particularly of the face, due to edema

---

*H. Hashimoto (1881-1934), Japanese surgeon.

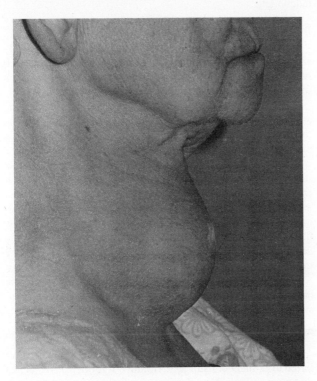

FIG. 18-9. Simple goiter. The goiter was congenital and has produced a smooth, rounded swelling of the anterior midline of the neck. *(Courtesy Curator of the Gordon Museum, Guy's Hospital, London, England.)*

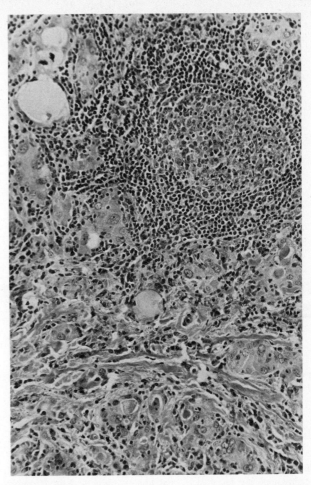

FIG. 18-10. Hashimoto's disease. There is atrophy of follicles where some of the cells are swollen by mitochondria (Hürthle cell change). A lymphoid follicle with a germinal center is present.

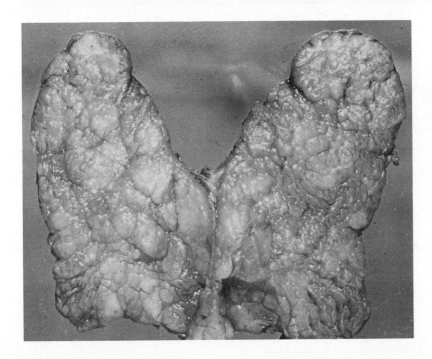

FIG. 18-11. Chronic thyroiditis. The thyroid is enlarged and lobulated due to the combination of expansion caused by the intense lymphocytic infiltration and fibrosis, producing the lobulated appearance. The appearance of the gland varies according to which feature is most prominent. *(Courtesy Curator of the Gordon Museum, Guy's Hospital, London, England.)*

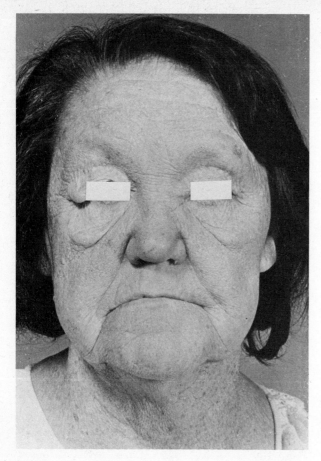

FIG. 18-12. Myxedema. Typical features are the heavy facies, dull expression, lax facial skin, and loss of eyebrow hair. *(Courtesy Curator of the Gordon Museum, Guy's Hospital, London, England.)*

associated with deposition of PREM (proteoglycan rich extracellular matrix) in the dermis.

Women are affected more than men in the ratio of at least 5:1. The thyroid may be enlarged or, less often, shrunken. The general features of myxedema are (1) physical and mental sluggishness, (2) intolerance of cold, (3) a deep or hoarse voice and slow speech, (4) increased body weight, (5) generalized myxedema, but most conspicuously, thickening and puffiness of the facial skin with thin eyebrows and sparse, coarse hair (Fig. 18-12), (6) bradycardia, and (7) constipation.

Angina and myocardial infarction are complications of long-standing myxedema as a result of hyperlipidemia (Chapter 11).

Primary hypothyroidism (adult myxedema)

This disorder, also termed *primary atrophic thyroiditis,* is the chief cause of myxedema after middle age. Its etiology is unknown but an autoimmune mechanism, similar to that in Hashimoto's disease is a likely cause and there is a considerable body of opinion that atrophic thyroiditis is the end result of Hashimoto's disease. However, since no transitional stage between the two diseases has been documented, they should still be regarded as separate entities. Circulating thyroid antibodies are present in most patients with atrophic thyroiditis.

Microscopically, there is replacement of thyroid parenchyma by hyaline fibrous tissue. Occasional follicles persist and show oxyphil change and there is a scanty infiltrate of lymphocytes and plasma cells.

The treatment of hypothyroidism and myxedema is with thyroxine or triiodothyronine which may need to be continued indefinitely.

Subacute granulomatous thyroiditis

This disorder also known as *de Quervain's disease* chiefly affects women and is thought to result from viral infection. It is usually preceded by an upper respiratory infection but in some patients a rising titer of mumps antibodies is found.

The onset is acute with a febrile illness and painful swelling of the thyroid. Sometimes there is transient hyperthyroidism followed by transient hypothyroidism before recovery takes place.

Microscopically, the thyroid gland shows lesions in different stages of development. Early lesions show necrosis of follicular epithelium and a neutrophil infiltrate. Later there is an increasing macrophage infiltration, with giant cell and granuloma formation in the site of follicular destruction. This is followed by fibrosis within and between the thyroid lobules. However, the damaged parenchyma regenerates and there is recovery after 2 to 3 months.

There is no specific treatment of proven value but in severe cases corticosteroids can be given to reduce the inflammation, swelling, and pain.

Subacute lymphocytic thyroiditis

This condition is frequently asymptomatic and has been referred to as silent or painless thyroiditis. It is often an incidental finding in goitrous thyroid tissue removed at surgery or autopsy. Symptomatic cases, as in granulomatous thyroiditis, initially show signs of hyperthyroidism followed by transient hypothyroidism and finally recovery. Women are more commonly affected often after middle age. One form of the disease affects postpartum women in whom antimitochondrial antibodies can be detected.

Microscopically, there are limited foci of lymphocytes and plasma cells which are mainly subcapsular in distribution but occasionally there is lymphoid follicle formation. There may be necrosis of thyroid follicles associated with a monocytic infiltrate. By contrast with chronic lymphocytic thyroiditis, Hürthle cell change is not seen.

Chronic fibrosing thyroiditis (Riedel's struma*)

This is a rare form of thyroiditis once considered a late stage of chronic lymphocytic thyroiditis, but now thought to be a separate entity. Fibrosing thyroiditis is more common in women and is characterized by enlargement of a pre-existing goiter, a stony hard thyroid which becomes fixed to surrounding tissues. Most patients are euthyroid, but with eventual replacement of the gland by fibrous tissue, hypothyroidism develops. In some patients, the fibrosclerotic process affects other sites, giving rise to mediastinal and retroperitoneal fibrosis.

Infections of the thyroid

Suppurative thyroiditis can result from infection by pyogenic bacteria or more chronic infection can result from tuberculosis or syphilis. All are rare.

As mentioned earler, granulomatous thyroiditis is thought to be viral in origin, but no specific viral infections of the thyroid have been identified.

---

*Bernhard Riedel (1846-1916), German surgeon.

Hyperthyroidism

The main type of hyperthyroidism is that associated with goiter and exophthalmos and known as Graves' (Basedow's) disease.* Other causes include toxic nodular goiter, toxic adenoma, and iatrogenic causes (overdose of thyroid hormone).

The sera of the majority of patients with Graves' disease contain autoantibodies against thyroid cell surface receptors for thyrotropin or thyroid stimulating hormone (TSH). Some antibodies against thyrotropin receptors induce hyperthyroidism by mimicking the stimulatory action of TSH. Others may block the binding of TSH to its receptors but overall the sera from 50% to 95% of patients with Graves' disease stimulate human thyroid gland activity. It is suggested therefore that several types of thyrotropin receptor antibodies exist. Some mimic the action of TSH, as mentioned earlier, and give rise to *hyper*thyroidism, whilst others cause *hypo*thyroidism by blocking TSH receptor binding. Knowledge of the thyroid stimulating autoantibody is however limited by the absence of an animal model for this disease.

Microscopically, there is generalized thyroid hyperplasia with great irregularity in size of the gland follicles, the epi-

*R.J. Graves (1797-1853), Irish physician; K.A. von Basedow (1799-1854), German physician.

thelium of which may be infolded (Fig. 18-13). The secretory cells are increased in height, whereas the colloid within the follicles is pale and "vacuolated." There are scattered foci of lymphocytes in the interstitial tissue, but there is conflicting evidence as to their function. Extracts of hyperthyroid tissue have reportedly shown a predominance of helper (CD4) lymphocytes, while tissue studies with monoclonal antibodies suggest the reverse, namely a predominance of suppressor/cytotoxic (CD8) lymphocytes. Further, even in patients with active disease, very few antigen-presenting (CD6) cells can be found. However thyroid cells in Graves' disease, apparently, express HLA-DR antigens with the result that there may be no need for antigen-presenting cells to stimulate helper T lymphocytes to form autoantibodies.

There is a significant association between Graves' disease and HLA B8 and an even stronger association with HLA-DR3.

Whatever the underlying mechanisms of Graves' disease however, the net effect is overproduction of thyroid hormone and this causes most of the main clinical effects.

Clinical aspects. The thyroid is usually diffusely enlarged (Fig. 18-14), and the increased vascularity may be sufficient to be felt as a thrill or may be audible through a stethoscope as a murmur.

The metabolic changes include (1) increased heat production causing sweating and heat intolerance, (2) weight loss, but increased appetite and diarrhea, (3) tachycardia, (4) anxiety, irritability, hyperkinesia, and tiredness, (5) fine tremor, particularly of the outstretched hands, and (6) arrythmias or cardiac failure, especially in older patients.

A serious complication of hyperthyroidism is therefore, cardiac disease which is mainly related to the severity and duration of the disease, and particularly affects older patients.

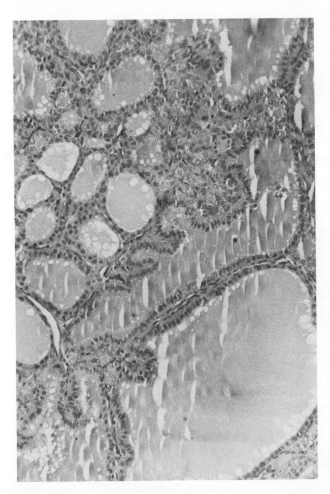

FIG. 18-13. Graves' disease. The thyroid follicles are lined by hyperplastic epithelium, which is columnar in places and forms papillary projections into follicles.

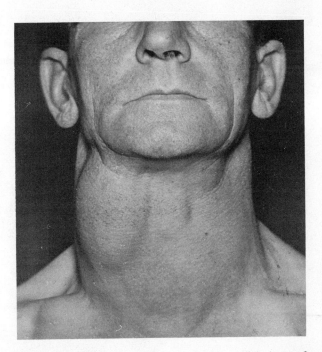

FIG. 18-14. Nodular goiter. Nodular goiter is a clinical term for irregular enlargement of the thyroid, which can be due to a variety of causes. In this case where there is gross englargement, particularly of the right lobe, it is probably caused by a tumor. Hyperthyroidism may develop later in a gland such as this. (*Courtesy Curator of the Gordon Museum, Guy's Hospital, London, England.*)

Another complication is ocular changes which can result from two separate mechanisms. The first is an increased sensitivity of the exophthalmic muscles to circulating catecholamines. This causes the staring appearance often seen in this disease and is alleviated by giving beta-blocking drugs. The second mechanism, responsible for exophthalmos (Fig. 18-15) is less clear but is thought to be immunologic, as retroorbital tissue is reported to have an affinity for both thyroglobulin and complexes of thyroglobulin with specific antibodies. The result can be protrusion of the eyes, so severe that ocular damage can result. This can take the form of conjunctivitis, corneal ulceration or optic atrophy. These ocular changes (ophthalmoplegia) can occasionally precede more typical signs of hyperthyroidism and typically persist despite effective treatment of the latter.

The eye signs include (1) exophthalmos, (2) edema of the eyelids, (3) lid lag when attempting to close the eyes or lid retraction, and (4) conjunctivitis.

Treatment. Thyroid hyperactivity can be reduced by surgery (partial thyroidectomy), irradiation by means of radioactive iodine, or antithyroid drugs.

Excessive adrenergic activity should be controlled by giving β-blocking agents, such as propranolol.

Tumors of the thyroid
Adenoma

Thyroid adenomas (Fig. 18-16) consist of follicular cells either in solid cords with minimal formation of small acini *(embryonal adenomas)* or, at the other extreme, of well-formed acini distended with colloid *(colloid adenomas)*. A less common variant contains large granular acidophilic cells (Hürthle cells) interspersed with poorly formed glandular tissue.

Adenomas can be functional and cause hyperthyroidism. The treatment is surgical excision.

Carcinoma of the thyroid

The thyroid is an uncommon site of cancer (Fig. 18-17) in most countries. It is also a recognized late complication of heavy doses of irradiation of the head and neck, but there is no evidence that goiter is a predisposing factor. Thyroid cancer

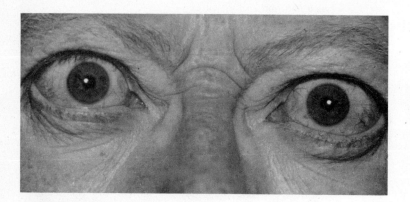

FIG. 18-15. Thyrotoxicosis (Graves' disease). The typical staring appearance is due to several changes, particularly protrusion of the eyes (proptosis) and retraction of the upper lids. The space between the upper and lower lids has thus become widened (widening of the palpebral fissure). *(Courtesy Curator of the Gordon Museum, Guy's Hospital, London, England.)*

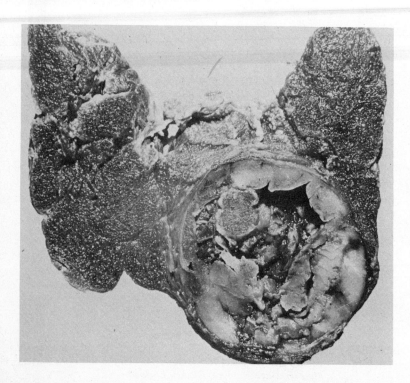

FIG. 18-16. Adenoma of the thyroid. This benign tumor is well circumscribed and shows central cystic change. *(Courtesy Curator of the Gordon Museum, Guy's Hospital, London, England.)*

accounts for 0.5% of cancer deaths in women and 0.2% in men, but appears to be increasing in frequency.

Pathology. The main types of thyroid carcinoma are papillary (60%), follicular (20%), anaplastic (15%) and medullary (5%). Of these, the first three arise from thyroid follicles, the last originates in the parafollicular or C cells.

Papillary carcinoma (Fig. 18-18) consists histologically, of fine branching papillae of thyroid cells with a vascular connective tissue core. The cells show all degrees of differentiation from a uniform cuboidal pattern to pleomorphism and loss of differentiation. Metastasis is usually through lymphatic channels to the regional cervical lymph nodes.

In *follicular carcinoma* (Fig. 18-19) the microscopic features are well-formed follicles, with nuclear enlargement, hyper-

chromasia and pleomorphism that can range from minimal to extreme (Fig. 18-20).

Anaplastic carcinomas as their name implies, have no definable pattern and the cells are either small, dark and featureless or variable in size and staining, sometimes showing several nuclei.

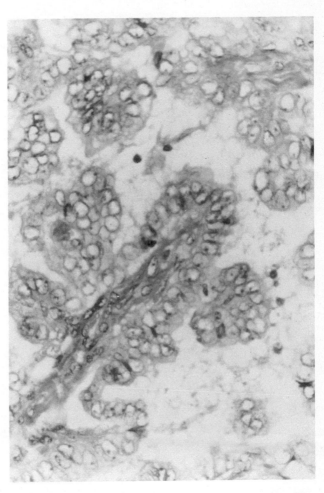

FIG. 18-18. Papillary carcinoma of the thyroid. Note the papillae lined by columnar cells containing the characteristic optically clear nuclei.

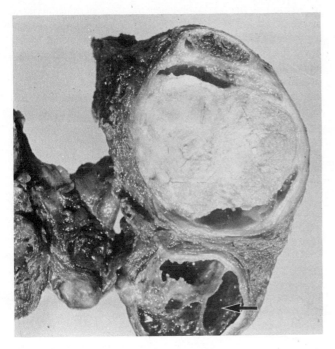

FIG. 18-17. Carcinoma of the thyroid. The main tumor mass is pale and relatively homogeneous. There are also cystic areas due to ischemic necrosis. The circumscribed appearance of the tumor is misleading. There is also a colloid cyst *(arrow)* below the tumor. *(Courtesy Curator of the Gordon Museum, Guy's Hospital, London, England.)*

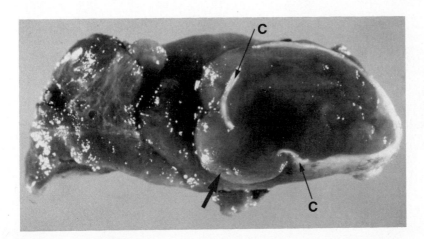

FIG. 18-19. Follicular carcinoma of the thyroid. The tumor is seen penetrating the capsule (*C*) and spreading out towards the large arrow. Capsular penetration is a sign of malignancy in thyroid neoplasms.

Capsular and/or blood vessel invasion are reliable criteria of malignancy in thyroid neoplasms (Figs. 18-19 and 18-20).

Medullary carcinomas (Fig. 18-21) arise from the calcitonin-producing, parafollicular or C cells. The cells are round or spindle-shaped and between them are varying amounts of amyloid (Fig. 18-22). These tumors produce large amounts of calcitonin (Fig. 18-23) and sometimes inappropriate products, such as ACTH or serotonin. They are also associated with preceding or coexisting C cell hyperplasia.

Medullary carcinomas may form part of the syndrome of *multiple endocrine adenomatosis II (MEA II)* associated with mucosal neurofibromas, particularly of the borders of the tongue.

Thyroid cancers vary widely in their behavior. Papillary and follicular carcinomas have the best survival; by contrast, the anaplastic type is highly malignant invades widely and metastasizes rapidly. The medullary carcinoma is usually slow growing and considerably less aggressive but can nevertheless metastasize.

Clinically, carcinomas of the thyroid may be detected as a nodule in a gland or in a goiter or cause pressure symptoms by pressing on the trachea or esophagus. A characteristic sign is hoarseness due to involvement of the recurrent laryngeal nerve.

The tumors are not usually functional but can cause hyperthyroidism. Occasionally, however, destruction of the remainder of the gland causes hypothyroidism.

Medullary carcinoma causes high plasma calcitonin levels, but these do not appear to affect calcium metabolism, and neither hypocalcemia nor skeletal defects are characteristic.

The treatment of choice is surgical excision.

Thyroglossal cysts

Thyroglossal cysts form as a result of an embryologic defect in which part of the tract joining the thyroid to the base of the tongue persists. The cyst forms very gradually as a result of accumulation of fluid. The lining of the cyst is usually squamous epithelium if it is high in the neck and close to the tongue, or it resembles thyroid acini if near the gland.

Clinically, a thyroglossal cyst often only becomes apparent in adult life and forms a swelling, often several centimeters in diameter, which typically moves in unison with the tongue and thyroid when the patient swallows.

Lingual thyroid

Thyroid tissue can persist in the tongue and may be the patient's only thyroid tissue. It is a rare developmental anomaly. The tongue may be enlarged and dark red and have an angiomatous appearance.

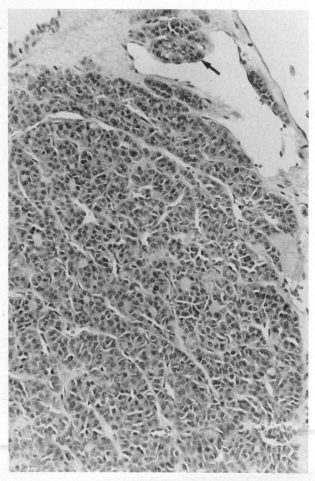

FIG. 18-20. Poorly differentiated thyroid follicular carcinoma showing vascular invasion by tumor cells *(arrow)*.

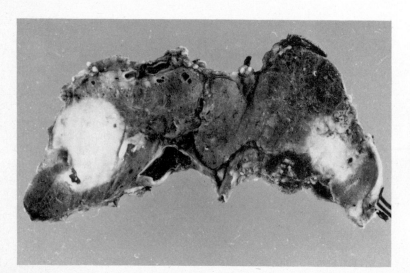

FIG. 18-21. Medullary carcinoma of the thyroid. There are two foci of carcinoma; one in each lobe at the anatomic site of highest concentration of C (parafollicular) cells.

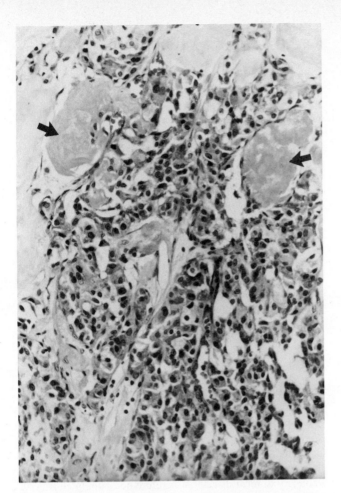

FIG. 18-22. Medullary carcinoma of the thyroid showing bundles of oval to polygonal tumor cells. The arrows indicate areas of amyloid in the intervening stroma.

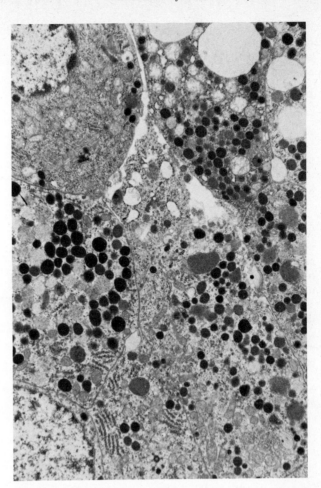

FIG. 18-23. Electron micrograph of thyroid medullary carcinoma showing calcitonin-containing granules of varying electron density.

THE PARATHYROIDS

Parathyroid hormone (PTH) maintains the plasma levels of ionized calcium within the normal range (see Chapter 17). PTH achieves this effect by (1) decreased excretion of calcium but increased phosphorus excretion in the urine, (2) mobilization of calcium from bone, (3) activation of vitamin D in renal tissue, and, to some extent (4) increased calcium absorption from the intestinal tract. As a result, blood calcium levels are raised and phosphorus levels may be depressed. Alkaline phosphatase levels are also increased. Disease of the parathyroids is uncommon.

Hypoparathyroidism

The most common cause is accidental removal of the glands during thyroidectomy. Occasionally the disease develops in early life. This may be the result of agenesis of the glands in DiGeorge's syndrome (Chapter 7). Alternatively it may be associated with circulating autoantibodies (both in the patient and in unaffected relatives) and sometimes with other autoimmune endocrine deficiencies, particularly Addison's disease. The polyendocrinopathy syndromes are discussed later.

Hypoparathyroidism may therefore, be (1) acute, due to accidental surgical removal, (2) of early onset in DiGeorge's syndrome, (3) autoimmune or (4) as an isolated phenomenon. The last three are grouped together as "idiopathic" hypopara-

thyroidism. Absence of parathyroid glands is incompatible with life.

Acute hypoparathyroidism

Acute hypoparathyroidism is the result of surgical removal of all parathyroid tissue. There is rapid drop in serum calcium levels and increased neuromuscular excitability, progressing to tetany or convulsions and sometimes death due to laryngospasm.

Treatment with calcium and a vitamin D analog is essential in this condition.

Idiopathic hypoparathyroidism

Tetany and convulsions are the most serious problems. Latent tetany can be elicited by tapping the facial nerve in front of the ear. This causes contraction of the facial muscles (Chvostek's sign*).

In hypoparathyroidism of early onset there may be hypercalcification of bones, cataracts, and, for less clear reasons, epithelial defects. These include hypoplasia of the teeth caused by defective enamel matrix formation and abnormalities of the fingernails.

The main findings are hypocalcemia and hypophosphatemia

---

*F. Chvostek (1835-1884), Austrian surgeon.

together with low serum parathormone levels. The basis of treatment is to raise the serum calcium level by giving calcium and vitamin D analogs, but there are risks from hypercalcemia or vitamin D intoxication.

Pseudohypoparathyroidism

Pseudohypoparathyroidism is the name given to a rare hereditary disorder characterized by features of hypoparathyroidism but hypersecretion of parathormone and parathyroid hyperplasia. It is mainly due to resistance to the hormone by receptors in the target tissues, particularly the skeleton and kidneys, but many features remain unexplained. Hypocalcemia and hypophosphatemia are essential features.

Clinical features include short stature and neck, a thickset body build, and multiple minor abnormalities of individual bones, particularly short fourth and fifth metatarsals and metacarpals. Unlike true hypoparathyroidism, soft tissue calcification, particularly of the basal ganglia, is common, but defects of teeth and nails are absent.

To confuse the matter still further, relatives of these patients often have skeletal and developmental defects without any evidence of parathyroid disease. This condition is called *pseudopseudohypoparathyroidism*, a term guaranteed to confound all but the most dedicated endocrine enthusiast!

Hyperparathyroidism

Primary hyperparathyroidism is a disorder of calcium and phosphate metabolism usually caused by a tumor of the parathyroids. Secondary hyperparathyroidism is a hyperplastic response to hypocalcemia, usually due to renal disease.

Primary hyperparathyroidism

By far the most common cause of primary hyperparathyroidism is a single adenoma. Occasionally multiple adenomas may be present and some of these may form part of MEA II (see Table 18-2). Hyperplasia of the parathyroids accounts for about 10% to 15% of cases, but only about 1% are carcinomas.

Pathology. Adenomas consist microscopically of closely packed chief cells, sometimes surrounded by a rim of normal or compressed atrophic tissue. Occasionally these tumors consist mainly of oxyphil cells.

Hyperplasia is characterized by increase in the size of the gland due to proliferation of chief cells. These are usually pale and vacuolated, but occasionally oxyphil or clear cells can predominate. The cells may be arranged as solid sheets or in cordlike or nestlike patterns.

Parathyroid carcinoma usually consists of solid sheets of cells, which may be enlarged chief cells, or other types, often separated by fibrous septa.

Clinical aspects. The effects of hyperparathyroidism are mainly (1) hypercalcemia, (2) bone resorption, and (3) renal calcinosis.

Renal effects (Fig. 18-24) include calcific deposits in the renal parenchyma or recurrent renal stones due to excretion of excessive amounts of calcium. Polyuria and polydipsia may be associated. The end result can be renal failure, which is the most important complication.

Bone resorption can produce the typical picture of *osteitis fibrosa cystica*, but this is now rare. The radiologic features are areas of radiolucency resembling multilocular cysts, particularly in the jaws. The lesions consist of vascular connective tissue containing great numbers of osteoclasts (Fig. 18-25). Resorption of bone can occasionally lead to pathologic fracture.

A more common type of skeletal change consists of thinning of bone trabeculae resembling osteoporosis (Fig. 18-26). Hypercalciuria results from the resorption of bone and is an important chemical finding. The serum alkaline phosphatase level is also raised, and urinary phosphorus excretion is increased. In spite of resorption of bones, ectopic calcification can develop in visceral organs. The most common complication is hypertension (16%), and later renal failure (11%) may develop.

Other effects of hypercalcemia include gastrointestinal symptoms (anorexia, nausea, and sometimes peptic ulcer), nervous and neuromuscular effects (lethargy, weakness, and sometimes psychiatric disturbances), and, in advanced cases, cataracts or calcification in the cornea.

Diagnosis depends on finding raised serum calcium and PTH levels. Hyperparathyroidism is one of the most common causes of hypercalcemia; other causes are discussed below. Investigation should also include tests of renal function and possibly a skeletal survey for bone lesions.

Treatment consists of removing the tumor(s) or hyperplastic tissue. The parathyroids may, however, be in abnormal sites, and finding them can be difficult.

Secondary hyperparathyroidism (renal osteodystrophy)

Severe renal disease can cause excessive calcium loss and interferes with vitamin D metabolism. Even in the absence of such effects, increased PTH secretion and parathyroid hyperplasia can develop. The mechanism of hyperparathyroidism secondary to renal disease is therefore not entirely clear.

Secondary hyperparathyroidism differs from the primary form in that, in spite of increased PTH secretion, patients are usually mildly hypocalcemic, and soft tissue calcification is more common and severe.

The abnormality of vitamin D metabolism causes rickets-like changes, especially in the epiphyses of growing bones, and skeletal deformities in children (renal rickets).

Hypercalcemia

Hypercalcemia most obviously can result from extensive bone resorption either as a direct result for example, of osteolytic neoplasms or secondarily to overactivity of parathyroid hormone however there is a variety of possible causes. The most common of these are malignant tumors and primary hyperparathyroidism.

Important causes of hypercalcemia are as follows*:
1. Increased intake or absorption
   a. Hypervitaminosis D
   b. Milk alkali syndrome
   c. Sarcoidosis
2. Increased calcium mobilization from the skeleton
   a. Hyperparathyroidism (primary)
   b. Malignant tumors secreting PTH-like hormones
   c. Widespread osteolytic neoplasms

---

*Several of the above main mechanisms may be operating *concomitantly* in some of these diseases, particularly those involving vitamin D or parathyroid hormone. Furthermore, *tumors* (other than those of the parathyroids) can cause hypercalcemia by secreting a variety of humoral mediators of bone resorption other than PTH-like peptides.

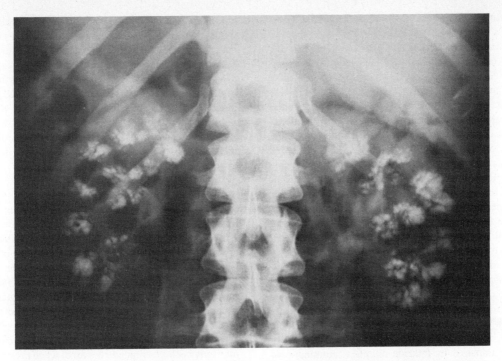

FIG. 18-24. This radiograph of the abdomen shows bilateral nephrocalcinosis in a patient with hyperparathyroidism.

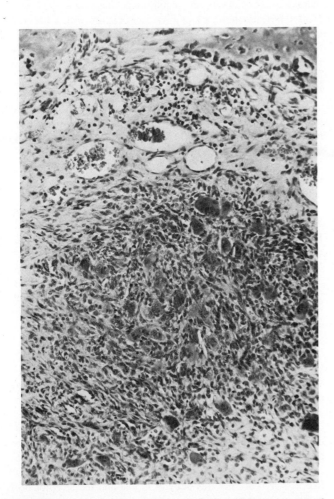

FIG. 18-25. "Brown tumor" of hyperparathyroidism. A cluster of osteoclasts is seen against a background of granulation tissue.

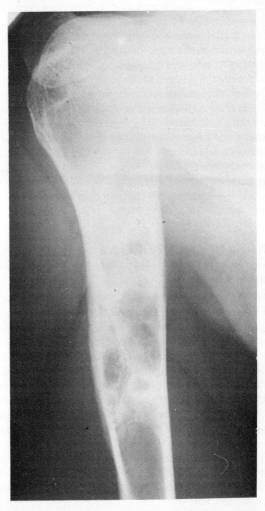

FIG. 18-26. Hyperparathyroidism. The appearance of multiple cysts (osteitis fibrosa cystica) is produced by foci of giant cells and fibrous tissue. *(Courtesy Dr AJ Bridge and Dr FL Ingram.)*

d. Hyperthyroidism
e. Paget's disease of bone (rarely)
3. Impaired calcium excretion
   a. Renal failure
   b. Thiazide-induced
   c. Aluminum associated

Pathogenesis. The main mechanisms can be summarized as (1) increased calcium intake or absorption, (2) increased calcium loss from the skeleton or (3) impaired renal excretion. More than one of these mechanisms can act concomittantly.

Increased calcium intake or absorption can result from hypervitaminosis D (Chapter 6) or the milk alkali syndrome (Chapter 16). Abnormal sensitivity to vitamin D is the probable cause of the hypercalcemia of sarcoidosis. Increased bone turnover or loss are features of hyperthyroidism or prolonged immobilization but oversecretion of parathyroid hormone (PTH) in hyperparathyroidism raises calcium levels by several mechanisms but including bone resorption. Some other tumors (particularly carcinoma of the lung or kidney) can cause hypercalcemia by secreting PTH-like peptides. Increased PTH secretion can also result from renal failure and secondary hyperparathyroidism. However the latter, unless severe, more usually is associated with hypocalcemia. Renal excretion of calcium can be impaired by thiazide diuretics, aluminum intoxication and the milk alkali syndrome, but these are rare causes of hypercalcemia.

Treatment of hypercalcemia is important particularly when symptomatic and is by control of the primary disease, where possible, and by decreasing intake or increasing renal excretion as appropriate. When renal function is adequate calcium excretion can be enhanced by giving sodium, since both are excreted together, fluids and the diuretic furosemide.

Clinically, hypercalcemia can be asymptomatic and a chance finding in routine biochemical investigation. Symptomatic hypercalcemia is characterized by anorexia and nausea, polyuria, weakness, and lethargy. This can progress to confusion or stupor and azotemia.

Severe hypercalcemia has a high mortality and death can result from cardiac arrhythmias and asystole. Chronic hypercalcemia can lead to renal calcinosis and sometimes renal failure.

PANCREATIC ISLET CELLS

Diabetes mellitus

Diabetes mellitus is the most common endocrine disease, and it is estimated that it affects more than 4 million Americans. It is characterized by abnormally elevated blood glucose levels and altered protein and lipid metabolism. These are due to a relative or absolute deficiency of insulin. Pathologic changes in blood vessels (atherosclerosis), especially those of the kidney and the retina, are also characteristic. Clear descriptions of diabetes mellitus date back to remote antiquity. The name derives from the sweet taste of the urine (Latin *mellis,* honey). This test for glycosuria is, however, somewhat less popular now.

Insulin, a double chain protein secreted by the beta-cells of the islets of Langerhans, stimulates carbohydrate metabolism (including glycogen storage), protein synthesis, amino acid uptake, and fatty acid synthesis.

Glucagon is a hormone produced by the alpha-cells. It rapidly mobilizes the liver glycogen and fatty acids from adipose tissue. Glucagon also releases glucose from storage sites so that its effects on the target organs oppose those of insulin.

Some now believe that excess glucagon activity, due possibly to a defect in the alpha-cells, may contribute to the pathogenesis of diabetes. Since glucagon release is mediated by a fall in the blood glucose level, some types of diabetes may result from failure of this feedback control. There may be genetic, immunologic, and viral factors responsible for the etiology of diabetes, which is not a single disease but a group of diseases as the classification given later indicates.

Genetic factors

The common types of diabetes show a strong familial distribution. The disease is common among close relatives; it is also more frequent in identical than in nonidentical twins. Nevertheless, because of the heterogeneous nature of diabetes there is no single clearly defined genetic pattern; juvenile onset (type I) disease for example has a different mode of inheritance from maturity onset (type II) diabetes. The inheritance of even a single type of diabetes may be polygenic and the problem is made more difficult by the facts that (1) *susceptibility* to diabetes is not detectable and (2) late onset diabetes in particular may only become clinically apparent when precipitated by some factor such as obesity, which increases insulin requirements.

A significant number of type I diabetics are HLA-DR3 or HLA-DR4, that is, persons who are HLA-DR3 or DR4 are at increased risk of developing insulin-dependent diabetes. These HLA types also have a significant association with other autoimmune diseases.

In maturity onset diabetes, genetic factors may be responsible for the decreased sensitivity of the target cells to insulin.

Immunologic mechanisms

Some types of diabetes (particularly type I and some of its variants) appear to be immunologically mediated. Microscopically, in type I disease there is a lymphocytic infiltration of the islets ("insulitis"). A majority of these cells are suppressor/cytotoxic (CD8) T cells and destruction of the β cells of the islets is highly specific in that other endocrine-producing islet cells are unaffected.

Type I diabetes can be associated with other autoimmune diseases as discussed later but even in isolated type I disease, IgG islet cell anticytoplasmic autoantibodies (ICAs) can be detected in up to 85% of cases at the time of diagnosis but, later, tend to disappear from the serum. Moreover in those with circulating ICAs, the disease tends to become more severe with the passage of time. Siblings of persons with type I diabetes may also have circulating ICAs and prospective studies have shown that all of those who developed diabetes have been ICA positive for several years beforehand.

Another autoantibody against islet cell surface antigens (ICSA) has also been identified but its importance in the development of diabetes is uncertain. Further, in different subtypes of type I diabetes there can be other autoantibodies such as those to insulin itself or to insulin receptors. For example, the latter are present in the rare syndrome of insulin-dependent diabetes associated with acanthosis nigricans, a skin disease discussed in Chapter 20. Insulin receptor antibodies mimic insulin by binding to the receptors and initially, have insulin-like activity but later this activity is lost and the receptor becomes resistant to insulin.

Cellular immunity probably plays an important role in "insulitis" as suggested by the histologic picture. Cellular immune mechanisms of islet cell destruction can be demonstrated in animals but they have not as yet been shown to play an essential role in human disease.

Much animal experimentation also suggests various immunologic mechanisms but their relevance to human disease remains uncertain. Currently the bulk of evidence is that anti-cytoplasmic IgG, β cell autoantibodies have the strongest associations with the development of type I diabetes, particularly in those persons who express the HLA DR3 or DR4 alleles.

Viruses

The relevance of viral infections to the etiology of diabetes mellitus remains controversial and largely epidemiologic. It has long been suspected that viruses may trigger autoimmune disease of various types and there is evidence that viruses can induce the development of HLA-DR (class II) molecules on β cells of the islets, which as a result become recognizable as antigens by T lymphocytes.

Viruses may also directly attack and destroy islet β cells. β cell destruction has for example been reported in a fatal case of cytomegalovirus infection in a child though it later appeared that the tissue damage had started before the infection. Congenital rubella is however a well recognized triggering factor and 20% of those affected develop diabetes later in life, particularly if they are HLA DR3 or DR4. There is an increased incidence of other autoimmune diseases, such as thyroiditis in these patients.

Coxsackie B viruses are also candidates as triggering factors and an extensive study in Europe and Australia found specific IgM responses to Coxsackie B strains (usually B4) in 30% of patients with recent onset type I diabetes and in only 6% of controls. By contrast there was no evidence of recent infection by mumps, cytomegalovirus or rubella.

Unlike type I diabetes, there is no convincing evidence of viral infections as triggering factors or of autoimmune mechanisms involved in late onset (type II) diabetes as discussed later.

Classification

As mentioned earlier diabetes mellitus is a heterogeneous group of diseases and a great variety of subtypes can be identified. The main types are the juvenile, insulin-dependent and the more common, maturity onset, non-insulin-dependent diseases. "Juvenile" and "maturity" are vague terms but are useful reminders that the more severe type of diabetes usually (but not always) has its clinical onset in childhood or adolescence while non-insulin-dependent diabetes mellitus usually has its onset in middle age.

In addition diabetes may be secondary to other clinically definable disease and a simple classification is as follows.
1. Insulin-dependent diabetes mellitus (IDDM; type I)
2. Non-insulin-dependent diabetes mellitus (NIDDM; type II)
3. Secondary diabetes mellitus (Cushing's diseases, acromegaly, etc.)

Pathogenesis

Diabetes mellitus is, in broad terms, the result of relative or absolute deficiency of insulin or failure of insulin activity and, as a consequence, inability to metabolize glucose normally. In the cases of juvenile onset (type I) diabetes, too little insulin is produced as a result of β cell destruction in the islets. In maturity onset (type II) diabetes, the response to insulin is decreased, partly because there is in most cases an excess of adipose tissue and also some degree of insulin resistance due to a post-receptor defect. In other types of diabetes there may be insulin receptor blockers or, in the rare hormone-induced types of diabetes, there is oversecretion of diabetogenic hormones, namely growth hormone (acromegaly) or glucocorticoids (Cushing's disease).

Hyperglycemia, glycosuria, and ketoacidosis. The essential feature of diabetes mellitus is hyperglycemia, usually associated with glycosuria, whereas ketoacidosis is a serious consequence of the metabolic derangement.

Hyperglycemia is the result of two factors: (1) impaired metabolism of glucose, especially in muscle and fat, and (2) overproduction of glucose by the liver as a result of the effect of lack of insulin on liver enzymes. Glucose released from the liver is (1) from dietary carbohydrate, (2) the result of mobilization of liver glycogen, and (3) due to increased gluconeogenesis. Impaired uptake of glucose by muscle also leads to loss of muscle glycogen and release of amino acids, which undergo gluconeogenesis.

Impaired metabolism of glucose as a result of obesity is less well understood. It may be partly the result of a relative deficiency of insulin. Alternatively, fat cells may be much enlarged and have inadequate insulin receptor sites in relation to their increased bulk. Too little insulin may therefore penetrate the fat cell membrane.

Impaired uptake of glucose by adipose tissue also causes impaired triglyceride synthesis and release of free fatty acids into the circulation. Some are metabolized by the liver to ketones, which are produced in excessive amounts.

Immediate effects of hyperglycemia and ketoacidosis are as follows. When the blood glucose level rises above the renal threshold, it is excreted in the urine. Glucose takes water with it, causing an osmotic diuresis and loss of fluid. Ketone bodies also accumulate in the blood and are excreted in the urine. Two of these ketones, acetoacetic and β-hydroxybutyric acid, are strong acids, and their excretion causes loss of buffer cations, particularly sodium and potassium. The result of loss of fluid and bases is progressive acidosis and dehydration. The pathogenesis of these complex metabolic changes is summarized in Fig. 18-27.

Pathology

Diabetes mellitus is frequently associated with or is the result of changes in the pancreas. As the disease progresses, it has increasingly severe effects on the blood vessels, kidneys, and the retina.

Changes in the β cells in juvenile-onset and maturity-onset diabetes can be shown by light and electron microscopy. Overall, there is a correlation between the amount of secretory tissue and degree of degranulation of the β-cells with the severity of juvenile diabetes. Fibrosis and occasionally lymphocytic infiltration of islet tissue is seen; particularly in juvenile diabetics who die soon after the onset of the disease.

Amyloid (Chapter 2) is often deposited around blood vessels and displaces secretory cells ('hyalinization' of the islets). Persistent hyperglycemia is associated with accumulation of glycogen in the β cells, which microscopically appear to be vacuolated.

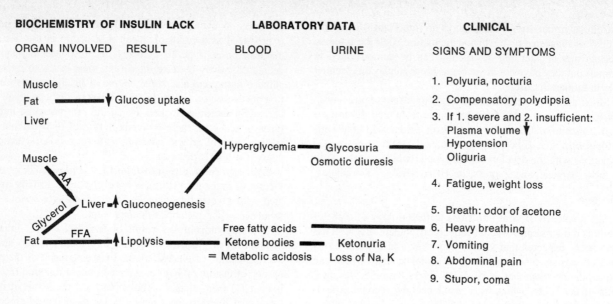

BIOCHEMISTRY OF INSULIN LACK   LABORATORY DATA   CLINICAL

ORGAN INVOLVED   RESULT   BLOOD   URINE   SIGNS AND SYMPTOMS

AA = Amino acids

FFA = Free fatty acids

FIG. 18-27. Pathogenesis of hyperglycemia, glycosuria, and ketoacidosis in diabetes mellitus. *AA,* amino acids; *FFA,* free fatty acids. *(From Steinke J and Soeldner JS: Diabetes mellitus. In Thorn GW et al, editors: Harrison's principles of internal medicine, ed 8, New York, 1977, McGraw-Hill Book Co. Copyright 1977 by McGraw-Hill Book Co. Used with permission of McGraw-Hill Book Co.)*

Complications

The numerous complications of diabetes mellitus include the following:

1. Ocular
   a. Retinopathy
   b. Cataracts
2. Renal
   a. Diabetic glomerulosclerosis
   b. Atherosclerosis and hypertensive damage
   c. Pyelonephritis
3. Neurologic
   a. Peripheral neuropathy
   b. Neuropathy of cranial nerves
   c. Autonomic neuropathy
4. Vascular
   a. Trophic changes or gangrene of the feet
   b. Coronary heart disease
   c. Cerebrovascular accidents
5. Infections
   a. Superficial, especially staphylococcal (boils) or candidosis
   b. Systemic, tuberculosis or deep mycoses
6. Dermatologic
   a. Infections
   b. Neuropathic or ischemic ulcers (especially of the legs)
   c. Fat atrophy or hypertrophy at insulin injection sites
   d. Xanthoma (yellowish foci of lipid), especially around the eyes

Ocular lesions. In patients who have been diabetic for at least 10 years, retinal lesions frequently develop. Microaneurysms form as a result of loss of mural cells (pericytes) of the capillaries. These changes form the specific retinal lesions of diabetes (diabetic retinopathy). In addition, the damaged vessel walls allow leaks of plasma or blood, visible as exudate or hemorrhages by ophthalmoscopy.

Diabetic retinopathy is the second most common cause of blindness in the United States and, it is predicted, will soon be the most common cause.

Renal disease. Renal disease is the chief cause of early death in childhood diabetes. The pathologic changes in the kidney consist of the characteristic basement membrane thickening of diabetic microangiopathy. In the mesangium the process can produce eosinophilic nodular thickenings (Fig. 18-28). This change is progressive and increases in severity with the duration of the disease (Kimmelstiel-Wilson disease).

Vascular disease. Diabetics are more susceptible to atherosclerosis than the normal population, as well as to a lesion of capillaries *(diabetic microangiopathy).*

Atherosclerosis in diabetics does not differ from the disease in nondiabetics but starts earlier and affects both sexes equally. Coronary heart disease and cerebrovascular accidents are significantly more frequent than in nondiabetics. Vascular disease is particularly severe in the lower leg and can cause gangrene (Fig. 18-29).

Diabetic microangiopathy is characterized by thickening of the basement membrane of the capillaries of the kidneys, eyes, and other sites.

Diabetic coma. Coma is a complication of severe diabetes as a result of lack of insulin due to (1) unsuspected diabetes mellitus, (2) inadequate insulin intake, or (3) infection with dehydration and increased need for insulin secondary to acute fluid loss.

Coma is gradual in onset, preceded by increasing lethargy caused by metabolic ketoacidosis (see Fig. 18-27) and asso-

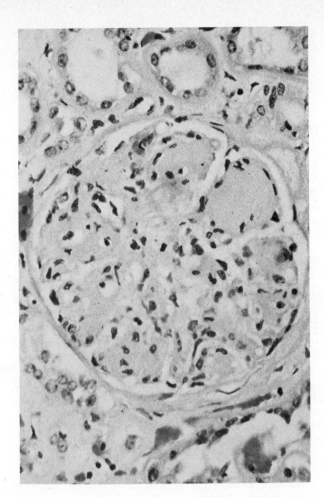

FIG. 18-28. Nodular diabetic (Kimmelstiel-Wilson) glomerulosclerosis showing typical hyaline mesangial nodules.

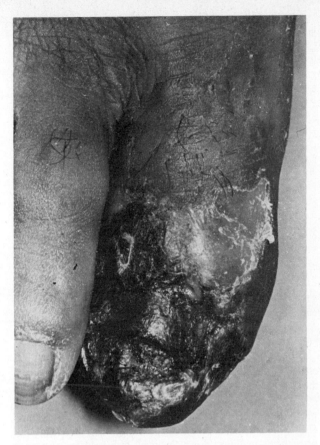

FIG. 18-29. Diabetic gangrene. The blackened necrotic appearance is typical. This is a common complication of ischemia secondary to severe atheroma of the arteries of the lower leg, which may have to be amputated as the disease progresses. *(Courtesy Curator of the Gordon Museum, Guy's Hospital, London, England.)*

ciated with characteristic air hunger with deep, labored breathing. Common early features are nausea and vomiting, often with abdominal pain, and are the result of sodium depletion. The breath has a fruity odor due to ketones. Dehydration causes a dry skin, soft eyeballs, and hypotension.

The urine typically contains large amounts of sugar and acetone, but output is low due to dehydration. There is severe hyperglycemia and azotemia due partly to dehydration but also to breakdown of tissue proteins.

The management of diabetic coma is based on the correction of dehydration, and electrolyte and acid-base abnormalities and the administration of insulin.

Hypoglycemic coma. Hypoglycemic coma is due to insulin overdose or failure to eat at the proper time after insulin has been taken. The relatively sudden lack of sugar available to the nerve cells causes rapid loss of consciousness.

Clinically, there is initially confusion, weakness, and dizziness and often nausea or vomiting. Consciousness is quickly lost but, unlike a fainting attack, is not regained when the patient is laid flat. If the dose of insulin was large, coma can progressively deepen.

Hypoglycemic coma is treated by the administration of oral or intravenous glucose, but to give insulin (as a result of confusing *hypo*glycemic for *hyper*glycemic coma) is likely to be fatal.

Clinical aspects

Juvenile-onset and maturity-onset diabetes generally produce distinct clinical pictures, but occasionally there are transitions between the two types.

Juvenile-onset diabetes is typically abrupt in onset with polyuria, polydipsia, and excessive appetite and eating (polyphagia). Weakness and relatively rapid deterioration of health can follow. Ketoacidosis can develop and result in coma (see Fig. 18-27).

In spite of modern treatment, the disease can be so severe as to result in early death from cardiovascular or renal failure. At the other extreme, the disease can be so mild as to cause no symptoms and be detectable only by hyperglycemia after meals and an abnormal glucose tolerance test. It may progress slowly in such cases.

In *maturity-onset diabetes* the patient is typically middle-aged and overweight. The onset is variable and sometimes insidious. Early symptoms may be polyuria, polydipsia, impaired sight, recurrent infections such as boils or vaginal candidosis, neuropathy with paresthesias or loss of sensation, or ulceration of the foot associated with loss of pulses and sensation.

Diagnosis

In severe cases the diagnosis may be obvious from the history and general clinical picture, including the complications. Nev-

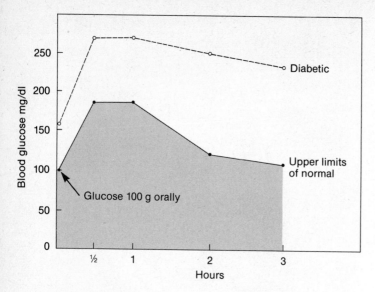

FIG. 18-30. Glucose tolerance test showing normal and diabetic curves.

ertheless, objective tests are needed to assess the severity of the disease and to detect complications.

In mild cases, the simplest screening test is to measure blood glucose levels, 1 to 2 hours after a heavy carbohydrate meal (Fig. 18-30). A level of 170 mg/dl or higher is very suggestive of diabetes mellitus. Since the renal threshold for glucose is variable, however, a blood glucose test (both after fasting and after a meal) and a glucose tolerance test are usually performed and the urine is tested for ketones. The glucose tolerance test is performed after the patient has been on a standard carbohydrate diet for 3 days. After a fasting blood glucose level is obtained, 100 g of glucose in solution is taken orally, and blood samples are taken at ½ hour and 1, 2, and 3 hours later for glucose estimation. The upper limits of normal and a typical diabetic response are shown in Fig. 18-30. A variety of factors, however, including age, intercurrent illness, and certain drugs, can influence the outcome of the test.

The principles of treatment of diabetes can be summarized as follows:
1. To correct the metabolic abnormality
2. To achieve and maintain ideal body weight
3. To try to prevent complications, particularly those involving the eyes, kidneys, and blood vessels

Juvenile diabetics and all diabetics who become ketotic need insulin. The adjustment of insulin dosage for the diabetic patient has, in the past, been dependent on measurements of blood and urine glucose. Estimation of blood levels of the glycosylated hemoglobin HbA_{1c} (Chapter 13) has however been shown to be a more reliable method on which to base insulin treatment. HbA_{1c} binds to glucose and acts as a cumulative indicator of diabetic control, since it remains circulating for the life of the erythrocyte. Mild cases of maturity-onset diabetes can be controlled by diet alone if the patient can be made to lose weight. If necessary, oral hypoglycemic agents, such as tolbutamide or phenformin, should also be given.

Prediabetes

For every patient with diabetes, there is probably another with asymptomatic disease, as shown by population screening tests. Blood glucose level and glucose tolerance tests are desirable for those who are particularly at risk of developing diabetes namely, (1) relatives of diabetics, (2) the obese, especially those over 45 years of age, and (3) women who give birth to large babies.

Islet cell tumors

Functional tumors of the islets of Langerhans can produce a variety of hormones and corresponding clinical effects. The main examples are insulin-producing tumors (insulinomas) of the β cells, which cause among other effects, hypoglycemia, and gastrinomas which cause gastric hypersecretion and severe peptic ulceration (Zollinger-Ellison syndrome). All are uncommon.

Beta-cell adenoma (insulinoma)

Insulinoma is the most common cause of fasting hypoglycemia in adults who are not taking insulin. Hypoglycemia can be acute or chronic, but symptoms typically develop in the early morning, when a meal has been missed, or after violent exercise. The fasting blood glucose level is low (less than 40 mg/dl), and immediate recovery follows administration of glucose.

Symptoms of acute hypoglycemia somewhat resemble drunkenness. There are disturbances of vision, slurred speech, a sense of unreality or detachment, and consciousness may be lost. Severe untreated cases can result in permanent brain damage.

Diagnosis is by detection of fasting hypoglycemia associated with high serum insulin levels.

Treatment is preferably surgical excision of the tumor or tumors, or subtotal pancreatectomy. If operative treatment fails or is not feasible, symptoms can be relieved by frequent carbohydrate snacks. Alternatively, streptozotocin can be used to suppress insulin production by a tumor of the islet cells.

THE THYMUS

The thymus is not known to produce hormones in the ordinary sense after puberty, but it plays an essential role in the processing of cells to produce T lymphocytes.

At least 10 thymic hormones have been described, including thymosin and lymphocyte-stimulating hormone. The biologic importance of these factors in humans has not, however, been established.

Thymosin has been studied in most detail, and in vitro it has been shown to induce immunologic maturation of T lymphocytes.

The thymus is colonized during intrauterine life by lymphocyte-forming cells, reaches its maximal development immediately after birth, and rapidly involutes after puberty.

Hyperplasia and tumors of the thymus are associated with a variety of diseases, particularly myasthenia gravis, red cell aplasia, and immune deficiencies. The pathology of diseases of the thymus is discussed here, but their immunologic effects and myasthenia gravis are discussed in more detail in Chapters 7 and 17, respectively.

Agenesis (DiGeorge's syndrome)

Agenesis of the thymus and parathyroids, and defective cell mediated immunity is discussed in Chapter 7.

TABLE 18-1. Polyendocrine deficiency syndromes (polyglandular autoimmune disease)

Endocrine or other disease	Type I	Type II
Addison's disease	100%	100%
Hypoparathyroidism	75%	—
Thyroiditis	10%	70%
Insulin-dependent diabetes	5%	>50%
Pernicious anemia	10%	1%
Gonadal failure	>15%	<5%
Malabsorption syndromes	>20%	—
Chronic mucocutaneous candidosis	75%	—

TABLE 18-2. Multiple endocrine adenoma (MEA) syndromes

	Type I	Type II	Type III
Pituitary adenoma	+++	—	—
Thyroid (medullary carcinoma)	++	+++	+++
Parathyroid adenoma	+++	++	—
Adrenal cortex adenoma	+++	+++	+
Pheochromocytoma	—	+	++
Pancreas islet cell tumor	+++	—	
Other features	Gastrinoma, multiple lipomas		Marfanoid features, mucosal and/or cutaneous neuromas

Thymoma

Thymomas are rare neoplasms of thymic epithelial (squamous) cells. They contain varying (and often large) numbers of nonneoplastic lymphocytes and should be differentiated from the even less common thymic lymphomas, in which lymphoid cells are the true neoplastic element.

The behavior of thymomas is variable, and some are invasive. The local effects of invasive thymomas are obstruction of the superior vena cava, involvement of esophagus or trachea, and pleural effusion due to involvement of the thoracic duct. The remote effects of thymomas are diverse, but the most important are (1) myasthenia gravis, (2) hemopathies, particularly pure red cell aplasia, (3) autoimmune disorders, and (4) defective cell-mediated immunity. These are discussed more fully in other chapters.

POLYENDOCRINE DEFICIENCY SYNDROMES (POLYGLANDULAR AUTOIMMUNE DISEASE)

The organ-specific autoimmune diseases mainly affect glandular organs and in particular endocrine glands. These diseases can be significantly more frequently associated in various patterns than would be dictated by chance. Two major syndromes associated with Addison's disease are recognized and their features are shown in Table 18-1. Type II appears to be considerably more prevalent than type I; nevertheless both syndromes are rare.

In type I disease, mucocutaneous candidosis is frequently associated and this appears to result from a limited defect of cellular immunity. Candidosis is not secondary to the glandular defects; it can be the first sign of the syndrome and precede overt endocrine deficiency by 10 or more years. Moreover replacement therapy for the endocrine deficiency has no effect on the candidal infection.

ENDOCRINE TUMOR SYNDROMES

These rare syndromes are due to functional tumors of many glands. They are often inherited as autosomal dominants, but sporadic cases are also seen. Their main features are summarized in Table 18-2. Clinically, their manifestations vary widely. The most common manifestations of Type I are (a) peptic ulcer, (b) hypercalcemia, (c) the local (Chapter 20) or endocrine effects of a pituitary tumor or (d) multiple lipomas. The islet cell tumors in this syndrome can produce a variety of peptides (see Chapter 14) with appropriate endocrine effects.

The most common manifestations of types II and III (sometimes termed IIa and IIb respectively) are pheochromocytoma and its complications and medullary carcinoma of the thyroid but type III differs strikingly in that there are multiple other morphologic abnormalities, such as Marfanoid features, oral and other mucosal neuromas and sometimes cutaneous neurofibromatosis.

Selected readings

Anon (LA): Insulin receptors, acanthosis nigricans, and insulin resistance, Lancet i:595, 1986.

Anon (LA): Testing anterior pituitary function, Lancet i:839, 1986.

Anon (LA): Hypoprolactinaemia, Lancet i:1356, 1987.

Anon (LA): Congenital adrenal hyperplasia, Lancet ii:663, 1987.

Banatvala JE, Schernthaner G, and Schober E et al: Coxsackie B, mumps, rubella, and cytomegalovirus specific IgM responses in patients with juvenile-onset insulin-dependent diabetes mellitus in Britain, Austria, and Australia, Lancet i:1409, 1985.

Barney PL: Pathology of thyroid cancer: summary and update, Laryngoscope 94:525, 1984.

Bodansky HJ, Grant PJ, and Dean BM et al: Islet-cell antibodies and insulin autoantibodies in association with common viral infections, Lancet ii: 1351, 1986.

Bloom SR and Polak JM: Somatostatin, Br Med J 295:288, 1987.

Brownlee M, Vlassara H, and Cerami A: Nonenzymatic glycosylation and the pathogenesis of diabetic complications, Ann Intern Med 101:527, 1984.

Burek CL and Rose NR: Cell-mediated immunity in autoimmune thyroid disease, Human Path 17(3):246, 1986.

Davidson MB: Review: pathogenesis of type 2 diabetes mellitus: an interpretation of current data, Am J Med Sc 292(1):35, 1986.

Davies RR and Johnston DG: Growth hormone releasing factors, J Royal Soc Med 80:3, 1987.

Eisenbarth GS and Rassi N: Polyglandular failure syndromes. In Davis PF, editor: Autoimmune endocrine disease, 1983, Wiley New York.

Flier JS and Underhill LH: Type I diabetes mellitus: a chronic autoimmune disease, N Engl J Med 314(21):1360, 1986.

Foulis AK: The pathogenesis of beta cell destruction in type I (insulin-dependent) diabetes mellitus, J Path 152:141, 1987.

Gerich JE: Intensive Insulin Therapy Symposium: Insulin-dependent diabetes mellitus: pathophysiology, Mayo Clin Proc 61:787, 1986.

Daughaday WH: Cushing's disease and basophilic microadenomas, N Engl J Med 310(14):919, 1984.

Hamburger JI: The various presentations of thyroiditis: diagnostic considerations, Ann Intern Med 104:219, 1986.

Hetzel BS: Iodine deficiency disorders (IDD) and their eradication, Lancet ii:1126, 1983.

Kahn CR: Insulin resistance: a common feature of diabetes mellitus, N Engl J Med 315(4):252, 1986.

Kao PC, Abboud CF, and Zimmerman D: Somatomedin C: an index of growth hormone activity, Mayo Clin Proc 61:908, 1986.

Klein I: Acromegaly and cancer, Ann Intern Med 101(5):706, 1984.

Lawton NF: Prolactinomas: medical or surgical treatment? Quarterly J Med 64(243):557, 1987.

Loriaux DL: The polyendocrine deficiency syndromes, N Engl J Med 312(24):1568, 1985.

McNicol AM: Pituitary adenomas, Histopathology 11:995, 1987.

Mellinger RC: The conundrum of Cushing's syndrome, Arch Intern Med 146:858, 1986.

O'Rahilly S, Spivey RS, and Holman RR et al: Type II diabetes of early onset: a distinct clinical and genetic syndrome? Br Med J 294:923, 1987.

Orth DN: The old and the new in Cushing's syndrome, N Engl J Med 310(10):649, 1984.

Pollett RJ: Principles of membrane receptor physiology and their application to clinical medicine, Ann Intern Med 92:663, 1980.

Pollett RJ: Insulin receptors and action in clinical disorders of carbohydrate tolerance, Am J Med 1983; Glipizide Symposium 15-22.

Raskin P and Rosenstock J: Blood glucose control and diabetic complications, Ann Intern Med 105:254, 1986.

Raskin P and Rosenstock J: Aldose reductase inhibitors and diabetic complications, Am J Med 83:298, 1987.

Rechler MM, Nissley SP and Roth J: Hormonal regulation of human growth, N Engl J Med 316(15):941, 1987.

Rojeski MT and Gharib H: Nodular thyroid disease, N Engl J Med 313(7):428, 1985.

Sakati S, Nakamura MD, and Miura K: Autoantibodies against thyroid hormones or iodothyronine, Ann Intern Med 103:579, 1985.

Semple CG: Hormonal changes in non-endocrine disease, Br Med J 293:1049, 1986.

Schimke RN: Genetic aspects of multiple endocrine neoplasia, Ann Rev Med 35:25, 1984.

Schimke RN: Multiple endocrine neoplasia, N Engl J Med 314(20):1315, 1986.

Sutton MG-St.J, Sheps SG, and Lie JT: Prevalence of clinically unsuspected Pheochromocytoma, Mayo Clin Proc 56:354, 1981.

Taylor R: Insulin receptors and the clinician, Br Med J 292:919, 1986.

Volpe R: Immunoregulation in autoimmune thyroid disease, N Engl J Med 316(1):44, 1987.

White PC, New MI and Dupont B: Congenital adrenal hyperplasia, N Engl J Med 316(24):1519, 1987.

White PC, New MI, and Dupont B: Congenital adrenal hyperplasia (second of two parts), N Engl J Med 316(25):1580, 1987.

CHAPTER 19

Diseases of the skin and mucous membranes

Diseases of the skin are common, and an enormous variety is recognized. Some of them also affect mucous membranes. Unfortunately, the subject of dermatology is difficult, mainly because diagnosis is often largely based on clinical criteria. An archaic terminology also clings to the subject.

Another factor complicating the pathology of skin diseases is the structure of the skin, particularly the presence of accessory organs such as hair follicles and sweat glands. These can become involved in or give rise to disease.

The skin consists of an epidermis of stratified squamous epithelium tightly bound to the connective tissue dermis. The structure of the oral mucous membrane is essentially similar, except that the skin keratinizes as part of its normal process of maturation, but keratinization is abnormal in the mouth. The accessory structures of oral epithelium are teeth and salivary glands.

Terminology

Erythema is a red area of skin level with the surrounding surface.

A *macule* is a flat area of skin in which there is a change in color (i.e., it cannot be felt with the finger) and which is less than a centimeter in diameter. A larger, colored area is called a *patch*.

A *papule* is a lesion raised sufficiently above the surface to be palpated and which measures approximately up to a centimeter in diameter. More extensive lesions are often called *plaques*.

A *vesicle* is a lesion of the epithelium less than 1 cm in diameter and filled with clear fluid—in lay terms, a blister. A larger lesion is called a *bulla* and may be several centimeters across.

An *ulcer* is an area of destruction of epithelium together with some of the underlying connective tissue.

An *erosion* is a lesion in which there is destruction of the epithelium only, exposing the underlying connective tissue. It is obviously difficult to distinguish between shallow ulcers and erosions. When these lesions are produced by scratching, they are often termed *excoriations*.

Squamous is the term given to the appearance of lesions that have adherent flakes of keratin, i.e., scaling.

There are many more clinical dermatologic terms, but one needs considerable experience to confidently identify the lesions. There is little purpose, therefore, in describing them further here.

In addition to the appearance of individual lesions, their *distribution* is often equally important in the diagnosis; both must always be considered. In smallpox, for example, the vesicles were characteristically peripheral in distribution, affecting the hands, feet, and face. In contrast, the vesicular lesions of chickenpox tend to be more central in distribution and affect the trunk more than the extremities.

In some cases skin lesions are highly localized, indicating a local cause. Thus dermatitis of the hands is commonly caused by contact with allergenic material. Other lesions can be even more localized and exactly reproduce the shape of a local cause, such as nickel dermatitis caused by a watchband. The local dermal environment, particularly the warm moist conditions in skin folds, may also favor infection. An inflammatory condition involving skinfolds is known as *intertrigo*.

The following terms are employed in histologic descriptions both in dermatology and stomatology.

Acanthosis is hyperplasia of the prickle cell layer. The thickening of this layer can be regular or irregular.

Hyperkeratosis is usually used as an abbreviation for hyperorthokeratosis, that is, a thickening of the cellular layer of mature keratin. When this happens, the underlying granular cell layer, where prekeratin is formed, becomes more prominent.

Parakeratosis is the overproduction of immature keratin so that nuclear remnants are present in the superficial cells. Granular cells are not present beneath parakeratotic hyperplasia. There is more rapid epithelial proliferation and failure of maturation.

Dysplasia, dyskeratosis, and *atypia* are terms for varying degrees of disorganization of epithelial maturation, as described in Chapter 9.

Spongiosis is the term given to the collection of fluid among the epithelial cells, which as a consequence become partially separated.

Vesiculation is a process in which there is a localized collection of fluid that may be either within the epithelium itself (intraepithelial vesiculation) or, alternatively, between the epithelium and the underlying connective tissue (subepithelial vesiculation).

The number of skin diseases is vast, and it is impossible to classify them completely.

If classified according to the clinical appearance, then diseases as diverse as psoriasis and intraepithelial carcinoma have to be grouped together. Moreover, many dermal diseases have a variety of clinical manifestations and therefore must be considered under several headings. Classification on the basis of etiology, on the other hand, is just as difficult because so many skin diseases are of unknown etiology. For better or worse, however, we have attempted to classify them by their etiology.

Heritable diseases of the skin and mucous membranes (genodermatoses)
Ectodermal dysplasia

Ectodermal dysplasia is a relatively common genodermatosis characterized by hypoplasia or agenesis of a wide variety of dermal appendages, including the teeth.

In typical cases the hair is fine and scanty, especially in the tonsural region. Sweat and sebaceous glands may be few or absent. When sweat glands are absent, heat control is defective and the disease is called *anhidrotic ectodermal dysplasia*. The nails may also be defective and the skin somewhat fragile. Either, or in extreme cases both, deciduous and permanent teeth may fail to form (anodontia). Failure of formation of the dentition leads to underdevelopment of the jaws. Teeth are more often reduced in number.

The facies is sometimes characterized by frontal bossing, a depressed nasal bridge, and, if the teeth are absent, a prematurely senile (nutcracker) profile (Fig. 19-1).

Epidermolysis bullosa

Epidermolysis bullosa is an uncommon bullous disease that shows different patterns of inheritance. The severity of the disease can vary greatly.

The severe form appears soon after birth. Milder forms do not become manifest until adolescence or later.

Vesicles, either subepidermal or intraepidermal, form in response to insignificant trauma and lead to disabling scarring. One characteristic effect is to transform the hands into fingerless stumps in severe cases (Fig. 19-2).

Dyskeratosis congenita

Dyskeratosis congenita is a rare disorder characterized by (1) dystrophy of the nails, (2) early loss of hair, (3) pigmentation of the skin, and (4) whitish areas of thickening of oral

and occasionally the anal mucosa (see Fig. 3-16) and (5) aplastic anemia in some cases.

The oral lesions may be inconspicuous but histologically show striking epithelial dysplasia. The risk of malignant change is high.

Ehlers-Danlos syndrome

Ehlers-Danlos syndrome is caused by defective cross-linking of the collagen molecule. There are now eight subtypes with different patterns of inheritance.

Clinically important features are hyperflexibility of joints, laxity of the skin (Fig. 19-3), and purpura (bruising). Typically the skin is thin and can be grossly stretched but returns to normal when released. Purpura is the result of excessive fragility of the connective tissue, but platelet defects are sometimes associated.

The severity of the different manifestations varies considerably among the subtypes (see Chapter 17).

Other effects sometimes include prolapse of the mitral valve (floppy mitral valve syndrome) and gaping of wounds. In later life weakness of the ligaments leads to arthritis. Mild forms of this syndrome appear to be common but are frequently unrecognized as such.

Neurofibromatosis

Neurofibromatosis is one of the phakomatoses (also termed neurodermatoses), which are genetically determined hamar-

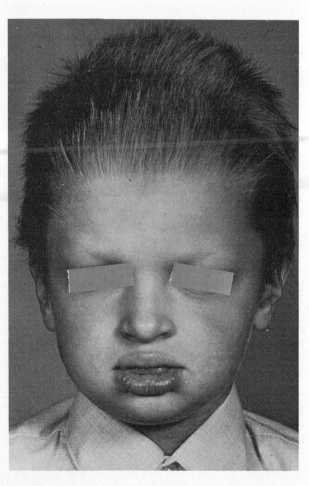

FIG. 19-1. Ectodermal dysplasia. The hair is fine, but in this boy only the eyebrow hair is absent. The pouting expression is the result of failure of formation of the teeth.

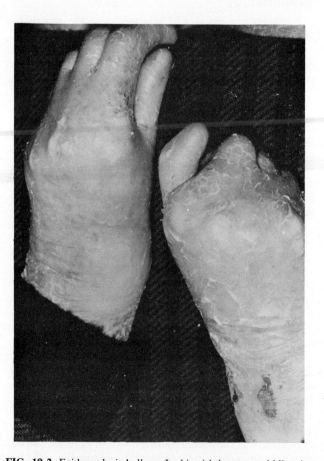

FIG. 19-2. Epidermolysis bullosa. In this girl the repeated blistering has left the skin of the hands and wrists covered by a tissue paper-like epithelium from which all the dermal appendages and the nails have been lost. Scarring has caused flexure contraction of the fingers, and the hands are being gradually reduced to functionless stumps.

tomatous (tumorlike) lesions of the skin (Fig. 19-4) and nervous system. Other members of this group are tuberous sclerosis, encephalofacial angiomatosis (Sturge-Weber syndrome*) and cerebroretinal angiomatosis (von Hippel-Lindau syndrome†). Neurofibromatosis is one of the most common autosomal dominant disorders, although over 50% of cases are the result of new mutations. The prevalence of the disease may approach 1 in 3,000 of the population, but many cases may be so mild as to inconspicuous.

Two forms of neurofibromatosis are recognized. The peripheral type (NF I) accounts for over 90% of cases and was described by von Recklinghausen‡ in 1882; the central type (NF II), which is characterized by bilateral acoustic neuromas (Chapter 20), accounts for the remainder. In addition, neurofibromatosis may be associated with pheochromocytoma in the multiple endocrine adenoma syndrome (Chapter 18) in which there are may be mucosal plexiform neuromas.

Peripheral and central neurofibromatosis appear to be genetically as well as phenotypically distinct. There is a loss of genes on chromosome 22 in bilateral acoustic neuromas, but this is not the case with cutaneous neurofibromatosis where the defective gene has not been identified. The essential features of the two different types of neurofibromatosis are often confused in all but the most recent publications.

---

*W.A. Sturge (1850-1919) and F. Parkes Weber (1863-1962), British physicians.
†E. von Hippel (1867-1939), German ophthalmologist; A. Lindau (b. 1892), Swedish pathologist.
‡F.D. von Recklinghausen (1833-1910), German pathologist.

The characteristic features of peripheral neurofibromatosis are multiple coffee-colored (café au lait) (macules which typically start to appear within the first year of life), cutaneous neurofibromas, and Lisch nodules. Lisch nodules are brownish, dome-shaped hamartomas of the iris; they are best seen by slit lamp examination, start to appear in early childhood, and in some series have been found in all affected adults (Chapter 18).

Clinically, the severity of the disease ranges from the inconspicuous to grossly disfiguring tumorous deformities or lethal complications. The skin tumors of neurofibromatosis start to develop at or near puberty, frequently cause itching while actively growing, and increase in number throughout life until in severe cases they form in hundreds or even thousands.

The café au lait spots resemble freckles but appear in sites shielded from sunlight, such as the axillae. In the absence of neurofibromas the diagnosis of the disease depends on finding multiple café au lait spots and Lisch nodules.

Microscopically, the cutaneous tumors of neurofibromatosis, particularly the grossly disfiguring masses in severe cases are plexiform neuromas. They consist of poorly organized mixtures of nerve fibrils usually unmyelinated and tangled, together with diffuse proliferation of spindle cells of neural origin, myxoid areas and, often, fat. Mast cells as in many other fibroproliferative disorders, are conspicuous and appear to contribute to the overgrowth of neural fibrous tissue. Preliminary reports

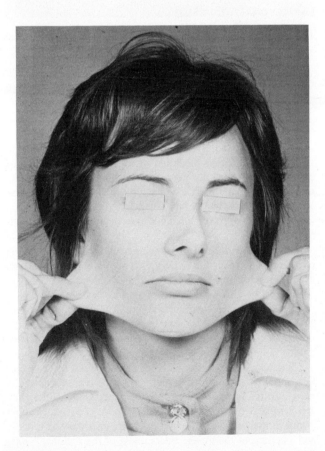

FIG. 19-3. Ehlers-Danlos syndrome. In this type of collagen defect there is hyperextensibility of the skin and joints. A brother of this patient was similarly affected.

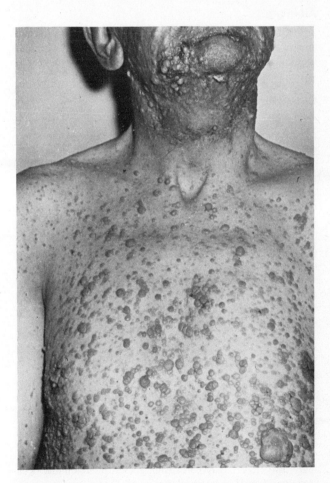

FIG. 19-4. Neurofibromatosis. In this disease, inherited as an autosomal dominant, skin tumors may sometimes be even larger or more numerous than in this case. Brownish (café-au-lait) pigmentation is typical, and intracranial glial cerebral tumors and a variety of other disorders may be associated (see Chapter 20).

have suggested that some patients with neurofibromatosis may show at least partial regression of the lesions as a result of long-term treatment with a mast cell membrane stabilizer (ketotifen).

In addition to plexiform neurofibromas, neurilemomas may also be present. Skeletal tissue can also be involved with resulting bone destruction and formation of tumorlike masses containing many giant cells.

The café au lait spots show melanin hyperpigmentation of both keratinocytes and melanocytes together with scattered abnormally large melanin granules (giant melanosomes) in most cases.

Serious complications include disfigurement, mental handicap, or other neurological complications such as epilepsy or spinal neurofibromas, skeletal abnormalities, malignant change in the neurofibromas and other sarcomas, and tumors of the central nervous system, in particular, gliomas of the optic nerves or chiasma. Acoustic neuromas, contrary to early descriptions, are rarely associated.

The "Elephant Man," made famous in a successful film, has long been regarded as a particularly severe case of neurofibromatosis. However, it now appears that he was an example of the much more rare *Proteus syndrome*, the many manifestations of which include assymetry of the limbs, partial gigantism of the hands and feet, plantar hyperplasia, macrocephaly and cranial hyperostoses, and overgrowth of long bones.

Albinism

In this genetic disease, there is failure of production of melanin and consequent lack of skin pigmentation. This renders the skin vulnerable to actinic damage and photodermatitis (see also Chapter 3).

Cutaneous angiomatosis

Vascular nevi of the skin may be isolated abnormalities or part of a syndrome such as the Sturge-Weber syndrome of angiomatosis within the distribution of the trigeminal nerve and of the leptomeninges of the same side, epilepsy or hemiparesis and, usually, mental defect.

These nevi are developmental anomalies and usually consist of grossly dilated vessels. There may be a genetic component in their etiology (as suggested by several syndromes of which they are a feature) and similar lesions can be induced by the drug thalidomide given during pregnancy and by the fetal alcohol syndrome.

Isolated nevi are rarely of clinical significance unless they are visible and disfiguring. Ugly angiomas of the face can be treated by means of skin grafting, liquid nitrogen cryotherapy, or laser-induced fibrosis.

Viral infections
Herpes simplex

Herpes is caused by the herpes simplex virus (HSV) and the usual manifestation of primary infection by the type I virus is an acute vesiculating stomatitis. HSV type II typically causes genital herpes (Chapter 23), which in the Western world is now considerably more common than herpetic stomatitis; increasingly also HSV I may be causing genital infection and occasionally, HSV II causes oral disease.

Herpetic stomatitis is relatively frequently seen as a consequence of the immune deficiency of AIDS and can be, but is not necessarily severe in these patients.

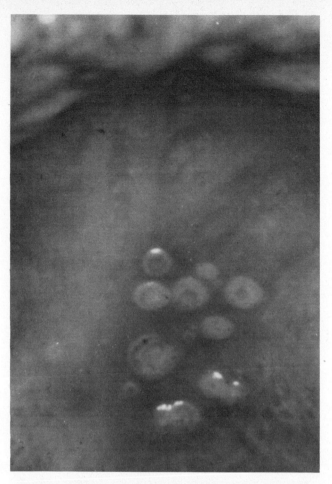

FIG. 19-5. Primary herpetic stomatitis. The sharply defined small vesicles on the palate are typical.

Pathology. The earliest detectable microscopic sign is the formation of vesicles, in the floor of which are epithelial cells showing the typical effects of viral damage. The roof of the vesicle is several cells thick and intact vesicles are often seen clinically. Infection, however, spreads through the full thickness of the epithelium. The damaged cells containing live virus, are shed to leave ulcers with sharply defined margins and a mixed inflammatory cellular infiltrate in the underlying connective tissue.

Herpetic stomatitis. This is the most common manifestation of primary infection due to HSV I. It is mildly contagious and usually develops in infancy or childhood. Many infections are subclinical or dismissed as "teething."

In poor urban communities, herpesvirus is usually disseminated among young children. In more affluent societies, the infection may not be acquired until much later. Herpetic stomatitis is now common in adults.

Clinically, herpetic stomatitis is characterized by vesiculation and ulceration affecting any part of the oral mucosa. The vesicles often form on the vault of the palate (Fig. 19-5). They are sharply defined, circular, dome shaped, and usually about 3 mm in diameter. The tongue is furred, and there is redness and swelling of the gums, enlargement of the regional lymph nodes, and fever.

Diagnosis can be made microscopically by identifying the

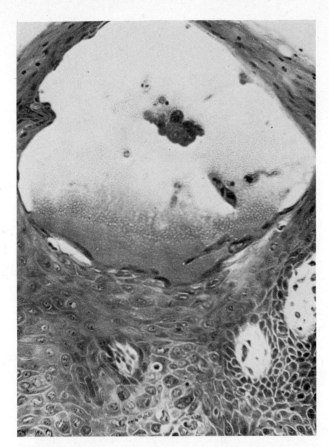

FIG. 19-6. Herpetic stomatitis. A typical vesicle, as seen here, shows the thick roof, a cluster of viral-damaged cells floating in the vesicle fluid, and nuclear changes in infected epithelial cells in the base.

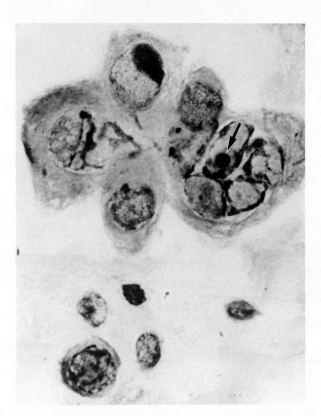

FIG. 19-7. Herpetic stomatitis. A smear of epithelial cells from a vesicle shows the distended nuclei with the chromatin pushed to the margins (ballooning degeneration). Several nuclei have divided, producing a giant cell. An inclusion body is shown *(arrow)*.

cellular abnormalities (ballooning degeneration and inclusion bodies) in smears from the lesion (Figs. 19-6 and 19-7). Although it is rarely necessary, the diagnosis can be confirmed by a rising titer of antibodies to HSV I.

After the primary infection, the virus can apparently persist in latent form in the trigeminal ganglia.

About 30% of patients who have herpetic stomatitis are susceptible to recurrences, known as *herpes labialis,* characterized by similar vesiculating lesions at the mucocutaneous junction of the lips.

Herpes labialis. Herpes labialis is precipitated by factors such as a febrile illness (hence, "fever blister"), exposure to sea air and sunshine, or menstrual disturbances (Fig. 19-8). These factors may reduce resistance, allowing reactivation of the virus.

The vesicles of herpes labialis weep exudate, rupture, and are followed by scabbing or may become secondarily infected. These lesions are also infective.

The current treatment of choice of herpetic infections is with acyclovir, which is highly effective against the Herpes simplex virus, but needs to be given early, preferably in the prodromal phase as viral destruction of the tissues is rapid.

Herpetic whitlow. Herpetic whitlow, an infection adjacent to the nail bed, causes vesiculation, painful inflammation, and ulceration that scabs over. It is an occupational hazard to health care workers particularly nurses and occasionally dentists, who acquire the infection by contact with a patient's herpetic infection.

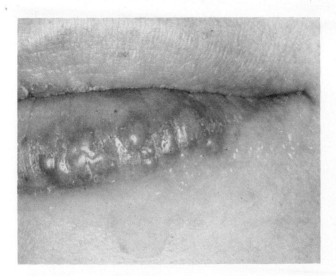

FIG. 19-8. Herpes labialis. The typical feature of this early lesion is the cluster of vesicles along the mucocutaneous border of the lower lip.

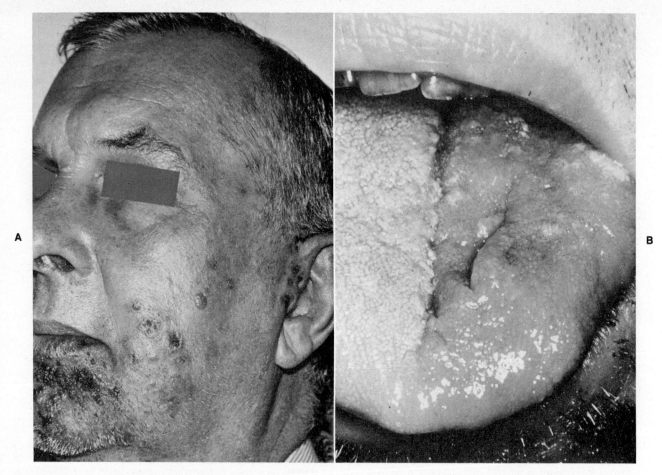

FIG. 19-9. A, Herpes zoster of the trigeminal area. The characteristic distribution along the dermatomes of the second and third divisions is seen. Some of the lesions are still in the vesicular stage; others are crusting over. **B,** Involvement of half the tongue in the same patient.

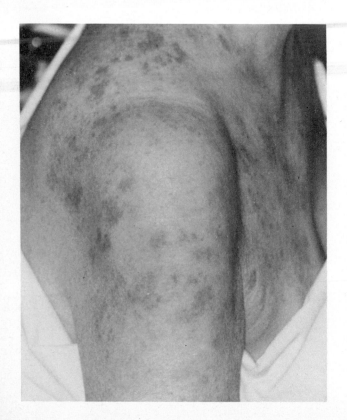

Herpes genitalis is a common sexually transmitted infection (Chapter 23), usually due to type 2 virus. It is clinically, (apart from the site) and pathologically, very similar to herpetic stomatitis.

Herpes zoster (shingles)

Herpes zoster is caused by varicella-zoster virus (VZV), which causes chickenpox in children, and zoster, usually after middle age. However, children or even infants can occasionally also develop zoster.

Zoster resembles herpes labialis in that it is the result of reactivation of a latent viral infection. VZV remains latent in sensory ganglia, and when reactivated results in a vesicular, inflammatory reaction in the area of skin supplied by the affected nerve. In descending order of frequency, thoracic, cervicofacial (Figs. 19-9 and 19-10), and lumbosacral nerves are involved.

In normal individuals, the precipitating factors are not known, although the frequency of the disease increases with advancing years. Zoster however, as mentioned earlier, can be

FIG. 19-10. Herpes zoster involving the upper cervical dermatome in a patient receiving corticosteroids. *(From McCracken AW and Cawson RA: Clinical and oral microbiology, Washington DC, 1982, Hemisphere Publishing Corp.)*

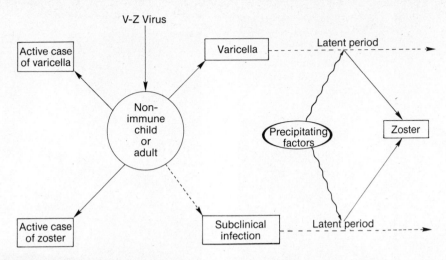

FIG. 19-11. Diagram of the pathogenesis of varicella-zoster. Zoster is the result of reactivation of previously acquired clinically apparent (chickenpox) or inapparent infection. *(From McCracken AW and Cawson RA: Clinical and oral microbiology, Washington DC, 1982, Hemisphere Publishing Corp.)*

a manifestation of immunodeficiency as in lymphoreticular malignancies, AIDS, or as a result of immunosuppression. In normal individuals and in patients who have underlying disease, zoster can be a generalized eruption.

The pathologic features of the cutaneous lesions in zoster are essentially the same as those described for herpes labialis; the pathogenesis is summarized in Fig. 19-11.

Clinically, particularly in older patients, pain can be the most prominent symptom, often persisting for long periods after the skin lesions have resolved. Severe cases and those, such as transplant and other immunodeficient patients, in whom the disease can be life threatening, should be treated with acyclovir. This drug has also been given prophylactically, to these high-risk patients, and as a consequence has significantly reduced the morbidity and mortality rates from zoster.

Chickenpox

The vesicular rash affects both skin and mucous membranes, as described in Chapter 8.

Hand-foot-and-mouth disease

This disease must be distinguished from foot and mouth (hoof and mouth) disease of cattle, which rarely affects humans.

Hand-foot-and-mouth disease is caused by a coxsackie-virus, usually types A10 or A16. It is exceedingly common and is highly contagious. Characteristically, it causes outbreaks in schools. It causes a mild illness characterized by a vesicular rash, particularly on the extremities (Fig. 19-12) and typically a vesicular stomatitis (Fig. 19-13). Both are mild, and patients may be unaware of the lesions.

The vesicles are intraepidermal with ballooning degeneration of the deeper cells followed by intercellular accumulation of fluid, which separates the cells and apparently causes the epithelium to disintegrate, forming an erosion.

The disease is self-limiting.

Viral warts

Warts (verrucae) are papilloma-like lesions of the skin or occasionally mucosal surfaces. They are discussed later.

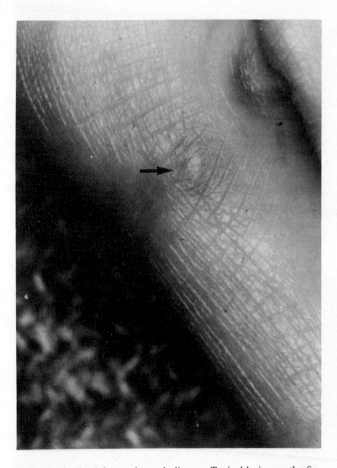

FIG. 19-12. Hand-foot-and-mouth disease. Typical lesion on the finger. Similar lesions may be present on the feet and the skin on other areas of the body. *(From McCracken AW and Cawson RA: Clinical and oral microbiology, Washington DC, 1982, Hemisphere Publishing Corp.)*

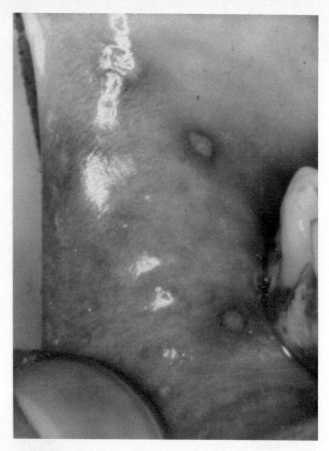

FIG. 19-13. Hand-foot-and-mouth disease. Recently ruptured intraoral vesicles. By contrast with herpetic stomatitis, lesions are typically few in number. *(From McCracken AW and Cawson RA: Clinical and oral microbiology, Washington DC, 1982, Hemisphere Publishing Corp.)*

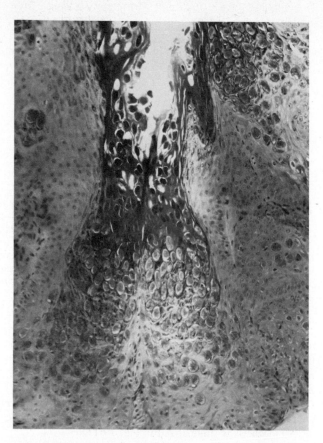

FIG. 19-14. Molluscum contagiosum. The lesion is umbilicated due to the dipping inward of the proliferating epithelium. The more superficial cells are distended by eosinophilic intracytoplasmic inclusion bodies, which extend up to the surface where they are shed.

Molluscum contagiosum

Molluscum contagiosum is another benign tumorlike lesion of the skin caused by a virus that is readily spread.

The virus causes proliferation of squamous cells. The rete ridges of the epidermis grow downward into the corium and compress the papillae into thin septa.

A goblet-shaped epithelial mass develops. A small tumor is thus formed with a central opening leading into a cavity, which mainly contains desquamated keratin and the molluscum bodies (Fig. 19-14). These are inclusion bodies that contain enormous numbers of the virus and appear microscopically as eosinophilic hyaline material that distends the epithelial cells.

Mollusca form minute painless nodules. These slowly increase in size to reach 1 cm or more in diameter. They are pale with a pearly white center, which can be expressed. They are highly infective, and the virus can be transmitted on garments, towels, or fingers.

Bacterial dermatoses
Erysipelas

Erysipelas is an acute infection of the skin and subcutaneous tissues due to a virulent beta-hemolytic *Streptococcus pyogenes*. The disease is characterized by fever, rapidly spreading redness, and swelling of the skin. In the past this infection had

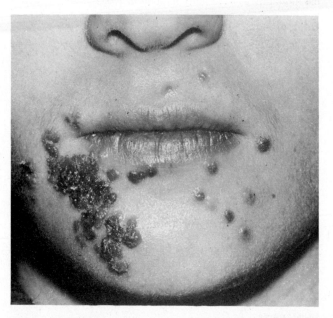

FIG. 19-15. Impetigo caused by *Staphylococcus aureus*. Note the characteristic "stuck on," crusted appearance of the lesions. *(From McCracken AW and Cawson RA: Clinical and oral microbiology, Washington DC, 1982, Hemisphere Publishing Corp.)*

an enormously high mortality. It is now rare, except in a few debilitated patients, and responds well to penicillin therapy.

Impetigo

The common type of impetigo is usually caused by *Staphylococcus aureus* or *Streptococcus pyogenes*. Impetigo is a disease of childhood and adolescence transmitted by contact and characterized by the formation initially of vesicles that develop into pustules in the superficial layers of the epidermis. The face is commonly affected (Fig. 19-15).

The disease responds to local and systemic antibiotics.

Furunculosis

A furuncle, or boil, is an infection of a hair (pilosebaceous) follicle by *Staphylococcus aureus*, which can be part of the patient's normal skin flora. Presumably, local resistance is unable to prevent inflammation. Diabetics are particularly susceptible. A local predisposing factor is pressure. Thus boils are prone to develop in the collar area.

A boil is a typical abscess with a central core of necrotic tissue surrounded by pus and by a wall of granulation tissue. Healing of the boil is characterized by discharge of pus on the surface, extrusion of the central core, and healing from the base by proliferation of granulation tissue.

A carbuncle is formed by the simultaneous infection of adjacent follicles and is characterized by suppurative inflammation and extensive necrosis of subcutaneous tissue.

Mycobacterial infections

Lupus vulgaris, the classic tuberculous disease of the skin, was rare even before the introduction of antituberculous drugs.

Currently the nontuberculous mycobacteria are more important. *M. scrofulaceum* and particularly *M. marinum* are occasional causes of chronic skin nodules that eventually ulcerate. The fingers, hands, and sometimes the feet are mainly affected. *M. marinum* infection is a hazard, particularly to those who dip their fingers in tropical fish tanks. The disease is also known as swimming pool granuloma.

Treatment is with antituberculous drugs.

Syphilis

Syphilis is discussed in more detail in Chapter 23. Dermal or mucosal lesions can be a feature of any of the stages.

Actinomycosis

Actinomycosis is caused by a filamentous bacterium. *Actinomyces israelii*, which lives as a commensal in the mouth but occasionally can give rise to infection. The organism appears to track through the subcutaneous tissues from the mouth and causes lesions in the soft tissue of the region of the angle of the jaw and the adjacent neck (Fig. 19-16). These lesions are characterized by a central mass of organisms that form a radiating pattern around which is a widespread and dense inflammatory infiltrate (Fig. 19-17) and peripherally a fibrous wall. The reaction is, however, unable to contain the infection, which progresses, forms chronic sinuses, and spreads further to form more lesions, until the skin and subcutaneous tissues are permeated by abscesses, sinuses, and fibrous tissue. The pus con-

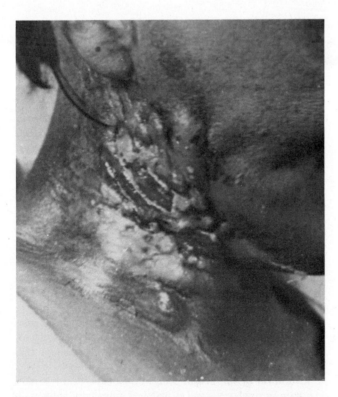

FIG. 19-16. Cervicofacial actinomycosis. This advanced case shows the typical puckering of the skin as a result of fibrosis around discharging foci of infection. *(Courtesy Curator of the Gordon Museum, Guy's Hospital, London, England.)*

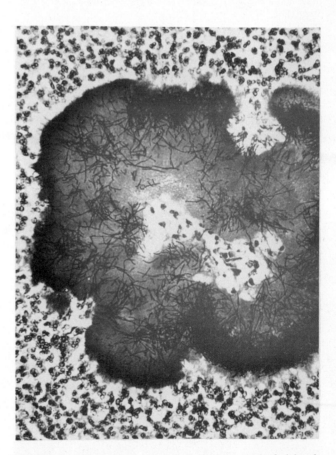

FIG. 19-17. Gram stain of "sulfur granule" from cervicofacial actinomycosis showing typical radiating gram positive branching filaments, surrounded by polymorphonuclear leukocytes. *(From McCracken AW and Cawson RA: Clinical and oral microbiology, Washington DC, 1982, Hemisphere Publishing Corp.)*

tains yellowish or yellow-gray granules, sometimes called sulfur granules. These are aggregations of the organism and are best seen if the pus is first washed with saline. Culture results and diagnosis are unlikely to be positive unless sulfur granules are obtained.

Actinomycosis responds to penicillin and other antibiotics, but surgery may also be needed.

Acne vulgaris

Acne, a common disease of adolescence, is a disorder of the pilosebaceous follicles with the formation of comedones (blackheads) and secondary inflammatory changes. It is not simply a bacterial disease, although bacteria play an important part in the pathogenesis.

Pathogenesis and pathology. Acne (Fig. 19-18) develops as a result of the following sequence of events:

1. Sebum secretion is increased as a result of raised circulatory androgen levels or hyperresponsiveness of the sebaceous glands to androgens.
2. Abnormal accumulation of keratin obstructs the pilosebaceous ducts.
3. The metabolism of the bacteria (particularly *Propionibacterium acnes*) in the follicles changes.
4. Mediators of inflammation are released.

The accumulation of sebum and epithelial debris in the follicles produces blackheads. Obstruction to discharge of the sebaceous glands often causes them to rupture and discharge their contents into the skin. This causes an inflammatory re-

action to the sebaceous fatty acids. This may progress to suppuration and necrosis of the gland. Discharge of pus is followed by healing and scarring.

Clinical aspects. Males are predominantly affected, and the disease usually subsides before the patient reaches the age of 30. By this time the lesions have sometimes caused considerable scarring and disfigurement.

The face, chest, and back are the main sites affected, and in the active stage of the disease these areas are studded with blackheads and in more severe cases erythematous nodules and pustules.

Antibiotics, particularly tetracycline, erythromycin, and clindamycin, either orally or topically, are effective in the vast majority of cases.

Lyme disease: erythema chronicum migrans

The rash of Lyme disease is characteristic and consists of enlarging red rings, which may be preceded by an itchy papule caused by the insect bite. The erythematous rim may be faint but slightly indurated and may encircle a limb. Lyme disease incidentally, gives rise, in Europe to somewhat different skin lesions from those seen in North America. Arthritis and cardiac complications are also less frequent in Europe.

Microscopically, erythema chronicum migrans is chiefly characterized by diffuse infiltration of the dermis by a mixture of lymphocytes, histiocytes and eosinophils at the site of the insect bite and mouth parts of the latter may also be present. Warthin-Starry stains may be positive for *Borrelia burgdorferi*. The erythematous rim is characterized only by a perivascular lymphocytic infiltrate. Since such appearances are not in themselves specific, diagnosis depends on the clinical features and serological confirmation of formation of antibodies to *B. burgdorferi*. (See also Chapter 17.)

Fungal infections

Fungal infections can be divided into (1) the superficial infections of the skin, hair, or nails by the *dermatophyte* group of fungi and (2) the deep mycoses. Dermatophyte infections are confined to the skin, and dermatophytes are divided into three genera—*Microsporum*, *Trichophyton*, and *Epidermophyton* (Table 19-1). The important fungus *Candida albicans* can produce both mucocutaneous lesions and also systematized infections. In contrast to the dermatophytes, *Candida albicans* predominantly affects mucosal surfaces, particularly that of the mouth; the skin is involved to a much lesser degree.

Ringworm (tinea)

Ringworm is a superficial infection by one of the dermatophytes involving the keratin of the skin, hair, or nails. Infection can be transmitted directly from person to person or can be acquired from domestic or farm animals or from inanimate objects.

Ringworm of the scalp (tinea capitis). Ringworm of the scalp is mainly a disease of childhood and causes rounded areas of scaling and hair destruction (Fig. 19-19). The entire hair-bearing area may occasionally be affected, and total baldness sometimes results.

Ringworm of the beard. Ringworm of the beard is most common in rural areas and is acquired from farm animals. It can also be transmitted by barber's implements (barber's itch).

There is suppurative inflammation, and pustules develop, at the apex of which a broken-off hair projects through a bead of pus.

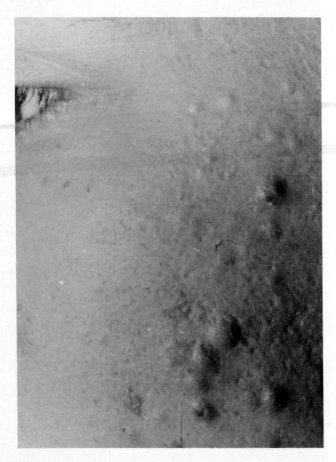

FIG. 19-18. Acne. Typical facial lesions in an adolescent. *(From McCracken AW and Cawson RA: Clinical and oral microbiology, Washington DC, 1982, Hemisphere Publishing Corp.)*

Ringworm of the feet. This type of ringworm, often known as athlete's foot, is easily acquired from moist bathmats, floorboards, or towels. The most common type is *intertriginous,* affecting the skinfold between the toes.

There is some doubt as to whether tinea alone causes athlete's foot. Fungi often cannot be isolated, and in many cases bacterial infection is present.

The affected skin becomes sodden and white and leaves a raw area when rubbed off. Vesicular and hyperkeratotic types are also described.

Candidosis

Candidosis (candidiasis) is caused by the yeastlike fungus *Candida albicans,* which produces filaments (hyphae or mycelium). The frequently used term *moniliasis* as a synonym is incorrect and obsolete because in current classification the *Moniliaceae* family are the dermatophyte genera discussed earlier.

Candida albicans causes a variety of diseases. The main forms of candidosis are (1) mucosal (and mucocutaneous), (2) cutaneous, and (3) systemic. These three variants remain distinct. Systemic candidosis only develops in special circumstances, such as a complication of open heart surgery, and will not be discussed here.

Thrush (acute candidosis). Oral thrush, a disease recognized even in early antiquity, is the most common and best known manifestation, particularly in the newborn. It is also common in immunodeficient patients (such as those receiving organ transplants) and is so common a feature of AIDS or its prodromes that HIV infection should be suspected when an adult male develops thrush for no apparent cause.

Plaques of thrush are produced by fungal hyphae invading the epithelium (Fig. 19-20), which shows a proliferative response. The plaque is widely infiltrated by inflammatory cells and exudate, which give it its soft and friable character. An inflammatory reaction is also present in the underlying dermis.

TABLE 19-1. Dermatophytes causing ringworm and related diseases*

Tinea capitis	Tinea corporis	Tinea barbae	Tinea cruris	Tinea unguium	Tinea pedis
M. canis	T. mentagrophytes	T. mentagrophytes	T. mentagrophytes	T. mentagrophytes	T. mentagrophytes
M. audouinii	M. canis	T. rubrum	T. rubrum	T. rubrum	T. rubrum
T. tonsurans			E. floccosum	E. floccosum	E. floccosum

*T., Trichophyton; M., Microsporum; E., Epidermophyton.

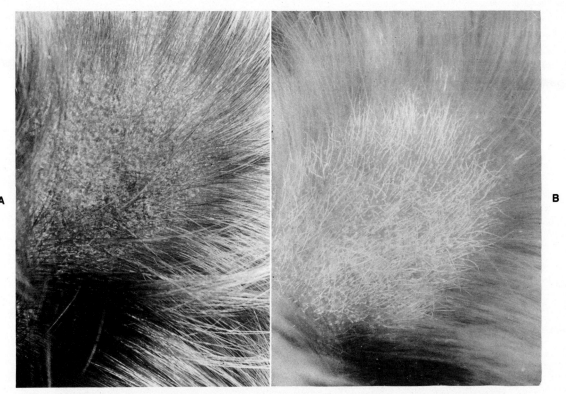

FIG. 19-19. Tinea capitis (scalp ringworm). **A,** The lesion is circular and shows loss of hair caused by destruction of hair follicles. **B,** Brilliant green fluorescence under Wood's (ultraviolet) light shows the fungus to be either *M. canis* or *M. audouinii,* both of which are common causes of tinea capitis. Few other dermatophyte infections of hairy skin fluoresce in this way. (*Courtesy Curator of the Gordon Museum, Guy's Hospital, London, England.*)

Clinically, thrush is characterized by cream-colored flecks or confluent plaques on the mucosa that can be wiped off, leaving a red area of mucosa beneath (Fig. 19-21).

Diagnosis is confirmed by microscopic examination of a smear that shows great numbers of tangled candidal hyphae.

Vulvovaginal thrush is also common. The lesions have the same appearance and pathology as those in the mouth. Unlike oral thrush, however, vaginal thrush typically affects otherwise healthy women and is frequently sexually transmitted.

Angular stomatitis (cheilitis). Macerated cracks at the angles of the mouth are a common feature of oral candidosis and are associated with any form of this infection. Angular stomatitis is frequently associated with candidal infection under dentures (denture stomatitis). The upper denture provides conditions that encourage the proliferation of the fungus and provide a reservoir of infection, which can spread outside the mouth.

Another cause of angular stomatitis is *Staphylococcus aureus*. Mixed candidal and straphylococcal infections can also develop.

Cutaneous candidosis. Candidosis can develop where the skin is kept abnormally moist. Favorable situations are skin folds (intertrigo) under the breasts or in the groin and under babies' diapers.

The skin is red and moist and tends to ooze serum; the lesion may have a raised margin.

Blastomycosis

North American blastomycosis is caused by *Blastomyces dermatitidis*. In spite of its name, this fungus primarily affects the lung but may also spread to involve the skin and bones.

Blastomycosis is most common in the southeastern United States and is caused by a rounded, thick-walled organism 5 to 15 μm in diameter. It reproduces by budding and can be found free in the tissues or within histiocytes.

In the skin the lesion begins as a small papule that gradually enlarges. The margins are raised, reddish violet, and studded with microabscesses. The center is depressed due to scarring. Histologically, microabscesses can be seen within the dermis

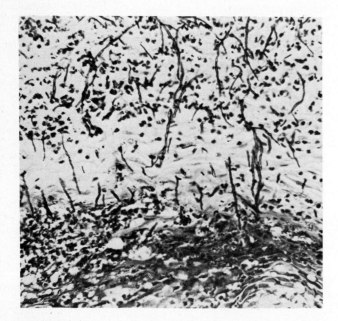

FIG. 19-20. Thrush (acute oral candidosis). Hyphae of *Candida albicans* are growing downward through the plaque and have been met by an acute inflammatory cellular exudate, which is most intense at the base of the plaque near the lower edge of the picture.

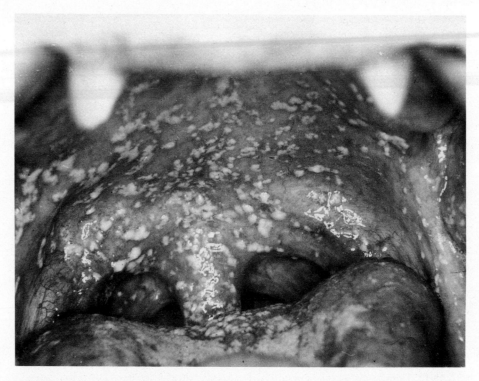

FIG. 19-21. Acute candidosis in a debilitated patient. Typical creamy plaques of thrush cover the whole palate and can readily be wiped off the underlying mucosa. *(From McCracken AW and Cawson RA: Clinical and oral microbiology, Washington DC, 1982, Hemisphere Publishing Corp.)*

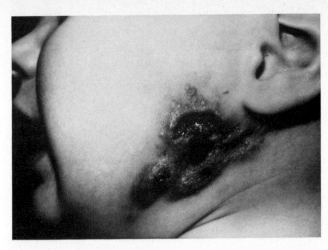

FIG. 19-22. Sporotrichosis. Cervicofacial lesions in a child. *(Courtesy David Whiting M.D.; From McCracken AW and Cawson RA: Clinical and oral microbiology, Washington DC, 1982, Hemisphere Publishing Corp.)*

surrounded by both acute and chronic inflammatory cells; small granulomatous lesions may also be seen.

The pulmonary infection may disseminate by the bloodstream. In addition to the skin and bones, any site including the central nervous system can be involved. Under these circumstances the infection is usually eventually fatal.

Sporotrichosis

Sporotrichosis is caused by *Sporotrichum schenckii*, a natural inhabitant of wood and plants. Infection is typically transmitted by a scratch from a thorn. Infection is followed by abscess formation with central necrosis and a surrounding granulomatous reaction (Fig. 19-22).

Clinically, dermal infection usually affects the arm and is characterized by formation of nodules followed by pustules and ulceration. Spread is typically along lymphatics (Fig. 19-23), forming a chain of nodules, until the regional lymph nodes are reached. These may remain persistently enlarged after the primary lesion has healed. The patient characteristically remains well, and dissemination of the infection is unlikely except in debilitated patients.

Pulmonary and systemic infections have also been described.

Diagnosis depends on identifying the spores. Treatment is by giving potassium iodide or, in severe cases, amphotericin.

Infestations
Scabies

Scabies, which was relatively uncommon in the last 30 years, has become epidemic worldwide.

Pathogenesis and pathology. Scabies is caused by a mite (*Sarcoptes scabei*) that causes disease by burrowing into the cornified layer of the epithelium to reach the stratum granulosum.

Within the burrow the female lays enormous numbers of eggs, which develop to adult form in a few days. After primary infestation, which is transmitted by close contact, there are no symptoms until several weeks later, when the patient becomes sensitized and there is itching and a rash. The common sites are on the hands and wrists.

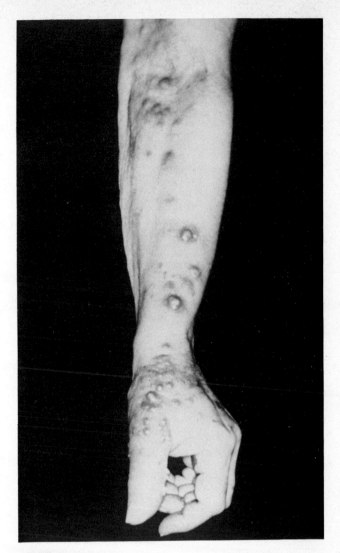

FIG. 19-23. Lymphocutaneous sporotrichosis. Lesions characteristically begin in the hand and progress up the arm via lymphatics. *(Courtesy William Sutker, M.D.; From McCracken AW and Cawson RA: Clinical and oral microbiology, Washington DC, 1982, Hemisphere Publishing Corp.)*

Clinical aspects. Formerly scabies was a disease of the dirty and neglected, but for unknown reasons it now affects all sections of the population.

The main symptom is itching, typically at night and especially of the hands. Lesions frequently become eczematous. The burrow, which is pathognomonic of the disease, consists of a short, sinuous, dirty looking line. More often the common lesion is a small excoriated papule.

The mite can be recognized microscopically in skin scrapings or in a biopsy specimen of skin.

Scabicides, such as crotamiton or sulfur, are moderately effective.

Mucocutaneous manifestations of immunodeficiency diseases

Mucocutaneous infections are common in immunodeficiency diseases such as AIDS. Some such as so-called hairy leuko-

TABLE 19-2. Mucocutaneous diseases associated with immunodeficiency or immunosuppression

Immunodeficiency	*Possible mucocutaneous diseases*
Primary	
DiGeorge's syndrome	Fungal and viral infections such as mucocutaneous candidosis
	Herpes simplex and zoster
Primary hypogammaglobulinaemia	Eczematoid skin infections
IgA deficiency	Eczema
	Lupus erythematosus
Wiskott-Aldrich syndrome	Eczema
	Purpura
	Infections
Ataxia telangiectasia	Telangiectasia
	Infections
C2 deficiency	Lupus erythematosus
Secondary	
Naturally acquired	
Diabetes mellitus	Staphylococcal and candidal infections particularly
Hodgkin's disease	Viral infections especially zoster
AIDS	See list below
Immunosuppressive treatment	Fungal and viral infections, especially zoster and candidosis
	Overgrowth of warts
	Severe dermatophytoses
	Skin lesions in systematized bacterial and mycotic infections particularly Pseudomonas and other gram-negative bacteria, and histoplasmosis
	Skin and lip cancer (in sunny climates)
	Kaposi's sarcoma, rarely
Graft-versus-host-disease	
Acute and subacute	Scarlatiniform rashes, lichen planus
Chronic	Pigmentation and fibrosis (resembling systemic sclerosis)
	Lichen planus

plakia (condyloma plana) (Chapter 14) are suspected of being of viral etiology.

Important mucocutaneous manifestations of immunodeficiency diseases are listed in Table 19-2.

Dermatologic features of HIV (AIDS and its prodromes)

Dermatologic diseases are often the presenting feature of AIDS; the main examples are Kaposi's sarcoma (Chapter 10) and opportunistic infections. The latter includes both nonspecific but florid variants of the common skin infections, such as tinea, as well as cutaneous manifestations of systemic infections such as histoplasmosis or other deep mycoses, which are otherwise rare.

Dermatologic and mucosal disease in AIDS or its prodromes are as follows:

1. Infections
   a. Herpes simplex
   b. Herpes zoster or varicella
   c. Molluscum contagiosum
   d. Tinea
   e. Infected seborrheic eczema
   f. Staphylococcal impetigo
   g. Chronic folliculitis
   h. Cutaneous lesions of deep mycoses (cryptococcosis, histoplasmosis, etc.)
   i. Oral thrush (candidosis)
   j. Oral hairy leukoplakia (?EBV)
2. Tumors
   a. Kaposi's sarcoma
3. Others
   a. Purpura
   b. Pigmentation (Addison's disease secondary to a deep mycosis)
   c. Major oral aphthae

Common cutaneous or mucocutaneous infections seen in AIDS or its prodromes include herpes simplex or zoster, molluscum contagiosum, staphylococcal impetigo, tinea infections, or seborrheic eczema. The last may be associated with pityrosporum infection and chronic folliculitis in which pityrosporum yeast forms can be seen microscopically in the hair follicles. However, Kaposi's sarcoma is the most common dermatologic feature of AIDS and is highly variable in its clinical appearances.

Other mucocutaneous manifestations of AIDS are as yet unclassifiable but cutaneous vasculitis and purpura are recognized complications. Oral lesions are common in AIDS, the most frequent being thrush (candidosis) and Kaposi's sarcoma. Other manifestations, are "hairy leukoplakia" (Chapter 14), which is associated with Epstein-Barr virus and appears to be specific to HIV infection, and major aphthae, which may prevent the patients from eating and accelerate their decline.

Mucocutaneous diseases that may be immunologically mediated

The term *eczema* may refer to an atopic disease particularly of infancy and characteristically associated with other atopic disorders such as asthma. Many other skin disorders, however, have similar appearances and may be termed eczematous dermatitis. Contact dermatitis has similar clinical appearances, but as the name implies is a reaction to many sensitizing materials, domestic or industrial, coming into direct contact with the skin.

Atopic (infantile) eczema

Atopic (infantile) eczema, like other atopic disease, is genetically determined and characterized by high IgE levels. However skin tests usually show an immediate (type I) reaction to many unrelated antigens and it is rarely possible to isolate a cause. Cell-mediated immunity appears often to be depressed and eczematous infants are susceptible to severe cutaneous viral infections by herpes simplex or zoster known as *Kaposi's varicelliform eruption*. Vaccination can cause a variant of this reaction termed *eczema vaccinatum*, which is potentially life threatening. Immunodeficiency diseases, particularly Wiskott-Aldrich syndrome (Chapter 7) are often also characterized by eczema but the most frequent association is congenital IgA deficiency.

Microscopically, there is spongiosis (intraepithelial edema), dilatation of blood vessels and perivascular, predominantly lymphocytic inflammatory infiltrates. The epithelial spongiosis may progress to microvesiculation and edema can also involve the underlying connective tissue. The epithelium becomes thickened (acanthosis) and parakeratotic.

Clinically, atopic dermatitis is characterized by intense pruritus (itching) and forms an erythematous area which becomes papulovesicular until its appearance is changed by scratching. The sites of predilection change with age; the cheeks are typically the first site affected but if it persists as it often does for 2 or 3 years, tends instead to involve the flexural surfaces of the limbs.

Like many other atopic diseases it is rarely possible to relieve eczema by finding and avoiding exposure to an allergen. Nevertheless, such a triggering agent should be sought, and occasionally the condition may resolve after exclusion of some item of diet. Otherwise, relief of itching with oral antihistamines or corticosteroid creams and prevention of superinfection are essential measures.

Contact dermatitis

Contact dermatitis is not mediated by IgE but is a type IV (cell-mediated) reaction. It shows pathologic features essentially similar to those of eczema, but, unlike the latter, the precipitating cause can be readily identified. If the cause is removed, the lesions resolve.

Substances that cause contact dermatitis may either be primary irritants or, alternatively, sensitizing agents. Primary irritants are substances such as acids, alkalis, or organic solvents that directly damage or irritate the skin when applied in high concentrations. Primary irritants can also act as sensitizing agents and can then cause reactions in much lower concentrations.

Sensitizing agents do not irritate normal skin but cause reactions in susceptible persons after continued exposure. Some of these sensitizing agents are allergens in their own right; enzymes used in some washing powders are examples. Others combine with epidermal protein in the skin to form a complete antigen. This antigen travels by lymphatic channels to the macrophage-monocyte system to stimulate an immune response. Thereafter, a reaction can develop whenever the substance comes into contact with the skin. Nevertheless, different parts of the body vary widely, both in their potential for developing contact dermatitis and in their response once contact dermatitis has developed. Sulfonamide ointments, for instance, are highly sensitizing when used on the skin but, by contrast, can be safely used in the eye.

Examples of industrial contact dermatitis include sensitivity to certain woods, mineral oils, photographic chemicals, and hairdressing chemicals. Domestic sensitizing agents include certain plants, cosmetics, washing powders, soap, and disinfectants. In medicine and dentistry causes of contact dermatitis include sulfonamides, antihistamine creams, streptomycin and related aminoglycoside antibiotics, procaine derivatives, and formalin.

Contact dermatitis develops first in exposed areas, particularly the fingers, but may spread across the back of the hands to the wrists and even the forearms. Other sites, particularly the eyelids, may be affected secondarily.

The reaction is eczematous and is characterized by redness, swelling, vesiculation, and oozing or scaling. Scratching often distorts the picture (see Fig. 7-4).

Diagnosis depends on identifying the sensitizing agent by means of a patch test. Avoidance of any further contact with the allergen is an effective preventive measure. If this is impossible, then the skin must be protected and a high standard of personal cleanliness maintained to remove the irritant before it can have an effect.

Urticaria

Urticaria (hives) is a common, intensely irritating rash characterized by wheal formation. The acute form can be an allergic (type I) reaction mediated by IgE, but there are many other possible causes of release of kinins and other vasoactive mediators which cause increased capillary permeability and wheal formation—i.e., urticaria is frequently not allergic in nature.

Triggering factors include exposure to cold or sunlight, insect bites, drugs and a variety of systemic diseases such as infections, the connective tissue disorders and lymphoreticular tumors.

Wheals are caused by increased capillary permeability, and by release into the skin and subcutaneous tissue of plasma which raises the skin surface. This reaction is mediated by histamine released by degranulation of sensitized mast cells coming into contact with IgE antibodies in many cases.

Causes include plant or jellyfish stings and drugs, particularly aspirin.

Angioedema (angioneurotic edema, giant urticaria)

Angioedema is characterized by massive escape of fluid into the tissues from blood vessels, causing large edematous swellings to develop suddenly. When the larynx is affected, the patient can be asphyxiated by edema of the glottis.

Angioedema in allergic subjects can be a reaction to sensitizing substances, which include foods such as eggs or vaccines prepared in egg cultures.

However, attacks may be without obvious cause. Antihistamines are moderately effective, but, when angioedema affects the glottis, intramuscular adrenalin must be given.

Hereditary angioedema

Hereditary angioedema is uncommon and is due to an inherited deficiency of C1 inactivator, which causes uncontrolled activation of the early stages of the complement system. There are recurrent attacks of angioedema often precipitated by trauma such as dental surgery. As with nonhereditary angioedema, laryngeal edema can be fatal. Diagnosis is made by finding abnormally low levels of C4. Treatment with plasminogen inhibitors, such as epsilon aminocaproic acid (EACA), is often beneficial, but danazol (an attenuated androgen) is at least as effective and has fewer side effects.

Drug eruptions

Skin reactions to drugs are common and include (1) urticaria, (2) toxic erythema and exfoliative dermatitis, often with exfoliative stomatitis, (3) eczematous, vesicular, and bullous reactions, (4) Stevens-Johnson syndrome, (5) lichen planus and lichenoid eruptions, (6) fixed eruptions, (7) purpura, (8) photodermatitis, and (9) lupus erythematosus.

Pemphigus vulgaris

Pemphigus vulgaris is an uncommon disease of skin and mucous membranes characterized by loss of attachment of the epithelial cells to one another and formation of vesicles and bullae. If untreated, the disease is fatal.

Histologically the epithelial cells just above the basal cell layer separate to form a cleft running roughly parallel to the lower border of the epithelium (Fig. 19-24). The epithelial cells become disconnected from their neighbors (acantholysis) and when thus released become compact and rounded. A vesicle forms, and the separated cells can be seen floating in the vesicle fluid. Rupture of vesicles causes widespread ulceration.

Pemphigus appears to be a well defined auto-immune disease in that there are antibodies both in the serum and localized to the interepithelial attachments, demonstrable by fluorescence microscopy (Fig. 19-25). Loss of epithelial intercellular ad-

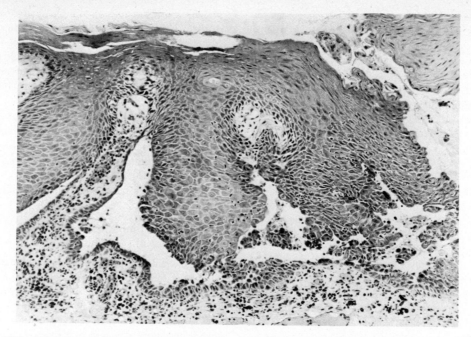

FIG. 19-24. Pemphigus vulgaris. An intraepithelial vesicle has formed following acantholysis (loss of cell contacts) between the suprabasal epidermal cells.

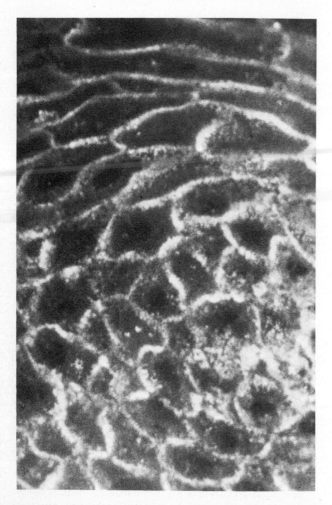

FIG. 19-25. Demonstration of IgG along the epidermal intercellular junctions in pemphigus vulgaris by immunofluorescence microscopy.

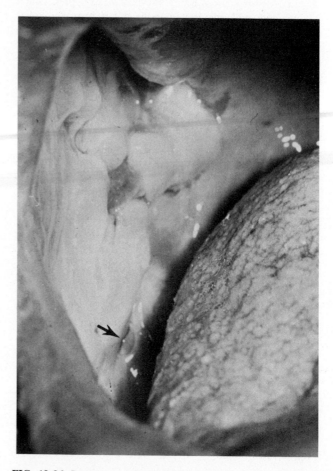

FIG. 19-26. Pemphigus vulgaris. The arrow points to the base of an intact vesicle; above, a ruptured vesicle has left an erosion in the center of the buccal mucosa. *(Courtesy Curator of the Gordon Museum, Guy's Hospital, London, England.)*

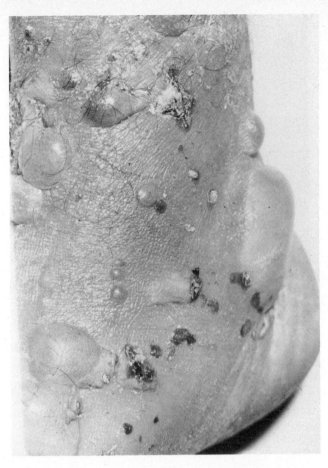

FIG. 19-27. Pemphigus vulgaris. There are many intact vesicles and crusted lesions left after their rupture on the skin. *(Courtesy Curator of the Gordon Museum, Guy's Hospital, London, England.)*

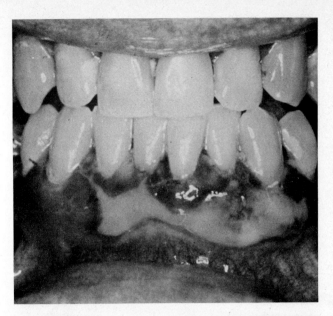

FIG. 19-28. Mucous membrane pemphigoid. The pale area in the gingivae is a typical collapsed bulla, which is surrounded by widespread inflammation. Shedding of the roof of the bulla will leave an extensive erosion.

herence appears to result from activation of proteases secondary to the antigen-antibody reaction.

Clinically, women are predominantly affected and the onset of the disease is frequently in early middle age.

Vesicles often first appear in the mouth (Fig. 19-26) but quickly rupture. Other mucous membranes such as the conjunctivae may be affected, but sooner or later vesiculation spreads to the trunk (Fig. 19-27) and limbs. If untreated, death results from widespread skin destruction with consequent loss of fluid, electrolyte disturbance, and often also, infection.

Immunosuppressive treatment, usually with corticosteroids and azathioprine, is life saving but the long-term complications of such treatment can be severe.

Mucous membrane pemphigoid (ocular or cicatricial pemphigoid)

Mucous membrane pemphigoid is an uncommon disease, usually affecting elderly persons, particularly women. Skin lesions are typically absent.

Microscopically and immunologically, this vesiculobullous disease is not distinguishable from bullous pemphigoid (discussed below). In essence it differs only in the distribution of the lesions. However bullous pemphigoid very occasionally also involves mucous membranes.

Clinically, there is bulla formation in the mouth (Fig. 19-28) or eyes or on other mucous membranes. The bullae rupture to leave erosions which in the eye in particular, heal by fibrosis

which can readily impair sight. Stenosis of the larynx or esophagus are less common consequences.

Microscopically, mucous membrane pemphigoid shows separation of the full thickness of the epithelium from the underlying connective tissue and later, increasingly dense, nonspecific inflammatory infiltration of the ulcerated surface. By immunofluorescence microscopy, immunoglobulin or more frequently the complement component C3 may be detectable along the epitheliomesenchymal junction at the level of the lamina lucida, but circulating autoantibodies are rarely a feature of this disease.

The disease is exceedingly indolent and may remain localized to the mouth, for instance, for several years before involving another site.

The response to topical corticosteroids is good, but systemic corticosteroids might have to be given to prevent ocular and other complications.

Bullous pemphigoid

Bullous pemphigoid is a disease mainly of the elderly and is characterized by the formation of large, tense subepithelial bullae on the skin. Deposition of immunoglobulins and complement components can be demonstrated along the basement membrane of the skin by immunofluorescence. A complement-fixing IgG antibody to skin basement membrane can be detected in the sera of about 70% of patients, but, in contrast with pemphigus vulgaris, the antibody titer is not related to the severity of the disease. The factors triggering these immunologic phenomena are unknown.

Bullae form as a result of detachment of the epithelium from the underlying connective tissue, possibly as a result of immunologically mediated damage to the basement membrane (Fig. 19-29). Superficial inflammatory changes are present, and eosinophils are prominent.

Bullous pemphigoid is a chronic disease particularly affecting flexor surfaces of the skin. The axillae, groins, and forearms are common sites.

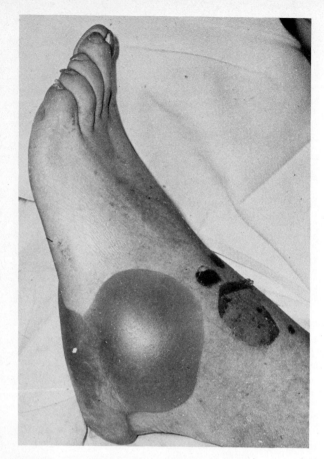

FIG. 19-29. Bullous pemphigoid. Very large tense bullae of the skin and absence of mucosal lesions are typical. *(Courtesy Curator of the Gordon Museum, Guy's Hospital, London, England.)*

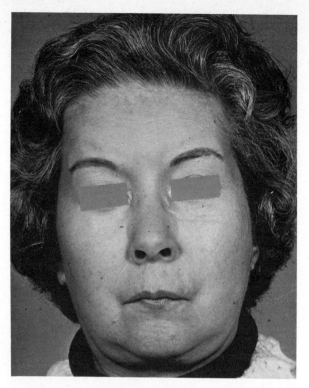

FIG. 19-30. Systemic sclerosis. The subepidermal fibrosis has smoothed out the skin surface, particularly around the eyes and mouth, where opening is limited as a result.

Oral lesions are rare, and clinically the disease is quite different from mucous membrane pemphigoid. Unlike the latter, bullous pemphigoid produces a significant mortality, especially in the elderly, if untreated. It responds well to immunosuppressive drugs.

A summary of the important vesiculobullous diseases of the skin is shown in Table 19-3.

Connective tissue diseases

The main examples of these disorders in which mucocutaneous lesions may be prominent are lupus erythematosus and systemic sclerosis (scleroderma). (See also Chapter 7.)

Discoid lupus erythematosus

Discoid lupus erythematosus has predominantly dermal manifestations and lacks the serologic abnormalities of SLE. The mucocutaneous lesions, however, are similar. Discoid lupus erythematosus is characterized by a rash that predominantly affects the face, neck, arms, scalp, and sometimes the oral mucous membrane. Raynaud's phenomenon and arthritis are often associated.

Pathology. The dermal lesions of discoid LE consist of irregular proliferation and thinning of the epithelium, edema at the dermoepidermal junction, thickening of the basement membrane with deposition of fibrinoid, and keratotic plugging. *Keratotic plugging* is the term given to the dipping inward of the keratinized layer to the underlying epithelium. The connective

tissue collagen appears hyaline, and there is also a thin and patchy infiltrate of chronic inflammatory cells.

Clinical aspects. The skin lesions are reddish and macular with a covering of thin adherent scales. Initially the lesions are typically circular (hence, "discoid"). They spread at their margins, however, and may coalesce but later heal with central scarring, often leaving an irregular, pale, depressed area.

The distribution is characteristically symmetric, and typically the lesions involve both cheeks and spread over the bridge of the nose to coalesce and form a bat-wing or butterfly pattern (see Fig. 7-7).

The oral lesions rarely have a well-defined shape but tend to be depressed and sometimes form linear or angular erosions surrounded by a whitish margin, sometimes resembling lichen planus. Biopsy is therefore necessary.

Systemic lupus erythematosus

The lesions on the skin and mucous membranes tend to be more acute and less well defined than in discoid LE. Essentially the same features may be present, but, in addition, acute necrotizing vasculitis is a typical feature.

Progressive systemic sclerosis (scleroderma)

Scleroderma (literally, hard skin) is the old name for progressive systemic sclerosis, a generalized disease characterized by the presence of excessive collagen formation in the subcutaneous tissues and also in organs such as the lungs and heart. The disease can endanger life.

Morphea is regarded as a localized form of scleroderma.

Pathology and pathogenesis. The main immunologic findings are antinuclear antibodies and, in a minority, rheumatoid factor, but their relationship to the disease is obscure.

TABLE 19-3. Important vesiculobullous diseases

	Pathogenesis	*Microscopic site of lesion*	*Gross distribution*
Genodermatoses			
Epidermolysis bullosa	Defect of adhesion of basal cells to one another or to basement membrane	Subepidermal	Oral mucosa and skin at sites of abrasion
Infective			
Herpes simplex	Destruction of epithelial cells by virus	Intraepithelial (middle layer)	Primary: intraoral Recurrences; labial (genital HSV II)
Herpes zoster	Destruction of epithelial cells by virus	Intraepithelial (middle layer)	Along dermatomes; dermal and mucosal in trigeminal area
Chickenpox	Destruction of epithelial cells by virus	Intraepithelial (middle layers)	Dermal and mucosal; spread outward from trunk
Smallpox	Destruction of epithelial cells by virus	Intraepithelial (middle layers)	Dermal and mucosal; spread typically downward from face and mouth
Hand-foot-and-mouth disease	Destruction of epithelial cells by virus	Intraepithelial (middle layers)	Mouth and extremities
Impetigo	Exudate under cornified layer	Intraepithelial (subcorneal)	Skin, especially face
Immunologically mediated			
Contact dermatitis	Cell mediated cytotoxic reaction and intercellular accumulation of exudate	Intraepithelial	Skin in area of contact with allergen only
Pemphigus vulgaris	Antibodies to intercellular attachments; loss of adhesion of epithelial cells	Intraepithelial, suprabasal destruction of intercellular attachments	Skin and mucosa
Mucous membrane pemphigoid	Antibody localized at basement membrane level; separation of full thickness of epithelium	Subepithelial	Mucosal; mouth and eyes especially; skin involvement minor and uncommon
Bullous pemphigoid	Antibody to skin basement membrane; separation of full thickness of epithelium	Subepithelial	Mainly skin
Unknown cause			
Stevens-Johnson syndrome (acute erythema multiforme)	Degeneration of superficial epithelial cells	Superficial intraepithelial	Mucosal (especially lips and mouth) and skin

There is deposition of excessive amounts of collagen in the subcutaneous tissues, lungs, joints, muscles, heart, and gastrointestinal tract. Lymphocytic infiltration or inflammatory changes are typically slight or absent.

Clinical aspects. Women are mainly affected, and in the majority Raynaud's phenomenon is the earliest symptom, associated with or soon followed by skin changes.

The affected skin is first edematous and then gradually becomes hard, smooth, and tightly adherent to underlying tissue (Fig. 19-30). Atrophy of dermal appendages follows. The hands and face may first be affected. Movement is increasingly severely impaired and may be made worse by involvement of joints and muscles. Muscle changes are essentially the same as those of polymyositis.

The lungs are usually involved, and the effects may include dyspnea, cough, or more severe symptoms.

Cor pulmonale may develop, but myocardial fibrosis alone can lead to cardiac failure in a minority.

Fibrosis of the gastrointestinal tract typically leads to dysphagia, constipation, and sometimes malabsorption. Renal disease is uncommon but potentially lethal.

The face may become immobile and masklike with thin lips and purse-string contracture of the mouth. Opening may be limited as a result of involvement of the joints and muscles. The intraoral tissues, particularly the tongue, may become stiff, and Sjögren's syndrome may be associated.

Treatment is symptomatic only, and less than 50% of patients survive for 5 or more years.

Morphea

Morphea is of unknown cause and is characterized by dermal changes similar to those of systemic sclerosis but localized in distribution and unassociated with systemic disease. Women are predominantly affected, and the onset is typically in early adult life.

The fibrosis causes scarlike bands or stripes and sometimes fixation of the skin to the underlying bone. When the face is affected, the skin is tightly bound to the underlying bone; morphea is the main cause of facial hemiatrophy. The scarlike lesion typically resembles a saber wound.

Dermatomyositis

For a discussion of dermatomyositis, see Chapters 7 and 17.

Stevens-Johnson syndrome (erythema multiforme exudativum)

Stevens-Johnson syndrome is an acute and typically recurrent vesicular bullous disease, which frequently (if not invariably) affects the lips and mouth (Fig. 19-31) and often the eyes (Fig. 19-32).

The syndrome is rarely a complication of drug treatment (particularly with the sulfonamides) and of infections caused by herpes simplex virus or *Mycoplasma pneumoniae*. The existence of these triggering factors has lead to the assumption that the disease is immunologically mediated; but if so, no immunologic mechanism or characteristic immunologic abnormalities have been identified. In many, if not the majority of cases, no triggering factor can be recognized.

Clinically, young adult males are chiefly affected. A characteristic, almost diagnostic feature is swelling, bleeding, and serosanguinous crusting of the lips. There are frequently widespread erosions in the mouth and intact or recently ruptured vesicles or bullae may be widespread on the skin. In severe attacks there is fever and malaise.

The characteristic rash of (nonbullous) erythema multiforme, consists of so-called target or iris lesions which are circular pinkish macules with a cyanotic center, about 1 cm across. In Stevens-Johnson syndrome, however, there is characteristically bulla formation in addition to other types of rash such as target lesions or widespread erythema. Conjunctivitis or ocular vesiculation is typically associated.

Microscopically, Stevens-Johnson syndrome is characterized by degeneration of keratinocytes and extensive eosinophilic colloid change. The latter is not specific but can progress to intraepithelial vesiculation, but more frequently vesiculation is subepithelial. There is a lymphohistiocytic infiltrate of very

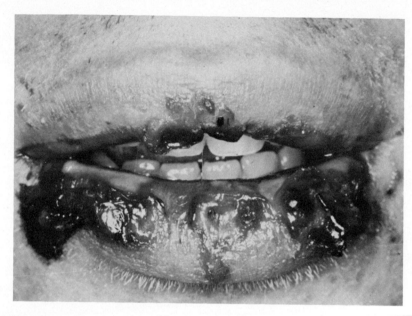

FIG. 19-31. Acute erythema multiforme. The swelling, bleeding, and crusting of the lips are the most constant and conspicuous features. *(From Cawson RA: Essentials of dental surgery and pathology, ed 4, Edinburgh, Scotland, 1984, Churchill Livingstone.)*

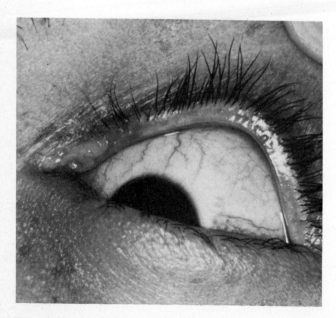

FIG. 19-32. Stevens-Johnson syndrome. There is conjunctivitis and small vesicles along the edges of the eyelids.

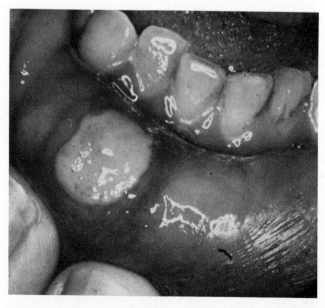

FIG. 19-33. Recurrent aphthous stomatitis. This well-demarcated rounded ulcer is typical of this common disorder.

variable intensity in the corium and sometimes also a perivascular mononuclear infiltrate more deeply. Paradoxically, perivascular leakage of immunologic products has been reported and immunologists usually classify this disease as a form of vasculitis. True vasculitis (Chapter 10) as a histologic feature is however absent.

Stevens-Johnson syndrome is usually self-limiting. Although there may be several attacks, often of increasing severity, the disease typically resolves spontaneously. Very rarely, it can be fatal usually as a result of renal damage or can cause impairment or loss of sight. There is no effective treatment; corticosteroids may ameliorate symptoms but do not prevent any of the severe complications.

Aphthous stomatitis (recurrent aphthae, canker sores)

Aphthae affect the mouth alone, unless they are a feature of Behçet's syndrome. They have been thought to be immunologically mediated but the evidence is conflicting. Otherwise healthy young persons are mainly affected. There is no association with the recognized immunologically mediated diseases and no consistently found immunologic abnormality is useful in diagnosis.

The etiology of this minor but troublesome disorder is therefore unknown. In a minority of cases there is an underlying hematinic deficiency; particularly in patients who have aphthae late in life, folate or vitamin B_{12} deficiency may be found. In a few women also, aphthae may be associated with the luteal phase of menstruation. Particularly severe aphthae can also be a feature of AIDS, but their relationship to the pathogenesis of this disease is unknown, since they are not a recognized feature of other major disorders of cell-mediated immunity.

Microscopically, the features of recurrent aphthae are nonspecific. Intercellular edema and intraepithelial microvesiculation may precede breakdown of the epithelium. The result is a ragged edged ulcer with a mixed inflammatory infiltrate with a predominance of neutrophils. In support of an immunopathogenesis, perivascular cuffing is said to be present but if so is inconspicuous; vasculitis is also said to be a feature but is not seen.

Clinically, aphthae may affect 10% or more of the population at some time. The onset is often during childhood or adolescence and the severity may increase at a variable rate over a long period. In the mildest cases, ulcers are small and recur only a few times in a year. At worst there can be ulcers several centimeters across (major aphthae) which persist for months and recur without remission. Healing may leave extensive scarring.

In most cases, the ulcers are round, shallow and usually 3 to 7 mm across (Fig. 19-33) and several may be present simultaneously. Healing usually starts after about a week but recurrence of ulcers at more or less regular intervals of weeks or months is typical. The course is often remittant and ultimately self-limiting after a period of years.

There is no cure for recurrent aphthae. A great variety of treatments have been used and include immunosuppressive and antiinflammatory drugs (particularly corticosteroids administered either topically or systemically), immunopotentiating agents and transfer factor among many others, but without consistent success. In any case any apparent benefit from such treatment is often no more than spontaneous remission or resolution which is characteristic of this disorder.

Behçet's syndrome

Behçet's syndrome* is an uncommon mucocutaneous disease comprising oral aphthae, genital ulceration and ocular lesions such as uveitis. However, almost any organ system can be affected. Skin lesions such as vesicles, pustules or erythema nodosum are common and thrombophlebitis or joint pain due to synovitis is frequently associated. In some cases there are neurologic or gastrointestinal disorders. The clinical picture is therefore highly variable, but oral and genital ulceration are the most consistently found features.

Young males are predominantly affected and there are wide geographic variations in incidence. The disease is uncommon or rare in Britain and the United States, for example, but common in Turkey. It is so common in Japan that the case incidence even within individual prefectures (administrative districts) has been mapped out.

A great variety of immunologic abnormalities have been reported, but there is no clear picture of any immunopathogenesis. Vasculitis has been reported in some cases. Immune complex damage has been proposed as a mechanism for the arthritis, which may be associated. Indeed the clinical features can be so protean that there are no absolute diagnostic criteria for Behçet's syndrome. Therefore the skeptic may cast doubt on the validity of the many reported laboratory abnormalities.

Lichen planus

Lichen planus is a common chronic disease of skin and mucous membranes. The cause is unknown but some features suggest that the disease may be immunologically mediated. For example, a similar disease can result from the administration of a variety of drugs such as antimalarials or gold salts. Although such lesions are frequently termed "lichenoid," they may not be distinguishable clinically or microscopically from the spontaneous disease. Furthermore, as described earlier, lichen planus is a characteristic feature of chronic graft-versus-host disease. In addition, the microscopic features of lichen planus have the appearance of a cell-mediated attack on the epithelium and T lymphocytes are prominent in the inflammatory infiltrate.

Despite such considerations, most cases of lichen planus are without apparent cause. There is no association with recognized autoimmune diseases, and any immunologic pathogenesis remains undefined.

Recently, human papilloma virus (HPV 16) DNA has been found in over 80% of cases of lichen planus but the significance of this finding is unclear.

Microscopically, lichen planus can have distinctive and characteristic histologic features. There may be parakeratosis and the deep surface of the epithelium shows a saw-tooth profile (Fig. 19-34). The basal cell layer is not identifiable as such and there is liquefaction degeneration at the dermoepidermal junction. In the corium there is a dense, bandlike infiltrate of mononuclear cells in which T lymphocytes may predominate.

Clinical aspects. The skin lesions (Fig. 19-35) consist of violaceous papules with a characteristic waxy-looking surface. Minute striae can be seen on close examination. The common sites are the flexor aspects of the extremities, the face, palms, and soles usually are not involved. The lesions usually cause intense itching, and asymptomatic mouth lesions are frequently associated.

---

*H. Behçet (1889-1945), Turkish dermatologist.

The characteristic oral lesion is a greatly magnified pattern of striae. These form well-defined bluish white lines often forming a lacelike pattern (Fig. 19-36). The characteristic sites are the buccal mucous membranes and the lateral part of the dorsum or margins of the tongue, frequently with a symmetric distribution.

The striae often cause no symptoms, but the red atrophic lesions and erosions are painful. The latter are often covered by a yellowish layer of fibrinous exudate where the epithelium has been destroyed.

Lichen planus responds well to the application of potent

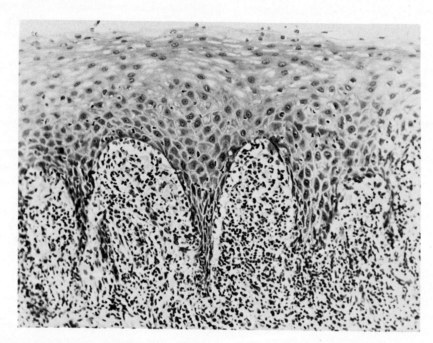

FIG. 19-34. Lichen planus. This shows the typical saw-tooth form of the epithelial ridges, liquefaction degeneration of the basal cell layer, and the mononuclear inflammatory exudate in the underlying connective tissue.

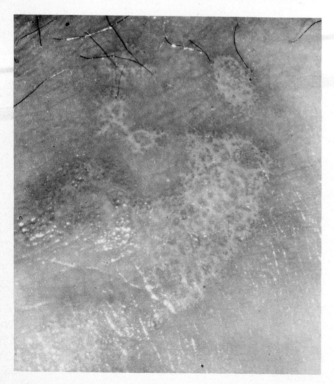

FIG. 19-35. Lichen planus of the skin. The lacelike pattern is typical but is usually on a much smaller scale than is seen here. (*Courtesy Curator of the Gordon Museum, Guy's Hospital, London, England.*)

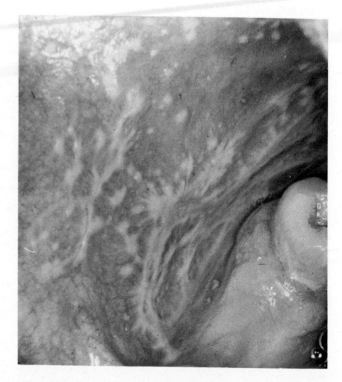

FIG. 19-36. Oral lichen planus. The lacelike pattern of white striae is often symmetrically distributed on both buccal areas. The lesions are gross in size compared with those on the skin, as seen in Fig. 19-35.

topical corticosteroids, but in severe cases these have to be given systemically.

Graft-versus-host disease

Graft-versus-host disease (GVHD) results from the transplantation of immunologically competent donor cells which can attack an immunodeficient host (Chapter 7). Cutaneous eruptions are typical features.

Acute GVHD starting within 100 days of engraftment is frequently characterized by a maculopapular pruritic rash which starts on the face or forearms but spreads to the trunk and limbs and may resemble lichen planus. In severe cases, generalized erythroderma, bulla formation, and desquamation may follow.

Microscopically, there is degeneration of keratinocytes with satelliting of mononuclear cells in the epithelium and, sometimes, a perivascular mononuclear cell infiltrate in the lamina propria.

Chronic GVHD starts more than 100 days after engraftment and has a high mortality. The mucocutaneous lesions are clinically indistinguishable from lichen planus and systemic sclerosis. The lichenoid lesions typically start in or are restricted to the mouth. Any skin involvement is similar in distribution to that in acute GVHD.

Microscopically, the lesions differ from spontaneous lichen planus (Fig. 19-34) only that the mononuclear infiltrate is slightly less dense and is associated with eosinophils. Globular or linear deposits of IgM and C3 at the basement membrane zone may be detectable by direct immunofluorescence microscopy.

In late chronic GVHD, the lesions resemble those of scleroderma (systemic sclerosis) but also affect the sites of predeliction for acute GVHD. Hyperpigmentation together with patchy depigmentation, and telangectasia are common. The histologic features are similar to those of systemic sclerosis described earlier.

Psoriasis

Psoriasis is a common disease and may affect 1% to 3% of the population. Chronic psoriasis was regarded as being associated with deep repressed emotional disturbance. The term "the heartbreak of psoriasis" so beloved by advertisers in the United States, may however be more accurate than skeptics might believe, but to distinguish cause from effect is a formidable task.

The cause of psoriasis, despite intensive investigation remains obscure. In any etiologic hypothesis, the following findings have to be taken in account: (1) there is sometimes a family history but no clear evidence of a genetic defect; (2) psoriasis genuinely seems in some patients to be a consequence of stress, not merely emotional but also physical such as infection or trauma; (3) lesions can first appear in or be exacerbated locally at a site of trauma (Koebner phenomenon*); (4) a strong systemic component is evident from the association of the cutaneous disease with arthritis (psoriatic arthropathy) (Chapter 17); (5) psoriasis is aggravated by hypocalcemia as discussed later; and (6) psoriasis can clear up on exposure to sunlight but has also been reported to respond to cyclosporine, which depresses T lymphocyte function.

Pathogenesis. The proliferative lesions of psoriasis do not show inflammatory changes. A major problem has been to find factors capable of inducing the epithelial hyperproliferation characteristic of the disease. Thus the turnover rate of normal

---

*H. Koebner (1838-1904), German dermatologist.

keratinocytes is 3 weeks, but is only 3 days in the case of psoriatic keratinocytes. Hyperproliferation of keratinocytes is associated with many of the pathologic findings in psoriasis, yet keratinocytes from psoriatic lesions have a normal rate of turnover when grown in tissue culture.

Dermal fibroblasts normally however play a major role in controlling the differentiation and function of epithelium. Psoriatic fibroblasts have been found to have increased biochemical activity and are also hyperproliferative. Moreover psoriatic fibroblasts, combined in tissue culture with normal epithelium, cause hyperproliferation of the latter; a diffusible fibroblast product seems likely to be responsible for the epithelial changes in psoriasis. The activity of a diffusible substance of this sort is suggested by the fact that the Koebner phenomenon can be prevented either by vascular occlusion or by injection of the patient's serum that had been collected during a remission.

Calcium may also play a role in that psoriasis may be aggravated by hypocalcemia and improvement may follow calcium replacement. Moreover calmodulin (an intracellular calcium receptor protein which activates phospholipase A2 and other proinflammatory mediators) is increased in psoriatic epidermis.

In addition, immunologic phenomena are associated as suggested by reports of response to cyclosporine mentioned earlier. Overall therefore recent findings in psoriasis suggest that epithelial proliferation is secondary to a fibroblast serum factor, but it is apparent that the etiologic mechanisms are complex.

Microscopically, typical findings (Fig. 19-37) are acanthosis with elongated, slender rete ridges, parakeratosis and absence of a granular cell layer, and collections of neutrophils (Munro abscesses) within the superficial epithelium. Macroscopic, sterile collections of neutrophils are characteristic of pustular psoriasis. In the corium there are dilated tortuous blood vessels which can be apparent clinically as erythema.

Clinically, lesions vary in severity and type. Most readily recognizable are plaques covered by fine silvery scales (Fig. 19-38). These start as small papules and can spread more or less extensively but the appearances are often changed by scratching.

Variants include guttate (droplike) psoriasis, which can follow streptococcal infections particularly in adolescents, pustular with deep-seated sterile abscesses, erythematous, flexural and others.

Psoriasis of the nails is common and can cause pitting or thickening and separation of the nail from its bed (oncholysis).

The treatments of psoriasis vary according to its type, severity, and response. If treatment is needed, the more troublesome lesions may respond to applications of salicylic acid, coal tar ointments, or anthralin (dithranol), which may be supplemented by exposure to ultraviolet B light. Severe disease unresponsive to other treatments may resolve after courses of photochemotherapy in which psoralens is given by mouth to sensitize the skin to long wave, ultraviolet A light. Hazards of the latter are skin burns, cataracts and possibly, skin cancer in the long term. As mentioned earlier, cyclosporine may also be effective and according to the type of psoriasis, improvement or clearance may follow in days or weeks.

Erythema nodosum

Erythema nodosum can be a manifestion of a wide variety of conditions, particularly infections such as primary tuberculosis. Other triggering causes include coccidioidomycosis, leprosy, syphilis, cat-scratch disease, measles, some vaccines

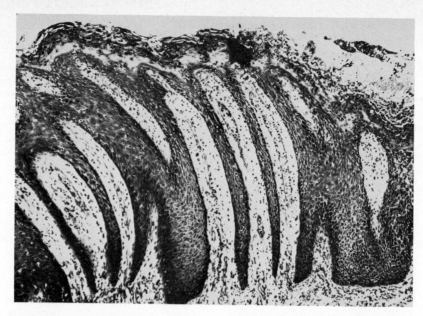

FIG. 19-37. Psoriasis. This biopsy specimen shows superficial microabscess formation and the characteristic elongation of the epithelial ridges.

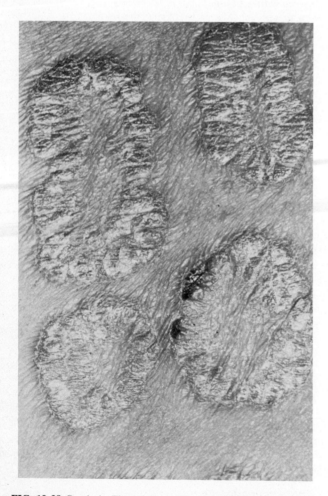

FIG. 19-38. Psoriasis. These typical lesions, unchanged by scratching, consist of rounded plaques with a raised margin. There is scaling of the surface and slight darkening caused by inflammation. *(Courtesy Curator of the Gordon Museum, Guy's Hospital, London, England.)*

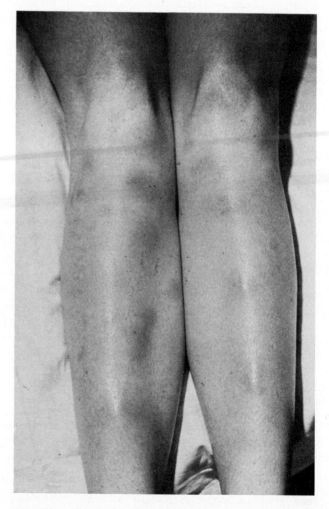

FIG. 19-39. Erythema nodosum. Extremely painful, tender, purple swellings are present on the anterior surface of the legs. In this case no underlying cause was found.

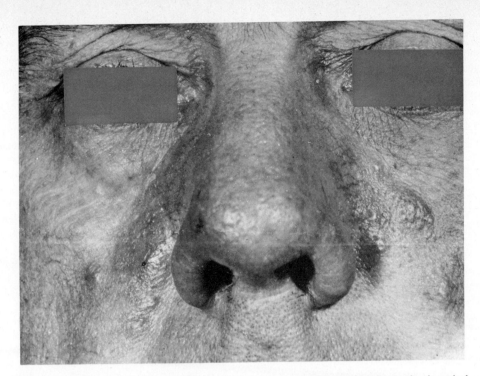

FIG. 19-40. Rosacea. The dusky thickening of the facial skin due to chronic inflammation is typical. The nose is more severely affected, and there may be incipient rhinophyma. *(Courtesy Curator of the Gordon Museum, Guy's Hospital, London, England.)*

or drugs or lymphomas, but in some cases no cause can be found.

Microscopically, the features are not diagnostic. Early there is patchy infiltration of the superficial corium with a mixture of cells in which neutrophils and lymphocytes usually predominate. Sometimes, radially arranged nodules of histiocytes form and later, noncaseating granulomas may be seen. Angiitis with thickening of the walls particularly of veins is also present in many but by no means all cases.

Clinically, women are predominantly affected, usually in the second decade. The lesions are typically on the shins and consist of red or purplish, raised tender areas (Fig. 19-39).

Erythema nodosum usually subsides after 3 to 6 weeks and its chief importance is as an indicator of underlying disease.

Rosacea

Rosacea is a common condition characterized by persistent facial erythema accompanied by edema or hyperplasia, producing papules or enlarged sebaceous glands.

The cause is unknown, and, although rosacea is often regarded as a sign of alcoholism, there is no foundation for this uncharitable assumption.

The pathologic features are dilatation of the facial blood vessels, edema, and a lymphocytic reaction.

Women are more frequently affected. The disorder most commonly becomes apparent between ages 30 and 50 but may start earlier in males.

The rash may affect the whole face but tends to spare the circumoral area (Fig. 19-40). The severity ranges from persistent erythema alone to a blotchy red appearance with edema, telangiectasis, thickening of the facial skin, and a papular eruption. In men, rhinophyma may be associated.

There is no specific treatment, but factors that exacerbate

the condition, such as exposure to sunlight, should be avoided. Small doses of tetracycline given for several months have been found to improve the condition in many cases.

Rhinophyma

Rhinophyma is a condition of chronic hyperplasia of the nasal sebaceous glands and connective tissue; minor inflammatory changes are associated. The cause is unknown, and the widespread belief that rhinophyma ("grog blossom"), especially when associated with rosacea, is a sign of alcoholism is unfounded.

Rhinophyma affects men almost exclusively and is a disease of middle age. The nose is at first erythematous and then gradually enlarges and becomes irregularly nodular.

There is no specific treatment for this disfiguring and distressing condition, and plastic surgery may be needed.

Tumors and tumorlike lesions of the skin (see also Chapter 9)

Both true neoplasms and developmental anomalies are included here. Developmental anomalies of the skin are often termed *nevi* and can be of epithelial or connective tissue origin. Pigmented nevi are particularly common.

The most important tumors of the skin are basal and squamous cell carcinomas and melanomas.

Warts (verrucae)

Warts are common tumorlike hyperplastic lesions of the skin, particularly common in childhood and adolescence. They are caused by papilloma viruses and transmissible by direct contact though not highly contagious. Warts are rarely spread to the oral mucosa from finger lesions.

Etiology. In recent years there has been intense interest in the papilloma virus group. These are of the papova *(pa*pilloma-*po*lyoma-*va*cuolating) virus group and at the time of writing, no fewer than 46 genotypes of human papilloma viruses (HPV) have been identified. The interest in these viruses resides not merely in their ability to give rise to warts but because of their possible role in carcinomas of the uterine cervix (Chapter 21) and possibly other sites. The potential for such change was first demonstrated in animals by Shope* in 1933. In humans there is an approximately 30% incidence of malignant change in the rare disease, epidermolysis verruciformis, which consists of multiple, persistent flat skin warts. Carcinomas in this disease contain DNA of HPV-5 or HPV-8. DNA from HPV-6 and the closely related HPV-11 have been cloned directly from anogenital warts, whilst HPV-16 DNA has been found in 84% of genital carcinomas. However in nearly 75% of cases the normal epithelium in the vicinity of genital carcinomas also contain HPV-16 DNA. HPV DNA has also been found to persist in latent form in normal laryngeal and oral as well as genital epithelium. Although HPV DNA has been found incorporated into the genome of cervical carcinoma cells in 80% to 90%, HPV DNA has not been found significantly more frequently in oral carcinomas than in nonmalignant tissue. Neither skin warts (apart from those of epidermolysis verruciformis) nor oral papillomas have any known premalignant potential.

Clinically, common warts (verruca vulgaris) consist of lo-

---

*R.E. Shope (1901-1966), American pathologist.

calized skin nodules with an irregular surface, usually of the same color as the surrounding skin and varying in size from one to 10 mm across (Fig. 19-41). Flat warts (verruca plana) mainly affect the face and the hands and are flat smooth and faintly pigmented. Plantar or palmar warts (verruca plantaris or palmaris) tend to be larger (up to 15 mm across) are heavily keratinized, deeply embedded (possibly because of pressure) and sometimes painful. Condyloma accuminatum (Chapter 21) affect the male or female genitalia, or perianal regions and are usually pinkish and cauliflower-like in form.

Microscopically, warts consist of a localized area of severe epithelial hyperplasia and (usually) hyperkeratosis; this hyperplasia gives the appearance in sections of folding or pleating of the epithelium. In addition, there is vacuolation of the cytoplasm of the keratinocytes, granular eosinophilic inclusions and deeply basophilic nuclei. Intranuclear viral particles can be shown by electron microscopy and, as mentioned earlier, HPV DNA can be demonstrated using DNA probes.

Basal cell carcinoma (rodent ulcer)

A basal cell carcinoma is a slow-growing, locally invasive tumor that very rarely metastasizes and usually begins late in life. They frequently develop in areas exposed to strong sunlight but also form in non-exposed areas.

Basal cell carcinomas arise from the pluripotential cells from which epithelial appendages develop.

Microscopically, basal cell carcinomas consist of a downgrowth of dense masses of small, compact darkly staining cells with little cytoplasm. At the margins of these downgrowing columns the cells are often arranged in a palisade fashion and tend to be more columnar in form. Pseudocystic change within the epithelial masses is common. Basal cell carcinoma does not affect the mouth or any other stratified squamous epithelium except that of the skin.

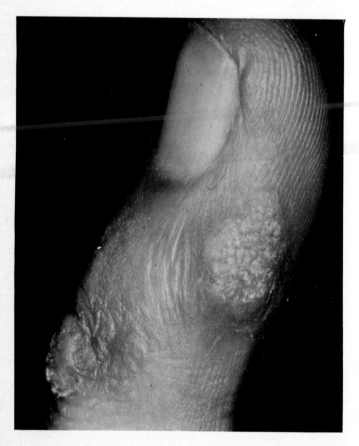

FIG. 19-41. Viral warts of the finger caused by papilloma virus. The patient had also implanted the infection and had similar lesions in the mouth.

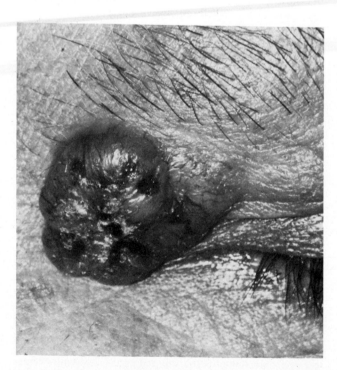

FIG. 19-42. Basal cell carcinoma. This relatively early lesion has the typical slightly nodular and translucent appearance. *(Courtesy Curator Gordon Museum, Guy's Hospital, London, England.)*

Clinically, men are more frequently affected than women, and the face is the most common site (Fig. 19-42). Exposure of fair-skinned people to strong sunlight is a causative factor in some parts of the world, such as the southern United States and Australia.

The tumor usually forms a slowly growing, firm, painless rounded, superficial nodule on the face that at first is often pale and translucent and has a pearly appearance. The center eventually becomes necrotic and forms a cratershaped ulcer with a raised, hard edge and a central brownish crust. If left untreated, the growth infiltrates deeper tissues and can destroy bone or the eye or expose the antrum. If destruction is sufficiently severe, the tumor may be untreatable because of the proximity of vital structures. The patient can then die from complications, such as secondary infection and bronchopneumonia.

Excision with or without radiotherapy is curative if the tumor is treated early.

Other epithelial (adnexal) skin tumors. A variety of benign tumors and their malignant counterparts arise from adnexal skin structures, such as sweat glands, sebaceous glands and hair follicles and include the trichoepithelioma, pilomatrixoma, hidradenoma, and many others. Some, as a result of their glandular origin may be difficult to distinguish from salivary gland tumors, whereas others have some resemblance to odontogenic tumors. The latter also arise from adnexal (dental) structures originating from the anterior oral epithelium which, in turn, is embryologically of the same origin as the skin ectoderm.

Intraepithelial carcinoma

Intraepithelial carcinoma (carcinoma in situ) is characterized by malignant change within the epithelium but absence of invasion of the underlying tissues. It occasionally affects the oral mucosa.

There are several varieties of intraepithelial carcinoma of the skin, which often form reddish patches, often with a scaling surface. They usually become invasive, sometimes only after many years. Examples are Bowen's disease of the skin, erythroplasia of the penis, and Paget's disease of the nipple.

Squamous cell carcinoma (see also Chapter 9)

Squamous cell carcinoma arises frequently in the face and the lower lip. Like all carcinomas, carcinoma of the skin is usually a disease of old age unless there has been early exposure to a carcinogenic factor, such as strong sunlight, x rays, mineral oils, coal tar and its products, or other chemicals.

Pathology. This neoplasm is a typical squamous cell carcinoma with irregular branching columns of epithelial cells growing into the dermis. The cells are usually clearly seen to be prickle cells, being large and polygonal and having intercellular bridges. In well-differentiated tumors, cell nests, that is, concentric layers of keratinized cells that stain red with eosin, can be seen deeply. Occasionally these neoplasms are less well differentiated, lack many of the details described, and tend to grow more rapidly. There is almost invariably an inflammatory reaction in the surrounding connective tissue.

Clinical aspects. A squamous carcinoma usually starts as a small nodule that grows to form a rounded swelling with a flat surface and usually raised only a few millimeters above the surrounding skin. The surface may be warty or scaly. A persistent scaling lesion of the lower lip, even if only 5 mm in diameter, is considered to be a squamous cell carcinoma until proved otherwise by biopsy.

Further development of the tumor causes an ulcer with hard, irregular, everted edges and a rough irregular floor from which there is usually a discharge or formation of a yellowish crust. If left untreated, the tumor invades and destroys adjacent tissues and metastasizes to the regional lymph nodes.

Treatment is by excision or radiotherapy, or both for more extensive lesions. The prognosis for localized tumors is good but deteriorates sharply once metastases have developed.

Keratoacanthoma

Keratoacanthomas are a heterogeneous group of tumorlike skin lesions, the most common of which is the solitary type. Like squamous cell carcinoma, which in many respects it resembles, the solitary keratoacanthoma usually develops in sundamaged skin. It begins as a florid downgrowth of contiguous follicular structures, giving rise over a period of weeks to a dome-shaped nodule with a dilated center plugged by cornified cells. The lesion typically undergoes *involution* over a period of 5 to 7 months, leaving a scar in its wake.

The exact cause of the keratoacanthoma remains unknown. Activation of the *h-ras* oncogene has been demonstrated in both keratoacanthomas and squamous cell carcinomas. It is possible that keratoacanthomas begin as squamous cell carcinomas but (for unknown reasons) rapidly involute. In many respects the natural history of keratoacanthomas is like that of common verrucae, and it is conceivable that papillomaviruses might play a role in their genesis.

Surgical excision is the recommended treatment, both to avoid the scarring that involution brings and to confirm the diagnosis histologically. In most cases, keratoacanthoma is readily distinguishable from squamous cell carcinoma, on ac-

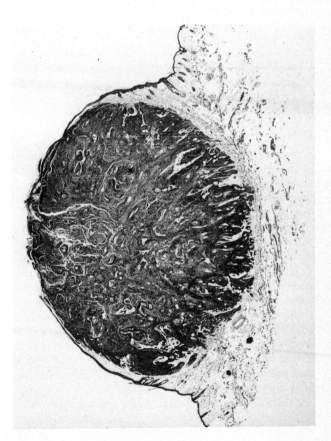

FIG. 19-43. Keratoacanthoma. The goblet shape and well-defined margin of the pseudoepitheliomatous hyperplasia can be seen.

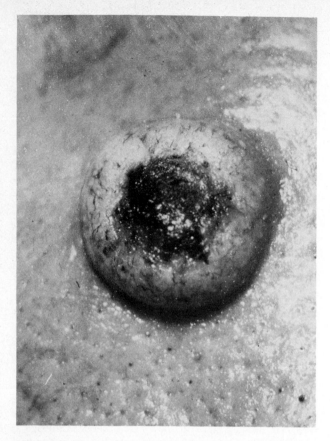

FIG. 19-44. Keratoacanthoma. The lesion is dome shaped and has a shallow central crater. *(Courtesy Curator of the Gordon Museum, Guy's Hospital, London, England.)*

count of its characteristic, symmetrical, crateriform shape (Figs. 19-43 and 19-44), and signs of involution, such as the presence of microabscesses within the epithelium. Occasionally, however, distinction may be difficult, and such cases warrant careful follow-up.

Melanomas and other pigmented tumors

Nevi and tumors characterized by abnormal proliferation of melanocytes are common.

Pigmented nevi (moles). A mole is a nevus (developmental growth disorder) and results from a benign proliferation of melanocytes (nevus cells) at the dermoepidermal junction.

Junctional nevi is the name given to lesions, common in children, in which clusters of melanocytes are seen clinging to the deep aspect of the epidermis. These lesions have a tendency to gradually undergo "maturation," in that clusters of melanocytes "drop off" into the underlying dermis and lose their connection with the epidermis. As adulthood is approached, proliferation of junctional melanocytes (junctional activity) gradually ceases, and all the nevus cells are seen lying in the dermis beneath a normal appearing epidermis. The latter are termed *intradermal nevi*, whereas those which show both intradermal nevus cell nests and junctional melanocyte proliferation are termed *compound nevi*.

Clinically these lesions consist of a pigmented area sometimes slightly raised above the surrounding surface. They do not need any treatment unless they show junctional activity persisting into adult life or start to increase in size, in which cases malignant transformation becomes a likelihood. Alter-

natively, they may be of such a size or in such a position that excision is required for cosmetic reasons.

Blue nevus. The blue nevus is a benign pigmented lesion that can occasionally affect the oral mucosa and must be distinguished from a melanoma.

Histologically there are interlacing bundles of elongated spindle-shaped cells, many of which contain large amounts of melanin. Unlike melanomas, the pigment-filled cells are usually well separated from the overlying epithelium, which shows no abnormality.

Lentigo. Lentigo is the name given to a pigmented lesion in which there is characteristic elongation of the rete ridges, a concentration of melanocytes along the basal cell layer, and melanin in the basal cells. Small numbers of melanin-containing cells (melanophages) and sometimes chronic inflammatory cells are also seen immediately beneath the epithelium in the dermis.

Lentigo typically appears in childhood but can develop at any time. Lentigines usually form minute (1 or 2 mm) brown or black macules and are distinguishable from freckles (ephelides) by the fact that they do not darken as a result of exposure to sunshine. They are usually isolated or few in number and often affect skin that is not normally exposed.

Malignant melanoma. Malignant melanomas form about 1% of all cancers but are the most common cause of death from skin cancer. Malignant melanoma is increasing in frequency particularly among fair-complexioned white populations exposed to strong sunlight as in the Southern United States and Northern Australia. Tanning with ultraviolet lamps may be an additional factor, but though exposure to ultraviolet radiation is a major risk factor for malignant melanoma, the latter can also arise in nonexposed areas of skin or even the oral cavity.

There is a complex relationship between vitiligo (areas of depigmentation of the skin) and melanoma. In many animals with depigmentation there is a high incidence of melanomas, but such melanomas have an unusually good prognosis or, in the case of the Sinclair swine, usually regress spontaneously. There is also evidence that melanomas in humans with vitiligo, have a better prognosis than those with normal skin pigmentation. Since vitiligo is caused by melanocyte destruction and is frequently associated with autoantibodies to melanocytes, it is tempting to suggest that these autoantibodies contribute to tumor cell destruction. However, such a suggestion remains unproven.

Most malignant melanomas (Fig. 19-45) arise in apparently normal skin, and a few arise in association with pre-existing (usually intradermal) nevi. Their association with so-called dysplastic nevi is controversial, mainly because there are no uniformly accepted criteria for the diagnosis of such lesions. Regardless of the setting, however, most melanomas begin as a proliferation of melanocytes in the lower epidermis, i.e. as malignant melanomas in situ. This phase, during which there is horizontal growth of melanocytes in the epidermis, is recognizable clinically as an irregularly shaped, poorly circumscribed, unevenly pigmented macule. With descent of neoplastic melanocytes into the dermis (vertical growth phase), the lesion loses its flat appearance and becomes raised in one or more places. At this stage in its development, the neoplasm acquires a metastatic potential, which increases progressively with increasing vertical growth (invasion).

Some classify malignant melanomas into four types (superficial spreading, lentigo maligna, nodular, and acral lentiginous), depending on their clinical setting and on certain mi-

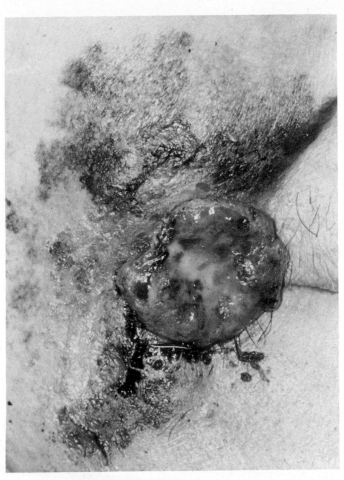

FIG. 19-45. Malignant melanoma. The tumor has produced an ulcerating mass, and the adjacent tissues are also widely stained with melanin from the tumor cells. *(Courtesy Curator of the Gordon Museum, Guy's Hospital, London, England.)*

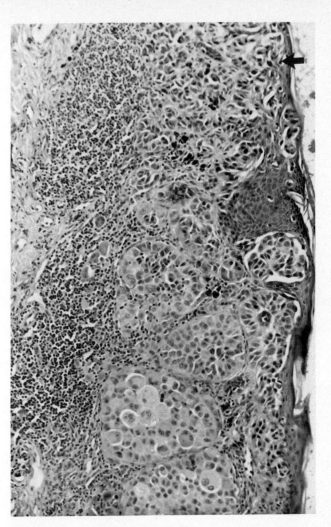

FIG. 19-46. Malignant melanoma of skin. Pleomorphic, neoplastic melanocytes in the form of single cells and as nests of varying sizes, have infiltrated the dermis and *(arrow)* the upper epidermis. Many small lymphocytes, indicative of an immunologic response, are seen among the tumor cells.

croscopic characteristics.* However, regardless of subtype, malignant melanomas of equal thickness or depth of invasion behave similarly and are treated clinically in the same way.

The prognosis of malignant melanoma depends largely on the depth of penetration of the tissues; this has to be graded as precisely as possible. Level I (Clark grading) refers to tumors confined to the epidermis and such tumors have little potential for metastasis; the most severe grade is level V where there is penetration through the full thickness of the epithelium and extension into subcutaneous tissues. In addition, it is desirable to measure the thickness of the tumor in millimeters (Bresslow thickness) as the prognosis deteriorates sharply in tumors over 0.7 mm thickness: however other variables such as mitotic

activity or the presence of satellite tumors or metastases affect the outcome.

When the cells of a malignant melanoma are filled with pigment and invasion is obvious, the diagnosis may be straightforward, but unpigmented malignant melanoma frequently presents diagnostic difficulties.

Clinical aspects. Any part of the body can be affected, but the face is the most frequent site. Malignant melanoma lacks the symmetry of a mole and may ulcerate (Fig. 19-45). The lesion is usually brown or black, but occasionally pigment is slight or absent and the tumor is reddish. Symptoms such as itching or bleeding are indicative of rapid growth, but the rate of growth is widely variable.

In the later stages a large pigmented area may develop, but usually ulceration and induration, indicative of deep infiltration, supervene before this can happen. Satellite tumors may appear near the primary growth. Spread to the lymph nodes may be an early or late feature, and thereafter hematogenous metastases may appear in liver, lung, or brain.

Malignant melanoma of the oral mucosa is uncommon. As with melanoma of the skin, there are superficially spreading and nodular invasive types that vary in prognosis accordingly.

---

*For example, malignant melanomas arising in sun-damaged skin are termed lentigo maligna melanomas, the in situ phase being called lentigo maligna. The more common, superficial spreading melanoma typically (but not exclusively) shows a scattering of single neoplastic cells at all levels of the epidermis (Fig. 19-46); because of the resemblance of this histologic pattern to that of Paget's disease of the skin, the superficial spreading melanoma is also called the "pagetoid" type.

Many are not recognized until a relatively advanced stage because symptoms are slight or absent.

Treatment of dermal and oral melanomas is the same.

Melanomas can be cured if excised before deeper infiltration has started. Deeper lesions have a poor prognosis, and metastases frequently appear after excision. Although chemotherapy or immunotherapy is used, the outlook is poor.

Cutaneous lymphomas

Mycosis fungoides. Mycosis fungoides is not a fungal infection but an uncommon, T cell lymphoma of the skin. Middle aged males are predominantly affected and characteristic features are an early eczema-like eruption, followed by multiple pruritic plaques and widespread cutaneous tumor nodules. Terms given to the various skin lesions of mycosis fungoides include parapsoriasis and erythroderma. Lymphoid tissue is involved late as may visceral tissue.

Microscopically, mycosis fungoides is characterized by a lymphocytic infiltration of the skin and in most cases the tumor lymphocytes bear the CD4 (T helper) marker. Infiltration is mainly of the corium but also of the epithelium, where clusters of lymphocytes form so-called Pautrier abscesses.* An unusual

---

*L.M. Pautrier (1876-1959), French dermatologist.

feature is the greatly convoluted (cerebriform) nuclei of some of the lymphocytes.

An association between HTLV I and mycosis fungoides has been reported as has the presence of the herpes simplex virus antigens and genome in early stage skin lesions. Prolonged remission of the disease has also been reported to result from treatment with acyclovir or α interferon; but such reports have not yet been widely confirmed. Unless such treatment is effective, the prognosis is poor.

*Sézary's syndrome.** This is another rare T cell lymphoma of the skin with affinities to mycoses fungoides but associated with leukemia-like presence of the tumor cells in the blood.

B cell lymphomas of the skin. Both primary and secondary deposits of the more common B cell lymphomas can affect the skin with variable clinical manifestations and prognoses.

Connective tissue tumors

Hemangioma. A hemangioma is a vascular hamartoma of the skin, often described by dermatologists as a "vascular nevus." Lay terms are *strawberry mark* and *port wine stain*. Hemangiomas consist of vast numbers of fine capillary channels and vasoformative tissue or they may be formed of thin-walled, blood-filled sinuses. When affecting the face hemangiomas often extend into the oral cavity and form a vascular swelling of the gums. Treatment of conspicuous lesions may be necessary for cosmetic reasons but is not entirely satisfactory.

---

*A. Sézary (1880-1956), French dermatologist.

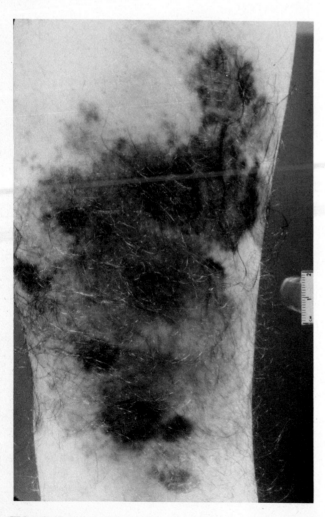

FIG. 19-47. Angiosarcoma of the leg. Several dark purple nodules are seen against the background of a large, poorly circumscribed, paler purple plaque.

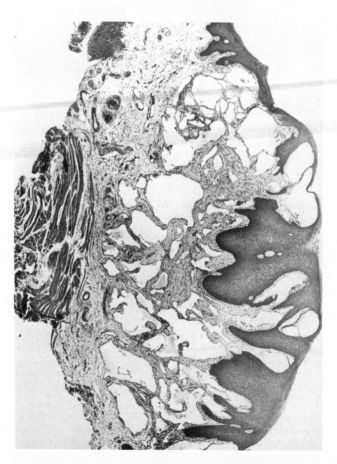

FIG. 19-48. Lymphangioma of the lip. The large lymphatic spaces can be clearly seen. *(From Cawson, RA: Essentials of dental surgery and pathology, ed 4, Edinburgh, Scotland, 1984, Churchill Livingstone.)*

Angiosarcomas of the skin (Fig. 19-47) are rare with the following exceptions:

1. Those which develop on the scalp and face of elderly patients
2. Those which are secondary to chronic intractable lymphedema

The latter type is usually seen in the arms of women following radical mastectomy with axillary lymph node excision. Both types are associated with early metastasis and short survival.

Lymphangioma. It is incorrect to classify these collections of lymph vessels (Fig. 19-48) as tumors. They are hamartomas, consisting of numerous normal lymph vessels or dilated lymph spaces and are found beneath the skin or mucosal surfaces. A more appropriate name for these benign lesions is lymphangiectasia.

Kaposi's sarcoma

Kaposi's sarcoma, formerly a rare tumor, is now a common feature of AIDS. In such patients the skin of the head and neck or the oral mucosa is frequently involved. This tumor appears clinically as a purplish macule or nodule. If such a lesion in an adult male is confirmed as Kaposi's sarcoma, this is virtually pathognomonic of AIDS unless the patient has had recent immunosuppressive treatment for an organ transplant. The disease is recognized as a rare complication of such treatment. The microscopic appearances of Kaposi's sarcoma are described in Chapter 10.

Vascular tumors, including Kaposi's sarcoma can sometimes be mistaken for *purpura* (Chapter 13). Furthermore, in patients with AIDS, purpura and Kaposi's sarcoma may coexist.

Granular cell tumor

Granular cell tumor is believed to be of neural origin with features that suggest Schwann cell differentiation. The tumor consists of large cells with finely granular cytoplasm. The granules have the ultrastructure of cytolysosomes. The granular cells form between or appear to replace muscle bundles. When situated immediately subepidermally, the overlying epithelium proliferates and can simulate remarkably closely a well-differentiated squamous cell carcinoma with deeply placed cell nests. This pseudoepitheliomatous hyperplasia has caused a few unfortunate patients to have radical treatment for a nonexistent carcinoma of the tongue. Once the granular cells have been noticed, however, the diagnosis becomes obvious (Figs. 19-49 and 19-50).

Clinically, the skin is the single most common site for these lesions, which can also affect the tongue, the digestive tract, and other sites. The appearance can range from a firm nodule 1 or 2 cm in diameter to a shallow depressed lesion resembling a scar. Most show little sign of neoplastic activity and excision is usually curative.

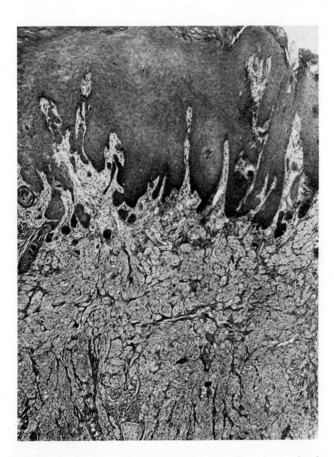

FIG. 19-49. Granular cell tumor of the tongue. There is pseudoepitheliomatous hyperplasia of the epithelium above the granular cells.

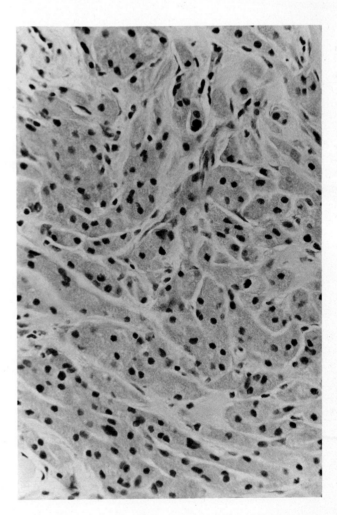

FIG. 19-50. Granular cell tumor of the skin. This high-power view shows the granular appearance of the cytoplasm.

Acanthosis nigricans

Acanthosis nigricans is a rare dermatosis that in adults is associated with visceral cancer (particularly with adenocarcinoma of the gastrointestinal tract in 50% to 60% of patients or occasionally with diabetes mellitus.

These dermal lesions consist of grayish-black warty plaques, whereas oral lesions typically consist of widespread velvety thickening of the mucosa.

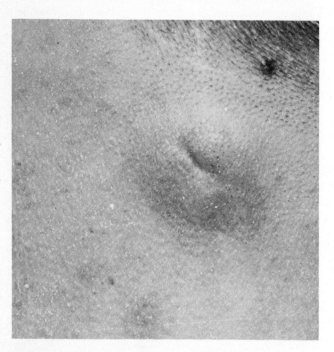

FIG. 19-51. Epidermal (sebaceous) cyst. The indentation on the surface of this rounded swelling is called a punctum.

Follicular cysts

A variety of cysts arise from the hair follicle. They are named according to the portion of the follicle the lining resembles. The most frequent variety is the *infundibular* type (incorrectly called "epidermal inclusion cyst" and "sebaceous cyst"), which keratinizes in the manner of the upper part of the follicle, the infundibulum. The *isthmus-catagen* type ("pilar cyst") has a lining identical to that of the isthmic (midportion) of the follicle and the involuting (catagen) follicle. Both kinds of cysts have a propensity for the head and neck region, the isthmus-catagen type usually developing in the scalp, and both contain foul-smelling keratin debris.

A less common type of follicular cyst is the *infundibular-matrix* cyst (pilomatricoma, or Malherbe tumor), the characteristic histologic appearance of which is due to the resemblance of much of the lining to the hair germ (matrix). The characteristic sheets of "ghost cells" formed by the matrical cells represents an abortive attempt at hair shaft formation. The contents of this and the isthmus-catagen cyst typically calcify.

Clinically, follicular cysts form painless, rounded, subepidermal rubbery swellings. There is sometimes a ductlike connection with the surface forming a characteristic indentation (punctum) (Fig. 19-51). Infection and inflammation may supervene but if not inflamed, the cysts can readily be excised.

Dermoid cysts (inclusion dermoids). Dermoid cysts are the result of enclavement of epithelium during development, particularly in the facial region. Their structure is that of an epidermal cyst, except that (1) the cyst wall contains dermal appendages, particularly hair follicles and sebaceous glands (Fig. 19-52), and (2) they are present at birth.

The most frequent site is near the outer canthus of the eye.

Implantation dermoid cysts. Implantation dermoids are cysts formed by epithelium embedded deeply in the subcutaneous tissues by an injury. In structure and clinical features these cysts are essentially similar to follicular cysts, infundibular type.

Sublingual dermoid cysts. Sublingual dermoids are also congenital anomalies resulting from enclavement of epithelium during closure of the pharyngeal arches. These cysts are most

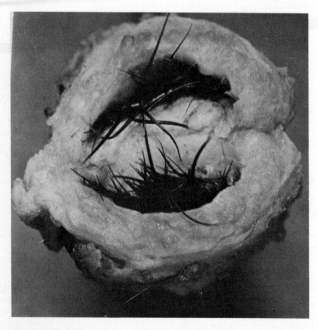

FIG. 19-52. Dermoid cyst. There are abundant hair follicles in the lining and hair growing into the cyst cavity. *(Courtesy Curator of the Gordon Museum, Guy's Hospital, London, England.)*

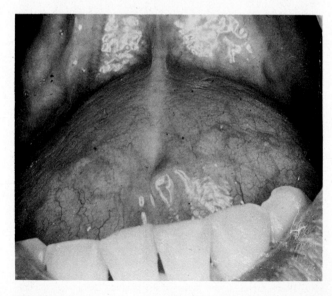

FIG. 19-53. Sublingual dermoid. This cyst, in the floor of the mouth, was filled with keratin.

frequently lined only by stratified squamous epithelium and filled with keratin (dermoid cyst). Alternatively, part of the lining may consist of ciliated respiratory epithelium, or dermal appendages, such as sebaceous glands, may be present in the cyst wall (epidermoid cyst).

Clinically, sublingual dermoids are in the midline, may be apparent at birth, and gradually fill the floor of the mouth as they expand (Fig. 19-53). Since a large bulk can be accommodated in this area, such a cyst may cause little disability until so large as to interfere with movement of the tongue. These cysts are typically of a puttylike consistency because of the semisolid keratin contents.

A sublingual dermoid cyst can also form deeply beneath the genial muscles, where it tends to push out the soft tissue below the chin rather than raise the floor of the mouth. These cysts should be removed surgically.

Selected readings

Breathnach SM and Katz SI: Cell mediated immunity in cutaneous disease, Human pathol 17:161, 1986.

Bunney MH: Viral warts: a new look at an old problem, Br Med J 293:1045, 1986.

Harper JI: Cutaneous graft versus host disease, Br Med J 295:401, 1987.

Howley PM: On human papilloma viruses, N Engl J Med 315:1089, 1987.

Kaplan AP and Buckley RH: Allergic skin disorders, JAMA 258:2900, 1987.

Maize JC and Ackerman AB: Pigmented lesions of the skin: Clinicopathologic correlations, Philadelphia, 1987, Lea & Febiger.

Matis WL, Triana A, and Shapiro R et al: Dermatologic findings associated with human immunodeficiency virus infection, J Am Acad Dermatol 17:746, 1987.

Millikan LE: Vesiculobullous skin disease with prominent immulogic features, JAMA 158:2910, 1987.

Nordlund JJ: Hypopigmentation, vitiligo, and melanoma, Arch Dermatol 123:1005, 1987.

Payne CMER: Psoriatic science, Br Med J 295:1158, 1987.

Rhodes AR, Weinstock MA, Fitzpatrick TB, et al: Risk factors for cutaneous melanoma, JAMA 258:3146, 1987.

Sison-Fonacier L and Bystryn JC: Heterogeneity of pemphigus vulgaris antigens, Arch Dermatol 123:1507, 1987.

Slater DN: Recent developments in cutaneous lymphoproliferative disorders, J Pathol 153:5, 1987.

Swerdlow AJ and Green A: Melanocytic naevi and melanoma: an epidemiologic perspective, Br J Dermatol 117:137, 1987.

Walker MM, Griffiths CEM, and Weber J, et al: Dermatologic conditions in HIV infection, Br Med J 294:29, 1987.

CHAPTER 20

Diseases of the nervous system

Damage to the brain inevitably has severe and far-reaching effects, which may include disturbance of consciousness, motor function, or sensation and mood changes or psychiatric disorders. Extensive damage to the brain is usually fatal. The most common causes of brain damage or disease are vehicular accidents and, mainly in later life, strokes or gradual cerebral degeneration caused by Alzheimer's and other diseases.

A wide variety of diseases can affect the brain, spinal cord, and peripheral nervous system, the complexity of which often necessitate highly specialized methods of investigation and treatment, in the fields of neurology and neurosurgery.

Once damaged, there is little functional repair possible in the brain. In such diseases as multiple sclerosis or cerebral tumors, effective treatment is difficult or impossible because of lack of knowledge of causative mechanisms or the extreme difficulties of brain surgery. Fortunately, one disease, acute poliomyelitis, which has unusually great potential for widespread and permanent damage to the nervous system, has been almost eradicated in the more developed parts of the world by the development of effective vaccines. By contrast, AIDS-related neurologic disease is an increasing problem.

Investigation of the nervous system

Clinical examination of nervous system function is especially important because physical signs help to localize the site of the lesion. Readily detectable defects resulting from nervous system disease include disturbance or loss of motor function, speech, vision, sensation, or level of consciousness.

Lumbar puncture and *examination of the cerebrospinal fluid* (CSF) may show abnormalities that include increased CSF pressure or the presence of blood, raised protein levels, leucocytes, or bacteria.

Radiologic examination includes: (1) conventional radiographs to detect fractures of the skull; (2) angiography to demonstrate occlusion or other abnormalities of the cerebral vessels, such as displacement by a tumor; (3) air encephalography in which air, injected into the subarachnoid space in the lumbar region, can show abnormalities such as change in size, displacement, or distortion (by a tumor, for example) of the ventricles and subarachnoid space; and (4) computerized assisted tomography (CT) scan, which produces a remarkably detailed image of a cross section of any part of the head. A CT scan will, for example, detect a cerebral hemorrhage only 1.5 cm in size.

Magnetic resonance imaging (MRI) is an important advance in investigative techniques for the nervous system. Not only does it allow (unlike CT scanning) imaging in different planes but also emphasizes the contrast between soft tissue lesions and normal tissues. Even gray and white matter are differentiated by MRI but it is less efficient for visualizing lesions involving the skull and a few other conditions, as calcified tissues produce no image. Otherwise, MRI is the method of choice of investigation of many lesions of the brain and cord.

In *electroencephalography* (EEG) electrodes are placed on several points on the head to show the electrical activity of different areas as waves of varying form and frequency. These rhythms are disturbed by such diseases as epilepsy and many organic brain lesions.

Microscopy is used for examination of cells in the CSF and for brain biopsies, particularly of tumors.

Anatomic aspects

The nervous system consists of (1) neurons (a nerve cell and axon that may be surrounded by a myelin sheath), which form the functional components of the brain, and (2) the glial cells and their processes, which support and maintain the neurons. The neuroglia comprises the oligodendroglia, astrocytes, and microglia. The microglia is part of the macrophage system (Chapter 7).

Diseases can affect any or all of these components and have many effects. As a result of the wide variety of functions of the different parts of the central nervous system, the clinical effects of a lesion often depend as much on its location as its size. An extensive lesion of the prefrontal cortex, for example, may have no apparent effect. By contrast, relatively little damage to the medulla oblongata can cause sudden death.

The skull. The skull protects the brain against injury, but at the same time it allows no expansion or displacement of the brain when a space-occupying lesion develops or excessive amounts of fluid accumulate. The resulting increased intracranial pressure can have serious or fatal effects.

Meninges. The coverings of the central nervous system are as follows:

1. The pia mater closely envelops the brain and spinal cord.
2. The dura mater closely adheres to the skull and vertebral column. The cranial cavity is also partially subdivided into compartments by extensions of the dura mater, as described later.
3. The arachnoid forms a thin spiderweb-like covering between the pia and dura mater.

The ependyma is the membranous lining of the ventricles and central canal of the spinal cord.

The CSF circulates between the arachnoid and pia mater in the subarachnoid space. The CSF is secreted by the choroid plexuses of the ventricles and reaches the subarachnoid space through the foramina in the roof of the fourth ventricle. The CSF is absorbed in the arachnoid granulations of the major sinuses and thereby removed by venous drainage. Obstruction to the escape of CSF leads to hydrocephalus.

Developmental disorders of the nervous system

A wide range of disorders can affect the nervous system, either as a result of genetic disease or as a result of intrauterine or perinatal injuries. These often result in mental deficiency as discussed later. Some important examples are as follows:

1. *Malformation of head, spine and related parts*
   a. Anencephaly, microcephaly, and macrocephaly
   b. Craniofacial syndromes
   c. Hydrocephalus
   d. Spina bifida
   e. Sturge-Weber syndrome
   f. Intrauterine infections
   g. Fetal alcohol syndrome
2. *Defective development of intellect and abnormalities of speech or motor function*
   a. Mental deficiency of all types
   b. Cerebral palsy
   c. Huntington's chorea
   d. Friedreich's ataxia
   e. Syringomyelia
3. *Hereditary disorders*
   a. Neurofibromatosis
   b. Tuberous sclerosis
   c. Inborn errors of metabolism
4. *Epilepsy*

Anencephaly, microcephaly, and macrocephaly

In anencephaly, microcephaly, and macrocephaly, the size of the brain is abnormal, and the microscopic architecture is also seriously disturbed. Therefore mental defect is characteristic.

Hydrocephalus

Hydrocephalus is characterized by excessive accumulation of CSF within the brain causing distention of the ventricular system and usually atrophy of the surrounding brain. The underlying causes are obstruction to the flow of CSF within the ventricular system or failure of absorption into the venous system. Theoretically, overproduction of CSF is also possible. In addition to the congenital type, hydrocephalus can also be *acquired* as a result for example of previous inflammatory disease or a tumor.

The effect of hydrocephalus depends to some extent on the site of obstruction; two subgroups of internal hydrocephalus can be distinguished.

1. *Obstructive*—Obstruction is at some point within the ventricular system and prevents the CSF from escaping into the subarachnoid space.
2. *Communicating*—Adhesions in the cisternae and subarachnoid pathways on the surface of the brain prevent the fluid from escaping behind the basilar cisternae.

In either case, the ventricular system is dilated, either in part or as a whole.

The effect of internal hydrocephalus is compression of the brain causing atrophy and thinning, usually with destruction of the normal architecture of the cortex.

Congenital hydrocephalus may be present at birth or become apparent sometime afterwards. The head gradually starts to distend a few weeks after birth until it becomes enormously enlarged, the sutures widely dilated, and the skin tightly stretched.

The Arnold-Chiari malformation* probably accounts for more than 60% of cases of hydrocephalus in infancy and consists of herniation of part of the cerebellum and medulla through the foramen magnum. This causes hydrocephalus with compression and atrophy of the surrounding brain substance.

Clinical aspects. The effects are variable. Typical features include mental retardation or dementia, nystagmus, ocular palsies, and spasticity of the legs. The treatment, when feasible, is a surgical shunt from the brain to the right atrium or peritoneum to allow the CSF to bypass the obstruction.

Other causes of hydrocephalus. Communicating hydrocephalus is caused by factors outside the ventricular system, particularly adhesions resulting from meningitis. Infections involving the arachnoid villi may make them impermeable to absorption. Subarachnoid hemorrhage sometimes also obstructs the arachnoid villi with fibrin and blood.

Obstruction to the flow of the CSF can also be caused by tumors compressing the ventricular system. In many cases, however, there is no obvious cause, and it is assumed that there is either overproduction of CSF or inadequate absorption.

Spina bifida

Spina bifida is basically a fusion defect of the vertebral column, particularly of the neural arches and spinal cord. The membranes and cord may protrude on the back.

The embryologic defect may be one of the following;

1. *Somatic ectodermal (cutaneous)*—The cutaneous defects include hypertrichosis (usually a tuft of long hair just above the buttocks), hypoplasia of the skin, or a congenital dermal sinus.
2. *Mesodermal defects*—Vertebral defects include split or absent spinous processes or clefts in the vertebral neural arch. Dural defects include failure of fusion.
3. *Neuroectodermal*—The neural tube may fail to close, and there may be intramedullary or extramedullary growth associated with failure of fusion.

Clinical aspects. Clinical effects depend on the extent of the defect. In its mildest form the defect is asymptomatic and marked only by a tuft of hair in the midline of the lower back. In the most severe type (araphia), the neural tube remains unclosed, and the defective spinal cord containing few nerve cells lies exposed on the infant's back. There is paraplegia, and usually fatal infection starts shortly after birth.

Meningocele. Meningocele consists of a protruding sac of meninges but no nervous tissue. The skin covering the sac and the cord is usually normal.

Meningomyelocele is a protrusion of the spinal cord, which is usually defective, through the vertebral defect in a sac covered by thin atrophic membranes. Symptoms, when present, typically include weakness of the legs, sensory impairment, and frequently disturbances of the bladder and rectal function. Other congenital anomalies may be associated. Rupture of the sac and infection can be rapidly fatal. Meningoceles and the milder meningomyeloceles can sometimes be repaired surgically.

Sturge-Weber syndrome

Sturge-Weber syndrome† is characterized by an angiomatous defect (hamartoma), which develops within the distribution of

---

*J. Arnold (1835-1915), German pathologist; H. Chiari (1851-1916), Austrian pathologist.
†W.A. Sturge (1850-1919), English physician; F. Parkes Weber (1863-1962), English physician.

the trigeminal nerve and also within the skull. When the ophthalmic division is affected, the occipital lobe of the brain is usually involved. When the vascular nevus is facial, the parietal and frontal lobes are usually affected.

Clinically, there are convulsions and mental defect. When the vascular nevus involves the face, it usually extends to the underlying oral mucosa and gums, which are red and sometimes hyperplastic.

Fetal alcohol syndrome

The fetal alcohol syndrome is caused by maternal alcoholism and is characterized by mental deficiency and abnormal facial development with eyes that slant downward laterally and an elongated lower half of the face.

Intrauterine infection

Intrauterine infections, particularly rubella, cytomegalovirus and toxoplasmosis, which are important causes of congenital malformations of the nervous system and of mental defect, have been described in Chapter 8.

Mental deficiency

There are many causes of defective mental development, some of which are associated with cranioskeletal defects; others are metabolic, and yet others are related to congenital infections, as discussed earlier. The more important examples are listed as follows and are discussed in this and other chapters.

1. Anencephaly, microencephaly, and macroencephaly
2. Hydrocephalus, including Arnold-Chiari syndrome
3. Down's syndrome (Chapter 3)
4. Cretinism (Chapter 18)
5. Intrauterine infections, including rubella, toxoplasmosis, and syphilis (Chapter 8)
6. Tuberous sclerosis
7. Sturge-Weber syndrome
8. Cerebral palsy
9. Kernicterus (Chapter 15)
10. Fetal alcohol syndrome
11. Inborn errors of metabolism, particularly phenylketonuria, the mucopolysaccharidoses, and Lesch-Nyhan syndrome (Chapter 3)
12. Simple mental defect*

Cerebral palsy

Cerebral palsy is the popular name given to abnormalities of motor function that have been present since birth or early childhood. The causes include intrauterine or perinatal injuries, including anoxia or ischemia of various parts of the brain and physical injury to the cord during difficult labor. There is often mental defect, but this is hard to assess when the child has difficulty in speaking as a result of impaired motor function (dysarthria).

Although there are many syndromes that can be included under this heading, the main types of cerebral palsy are as follows.

Spastic type. There may be spasticity of both legs with little or no involvement of the arms (spastic diplegia), or both arms and legs may be affected with the arms more severely than the legs. The effects are sometimes asymmetrical. Strabismus (squint), convulsions, and mental retardation are common.

Athetosis. Athetosis is characterized by involuntary jerking movements, often of a wriggling character; it is sometimes accompanied by grimacing. Athetosis is slightly more common than pure spasticity, although the two are often combined in some degree, and probably accounts for about 45% of affected children. The incidence of mental retardation is particularly high in this type.

Ataxia. Ataxia is characterized by loss of neuromuscular coordination as a result of cerebellar damage and usually causes loss of balance or an unsteady gait, with poor control over voluntary movements. It affects only about 10% of those with cerebral palsy.

Huntington's disease

Huntington's disease* is inherited as an autosomal dominant and was first described in the 19th century among a family living in Long Island, New York.

Pathology. The underlying disorder appears to be a deficiency of cerebral transmitter enzymes. There is atrophy of several parts of the brain, particularly the caudate nucleus. Microscopically, there is severe loss of nerve cells and reactive gliosis.

Clinical aspects. Huntington's disease appears in middle adult life and is characterized by chorea—irregular involuntary movements that cause disturbances of speech and gait, usually associated with progressive dementia. Progress of the disease is slow, but life is often ended by intercurrent infection or, sometimes by suicide.

Recently, linked DNA markers for the locus for Huntington's disease have been identified, permitting genetic counselling for affected families.

Friedreich's ataxia

Friedreich's ataxia† is usually inherited as an autosomal recessive trait. The main pathologic feature is degeneration of many tracts of the spinal cord extending up to the brain stem. Degenerative heart disease with myocardial hypertrophy and interstitial fibrosis may be associated.

Following are the clinical features:
1. Onset typically in late childhood
2. Staggering gait and unsteadiness while standing
3. Clumsiness and tremor
4. Muscle weakness and atrophy, skeletal deformities, and sensory loss
5. Early death, often from myocardial disease

Syringomyelia and syringobulbia

Syringomyelia is a rare developmental anomaly characterized by gliosis and the formation of cavities that extend from the central canal of the spinal cord, usually in the lower cervical segments. The effect is to cause atrophy and degenerative changes, particularly of the tracts passing upward and downward in the spinal cord.

Clinically, symptoms usually begin in the second or third decade. Loss of sensation allows burns, injuries, or infections to progress unnoticed. Later involvement of the anterior horn cells causes weakness or paralysis of the hands. Damage to sympathetic fibers causes vasomotor disturbances.

Syringobulbia involves the medulla. The effects include loss of pain and temperature sensation in the distribution of the

---

*Simple mental defect is the term given to failure of intellectual development without other abnormality.

*G. Huntington (1851-1916), American physician.
†N. Friedreich (1852-1882), German neurologist.

trigeminal nerve. Anesthesia and paralysis of the face may be associated, and atrophy and fasciculation of the tongue are among the most common signs. The respiratory or cardiovascular centers are usually not significantly affected.

Neurofibromatosis (von Recklinghausen's disease*)

Neurofibromatosis is inherited as a simple dominant trait. Tumors of the nerve sheath (neurilemomas or neurofibromas) sometimes form in vast numbers (Chapter 19). Glial tumors often complicate cutaneous neurofibromatosis while bilateral acoustic neuromas are characteristic of the central type of neurofibromatosis, as discussed later in this chapter.

Tuberous sclerosis

Tuberous sclerosis is inherited as a simple dominant trait and is characterized by convulsions, mental defects, and adenoma sebaceum. These tumorlike lesions are not adenomas but fibromas, which are characteristically distributed in a butterfly pattern across the cheeks, nose, and forehead. The brain lesions consist of areas of malformed cortex with extensive gliosis. Atypical glial cells and bizarre neurones may be seen.

These patients develop extracranial tumors, typically rhabdomyomas of the heart, or hamartomas in the kidney, liver, adrenal glands, and pancreas.

Epilepsy

Epilepsy is a common disease characterized by disturbances of consciousness with or without convulsions. In the majority of cases, epilepsy is idiopathic and apparently developmental. Secondary epilepsy, which develops in adult life, is typically, a consequence of a cerebral lesion such as a tumor or an abscess.

Idiopathic epilepsy may be caused by birth injury. The immediate cause of a seizure is sudden electrical discharge from neurons of the damaged areas of cortex. This also causes almost immediate disturbances of sensation and loss of consciousness.

Clinically, epilepsy is of three main types: major epilepsy (grand mal), minor epilepsy (petit mal, absence seizures), and temporal lobe epilepsy.

Major epilepsy. Major epilepsy is characterized by recurrent convulsions which follow a regular pattern. There is sudden loss of consciousness and usually a cry caused by contraction of the muscles of the chest and expulsion of air against the closed glottis, and the patient falls to the ground. The limbs become rigid (tonic spasm); there are then violent jerking movements (clonic spasm) and sometimes incontinence.

The violence of the convulsion may be such that the patient injures himself. The convulsion is transient but leaves the patient in a state of coma for 5 to 30 minutes, followed by confusion, drowsiness, and headache.

Minor epilepsy. Petit mal (minor) epilepsy usually affects children from the age of about 4 years until adolescence. It consists of a sudden but brief loss of consciousness, which comes without warning. The alternative names of *absence* and *absence fit* are particularly appropriate. Little or no motor activity accompanies the seizure, which is so brief that the patient does not usually fall. Usually little more is seen than blinking and a sudden, obvious loss of contact with the surroundings.

Temporal lobe epilepsy. Temporal lobe epilepsy is characterized predominantly by disturbances of consciousness often with mental disorder and, sometimes, behavioral problems.

---

*F.D. von Recklinghausen (1833-1910), German pathologist.

Henry James gives a graphic picture of the effects of temporal lobe epilepsy, which accounts for the narrator's strange feelings and visions in his novel *The Turn of the Screw.*

Acquired diseases of the nervous system
Disturbance of consciousness

Coma is a state of unconsciousness with loss of responsiveness to stimuli. A patient can readily be aroused from normal sleep, but in deep coma no reactions can be obtained and reflex activity is lost. Consciousness may be lost immediately (particularly as a result of a head injury) or slowly (as in the case of a tumor) and preceded by confusion and stupor.

Some of the many causes of coma are listed as follows:
1. Toxic and metabolic (systemic) causes
   a. Intoxication (alcohol, barbiturates, opiates)
   b. Metabolic disease (diabetic acidosis, uremia, Addisonian crisis, hepatic coma, hypoglycemia)
   c. Severe systemic infection (pneumonia, typhoid fever, malaria)
   d. Hypoxia
   e. Acute hypotension (circulatory collapse from any cause)
   f. Hypertensive encephalopathy
   g. Hyperthermia and hypothermia
   h. Reye's syndrome
2. Disease of the central nervous system (CNS)
   a. Trauma
   b. Hemorrhage, including subarachnoid, epidural, or subdural bleeding
   c. Cerebral infarction as a result of thrombosis or embolism
   d. Cerebral abscess
   e. Bacterial or viral meningoencephalitis
   f. AIDS (infections and other causes)
   g. Tumors
   h. Raised intracranial pressure from any cause
   i. Epilepsy

These causes differ mainly in the nature of the associated signs, which are discussed in more detail in this and other chapters. There may be multiple causes and (for example) up to 60% of all patients admitted in coma are alcoholics who often have also had a head injury.

Pathology. When neurons are damaged by any of these causes, they first lose their affinity for stains. Later the cell body becomes swollen and rounded, and the nuclear chromatin and Nissl substance (endoplasmic reticulum) fade. Death of the cell causes the neurons to shrink and become angular with pyknotic nuclei and strongly eosinophilic cytoplasm. The myelin sheaths and axon cylinders disintegrate, and the oligodendroglia, which normally clusters around the neurons, also disappears. There is infiltration by polymorphonuclear leukocytes, which become replaced later by histiocytes and compound granular cells (microglia). These gradually remove necrotic debris and become foamy in appearance by ingestion of fatty breakdown products.

Effects on function. The first group of conditions, namely, toxic and metabolic disorders, cause no focal or localizing neurologic signs. However, when there is disease of the CNS itself, sensory or motor disturbances may indicate the site of the lesion. In some of these diseases white cells and bacteria or blood may also appear in the CSF.

Intoxications, whether the result of exogenous agents or disorders of metabolism and severe infections, have essentially similar effects and will not be discussed further here.

Trauma, hemorrhage, infarction, abscess, encephalomyelitis, and tumors of the brain are discussed later.

Anoxic encephalopathy

Following are the main causes of anoxic encephalopathy:
1. Severe hypotension
    a. Shock syndrome
    b. Cardiac arrest
    c. Severe bradycardia
2. Hypoxia
    a. Respiratory failure
    b. Anesthetic accidents
    c. Strangulation or other causes of airway obstruction

Cardiac failure, anemia, or widespread atherosclerosis can be contributory, and several of these factors may be combined.

The severe effects of cerebral anoxia are a result of the sensitivity of neurons to lack of oxygen and the fact that the brain needs an enormous blood supply for normal function. The brain takes 20% of the cardiac output although it accounts for only 2% of the total body weight. Even transient anoxia can cause cerebral damage, while anoxia for more than a few minutes can cause total destruction of intellect and dementia.

Pathology. Transient hypoxia causes minor disturbances of function but no detectable morphologic changes. Total oxygen deprivation for more than a few minutes causes no anatomic changes (other than ultrastructural changes) because death intervenes before these can develop.

Detectable effects of hypoxia are edema of the brain and loss of demarcation between gray and white matter. Damage is sometimes patchy, possibly because of atherosclerosis of some of the vessels. This exacerbates the hypoxia locally. Cell injury becomes visible by light microscopy after 12 hours. In severe cases there are large areas of necrosis of neurons, which are later replaced by glial scars if the patient survives.

Clinical aspects. Anoxia causes coma within less than a minute, but if the circulation and oxygenation of the blood are restored within 3 to 5 minutes, recovery should be complete. Severe hypoxia causes coma with fixed, dilated pupils, inert or rigid limbs, unresponsiveness to all stimuli, and abolition of brain stem reflexes. An electroencephalogram shows no electrical activity: this is termed *brain death.*

The effects of acute cerebral hypoxia are particularly important in anesthesia because they can be readily caused by impaired oxygenation. Because the patient is already unconscious, the effects of anoxia are less obvious. In these circumstances there is often a combination of contributory factors. The anesthetic agent can depress respiration, but there may also be partial (often unnoticed) respiratory tract obstruction. The patient may also have atherosclerotic changes that impair the cerebral circulation. As a consequence, some patients can die, and others can be reduced to a vegetative state as a result of widespread cortical damage.

Vigilant supervision of all patients undergoing anesthesia is therefore, essential. Special care must be taken to ensure that the patient is breathing fully and effectively, that oxygen supplies are adequate, and that no signs of hypoxia, however slight, be allowed to develop.

Raised intracranial pressure

Because of the rigidity of the skull, any increase in the volume of its contents causes a rise of intracranial pressure. This, in turn, tends to impede the venous return from the brain and to further increase the CSF pressure. Cerebral blood flow is thus reduced, but the increased CSF pressure causes a reflex rise in systemic blood pressure in an attempt to maintain an adequate cerebral flow.

Causes of raised intracranial pressure include the following:
1. *Space-occupying lesions*—Hematoma, abscess, and tumor are examples.
2. *Displacement of part of the brain and herniation* (as discussed later) into another compartment
3. *Edema of the brain*—This is most often a consequence of traumatic injury or vascular lesions of the brain. Tumors can cause edema out of proportion to their size.
4. *Obstruction to the flow of cerebral spinal fluid*—Causes include blockage of the aqueduct of Sylvius or adhesions that are the result of meningitis in the subarachnoid space and obstruct the outflow from the ventricles.

Effects of raised intracranial pressure. The effects of raised intracranial pressure depend on the rate of increase of pressure and include the following:
1. Papilledema or bulging of the optic disc with engorgement of its vessels, which can be seen by ophthalmoscopy
2. Headache
3. Vomiting
4. Impaired consciousness
5. Rising systemic blood pressure and reflex slowing of the pulse
6. Herniation of the brain

It is essential to try to relieve the causes of increased intracranial pressure if possible. Lumbar puncture must be very carefully performed. However, it is usually contraindicated because it can precipitate herniation, compression of the medulla, and death.

Herniation of the brain

Herniation is the name given to displacement of part of the brain from one dural compartment to the other. It is a serious consequence of raised intracranial pressure.

Effects of herniation. The effects of herniation depend on the direction of displacement and are of three main types: (1) a large lesion above the tentorium can force part of the brain through the incisura causing compression of the mid-brain; (2) an overall increase in intracranial pressure or a lesion in the posterior fossa can force part of the cerebellum through the foramen magnum causing compression of the medulla and, usually, immediate death; and (3) swelling of one hemisphere can displace the cerebral peduncles laterally against the edge of the tentorium. Herniation can also compress brain substance or blood vessels against the margins of the dura.

Traumatic lesions of the brain

Head injuries with damage to the brain are common. Motor vehicle accidents are the main cause. Among patients with head injuries over 12% die within 2 days, while approximately 50% have persistent aftereffects such as paralysis, loss of speech, impaired vision, epilepsy, or disturbances of personality. Males between the ages of 10 and 40 are mainly affected.

Mechanisms of nonpenetrating brain injuries

The effects of nonpenetrating brain injury are variable and depend on the location, nature, and force of the injury. In most cases several lesions are combined. Brain injury results because the brain is heavier and has much greater inertia than the skull. As a consequence, a blow to the head causes rapid acceleration and deceleration of the skull. The brain accelerates less rapidly so that the skull is driven against the brain. This can happen so violently that the brain is pulled away from the skull at the side opposite to the blow, tearing the meninges and blood vessels.

If the blow is still more severe, the greater momentum causes the brain to be driven against the skull on the side opposite to the blow (contrecoup lesion). There are often also rotational forces that cause shearing of structures within the brain.

Blunt injuries of this sort almost invariably cause loss of consciousness. Maxillofacial trauma is often associated with injuries to the skull, and in such accidents it is essential to decide whether there has been brain injury and assess its severity. On the other hand, because of the relative weakness of the maxillofacial structure, fractures of the facial skeleton can often absorb much of the force of a blow and, thus, prevent injury to the brain.

Concussion

A blow to the head severe enough to cause loss of consciousness, however transient, always causes brain damage. During the period of unconsciousness, reflexes may be suppressed, respiration impaired or stopped, and there may be slowing of the heart and a fall in blood pressure.

In most cases, consciousness returns after some minutes or at most 24 hours, but there is usually loss of memory of the injury and the events immediately beforehand (retrograde amnesia). Headache, irritability, insomnia, and personality changes can persist for months (postconcussional syndrome).

The single most important aspect of the immediate management of injured comatose patients is to make sure that they can breathe. Many, particularly those with maxillofacial injuries, die of respiratory obstruction before they reach the hospital.

Contusion is bleeding into brain tissue without gross disruption of its structure and is in effect a bruise of the brain. A contusion causes a wedge-shaped area of bleeding with ischemic necrosis at the center and is eventually replaced by a scar. In severe cases the leptomeninges are also torn, causing adhesion of the brain to the overlying dura.

Laceration is a tear in the brain tissue, often with severe destruction of neurons and bleeding.

Concussion, contusion, and laceration are often not distinguishable clinically. The effects vary with the site and extent of the damage, but posttraumatic epilepsy affects 20% to 40% of patients and is particularly likely to result from a meningocerebral cicatrix (scar).

Brain damage in boxers. Boxers are at risk from progressive brain damage as a result of repeated concussions (knockouts) with permanent effects as described in the previous section. Occasionally, a boxer may suffer an epidural hematoma or a more massive, acute hemorrhage which may be immediately fatal.

Nevertheless persistently repeated light jabs to the head, without loss of consciousness, appear to be the more important cause of the characteristic brain lesions seen in boxers and the severity of chronic brain damage correlates better with the number of bouts fought than the number of knockouts. The summation of these effects creates the punch-drunk boxer.

The punch-drunk syndrome comprises such features as intellectual impairment, slurred speech, and defective coordination of movement. Deterioration continues long after retirement.

Microscopically, many neurones are lost particularly in parts of the cerebral cortex, brain stem and cerebellum. Neurofibrillary tangles similar to those seen in Alzheimer's disease (p. 513) also form and cells of the substantia nigra are also damaged. In addition to loss of Purkinje cells in the cerebellum, the ventricles become enlarged and the falx cerebri may be split or torn.

Signs of such damage can be found in young amateur boxers long before overt signs of brain damage appear. Sequential magnetic resonance imaging scans should clarify the way in which brain damage develops in boxers.

Cerebrovascular disease
Epidural hematoma

Epidural hematoma is a consequence of bleeding between the skull and dura. The usual cause is a fracture that tears the middle meningeal artery or one of its branches. The hematoma forms a mass, which compresses part of the brain and causes increasing intracranial pressure as it expands.

Clinically, the typical story is of a heavy blow with loss of consciousness. There is usually then a period of apparent recovery (lucid interval) followed by signs of increasing intracranial pressure. If the clot is not removed, death from respiratory arrest follows.

A radiograph showing a fracture line crossing the line of the middle meningeal artery is strongly suggestive of epidural hemorrhage. A CT scan will confirm the diagnosis. The treatment is to drill through (trephine) the skull to drain the clot and to ligate the bleeding vessel.

Subdural hematoma

Bleeding between the dura and the leptomeninges may be acute or chronic. *Acute* subdural hematoma (Fig. 20-1) is often the result of an injury causing a tear in the arachnoid and may be associated with laceration or contusion of the brain.

Clinically, there is a latent interval after the injury followed by progressive deterioration of consciousness and the development of symptoms somewhat similar to those of an epidural hematoma. After coma has developed, up to 50% of patients die.

The main principles of management are to localize the lesion and to evacuate the clot through burr holes. The results are variable and depend on the degree of cerebral damage.

Chronic subdural hematoma can be caused by very mild injury. Nevertheless, the veins between the pia mater and the dura mater are torn. Leakage of blood into the subdural space is very slow. There is a fibroblastic response, and eventually the hematoma becomes enclosed in scar tissue or, occasionally, resorbed.

Clinically, the head injury, especially in an elderly person, may be so slight as to have been forgotten. After several weeks headache, dizziness, slowness of thinking or confusion, and disturbance of consciousness develop. There may be localizing signs such as hemiparesis or aphasia (loss of articulate speech). The picture can, therefore, resemble that of drug intoxication, a brain tumor, or a stroke.

Evacuation of the hematoma usually leads to rapid and complete recovery. If untreated a chronic subdural hematoma eventually causes increasing intracranial pressure, herniation of the brain, and death.

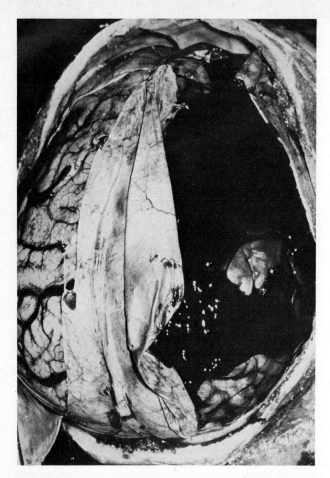

FIG. 20-1. Massive subdural hematoma. A large blood clot entirely fills the subdural space on the right side of the brain. The hemorrhage was the result of a head injury. *(Courtesy Curator of the Gordon Museum, Guy's Hospital, London, England.)*

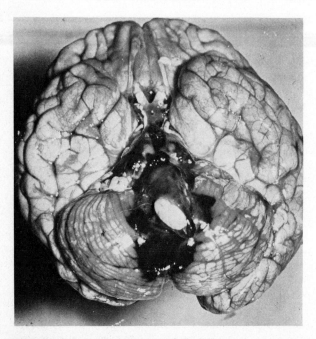

FIG. 20-2. Subarachnoid hemorrhage around the base of the brain caused by rupture of a berry aneurysm of the circle of Willis. *(Courtesy Curator of the Gordon Museum, Guy's Hospital, London, England.)*

Cerebral hemorrhage and other vascular injuries

The brain can be damaged by hemorrhage into its substance or by acute ischemia, a common tragedy known as *stroke*. Strokes are one of the leading causes of death or of severe disability in the United States today. Because atherosclerosis and, particularly, hypertension are usually important contributory factors, strokes mainly affect those of middle age or over. The main types are as follows:

1. Subarachnoid hemorrhage
2. Cerebral hemorrhage
3. Cerebral infarction (thrombosis or embolism)

Subarachnoid hemorrhage

Bleeding into the subarachnoid space accounts for about 10% of cerebrovascular accidents (strokes). The most common cause is rupture of a berry-shaped aneurysm of the circle of Willis (Fig. 20-2). A berry aneurysm results from a localized developmental deficiency of the muscle layer and internal elastic membrane. The vessel wall may therefore consist of little more than the intima at this point; this allows a small saccular aneurysm to form.

Berry aneurysms may reach a centimeter or more in diameter but do not necessarily cause any ill effects. Factors contributing to rupture are hypertension, atherosclerosis, and, often, acute physical or emotional strain.

Rupture of a berry aneurysm causes hemorrhage into the subarachnoid space in its immediate neighborhood. Hemorrhage may, however, be so severe as to burst through the brain substance into the cerebral ventricle.

Clinical aspects. Berry aneurysms rarely cause symptoms except in unusual cases when one grows large enough to press on the third cranial nerve to cause a painful palsy. Such symptoms may precede rupture of the aneurysm.

Aneurysmal subarachnoid hemorrhage typically affects those between 40 and 60 but is the only important cause of strokes in the young. Women are more frequently affected than men.

The typical symptoms are sudden, excruciating headache, quickly followed by coma. If the blood penetrates into a ventricle, death follows within minutes or hours.

If the aneurysm has been leaking slowly, headache and minor neurologic disturbances precede the stroke. Unlike other types of stroke, localizing signs, such as hemiplegia, are rare, but blood is present in the CSF.

Subarachnoid hemorrhage can be confirmed by a CT scan.

Complications. In those that survive the chief complications are rebleeding, cerebral ischemia or hydrocephalus.

Cerebral ischemia is particularly likely in those who survive severe hemorrhages and is the result of arterial spasm which may follow the formation of clot in the subarachnoid space in the region of the major cerebral vessels. In about 65% of cases cerebral ischemia leaves permanent neurologic damage or is fatal.

Hydrocephalus results from occlusion of the subarachnoid space by organizing clot. Failure of clinical improvement and development of a vegetative state are typical effects, but can sometimes be relieved by insertion of a ventriculoperitoneal shunt.

Prognosis. Early diagnosis preferably confirmed by a CT scan is essential. Treatment is highly specialized and may be medical or surgical by clipping the artery. More than a third of patients either die suddenly or within a few days from severe brain damage. About 25% of the survivors may die from recurrent hemorrhage or cerebral ischemia within the following 3 weeks.

Strokes

Cerebral hemorrhage. Cerebral hemorrhage mainly affects those over middle age, particularly those with longstanding uncontrolled hypertension and atherosclerosis. It is a violently sudden event with a high mortality rate as a result of the widespread damage to the brain. Cerebral hemorrhage is the cause of a little over 10% of strokes, but it is the most lethal type.

Pathogenesis and pathology. Most patients are severely hypertensive, and, broadly speaking, the higher the blood pressure, the greater the risk of cerebral hemorrhage. Atherosclerosis is usually also present. A hemorrhagic diathesis is another cause, and intracranial bleeding is one of the most frequent fatal complications of uncontrolled hemophilia. The source of bleeding is often the lenticulostriate branch of the middle cerebral artery.

Bleeding into the brain substance destroys and tears the tissue apart, forming a lesion that expands as bleeding progresses (Fig. 20-3). A large rounded collection of blood with irregular margins is thus formed. The remainder of the brain is distorted, and there is massive cerebral edema. The hemorrhage often ruptures into the ventricular system so that the CSF becomes bloody.

In those who survive, there is rapid exudation of polymorphonuclear leukocytes. Later, microglia begin to appear and become filled with hemosiderin. After about 10 days, fibroblasts from the damaged blood vessels and astrocytes start to form scar tissue. Large lesions can ultimately be converted into cystic scars.

Cerebral infarction. Cerebral infarction probably now accounts for more than 60% of cerebrovascular accidents. Thrombosis is the most common cause. The true incidence of embolism is not known because published figures are contradictory.

Cerebral defenses against ischemia. Several mechanisms, some of which are not understood, help to counteract reduction in cerebral flow. There is widespread intracerebral vasodilatation stimulated by a low oxygen or high carbon dioxide tension in the blood. A network of anastomoses also provides collateral vessels. These protective mechanisms usually limit an infarct to less than the whole area normally supplied by the occluded vessel.

Factors that affect the severity of the effects of ischemia are as follows:
1. Acuteness of onset
2. State of the vessels
3. Level of oxygenation of the blood

Sudden ischemia by an embolus, for example, is likely to cause an infarct, while gradual reduction of the local blood supply by atherosclerosis alone, although it ultimately impairs cerebral function, does not by itself cause infarction.

Cerebral thrombosis. Cerebral thrombosis is one of the most important complications of hypertension and atherosclerosis. For unknown reasons the risk factors are not the same for infarction of the brain as for the heart. Hypertension shows a closer association with brain infarction, while hyperlipidemia is more closely correlated with myocardial infarction.

The most frequent cause of cerebral infarction is thrombosis on an atheromatous plaque. Occlusion develops relatively slowly, and a collateral blood supply sometimes develops. Even so infarction often develops in the most distal areas where the pressure drop is greatest. In other arteries that have no major collaterals, such as the middle cerebral artery, obstruction usually causes widespread infarction.

Occasionally atherosclerotic lesions can lead to infarction, especially in an elderly patient, if for example sudden hypotension or a cardiac arrhythmia reduces the blood supply to the area.

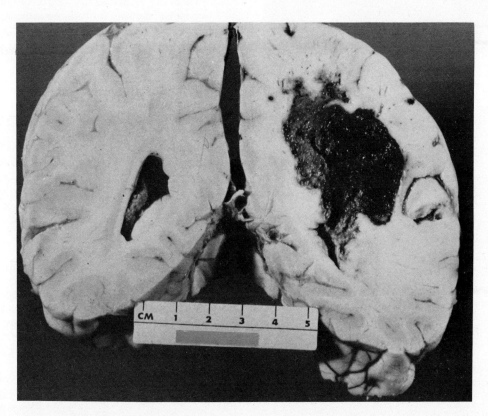

FIG. 20-3. Massive cerebral hemorrhage in a patient with severe hypertension.

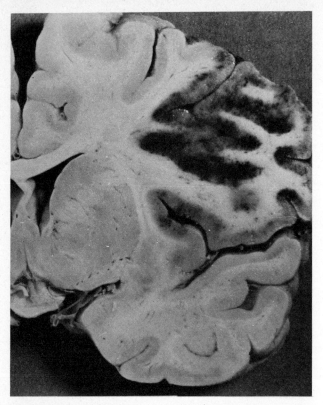

FIG. 20-4. Recent cerebral infarct. An area of the motor cortex shows intense congestion and small areas of hemorrhage. *(Courtesy Curator of the Gordon Museum, Guy's Hospital, London, England.)*

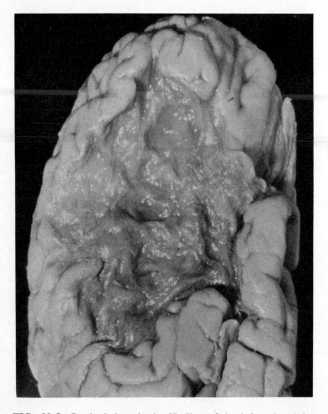

FIG. 20-5. Cerebral thrombosis. Healing of the infarct has left a shrunken and scarred area of brain. *(Courtesy Curator of the Gordon Museum, Guy's Hospital, London, England.)*

Grossly, an infarct of the brain is usually purplish as a result of leakage of red cells into the area. The gray matter also becomes dull and less translucent (Fig. 20-4). Demarcation between the gray and white matter disappears, and after a few days the infarcted area softens. During the following weeks, the necrotic tissue gradually liquefies and is eventually removed. At the same time, glial and fibroblastic proliferation at the periphery defines the extent of the damage. Finally, all that is left is a cystic space with a ragged wall of scar tissue (Fig. 20-5).

Cerebral embolism. The embolus most often originates from thrombus formed in a fibrillating atrium. Other sources are mural thrombus formed after a myocardial infarct or, rarely, vegetations of infective endocarditis or fat embolism from fracture of a long bone.

Smaller vessels are usually obstructed by emboli rather than by thrombosis, and the middle cerebral artery is most frequently affected. The occlusion is, however, more abrupt and complete, and as a consequence the infarct is more extensive than that resulting from thrombosis. Microscopic changes within the infarct are the same whether an embolus or thrombus is the cause.

Clinical aspects of strokes. Men and women are affected approximately equally. Victims are usually past middle age. Younger patients are more likely to have embolic strokes.

Clinically, cerebral hemorrhage, thrombosis, and embolism are often indistinguishable. They differ mainly in the rapidity of onset. The effects depend mainly on the size and site of the lesion, and these can be summarized as follows:

1. *Loss of consciousness*—This may be immediate and, particularly after cerebral hemorrhage, can progress to coma and death.
2. *Hemiplegia* and other localizing signs—Loss of voluntary movement of the side of the body opposite to the lesion is common. The destroyed neurons do not regenerate, but a considerable degree of clinical recovery is possible. Sensory loss may be associated.
3. *Loss of speech* (aphasia)
4. *Raised intracranial pressure*—This is a consequence of continued bleeding and edema after a cerebral hemorrhage.
5. *Blood in the CSF*—This is found mainly after cerebral hemorrhage.

Typical clinical features of the different types of strokes are summarized in Table 20-1.

Transient ischemic attacks. Transient ischemic attacks are repetitive disturbances of neurologic function. There may be hemiplegia or aphasia, but the attacks last only a few minutes or less and repeat the same pattern each time. Function is normal between attacks, but cerebral thrombosis usually eventually follows.

Migraine

Migraine is an important cause of headache. It appears to be biochemically mediated.

Etiology and pathogenesis. The etiology of migraine is unknown but the attack appears to be mediated by the vasoactive agent serotonin. The attack begins with transient vasoconstriction followed by dilatation and stretching of the walls of blood vessels at the base of the brain, especially the external carotid, causing pain.

Attacks often appear to be precipitated by fatigue, stress, or dietary indiscretions. Hereditary factors may also be important.

TABLE 20-1. Typical clinical features of strokes

	Hemorrhage	Thrombosis	Embolism
Prodromal signs	None	Transient ischemic attacks	None
Onset	Sudden	Relatively gradual and variable	Instantaneous
First symptom	Headache in 50%, vomiting	Variable, often ill-defined	Headache often
Development	Rapid hemiplegia and aphasia	Gradual, irregularly intermittent	Almost instantaneous
Associated disease	Hypertension	Hypertension	Atrial fibrillation or other sources of emboli
	Atherosclerosis (hemorrhagic disease occasionally)	Atherosclerosis	
Outcome	75% die within a month	Ranges from minimal dysfunction to death within a week	Recurrence in 80%
Cause of death	Massive cerebral damage or cerebral edema and herniation of brain stem or from other effects of associated disease; myocardial infarction is especially common after cerebral thrombosis		

Clinically, typical migraine is characterized by a defined sequence of events. There is an aura—typically a hallucination of a zigzag pattern of light. Nausea is common, and there is sometimes vomiting and malaise. The headache gradually increases in severity and usually spreads to involve one side of the head (hemicrania). Photophobia is also common. The headache can last for 12 to 24 hours or more. There are many migraine variants, and the vascular disturbance can occasionally be so severe as to cause temporary hemiplegia or aphasia.

Migraine can be aborted in many cases by the use of ergotamine, which has a vasoconstricting effect. Clonidine, which stabilizes the response of vessels to vasoactive substances, or beta blockers are effective prophylactic agents.

Infections of the central nervous system

Infections of the central nervous system are often limited to the membrane of the brain (meningitis). The parenchyma of the brain may be affected generally (encephalitis) or locally (brain abscess). Membranes and parenchyma are involved together in meningoencephalitis.

As a broad generalization viral meningitis is usually a mild disease; by contrast bacterial meningitis and viral encephalitis are typically severe, potentially lethal infections.

A great variety of infections of the central nervous system result from the immunodeficiency characteristic of AIDS. In addition, brain cells have receptors for the human immune deficiency virus so that a variety of syndromes can result from infection of the brain by this virus as discussed later.

Suppurative meningitis

Etiology and pathogenesis. The chief causes of suppurative meningitis are *Haemophilus influenzae, Neisseria meningitidis* (meningococcus), *N. gonorrhoeae,* and *Streptococcus pneumoniae.* The causative organisms differ in different age groups (Table 20-2).

Overall, *H. influenzae* is by far the most common cause of acute meningitis in childhood; the age of highest incidence is at 6 or 7 months. Much less frequently, but next most commonly, meningococci and pneumococci are the cause. From 10 years of age into early adult life, meningococci and pneumococci are the main causes. Meningococcal meningitis was a serious problem in United States Army recruits before the introduction of an effective vaccine.

In later adult life, the pneumococcus becomes increasingly

TABLE 20-2. Important causes of suppurative meningitis

Age	Bacteria		
Neonatal period	Group B streptococci	*Escherichia coli*	*Listeria monocytogenes*
1 to 10 years	*Haemophilus influenzae*	*Neisseria meningitidis*	*Streptococcus pneumoniae*
11 to 20 years		*N. meningitidis*	*S. pneumoniae*
30 to 60 years			*S. pneumoniae*
60 years +	Gram-negative bacilli	Various streptococci	*S. pneumoniae*

important, particularly in those with impaired resistance as a result of alcoholism, splenectomy, or other causes.

The meningococcus is carried in the nasopharynx and sometimes causes epidemics. Spread of the organism to the meninges is by the bloodstream.

In some parts of the world, including Britain, the incidence of meningococcal meningitis has been increasing slowly but this seems to be part of a regular cyclic variation in its incidence. In Britain many of the outbreaks have been due to the hitherto uncommon B 15 strain.

Meningococcal infection (group A) is also being increasingly imported by travellers from the Middle East.

Meningitis caused by *H. influenzae* usually follows upper respiratory tract infection or middle ear infections. Pneumococcal meningitis is usually preceded by pneumonia or an upper respiratory tract infection. Meningitis can also originate from sinusitis, otitis media, and mastoiditis.

A variety of opportunistic infections can develop in patients receiving immunosuppressive treatment, with AIDS or who are debilitated by neoplastic disease. Maxillofacial fractures involving the cribriform plate of the ethmoid, with tearing of the overlying dura and leakage of CSF can also result in meningitis.

Pathology. Infection spreads through the subarachnoid space and therefore involves the cerebral and spinal meninges and the ventricular system. The infection provokes an acute inflammatory reaction in the pia mater and arachnoid so that pus accumulates in this space (Fig. 20-6). Neutrophils predominate in the early stages. Later the exudate may become fibrinous and contain mononuclear cells. The infection can (1) damage structures within the subarachnoid space, particularly cranial and spinal nerve roots, (2) cause thrombophlebitis of the dural

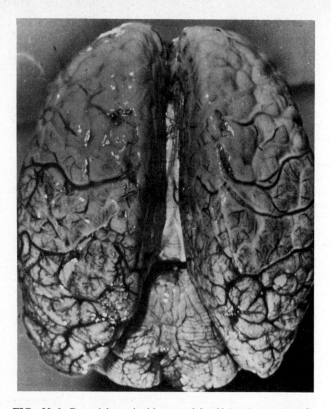

FIG. 20-6. Bacterial meningitis caused by *Neisseria meningitidis.* There is intense inflammation of the meninges and collection of pus in the subarachnoid space. *(Courtesy Curator of the Gordon Museum, Guy's Hospital, London, England.)*

sinuses or bridging veins, (3) interfere with the flow of CSF from the ventricles, and (4) cause adhesions to form between the meninges and the brain later (Fig. 20-7).

Meningococcal septicemia (with or without meningitis) also causes purpura (spotted fever). Widespread disseminated intravascular coagulation may develop.

Clinical aspects. The patient may already have an infection such as pneumonia. The onset of meningitis is marked by severe headache, drowsiness, stupor or coma, and occasionally convulsions. An important clinical sign is stiffness of the neck.

Meningococcal infection (Fig. 20-8) should be suspected when meningitis develops in an apparently fit person and particularly during an outbreak. A purpuric rash is a characteristic feature; fulminating septicemia can cause vasomotor collapse, shock, and death, as 10% to 20% of patients with meningococcemia have acute adrenocortical failure as a result of bleeding into the adrenal cortex (Waterhouse-Friedrichsen syndrome) (Chapter 18).

The mortality rate of hemophilus or meningococcal meningitis has remained at 5% to 15% for many years. Pneumococcal meningitis has a high mortality rate in alcoholics or patients with other diseases, particularly pneumonia and endocarditis.

Diagnosis depends mainly on the gram-stained smear and culturing the organism from a specimen of CSF. Vigorous antibiotic treatment should then be started. If this is promptly done, the overall mortality rate is low, but about 20% of patients have permanent neurologic damage especially after *H. influenzae* infections. Such damage may include hydrocephalus, cranial nerve injuries (blindness, deafness, or palsies), seizures, or mental retardation.

Where there is a risk of spread of meningococcal infection,

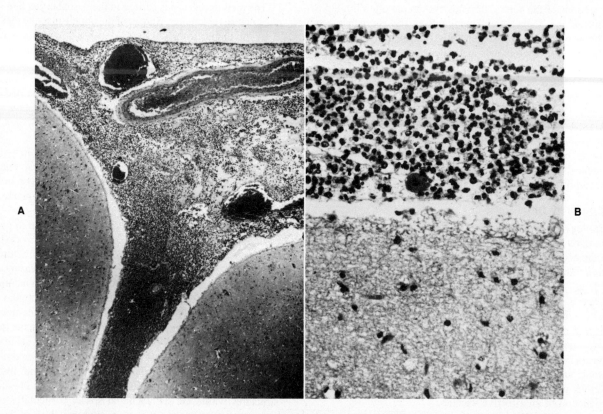

FIG. 20-7. Acute bacterial meningitis. **A,** The subarachnoid space is filled with pus and several small vessels are thrombosed. **B,** Higher magnification shows that the inflammatory reaction is present only in the meninges *(top)* and not in the brain substance *(bottom).*

antibiotic prophylaxis may be indicated. For this purpose rifampicin is suitable, particularly for otherwise resistant meningococci such as group A.

Granulomatous meningitis

Granulomatous meningitis is usually caused by *Mycobacterium tuberculosis* or, more frequently now as a result of the AIDS epidemic, *Cryptococcus neoformans.*

Tuberculous meningitis is usually secondary to pulmonary infection or is a feature of miliary infection. Cryptococcal meningitis is usually also secondary to pulmonary infection and is the most important extrapulmonary complication. It is particularly likely to affect patients debilitated by AIDS, lymphoma, Hodgkin's disease, or immunosuppressive treatment.

Clinically, granulomatous meningitis is relatively slow in onset with malaise, headache, and low-grade fever together with the development of signs of meningeal irritation.

Lyme disease

This infection by *Borellia burgdorferi* usually causes arthritis (Chapter 17) as its most prominent and persistent effect. However symptoms of meningeal irritation may accompany the characteristic rash. Months or weeks later a small minority of patients develop neurologic abnormalities such as self-limiting meningitis with fluctuating symptoms, cranial neuritis (particularly bilateral facial palsy) and radicular neuritis (intense pain resembling referred pain and radiating widely within the distribution of the nerve root). The CSF shows a mild lymphocytosis and raised protein levels.

Brain abscess

Most of these focal suppurative intracranial infections are secondary to chronic ear, sinus, or pulmonary infections. Ap-proximately 50% of brain abscesses are secondary to disease of the middle ear and mastoid. Most of the remainder are metastatic infections from a primary source in the lung such as bronchiectasis, empyema, or lung abscess. Other sources of infection may be the mouth, skin, or bone. Patients with congenital heart disease, particularly those with left to right shunts, are also at risk. In up to 10% of cases the source of infection cannot be found. Cerebral abscess is very rarely a consequence of infective endocarditis.

Etiology and pathology. Approximately one third of brain abscesses are caused by anaerobic bacteria such as *Bacteroides* species or peptostreptococci. In another third, anaerobes are associated with aerobic bacteria while the remainder are due to aerobic bacteria.

The pathologic process is essentially that of abscess formation anywhere, that is, necrosis, edema, and intense infiltration with leukocytes. Destruction and liquefaction of brain substance causes formation of an abscess, which becomes surrounded by a wall of granulation tissue (Fig. 20-9). A dense capsule may eventually be formed by fibrosis and gliosis.

Clinical aspects. An established cerebral abscess characteristically produces the signs and symptoms of increased intracranial pressure and localizing signs such as hemiparesis, hemianopia, and seizures.

A brain abscess can be visualized by radiographic scanning techniques unless it is very small. An electroencephalogram can also be used to localize the site of an abscess. Sometimes, however, surgical exploration is needed to confirm the diagnosis.

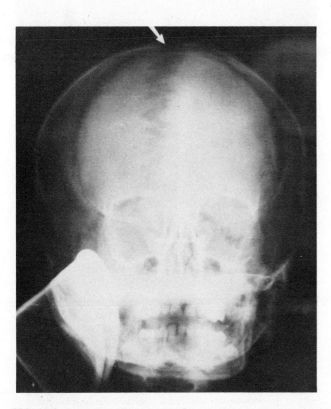

FIG. 20-8. Separation of the sutures of the skull *(arrow)* by increased intracranial pressure in meningococcal meningitis.

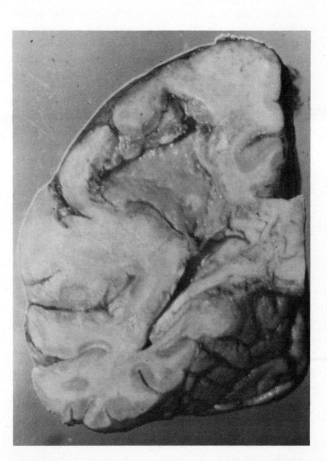

FIG. 20-9. A large brain abscess. The source of the infection was pulmonary infection; the patient had severe bronchiectasis. *(Courtesy Curator of the Gordon Museum, Guy's Hospital, London, England.)*

Treatment is by adequate doses of appropriate antimicrobial drugs immediately after the diagnosis has been confirmed, followed when necessary by aspiration or drainage. In spite of advances in diagnosis and treatment, the mortality rate remains between 30% to 40%.

Viral meningitis

Infection of the meninges can be caused by several different viruses. In the United States the main causes are coxsackieviruses A and B and echoviruses. In meningitis caused by these agents, there is little involvement of brain tissue, and the infections (unlike bacterial meningitis) are generally mild and self-limiting. Viral meningitis is often called *aseptic* because bacterial cultures are sterile.

Pathogenesis and pathology. Infection by enteroviruses is acquired by ingestion of the viruses, which reach the nervous system by way of the intestinal lymphatics and bloodstream. The meningeal vessels become engorged and dilated, but there is little inflammatory cellular exudate. Typically, when the cerebrospinal fluid is examined, only a few hundred lymphocytes per cubic micrometer are found.

Clinical aspects. The disease is characterized by fever, followed by severe headache, neck stiffness, and photophobia. A transient erythematous rash may appear especially in echovirus infections. In nearly all cases there is resolution of the meningitis with no apparent sequelae. In a few cases transient muscle paralysis caused by coxsackie viruses A7 and A9 may develop. There is no specific treatment available.

Encephalitis (meningoencephalitis)

Inflammation of the brain can also be caused by viruses, but these differ from those which cause viral meningitis and the effects are severe. However, it should be noted that some degree of meningitis is frequently associated with encephalitis, although the latter dominates the clinical picture. *Meningoencephalitis* is, therefore, a better term for these diseases.

The viruses that cause meningoencephalitis are the arboviruses, *Herpes simplex,* varicella-zoster virus, rabies virus, certain enteroviruses, and mumps virus. Rarely, encephalitis is associated with influenza and vaccinia viruses. Poliomyelitis in which there is inflammation of the spinal cord and/or brain, is a unique form of encephalomyelitis in that only motor nerve cells are involved.

The incidence and causes of encephalitis vary widely from country to country and within different areas of the United States. In 1975, for example, over 4000 cases of encephalitis were reported in the United States (Table 20-3). The arboviruses, particularly St. Louis encephalitis virus, were the most important single cause and accounted for 49% of the total.

TABLE 20-3. Cases of encephalitis reported in 1975 in the United States*

Causes	Percentage (%)
Arboviruses	49.0
Enteroviruses	3.2
Childhood infections, especially mumps	5.5
Associated with respiratory tract infections	0.3
Other viruses (mostly *Herpes simplex*)	2.3
Undetermined causes	39.7

*Total cases reported, 4308.

St. Louis encephalitis. The highest incidence of St. Louis encephalitis is in the late summer and early fall and particularly affects infants and elderly. The infection is mosquito-borne, and the reservoirs of infection are birds, including poultry.

Pathology. There is nonsuppurative inflammation with edema, hyperemia, and occasional petechiae. The meninges are infiltrated by mononuclear cells, and there are focal accumulations of inflammatory cells and a glial reaction in the brain substance (Fig. 20-10). Characteristic degenerative changes develop in the neurons. The effects are most severe in the thalamus and brain stem and both gray and white matter are involved. There is usually a leukocytosis in the blood and a lymphocytosis in the CSF.

Clinical aspects. The infection may be mild or asymptomatic and detectable only by the development of antibodies. In more severe cases there is often prodromal lassitude, malaise, headache, high fever, stiff neck, confusion, and blurring of vision. Neck rigidity and increased reflexes develop, and there may be signs of involvement of the motor tracts of the cord or of various cranial nerves. There may be coarse tremors of the fingers and tongue together with apprehension, confusion, and delirium. In fatal cases there is a persistently high temperature, stupor, and coma. In 1975 the mortality rate was 7%, but it has been as high as 25% in earlier epidemics. The diagnosis can be confirmed by the rising titer of antibodies.

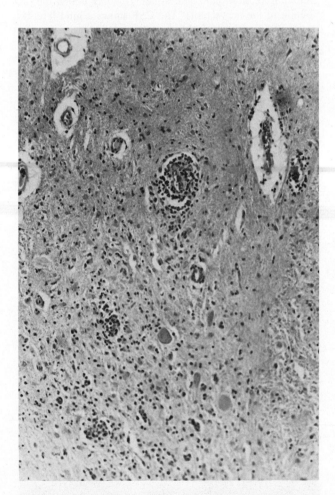

FIG. 20-10. The histologic features of viral encephalitis include widening of the perivascular spaces and a perivascular lymphocytic infiltrate (perivascular cuffing).

Rabies

Rabies is spread by dogs, many other domestic and wild animals, and bats. Infection is usually the result of a bite, but contact with infected saliva or inhalation of dust from bat droppings can also transmit the infection.

In spite of the thousands of cases of rabies detected each year among animals, human infection is surprisingly rare in the United States, although it appears that some cases are misdiagnosed. Thus in two dramatic incidents, rabies was inadvertently transmitted with fatal results by means of corneal transplants. The donors, who died of unknown causes, were later found to have had rabies.

The pathologic changes in rabies are those of an encephalitis, with viral invasion of neurons. The characteristic histologic finding is the Negri body, an eosinophilic cytoplasmic inclusion (Fig. 20-11). Acute viral myocarditis has also been described and may partly account for the fatal outcome of most cases of rabies.

The incubation period can be several months. The onset is then nonspecific with headache, fever, and malaise. If the disease has been caused by a bite by a rabid animal, there are paresthesias around the wound. The characteristic effect of rabies infection is extreme hypersensitivity of the central nervous system to slight stimuli, which cause violent neuromuscular excitability, uncontrollable muscle spasms, or convulsions.

This well-known picture does not develop in the paralytic form of rabies, which is rare and not readily recognizable as such.

There are disturbances of consciousness, confusion, and hallucinations, at first with lucid intervals, until the patient lapses into coma. The disease is virtually uniformly fatal with an average survival of about 4 days after the onset of symptoms.

There is no effective treatment for the fully developed disease but because of the long incubation period, immunization after infection may effectively prevent development of the disease. Human diploid cell vaccine should be given on suspicion to anyone who has been in contact with a rabid animal even if there is no obvious wound.

Herpetic encephalitis

Herpetic infection is common, but encephalitis is a rare complication. Nevertheless the herpes simplex virus is the most common cause of encephalitis in temperate climates. About 15% of patients who develop the disease may give a history of recurrent herpes labialis. In other cases herpetic encephalitis appears to be a primary infection, but though the route by which the virus reaches the brain in either case is speculative, hematogenous spread seems the most probable. The pathologic effects are unusual and consist of patches of necrosis, inflammation, and thrombosis of related blood vessels, usually in the temporal and parietal lobes. Typically, neurons and glial cells contain nuclear eosinophilic inclusion bodies.

The clinical effects are highly variable. Early symptoms are sometimes mistaken for drunkenness or psychosis and include disorientation, personality changes, hallucinations, and ataxia. Other effects include stupor, seizures, skeletal and cranial nerve paralysis, and sensory loss. Coma is often preterminal.

The diagnosis can only be confirmed with certainty, in the early stages, by brain biopsy.

Herpetic encephalitis if not treated early is frequently fatal and in those that survive, permanent neurologic damage is common. The prognosis of herpetic encephalitis has improved considerably as a result of the introduction of acyclovir. Intravenous administration of acyclovir on suspicion has largely eliminated the need for brain biopsy and has significantly reduced both the mortality and disability among survivors.

Poliomyelitis

Poliomyelitis is an acute viral infection that is predominantly asymptomatic but can cause widespread paralysis and sometimes death. It is presently uncommon in countries where mass immunization has been practiced.

Etiology. Poliovirus is a typical enterovirus; three serotypes are known and the virus can remain viable in water or sewage for several months. Epidemics have broken out from time to time in various parts of the world and in areas of poor sanitation, antibodies usually develop in early childhood, but in more highly developed communities, immunity may not be acquired until adolescence or not at all. The disease is mainly transmitted by human carriers. The intestinal tract is the main source from which the virus spreads, and the infection has a fecal-oral mode of transmission.

Pathogenesis and pathology. The pathogenesis of poliovirus infection is decribed in Chapter 8 (see also Fig. 8-10).

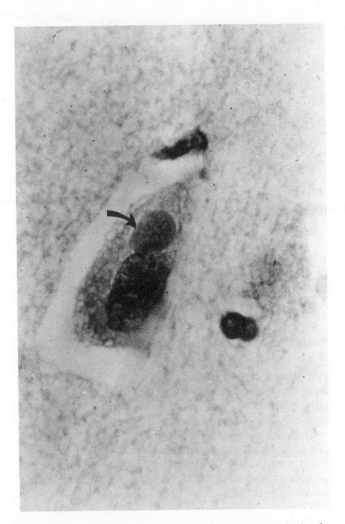

FIG. 20-11. A section from the hippocampal area of the brain of a rabid dog. A neuron containing the typical cytoplasmic inclusion body (Negri body) of rabies is shown *(arrow). (From McCracken AW and Cawson RA: Clinical and oral microbiology, Washington DC, 1982, Hemisphere Publishing Corp.)*

Microscopically, poliomyelitis causes degeneration and destruction of the cells of the anterior horns of the spinal cord, the motor nuclei of the cranial nerves, and the Betz cells of the motor cortex (Fig. 20-12). An inflammatory reaction with a lymphocytic infiltrate surrounds the damaged or necrotic neurons.

Four main areas of the central nervous system may be affected, causing the following types of paralytic disease:

1. *Spinal poliomyelitis* may involve any segment of the cord alone or several in combination.
2. *Bulbar poliomyelitis* involves cranial nerves and sometimes the cardiorespiratory center, causing respiratory tract paralysis.
3. *Bulbospinal poliomyelitis,* as the name implies, involves both medulla and cord. Paralysis of any of the muscles supplied by the spinal or cranial nerves and also cardiorespiratory paralysis can result.
4. *Polioencephalitis* may be the sole manifestation or may be combined with bulbar or spinal paralytic disease. The sensory neurons are not involved; this suggests that there are specific receptors for polioviruses on the surface of motoneurons only.

Clinical aspects. The incubation period varies from 3 to 35 days, and there are four types of infection:

1. Subclinical (inapparent) infection accounts for 95% of cases.
2. "Minor illness" consists of influenza-like symptoms only.
3. Nonparalytic poliomyelitis consists of "minor illness" together with signs of meningeal irritation and lymphocytosis in the CSF.
4. Paralytic poliomyelitis.

Paralytic poliomyelitis starts with symptoms similar to those of the nonparalytic forms; but muscular weakness (paresis) or paralysis often develops within 2 days and is preceded by severe cramping pain in the muscles (Fig. 20-13). Common effects are paresis of one or several limbs and in the worst cases, usually in those patients over 16 years old, respiratory tract paralysis. The extent of muscular paralysis tends to increase with the patient's age.

Bulbar poliomyelitis is characterized by cranial nerve paralysis and involvement of the medulla. The incidence varies widely, but approximately 85% of patients who have had tonsillectomy within 30 days of the onset of the disease develop bulbar infection.

Respiratory paralysis can result either from damage to the respiratory center or from paralysis of the thoracic muscles and diaphragm without involvement of the medulla.

The overall mortality rate is about 5% and is highest in adults. The fatality rate of bulbospinal poliomyelitis varies between 25% and 75%. Among patients with paralytic disease, some muscle function usually returns.

In the United States live attenuated strains of poliovirus are given by mouth (Sabin vaccine*). These colonize the gastrointestinal tract and stimulate antibody production. The level of protection is over 90%. Of the three attenuated types used for immunization, type 3 can apparently regain neurovirulence and cause paralytic disease in the nonimmune recipients of the vaccine or, more often, their nonimmune contacts. Killed (Salk**) vaccines have been equally successful in other countries in controlling poliomyelitis.

---

*A.B. Sabin (b. 1906), American microbiologist.

**J.E. Salk (b. 1914), American microbiologist.

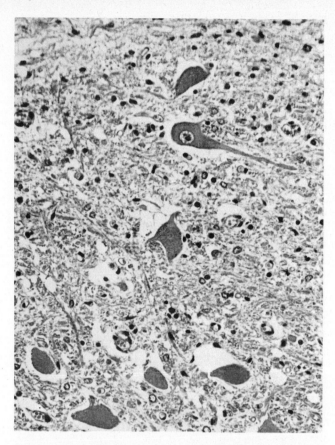

FIG. 20-12. Poliomyelitis. Section of anterior horn of cord showing destructive effects of poliovirus on motoneurons, many of which have lost their nuclei. *(From McCracken AW and Cawson RA: Clinical and oral microbiology, Washington DC, 1982, Hemisphere Publishing Corp.)*

Bulbar palsy

Bulbar palsy is the name given to weakness or paralysis of muscles supplied by the medulla. These are the tongue, pharynx, larynx, sternomastoid, and upper trapezius. Acute bulbar palsy can be the result of poliomyelitis or diphtheria. A chronic form of the disease is progressive bulbar palsy (a rare degenerative motor system disease) or can be due to tumors or aneurysms of the posterior fossa.

Postinfectious encephalomyelitis

Postinfectious encephalomyelitis is an uncommon complication of several viral infections, including mumps and rubella or less commonly, influenza. It is thought to be immunologically mediated and is characterized by scattered foci of demyelination throughout the brain and cord.

Clinically, the onset is usually within a week after the start of a viral infection. Headache and fever may be followed by stupor, convulsions, and severe neurologic impairment. The disorder is usually transient and self-limiting, but after measles the mortality rate may be up to 20%.

Reye's syndrome

Reye's syndrome* is a rare cause of encephalopathy and liver damage in childhood. It is frequently fatal and survivors

---

*R.D.K. Reye (1912-1977), Australian pathologist.

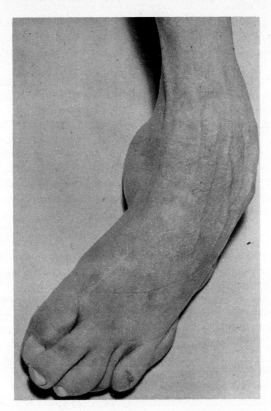

FIG. 20-13. Peripheral nerve paralysis in poliomyelitis. Because of lower motor neuron destruction, the patient has paralysis of the peroneal muscles, resulting in a club foot. *(Courtesy Curator of the Gordon Museum, Guy's Hospital, London, England.)*

may have permanent neurologic damage. Its current importance is its epidemiologic association with the administration of aspirin to children, particularly those who have a viral infection (Chapter 15).

Pathologic changes include cerebral edema and abnormalities of mitochondrial structure and function, best seen in the liver. Biochemical findings include hyperammonemia, hypoglycemia, raised aspartate aminotransferase levels and prolonged prothrombin time.

Liver failure with intense fatty change and glycogen depletion accounts for the mortality rate of about 30%.

Guillain-Barré syndrome (infective or idiopathic polyneuritis)

Guillain-Barré syndrome* essentially comprises (1) motor weakness, (2) abolition of tendon reflexes, (3) absence of pain and tenderness in muscles, and (4) an increase in CSF protein without a corresponding increase in cells. It is thought to be an immunologically mediated disorder similar to postinfectious encephalitis. A variety of infections, especially viral, and vaccination can precede the disease. Many cases followed the vaccination program against swine influenza in the United States in 1976.

Microscopically, there is segmental demyelination of spinal nerve roots and peripheral nerves together with inflammatory changes.

*C. Guillain (1876-1961), French neurologist; J.A. Barré (1880-1967), French neurologist.

Clinically, persons of any age can be affected, and the picture can range from bilateral facial palsy with minor motor and sensory loss in the limbs, to fulminating disease with raised intracranial pressure, quadriplegia, and respiratory paralysis. Sudden respiratory paralysis develops in 10% to 20% of cases and is fatal unless immediate mechanical ventilation can be given.

The disease usually reaches peak severity within about a week, then gradually subsides after about 3 weeks. The majority of patients recover slowly, but between 10% and 30% have severe residual disabilities after a year.

Chronic "slow virus" encephalitis

Slow virus infections are discussed in Chapter 8.

Neurosyphilis

Syphilis (Chapter 23) can affect the nervous system in the tertiary stage, but this is now rare in treated syphilis. There may be an interim phase of asymptomatic syphilitic meningitis a few years after the primary lesion. This is characterized by lymphocytosis and reactive serologic tests in the CSF. Later, if symptomatic neurosyphilis develops, it takes one of the following forms.

Meningovascular neurosyphilis. Meningovascular neurosyphilis is characterized by mononuclear infiltration of the leptomeninges, particularly in the region of the optic chiasma and brain stem. There is typical syphilitic endarteritis and occasionally gumma formation. The early symptoms are highly variable, but the late effects may be hydrocephalus or paralysis of the second, third, and eighth cranial nerves.

Paretic neurosyphilis. Paretic neurosyphilis is characterized by widespread destruction of nerve cells, which causes atrophy of the entire brain. Microscopically, there is perivascular inflammation and transformation of the microglia into rod cells. This type of syphilis begins insidiously with subtle mental disturbance and progresses to severe personality changes, complete dementia, and widespread paralyses (general paralysis of the insane, GPI).

Tabes dorsalis. Tabes dorsalis (locomotor ataxia) is characterized predominantly by atrophy of the posterior nerve roots in the lumbar region and sometimes also of the optic nerves. Clinically, tabes dorsalis is characterized by sudden, lightning-like attacks of pain and paresthesias of the leg or trunk. There is also loss of normal pain sensation, vibration sense, and deep proprioceptive reflexes. These cause the peculiar tabetic gait where the most obvious feature is the way in which the feet are slapped onto the ground because any sense of their position is lost. The pupils are also fixed, unequal, and unresponsive to light (Argyll Robertson pupils*).

Acquired immune deficiency syndrome (AIDS)

As mentioned earlier a variety of infections of the nervous system are well recognized features of AIDS. Important examples are listed as follows:

1. Infections
   a. Viral (proven or probable)
      (1) Herpetic encephalitis
      (2) Varicella zoster encephalitis
      (3) Progressive multifocal leukoencephalopathy
      (4) Subacute encephalitis†‡

*D.M.C.L. Argyll Robertson (1837-1909), Scottish ophthalmic surgeon.
†Probably caused by HIV itself.
‡The most common of the reported infections.

(5) "Aseptic meningitis"*†
(6) Viral myelitis
b. Bacterial, fungal or parasitic
(1) *Toxoplasma gondii*†
(2) *Cryptococcus neoformans*†
(3) *Candida albicans*
(4) Coccidioidomycosis
(5) *Aspergillus fumigatus*
(6) *Treponema pallidum*
(7) Mycobacterioses (tuberculous or nontuberculous)
(8) Other bacteria rarely
2. Tumors
a. Lymphoma
b. Kaposi's sarcoma

In addition, the human immune deficiency virus itself can infect the brain, either in association with typical features of AIDS or in the absence of overt immunodeficiency. *AIDS encephalopathy* can take many forms. It has been estimated that in about 10% of cases, neurologic symptoms precede any others; in about 49% of cases they are associated with signs of immunodeficiency while in the remainder they appear after the typical manifestations of AIDS. Overall, subacute encephalitis is found in 90% of patients at autopsy. The virus has been isolated from the brains of patients who have died with AIDS-related dementia and has also been isolated, in one series, from the CSF of 30 of 48 seropositive persons with or without neurologic disease. It has also been reported that noncytocidal variants of the AIDS virus, which do not kill CD4 (helper) lymphocytes, have been isolated from patients with neurologic disease.

Clinically, the effects may be acute, subacute or chronic. Acute manifestations tend to coincide with the appearance of antibodies to HIV and take the form of acute encephalopathy, meningitis or acute neuropathy. Encephalopathy is generally associated with fever, malaise, mood changes, and sometimes epileptiform fits. Neuropathy is frequently manifested as facial palsy associated with sensory and motor impairment in the limbs. Gradual improvement may take place in the ensuing months.

Subacute encephalitis is the most common neurologic effect of AIDS. Typical features are increasingly severe confusion and a state resembling psychological depression (as a reaction to the illness), accompanied by fever and mild metabolic abnormalities. Progressive multifocal leukoencephalopathy has also been reported. In the late stages the patient becomes bedridden, incontinent, and demented.

In this syndrome there is pleocytosis and a rise in protein concentration in the CSF, while CT scans show cerebral atrophy, indicated by dilated ventricles and prominent cortical sulci. Microscopically, the white matter stains abnormally and appears pale, and there is vacuolar myelopathy of the cord which appears as a bubbly change in the myelin sheaths. Virus is usually detectable in macrophages and giant cells, and may also be present in brain endothelial cells.

Other reported changes include infarcts resulting from vascular occlusion or intracranial hemorrhage, central pontine myelinosis and foci of necrotizing leukoencephalopathy in pontocerebellar fibers.

In children with HIV infection, 75% develop encephalopathy. The effects include microcephaly, cognitive defects and pareses. Calcification of the basal ganglia is common and may be associated with abnormalities of the white matter and atrophy.

Overall, however, the degree of nervous system dysfunction is disproportionately great for the amount of detectable structural damage.

Currently, the mechanisms of brain damage by the AIDS virus are unclear. The virus may attack brain cells directly by binding to the CD4 receptor or may have an indirect action mediated by infected macrophages. There is evidence that the virus directly infects glial cells but, alternatively or in addition it may inhibit the action or formation of peptides necessary for the maintenance or survival of nervous tissue.

Viral budding from glial cells has been reported and it seems likely that infection is maintained by release of virus from macrophages. However, very little HIV is found in the brain, compared with the amount detectable in the immune system and its detection by electron microscopy is laborious.

It may be noted that another retrovirus, HTLV I also causes neurologic disease in humans, namely tropical spastic paresis, a common disease resembling multiple sclerosis, in the tropics. Closely related retroviruses cause neurologic disease in animals. The visna virus of sheep, however causes brain damage secondary to inflammation and does not attack the immune system.

In addition to brain infection by the AIDS virus itself, other agents such as cytomegalovirus may be associated and complicate the picture. The manifestations of neurosyphilis are also modified by AIDS and there can be infection of the brain by several different microbes simultaneously. Central nervous system infections and tumors seen in AIDS are listed on p. 509-510.

Degenerative and demyelinating disease of the CNS
Parkinson's disease (paralysis agitans)

Parkinson's disease* is common and of unknown cause. The incidence of the disease increases with age. It is characterized by impaired initiation and fine control of muscular activity. Paralysis is not a typical feature despite the name of the disease.

A similar clinical disorder can be the result of a variety of causes including the aftereffects of encephalitis, atherosclerotic infarcts, poisoning with manganese or carbon monoxide, and, in a minority of cases, drug treatment, particularly with phenothiazine tranquilizers.

Pathogenesis and pathology. Parkinson's disease is a disorder of extrapyramidal function; the basic mechanism is an imbalance between cholinergic and dopaminic activity. The reduced dopaminic activity is associated with degenerative changes in the basal ganglia, and it has become apparent that the symptoms of Parkinson's disease result solely from cell death in the substantia nigra. This finding results from the observation in 1982, of severe Parkinson's disease in drug addicts who had been injecting "synthetic heroin" produced locally. A report had also been published in 1979, of a student who had developed parkinsonian symptoms as a result of using a meperidine-like drug, methylphenyl-propionoxy-piperidine (MPPP) contaminated with methylphenyl-tetrahydropyridine (MPTP). This student finally died of an overdose and at au-

---

*Probably caused by HIV itself.
†The most common of the reported infections.

---

*James Parkinson (1755-1824), English physician.

topsy, severe depletion of the cells of the substantia nigra was found. In a long and complex story full of ironies it was later found that MPTP is oxidized to a more toxic compound, methylphenylpyridium ion MPP+. One of the enzymes involved in this process is monoamine oxidase and trials of selective monoamine oxidase inhibitor drugs have suggested that these may improve some cases of Parkinson's disease.

However, it is not clear how important is the role of MPTP in Parkinson's disease in general, although it does at least suggest that environmental factors could contribute to the causation of the disease. Currently the chief importance of these findings is to confirm that the selective damage to the substantia nigra alone will produce all the features of Parkinson's disease including even the oily skin.

Other evidence for environmental factors in the etiology of neurologic disease is the exceptionally high incidence of the latter in Guam in the Marianas, where flour is made from the seeds of cycads (a primitive fern-like tree). In Guam neurologic disease takes a variety of forms and may be Parkinson-like or sometimes resemble Alzheimer's disease.

Microscopically, the most striking changes in Parkinson's disease are seen in the substantia nigra where most of the neurons disappear and are replaced by glial cells. The normal pigment of this part of the brain is taken up by phagocytes. Round eosinophilic intracytoplasmic inclusions (Lewy bodies) appear in the residual neurons. The changes are less severe in other parts of the basal ganglia and consist of nonspecific degenerative changes.

Clinical aspects. Typical features of idiopathic Parkinson's disease include the following:

1. Onset in middle or old age
2. Coarse tremor of a hand or leg suppressed by active movement
3. Reduced spontaneous movements (akinesia), stiffness of muscles, immobile (masklike) facial expression, and monotonous voice
4. Stooping posture and quick shuffling gait

Secondary Parkinson's disease or parkinsonian manifestations such as those caused by drugs, all develop at a much earlier age. The only exception is atherosclerotic Parkinson's disease which typically manifests itself in old age.

Levodopa, a precursor of dopamine, is able to cross the blood brain barrier and is effective in the control of Parkinson's disease. Selegeline, a selective monoamine oxidase inhibitor, enhances the effects of levodopa and may possibly inhibit the formation of MPP in those with MPTP-induced disease. Secondary parkinsonism, however, may be worsened by levodopa and responds to drugs which block the action of acetylcholine.

Apart from side effects and the fact that treatment has to be for the remainder of the patient's life, the chief limitation of levodopa is that after a time it may become less effective and does not control the progress of the disease. Currently, though it is controversial, there is great interest in reports that implantation into the brain of adrenal tissue (as a source of dopamine) is effective in controlling Parkinson's disease and may possibly obviate the need for drugs.

Multiple sclerosis

Multiple sclerosis (MS) is the most common chronic neurologic disease. It is characterized by episodes of weakness and paralysis, which can progress to complete disability and incapacity after several years. The basic lesions consist of patches of demyelination throughout the central nervous system.

Etiology. The etiology of multiple sclerosis is unknown but viruses and abnormal immune responses are currently favored. Several aspects of the epidemiology are however firmly established. The disease is rare in the warmer climates directly above and below the equator, but thereafter it becomes more common as the latitude increases. The prevalence of multiple sclerosis is, for example, six times higher in Winnipeg than in New Orleans. Furthermore, if an adult moves from a high-risk to a low-risk area, the high level of risk is maintained.

However, the risk is lessened by migration from a high-risk area before the age of about 15, although it has been argued that there are too few cases on which to base firm conclusions about the effect of age and level of risk. A factor complicating this geographical risk factor is that some races such as the Japanese and Blacks are considerably less susceptible to the disease, but even these groups may show some North-South gradient of incidence.

A familial pattern is recognizable, but no consistent genetic pattern is evident and the vulnerability of close relatives to the disease is also consistent with exposure to an environmental factor. However, persons who are HLA B7 have a twofold to threefold greater risk of acquiring the disease while Northern Europeans who are HLA DR2 have a fourfold to fivefold greater risk. In persons of Mediterranean origin an increased susceptibility is associated with HLA DR4. The level of risk is yet further increased in those who also carry the GM marker. The latter is located in the gene region that codes for immunoglobulin production. Further evidence of genetic factors is that the concordance rate for identical twins may be as high as 40%.

Infective agents suspected of precipitating MS are chiefly the paramyxoviruses such as the measles and canine distemper viruses and there have been reports of the recovery of paramyxovirus-like particles from the brain of these patients. Immunologic findings suggestive of a viral cause are (1) increased titers of measles antibodies in the serum and CSF and (2) production of some of these antibodies in the brain.

Evidence for the contribution of canine distemper virus is the high incidence of MS in the Orkney and Shetland islands where the virus is thought to have been imported earlier, and an outbreak of MS in Iceland after an epidemic of canine distemper. Other candidate infective agents are prions (proteinaceous infective particles) which are thought to cause a somewhat similar disease, scrapie, in sheep and Creutzfeld Jacob disease and kuru in man. As mentioned earlier, tropical spastic paresis which has some resemblance to multiple sclerosis but is a common disease in the tropics is caused by the retrovirus, HTLV I.

Whether or not viruses are the triggering agent of MS, a great variety of immunologic abnormalities have been reported and the lesions have some histologic similarity to those of allergic encephalitis and postinfectious encephalomyelitis. Antibodies are produced in the nervous system and oligoclonal bands, suggestive of persistent viral infection, are detectable in the CSF of 65% to 95% of patients with multiple sclerosis. Popular hypotheses are that myelin destruction may be an innocent bystander phenomenon as a result of cross-reacting viral antibodies or that myelin may be induced to express self antigens to which T lymphocytes respond.

However, it should not be assumed that multiple sclerosis is a "typical" autoimmune disease or that the immunologic abnormalities are necessarily causative rather than secondary phe-

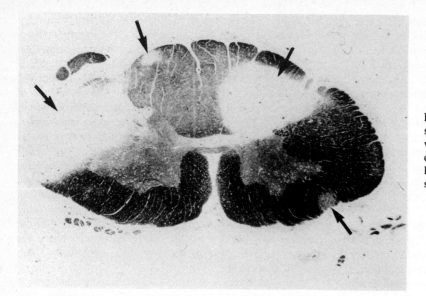

FIG. 20-14. Multiple sclerosis plaques. Transverse section of the cervical spinal cord stained for myelin, which stains black. Two large and two small well-demarcated areas of myelin loss are present. The large plaques in the posterolateral quadrants can be seen with the naked eye (Loyez stain).

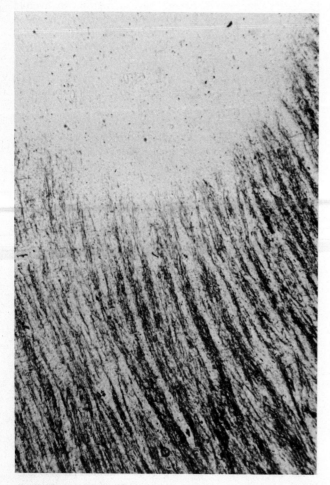

FIG. 20-15. Multiple sclerosis. Histologic section through a multiple sclerosis plaque, showing the sharply demarcated area of demyelination *(above)*. The demyelinated axons pass through the lesion but are not stained in this preparation (Loyez stain). *(Courtesy of Professor Sydney Liebowitz.)*

nomena. Corticosteroids or other immunosuppressive treatment, for example, in MS are of little benefit and do not arrest the progress of the disease.

In summary, the etiology of multiple sclerosis appears to be multifactorial; there is a genetic component conferring susceptibility and the geographic epidemiology suggests an environmental agent. The evidence implicating viruses as direct or indirect causes of the disease is little more than circumstantial. Although there is no doubt that a great variety of immunologic abnormalities can be detected, their role in causing tissue damage is as yet unproven.

Pathology. The characteristic feature is scattered plaques of demyelination mainly in the white matter (Fig. 20-14). These form yellowish or pinkish edematous areas when fresh, but later become grayish and firm.

Microscopically, plaques show loss of myelin sheaths (Fig. 20-15) and oligodendrocytes. Axons are usually preserved but may degenerate in severe, long-standing disease. In early active lesions many compound granular cells can be seen engulfing the degenerating myelin. Lymphocytes and plasma cells surround blood vessels (perivascular cuffing). Older lesions are characterized by increasing gliosis, especially around the periphery, and diminution of inflammatory infiltrate.

Clinical aspects. The onset of multiple sclerosis is usually in early adult life, and the course is highly variable, unpredictable, and erratically remittant. Typical features are as follows:

1. The onset is characteristically highly capricious. Transient visual disturbance or blindness and weakness or paralysis of a limb with complete, although temporary, recovery are common features.
2. Later nystagmus, disturbance of gait, irregular ("scanning") speech, tremors, and loss of muscular coordination develop as a result of cerebellar involvement.
3. Ultimately there is widespread paralysis, and often urinary incontinence may develop.

A few patients die within a few months. However, in persons over age 25, more than 60% remain mobile or even able to carry out their normal work. The disease can, however, reduce a young person to a paralyzed, bedridden, and incontinent invalid, suffering painful spasms of the limbs and episodes of infection. There is no reliably effective treatment.

The great variety of treatments that have been claimed to benefit patients with multiple sclerosis attests to the lack of knowledge about the causation of the disease.

Alzheimer's disease

Alzheimer's disease* is the most common cause of senile and presenile dementia. It is estimated to affect up to 3 million Americans, or 10% to 15% of those over 65 and up to 20% of those over 80. Insidious loss of memory and intellect soon prevent the performance of the simplest everyday tasks, such as combing the hair, and are followed by confusion and disorientation.

Motor, sensory (apart from early olfactory loss) and visual functions are however, little affected and the initial disabilities result from the patient's loss of ability to carry out even simple tasks. Mental and physical deterioration are progressive and relentless.

Precise diagnosis of Alzheimer's disease is difficult but may be assisted by magnetic resonance imaging to distinguish it from important organic causes of dementia, listed as follows:

1. Alzheimer's disease
2. Vascular (multi-infarct), Binswanger type
3. Alcoholic
4. Metabolic (hypoxia, hypoglycemia, hypo- or hyperthyroidism, hyperparathyroidism, hypo- or hypercalcemia, hepatic)
5. Tumors
6. Hydrocephalus (idiopathic, posthemorrhagic or posttraumatic)
7. Huntington's disease
8. Drug-induced (usually mild and reversible)
9. Infection (AIDS, syphilis rarely, Creutzfeld Jacob disease, progressive multifocal leukoencephalopathy)

Etiology and pathology. Although the majority of cases are sporadic, a genetic component in Alzheimer's disease is discernable. There is a familial susceptibility in those who develop the disease in middle age and a rare, autosomal dominant form of the disease. Moreover, the sporadic and familial forms of this disease are not distinguishable clinically or pathologically.

Similar changes in the brain also develop in patients with Down's syndrome after the age of 40. A link between the latter and Alzheimer's disease is a defect in a gene on chromosome 21, where the amyloid protein gene is also located. Duplication of this gene appears to be a major factor in the etiology. This is strongly suggested by the finding that there is linkage between the markers for familial Alzheimer's disease and the amyloid protein gene on chromosome 21. Sporadic Alzheimer's disease may therefore result from incomplete penetrance of the gene for the familial type of disease. However, it is as yet unclear whether the excess amyloid protein is synthesized in the brain and whether its formation is the fundamental cause of the disease.

In addition to genetic factors affecting amyloid production it seems likely that environmental factors (as yet unidentified) are also involved.

Microscopically, the cortex in Alzheimer's disease shows clumps of nerve cell fibers termed *neurofibrillary tangles* consisting of protein filaments twisted into a double helix (paired helical filaments). In addition dying nerve fibers (*neuritic plaques*) are clustered around deposits of amyloid which is also deposited around blood vessels (Fig. 20-16). Alzheimer's disease is now recognized as the most common cause of amyloi-

*A. Alzheimer (1864-1915), German psychiatrist and neurologist.

dosis. In regions of brain damage, normal RNA and protein synthesis are greatly decreased.

The number of neuritic plaques correlates with the severity of dementia but neurofibrillary tangles are found in other diseases such as postencephalitic Parkinson's disease. Areas of such damage adjacent to the hippocampus appear to be the cause of loss of memory by blocking the normal input and output. This appears to result from a deficiency of the neurotransmitter acetylcholine in both the cortex and hippocampus. The worst affected areas are the temporal, parietal and frontal lobes.

Prognosis and management. Incontinence and death, usually within 5 to 15 years, are the outcome of Alzheimer's disease. There is no specific treatment but cholinergic drugs such as THA (tetrahydroaminoacridine), a cholinesterase inhibitor are thought to benefit some patients. Otherwise Alzheimer's disease presents a prolonged period of nursing care and distress for the rest of the family.

Vascular (Binswanger-type*) dementia

Senile dementia has long been ascribed to cerebral atherosclerosis. This, however, does not seem to be the case, as modern imaging techniques have shown that one of the most common causes of dementia in the elderly, second only to Alzheimer's disease, is the production of multiple small infarcts

*O.L. Binswanger (1852-1929), German psychiatrist.

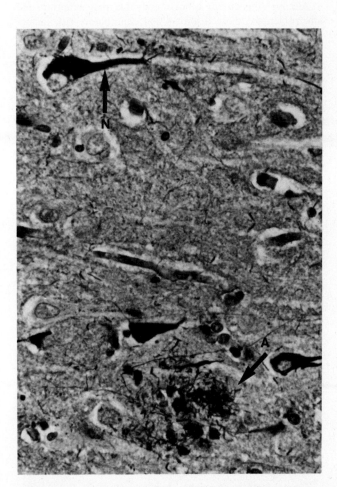

FIG. 20-16. Alzheimer's disease. Section of brain showing two characteristic microscopic features: (1) neurofibrillary tangles *(N)* and (2) deposition of amyloid *(A)*. (*Courtesy Charles W. White III, M.D.*)

particularly in the periventricular areas (ischemic periventricular leukoencephalopathy). Typical changes may be found in more than a third of all cases of dementia at autopsy. Vascular dementia and Alzheimer's disease are also frequently associated in the elderly.

Clinically, vascular dementia becomes common after the age of fifty; asymptomatic radiologic signs may be detected, but there is a wide clinical spectrum. This may include deterioration of memory, initiative and intellect, focal deficits, personality changes, disordered gait, urinary incontinence or pseudobulbar palsy and dementia. Such abnormalities are insidious in onset and relentlessly progressive. A history of repeated small strokes is common.

Pathology. At autopsy, the early naked-eye changes are slight. Microscopically, early lesions show partial loss of myelin and oligodendroglia, astrocytosis, and hyaline sclerosis of penetrating medullary arteries terminating in occlusion. Later there are periventricular ischemic infarctions with loss of myelin and axons, and reactive astroglial proliferation. The resultant periventricular softening, if widespread, can lead to ventricular dilatation.

The distribution of these changes results from the fact that the blood supply of the periventricular white matter depends on long penetrating arteries arising almost entirely from the surface of the brain. These are subject to selective narrowing and vulnerable to hypotensive episodes from any cause (including overtreatment of hypertension) leading to hypoperfusion of this area.

Although this disease is not directly due to hypertension and atherosclerosis, these disorders and contributory risk factors (particularly smoking) accelerate the deterioration in Binswanger type dementia. Removal of these risk factors and prevention of anything contributing to hypotension in the elderly can bring significant improvement and delay deterioration.

Tumors of the nervous system

Intracranial tumors can be primary or more commonly metastatic. Primary intracranial tumors can arise from cerebral tissues, from the meninges, skull or any other associated tissues.

Intrinsic (cerebral) tumors are usually malignant but rarely spread outside the central nervous system. Nevertheless, even histologically benign tumors have a poor prognosis because they can seriously damage cerebral function. Surgery is also difficult because of such factors as the nature of the tissue and the difficulties in defining the tumor margins. Brain tumors account for approximately 2% of all cancer deaths, but they are second only to acute leukemia as causes of cancer deaths in children.

The main types of cerebral tumors are as follows:
1. Gliomas (These are by far the most common type and include the astrocytoma, oligodendroglioma and ependymoma.)
2. Medulloblastoma
3. Meningioma
4. Neurilemoma
5. Pituitary tumors including craniopharyngioma
6. Metastatic tumors

Clinical aspects of cerebral tumors

Typical features of cerebral tumors include the following:
1. *Localizing signs*—These depend on the site of the tumor; those affecting the motor cortex, for example, typically cause convulsions or paralyses. The onset of epilepsy after the age of 25 is a typical sign. Other examples of focal signs are loss of coordination of movement as a result of a cerebellar tumor, visual field defects due to a tumor in the pituitary region, or loss of the sense of smell due to a tumor in the frontal region.
2. *Signs of raised intracranial pressure*—Intracranial pressure is increased as a direct effect of the size of the tumor or the latter can give rise to cerebral edema or obstructive hydrocephalus.

Signs and symptoms of raised intracranial pressure include (1) headache, (2) vomiting, (3) drowsiness, and (4) visual disturbances.

Persistent vomiting can be an early sign, but drowsiness is indicative of severely raised intracranial pressure; it is sometimes associated with mild pyrexia and stiffness of the neck. Visual disturbances may be associated with papilledema which is attended by the risk of optic atrophy and permanent blindness.

In addition, there can be intellectual deterioration, loss of memory or personality changes the causes of which may not be obvious.

Diagnosis of a cerebral tumor, its site and nature depend on careful clinical examination for localizing signs of other causes of the symptoms, CT or MR imaging or both, radiographs of the skull, brain biopsy, and chest radiographs to exclude a primary bronchial tumor.

Pathologic features and behavior

The usual gross features are a grayish or pinkish mass which infiltrates, displaces, and distorts the surrounding brain tissue.

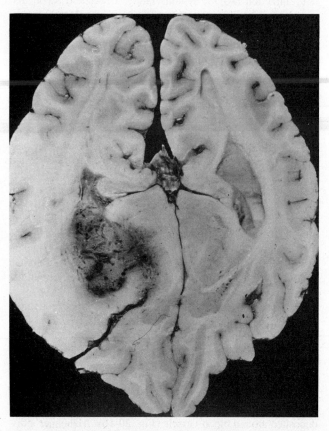

FIG. 20-17. Cerebral astrocytoma. Note the diffuse margins of the tumor as it invades the surrounding brain. *(Courtesy Curator of the Gordon Museum, Guy's Hospital, London, England.)*

Astrocytomas are the most common type of glioma (Figs. 20-17 and 20-18) and account for nearly 40% of cases. They most often affect young adults and usually originate in a cerebral hemisphere or less often the posterior fossa, particularly in children. Microscopically, the tumor consists of a relatively homogeneous collection of astrocytes with prominent nuclei. Despite the uniform cell pattern the behavior of the disease is variable.

Astrocytomas are slowly invasive and the history is typically of several months duration. Recurrence of cerebral astrocytomas after removal is common but posterior fossa tumors are potentially curable. The 5-year survival rate is up to 50%.

Glioblastoma multiforme (malignant astrocytoma; high grade astrocytoma) accounts for approximately 30% of gliomas. They are highly malignant tumors and usually affect those between the ages of 40 to 60.

Microscopically, the tumor cells are highly pleomorphic with bizarre hyperchromatic nuclei and mitoses are common. Multinucleated giant cells, angiomatoid proliferation, foci of hemorrhage, and necrosis with cyst formation are also typical features.

These tumors grow rapidly and the history is usually only of one or two months; death after a few months as a result of recurrence after treatment is common. They are not radiosensitive and the 1-year survival rate is less than 20%.

Oligodendroglioma accounts for less than 5% of gliomas. Adults are affected and the history is frequently very long so that symptoms may be present for several years. A characteristic radiographic feature is the presence of concentric, lobulated calcifications.

Microscopically, this tumor consists of sheets of oligodendrocytes in a scanty vascular connective tissue stroma. The cell membranes and nuclei stain strongly but the cytoplasm does not. The typical appearance is therefore of small dark spots in the centers of a network of cell membranes. In addition, as mentioned earlier, calcifications are present.

Oligodendrogliomas usually grow very slowly and survival for several years after treatment is possible. The 10-year survival rate is over 50% but these tumors eventually become more malignant in behavior and are often ultimately fatal.

Ependymomas mainly affect children and young adults and account for just over 5% of gliomas. They arise in the ventricular system and in particular in the fourth ventricle or sometimes from the lower end of the cord.

Microscopically, the pattern is highly variable but typically there are rosettes of ependymal cells arranged around blood vessels. Ependymomas may spread throughout the ventricular system.

The behavior of these tumors is also variable. However, because of their usual site of origin, they tend to cause hydrocephalus and obstruct the flow of CSF with serious consequences.

Removal is difficult and recurrence after removal is common. Radiotherapy may be beneficial and the 5-year survival rate is over 30%.

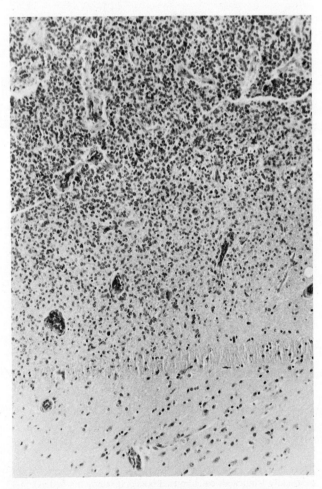

FIG. 20-18. Astrocytoma. There is gradual transition from apparently normal brain tissue *(below)* to highly cellular astrocytoma *(above)*.

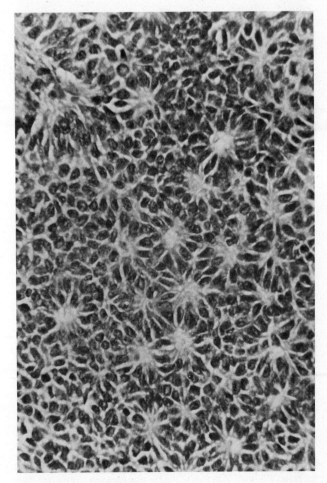

FIG. 20-19. Rosette formation is often a characteristic histologic feature of the medulloblastoma.

Medulloblastoma accounts for about 10% of gliomas and predominantly affects children and adolescents. It commonly arises in the roof of the fourth ventricle, forming a gray fleshy mass which typically hangs down into and obstructs the ventricle, and infiltrates the cerebellum.

Microscopically, the medulloblastoma is highly cellular, consisting of small darkly staining cells with little cytoplasm and a tendency to form rosettes arranged round blood vessels (Fig. 20-19).

Medulloblastomas are highly malignant and may spread throughout the pathway of the CSF and, unlike most other primary cerebral tumors may spread outside the central nervous system. Without treatment, patients are likely to die within a year but the tumor is highly radiosensitive. Surgery combined with vigorous radiotherapy to the whole central nervous system has been reported to give a 5-year survival rate between 40% and 70%.

Meningioma

Meningiomas are the most important benign tumors of the central nervous system, nevertheless they can be difficult to remove and may undergo malignant change. They usually arise from arachnoid cells, particularly from the arachnoid villi, and intracranial meningiomas are therefore common along the major dural sinuses. Meningiomas can also arise from any dural structure such as the falx or tentorium, or within the spinal canal particularly in the thoracic region. They are uncommon before the age of 40.

Meningiomas usually form firm circumscribed masses attached to the dura and are sometimes multiple. They are encapsulated and compress the brain substance (Fig. 20-20). Calcification is common and meningiomas also characteristically provoke an osteoblastic reaction in the adjacent bone to produce a localized thickening of the bone of the skull.

Microscopically, there are several patterns, but the most readily recognized, is the arrangement of the cells in whorls often surrounding laminated calcified, *psammoma* bodies (Fig. 20-21). The latter are particularly common in the spinal canal and form by calcification of an obliterated capillary. More common however are sheets of poorly defined polygonal cells which appear syncytial, but those arising in the posterior fossa tend to be fibrous in nature. Meningiomas are well vascularized, so much so that they sometimes appear to be angioblastic. Rarely, meningiomas, especially the angioblastic type, may undergo malignant change, characterized by pleomorphic, hyperchromatic nuclei, mitoses and abnormally large cells. These tumors invade the brain but rarely metastasize.

Meningiomas may recur after resection but this is probably because of incomplete removal but even microscopically benign meningiomas may occasionally invade the adjacent bone.

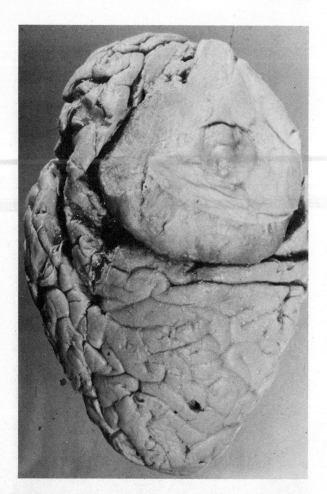

FIG. 20-20. A large meningioma that caused severe compression of the brain. *(Courtesy Curator of the Gordon Museum, Guy's Hospital, London, England.)*

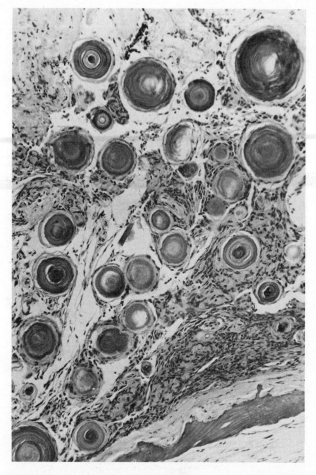

FIG. 20-21. A feature of many meningiomas is the presence of concentrically laminated, calcium-rich bodies (psammoma bodies).

Neurilemoma (schwannoma)

The neurilemoma is a benign tumor arising from the connective tissue (Schwann cells) of the axonal sheath of cranial nerves or spinal nerve roots. The most common and important type in the central nervous system is the so-called *acoustic neuroma* arising from the vestibular branch of the eighth nerve in the cerebropontine angle. Neurilemomas are also relatively common in the spinal cord and can arise from peripheral nerves anywhere in the body.

Microscopically, neurilemomas typically consist of elongated spindle cells which are regularly arranged and often with rows of nuclei side by side in a palisaded arrangement (Figs. 20-22 and 20-23). This is termed *Antoni A tissue;* it is usually associated with Antoni B tissue consisting of shorter spindle-shaped cells or elliptical cells in a mucinous matrix together with wavy delicate bundles of collagen fibers.

Clinically, an acoustic neuroma gives rise to a highly characteristic clinical picture as the trigeminal, facial, glossopharyngeal, and vagus nerves are displaced or stretched over the tumor. Typical results are tinnitus (ringing in the ears), deafness and rotational vertigo (a sensation of dizzily spinning). Further growth of the tumor can cause postauricular pain, disturbance of balance, twitching or weakness and paresthesia of the face, together with difficulty in speaking or swallowing. Neurilemomas occasionally form on the fifth or vagus nerves.

Current imaging techniques enable neurilemomas to be localized precisely. They are slow-growing tumors and can be completely removed in about two thirds of all cases, but the operative difficulties can be formidable.

Nervous system tumors in neurofibromatosis

Bilateral acoustic neuromas are the main manifestation of the central type of neurofibromatosis (NF II) which accounts for less than 10% of cases but like the peripheral type (NF I, described in Chapter 19) is also heritable as an autosomal dominant trait.

Some acoustic neuromas are neurofibromas rather than neurilemomas. Other tumors of the central nervous system of various kinds but particularly gliomas, also tend to be associated with central type neurofibromatosis and account for its severe morbidity and mortality. Skin lesions tend to be minimal or absent.

Neurofibromas of peripheral nerves are the characteristic feature of NF I (von Recklinghausen's disease) but an important complication of the latter is optic glioma. This typically appears in childhood, causing deterioration of vision or protrusion of the eye. Other features of gliomas have been discussed earlier.

An uncommon complication of peripheral neurofibromatosis is neurofibromas of the spinal cord. These cause a variety of compression effects, but they are usually amenable to surgery

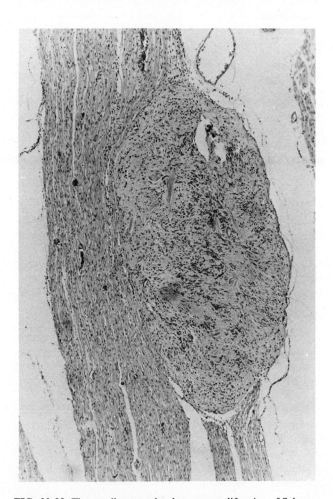

FIG. 20-22. The neurilemoma develops as a proliferation of Schwann cells which has displaced the nerve fibers to one side.

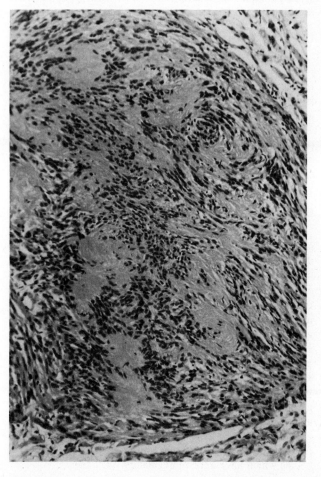

FIG. 20-23. Neurilemoma showing the palisading of Schwann cell nuclei. The intervening paler areas consist of interdigitating Schwann cell processes.

if treatment is not delayed. Acoustic neuroma is rarely associated with peripheral (von Recklinghausen's) neurofibromatosis, but until recently there has been considerable confusion between these different diseases.

Pituitary tumors

Adenomas are the most common type of pituitary tumor and are discussed in Chapter 18 because their endocrine effects usually dominate the clinical picture. Nonfunctional pituitary tumors compress the rest of the gland (causing hypopituitarism) and the optic chiasma (causing impairment of sight). If large enough they can give rise to signs typical of any cerebral tumor.

Craniopharyngioma

Craniopharyngiomas are uncommon tumors that arise from epithelial remnants in the region of the pituitary stalk. These cellular remnants are derived from Rathke's pouch an upgrowth from the primitive stomadeum and as a consequence, craniopharyngiomas may resemble odontogenic tumors microscopically.

Craniopharyngiomas are usually well encapsulated and either solid or cystic. One variant, can resemble the ameloblastoma (Chapter 17) or may contain many ghost cells (effete epithelial cells which have lost their nuclei) and so resemble the calcifying odontogenic cyst.

Craniopharyngiomas are generally benign in behavior but can, by compressing adjacent structures, cause hypopituitarism or visual defects.

Cerebral tumors in AIDS

As mentioned earlier, otherwise rare cerebral tumors, namely primary lymphomas and Kaposi's sarcoma are a recognized feature of AIDS. Cerebral Kaposi's sarcoma is virtually unknown in normal persons in whom primary cerebral lymphomas are also uncommon.

Clinically, the effects of AIDS-related cerebral tumors depends on their site but is likely in most cases to be complicated by other features of the disease and in particular AIDS encephalopathy which may be associated. The prognosis is inevitably poor.

Extracranial neural tumors

Paragangliomas. Paragangliomas are uncommon tumors arising from that part of the neural crest which gives rise to the collateral sympathetic system. The main example of a functional tumor originating from this tissue is the pheochromocytoma (Chapter 18) but the paragangliomas in general arise from the chemoreceptor cells in four main sites. These are the jugulotympanic, vagal, carotid body and laryngeal paragangliomas. Earlier classifications depended on the chromaffin reaction but this is not a reliable indicator of catecholamine secretion as nonfunctional paragangliomas synthesize small amounts of the latter as indicated by their affinity for silver stains.* Paragangliomas were also in the past confused with glomus tumors and the old name occasionally clings to them, as in the case of the "glomus jugulare" (jugulotympanic paraganglioma). True glomus tumors (Chapter 10) are, however, formed from modified vascular smooth muscle cells of glomus bodies which have a thermoregulatory function.

The carotid body tumor is the most common type of paraganglioma and arises behind the bifurcation of the common carotid artery, where the normal carotid body lies. It is most frequent in adults and forms a slowly growing painless mass just below the angle of the jaw; occasionally symptoms such as hoarseness are caused by pressure on adjacent structures. Up to 5% of carotid body tumors are bilateral but there also appears to be a familial trait in which approximately a third of cases are bilateral.

Microscopically, carotid body tumors typically consist of epithelium-like cells arranged in nests (cell balls, *zellballen*), which are demarcated by a delicate connective tissue stroma, or in short cords and resembling a carcinoid tumor. The individual cells have large nuclei and typically, a granular or, less often, a vacuolated cytoplasm. Although the appearance may be adenomatoid, the nature of the tumor can be confirmed by positive silver (Grimelius) staining and negative staining for glycogen.

Carotid body tumors are usually benign but may be difficult to resect completely because of their intimate relation and attachment to the carotid artery. Metastasis is uncommon and the histologic features are not a reliable guide to behavior. These tumors have rarely been reported to be functional and cause hypertension.

Jugulotympanic paragangliomas are even more uncommon than carotid body tumors but are nevertheless the most common tumors of the middle ear. The jugular bulb is the other main site of origin.

Clinically, women usually of middle age are chiefly affected but the symptoms depend on the site of origin of the tumor. Those arising in the temporal bone tend to cause deafness, tinnitus, or dizziness; later a hemorrhagic mass may appear in the external auditory canal. Tumors arising from the jugular bulb may involve the middle ear but generally tend to grow upward toward the base of the skull to cause erosion of the bone and cranial nerve palsies.

Microscopically, jugulotympanic paragangliomas are essentially similar to carotid body tumors except that the cell nests are usually more variable in size and they are frequently highly vascular.

Middle ear paragangliomas can be removed by radical mastoidectomy but spread of these tumors to the base of the brain may make resection difficult. In such cases supervoltage irradiation is effective. Metastasis is rare.

Other paragangliomas are rare. They show, with minor variations, similar structural features to carotid body tumors. Some, however, are more aggressive or metastasize more frequently.

Neuroblastoma

Neuroblastomas are important causes of childhood cancers. They also arise from the sympathetic chain at virtually any point but their most common site is the adrenal medulla and only rarely cerebral. They are frequently functional (95% contain catecholamine metabolites) and highly malignant.

Clinically, the most common picture is that of a rapidly growing abdominal tumor with fever, malaise, and loss of weight. Metastases are frequently to bone, causing severe pain, and, virtually peculiar to this tumor, to the orbit. Raised serum or urinary levels of catecholamine metabolites are helpful in confirming the diagnosis.

Microscopically, neuroblastomas consist of sheets of small dark round cells resembling lymphocytes but like retinoblas-

---

*In this case the Grimelius silver staining method.

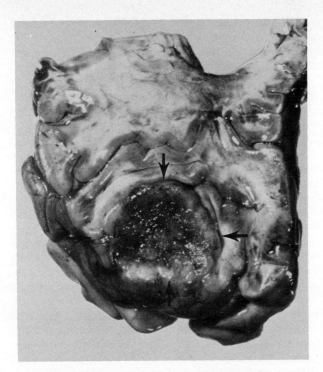

FIG. 20-24. Metastatic carcinoma *(arrows)* in the brain. The primary tumor was in the bronchus. In contrast to many primary neoplasms of the brain, the tumor tissue is obviously demarcated from the surrounding brain. *(Courtesy Curator of the Gordon Museum, Guy's Hospital, London, England.)*

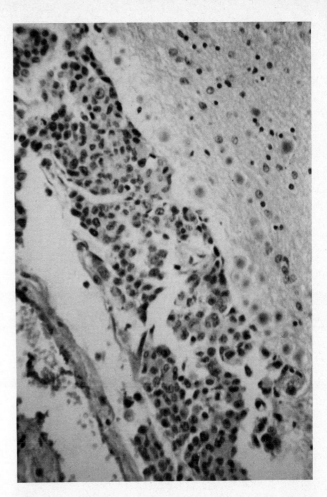

FIG. 20-25. Metastatic carcinoma of the lung infiltrating the meninges.

tomas (see below), sometimes showing a rosettelike arrangement. Differential diagnosis on histologic grounds is therefore difficult especially as similar-appearing tumors also express neural markers.

The prognosis is poor especially as many tumors have metastasized at the time of diagnosis, and its relationship to specific oncogenes is discussed in Chapter 9. Multiagent chemotherapy is then the only feasible approach, but it has been reported that proliferation of the tumor may be retarded by retinoic acid, which induces maturation of the cells in vitro. Spontaneous remission has rarely been reported but particularly in young infants.

Retinoblastoma

Retinoblastomas are highly malignant tumors which arise from primitive retinal cells, usually within the first two years of life.

Clinically, retinoblastomas may spread forward through the orbit and perforate it, or more frequently spread backward to the brain and cause death before widespread metastases develop. The latter are rarely seen. Genetic abnormalities associated with sporadic and familial forms are discussed in Chapter 9.

Microscopically, retinoblastomas have similar appearances to neuroblastomas but may show more conspicuous rosette formation. Many of the neural markers are also shared by these tumors so that differential diagnosis may be difficult. As mentioned in Chapter 17, Ewing's sarcoma though it usually gives rise to a quite different clinical picture, resembles neuroblastoma and retinoblastoma microscopically and also carries neural markers.

Metastatic tumors of the central nervous system

Metastatic tumors are second only to cerebrovascular disease as a cause of endogenous neurologic disease (Fig. 20-24). The main sources of cerebral metastases are carcinomas of the lung (Fig. 20-25), breast, gastrointestinal tract, and kidney. Symptoms of a cerebral tumor are sometimes the first indication of a primary lesion elsewhere. Metastases in the brain are usually multiple, rounded, and appear well demarcated. The histologic appearances are those of the primary tumor.

Diseases of the peripheral nerves

The peripheral nerves are subject to traumatic injury, inflammatory and degenerative disease, collectively termed peripheral neuropathies, and tumors particularly neurofibromas.

Peripheral neuropathies

Whereas diseases of the central nervous system such as poliomyelitis, have conspicuous peripheral effects, there is an enormous variety of causes of diseases of the peripheral nerves themselves. These peripheral neuropathies typically give rise to pain or paralyses or both, within their area of distribution. Probably the most clinically obvious type of peripheral (or more strictly, cranial) neuropathy is that of Bell's (facial) palsy in which pain is an early symptom in about 40% of cases. Like many other peripheral neuropathies the cause of Bell's palsy is unknown but is possibly viral in origin as discussed earlier. Peripheral neuropathy may affect only one nerve trunk (usually as a result of trauma) or many (polyneuropathy).

Etiology and pathology. Types of peripheral neuropathy are listed as follows:
1. Hereditary neuropathies
    a. Charcot-Marie-Tooth disease
    b. Refsums's disease
    c. Dejerine-Sottas disease
2. Toxic
    a. Alcohol
    b. Arsenic and heavy metals
    c. Gold compounds and some other drugs
3. Metabolic
    a. Diabetic
    b. Uremic
    c. Vitamin deficiencies
4. Infective or postinfective
    a. Herpes zoster
    b. Diphtheria
    c. Leprosy
    d. Guillain-Barre syndrome
5. Neuropathies associated with tumors
6. Unknown cause
    a. Bell's (seventh nerve) palsy
    b. Acute brachial neuritis
7. Trauma (localized neuropathy)

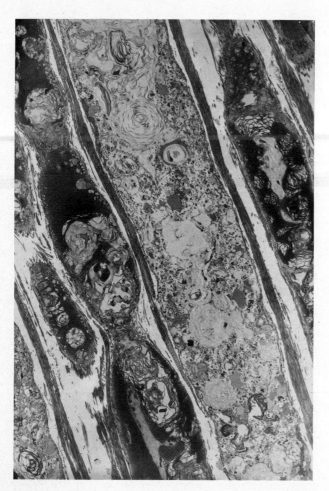

FIG. 20-26. Peripheral neuropathy. Electron micrograph showing disorganization of myelin sheaths.

Their pathogenesis is often obscure. In spite of their variety, however, there are common pathologic features namely, (1) degeneration of axons (wallerian degeneration), (2) patchy loss of the myelin sheath (segmental demyelination), or (3) both.

Wallerian degeneration is a result of injury to a neuron or axon. It is characterized by fragmentation and eventually complete loss of the distal part of the axon accompanied by breakdown of the myelin sheath. Destruction of an axon causes degeneration to spread back to the cell body.

Segmental demyelination, which is patchy loss of the myelin sheath, is usually associated with impaired function of the neuron, but the axon remains intact for a time. Demyelination is believed to result from damage to the Schwann cells, but it is often temporary. Remyelination may follow, and function can be completely restored.

Demyelination usually precedes wallerian degeneration and is thought, therefore, to be a more sensitive index of neuronal damage. In many cases, however, both processes are seen together.

In generalized disorders affecting neurons, the effects are most severe in the most distal parts of the longest neurons. The increasing vulnerability with distance from the nerve cell suggests that the latter may be a source of nutrients and protein synthesis.

The characteristic feature of progressive peripheral neuropathies (Fig. 20-26) is, therefore, wallerian degeneration spreading proximally from the most distal part of the neurons.

Clinical aspects. The main features of peripheral neuropathy are sensory loss, pain, motor weakness, and diminution or loss of tendon reflexes. The feet tend to be affected first, since the longest neurons generally suffer the most severe damage.

Although this is the general clinical pattern, it varies greatly in the individual diseases.

Diseases of the cranial nerves
Trigeminal neuralgia (tic douloureux)

The cause of this excruciatingly severe pain in the distribution of the trigeminal nerve is not known. It is thought to be a disorder affecting the nucleus of the spinal root of the fifth nerve. On the other hand, the fact that the drugs most effective in controlling the pain are anticonvulsants suggests that this disorder may have some features in common with epilepsy. In epilepsy the neurons are hypersensitive and remain in a persistent stage of partial depolarization. Their cytoplasmic membranes have an increased permeability, which makes them susceptible to a variety of stimuli. The event that initiates an epileptic seizure is a sudden electrical discharge of a group of cortical neurons. Trigeminal neuralgia might be regarded in some ways, therefore, as a sensory equivalent of epilepsy.

Clinical aspects. Trigeminal neuralgia mainly affects elderly people and is not seen before middle age. The characteristic features are as follows:
1. Sudden paroxysms of excruciatingly severe pain—The pain usually lasts for only a few seconds, but the paroxysms can recur in quick succession. The pain is so intense that the patient winces (hence the term *tic*); it often brings tears to the patient's eyes and may make the patient suicidal. There are often remissions for varying periods.
2. Pain is felt only within the area of distribution of the trigeminal nerve.
3. Trigger zones are present on the face or within the mouth, where light contact precipitates an attack. There is no

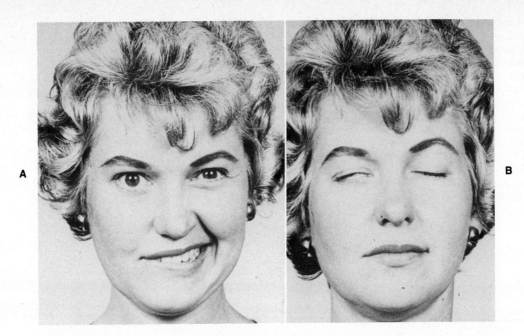

FIG. 20-27. Bell's palsy. **A,** When the patient attempts to smile, the mouth fails to move on the affected side, which remains expressionless. **B,** When the patient attempts to shut her eyes, the lids on the affected side fail to close completely, but the eye rolls upward normally. *(From Cawson RA: Essentials of dental surgery and pathology, ed 4, Edinburgh, Scotland, 1984, Churchill Livingstone.)*

sensory loss, and there are no detectable abnormalities on investigation.

Diagnosis of this disease depends on the recognition of the clinical criteria described and is often confirmed by the response to anticonvulsant drugs. Section of the root of the trigeminal nerve between the ganglion and brain stem is needed if medical treatment fails.

Facial (Bell's) palsy

Bell's palsy is of unknown cause, but it appears to result from an inflammatory process, thought to be viral, in or around the facial nerve in the region of the stylomastoid foramen or facial canal. There is sometimes mild pleocytosis in the CSF, which also suggests infection or inflammation.

Clinical aspects. Bell's palsy affects adults. The onset is acute, sometimes starting with pain behind the ear or in the region of the ramus of the mandible. Paralysis of the muscles of facial expression of one side usually develops in a matter of hours (Fig. 20-27). The corner of the mouth droops, skinfolds are obliterated, and the eye will not close. When the patient tries to smile, the corner of the mouth on the affected side fails to lift symmetrically with that on the normal side. Sagging of the lower lid allows the punctum to fall away from the conjunctiva, allowing tears to spill over the cheek. In severe cases saliva may dribble from the drooping corner of the mouth.

Complications develop if recovery is incomplete. These include facial spasms or attempts at regeneration of the seventh nerve, which may allow abnormal connections to form. Thus attempts to close the eyelids may cause retraction of the angle of the mouth. In other cases activity of the facial muscles may cause secretion by the lacrimal glands (crocodile tears) when eating.

About 80% of patients recover within a few weeks. But those who do not are left with a disfiguring and distressing disability. The disease may respond well to a short intensive course of corticosteroid therapy in the early stages and which

is presumed to lessen inflammatory swelling and compression of the facial nerve.

Other causes of facial paralysis

Other causes of facial paralysis include the following:
1. Tumors invading the temporal bone
2. An acoustic neuroma pressing on the facial nerve
3. Malignant tumors of the parotid gland
4. Herpes zoster affecting the geniculate ganglion (Ramsay Hunt syndrome)
5. Vascular lesions or tumors in the pons
6. Acute polyneuritis
7. Melkersson-Rosenthal syndrome

Melkersson-Rosenthal syndrome is a rare cause of facial palsy and also unusual in that it affects adolescents. Histologically, sarcoidlike follicles may be found in the thickened lip or facial tissues. The syndrome consists of (1) recurrent facial paralysis, eventually becoming permanent, (2) swelling of the lower lip, and (3) rarely plication of the tongue (scrotal tongue).

Selected readings

Anders KH et al: The neuropathology of AIDS, Am J Pathol 124:537, 1986.

Anon (LA): Alzheimer's disease, Down's syndrome and chromosome 21, Lancet ii:1011, 1987.

Anon (LA): Brain transplant for Parkinson's disease, Lancet i:1012, 1987.

Anon (LA): Reye's syndrome and aspirin: epidemiological associations and inborn errors of metabolism, Lancet ii:429, 1987.

Ellison GW et al: Multiple sclerosis, Ann Intern Med 101:514, 1984.

Foster JB: Subcortical dementia, Br Med J 292:1035, 1986.

Gabuzda DH and Hirsch MS: Neurologic manifestations of infection with human immunodeficiency virus, Ann Intern Med 107:383, 1987.

Hollander H and Levy JA: Neurologic abnormalities and recovery of human immunodeficiency virus from cerebrospinal fluid, Ann Intern Med 106:692, 1987.

Katzman R: Alzheimer's disease, N Engl J Med 314:964, 1986.

Larner AJ: Aetinological role of viruses in multiple sclerosis: a review, J Soc Med 79:412, 1986.

Lewin R: Trail of ironies to Parkinson's disease, Science 224:1083, 1984.

Martyn CN: Neurological clues from environmental neurotoxins, Br Med J 295:346, 1987.

Morrison KE: Brain transplantation—still a fantasy? (discussion paper), J R Soc Med 80:441, 1987.

Mozar HN, Bal DG, and Howard JT: Perspectives on the etiology of Alzheimer's disease, JAMA 257:1503, 1987.

Prusiner SB: Prions and neurodegenerative diseases, N Engl J Med 317:1571, 1987.

Rhodes RH: Histopathology of the central nervous system in the acquired immunodeficiency syndrome, Hum Pathol 18:636, 1987.

Sharer LR et al: Pathologic features of AIDS encephalopathy in children: evidence for LAV/HTLV-III infection of brain, Hum Pathol 17:271, 1986.

Sitrin MD et al: Vitamin E deficiency and neurologic disease in adults with cystic fibrosis, Ann Intern Med 107:51, 1987.

Steiner RE: Nuclear magnetic resonance imaging, Br Med J 294:1570, 1987.

Van Horn G: Dementia, Am J Med 83:101, 1987.

CHAPTER 21

Diseases of the female genital system and breast

The major portion of the female genital tract, from the fallopian tubes to the vagina, develops from the mullerian (paramesonephric) ducts. These paired structures arise as zones of thickening and invagination of the celomic epithelium on the lateral aspects of the intermediate mesoderm at about the fortieth day of embryonal life. The urogenital sinus epithelium advances cranially and replaces the paramesonephric epithelium of the vagina to the level of the ectocervical os by the nineteenth week of fetal development.

Congenital malformations of the uterus

Clinically important congenital uterine abnormalities are uncommon. Among the more frequently encountered are *mullerian duct fusion defects* (i.e., malformations resulting from partial or complete failure of the mullerian ducts to fuse at the appropriate positions along their length). Anomalies of this kind (Fig. 21-1) may present as infertility or be associated with habitual abortions. However, there are numerous other conditions of the female genital tract that may cause infertility. Several of these are discussed in this chapter, and the more common ones are listed in the accompanying box.

Disorders of the vulva

The vulva, which is almost entirely covered by skin, may be involved by the same inflammatory and neoplastic processes that affect skin elsewhere. However, several lesions are peculiar to or have a special predilection for this site.

Bartholin's duct cysts

Bartholin's duct cysts develop as a consequence of obstruction to the ducts draining the paired Bartholin's mucous glands at the introitus. The obstruction is usually caused by repeated episodes of inflammation and the resulting cysts are liable to be reinfected. Chlamydia and gonococci are among the organisms most commonly infecting Bartholin's glands. Clinically, the Bartholin's duct cyst presents as a firm swelling in the labium major. Surgical excision is the treatment of choice.

Lichen sclerosus et atrophicus

Lichen sclerosus et atrophicus is a skin condition that affects both sexes, of all ages, and all areas of the body. The main incidence is in the anogenital area of middle-aged women, where itching and pain are common symptoms. It has a typical clinical appearance, with ivory papules that coalesce into crinkly atrophic plaques. Microscopically, the epidermis is thin and there is a subepidermal zone of amorphous hyalinization above a deeper band of inflammatory cells. The etiology is obscure, although a possible autoimmune basis and an association with infection by *Borrelia* spirochetes has been postulated.

FEMALE CAUSES OF INFERTILITY	
Abnormality	*Examples*
Congenital malformations	Bilateral ovarian agenesis
Chromosomal anomalies	Turner's syndrome
Endocrine disorders	Polycystic ovary disease
Endometriosis	
Iatrogenic causes	Asherman's syndrome (absent endometrium following vigorous curettage)
Immunologic causes	Serum/cervix mucus anti-sperm antibodies
Inadequate cervical secretions	Drug effects
Pelvic inflammatory disease	Chlamydial infection, gonorrhea, tuberculosis
Pregnancy disorders	Abortion, tubal pregnancy
Sexual dysfunction	

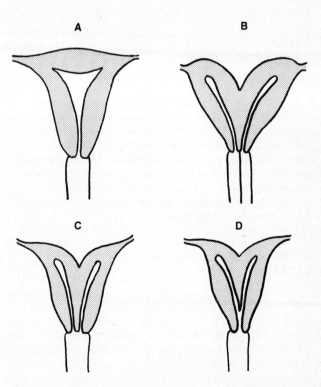

FIG. 21-1. Anomalies caused by varying degrees of incomplete fusion of lower mullerian ducts. **A,** Normal uterus and vagina. **B,** Double uterus and vagina. **C,** Double uterus (didelphys). **D,** Bicornuate uterus.

Herpes simplex infection

Herpes simplex infection of the vulva is acquired by sexual contact and presents clinically as a painful, recurrent ulcerative vulvitis. It is discussed further in Chapter 23.

Vulvar condylomas

Human papillomaviruses, which are transmitted by sexual contact, may involve any part of the lower genital tract. Viral infection may either produce no clinical manifestations or may result in a spectrum of epithelial lesions, some of which (depending to some extent on the viral strain involved) may progress to squamous cell carcinoma. The best known manifestation of papillomavirus infection in the vulva is the genital wart (condyloma acuminatum), a papillary or verrucous growth which is often multiple. Papillomaviruses may also give rise to flat (i.e., nonpapillary) condylomas. The cellular changes produced by these viruses, and the evidence for their role in carcinogenesis, are discussed later.

Hydradenoma papilliferum

Hydradenoma papilliferum is an uncommon benign skin adnexal tumor that has a predilection for the anogenital region. It forms a solitary dermal nodule that occasionally ulcerates and gives rise to a projecting red mass that may clinically resemble a carcinoma.

Squamous cell carcinoma of the vulva

Squamous cell carcinoma of the vulva is an uncommon entity, accounting for only 1% of all malignant tumors in the female. The disease presents most frequently in the sixth decade, usually as a nodule or ulcer involving the labium major. It begins as an intraepithelial neoplastic process (vulvar intraepithelial neoplasia, or VIN), with or without papillomavirus-associated cellular changes. There is an early phase of limited invasion (microinvasion), which shows little metastatic potential which may progress to carcinoma with spread to inguinal lymph nodes. Metastasis outside the pelvis is rare. Radical vulvectomy may be curative.

Extramammary Paget's disease

Extramammary Paget's disease is a rare condition of the anogenital region characterized by intraepithelial (usually intraepidermal) spread of cells from an underlying, often clinically occult, adenocarcinoma. The presence of scattered cancer cells in the epidermis results in a clinical picture that mimics dermatitis. The prognosis is that of the underlying carcinoma, which may originate in sweat glands or, less commonly, the cervix or rectum. (Paget's disease of the nipple is described under "Disorders of the Breast.")

Disorders of the vagina
Vaginitis

Vaginitis is often *noninfective* and is a result of factors such as trauma, foreign bodies, or chemical irritants. When plasma estrogen levels are low (i.e., before the menarche, during lactation or after the menopause), the vaginal epithelium becomes thin and *atrophic* vaginitis may develop. *Infective vaginitis* is usually caused by the following:

1. *Candida albicans*
2. *Trichomonas vaginalis*
3. *Gardnerella vaginalis*
4. *Neisseria gonorrhoeae*
5. *Herpesvirus hominis* type 2

Candida vaginitis is usually associated with inflammation, a "cottage cheese" discharge and white mucosal patches containing fungal elements. *Trichomonas vaginitis* (Chapter 23) is usually, though not invariably, sexually transmitted. The flagellate protozoon causing the infection is easily demonstrated in vaginal smears. *Gardnerella vaginitis* is sexually acquired and is characterized by a malodorous, thin, greyish vaginal discharge. Cytologic smears typically contain squamous epithelial cells, the so-called "clue cells," that are recognized by the fact that their surfaces appear completely carpeted by the causative bacteria. *N. gonorrhea* is incapable of producing a true vaginitis in adult women because the thick vaginal squamous epithelium is resistant to the organism. In children, however, a chronic vaginitis may result. *Herpetic vaginitis* is present in most cases of herpes infection of the vulva but is often overshadowed by the vulval lesions and hence overlooked.

Toxic shock syndrome is discussed in Chapter 8.

Vaginal neoplasms

Primary malignancy of the vagina is rare. The usual tumor is a typical *squamous cell carcinoma*. Like other squamous cell carcinomas of the lower female genital tract, this neoplasm is preceded by characteristic intraepithelial changes (vaginal intraepithelial neoplasia), and human papillomaviruses have been implicated in its pathogenesis. In recent years there has been a significant increase in the United States of *clear cell adenocarcinoma* of the vagina, which exclusively affects young girls exposed prenatally to diethylstilbestrol (DES). The precursor lesion for this cancer appears to be vaginal adenosis. Another rare malignant neoplasm is *embryonal rhabdomyosarcoma*, a highly malignant neoplasm which develops in the first five years of life and which typically appears as a large, lobulated mass resembling a bunch of grapes that frequently protrudes from the vaginal orifice. Sarcoma botryoides is an older term used to describe the typical gross appearance.

Disorders of the cervix
Cervicitis

Nonspecific cervicitis. Infiltrates of plasma cells, lymphocytes, eosinophils and histiocytes, concentrated beneath the surface epithelium, are present to some degree in every multiparous woman and are considered normal. Significant inflammation of the cervix, however, may accompany prolapse or cervical polyps and is sometimes seen in women using intrauterine contraceptive devices or following surgery or irradiation.

Cervical inflammation due to infection is relatively uncommon. Among the infectious agents most commonly causing cervicitis is *Chlamydia trachomatis,* which typically elicits an inflammatory response characterized by the formation of lymphoid follicles with germinal centers ('follicular cervicitis'), a pattern of inflammation analogous to the conjunctival follicular hyperplasia seen in trachoma. The organism replicates within lysosomes in cervical columnar epithelial cells, producing basophilic cytoplasmic inclusions. Although most patients with chlamydial cervicitis are asymptomatic, the infected cervix is important as the source of infection of the endometrium and fallopian tubes, transmission to a male partner and to the fetus and neonate. Infection with *Chlamydia trachomatis* is now recognized as the most common sexually transmitted disease in the Western world. It is highly susceptible to tetracycline.

Cervical polyps

These are common, benign lesions usually arising in the endocervix, most commonly between the fourth and sixth decades of life. They may be pedunculated or sessile and are composed of endocervical glandular epithelium and vascular stroma. They may cause intermenstrual or postcoital bleeding, but are frequently asymptomatic. Large polyps commonly protrude from the external cervical os.

Carcinoma of the cervix

Carcinoma, usually of squamous cell type, is by far the most important disease of the uterine cervix. Beside being one of the most common pelvic gynecologic cancers, it is also the most preventable because it is preceded by a series of treatable, localized epithelial lesions that may be present for several years before the invasive stage is reached. The ease of clinical examination of the cervix permits large-scale screening of women by means of exfoliative smears. The development of this technique by Papanicolaou* in the early 1940s was a major breakthrough in the early detection of cancer.

---

*G.N. Papanicolaou (1883-1962), Greek-American cytologist.

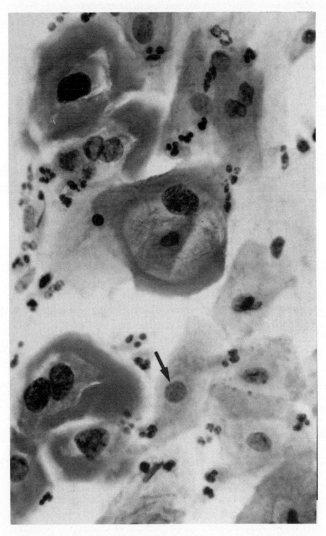

FIG. 21-2. Cytologic smear demonstrating several koilocytes. Note the accompanying nuclear enlargement and hyperchromasia. *Arrow* indicates a normal intermediate cell nucleus for comparison.

Etiology and risk factors. Cancer of the cervix and its precursor lesions have the epidemiologic characteristics of a venereal disease and are not found in virgins. There is strong, although still largely circumstantial, evidence linking cancer of the cervix to human papillomavirus (HPV) infections. In over 90% of cases papillomaviral antigens can be demonstrated with special techniques in the cells of cervix cancer and its precursor lesions. At least 46 HPV genotypes have been identified to date; those commonly demonstrated in cervix cancers are types 16, 18, or 31. Types 6 or 11 are demonstrable in condylomas of the cervix, but are seldom demonstrated in lesions progressing to cancer.

Those females most at risk for the development of cervix cancer are those who have had frequent sexual contact with multiple male partners, commencing early in the reproductive years. This appears to be due to the great susceptibility of the metaplastic cells at the adolescent squamocolumnar junction to the carcinogenic effects of the virus. The male sexual partners of females infected with papillomaviruses also tend to harbor the virus(es), commonly in the prepuce or urethra.

Pathogenesis and pathology. Most, if not all, cancers of the cervix, appear to start as papillomavirus-induced lesions, called *condylomas,* which tend to be flat rather than papillary or verrucous. The pathognomonic cellular change is *koilocytosis.* The koilocyte, which is present in smears and in biopsy specimens, has a large, irregular, cave-like vacuole in a perinuclear location, sharply demarcated from the densely staining cell periphery (Fig. 21-2). In type 6 or 11 HPV lesions the viral DNA is episomal and is not integrated into the host cell genome. The nuclear DNA tends to remain largely euploid (diploid), and these lesions tend to persist as pure condylomas, or to regress. In type 6 or 11 lesions, koilocytosis is associated with degenerative nuclear changes due to viral proliferation within the nucleus.

In lesions caused by type 16, 18, or 31 papillomaviruses the viral DNA is integrated into the genome of the host cell, and the purely condylomatous appearance becomes overshadowed by the changes of *cervical intraepithelial neoplasia (CIN)** (Fig. 21-3). The squamous epithelial cells in CIN develop nuclear DNA aneuploidy and nuclear enlargement, often with coarse clumping of the chromatin. With increasing severity (CIN grades I through III), there is increasing loss of cytoplasmic differentiation, starting at the base of the epithelium; ultimately cells at virtually all levels in the epithelial layer have scanty cytoplasm and a high nuclear-cytoplasmic ratio. Koilocytotic changes may still be evident in many cases of CIN, particularly early in its evolution. If left untreated, type 16 or 18 lesions tend to progress to invasive cancer. The rate of progression from initial infection to invasive cancer is variable, ranging from less than a year to as much as 20 years.

Human papillomavirus infections are also associated with the development of cervical adenocarcinoma, although this form of cancer is less commonly seen in the cervix than squamous cell carcinoma. Human papillomavirus antigens of different types may also be demonstrated in many women in cervical epithelia that appear histologically normal. This suggests that factors other than mere infection by the virus, for example, cigarette smoking or coinfection with herpesvirus, may be required in promoting carcinogenesis.

---

*An alternative to the CIN terminology is the dysplasia-carcinoma terminology, in which mild and moderate dysplasia are equivalent, respectively, to CIN grades I and II. Severe dysplasia and carcinoma-in-situ are both equivalent to CIN III.

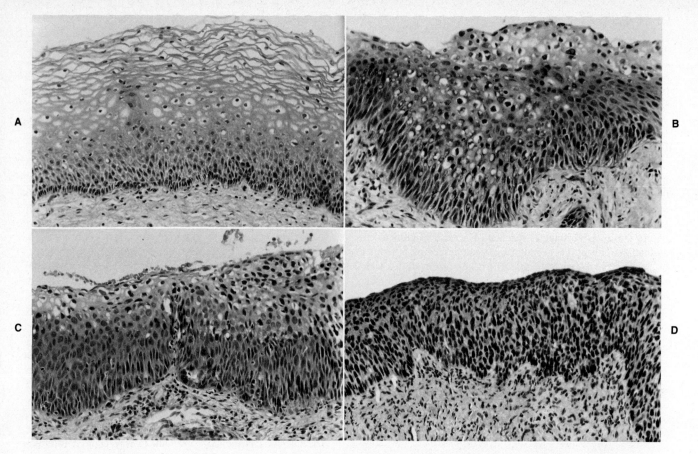

FIG. 21-3. Spectrum of epithelial appearances ranging from normal to CIN III. **A,** Normal squamous epithelium. **B,** CIN I. Abundant koilocytes are apparent. **C,** CIN II. Fewer koilocytes are seen. **D,** CIN III. Koilocytes are absent.

Spread of cervical carcinoma. Lesions up to and including the stage of microinvasion behave in an indolent fashion, do not metastasize, and are asymptomatic. After invasion has proceeded *beyond 3 mm,* metastasis is likely, and the outlook for the patient changes drastically. At first the spread of invasive cervical carcinoma is local. Infiltration of the underlying stroma produces a tumor mass that may ulcerate and cause vaginal bleeding. Ulceration also predisposes to infection and a foul-smelling vaginal discharge. The tumor eventually grows through the cervical wall to invade the ureters, bladder, rectum, vagina, and the upper portions of the uterus. Invasion of the ureters produces urinary tract obstruction with resultant hydronephrosis, pyelonephritis, and renal failure, which is the most common cause of death in cervical cancer. Necrosis and liquefaction of tumor tissue connecting the vagina with the bladder and rectum may lead to the development of rectovaginal and vesicovaginal fistulae.

Initially there is lymphatic spread to the pelvic lymph nodes and later to the paraaortic lymph nodes. Blood-borne metastasis is usually to the skeleton, lungs, and liver.

Detection and treatment of lesions preceding invasive cervix cancer. CIN tends to be symptomless and is usually detected on cytologic ("Pap") smears. The American Cancer Society and the American College of Obstetricians and Gynecologists jointly recommend that all women who are, or who have been sexually active, or have reached the age of 18 years, have an annual Pap test and pelvic examination; after a woman

has had three or more consecutive satisfactory normal annual examinations, the Pap test may be performed less frequently at the physician's discretion. A representative cellular sample of the cervix is obtained by scraping the ectocervix and sampling the endocervical canal by means of aspiration or by use of a cotton swab. Endocervical sampling is important because the more advanced epithelial lesions of the cervix tend to develop farthest from the ectocervical os.

Where the appearance of the smears is sufficiently atypical to suggest cervical intraepithelial neoplasia or carcinoma, colposcopy is performed (i.e., the examination of the cervical mucosa with a magnifying lens); different classes of mucosal lesions are recognized by their typical vascular patterns, and biopsies of the most advanced lesions are taken. If the lesion extends into the endocervical canal and its limits cannot be visualized, a cone biopsy of the cervix, encompassing the endocervical canal, is frequently performed. Epithelial lesions of lesser degree than invasive cancer may be treated with local cryotherapy or CO_2 laser therapy. In cases where the severity or the extent of the lesion is great or is in doubt or where preservation of fertility is not important, a total hysterectomy may be carried out.

Diagnosis and treatment of invasive cervix cancer. Invasive cancer often causes either bleeding or vaginal discharge and the tumor may be obvious on clinical examination. A simple punch biopsy can confirm the clinical diagnosis. Usually where the cancer appears to be limited to the reproductive organs, a hysterectomy, together with removal of regional lymph nodes (radical hysterectomy) is carried out in an effort to contain the disease. Irradiation may be employed as an adjunct to surgery.

Disorders of the endometrium
Endometritis

Acute endometritis is rare and may develop after abortion or delivery or as an ascending chlamydial or gonococcal infection. *Chronic nonspecific endometritis* is more common and results from the presence of retained products of conception, intra-uterine contraceptive devices, or as a result of spread from chlamydial cervicitis or a chronically inflamed fallopian tube. *Tuberculous endometritis* is usually associated with tuberculous salpingitis and is not uncommonly seen as a cause of infertility in underdeveloped countries. *Actinomycosis* of the endometrium is sometimes seen in women following prolonged insertion of an intrauterine contraceptive device. Endometritis may present as abnormal uterine bleeding.

Endometrial polyps

The term *endometrial polyp* refers to a focal, circumscribed overgrowth of the mucosa, usually the basal portion, which protrudes into the endometrial cavity. A possible explanation of its development is that a nonresponsive focus of endometrium does not detach during menstruation and continues to grow with each menstrual cycle. These polyps can develop at any age after puberty but are most commonly seen during the fifth and sixth decades. They arise most frequently in the fundus and may be pedunculated or sessile. Histologically, they are composed of fibrous stroma containing thick-walled blood vessels and glands which usually do not share in the normal cyclical activity of the endometrium and are frequently atrophic and cystic. Endometrial polyps present as abnormal uterine bleeding and are a common finding in perimenopausal women. Malignant change in a polyp is uncommon.

Endometrial carcinoma

Endometrial cancer is twice as common as cervical cancer, with 36,000 new cases reported in the United States for 1986 as opposed to 14,000 for cervical cancer. It is the sixth most common cause of cancer death among women, with a peak incidence in the sixth and seventh decades of life. Most are adenocarcinomas; some are adenosquamous carcinomas.

Pathogenesis. Currently two types of endometrial carcinoma are recognized. One type develops in association with generalized endometrial hyperplasia in patients subjected to long-term estrogenic stimulation of the endometrium (*estrogen-dependent* type), and, on assay, is found to consist of estrogen receptor-positive cells. The other is *estrogen-independent* and develops focally either in an atrophic or focally hyperplastic endometrium and is estrogen receptor-negative. The average age of patients with estrogen-independent cancers is slightly higher than those with the estrogen-dependent type.

The role of hyperestrogenism as a major risk factor for endometrial carcinoma is understandable when estrogen's physiologic effects on the endometrium are considered. During the follicular phase of the menstrual cycle, estrogen secreted by the ovarian follicular lining cells causes the endometrial glands and stroma to proliferate (proliferative endometrium). Following ovulation, progesterone secreted by the corpus luteum opposes the proliferative effects of estrogen, and induces secretory changes (secretory endometrium). Any condition resulting in

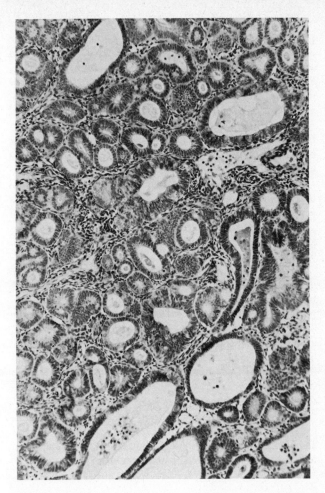

FIG. 21-4. Endometrial hyperplasia with atypia. Note gland budding with extreme crowding.

long-term high estrogen levels unopposed by progesterone can thus be expected to cause *endometrial hyperplasia.* If this condition persists, there may be gradual development of cytologic and architectural atypia involving the hyperplastic epithelium (Fig. 21-4), with progression to *carcinoma-in-situ* and, ultimately, infiltrating carcinoma.

Hyperestrogenism may be caused by the following:
1. Chronic anovulation which, in younger women, may be due to polycystic ovary disease
2. Estrogen-secreting tumors (e.g., granulosa cell or theca cell tumors of the ovary)
3. Obesity (increased conversion of androstenedione to estrone by fat cells)
4. Nulliparity (absence of the progesterone dominance caused by pregnancy and lactation)
5. Prolonged estrogen therapy

The risk of developing endometrial carcinoma increases with estrogen levels and duration and remains for up to ten years after estrogen levels have been brought under control. Progesterone decreases the risk of endometrial carcinoma by preventing hyperplasia of the endometrium, and combination oral contraceptives used for 12 months or longer confer protection against endometrial cancer for at least 15 years after cessation of oral contraceptive use.

Spread and prognosis. The estrogen-dependent carcinomas are better differentiated, of lower nuclear grade, and less biologically aggressive than their estrogen-independent counterparts. Because hyperplastic endometrium tends to disintegrate and cause irregular or excessive bleeding, estrogen-dependent carcinomas are discovered earlier in the course of the disease. Estrogen independent-carcinomas, by contrast, frequently remain asymptomatic until the myometrium has been deeply invaded (Fig. 21-5) or the tumor has metastasized.

Overall, mortality from endometrial cancer is lower than that from cervical cancer, because most endometrial cancers have not metastasized at the time of diagnosis. At presentation up to 80% of patients with endometrial cancer are in stage I (disease confined to the uterine corpus), which has a 5-year survival of about 80%. Invasion of the wall of the body of the uterus is a relatively slow process and, in addition, does not involve vulnerable structures such as the ureters. Overt symptoms usually appear long before the cancer has penetrated or spread beyond the uterine wall.

Clinical aspects. The first sign of endometrial hyperplasia is usually menorrhagia (excessive menstrual bleeding), which may start relatively early in the disease. Many cases of hyperplasia are detected and treated before adenocarcinoma can develop. Carcinoma of the endometrium, on the other hand, usually causes metrorrhagia (intermenstrual or postmenopausal bleeding) as a result of ulceration. Early detection of non-estrogen-related cancers may be accomplished in some instances by screening all asymptomatic postmenopausal women with appropriate cytologic methods.

Endometrial hyperplasia without atypia may be reversible by treatment with progestogens, whereas atypical hyperplasias and carcinomas require hysterectomy and, in selected cases, radiotherapy may be indicated for carcinoma. Deep myometrial

invasion, poor tumor differentiation, and DNA aneuploidy are useful predictors of distant metastases and a poor prognosis.

Stromal and mixed mullerian neoplasms of the endometrium

While endometrial stromal tumors clearly originate in the endometrium, the site of origin of mixed mullerian (mixed mesodermal) tumors is often less obvious; most, however, develop in the endometrium. Both types of tumor are uncommon and can be benign or malignant. The malignant varieties, collectively classified as *endometrial sarcomas*, are subclassified according to (1) whether they are pure (i.e., contain only one cellular component) or mixed, and (2) whether they are homologous and contain only cell types normally found in the uterus, or heterologous (i.e., contain cell types normally alien to the uterus). For example, an endometrial stromal sarcoma is a pure homologous tumor, while a carcinosarcoma containing striated muscle or cartilage is a mixed heterologous neoplasm. Mixed mullerian tumors and high-grade stromal sarcomas are highly malignant neoplasms that tend to metastasize early. Most cases present as postmenopausal bleeding.

Disorders of the myometrium
Adenomyosis

Adenomyosis refers to the presence of endometrial glands and stroma, focally or diffuse, deep *within* the myometrium, probably due to ingrowth of the basal layer of the endometrium. In the pre-menopausal uterus there is characteristically hypertrophy of smooth muscle around these foci. By contrast, endometriosis, discussed later, refers to ectopic endometrial glands and stroma present *outside* the myometrium; it is usually not associated with adenomyosis.

Patients with adenomyosis may be asymptomatic or may suffer from dysmenorrhea or irregular uterine bleeding.

Smooth muscle neoplasms

Myometrial smooth muscle tumors are among the lesions most frequently encountered in gynecologic practice. They are usually benign.

Leiomyomas (fibroids) are benign smooth muscle tumors and are found in approximately 20% of women older than 30 years. Leiomyomas appear to begin developing in early life, but because they tend to grow slowly, often do not cause symptoms until middle age. They contain more high-affinity estrogen-receptors than neighboring normal uterine muscle and depend on estrogen for growth. The estrogen dependence of these neoplasms is further reflected in their tendency to undergo degenerative changes or involution after the menopause. However, this same hormonal dependence sometimes causes them to enlarge during pregnancy and obstruct labor.

Grossly, fibroids appear as round, well-circumscribed, non-encapsulated tumors that are very often multiple and sometimes extremely large (Fig. 21-6). Examples weighing more than 50 kg have been reported. Their cut surface characteristically bulges and is composed of glistening white tissue with a typically whorled appearance. Some tumors have a stroma in which proteoglycans predominate and which give the cut surface a myxoid or pseudocystic appearance. Areas of calcification are common.

Histologically, fibroids consist of an interlacing arrangement of spindle-shaped smooth muscle cells separated by stroma in which either collagen or, less commonly, proteoglycans, predominate.

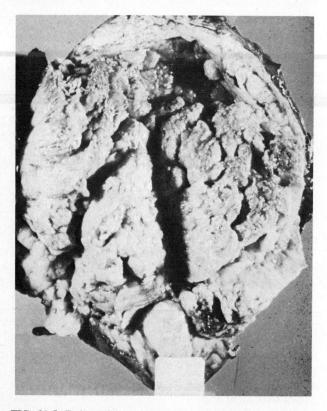

FIG. 21-5. Endometrial carcinoma filling and expanding the uterine cavity. There is also deep infiltration of the myometrium.

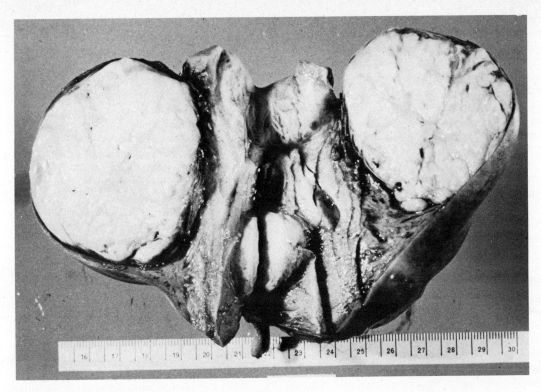

FIG. 21-6. Hysterectomy specimen showing several intramural leiomyomas. Note the sharp demarcation of these benign neoplasms from the surrounding myometrium.

The main clinical features of leiomyomas are the following:
1. Bleeding—menorrhagia or metrorrhagia
2. Pelvic obstruction causing complicated labor, or ureteric obstruction causing retention of urine
3. Abdominal swelling with large tumors

Management of patients with symptomatic uterine leiomyomas has traditionally been surgical—myomectomy for women desirous of children or hysterectomy for those whose families are complete. The administration of hormones to induce a hypoestrogenic state may considerably reduce tumor vascularity and simplify surgery.

Leiomyosarcomas are the most common uterine sarcoma but are nonetheless rare, accounting for approximately 3% of uterine malignant neoplasms. They appear to arise *de novo* and not in pre-existing leiomyomas, and unlike leiomyomas they tend to develop after the menopause. The typical leiomyosarcoma is a bulky, fleshy mass with hemorrhage and necrosis. Microscopically, leiomyosarcomas are highly cellular neoplasms with a high mitotic rate. The overall 5-year survival rate is only about 20%; there is rapid pelvic and intraabdominal spread, and blood-borne metastases develop in the lungs, pleura, kidneys, and liver.

Disorders of the fallopian tubes

Inflammation of the fallopian tubes* is common, while tumors are rare. Another common condition is tubal pregnancy, which is discussed later.

Salpingitis (inflammation of the fallopian tubes) is the most prominent feature of the syndrome of *pelvic inflammatory disease*. This syndrome comprises inflammation that involves al-

---
*Gabriello Fallopio (1523-1562), Italian anatomist.

most the entire female genital tract and is usually secondary to ascending bacterial infection. The most common causes are pyogenic bacteria, particularly *Neisseria gonorrhoeae,* and *Chlamydia trachomatis*. Most cases follow sexual transmission of the causative agents, and pelvic inflammatory disease can also follow childbirth or abortion. In most cases the tubes and ovaries on both sides and the pelvic peritoneum are affected.

In the fallopian tubes there is exudation of fibrin and pus, which reaches the pelvic peritoneum and the ovaries. Organization of this exudate results in the formation of fibrous adhesions involving tubal fimbriae, pelvic peritoneum, and ovaries, and the fallopian tubes become sealed off from the peritoneal cavity. This results in distention of the fallopian tube with pus to produce a *pyosalpinx*. Eventually absorption of the pus may leave the tube distended with a watery, serous fluid (hydrosalpinx). Adhesion of tubal mucosal plicae produces stenosis of the lumen. Adhesion of tube and ovary converts them into a single, inflamed mass (tuboovarian abscess).

Pelvic inflammatory disease commonly produces pelvic discomfort and dysmenorrhea. Tubal pregnancy may result from trapping of a fertilized ovum in a partially obstructed tube. Sterility invariably follows total tubal obstruction. Pelvic inflammatory disease is difficult to control with antibiotics alone, and surgery is often necessary.

Disorders of the ovaries
Nonneoplastic disorders of the ovary

Aside from its frequent involvement in pelvic inflammatory disease and endometriosis, the ovary is the site of several disorders characterized by abnormal hormone stimulation of, or abnormal hormone production by, stromal and/or follicle-derived elements.

Solitary follicular cyst. This common cyst usually develops during the reproductive years. It is thought to result from continuous gonadotropin stimulation of a developing follicle without the midcycle surge of luteinizing hormone that normally triggers ovulation. Solitary follicular cysts may be associated with menstrual irregularities or may rupture causing acute abdominal pain with hemoperitoneum. In most cases, however, they involute spontaneously or after the administration of oral contraceptives. Occasionally a solitary follicular cyst forms after the menopause and causes uterine bleeding by secreting estrogen.

Corpus luteum cysts. Many corpora lutea become cystic and often there is hemorrhage into the cyst cavity. Corpus luteum cysts may be associated with menstrual irregularities or amenorrhea, and, like follicular cysts, may rupture with resulting intraabdominal hemorrhage. The latter is a well recognized complication of anticoagulant therapy.

Polycystic ovary disease (Stein-Leventhal syndrome*), stromal hyperplasia, and stromal hyperthecosis. Several clinical syndromes, characterized by the effects of androgen excess, estrogen excess, or both, are attributed to changes in the ovarian follicles, stroma, or both. Recognition of these associations has spawned a host of confusing clinical and pathologic terms, including those listed above. Experience has demonstrated, however, that these disorders overlap considerably and are best viewed as part of a continuum rather than constituting distinct entities. They are important causes of anovulation, amenorrhea, endometrial hyperplasia, hirsutism, and infertility.

Ovarian neoplasms

Many histologically distinct neoplasms arise in the ovary*:
1. Common epithelial tumors
   a. Serous tumors
   b. Mucinous tumors
   c. Endometrioid tumors
   d. Clear cell (mesonephroid) tumors
   e. Brenner tumors
   f. Mixed epithelial tumors
   g. Undifferentiated carcinoma
   h. Unclassified epithelial tumors
2. Sex-cord-stromal tumors
   a. Granulosa-stromal cell tumors
      (1) Granulosa cell tumor
      (2) Thecoma-fibroma group
   b. Sertoli-Leydig tumors (androblastomas)
   c. Gynandroblastoma
   d. Sex cord tumor with annular tubules
   e. Unclassified
3. Lipid (lipoid) cell tumors
4. Germ cell tumors
   a. Dysgerminoma
   b. Endodermal sinus tumor (yolk sac tumor)

---

*I.F. Stein (1887-1981), American gynecologist; M.L. Leventhal (b. 1904), American gynecologist.

*World Health Organization, 1973, and Young and Scully, 1982, (abbreviated).

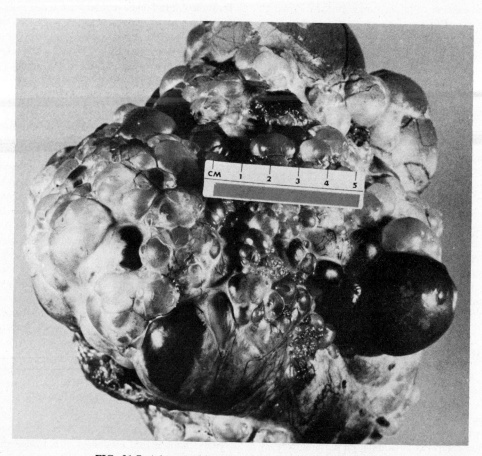

FIG. 21-7. A large multilocular serous cystadenoma of the ovary.

c. Embryonal carcinoma
d. Polyembryoma
e. Choriocarcinoma
f. Teratomas
g. Mixed forms
5. Gonadoblastoma
   a. Pure
   b. Mixed with dysgerminoma or other form of germ cell tumor
6. Soft tissue tumors not specific to ovary
7. Unclassified tumors
8. Secondary (metastatic) tumors
9. Tumorlike conditions

Primary tumors may arise from any of the three ovarian cellular components: (1) surface (celomic) epithelium, (2) sex-cord or stromal cells, and (3) germ cells. Seventy-five to 80% of ovarian neoplasms are benign. The vast majority of ovarian cancers are of the common celomic epithelial types; malignant germ cell and sex-cord stromal neoplasms are relatively rare. The main signs and symptoms of ovarian tumors are a result of their size, hormonal secretions, and malignant behavior. Ovarian tumors are treated by surgical removal, chemotherapy, and radiotherapy or by combinations of these methods.

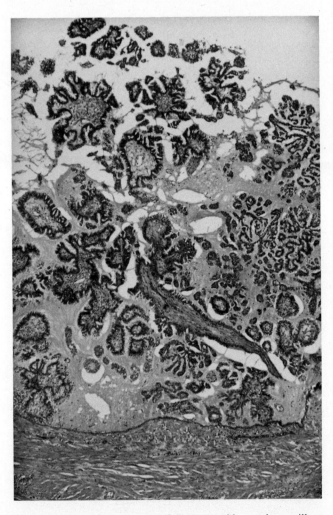

FIG. 21-8. Serous cystadenoma of the ovary with complex papillary folds lining a cystic space.

Celomic epithelial neoplasms. These tumors develop from invagination of surface epithelium into the ovarian stroma. They include benign neoplasms (cystadenomas) (Fig. 21-7), malignant neoplasms (cystadenocarcinomas) and "borderline" types (tumors of low malignant potential). The epithelium may show any of the mullerian lines of differentiation, but is generally either of serous (tubal), mucinous (endocervical), or endometrial type, and combinations of these are sometimes seen. The epithelium lines one or more cystic cavities, separated by varying quantities of stroma. Papillary folding of the epithelium (Fig. 21-8) is common, and psammoma bodies, probably resulting from tumor cell apoptosis, are often found in serous neoplasms. Depending on the type of epithelium, the cystic spaces contain either mucus or serous fluid. Malignant varieties may be partly or almost completely solid, rather than cystic. Serous neoplasms are frequently bilateral.

Cystadenomas. Benign epithelial ovarian neoplasms, or cystadenomas, are among the largest of all human neoplasms. The most extreme example, worthy of the *Guinness Book of World Records,* is a mucinous cystadenoma that weighed 328 pounds and had to be "transported in a wheelbarrow"! Most, however, are between 10 and 30 cm in diameter. *"Borderline" neoplasms* show varying degrees of epithelial stratification and nuclear atypia and may involve sites beyond the ovary, mainly the peritoneum. They are distinguished from frank carcinomas by the absence of an invasive growth pattern, and generally by an indolent clinical course.

Cystadenocarcinomas. The common epithelial cancers of the ovary, or cystadenocarcinomas, are the leading cause of death due to genital cancers in American women. The estimated annual number of deaths (11,500 in 1984) exceeds that from cancer of the uterine cervix (7,000) and endometrium (3,000) combined. Unlike benign epithelial tumors of the ovary, which may be found at any age, with a peak incidence in the fourth and fifth decades, ovarian epithelial cancers most commonly present in the fifth to seventh decades.

These neoplasms appear to be estrogen-related and it has been found that the risk of ovarian cancer rises steadily with "ovulatory age." This is the total time in a woman's life during which her ovarian cycle is not suppressed by pregnancy, lactation, or oral contraceptive administration. Asymptomatic mumps also appears to be associated with an increased risk, and epithelial cancers of the ovary can be familial.

Malignant epithelial tumors of the ovary present as bulky, partially cystic or solid neoplasms. Microscopically, most show a serous epithelial type differentiation, with a papillary architecture being typical of the more differentiated serous cystadenocarcinomas. These cancers are often associated with ascites.

Prognosis and management are closely linked to the degree of spread (stage). Cancers limited to the ovary (stage I) may be amenable to surgery alone, but higher stage lesions may require chemotherapy (to which there may be an excellent response), and sometimes radiotherapy. Tumors which have spread to the extrapelvic peritoneum, retroperitoneal lymph nodes, liver, or to sites outside the abdomen unfortunately account for almost 60% of cases at the time of diagnosis and are associated with only a 10% 5-year survival compared with 65% for stage I cancers. Degree of differentiation, nuclear grade, and possibly DNA cytometry, are also of value in predicting prognosis and selecting therapy.

Germ cell neoplasms. Tumors derived from ovarian germ cells may be *dysgerminomas,* which show no evidence of either embryonic or extraembryonic differentiation; germ cell neoplasms may show minimal differentiation into primitive embryonic-type cells to form the embryonal carcinoma. They may differentiate further as follows:

1. Embryonic: teratoma (Fig. 21-9)
2. Extraembryonic
    a. Trophoblastic: choriocarcinoma (Fig. 21-10)
    b. Yolk sac: yolk sac tumor.

Many germ cell tumors are, however, combinations of these.

The most common ovarian germ cell neoplasms are dysgerminomas and mature cystic teratomas. The *dysgerminoma* is formed of cells resembling primordial germ cells, commonly arranged in groups separated by fibrous septa. This neoplasm is typically found in adolescent girls and young women, is bilateral in about 10% to 15% of cases, and is generally hormonally inactive. Like the testicular seminoma, to which it is histologically identical, the dysgerminoma is very radiosensitive and is associated with an 80% 5-year survival. *Mature cystic teratomas,* the common "dermoid cysts" of the ovary, account for about 15% of ovarian neoplasms and are bilateral in 10% of cases. Typically they are cystic masses usually containing thick sebaceous material and hair, and teeth, cartilage, bone, brain, or thyroid tissue may be present in the lining. Malignant change is only seen in 1% to 2% of cases, usually in the postmenopausal years.

Sex cord-stromal neoplasms. The granulosa cells and Sertoli cells* are believed to be derived from the primitive sex cords of the embryonic gonad. These cells, together with the theca and Leydig cells† of the gonadal stroma, are the principal constituents of this group of ovarian neoplasms, in which they may be found as a single cell population or in any combination.

Granulosa-theca cell neoplasms account for approximately 5% of ovarian neoplasms, and are bilateral in about 5% of cases. Grossly, they frequently have a cut surface with extensive hemorrhage and cystic change. Microscopically, they resemble an overgrown follicle wall (Fig. 21-11). These neoplasms typically secrete estrogens, causing endometrial hyperplasia. About 25% behave in a malignant manner.

Fibrothecomas account for a further 5% of ovarian neoplasms, and 10% are bilateral. Grossly, they form solid, spherical, well-circumscribed yellow-white masses. Microscopically, fibroblast-like stromal cells, a variable proportion of which are luteinized, form the cellular constituents. These neoplasms, which sometimes secrete estrogens, are exceptional in that they are an example of a benign tumor which may be associated, for unknown reasons, with ascites and hydrothorax *(Meig's syndrome).*

---

*E. Sertoli (1842-1910), Italian histologist.
†F. von Leydig (1821-1902), German anatomist.

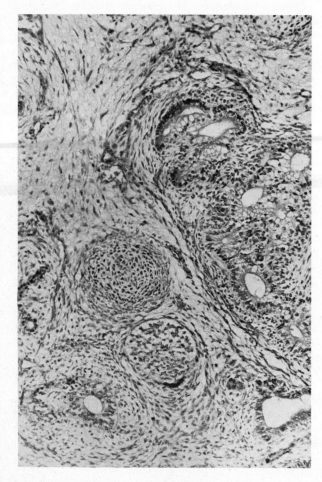

FIG. 21-9. Immature ovarian teratoma. Islands of developing cartilage and duct-like structures resembling the primitive gut are apparent.

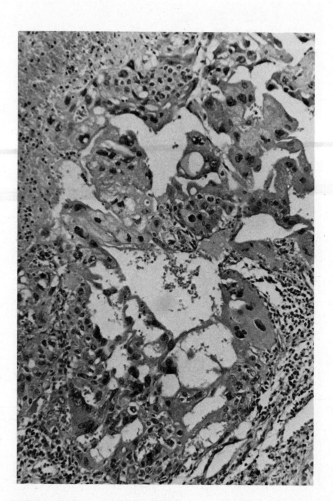

FIG. 21-10. Choriocarcinoma. Note the typical plexiform arrangement of cyto and syncytiotrophoblastic cells.

Sertoli-Leydig cell tumors (arrhenoblastoma, androblastoma). These are rare neoplasms that resemble the fetal testis and which commonly secrete androgens and cause virilization.

Metastatic neoplasms of the ovary. The ovary is a common site for metastases, particularly from carcinoma of the breast, gastrointestinal tract, and uterus. They sometimes produce large masses that may closely mimic primary carcinomas of the ovary. *Krukenberg tumors** are signet-ring cell adenocarcinomas that are usually metastatic and of gastric origin. Typically they are bilateral and form smooth-surfaced, solid ovarian masses.

Endometriosis

Endometriosis is the presence of ectopic or displaced endometrial glands and stroma outside the confines of the uterine corpus.

The most common site is the ovary; others include the pelvic peritoneum, especially the pouch of Douglas.† Implantation of endometrial tissue in surgical wounds may account for endometriosis developing in abdominal or episiotomy scars. Foci of endometriosis may reach up to 10 cm in diameter. They usually

---

*F. Krukenberg (1871-1953), German pathologist.
†J. Douglas (1675-1742), Scottish anatomist.

respond to menstrual hormonal stimuli, resulting in cyclical bleeding. This, in turn, leads to gradual development of blood-filled cavities in affected tissues. Bleeding leads to the development of fibrous adhesions and deposition of iron pigment which accumulates in the extravasated blood, and gives it a characteristic chocolate brown color ("chocolate" cysts) (Fig. 21-12).

Endometriosis tends to cause dysmenorrhea. Dense adhesions of ovaries or fallopian tubes may cause sterility. Hormonal therapy can suppress symptoms, but hysterectomy may be required. Endometriosis occasionally undergoes malignant change.

Etiology and pathogenesis. There are three main theories regarding the development of endometriosis. However, more than one of these mechanisms may be responsible.

Endometriosis may be a systemic, autoimmune disorder involving both humoral and cellular immune mechanisms. Retrograde menstruation with transport of shed endometrial fragments to ectopic locations, is probably the most common mechanism for development of endometriosis and is common to all menstruating females. Implantation or rejection of ectopic endometrial fragments may be under the control of the cell-mediated arm of the immune system, and endometriosis may reflect a deficiency in cell-mediated immunity, allowing implantation of these fragments. There is a high frequency of autoantibodies against endometrial and ovarian tissues in women with endometriosis. This may be in response to ectopic endometrial growth and may explain the infertility and greater

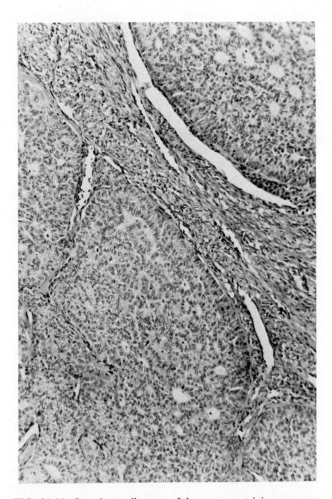

FIG. 21-11. Granulosa cell tumor of the ovary containing numerous Call-Exner bodies (pseudolumina).

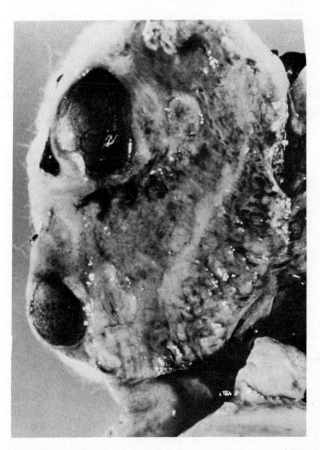

FIG. 21-12. Endometriosis affecting the ovary. The ovary has been sectioned to show blood filled cysts characteristic of this condition.

miscarriage rates that are features of even mild endometriosis.

Endometriosis may be a defect of differentiation or migration of the mullerian duct system during embryonic development, with the result that there is displaced mullerian tissue in the adult.

Endometriosis may arise through metaplasia of the celomic epithelium foci.

Disorders of pregnancy

The major pregnancy disorders are (1) ectopic pregnancy, (2) gestational trophoblastic disease, and (3) abortion.

Ectopic pregnancy

Ectopic pregnancy follows implantation of a fertilized ovum in any tissue other than the endometrium. The most common site is the fallopian tube, usually following partial tubal occlusion as a result of inflammation (Fig. 21-13). Other sites include the cervix, ovary, and pelvic peritoneum.

In tubal pregnancy the wall of the organ is penetrated by chorionic villi, but it is too thin to sustain the development of a complete placenta. The result is that rupture with hemorrhage into the tubal lumen and peritoneal cavity usually takes place during the second month of pregnancy, and the embryo dies. An emergency salpingectomy is generally required in order to control the bleeding. In rare instances the pregnancy may progress to full term with delivery of the fetus by laparotomy.

Gestational trophoblastic disease

The term *gestational trophoblastic disease* is used to distinguish trophoblastic proliferations that follow pregnancy from gonadal and extragonadal germ cell neoplasms unrelated to pregnancy. The best known example of the latter is choriocarcinoma, which may develop in both males and females. Only the more common examples of gestational trophoblastic disease are discussed here.

Hydatidiform mole. (Lt, hydatis, a drop of water). Two types of hydatidiform mole are recognized, the complete mole and the partial mole.

The *complete mole* looks very like a "bunch of grapes" and is formed of strings or clusters of vesicular villi measuring from 1 mm to 3 cm in diameter. All villi show some degree of distension and no fetus or normal placental tissue is present. Histologically, all villi appear edematous, distended, and show varying degrees of central cavitation. Fetal vessels are absent. The definitive feature is, however, trophoblastic hyperplasia of varying degrees.

The *partial mole* differs from the complete mole in that only scattered villi show vesiculation. Trophoblastic hyperplasia is an inconstant feature. A fetus, often abnormal, is commonly present and the villi contain fetal vessels.

Both complete and partial moles may sometimes penetrate the myometrium or its blood vessels. Lesions of this type, termed *invasive moles,* may spread to distant sites such as the lungs or the brain via the bloodstream. The trophoblastic component is more atypical than in regular hydatidiform moles. These "metastases," unlike those of a malignant tumor, tend to regress spontaneously. They may occasionally lead to infarction in distant sites or to hemorrhage caused by the natural ability of trophoblast to invade vessels.

Choriocarcinoma. This malignant tumor of trophoblast follows a complete hydatidiform mole in 60% of cases, an abortion in 30% and a normal pregnancy in 20%. The time between the

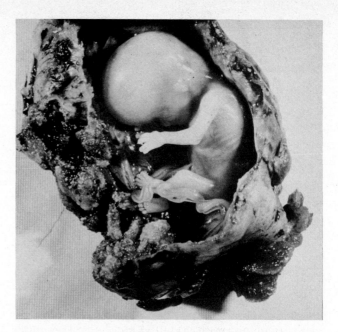

FIG. 21-13. Ectopic pregnancy. In this case the pregnancy developed in the fallopian tube. Surgical removal was necessary because of rupture of the tube and intra-abdominal hemorrhage.

preceding pregnancy and the development of a choriocarcinoma varies from a few months to 15 years. A choriocarcinoma forms single or multiple hemorrhagic nodules within the uterus which histologically show central necrosis with a surrounding core of viable tumor tissue. The neoplasm shows the dimorphic pattern of the early implanting blastocyst, namely central cores of cytotrophoblast surrounded by a peripheral rim of syncytiotrophoblast (see Fig. 21-10). Villi are not seen.

Clinical aspects. Hydatidiform moles are characterized by disproportionate enlargement of the uterus during early pregnancy and a bloody or brown discharge that continues until evacuation of the mole. It is often associated with toxemia of pregnancy (albuminuria, edema, hypertension). Moles can persist or invade the uterus, and up to 5% of complete moles are estimated to develop into choriocarcinoma. Partial moles may evolve into persistent or invasive trophoblastic disease and should be followed up in exactly the same way as complete moles (i.e., by monitoring the serum human chorionic gonadotropin (hCG) levels). No case of choriocarcinoma arising from partial mole has, however, been authenticated to date. Persistent trophoblastic disease and choriocarcinoma respond well to chemotherapy, particularly methotrexate, even in patients with metastases.

Pathogenesis of hydatidiform moles and choriocarcinoma. As a result of chromosomal studies complete moles are now known to have exclusively paternal chromosomes and thus constitute total allografts in the mother as do the choriocarcinomas arising from their trophoblast. Their development may be due to the fertilization of an "empty egg" by either one or two spermatozoa, depending on the karyotype of the mole. It is postulated that the totally homozygous state "uncovers" recessive lethal genes that first cause the early demise of the embryo proper, and may later also "uncover" a rare recessive oncogene responsible for choriocarcinoma. Partial hydatidiform moles, by contrast, may contain a set of maternal chromosomes in addition to two sets of paternal chromosomes.

Cases with a maternal chromosomal complement may have a less aggressive potential.

Abortion

Abortion is the termination of pregnancy before viability of the conceptus. It may be induced or spontaneous. Induced, or therapeutic, abortion is a highly controversial subject beyond the scope of this textbook. The term *miscarriage* is commonly used as a synonym for spontaneous abortion.

The incidence of spontaneous abortion is generally underestimated. Subclinical loss of fertilized ova is a common event, and probably only 50% of fertilized ova survive. Clinically apparent spontaneous abortions take place in a minimum of 15% of all pregnancies. The most common identifiable causes are intrauterine infections, teratogenic drugs taken during early pregnancy, or chromosomal anomalies. Spontaneous abortions are further classified as either early or late.

Approximately 80% of *early spontaneous abortions,* i.e., those taking place during the embryonic stage of pregnancy, are morphologically abnormal. Most of these are *growth-disorganized embryos (GDEs)* ("blighted ova"), in which the chorionic sac either appears empty or contains a severely malformed embryo. A high percentage of GDEs are associated with chromosomal anomalies, such as trisomy, monosomy, or polyploidy. Abortions of this type, especially when recurrent, can sometimes be linked to chromosomal abnormalities in one or both parents, and karyotyping followed by genetic counseling is indicated in such cases. The remaining 20% of early spontaneous abortions are normally developed embryos, suggesting either a hormonal imbalance (abnormal function of corpus luteum or endometrium) or placental infection as the cause.

Fetal morphologic abnormalities, or chromosomal anomalies, in *late spontaneous abortions* (i.e., those taking place in the fetal stage of development) are seen in only a quarter of cases. Late abortions are more commonly the result of intrauterine infections such as bacterial or fungal villitis or chorioamnionitis.

Disorders of the breast

The adult female breast consists largely of fibroadipose stroma supporting a system of ducts that comprises no more than about 10% of the bulk of the organ. The ducts extend from the nipple to deeper in the breast, where they terminate as little branched clusters termed lobules (Fig. 21-14). Unless pregnancy supervenes, the ducts have no significant secretory function. During pregnancy there is extreme hyperplasia of intralobular ducts, which assume a milk-secreting function during lactation. Secretion of milk is aided by the myoepithelial cells of the breast lobules.

The breast is a target organ for sex steroid hormones such as estrogen and progesterone, and *both ducts and stroma respond to menstrual cyclical hormonal stimuli*. Thus epithelial proliferation, alternating with partial lobular destruction by apoptosis, takes place throughout reproductive life. These events are accompanied, respectively, by lobular stromal expansion (with an increase in proteoglycan content), and stromal collapse and condensation. From the third or fourth decade of life, the balance of the cyclical changes gradually tips in favor of both lobular epithelial and stromal loss, with a relative increase in breast fat content.

In the study of breast diseases, attention is mainly directed

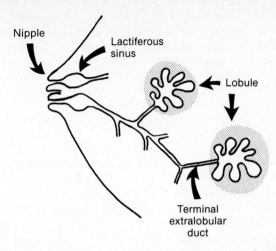

FIG. 21-14. Diagram depicting the basic structural units of the female breast.

toward one distressingly common and potentially lethal entity—carcinoma arising from the ductal epithelium. Most other breast lesions are important mainly because, clinically or histologically, they mimic carcinoma, or are important indicators of increased risk for carcinoma.

Most clinically important breast conditions present either as lumps in the breast, or as suspicious shadows detected by mammographic screening.

Fibrocystic disease complex

In the breast there is a spectrum of extremely common processes which can be considered as exaggerated proliferative or involutional responses of ducts and/or stroma to hormonal stimuli. These processes, which may be seen alone or in varying combinations, are the following:

1. Epithelial hyperplasia in lobular or extralobular ducts (epitheliosis, papillomatosis)
2. Increased numbers of lobular ducts (adenosis)
3. Cyst formation, with or without apocrine metaplasia
4. Fibrosis

One or more of these processes may be seen in up to 90% of breasts examined at autopsy. Minor ones, especially if asymptomatic, are therefore probably best regarded as variations of normal. When pronounced, however, some may give rise to symptoms, such as a breast mass, and the term "fibrocystic disease" is traditionally employed under such circumstances. In addition, some variants have been shown to be associated with an increased risk of breast carcinoma. Each of these processes is considered in more detail below.

Ductal epithelial hyperplasia

Ductal epithelial hyperplasia is characterized by an intraductal proliferation of epithelial cells leading to partial or total obliteration of the lumen. The proliferating cells form varying patterns of solid masses, gland-like (cribriform) structures, or papillary fronds with fibrovascular cores. The microscopic appearances are, in most cases, readily distinguishable from in situ carcinoma (intraductal carcinoma and lobular carcinoma in situ). In cases where the hyperplastic epithelium appears cytologically or architecturally atypical, but where the features fall short of those of in situ carcinoma, the term *atypical hyperplasia* (ductal or lobular) is used. Atypical hyperplasia has been found to be associated with a moderately increased risk for the subsequent development of invasive breast carcinoma.

Ductal epithelial hyperplasia, when moderate or florid, but lacking any atypical features, has been found to approximately double the risk for invasive breast cancer. The term *proliferative fibrocystic disease* is applied to this process to distinguish it from those which have no proven association with any increased risk for carcinoma, such as adenosis, cysts, and fibrosis.

Adenosis

Adenosis is an abnormal proliferation of intralobular ducts leading to an increase in tubular profiles (Fig. 21-15). When this is accompanied by a prominent increase in intralobular collagen, the term *sclerosing adenosis* is applied. (See Fig. 21-12.)

Cysts

Cysts (Fig. 21-16) are presumed to arise from distended ducts and are usually multiple. They appear blue to the naked eye and may be microscopic or grossly visible. Apocrine metaplastic cells are often found lining cysts. Larger cysts may be "cured" by needle aspiration of their fluid contents.

Fibrosis

Most of the changes described above show some degree of associated fibrosis. However, the term *focal fibrosis* (fibrous mastopathy) is employed in cases with a tumorlike mass due mainly to the production of comparatively acellular fibrous tissue encompassing atrophic ducts.

Breast neoplasms

The majority of the important breast neoplasms are either (1) epithelial or (2) of mixed connective tissue-epithelial type. Most of the epithelial neoplasms are carcinomas, and most of the mixed neoplasms are fibroadenomas. The bulk of the discussion that follows is on these entities. A histologic classification of breast neoplasms follows*:

  A. Epithelial tumors
    1. Benign
      a. Intraductal papilloma
      b. Adenoma of the nipple
      c. Adenoma
        (1) Tubular
        (2) Lactating
    2. Malignant
      a. Noninvasive
        (1) Intraductal carcinoma
        (2) Lobular carcinoma *in situ*
      b. Invasive
        (1) Invasive ductal carcinoma
        (2) Invasive ductal carcinoma with a predominant intraductal component

*Modification of World Health Organization classification, 1982.

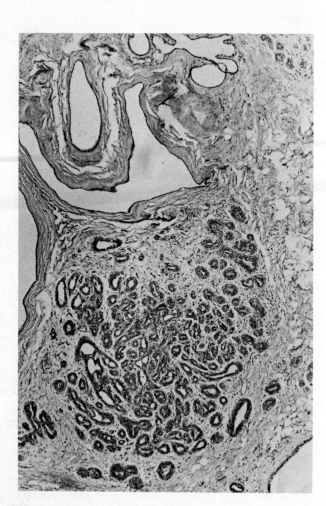

FIG. 21-15. Fibrocystic disease of the breast. A lobule showing an increase in ductal profiles (adenosis) is seen.

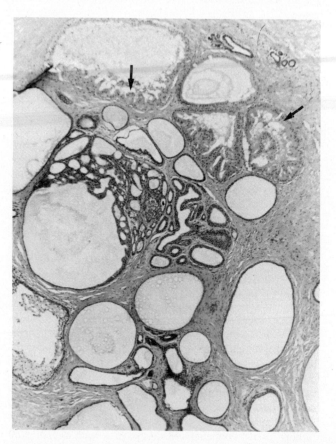

FIG. 21-16. Fibrocystic disease of the breast. There is cystic dilatation of several ducts, some of which show apocrine metaplasia *(arrows)*.

(3) Invasive lobular carcinoma
(4) Mucinous carcinoma
(5) Medullary carcinoma
(6) Papillary carcinoma
(7) Tubular carcinoma
(8) Adenoid cystic carcinoma
(9) Secretory (juvenile) carcinoma
(10) Apocrine carcinoma
(11) Carcinoma with metaplasia
    (a) Squamous type
    (b) Spindle-cell type
    (c) Cartilaginous and osseous type
    (d) Mixed type
  c. Paget's disease of the nipple
B. Mixed connective tissue and epithelial tumors
  1. Fibroadenoma
  2. Phyllodes tumor (cystosarcoma phyllodes)
  3. Carcinosarcoma
C. Miscellaneous tumors
  1. Soft tissue tumors
  2. Skin tumors
  3. Tumors of hematopoietic and lymphoid tissues
D. Unclassified tumors

Carcinoma of the breast

Breast carcinoma is the most common cancer found in women, accounting for more than a quarter of all cancers among females in the United States where 120,000 new cases of breast carcinoma are detected annually in women, and about 900 in men. It is estimated that about one in every 10 women will develop breast cancer and one out of four will die as a consequence of it. The incidence of breast cancer is increasing at a rate of about 2% per annum. This may be partly attributable to better detection and diagnosis of breast abnormalities. While breast cancer is found most frequently in women over age 50, a small but significant percentage is seen, tragically, in much younger women.

Etiology and risk factors. Women who have a family history of breast cancer are extremely vulnerable, especially when a mother, daughter or sister has had the disease. The risk increases further if that relative developed breast cancer before age 50, or the disease was bilateral. Breast cancer appears to be related, at least in part, to relative hyperestrinism. Thus women in developed Western countries, who on the average have fewer and later pregnancies and are exposed to the effects of unopposed estrogen secretion for longer periods of their lives, show a far higher incidence of breast carcinoma than women in underdeveloped countries.

It has been consistently shown that a higher risk of breast cancer is associated with even moderate consumption of alcohol, there being a 40% to 60% higher risk in moderate drinkers than in non-drinkers. Dietary factors, in particular a high fat intake, increases the risk of developing breast cancer, and obese women are more prone to the disease. Exposure to the effects of radiation also puts women at greater risk, and the disease can appear after a latent period of 10 to 15 years.

Pathogenesis and pathology. All forms of breast carcinoma arise from the duct epithelium. Approximately 90% arise from the large, extralobular ducts (ductal carcinoma), and 10% arise from the smaller, intralobular ducts and terminal extralobular ducts (lobular carcinoma). Ductal (Fig. 21-17) and lobular forms of *carcinoma in situ* are recognized as lesions preceding the development of infiltrating carcinoma.

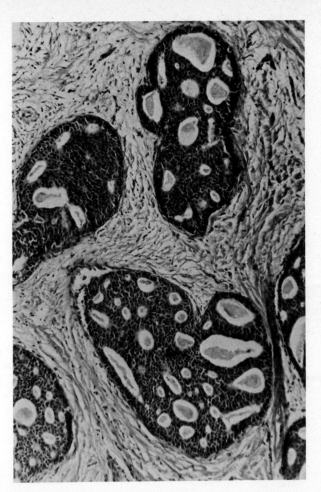

FIG. 21-17. Intraductal (in-situ) breast carcinoma of cribriform type. The ducts are distended by small, uniform cells lining "punched out" lumina.

Infiltrating breast carcinoma. Infiltrating breast carcinoma may take several forms. In the majority of cases, the invasive tumor cells appear as cords or sheets of cells sometimes with duct lumen formation. The induction of a dense, collagen-rich tumor stroma (Fig. 21-18) is common, and such tumors are hard and are called *scirrhous carcinomas* (Chap. 2). When cut, they have the consistency of an unripe pear and appear as a translucent grey-white mass (Fig. 21-19), usually less than 4 cm in diameter, with numerous processes extending into the surrounding tissue. This crablike appearance of the tumor gave rise to the word cancer (literally, a crab) for malignant disease.

Biology of breast carcinoma. It is widely believed especially by the lay public that the earlier a breast cancer is detected, the more likely is its cure. Indeed, overemphasis on early detection as a means of wiping out breast cancer has led to many malpractice suits alleging that diagnostic delay was responsible for a lethal outcome. However, in most instances the outcome is determined by the biologic nature of the cancer.

About 60% of breast carcinomas are slow growing and associated with long survival, whereas the other 40% are fast growing and associated with short survival. Early detection, by regular self-examinations and periodic mammography, may, indeed, help improve the prognosis for patients with slow-growing carcinomas. Regrettably, however, the fast growing carcinomas will usually have undergone systemic spread (occult

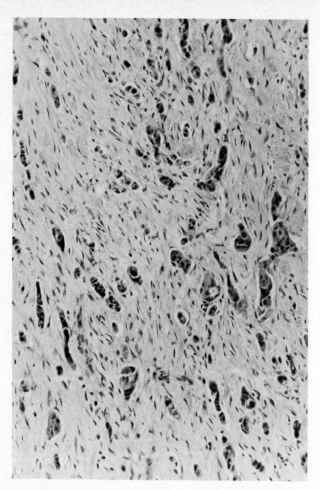

FIG. 21-18. Infiltrating scirrhous breast ductal carcinoma. The neoplastic cells tend to form narrow cords and are separated by an abundant, collagen-rich fibrous stroma (desmoplastic phase of connective tissue activation).

or overt) by the time they become clinically or radiologically detectable in the breast, and death from progressive disease usually follows within less than 5 years following diagnosis.

Unlike most other cancers, such as those of the endometrium, cervix, ovary, colon, stomach, or lung, absence of clinical disease after five years following apparent eradication of breast

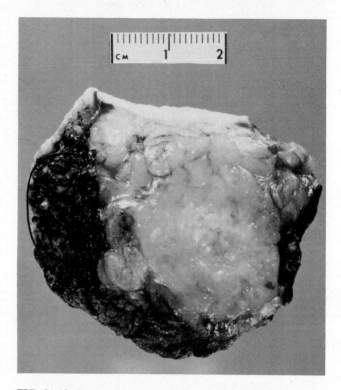

FIG. 21-19. Section through a breast lumpectomy specimen showing a pale, translucent carcinoma. The opaque streaks seen centrally are foci of elastosis.

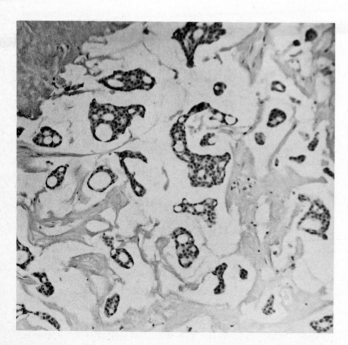

FIG. 21-20. Colloid (mucous) carcinoma of the breast. Clusters of lumen-forming tumor cells are seen lying in clear pools of mucus. (*Courtesy Curator of the Gordon Museum. Guy's Hospital, London, England.*)

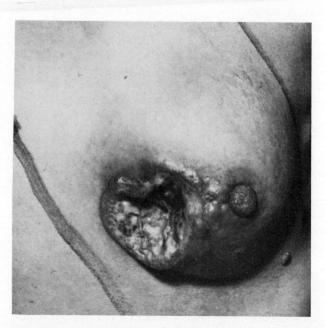

FIG. 21-21. A large ulcerating carcinoma of the breast. Note also the retraction of the nipple.

cancer does not necessarily imply cure of this disease. The reason is that some of the less aggressive breast cancers can spread systemically early in their evolution, only becoming clinically apparent as metastases many years later.

Several methods are used in an attempt to predict the biologic behavior of breast cancers.

Routine histologic study of the excised cancer. Five histologic subtypes, which are slightly more common in older patients, are characteristically associated with slow growth; these are *adenoid cystic carcinoma, tubular carcinoma, papillary carcinoma, mucinous (colloid) carcinoma* (Fig. 21-20), and *medullary carcinoma*. In most other types of breast carcinomas the size of the tumor, the degree of nuclear atypia (nuclear grade) and the presence or absence of invasive tumor necrosis and lymphatic or blood vessel invasion may be useful pointers.

Estrogen and progesterone receptor assays. Estrogen and progesterone receptor assays have prognostic value, and tumors rich in these receptors are more likely to respond to endocrine therapy than those in which they are lacking. Receptor-positive neoplasms are usually better differentiated, of lower nuclear grade, and slower growing than receptor-negative ones.

Flow cytometry. Flow cytometry can determine both the percentage of cells in the S phase (DNA synthetic phase) of the cell cycle (which indicates the growth rate of the tumor cells), as well as assessing the DNA ploidy. This technique is more accurate and reproducible than microscopic methods in predicting the biologic behavior of a neoplasm.

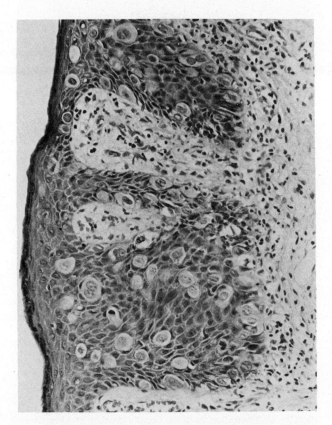

FIG. 21-22. Paget's disease of the nipple. Carcinoma cells with abundant pale cytoplasm lie scattered in the nipple epidermis.

Stage. The presence or absence of axillary lymph node metastases is of great clinical importance. If the tumor is of the slow growing variety, the presence of nodal metastases may be compatible with long patient survival following mastectomy.

Patterns of spread of breast carcinoma. Cancer of the breast may spread locally, via lymphatic channels, or via the bloodstream.

Local spread. Invasion of the pectoral muscles and deep fascia causes the tumor to become "fixed" to the chest wall, making resection impractical. Adherence to the overlying skin produces retraction or dimpling of the skin and the nipple (Fig. 21-21). Where carcinoma arises in ducts near the nipple, the carcinoma may extend to the epidermis and produce a lesion resembling dermatitis of the nipple. This is called Paget's disease of the nipple and is confirmed histologically by the demonstration of large, round tumor cells in the epidermis around the nipple (Fig. 21-22).

Lymphatic spread. In approximately two thirds of cases breast cancer has undergone lymphatic spread by the time it is clinically detected. Sixty percent of breast carcinomas arise in the upper, outer breast quadrant and spread predominantly to axillary lymph nodes. Mastectomy, which may or may not include the pectoral muscles, is an attempt to remove the breast, tumor, and axillary nodes and, thus, theoretically to prevent further spread of the disease. The degree of axillary node involvement correlates with the prognosis. Breast cancers that arise in the medial quadrants have a greater tendency to spread to the internal thoracic lymph nodes and are therefore, less amenable to this type of surgery.

The name *inflammatory carcinoma* is applied when dermal lymphatic blockage by carcinoma cells causes increasing breast size, pain, warmth, edema (Fig. 21-23) and skin redness. This clinical picture is usually associated with a poor prognosis.

Blood spread. Spread through the bloodstream is usually a late event but, as previously pointed out, takes place early in some breast cancers. The skeleton is the site of metastases in a high percentage of cases. Patients with blood-borne metastases have inoperable disease, and treatment is palliative.

Detection, diagnosis, and treatment of breast carcinoma. Although there are exceptions, the prognosis for women with breast cancer is related to tumor size and the presence or absence of metastases at the time of detection. The American Cancer Society has accordingly recommended guidelines for the screening of asymptomatic women in an attempt to find breast cancer at an early, potentially curable stage:

1. Monthly breast self-examinations starting at age 20
2. Professional physical examination of the breast at 3-year intervals between the ages of 20 and 40, and annually thereafter
3. A baseline mammogram between the ages of 35 and 40, followed by annual or biennial mammograms from 40-49, and annual mammograms from age 50

Cancer that produces a breast lump is usually invasive (see Fig. 21-19). The value of mammography by low-dose x-ray examination is its ability to detect very small, nonpalpable cancers, including in situ cancers. Foci of dystrophic calcification are common in these lesions and show up on x-rays (Fig. 21-24). It should be noted that foci of calcification are also very commonly seen in breasts with benign lesions, although the pattern of calcification may differ. Following detection of calcification on mammography, breast biopsy (fine needle aspiration, cutting needle, or open biopsy) is performed to make a definitive diagnosis.

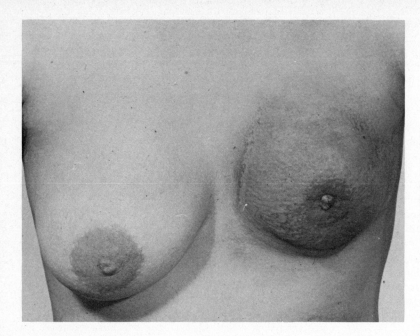

FIG. 21-23. Carcinoma of the breast. The lymphatics of the left breast have been infiltrated with tumor resulting in superficial lymphatic blockage and edema, which give the skin of the breast the appearance of an orange skin (peau d'orange). In addition, the contraction of the fibrous stroma of the tumor has caused elevation and contraction of the nipple.

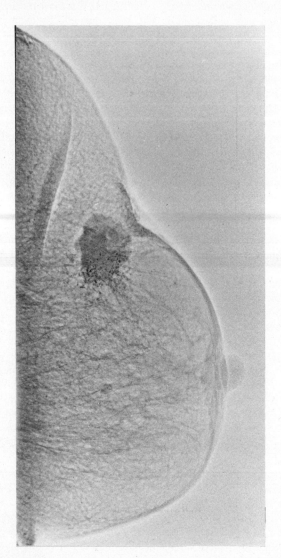

FIG. 21-24. Xeroradiograph of the breast shows an irregular stellate mass, retraction of the skin, and punctate calcification indicating the presence of a carcinoma.

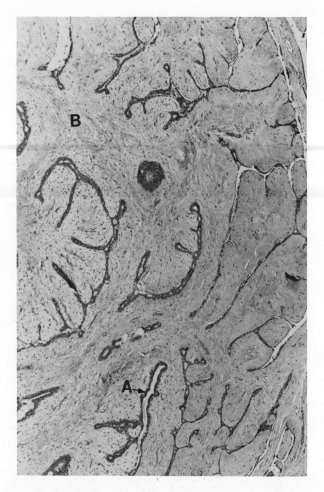

FIG. 21-25. Fibroadenoma of the breast consisting of a proliferation of ducts *(A)* and accompanying fibrous stroma *(B)*.

Smaller, low-grade cancers are generally treated either by simple removal of the tumor (lumpectomy), followed by local irradiation, or by mastectomy. Higher grade or larger lesions generally require, in addition to surgical removal, adjuvant chemotherapy, and anti-estrogenic agents may be employed for estrogen-receptor positive tumors. Much controversy surrounds the management of patients with in-situ cancers, which are multicentric or bilateral in a significant percentage of cases, mainly because the natural history of such lesions in individual cases is presently largely unknown.

Mixed connective tissue and epithelial neoplasms

Fibroadenoma. The fibroadenoma, in its typical form, is a well circumscribed mass resulting from proliferation of lobular ducts, accompanied by a striking increase in intervening fibrous stroma (Fig. 21-25). Fibroadenomas arise predominantly between the ages of 15 and 25, but they may not be diagnosed until later in life, when they are more easily palpated. They show lactational changes during pregnancy and involution along with the rest of the breast towards the menopause. Most of these lesions, which are, in essence, greatly hyperplastic breast lobules rather than true neoplasms, grow to 1 or at most 2 cm in diameter and their size does not change thereafter. Exceptionally, especially in adolescents, fibroadenomas may grow to a very large size (*giant fibroadenoma*).

Phyllodes tumor (cystosarcoma phyllodes). Phyllodes tumors are fairly well circumscribed, usually large neoplasms composed of connective tissue and epithelial elements. They resemble fibroadenomas, but their connective tissue is much more cellular. They may also contain myxoid, adipose, osseous, and chondroid foci. Based on stromal cellularity, stromal overgrowth, nuclear atypia, frequency of mitoses, and the presence or absence of infiltrative margins, phyllodes tumors are separated into benign, and malignant types. Either of these may recur locally following incomplete removal, but metastases (usually blood-borne) are generally limited to the histologically malignant variety.

Inflammatory and miscellaneous disorders of the breast

Acute mastitis. Acute mastitis is common in the lactating woman and usually takes the form of a breast abscess that develops following the entry of pyogenic bacteria into the breast via a cracked nipple. It heals readily following incision and drainage.

Duct ectasia. In duct ectasia, also known as periductal mastitis and plasma cell mastitis, there is progressive dilatation of the mammary duct system usually in the subareolar region. Debris and lipids characteristically fill the lumen. The periductal stroma is infiltrated by inflammatory cells and, as the disease progresses, it becomes more and more fibrotic. When the continuity of the epithelial lining is broken, lipid material enters the stroma and provokes a foreign body reaction. Clinically, the presence of a subareolar mass, perhaps associated with nipple retraction, may cause confusion with breast carcinoma. An association of duct ectasia with pituitary adenomas suggests a possible endocrine basis for this disease.

Fat necrosis. Fat necrosis is most likely to develop in older women with large, pendulous breasts. It may apparently result from trauma or be without obvious cause. There is repair by fibrous tissue that may result in the formation of a firm lump, which clinically mimics a scirrhous carcinoma.

Gynecomastia. Gynecomastia is a condition of the male breast characterized by unilateral or bilateral breast enlargement and, histologically, a proliferation of ducts and increased periductal stroma which may have a myxoid appearance. Epithelial hyperplasia may be observed, but there is no evidence of an increased predisposition to the development of carcinoma. This common disorder can be caused by the following:

1. Androgen-deficiency states (e.g., aging and hypogonadism)
2. Estrogen-excess states (e.g., obesity, liver cirrhosis, and some testicular tumors)
3. Unknown mechanisms, as in the case of gynecomastia associated with the use of digitalis derivatives

Selected readings

Anon: Human papillomaviruses and cervical cancer: a fresh look at the evidence, Lancet i:725, 1987.

Azzopardi JG: Problems in breast pathology, Philadelphia, 1979, WB Saunders Co.

Barber HRK et al: Symposium on endometrial carcinoma: classification, grading, and staging, Pathol Annu 20(2):507, 1985.

Deligdisch L and Holinka CF: Endometrial carcinoma: two diseases? Cancer Detection and Prevention 10:237, 1987.

Dressler LG et al: DNA flow cytometry and prognostic factors in 1331 frozen breast cancer specimens, Cancer 61:420, 1988.

Fox H, editor: Haines and Taylor, Obstetrical and gynaecological pathology, ed 3, Edinburgh, 1987, Churchill Livingstone.

Fox H and Buckley CH: Atlas of gynecological pathology, Philadelphia and Toronto, 1983, JB Lippincott Co.

Gleicher M et al: Is endometriosis an autoimmune disease? Obstet Gynecol 70:115, 1987.

Harris JR et al, editors: Breast diseases, Philadelphia, 1987, JB Lippincott Co.

Hendrickson MR and Kempson RL: Surgical pathology of the uterine corpus, Philadelphia, 1980, WB Saunders Co.

Koss LG: Cytologic and histologic manifestations of human papillomavirus infection of the female genital tract and their clinical significance, Cancer 60:1942, 1987.

Kurman RJ, editor: Blaustein's pathology of the female genital tract, ed 3, New York, 1987, Springer-Verlag.

Lauchlan SC: Metaplasias and neoplasias of mullerian epithelium, Histopathology 8:543, 1984.

Osborne MP: The biologic basis for breast cancer treatment options, Am Coll Surg Bull 71:4, 1986.

Page DL: Cancer risk assessment in benign breast biopsies, Hum Pathol 17:871, 1986.

Perrin EVDK, editor: Pathology of the placenta, New York, 1984, Churchill Livingstone.

Richardson GS, Scully RE, Nikrui N, and Nelson JH, Jr: Common epithelial cancer of the ovary, N Engl J Med 312:415, 1985.

Richart RM: Causes and management of cervical intraepithelial neoplasia, Cancer 60:1951, 1987.

Roebuck EJ: Mammography and screening for breast cancer, B Med J 292:223, 1986.

Urban JE: Breast cancer 1985: What have we learned? Cancer 57:636, 1986.

Wells M and Brown LJR: Glandular lesions of the uterine cervix: the present state of our knowledge, Histopathology 10:777, 1986.

Wilkinson EJ: Pathology of the vulva and vagina, New York, 1987, Churchill Livingstone.

Winkler B and Crum CP: *Chlamydia trachomatis* infection of the female genital tract: pathogenetic and clinicopathologic correlations, Pathol Annu 22(1):193, 1987.

CHAPTER 22

Diseases of the male genital system

This chapter deals with the more common nonsexually transmitted diseases of the prostate glands, testes, spermatic cord, scrotum, and penis. Sexually transmitted diseases which can involve many of these structures are discussed in Chapter 23.

Disease of the prostate gland
Anatomy

The prostate gland lies at the base of the bladder and is composed of five lobes: anterior, posterior, median, and two lateral lobes. The gland is 2.5 cm to 3.8 cm (1 to 1½ inches) in diameter, weighs about 20 g, and consists of glandular and fibromuscular tissue. The glandular portion of the prostate is lined by cuboidal epithelium, which produces a mucoid secretion. The gland is traversed by the prostatic urethra.

The important diseases of the prostate are as follows:
1. Prostatitis
2. Nodular hyperplasia
3. Carcinoma

Prostatitis

A variety of organisms can cause acute inflammation of the prostate. Most of these are either sexually transmitted infections, especially gonorrhea and chlamydial disease, or are conveyed to the prostate by the passage of clinical instruments, such as catheters or cystoscopes through the urethra. Occasionally, prostatic infection is the result of bloodborne dissemination of staphylococcal or tuberculous infection.

Acute prostatitis is characterized by multiple small abscesses in the gland. Clinically, there is dysuria and deepseated perineal pain.

Chronic prostatitis may follow unresolved acute inflammation with the development of fibrosis and lymphocytic infiltration of the gland. Symptoms of chronic prostatitis are similar to those of the acute form but they are generally less severe.

Tuberculous prostatitis is the result of spread to the prostate gland of tuberculosis elsewhere in the genitourinary system. The pathologic changes (caseating granulomas) are typical of tuberculous infection. Clinically there may be sufficient inflammatory enlargement of the gland to cause urinary obstruction.

Nodular hyperplasia

Nodular hyperplasia is a common prostatic disease found almost exclusively in men over the age of 50. It is present to some degree in most elderly males, and about 5% to 7% of these will develop clinical symptoms. A synonymous, but inaccurate term, *prostatic hypertrophy* is sometimes used to describe this condition. The abnormality, however, is a true hyperplasia (i.e., cellular proliferation) not hypertrophy. The hyperplastic process mainly involves the median and lateral lobes. It is thought to be due to the effects of adrenocortical estrogens

acting on prostatic glandular tissue. Normally this effect is opposed by testicular androgens, but in the presence of decreased secretion of these hormones, the estrogens are able to act unopposed.

The pathologic features in the median and lateral lobes consist of hyperplastic nodules of proliferating but benign glandular epithelium (Fig. 22-1). This hyperplastic process compresses the remainder of the gland into a peripheral rim of tissue. Within the glands, *corpora amylacea,* which are small concentric hyaline bodies, are frequently present. Their significance is not known. The effects of the hyperplastic process are as follows:
1. Enlargement of the gland to four or five times its normal size
2. Obstruction to the outflow of urine from the bladder by enlarging lateral lobes and/or plugging of the urethra by upward growth of the enlarging median lobe

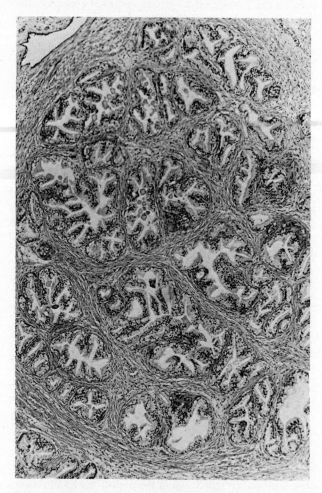

FIG. 22-1. Benign nodular hyperplasia of the prostate gland. A typical nodule consisting of large benign glands is shown.

The effects of obstruction (Fig. 22-2) if unrelieved are the following:

1. Hypertrophy of the muscular bladder wall
2. Hydroureter (dilatation of the ureter)
3. Bilateral hydronephrosis (Fig. 22-3)
4. Predisposition to urinary tract infection

It has been claimed that patients with nodular hyperplasia are more likely to develop cancer, but there is little valid evidence to support this opinion.

Clinically, prostatic hyperplasia affects the patient's ability to control his bladder function. Urinary frequency, dribbling and nocturia are also common. The symptoms of urinary tract

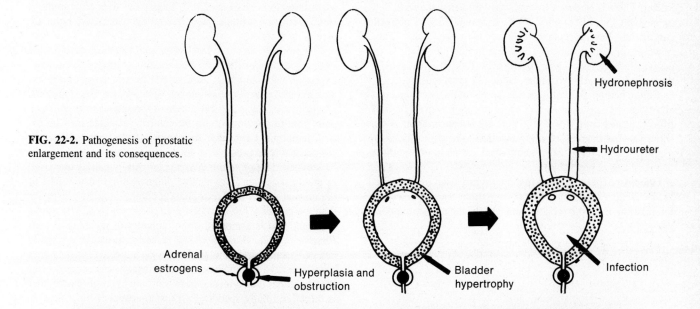

FIG. 22-2. Pathogenesis of prostatic enlargement and its consequences.

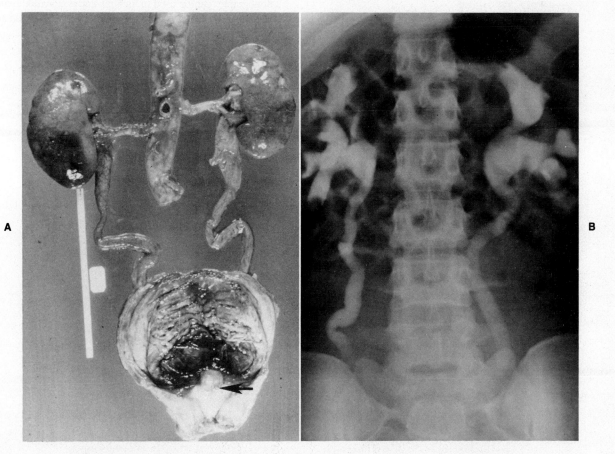

FIG. 22-3. A, Prostatic hyperplasia and its consequences. The middle lobe of the prostate *(arrow)* is prominently enlarged causing urinary obstruction. There is, as a result, hypertrophy of the bladder wall, bilateral hydroureter, and hydronephrosis. **B,** Bilateral hydronephrosis and hydroureter. The radiopaque dye has outlined the grossly dilated ureters and renal pelves, which have resulted from chronic prostatic obstruction.

infection may be superimposed. Treatment is resection of the prostate.

Carcinoma of the prostate

This common malignancy is third only to lung and colo-rectal cancers as a cause of cancer deaths in males. In 1985, in the United States more than 25,000 men died from prostatic cancer. There is evidence from autopsy studies that almost 50% of all men over the age of 50 have minute foci of prostatic cancer, and this percentage increases with age. The disease, however, becomes clinically apparent in only one sixth of the cases. Nevertheless, each year nearly 100,000 men will be diagnosed in the United States as having prostatic cancer.

Unlike benign nodular hyperplasia, prostatic carcinoma usually originates in the posterior lobe. It may however, be multifocal. Microscopically, the tumors are adenocarcinomas that show varying degrees of differentiation. The tumor cells are usually cuboidal and form acini lined by single or multiple layers of cells (Fig. 22-4).

One histologic grading system* currently used in the United States assigns a number (1 to 5) to denote the degree of differentiation of (a) the predominant and (b) the next-to-predom-

*Gleason DF and Mellinger GT: Prediction of prognosis of prostatic adenocarcinoma by combined histological grading and clinical staging, J Urol 111:58, 1974.

inant pattern present in the tumor. These numbers are then added: the higher the total (2 to 10) the less differentiated is the tumor and the poorer the survival rate.

A few rare malignant tumors of the prostate are of transitional or other cell types.

Prostatic carcinoma spreads both locally and distantly. Invasion of the capsule is followed by spread to local lymphatics. Metastases to bone (Fig. 22-5), lungs, and liver are common. Bony metastases, often characterized by sclerosis of bone are especially frequent.

Symptoms of prostatic carcinoma, unfortunately develop late in the disease. For this reason, palpation of the prostate gland by rectal examination is an essential part of any clinical examination of men, especially over 50 years old. The symptoms are the result of urinary obstruction or metastases to bone. Back pain from tumor deposits in the lumbar vertebrae may be the first symptom. Clinically, the diagnosis is suggested by palpation of a hard prostatic mass.

Measurement of *serum acid phosphatase* which is increased in prostatic cancer is a valuable diagnostic aid. About half of the normal serum acid phosphatase comes from sources other than the prostate; but *prostatic acid phosphatase (PAP)* can be measured and is a more specific indicator of prostatic cancer. *Prostate-specific antigen (PSA),* a serine protease originally isolated from seminal fluid, has recently been described as a more sensitive plasma marker for prostatic cancer. However, PSA like PAP is also increased in prostatic hyperplasia. Neither is therefore totally specific for prostatic cancer.

Sonography can be used to localize and delineate the tumor, and the histologic diagnosis made by transperineal or transrectal needle biopsy. Radiologic skeletal survey is used to determine

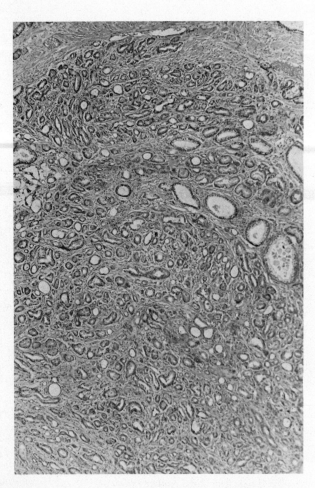

FIG. 22-4. Well-differentiated prostatic adenocarcinoma. There is florid proliferation of neoplastic glands, which are characteristically small.

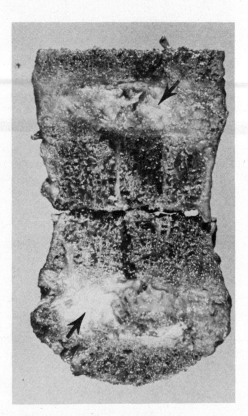

FIG. 22-5. Metastatic carcinoma from the prostate gland. The secondary deposits appear as dense white areas *(arrows)* in the sectioned lumbar vertebrae.

if bony metastases are present. It is also customary to stage the disease based on its extent as assessed by clinical, surgical, and radiologic findings. Treatment can then be based on the particular stage (A through D). The current treatment of prostatic carcinoma presents so many problems that a leading authority in the field has written, "I don't know how to treat carcinoma of the prostate."* Nevertheless, the treatment of choice is usually radical prostatectomy. When metastases are present, orchidectomy, estrogen therapy, or suppression of androgens by drugs or surgery is used to supplement prostatectomy.

Diseases of the testis, epididymis, and spermatic cord

Cryptorchidism is the failure of normal descent of the testes into the scrotum. It may be unilateral or bilateral. The testes may be found along the line of the gubernaculum testis, usually in the inguinal canal or within the abdominal cavity. If the testes fail to descend before puberty, either naturally or by surgical treatment, testicular atrophy results. Since 10% of cases of testicular cancer develop in undescended testes, it is usual practice to perform orchidectomy if the testes have not entered or been placed surgically in the scrotum by the age of 10 or 11.

Hydrocele, hematocele, and spermatocele

A *hydrocele* is an abnormal collection of fluid within the tunica vaginalis, which is a mesothelial-lined sac attached to the testes and derived from the peritoneum. Hydrocele fluid is usually clear and colorless and may collect following trauma or infection or may be associated with testicular malignancy. In many cases, however, the cause of the hydrocele is not apparent.

The presence of blood in the tunica vaginalis is called a *hematocele*. It is frequently the result of trauma.

As a result of blockage of tubules in the epididymis, a small cyst containing spermatozoa may develop. This is known as a *spermatocele*.

Varicocele

The veins of the pampiniform plexus, which surrounds the spermatic cord, may become elongated and dilated forming a *varicocele*. This results from increased venous pressure or more often from unknown causes (idiopathic varicocele). If a varicocele causes symptoms it can be surgically removed.

Orchitis and epididymitis

The following are the main causes of *acute* testicular inflammation (orchitis):
1. *Neisseria gonorrhoeae*
2. *Staphylococcus aureus*
3. Gram-negative enteric bacilli
4. *Salmonella typhi*
5. Mumps virus

Acute epididymitis without orchitis is usually the result of spread of gonococcal infection via the spermatic cord. Orchitis may occasionally result from epididymal spread of infection, but it is more commonly due to hematogenous spread of bacteria or viruses. Of these mumps is the most important. About 20%

---

*Stamey TA: Cancer of the prostate: an analysis of some important contributions and dilemmas, Monographs in Urology 3:65, 1982.

of postpubertal males with mumps develop epididymoorchitis. The disease is bilateral in one fourth of these patients. Although mumps can cause some degree of testicular atrophy, sterility is rare.

Granulomatous inflammation of the epididymis is usually due to hematogenous dissemination of tuberculosis. The disease seldom spreads to involve the testis, despite extensive caseous necrosis of the epididymis.

Syphilitic involvement of the testis is seen in the late stages of the disease. The testis becomes hard, but painless due to the presence of *gummatous necrosis* (Chapter 23).

Chronic granulomatous orchitis, which histologically resembles tuberculosis but does not yield any microorganisms on culture is sometimes found in men over the age of 50 years. The cause is not known.

Infarction of the testis can result from twisting (torsion) of the spermatic cord, unless the torsion is rapidly relieved by surgery.

Testicular tumors

Malignant neoplasms of the testis account for about 1% of all malignant neoplasms, but nearly 90% of testicular tumors are malignant. A classification of testicular germ cell tumors based on that of the World Health Organization follows:
1. Tumors of one histologic type
   a. Seminoma
   b. Embryonal carcinoma
   c. Yolk sac tumor
   d. Choriocarcinoma
   e. Teratomas
2. Tumors of more than one histologic type
   a. Embryonal carcinoma and teratoma (teratocarcinoma)
   b. Choriocarcinoma and any other type
   c. Other combinations

Other than a few cases of testicular lymphoma, virtually all testicular malignancies arise from germ cells. The sex-cord-stromal tumors of the testis, such as the Leydig or Sertoli cell tumors, are rare and are almost invariably benign.

Apart from maldescent of the testis previously mentioned, little is known of factors which predispose to testicular cancers. Seventy-five percent of all cases are between 20 and 49 years of age.

Pathogenesis. Recently, using testicular biopsy and refined histologic techniques, the condition of *carcinoma in situ* of the testis has been recognized. The main histologic feature is in the spermatogonia, in which there is nuclear atypia and excessive mitotic activity. Progression to malignant germ cell neoplasms from carcinoma in situ has been noted in as many as 50% of one group of infertile men who have been followed by testicular biopsy. Since the germ cells (gonocytes) involved are not true epithelial cells, the term *carcinoma in situ* is inappropriate and *gonocytoma in situ* has been proposed. The significance of recognizing *in situ* testicular cancer has still to be assessed.

Seminoma. This is the most common testicular tumor. It has a characteristic gross appearance, usually being of moderate size, with a homogeneous, light yellow cut surface. Microscopically, the tumor cells are arranged in sheets or cords and resemble spermatogonia, with large, polygonal nuclei, prominent nucleoli, and a clear cytoplasm. Tumor cells are separated by a delicate fibrous stroma in which lymphocytic infiltrates are usually seen (Fig. 22-6). Metastases to retroperitoneal lymph nodes are a relatively late development. This slow rate

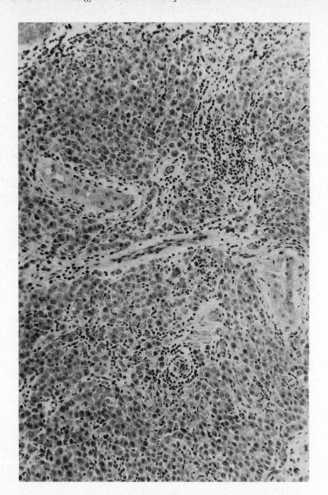

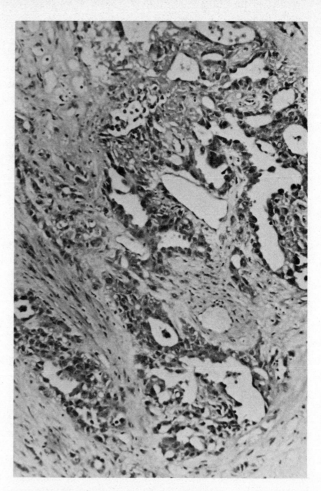

FIG. 22-6. Testicular seminoma. Groups of uniform tumor cells are separated by a fine stroma that contains collections of lymphocytes. The remains of two seminiferous tubules are visible.

FIG. 22-7. Embryonal carcinoma of the testis. The invasive tumor cells are forming glandular structures characteristic of this tumor.

of spread, together with the sensitivity of the tumor to radiation, makes the prognosis in seminoma relatively good, with an overall 85% to 100% 5-year survival rate.

Embryonal carcinoma. *Embryonal carcinoma* (Fig. 22-7) is a tumor composed of primitive cells similar to those of the seminoma, but with a tendency to mimic the architecture of the primitive embryo, with the formation of cleft-like or gland-like structures. Grossly, the tumor has a more varied cut surface than the seminoma with frequent foci of hemorrhage or necrosis. The prognosis is considerably worse than that of the seminoma, with an average 5-year survival of 50%.

Yolk sac tumor. The yolk sac tumor is, in pure form, a neoplasm of young children, in whom it has a somewhat better prognosis than when found in adults. It consists of primitive epithelial and mesenchymal elements that form structures interpreted as an attempt to form yolk sacs. Using immunohistologic techniques, α-fetoprotein (Chapter 15) can be demonstrated in the cytoplasm of some tumor cells.

Choriocarcinomas. Choriocarcinomas are highly malignant tumors that are often small, with no resulting testicular enlargement. They are usually hemorrhagic and partially necrotic. The syncytiotrophoblastic cell components have been shown by immunocytochemistry to contain chorionic gonadotropin.

Teratomas. The *mature* teratoma, as its name suggests, contains a variety of well-differentiated tissues from the three germ cell layers. Fat, cartilage, and mature epithelia are commonly found, and the tumor contains both cystic and solid areas (Fig. 22-8). However, in patients over 5 years of age, occult foci of embryonal carcinoma (from which such tumors are believed to develop), may be present, and can metastasize to kill the patient. Teratomas in those under 5 years of age appear to arise differently and are associated with a good prognosis. Some teratomas contain, in addition to mature elements, varying quantities of tissues resembling those found in the embryo. The prognosis of these rare variants, termed *immature teratomas,* is uncertain but should probably remain guarded.

Of the testicular germ cell tumors composed of more than one histologic type, *teratocarcinoma* (combined embryonal carcinoma and teratoma) is the most common. The prognosis of combined (mixed) germ cell tumors varies with the components present, the worst outcome being associated with those containing choriocarcinoma.

Clinically, patients with testicular tumors usually present with testicular enlargement. Occasionally, the initial findings may result from distant metastases from an unsuspected choriocarcinomatous component. Clinical staging, based on local, lymphatic, and distant spread of the tumor is being used in-

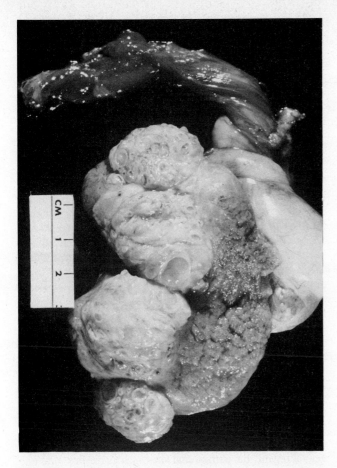

FIG. 22-8. Teratoma of the testis. A variety of tissues is present in the tumor: some solid, some papillary, some cystic. Histologically, the tumor appeared benign.

creasingly as a guide to treatment, and serum α-fetoprotein or chorionic gonadotropin levels may be used to monitor patients in appropriate cases. Treatment of testicular cancer using combinations of surgical removal, radiotherapy, and chemotherapy have had considerable success. Extremely good results have been achieved with seminoma and mature teratoma, with 10-year survival in greater than 90% of cases. Treatment of other forms of testicular malignancy has not yielded such good results. Improved survival rates, however, have been reported especially where there is little or no spread of the tumor (stage I).

Diseases of the penis

Congenital defects of the penis are mostly caused by failure of closure of the penile urethra resulting in the urethra opening abnormally at some point along the underside of the penis (hypospadias). *Squamous carcinoma* of the penis is a disease of elderly men. It is found predominantly in those who have not been circumcised. Chronic irritation is thought to predispose to the disease, but infection by human papilloma viruses appears to have an important causative role.

Bowen's disease is a variety of intraepidermal squamous carcinoma that may be found in various sites in the skin, including the penis. There is thought by some to be an association with cancers in other parts of the body, especially of the gas-

trointestinal tract; however, these cancers do not become apparent for some years following the appearance of Bowen's* disease. The lesion is a hyperkeratotic reddish area of the skin. Microscopically, there is loss of polarity of the epidermal cells, sometimes described as a "windswept" appearance. The cells are large, and the nuclei are hyperchromatic. Dyskeratotic cells are typically present. Mitotic figures are seen at all levels of the epidermis.

Occasionally, a disease resembling Bowen's disease, called erythroplasia of Queyrat† may precede the development of penile carcinoma.

Penile carcinoma is usually an ulcerative squamous cell tumor and spread to the regional lymph nodes is a relatively late event. The treatment is primarily surgical.

Condyloma acuminatum, caused by papilloma virus is considered in Chapter 21. It is the most common benign tumor of the penis.

Male infertility

A consideration of male infertility is beyond the scope of this text; however, many diseases discussed in this and other chapters may play a role in this condition and the main causes are listed as follows:

1. Genital abnormalities
   a. Congenital anomalies
      (1) Hypospadias
      (2) Epispadias
   b. Acquired abnormalities
      (1) Varicocele
      (2) Trauma (including urogenital surgery)
      (3) Infections
         (a) Sexually transmitted (e.g., gonorrhea)
         (b) Non-sexually transmitted (e.g., tuberculosis)
2. Abnormalities of fertilization
   a. In sperm-cervical mucus interaction
   b. In sperm-ovum interaction
3. Extragenital disorders
   a. Endocrine disorders
   b. Spinal cord injuries
   c. Neurologic disease
4. Sexual dysfunction

---

*John T. Bowen (1857-1941), American dermatologist.
†August Queyrat (1872-1940), French dermatologist.

Selected readings

Del Regato JA: Cancer of the prostate (2 parts), JAMA 235:1717, 1976.
Editorial: Carcinoma of the penis, Med J Aust 2:1035, 1973.
Editorial: Carcinoma-in-situ of the testis, Lancet 2:545, 1987.
Huben RP and Murphy GP: Prostatic cancer: an update, CA 36:274, 1986.
Javadpur N: The role of biologic tumor markers in testicular cancer, Cancer 45:1755, 1980.
Kirk D: Prostatic carcinoma, Br Med J 290:875, 1985.
Krabbe S, Skakkebaek NE, and Berthlesen JG et al: High incidence of undetected neoplasia in maldescended testes, Lancet 1:999, 1979.
Weissbach L and Widman T: Familial tumors of the testis. Eur Urol 12:104, 1986.

CHAPTER 23

Sexually transmitted diseases

The most important and most common sexually transmitted diseases (STDs) are syphilis, gonorrhea, nongonococcal urethritis (NGU), acquired immunodeficiency syndrome (AIDS), herpes genitalis, candidosis, and trichomoniasis. Chancroid, lymphogranuloma venereum, and granuloma inguinale are much less common and will be considered only briefly (Table 23-1). Acquired immunodeficiency syndrome is discussed fully in Chapter 7.

Several other common infectious agents may sometimes be transmitted by sexual contact, but this is not their usual mode of transmission. These include hepatitis B, cytomegalovirus, and Epstein-Barr virus; infestation by scabies mite *(Sarcoptes scabei)* and crab lice *(Phthiris pubis)* can also take place during sexual contact.

It is important to remember that a patient can have two or more simultaneously transmitted infections. In practice, irrespective of which infection is suspected, serologic tests for syphilis should be performed so that this important disease does not pass unnoticed.

Syphilis

Syphilis is a sexually transmitted spirochetal disease that is remarkable for its great variety of clinical manifestations. Syphilis today remains, as it has for centuries, a major worldwide health problem. Despite the availability of penicillin, the number of reported cases in the United States over the last ten years has remained fairly constant between 21,000 and 29,000 reported cases. This, however, means that in reality about 80,000 people are infected each year because most cases go unreported.

Etiology

Syphilis is caused by the spirochete *Treponema pallidum*. This bacterium is slender and motile and can be seen only by darkfield or fluorescence microscopy or when impregnated with silver stain. It is 6 to 14 μm in length with 6 to 12 regular coils. Although *T. pallidum* has not been successfully cultivated in vitro, and therefore does not strictly fulfil Koch's postulates, the evidence for its etiologic role in syphilis is overwhelming. The detection of antibodies in syphilis by a variety of serologic methods is the single most important means of investigating the disease.

Pathogenesis

Infection by *T. pallidum* is usually sexually acquired, but it may also be congenitally transmitted. Acquired infection takes place through the skin or mucous membranes, and it seems likely that minute abrasions of the epithelial surface permit penetration of the organism. Congenital infection is transmitted from an infected mother to the fetus by way of the placenta.

After *T. pallidum* has entered the body, it is probably disseminated throughout the body in a matter of hours or days.

Thus almost from the very start, syphilis is a *generalized disease*. It is, however, convenient and traditional to describe the disease in stages, each with its typical local and/or systemic manifestations. In the periods between these stages, the disease continues to be active, despite the absence of overt clinical manifestations. The stages of syphilis are primary, secondary and late or tertiary syphilis. There is also the important latent form of syphilis in which there is no physical evidence of disease but serologic tests are reactive (positive). *T. pallidum* is readily transmitted in the primary and secondary stages of syphilis but patients with late or latent syphilis are not infectious.

Primary syphilis. Following an incubation period of about 3 weeks, the primary stage of syphilis develops. It is characterized by (1) the syphilitic *chancre* and (2) regional lymphadenopathy. The chancre is the lesion present at the site of entry and initial multiplication of the spirochete (Fig. 23-1). Typically, it is single, hard, and painless, but there are frequent exceptions to this description. The chancre is usually on the genital organs, but extragenital sites such as the lips, oral mu-

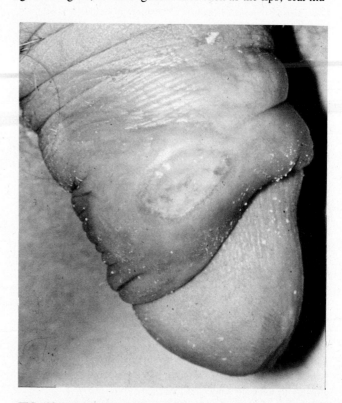

FIG. 23-1. Primary syphilitic chancre. The lesion is typically hard and painless; the surrounding skin shows inflammatory edema. *Treponema pallidum* can be observed by darkfield microscopic examination of exudate from the lesion. *(Courtesy Curator of the Gordon Museum, Guy's Hospital, London, England.)*

TABLE 23-1. Sexually transmitted infections

Disease	Infectious agent	Pathology	Usual clinical findings	Complications	Remarks
Syphilis	*Treponema pallidum*	Endarteritis; periarteritis; chronic inflammation	Primary: chancre Secondary: mucocutaneous eruptions Late: cardiovascular and neurosyphilis Latent: none	Mainly from effects of late syphilis	Extragenital infections common; may be transmitted congenitally
Gonorrhea	*Neisseria gonorrhoeae*	Pyogenic inflammation	Urethritis (male) Cervicitis (female)	Abscess formation; spread to joints, CNS, and heart via bloodstream	Asymptomatic infection common in women; may be transmitted to infants during delivery
Nongonococcal urethritis (NGU)	*Chlamydia trachomatis* (most cases) or *Ureaplasma urealyticum*	Acute urethral pyogenic inflammation	Urethritis (male)	Rare	Asymptomatic inflammation usual in women
Herpes genitalis	*Herpesvirus hominis*	Epithelial giant cells with intranuclear inclusions; acute inflammation	Genital vesicular lesions (male and female) often recurrent	Rare in adults	High risk to infants during delivery if mother has active herpes genitalis
Candidosis	*Candida albicans*	Acute pyogenic inflammation; yeasts with pseudohyphae	Vulvovaginitis (female) Balanitis (male)	Rare	
Trichomoniasis	*Trichomonas vaginalis*	Acute inflammation; protozoa present in exudate	Vaginitis with leucorrhea	Rare	Males usually asymptomatic
Chancroid	*Haemophilus ducreyi*	Acute inflammation	Painful genital ulceration and lymphadenopathy (both sexes)		Increased risk of transmission of AIDS among patients with chancroid
Granuloma inguinale	*Calymmatobacterium granulomatis*	Chronic inflammation with fibrous scarring and epithelial hyperplasia	Genital or perianal ulceration; inguinal soft tissue swellings (pseudobuboes)	Rarely generalized infection	
Lymphogranuloma venereum	*C. trachomatis* (serotypes L1, L2, and L3)	Lymph nodes show granulomatous inflammation; stellate abscesses	Painless, tiny genital lesion; severe inguinal lymphadenopathy	Severe chronic pelvic inflammation (females); generalized infection (both sexes)	
Acquired immunodeficiency syndrome	HIV-1, HIV-2*	Suppression of T4 helper lymphocyte function	Fever, weight loss, lymphadenopathy, dyspnea, diarrhea, ± Kaposi's sarcoma	Severe opportunistic infections with numerous complications	Involvement of CNS and eyes, now known to be common

*HIV, Human immunodeficiency virus.

cosa and anus are well recognized. The chancre heals spontaneously within 3 to 6 weeks, an event which can easily lull the uninformed into a dangerous sense of false security. In women, uterine cervical chancres are painless and self-healing and may never be detected. Chancres of the oral cavity are highly infectious; on the lip their raised indurated edge may resemble carcinoma. During the primary stage serologic tests begin to convert to being reactive.

Secondary syphilis. The manifestations of secondary syphilis develop about 6 to 8 weeks following the appearance of the primary chancre. This stage of the disease is characterized by rashes, mucosal lesions, and systemic symptoms. The rash consists of reddish-brown or copper-colored macules which may be widespread or confined to the palms and soles (Fig. 23-2). About 30% of patients with secondary syphilis develop lesions of the oral mucous membranes known as *mucous patches* (Fig. 23-3). They are painless erythematous areas that develop into grayish-white erosions or patches. Other lesions

may be irregularly linear and are called "snail-track" ulcers. These lesions teem with spirochetes and are highly contagious. A typical secondary lesion is *condyloma latum,* a flat papular lesion found in moist areas of skin such as the perianal region. During the secondary stages generalized lymph node enlargement and episodes of fever may appear. Secondary syphilitic lesions usually resolve spontaneously, but by this time virtually all patients will have reactive serologic tests for syphilis.

Without treatment about two thirds of patients who develop secondary syphilis will remain asymptomatic following the secondary stage. These patients have *latent syphilis* and they can only be detected by serologic tests. The remaining one third, if untreated eventually develop serious disease of the central nervous system (neurosyphilis) or cardiovascular system. This is known as *late* (formerly tertiary) syphilis.

Late syphilis. Many years can elapse between initial infection and the development of late syphilis. The characteristic lesion of late syphilis is the *gumma,* which is described later.

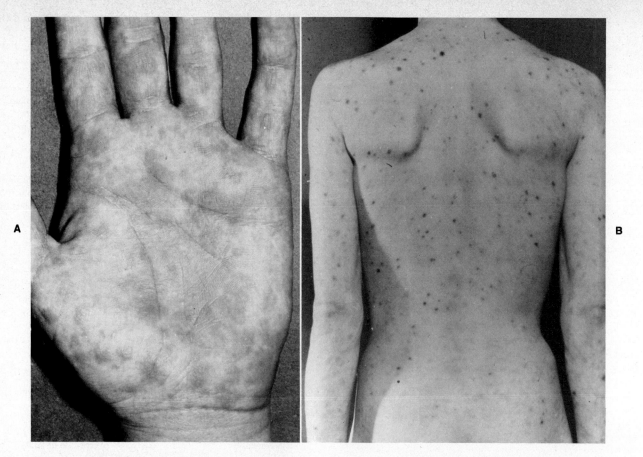

FIG. 23-2. A, Typical copper colored macular rash on the hands in secondary syphilis. *(Courtesy Curator of the Gordon Museum, Guy's Hospital, London, England.)* **B,** Typical copper colored macular rash on the trunk in secondary syphilis. *(From McCracken AW and Cawson RA: Clinical and oral microbiology, Washington DC, 1982, Hemisphere Publishing Corp.)*

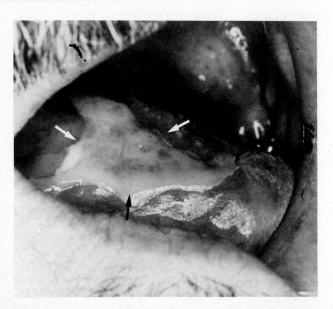

FIG. 23-3. Secondary syphilis. A triangular-shaped mucous patch *(arrowed)* covers a large area on the dorsum of the tongue. *(From McCracken AW and Cawson RA: Clinical and oral microbiology, Washington DC, 1982, Hemisphere Publishing Corp.)*

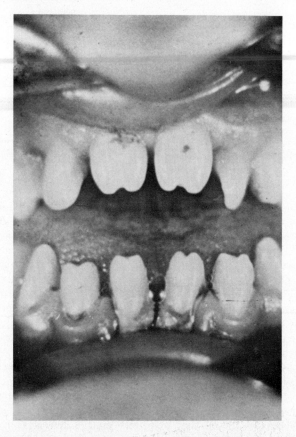

FIG. 23-4. Congenital syphilis. The incisors (Hutchinson's teeth) show the typical notches and taper toward the incisal edges. *(Courtesy Curator of the Gordon Museum, Guy's Hospital, London, England.)*

The nervous system diseases caused by syphilis are tabes dorsalis, meningovascular syphilis, and generalized paresis of the insane (GPI) (Chapter 20). The main cardiovascular disease in late syphilis is aortic aneurysm (Chapter 10).

Congenital syphilis. Infants infected in utero may develop congenital syphilis as a result of undetected primary or secondary syphilis in the mother. Congenital syphilis may be detectable by the following:

1. *At birth*—The affected infant has a variety of mucocutaneous lesions and usually a mucoid nasal discharge as a result of involvement of the nasopharyngeal mucosa. Bones and viscera may also be involved and syphilitic pneumonia (pneumonia alba) is sometimes present. Up to 40% of syphilitic infants are stillborn.
2. *Later in life*—A variety of syphilitic stigmata, many of which are oro-facial or dental abnormalities are seen. These include Hutchinson's teeth (Fig. 23-4), "saddle" nose (Fig. 23-5), and Moon's molar teeth in which the cusps on the occlusal surfaces are dome shaped or maybe replaced by nodules so that the tooth resembles a mulberry (mulberry molars).
3. *Only by reactive serologic tests*—About two thirds of congenital syphilitic patients have no evidence of the disease other than reactive serologic tests.

Pathology

The basic pathology of syphilitic lesions is the same irrespective of site, the stage of the disease, or the appearance of the lesions. The main changes are in the small arteries, in which the endothelial cells swell and proliferate, partly occluding the vessel. This process is known as *endarteritis,* and its effect is to reduce blood flow through the affected vessels. An inflammatory mononuclear infiltrate rich in plasma cells surrounds the damaged vessels, and the term *periarteritis* is applied to this inflammatory process. Thus the underlying pathology of syphilitic lesions is endarteritis and periarteritis.

In late syphilis an additional element, a form of tissue necrosis, is added as a consequence mainly of the vascular changes. Because of its rubbery texture, the term *gummatous necrosis* is applied, and the lesions are known as *gummas.* Gummas are most frequently found in the skin and bones, but they can affect almost any part of the body. They may be the sole manifestation of late syphilis, and when this happens, the term *benign gummatous syphilis* has been applied. Healing of a gumma is by absorption of the necrotic center and progressive fibrous proliferation. This in turn leads to scarring and distortion of soft tissues or to perforation or deformity of bone (Fig. 23-6).

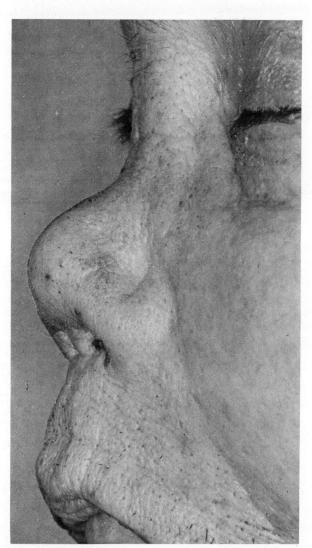

FIG. 23-5. The saddle nose of congenital syphilis. *(Courtesy Curator of the Gordon Museum, Guy's Hospital, London, England.)*

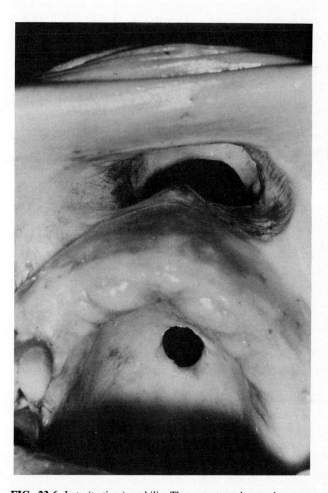

FIG. 23-6. Late (tertiary) syphilis. There are two abnormal communications between the mouth and nasal cavity caused by perforation of the maxilla and hard palate as a result of gumma formation. *(Courtesy Curator of the Gordon Museum, Guy's Hospital, London, England.)*

Serology of syphilis

Syphilis is often asymptomatic, but it is potentially deadly. Because many cases can be diagnosed only by serologic methods, the serology of syphilis has been of the greatest clinical importance since August Wassermann* introduced the complement fixation test for syphilis which bears his name, in the early 1900's.

Antibodies in syphilis. Infection by *T. pallidum* results in the production of two antibodies: (1) Wassermann antibodies and (2) treponemal antibodies.

Wassermann antibodies react in a variety of serologic procedures with a cross-reacting antigen called *cardiolipin*. This is an extract of mammalian heart that is rich in mitochondrial membranes, and to which lecithin and cholesterol have been added to amplify the antigen-antibody reaction. The standard test for Wassermann antibodies is the Venereal Disease Reference Laboratory (VDRL) test. The rapid plasma reagin (RPR) circle card test is a simpler and more rapid procedure, and has the same significance as the VDRL test.

Syphilis is by far the most common disease that gives a reactive (positive) VDRL or RPR test, but reactive (false positive) results are also obtained in diseases other than syphilis. These include infectious mononucleosis, mycoplasmal infections, brucellosis, chickenpox, and systemic lupus erythematosus. When a reactive VDRL or RPR test is the result of a disease other than syphilis it is called a *false positive reaction*. Thus, the correct interpretation of a reactive VDRL or RPR test is that the patient is likely to have syphilis, but there is a chance that he may have a disease other than syphilis. When syphilis is adequately treated the VDRL and RPR usually become nonreactive although this may take as long as 1 to 2 years.

Treponemal antibodies that react with surface antigens of *T. pallidum* appear quickly after primary infection and as a rule persist for life. Several methods have been devised to detect treponemal antibodies. Two procedures are in common use in the United States: the FTA-ABS test† and the MHA-TP test‡. The latter test is simpler and much less prone to subjective error; however, the significance of the test results is the same. *When either of these tests are* performed *on patients who are known to have a reactive VDRL or RPR test,* a reactive FTA-ABS or MHA-TP test indicates *active syphilis*. A nonreactive test in the presence of a reactive VDRL test indicates a false positive reaction. The interpretation of the combined results of VDRL/RPR and FTA-ABS/MHA-TP tests is shown in Table 23-2.

Clinical aspects

The great importance of syphilis is, first, the risk of serious cardiovascular or neurologic damage if the disease is not detected early and treated; second, if untreated, spread of infection to sexual partners during the primary and secondary stages is highly likely; third, women with active syphilis during pregnancy can transmit the infection to the developing fetus.

The clinical diagnosis of syphilis is often difficult even for experts, because of the great variety of signs and symptoms. The diagnosis can only be confirmed in the laboratory. In pri-

---

*1886-1926, German bacteriologist.

†FTA-ABS stands for fluorescent treponemal antibody absorbed test. "Absorbed" refers to a stage in the test in which interfering antibodies are absorbed from the test serum using extracts of *Treponema reiteri*.

‡MHA-TP is the microhemagglutination *Treponema pallidum* test.

TABLE 23-2. Interpretation of serologic tests for syphilis

RPR* or VDRL†	MHA-TP or FTA-ABS‡	Interpretation
Reactive	Reactive	Active syphilis
Nonreactive	Nonreactive	No serologic evidence of syphilis
Reactive	Nonreactive	False positive reaction caused by other diseases
Nonreactive	Reactive	Usually past treated syphilis; occasionally very early syphilis

*Unsuitable for testing cerebrospinal fluid.
† With rare exceptions, such as in some cases of subarachnoid hemorrhage, a reactive VDRL test on cerebrospinal fluid is a diagnostic for active neurosyphilis.
‡ Performing MHA-TP or FTA-ABS without RPR or VDRL tests is not advisable; as many as 15% of results can be false positives.

mary, secondary and sometimes in congenital syphilis, the diagnosis can be made from a chancre or a mucocutaneous lesion. Errors, however, are easily made especially in the mouth where other spirochetes such as *T. microdentium* are normally present. Because of these difficulties and the absence of treponemes in late and latent syphilis, serologic tests are of paramount importance in diagnosis.

The specific treatment for all stages of syphilis is penicillin. The long term effectiveness of alternative antibiotics such as erythromycin and chloramphenicol, has not been clearly established.

Gonorrhea

Gonorrhea is a sexually transmitted bacterial infection. It is an enormous public health problem worldwide because of the large numbers of cases reported each year and the potential for serious consequences in untreated disease. The number of cases of gonorrhea in the United States is estimated at around 3 million a year. Ninety percent of patients are under 30 years of age.

Etiology

The causative organism is *Neisseria gonorrhoeae* (gonococcus), which is a fastidious gram negative diplococcus. It is commonly kidney-shaped and usually observed within the cytoplasm of polymorphonuclear leukocytes. The organism has some properties which are thought to be important in the pathogenesis of gonorrhea:

1. It has hairlike projections of its cell membrane called pili, by which it attaches to the mucosal cell to initiate infection.
2. It produces an enzyme that cleaves secretory IgA molecules. Because IgA is thought to be the important protective antibody against infections of mucosal surfaces, its destruction by *N. gonorrhoeae* may account for the ability of the bacterium to cause repeated infections.
3. It is capable, as are other gram-negative organisms, of releasing endotoxin and other toxic products that may enhance mucosal damage.

Pathogenesis and pathology

N. gonorrhoeae can infect the urethral, endocervical, anal, and pharyngeal mucosae and the conjunctival sac. The latter is usually infected during birth when the mother has gonococcal cervicitis. This causes purulent conjunctivitis in the newborn infant *(ophthalmia neonatorum)*.

In the mucosal sites, the bacterium proliferates and spreads to contiguous organs. In some instances, hematogenous spread to many sites in the body may take place.

The most frequent site of infection in males is the urethra. Untreated infection spreads locally to the periurethral glands and the epididymis, but the testes themselves are seldom involved.

In women endocervical infection progresses to salpingitis, often skipping the intervening endometrium. Infection may then spread to involve areas of the pelvic peritoneum. Gonorrhea is, therefore, one of several important causes of *pelvic inflammatory disease (PID)*. Bloodborne spread of gonococcal infection is more likely in women and can give rise to septic arthritis, meningitis, or endocarditis.

The pathologic process in gonorrhea is acute pyogenic inflammation. Abscess formation may develop in the periurethral glands in untreated males and within the fallopian tubes (pyosalpinx) or Bartholin's glands* in females. As with syphilis there is no protective immunity.

Clinical aspects

The most common complaint in men with gonorrhea is a purulent urethral discharge (the clap) accompanied by painful urination. In women cervicitis with a purulent vaginal discharge is common, but many women have few or no symptoms. Spread of infection in women leads to menstrual disorders and symptoms referrable to the fallopian tubes and ovaries. Inflammation can cause obliteration of the fallopian tubes leading to sterility. Anorectal infection caused by direct spread of infected secretions is the rule in women with genital tract infection. As a result, anorectal cultures in women have a higher positive yield than genital cultures.

Largely as a result of homosexual relationships, pharyngeal, and anal infections are now common. Sites of involvement in oral gonorrhea include lips, tongue, and buccal mucosa, but the pharynx and tonsils are the most common intraoral sites. Gonococcal pharyngitis is characterized by severe, painful exudative or ulcerative tonsillitis with inflammatory enlargement of the cervical lymph nodes, but more frequently is asymptomatic.

The diagnosis of gonorrhea can be made by examination of smears of pus stained by gram stain or fluorescent antibody. However, reliance on staining methods alone will result in failure to detect significant numbers of asymptomatic women. The rate of diagnosis in this group is greatly enhanced by special methods of handling and culturing samples on special media such as Martin-Lewis medium. By these methods up to 6% of all asymptomatic women attending clinics and emergency rooms have been shown to have gonorrhea.

There are no reliable serologic tests comparable to those for syphilis, but there is a great need for such a test. The antibiotic treatment for most cases of gonorrhea is amoxacillin. Alternative drugs may be required because of penicillin allergy or because a minority of strains, about 1% to 2% in the United States, have become resistant to penicillin. In these situations, ceftriaxone or spectinomycin are suitable alternative drugs.

Nongonococcal urethritis

Nongonococcal urethritis is an extremely common sexually transmitted disease which closely resembles gonorrhea in its behavior. *N. gonorrhoeae*, however, is not the cause.

Etiology

Most cases of nongonococcal urethritis (NGU) are caused by *Chlamydia trachomatis*. This is an obligate intracellular bacterium belonging to the same genus that causes psittacosis, lymphogranuloma venereum, trachoma and inclusion conjunctivitis. This group of organisms is typified by the appearance of basophilic inclusions in the cytoplasm of infected cells. NGU is the most common of a wide range of clinical manifestations due to *C. trachomatis*.

C. trachomatis has been isolated from many cases of NGU and specific antibodies to the organism have been shown to develop during the course of the disease. This organism cannot be isolated from all cases, however. From some, the mycoplasma *Ureaplasma urealyticum* can be recovered. Although the evidence that ureaplasma can cause NGU is not so complete as that for *C. trachomatis*, it seems likely that about 10% to 15% of cases of NGU are due to ureaplasma.

Pathogenesis and pathology

The mechanisms by which chlamydia cause cell damage are only partly understood. A heat labile factor which has cytotoxic effects and which can be neutralized by specific antibody has been described. There is also indirect evidence that chlamydial infection stimulates cell-mediated immunity.

Mucosal involvement in *C. trachomatis* infection is characterized by patchy inflammation and ulceration and the presence of inclusion bodies in some of the epithelial cells. In acute infections, there is a purulent or mucopurulent exudate while in more chronic infections, the submucosa contains collections of macrophages and lymphocytes.

Although urethritis and cervicitis are respectively, the most common clinical effects in men and women, the disease may spread to other sites. In men, prostatitis, epididymitis or Reiter's syndrome (urethritis, conjunctivitis, arthritis) may develop, while in women the fallopian tubes and bladder may become infected. Some cases of Fitz-Hugh-Curtis syndrome* due to perihepatic inflammation have been attributed to spread of infection from the fallopian tubes. Many cases of chronic pelvic inflammatory disease are now being attributed to *C. trachomatis*. Infection may also be transmitted to infants during birth, often resulting in conjunctivitis or less commonly, in pneumonia.

Clinical aspects

Many infections by *C. trachomatis* are asymptomatic and go undetected for long periods, especially in women. In many countries including the United States and Great Britain, NGU is the most common of all sexually transmitted diseases in men. The symptoms of acute infection, usually urethritis in men and cervicitis in women, are very similar to those described for acute gonorrhea, but the diagnosis is suggested when the patient fails to respond to penicillin. Culture-negative urethritis may also suggest NGU, but because gonorrhea may be present in the same patient, isolation of *N. gonorrhoeae* does not exclude

---

*Thomas Bartholin (1618-1680), Danish anatomist.

*Fitz-Hugh-Curtis syndrome: upper right quadrant pain with friction rub over the liver.

NGU. *C. trachomatis* can be grown in cell culture from epithelial scrapings from the urethra or cervix. The diagnosis of NGU is confirmed when the disease responds to treatment with tetracycline. Cases of NGU which do not respond to tetracycline are treated with spectinomycin, under the assumption that *U. urealyticum* is the cause.

Herpes genitalis
Etiology

Herpes genitalis is caused in the majority of cases by *Herpesvirus hominis* type 2 (HSV-2); a minority of cases is caused by type 1 (HSV-1). It is now recognized as one of the most common sexually transmitted diseases.

Pathogenesis and pathology

When a nonimmune person is infected by HSV-2, the resulting infection is usually asymptomatic, but in some instances an acute primary inflammatory reaction characterized by multiple vesicles develops in the genital mucous membranes. After primary infection has taken place, some patients experience recurrent herpetic infections as a result of reactivation of the virus from its latent state in the sacral nerves. Recurrent attacks are similar to primary attacks, but they are less severe and less extensive and are not accompanied by constitutional symptoms that often accompany primary infections. Because recurrences develop in the presence of circulating antibodies to HSV-2, it is clear that humoral immunity is ineffective in preventing recrudescent infection.

HSV-2 causes changes in the epithelial cells identical to those seen in HSV-1 infections, namely formation of multinucleate giant cells in which eosinophilic nuclear inclusions are present.

The vesicles (Fig. 23-7) in which these changes are seen are usually multiple. In women they are present on the cervix, the vaginal wall, and the labia; in men they are usually on the glans. These lesions resolve in 7 to 10 days unless secondarily infected.

Clinical aspects

Genital herpes, particularly in its recurrent form, not only causes pain and irritation in the genital organs, but because of

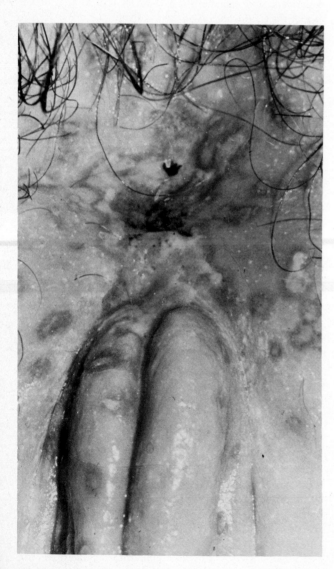

FIG. 23-7. Herpetic vulvovaginitis. Numerous painful, vesicular lesions are present as a result of primary infection by *Herpesvirus hominis* type 2. (*Courtesy Curator of the Gordon Museum, Guy's Hospital, London, England.*)

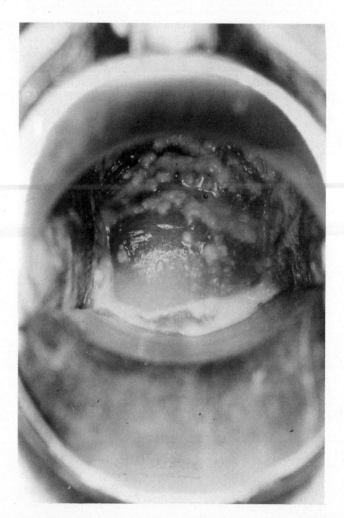

FIG. 23-8. Acute vaginitis caused by *Candida albicans*. Viewed through an endoscope, the cervix is acutely inflamed with a white exudate, which is typical of this infection. (*Courtesy Curator of the Gordon Museum, Guy's Hospital, London, England.*)

its repetitive nature and failure to respond to treatment, it can cause a great deal of anxiety among its victims.

The diagnosis is readily made by microscopic examination of smears prepared from the floor of freshly opened vesicles. The demonstration of typical inclusion bearing cells is sufficient for diagnosis. The virus is readily isolated in cell culture, but this and serotyping are seldom necessary.

Treatment of the disease is still unsatisfactory. The antiviral drug acyclovir has limited use in genital herpes; it is most effective in reducing the duration and severity of primary herpetic infection. Long term administration of acyclovir has been shown to suppress recurrences.

Herpes genitalis in pregnant women is a serious threat to infants during delivery, since there is a high risk of infection in the baby resulting in generalized herpes. When the disease is active at the time of delivery, exposure of the infant is avoided by performing a caesarean section.

Trichomoniasis
Etiology

Trichomoniasis is a genital infection, usually sexually transmitted and caused by *Trichomonas vaginalis,* a flagellate protozoon which inhabits the male and female genital tracts. Unlike most other flagellate protozoa found in humans, *T. vaginalis* exists only in the active trophozoite form and does not form a cystic stage.

Pathogenesis and pathology

Trichomoniasis in women is usually symptomatic. The protozoa proliferate on the mucosal surface and induce an acute inflammatory reaction with exudation of polymorphonuclear leukocytes. This creates a purulent vaginal discharge (leukorrhea). The inflammation persists for several weeks or months but eventually subsides spontaneously, although the parasite can still be detected in vaginal secretions.

In men, infection is often asymptomatic or limited to a mild persistent urethritis.

Clinical aspects

Trichomoniasis is a common sexually transmitted infection. In some European countries it is the most common genital tract infection in women. Trichomonal infection is characterized by a vaginal discharge and severe itching and burning sensations. The diagnosis can be made by microscopic examination of wet or stained preparations of vaginal secretions. However, a much higher positive yield is obtained if cultures on specially enriched

media are performed. The disease responds very readily to metronidazole.

Candidosis

Candidal vulvovaginitis is now among the most common sexually transmitted diseases (Fig. 23-8). The lesions are essentially the same as those of oral thrush (Chapter 14), but unlike the latter they can cause intense itching and distressing irritation.

The reason that candidal vaginitis is much more common than oral candidosis in otherwise healthy women is not known, but the widespread use of oral contraceptives that affect the cellular metabolism of vaginal epithelium is thought to be a factor.

Candidal vaginitis can be treated with antifungal drugs such as nystatin. Some cases are, however, exceedingly resistant to treatment for reasons that are unclear. Reinfection from an infected sexual partner is a common event.

Sexually transmitted diseases and cancer of the uterine cervix

The association of Herpesvirus hominis type 2 and human papilloma virus with cancer of the uterine cervix are discussed in Chapter 21.

Selected readings

Brown ST: Serologic response to syphilis treatment, JAMA 253:1296, 1981.

Burnham RC: Mucopurulent cervicitis, N Engl J Med 311:1, 1984.

Corey L, Adams H, and Brown Z et al: Genital herpesvirus infections: clinical manifestations, course, and complications, Ann Intern Med 98:958, 1983.

Kuberski T: Granuloma inguinale, Sex Transm Dis 7:29, 1980.

McCracken AW: Laboratory diagnosis of sexually transmitted diseases. In Spittell JA, Jr., editor: Clinical medicine, vol 1, Philadelphia, 1985, Harper & Row.

Mercola L: Congenital syphilis revisited, Am J Dis Child 139:575, 1985.

Rockwell DH: The Tuskegee study of untreated syphilis, Arch Intern Med 114:792, 1963.

Schachter JS, Hill EG and King EB, et al: Chlamydia trachomatis and cervical neoplasia, JAMA 248:2134, 1982.

Terho P: Chlamydia trachomatis and genital infections: a general review, Infection 10:1, 1982.

Tice AW, and Rodriguez MVL: Pharyngeal gonorrhea, JAMA 246:2717, 1981.

Glossary

Amyloid A term applied to a variety of filamentous proteins which, because they share a β-pleated secondary structure, stain orange with Congo Red. Amyloid deposits are generally found in an extracellular location.

Amyloidosis Disease resulting from amyloid deposition.

Anaplasia A term used to indicate either lack of cytoplasmic differentiation in malignant neoplasms or the presence of exaggerated nuclear features of malignancy. Recently, there has been a trend towards restricting its use to the latter meaning, and applying the term *undifferentiated* to the former.

Aneuploidy *Chromosomal aneuploidy* is a karyotypic abnormality consisting of the presence of too many or too few copies of a specific chromosome(s) in a cell population. *DNA aneuploidy* is the presence of a population of cells with nuclear DNA in quantities greater or less than the normal diploid amount as measured by flow cytometry. Aneuploidy implies that chromosomes or DNA are not present in amounts representing exact multiples of the normal haploid number.

Apoptosis A form of cell death different from necrosis. Apoptosis is seen under both physiologic and pathologic circumstances and involves condensation, fragmentation and subsequent phagocytosis of scattered, single cells. Unlike necrosis, apoptosis is an energy-dependent process involving the activation of endogenous endonucleases.

Atrophy The wasting away or diminution in size of a cell, tissue, organ, or part thereof.

Atypia A term applied to cells with large, hyperchromatic, and pleomorphic nuclei.

Autolysis Breakdown of a cell by its own (lysosomal) enzymes.

Autophagy Sequestration of cellular material or organelles in membrane-bound vesicles, with subsequent intralysosomal digestion.

Basal lamina (external lamina) A discrete layer of extracellular matrix components lying near and parallel to cell surfaces that face toward the stroma.

Benign Literally, innocuous; when applied to tumors it implies an inability to metastasize.

Calculus (stone) A solid mass consisting of precipitated material that forms in the lumen of a secretory (or excretory) duct system.

Cell coat The carbohydrate-rich layer on the outer surface of the plasma membrane.

Cell swelling The appearance usually assumed by cells prior to necrosis. Theoretically reversible.

Centriole A paired microtubular organelle that functions as the site where the formation of cilia and the mitotic spindle commences.

Chromatin A complex of DNA and proteins. Only the latter component, which consists chiefly of histones, stains with hematoxylin and is therefore visible in routine histologic and cytologic slides.

Chromosome Structure consisting of chromatin strands, which become extremely compact during cell division.

Cilium A strongly motile microtubular organelle projecting from the cell surface.

Connective tissue activation A common, nonspecific response of connective tissue to injury, resulting in an increase in connective tissue cells and matrix.

Cyst An epithelial-lined round or oval space.

Cytocavitary network A system of communicating vesicles and sacs of diverse function found in all eukaryotic cells. The contents of the system are either directly or indirectly in communication with the extracellular environment.

Cytoskeleton Complex cellular network of microtubules and filaments, involved in cell movement and the maintenance of cell structure.

Desmoplasia An increase in fibrous stroma. The late phase of connective tissue activation.

Desmosome Probably the toughest kind of intercellular junction. Tonofibril bundles connect with the plasma membrane on either side of the junction.

Differentiation The acquisition of cytoplasmic structures aimed at specialized functions.

Dysplasia Literally, abnormal growth. The term has variable meanings depending on the context in which it is used. In connection with epithelia, the term is used for cellular changes of the kind that precede invasive cancer.

Dystrophic calcification Pathologic calcification other than that resulting from hypercalcemia.

Endocytosis The passage of material from outside the cell into the cytocavitary network.

Endoplasmic reticulum Part of the cytocavitary network. Two forms are seen, that is, the ribosome studded rough (granular) type, involved in glycoprotein synthesis, and the smooth (agranular) type, involved in other functions, such as steroidogenesis.

Euchromatin A term, now falling into disuse, used to refer to finely dispersed chromatin, thought to be transcriptionally active.

Eukaryote Organism (unicellular or multicellular) whose cells contain a true nucleus.

Exocytosis The reverse of endocytosis.

Exon Part of the gene that transcribes to mature mRNA after the intervening sequences (introns) are spliced out.

Fibronectin A family of extracellular, noncollagenous glycoproteins that function in connection with blood clotting and cellular locomotion.

Fibrinoid change A microscopic appearance in which tissue assumes the staining properties of fibrin.

Fibrosis An abnormal increase in fibrous stroma. Results from connective tissue activation and/or diminished enzymatic lysis of extracellular matrix.

Gangrene Extensive tissue necrosis, typically associated with putrefaction.

Gap junction A form of cell junction permitting the rapid intercellular passage of electrolytes.

Gene Chromosomal unit specifying the production of a distinct protein (e.g., an enzyme) or RNA.

Glycocalyx The cell coat.

Golgi complex That part of the cytocavitary network that enzymatically modifies and packages glycoprotein products received from the rough endoplasmic reticulum.

Granulation tissue Highly vascular, proteoglycan-rich connective tissue that contains inflammatory cells and forms in response to tissue injury or destruction. An example of the lytic phase of connective tissue activation.

Granulomatous inflammation A form of inflammatory response in which epithelioid histiocytes, in the form of nodular aggregates, predominate.

Heterochromatin A term, now falling into disuse, used to refer to compact, darkly staining chromatin, thought to be transcriptionally inactive.

Hyalin A nonspecific term for any structure with a hyaline appearance.

Hyaline Having a homogeneous and eosinophilic microscopic appearance.

Hyperplasia An increase in the absolute number of cells of a tissue, organ, or part. Generally employed in connection with nonneoplastic phenomena.

In situ Not involving stromal infiltration or metastasis.

Intron Intervening sequence of DNA, located within a gene, that is not transcribed into mature mRNA.

Karyolysis Enzymatic lysis of the nucleus. Usually a part of the autolytic process.

Karyorrhexis Fragmentation of clumped chromatin. A feature of both apoptosis and necrosis.

Karyotype Chromosome set of a cell, clone, or species.

Lysosome A vesicle rich in hydrolytic enzymes and involved in intracellular digestion. Part of the cytocavitary network.

Malignant Literally, acting maliciously. When used in reference to neoplasms the term implies a metastatic capability.

Matrix vesicle An extracellular membrane-bound vesicle that functions as the initial site of apatite crystal deposition in many calcifying tissues.

Metastatic calcification Pathologic calcification resulting from hypercalcemia.

Microfilament A synonym for actin filament.

Micropinocytosis A form of endocytosis involving transport of material into the cell in tiny vesicles (micropinocytotic vesicles).

Microvillus A cylindrical plasma membrane projection that functions mainly to increase the cell surface area.

Mitochondrion The organelle of eukaryotic cells that generates ATP for energy-dependent activities.

Necrobiosis Outmoded term usually used to indicate physiologic cell death.

Necrosis Localized cell death involving tracts of contiguous cells and which (unlike apoptosis) invariably indicates a disease process.

Nucleolus The site of ribosomal RNA synthesis in the nucleus.

Nucleosome Repeating unit of chromatin consisting of 200 base pairs of DNA coiled around a histone octamer.

Nucleus The chromatin-housing portion of the eukaryotic cell.

Phagocytosis A form of endocytosis involving transport of particulate matter into the cell in large vesicles termed phagosomes.

Pigment A colored substance visible in both stained and unstained tissue. Pigments may either be produced in the body or introduced from without.

Pinocytosis Ingestion of liquids and soluble materials by the cell.

Prokaryote Organism that lacks a true nucleus.

Pyknosis Nuclear chromatin clumping resulting in the nucleus appearing as a body exhibiting dense staining with hematoxylin.

Recombinant DNA technology Array of techniques that facilitate the manipulation and duplication of pieces of DNA for industrial, medical, and research purposes. Also termed genetic engineering.

Reticulin Extracellular matrix components that strongly bind silver stains.

Ribosome An RNA particle that functions as the "workbench" where amino acids are linked together to form proteins.

Sclerosis Literally, hardness. The term is vague unless qualified by appropriate adjectives or prefixes (e.g., progressive systemic sclerosis, glomerulosclerosis, atherosclerosis).

Sex chromatin A transcriptionally inactive X-chromosome in a female cell and seen as a compact mass of chromatin on the inner aspect of the nuclear membrane. Also called a Barr body.

Tight junction A watertight form of intercellular junction involving actual fusion of plasma membranes. It is usually located toward the apical portion of lumen-forming cells.

Tonofibril A sheaflike bundle of intermediate filaments.

Transcription Process by which an RNA molecule is polymerized on a DNA template with the aid of RNA polymerases.

Translation Process by which a protein is synthesized from amino acids according to a sequence encoded in the mRNA.

Tumor A swelling. Incorrectly used as a synonym for neoplasm, which does not necessarily imply swelling (tumor formation).

Index

Page numbers in *italics* indicate illustrations;
page numbers followed by t indicate tables.